a Lange medical book

QUICK ANSWERS
to Medical Diagnosis
& Treatment

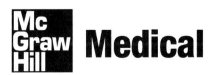 **Medical**

New York   Chicago   San Francisco   Lisbon   London   Madrid   Mexico City   Milan
New Delhi   San Juan   Seoul   Singapore   Sydney   Toronto

Quick Answers to Medical Diagnosis & Treatment

Copyright © 2009 by The McGraw-Hill Companies, Inc. All rights reserved. Printed in the United States of America. Except as permitted under the United States Copyright Act of 1976, no part of this publication may be reproduced or distributed in any form or by any means, or stored in a data base or retrieval system, without the prior written permission of the publisher.

1 2 3 4 5 6 7 8 9 0   QPD/QPD   12 11 10 9

ISBN 978-0-07-159999-3
MHID 0-07-159999-1

Notice

Medicine is an ever-changing science. As new research and clinical experience broaden our knowledge, changes in treatment and drug therapy are required. The authors and the publisher of this work have checked with sources believed to be reliable in their efforts to provide information that is complete and generally in accord with the standards accepted at the time of publication. However, in view of the possibility of human error or changes in medical sciences, neither the authors nor the publisher nor any other party who has been involved in the preparation or publication of this work warrants that the information contained herein is in every respect accurate or complete, and they disclaim all responsibility for any errors or omissions or for the results obtained from use of the information contained in this work. Readers are encouraged to confirm the information contained herein with other sources. For example and in particular, readers are advised to check the product information sheet included in the package of each drug they plan to administer to be certain that the information contained in this work is accurate and that changes have not been made in the recommended dose or in the contraindications for administration. This recommendation is of particular importance in connection with new or infrequently used drugs.

This book was set in Garamond by Silverchair Science + Communications, Inc.
The editor was Ruth Weinberg.
The production supervisor was Phil Galea.
The text was designed by Eve Siegel and the cover by Mary McKeon.
Quebecor World Dubuque was printer and binder.

This book is printed on acid-free paper.

QUICK ANSWERS
to Medical Diagnosis & Treatment

INTRODUCTION

Quick Answers to Medical Diagnosis & Treatment provides practical, expert information on diagnosis and management when you just have a few minutes. It is a single-source reference designed for quick and easy access to the information you need in the clinical setting.

Structured alphabetically, it presents each topic with just the right amount of information to give you the key diagnostic and treatment features of more than 500 diseases. The bulleted format promotes rapid comprehension so that you can immediately apply what you learn from this quick consult.

Each disease entry includes:
• **Key Features:** Essentials of diagnosis and general considerations
• **Clinical Findings:** Symptoms and signs and differential diagnosis
• **Diagnosis:** Laboratory tests, imaging studies, and diagnostic procedures

And, most also include:
• **Treatment:** Medications, surgery, and therapeutic procedures
• **Outcomes:** Complications, prognosis, when to refer, and when to admit
• **Evidence:** Up-to-date clinical guidelines, targeted references, and web sites for clinicians and patients

Supplementing this is a section of pertinent tables and figures that display specific diagnostic and treatment options to help you find the best solutions to immediate clinical problems. Using selected tables, you can quickly pinpoint individual drugs and dosages.

Content is derived from *Current Medical Diagnosis & Treatment (CMDT)*, the leading medicine textbook for hospital and out-patient settings, now in its 48th edition.

Used alone or as a complement to *CMDT,* you will find practical clinical solutions to more than 500 disorders are just seconds away.

McGraw-Hill wishes to acknowledge the contributions made by the authors of *Current Consult Medicine 2007*, whose work forms part of the topics in *Quick Answers* but who are not authoring current topics.

We are also grateful to Maxine A. Papadakis and Stephen J. McPhee, who acted as consultants to this edition.

Authors of content adapted from chapters in *Current Medical Diagnosis & Treatment 2008*:

Daniel C. Adelman, MD

Michael J. Aminoff, MD, DSc, FRCP

Robert B. Baron, MD, MS

Thomas M. Bashore, MD

Timothy G. Berger, MD

Henry F. Chambers, MD

Catherine K. Chang, MD

Mark S. Chesnutt, MD

Peter V. Chin-Hong, MD

William R. Crombleholme, MD

Stuart J. Eisendrath, MD

Paul A. Fitzgerald, MD

Lawrence S. Friedman, MD

Masafumi Fukagawa, MD, PhD

Armando E. Giuliano, MD

Ralph Gonzales, MD, MSPH

Christopher B. Granger, MD

B. Joseph Guglielmo, PharmD

B. Joseph Guglielmo, PharmD

Richard J. Hamill, MD

G. Michael Harper, MD

David B. Hellmann, MD, MACP

Patrick Hranitzky, MD

John B. Imboden, Jr., MD

Robert K. Jackler, MD

Richard A. Jacobs, MD, PhD

Richard A. Jacobs, MD, PhD

C. Bree Johnston, MD, MPH

Christopher J. Kane, MD

Michael J. Kaplan, MD

Mitchell H. Katz, MD

Jeffrey L. Kishiyama, MD

Hoonmo Koo, MD

Kiyoshi Kurokawa, MD, MACP

C. Seth Landefeld, MD

Jonathan E. Lichtmacher, MD

Charles A. Linker, MD

Lawrence Lustig, MD

H. Trent MacKay, MD, MPH

Umesh Masharani, MB, BS, MRCP (UK)

Kenneth R. McQuaid, MD

Maxwell V. Meng, MD

Brent R. W. Moelleken, MD, FACS

Gail Morrison, MD

James A. Murray, DO

Kent R. Olson, MD

Maxine A. Papadakis, MD

Susan S. Philip, MD, MPH

Thomas J. Prendergast, MD

Reed E. Pyeritz, MD, PhD

Joseph H. Rapp, MD

Paul Riordan-Eva, FRCS, FRCOphth

Philip J. Rosenthal, MD

Hope Rugo, MD

Rajabrata Sarkar, MD, PhD

Joshua Schindler, MD

Wayne X. Shandera, MD

Samuel A. Shelburne, MD

Marshall L. Stoller, MD

Michael Sutters, MD

Suzanne Watnick, MD

Andrew R. Zolopa, MD

Topics
A–Z

Abdominal Aortic Aneurysm

KEY FEATURES

ESSENTIALS OF DIAGNOSIS

- Most aortic aneurysms are asymptomatic until rupture, which is catastrophic
- Aneurysms measuring 5 cm are palpable in 80% of patients
- Back or abdominal pain with aneurysmal tenderness may precede rupture
- Hypotension
- Excruciating abdominal pain that radiates to the back

GENERAL CONSIDERATIONS

- The aorta of a healthy young man measures approximately 2 cm
- An aneurysm is considered present when the aortic diameter exceeds 3 cm
- Aneurysms rarely cause problems until diameter exceeds 5 cm
- 90% of abdominal atherosclerotic aneurysms originate below the renal arteries
- Aortic bifurcation is usually involved
- Common iliac arteries are often involved

DEMOGRAPHICS

- Found in 2% of men over age 55
- Male to female ratio is 8:1

CLINICAL FINDINGS

SYMPTOMS AND SIGNS

- Most asymptomatic aneurysms are discovered as incidental findings on ultrasound or CT imaging
- Symptomatic aneurysms
  - Mild to severe midabdominal pain due to aneurysmal expansion often radiates to lower back
  - Pain may be constant or intermittent, exacerbated by even gentle pressure on aneurysm sack, and may also accompany inflammatory aneurysms
- Inflammatory aneurysms occur when an inflammatory peel surrounds the aneurysm and encases the retroperitoneal structures, which include the duodenum and, occasionally, the ureters
- Ruptured aneurysms
  - Severe pain

- Palpable abdominal mass
- Hypotension
- Free rupture into the peritoneal cavity is lethal
- Most aneurysms have a thick lining of blood clot, which can break away and occlude blood flow in a small peripheral artery (embolism)
- Although this phenomenon is rare, multiple localized areas of poor peripheral blood flow (blue toe syndrome) should prompt a search for an aneurysm

DIAGNOSIS

LABORATORY TESTS

- Even with a contained rupture, there may be little change in routine laboratory findings
- Hematocrit will be normal, since there has been no opportunity for hemodilution
- Aneurysms are associated with cardiopulmonary diseases of elderly male smokers, which include
  - Coronary artery disease
  - Carotid disease
  - Renal impairment
  - Emphysema
- Preoperative testing may indicate the presence of these comorbid conditions

IMAGING STUDIES

- Abdominal ultrasonography
  - Study of choice for initial diagnosis
  - Useful in screening 65- to 74-year-old men, but not women, who have a history of smoking
  - Repeated screening does not appear to be needed
- Abdominal or back radiographs: curvilinear calcifications outlining portions of aneurysm wall may be seen in approximately 75% of patients
- CT scans
  - Provide a more reliable assessment of aneurysm diameter
  - Should be done when the aneurysm nears the diameter threshold for treatment
- Contrast-enhanced CT scans
  - Show the arteries above and below the aneurysm
  - Visualization of this vasculature is essential for planning repair

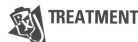 TREATMENT

EMERGENCY REPAIR

- If the rupture and bleeding are confined to the retroperitoneum, both the low blood pressure and retroperitoneal containment may arrest blood loss long enough for the patient to undergo urgent operation
- Endovascular repair represents the best opportunity for survival because the retroperitoneal blood clot is left intact
- Patients who have free rupture of the aneurysm into the peritoneum do not survive long enough to undergo surgical repair

ELECTIVE REPAIR

- Generally indicated for aortic aneurysms > 5.5 cm in diameter or aneurysms that have undergone rapid expansion (> 5 mm in 6 months)

SURGERY

- Not indicated when inflammatory aneurysm is present unless retroperitoneal structures, such as the ureter, are compressed
- Interestingly, the inflammation that encases an inflammatory aneurysm recedes after either endovascular or surgical aneurysmal repair
- Open surgical aneurysm repair
  - Graft is sutured to the non-dilated aorta above and below the aneurysm
  - This involves an abdominal incision, extensive dissection, and interruption of aortic blood flow
  - Mortality rate is low when the procedure is performed in good risk patients in experienced centers
  - Older, sicker patients may not tolerate cardiopulmonary stresses of the surgery

ENDOVASCULAR REPAIR

- Stent-graft is used to line the aorta and exclude the aneurysm
- Anatomic requirements to securely achieve aneurysm exclusion vary according to performance characteristics of the specific stent-graft device
- In general, successful attachment requires a segment of non-dilated aorta (neck) between the renal arteries and the aneurysm to be at least 15 mm in length
- Device insertion requires iliac arteries to be at least 7 mm in diameter

- Endovascular techniques have improved outcomes, so some experts recommend treating smaller aneurysms
- Studies are ongoing to determine whether this may be appropriate

 OUTCOME

COMPLICATIONS

- Myocardial infarction
- Routine infrarenal aneurysms
- Respiratory complications are similar to those seen in most major abdominal surgery
- Gastrointestinal hemorrhage

PROGNOSIS

- Open elective surgical resection
  - Mortality rate is 1–5%
  - Of those who survive surgery, about 60% are alive at 5 years
  - Myocardial infarction is leading cause of death
- Endovascular aneurysm repair
  - May be less definitive than open surgical repair
  - In high-risk patients, endovascular approach reduces perioperative morbidity and mortality
  - Prognosis depends on how successfully aneurysm has been excluded from the circulation
- Mortality rates among patients with large aneurysms who have not undergone surgery
  - 12% annual risk of rupture in aneurysms ≥ 6 cm in diameter
  - 25% annual risk of rupture in aneurysms ≥ 7 cm diameter

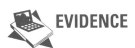 **EVIDENCE**

PRACTICE GUIDELINES

- Brewster DC et al. Guidelines for the treatment of abdominal aortic aneurysms. Report of a subcommittee of the Joint Council of the American Association for Vascular Surgery and Society for Vascular Surgery. J Vasc Surg. 2003 May;37(5):1106–17. [PMID: 12756363]

INFORMATION FOR PATIENTS

- Cleveland Clinic: Abdominal Aortic Aneurysm
- MedlinePlus: Abdominal Aortic Aneurysm

- MedlinePlus: Abdominal Aortic Aneurysm interactive tutorial

REFERENCES

- Blankensteijn JD et al; Dutch Randomized Endovascular Aneurysm Management (DREAM) Trial Group. Two-year outcomes after conventional or endovascular repair of abdominal aortic aneurysms. N Engl J Med. 2005 Jun 9; 352(23):2398–405. [PMID: 15944424]
- Fleming C et al. Screening for abdominal aortic aneurysm: a best-evidence systematic review for the U.S. Preventive Services Task Force. Ann Intern Med. 2005 Feb 1;142(3):203–11. [PMID: 15684209]
- Hellmann DB et al. Inflammatory abdominal aortic aneurysm. JAMA. 2007 Jan 24;297(4):395–400. [PMID: 17244836]
- McFalls EO et al. Coronary-artery revascularization before elective major vascular surgery. N Engl J Med. 2004 Dec 30;351(27):2795–804. [PMID: 15625331]
- Prinssen M et al; Dutch Randomized Endovascular Aneurysm Management (DREAM) Trial Group. A randomized trial comparing conventional and endovascular repair of abdominal aortic aneurysms. N Engl J Med. 2004 Oct 14;351(16):1607–18. [PMID: 15483279]

Abortion

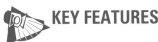 **KEY FEATURES**

ESSENTIALS OF DIAGNOSIS

- In the United States, 87% of abortions are performed before 13 weeks' gestation and only 1.4% after 20 weeks
- If abortion is chosen, every effort should be made to encourage an early procedure

GENERAL CONSIDERATIONS

- The abortion-related maternal mortality rate has fallen markedly since the legalization of abortion in the United States in 1973
- While several state laws limiting access to abortion and a federal law banning a rarely-used variation of dilation and evacuation have been enacted, abortion remains legal and available until fetal viability under Roe v. Wade
- The long-term sequelae of repeated induced abortions are uncertain regarding increased rates of fetal loss or premature labor
- Adverse side effects can be reduced by performing abortion early with minimal cervical dilation or by the use of osmotic dilators to induce gradual cervical dilation

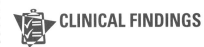 **CLINICAL FINDINGS**

SYMPTOMS AND SIGNS

- Pregnancy at less than the gestational age of viability

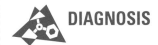 **DIAGNOSIS**

LABORATORY TESTS

- Determine if patient is Rh positive or negative
- Pregnancy test

DIAGNOSTIC PROCEDURES

- Establish date of last menstrual period (LMP) by pelvic examination or ultrasound

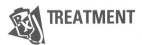 **TREATMENT**

MEDICATIONS

- Mifepristone/misoprostol
  - Day 1: Mifepristone (RU 486), 600 mg as a single dose; FDA-approved oral abortifacient
  - Day 3: Misoprostol (a prostaglandin) 400 mcg PO in a single dose
  - Combination 95% successful in terminating pregnancies of up to 9 weeks' duration with minimum complications
- Although not approved by the FDA for this indication, a combination of intramuscular methotrexate, 50 mg/m^2 of body surface area, followed 7 days later by vaginal misoprostol, 800 mcg, is 98% successful in terminating pregnancy at 8 weeks or less
  - Minor side effects of nausea, vomiting, and diarrhea are common
  - There is a 5–10% incidence of hemorrhage or incomplete abortion requiring curettage, but there are no known long-term complications

THERAPEUTIC PROCEDURES

- Abortion in the first trimester is performed by vacuum aspiration under local anesthesia
- A similar technique, dilation and evacuation, is generally used in the second trimester, with general or local anesthesia
- Techniques using intra-amniotic instillation of hypertonic saline solution or various prostaglandin regimens, along with osmotic dilators, are also occasionally used after 18 weeks from the LMP but are more difficult for the patient

 OUTCOME

COMPLICATIONS

- Retained products of conception (often associated with infection and heavy bleeding)
- Unrecognized ectopic pregnancy; immediate analysis of the removed tissue for placenta can exclude or corroborate the diagnosis of ectopic pregnancy
- Women with fever, bleeding, or abdominal pain after abortion should be examined; use of broad-spectrum antibiotics and reaspiration of the uterus are frequently necessary
- Endometritis and toxic shock caused by *Clostridium sordellii* following medical abortion (rare)

PROGNOSIS

- Legal abortion has a mortality rate of < 1:100,000
- Rates of morbidity and mortality rise with length of gestation

WHEN TO ADMIT

- Hospitalization is advisable if acute salpingitis requires IV administration of antibiotics
- Complications following illegal abortion often need emergency care for hemorrhage, septic shock, or uterine perforation

PREVENTION

- Contraception should be thoroughly discussed and provided at the time of abortion
- Prophylactic antibiotics are indicated; for instance
  – A one-dose regimen of doxycycline, 200 mg PO 1 h before the procedure
  – Many clinicians prescribe tetracycline, 500 mg PO QID, for 5 days after the procedure for all patients as presumptive treatment for *Chlamydia*

- Rh immune globulin should be given to all Rh-negative women following abortion

 EVIDENCE

PRACTICE GUIDELINES

- National Abortion Federation Clinical Policy Guidelines, 2006.
- ACOG. ACOG practice bulletin: Clinical management guidelines of Obstetrician-Gynecologists. Number 67, October 2005. Medical management of abortion. Obstet Gynecol. 2005 Oct; 106(4):871–82. [PMID: 16199653]

WEB SITES

- National Abortion Federation: Professional Education Resources
- Kaiser Family Foundation Fact Sheet: Abortion in the U.S.

INFORMATION FOR PATIENTS

- American College of Obstetricians and Gynecologists (ACOG)
- ACOG: Pregnancy Choices
- ACOG: Induced Abortion
- MedlinePlus: Abortion

REFERENCES

- Fischer M et al. Fatal toxic shock syndrome associated with *Clostridium sordellii* after medical abortion. N Engl J Med. 2005 Dec 1;353(22):2352–60. [PMID: 16319384]
- Grimes DA et al. Induced abortion: an overview for internists. Ann Intern Med. 2004 Apr 20;140(8):620–6. [PMID: 15096333]

Abortion, Recurrent

 KEY FEATURES

- Defined as loss of three or more previable (< 500 g) pregnancies in succession
- Women with three previous unexplained losses have a 70–80% chance of carrying a subsequent pregnancy to viability

 CLINICAL FINDINGS

- Occurs in 0.4–0.8% of all pregnancies
- Clinical findings are similar to those in spontaneous abortion

 DIAGNOSIS

- Preconception therapy aims to detect maternal or paternal defects contributing to abortion; these are found in about 50% of couples
- Polycystic ovaries, thyroid abnormalities, and diabetes should be ruled out
- Hypercoagulable states should be ruled out
- Endometrial extra tissue should be examined to determine the adequacy of its response to hormones in the postovulatory phase
- Hysteroscopy or hysterography can exclude uterine abnormalities
- Chromosomal analysis of partners identifies balanced translocations in 5% of couples

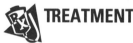 **TREATMENT**

- Early prenatal care and frequent office visits are routine
- Complete bed rest is justified only for bleeding or pain
- Empiric sex steroid therapy is contraindicated

Abortion, Spontaneous

 KEY FEATURES

ESSENTIALS OF DIAGNOSIS

- Intrauterine pregnancy < 20 weeks
- Low or falling levels of human chorionic gonadotropin (hCG)
- Bleeding or midline cramping pain, or both
- Open cervical os
- Complete or partial expulsion of products of conception

GENERAL CONSIDERATIONS

- Defined as termination of gestation prior to the 20th week of pregnancy
- 75% of cases occur before the 16th week, with 75% of these before the 8th week
- Almost 20% of clinically recognized pregnancies terminate in spontaneous abortion
- More than 60% of cases result from chromosomal defects
- About 15% of cases arc associated with
  - Maternal trauma
  - Infection
  - Dietary deficiency
  - Diabetes mellitus
  - Hypothyroidism
  - The lupus anticoagulant-anticardiolipin-antiphospholipid antibody syndrome
  - Anatomic malformations
- There is no evidence that psychic stimuli such as severe fright, grief, anger, or anxiety can induce termination
- There is no evidence that electromagnetic fields are associated with an increased risk of termination
- It is important to distinguish women with incompetent cervix from more typical early abortion, premature labor, or rupture of the membranes

DEMOGRAPHICS

- Predisposing factors
  - History of incompetent cervix
  - Cervical conization or surgery
  - Cervical injury
  - Diethylstilbestrol exposure
  - Anatomic abnormalities of the cervix

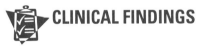 **CLINICAL FINDINGS**

SYMPTOMS AND SIGNS

- **Incompetent cervix**
  - Classically presents as "silent" cervical dilation (without contractions) between weeks 16 and 28
- **Threatened abortion**
  - Bleeding or cramping without termination
  - The cervix is not dilated
- **Inevitable abortion**
  - The cervix is dilated and membranes may be ruptured
  - Passage of products of conception has not occurred but is considered inevitable
- **Complete abortion**
  - The fetus and placenta are completely expelled
  - Pain ceases, but spotting may persist

- **Incomplete abortion**
  - Some portion of the products of conception remain in the uterus
  - Cramps are usually mild; bleeding is persistent and often excessive
- **Missed abortion**
  - The pregnancy has ceased to develop, but the conception has not been expelled
  - There is brownish vaginal discharge but no free bleeding
  - Symptoms of pregnancy disappear

DIFFERENTIAL DIAGNOSIS

- Ectopic pregnancy
- Hydatidiform mole
- Incompetent cervix
- Anovular bleeding in a nonpregnant women
- Menses or menorrhagia
- Cervical neoplasm or lesion

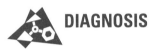 **DIAGNOSIS**

LABORATORY TESTS

- Falling levels of hCG
- Complete blood count should be obtained if bleeding is heavy
- Rh type should be determined and Rho(D) Ig given if the type is Rh negative
- All recovered tissue should be preserved and assessed by a pathologist

IMAGING STUDIES

- Ultrasound can identify the gestational sac 5–6 weeks from the last menstrual period, a fetal pole at 6 weeks, and fetal cardiac activity at 6–7 weeks
- With accurate dating, a small, irregular sac without a fetal pole is diagnostic of an abnormal pregnancy

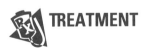 **TREATMENT**

MEDICATIONS

- Antibiotics should be used only if there is evidence of infection
- Hormonal treatment is contraindicated in **threatened abortion**
- Prostaglandin vaginal tablets (misoprostol) may be used in termination of **missed abortion**

SURGERY

- **Incomplete or inevitable abortion** is treated with prompt removal of any

remaining products of conception to stop bleeding and prevent infection

THERAPEUTIC PROCEDURES

- **Threatened abortion**
  - Can be treated with bed rest for 24–48 h with gradual resumption of activities
  - Abstinence from coitus and douching
- **Inevitable** or **missed abortion**
  - Requires evacuation
  - Dilation with laminaria insertion and aspiration is preferred for missed abortion, though prostaglandin tablets are an alternative
- **Incompetent cervix**
  - Treated with cerclage and restriction of activities
  - Cervical cultures for *Neisseria gonorrhoeae, Chlamydia*, and group B *Streptococcus* should be obtained before the procedure

 OUTCOME

FOLLOW-UP

- With recurrent first-trimester losses (three or more) chromosomal analysis of tissue may be informative

COMPLICATIONS

- Retained tissue and prolonged bleeding can occur with prostaglandin use

WHEN TO REFER

- Missed abortion
- Inevitable or incomplete abortion

WHEN TO ADMIT

- Vital signs unstable from excessive bleeding
- When evacuation of uterine contents cannot be done as an outpatient

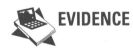 **EVIDENCE**

PRACTICE GUIDELINES

- ACOG practice bulletin. American College of Obstetricians and Gynecologists. Management of recurrent pregnancy loss. Number 24, February 2001. (Replaces Technical Bulletin Number 212, September 1995.) American College of Obstetricians and Gynecologists. Int J Gynaecol Obstet. 2002;78:179. [PMID: 12360906]

INFORMATION FOR PATIENTS

- American College of Obstetricians and Gynecologists: Early Pregnancy Loss: Miscarriage and Molar Pregnancy
- March of Dimes: Miscarriage
- MedlinePlus: Miscarriage
- Torpy JM. JAMA patient page. Miscarriage. JAMA. 2002;288:1936. [PMID: 12377095]

REFERENCES

- Aleman A et al. Bed rest during pregnancy for preventing miscarriage. Cochrane Database Syst Rev. 2005 Apr 18;(2):CD003576. [PMID: 15846669]
- Trinder J et al. Management of miscarriage: expectant, medical, or surgical? Results of randomised controlled trial (miscarriage treatment (MIST) trial). BMJ. 2006 May 27;332(7552):1235–40. [PMID: 16707509]

Acanthamoeba Infections

 KEY FEATURES

ESSENTIALS OF DIAGNOSIS

- Acute meningoencephalitis or chronic granulomatous encephalitis after contact with warm fresh water
- Keratitis, particularly in contact lens users

GENERAL CONSIDERATIONS

- Free-living amebas of the genus *Acanthamoeba*
- Found in soil and in fresh, brackish water

Granulomatous amebic encephalitis

- Caused by *Acanthamoeba* species and *Balamuthia mandrillaris*
- More chronic than primary amebic meningoencephalitis (see Amebic Meningoencephalitis, Primary)
- Neurologic disease
  - May be preceded by skin lesions, including ulcers and nodules
  - Develops slowly after an uncertain incubation period

Keratitis

- Painful, sight-threatening corneal infection

- Associated with corneal trauma, most commonly after use of contact lenses and contaminated saline solution

 CLINICAL FINDINGS

SYMPTOMS AND SIGNS

Granulomatous amebic encephalitis

- Headache
- Meningismus
- Nausea, vomiting
- Lethargy
- Low-grade fevers
- Focal neurologic findings, mental status abnormalities

Keratitis

- Progresses slowly, with waxing and waning clinical findings over months
- Severe eye pain
- Photophobia
- Tearing
- Blurred vision

DIFFERENTIAL DIAGNOSIS

- Many cases of *Acanthamoeba* keratitis are misdiagnosed as viral keratitis

 DIAGNOSIS

LABORATORY TESTS

Granulomatous amebic encephalitis

- Cerebrospinal fluid
  - Shows lymphocytic pleocytosis with elevated protein levels
  - Amebas not typically seen
- Diagnosis can be made by biopsy of skin or brain lesions
- Lumbar puncture is dangerous due to increased intracranial pressure

Keratitis

- Lack of response to antibacterial, antifungal, and antiviral topical treatments and potential use of contaminated contact lens solution are suggestive of the diagnosis
- Ocular examination shows corneal ring infiltrates, but these can also be caused by other pathogens
- Diagnosis can be made by examination or culture of corneal scrapings
- Available diagnostic techniques include
  - Examination of a wet preparation for cysts and motile trophozoites
  - Examination of stained specimens
  - Evaluation with immunofluorescent reagents, culture of organisms, and polymerase chain reaction

IMAGING STUDIES

- CT and MRI show single or multiple nonspecific lesions in patients with encephalitis

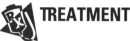 TREATMENT

MEDICATIONS

Granulomatous amebic encephalitis

- Some patients have been treated successfully with various combinations of
  - Flucytosine
  - Pentamidine
  - Fluconazole or itraconazole
  - Sulfadiazine
  - Trimethoprim-sulfamethoxazole
  - Azithromycin
- However, no treatment has been proved effective

Keratitis

- Can be cured with local therapy
- Topical propamidine isethionate (0.1%), chlorhexidine digluconate (0.02%), polyhexamethylene biguanide, neomycin-polymyxin B-gramicidin, miconazole, and combinations of these agents have been used successfully
- Oral itraconazole or ketoconazole can be added for deep keratitis
- Drug resistance has been reported
- Use of corticosteroid therapy is controversial

THERAPEUTIC PROCEDURES

- Debridement and penetrating keratoplasty have been performed in addition to medical therapy
- Corneal grafting can be done after the amebic infection has been eradicated

 OUTCOME

PROGNOSIS

- With early treatment, many patients can expect cure and a good visual result
- Untreated encephalitis can lead to death in weeks to months
- Untreated keratitis can progress slowly over months and can lead to blindness

WHEN TO REFER

- All patients with keratitis should be referred to an ophthalmologist

WHEN TO ADMIT

- All cases of encephalitis

PREVENTION

- Prevention of keratitis requires immersion of contact lenses in disinfectant solutions or heat sterilization
  - Lenses should not be cleaned in homemade saline solutions
  - Lenses should not be worn while swimming

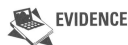 EVIDENCE

PRACTICE GUIDELINES

- National Guideline Clearinghouse

WEB SITE

- Centers for Disease Control and Prevention—Division of Parasitic Diseases

INFORMATION FOR PATIENTS

- Centers for Disease Control and Prevention

REFERENCES

- Driebe WT Jr. Present status of contact lens-induced corneal infections. Ophthalmol Clin North Am. 2003 Sep; 16(3):485–94. [PMID: 14564769]
- Marciano-Cabral F et al. *Acanthamoeba* spp. as agents of disease in humans. Clin Microbiol Rev. 2003 Apr;16(2):273–307. [PMID: 12692099]
- Vargas-Zepeda J et al. Successful treatment of *Naegleria fowleri* meningoencephalitis by using intravenous amphotericin B, fluconazole and rifampicin. Arch Med Res. 2005 Jan–Feb;36(1):83–6. [PMID: 15900627]

Acetaminophen Overdose

 KEY FEATURES

ESSENTIALS OF DIAGNOSIS

- Toxic dose: > 140 mg/kg, not to exceed > 7 g (acute) or > 4–6 g/day (chronic)
- Nausea, vomiting early after acute ingestion
- Hepatic necrosis evident after 24–36 h
- Fulminant hepatic failure can occur

 CLINICAL FINDINGS

- Early: nausea and "exploding head" sensation
- After 24–36 h: elevated transaminases, evidence of hepatic dysfunction, and fulminant hepatic failure
- Massive overdose (eg, levels > 600 mg/L) can cause coma, hypotension, metabolic acidosis soon after ingestion

 DIAGNOSIS

- Elevated serum acetaminophen level (> 150–200 mg/L at 4 h or 75–100 mg/L at 8 h)
- Chronic excessive dosing may produce only moderately elevated levels
- Elevated hepatic transaminases, prothrombin time/INR, bilirubin
- Poor prognosis
  - Hepatic failure with metabolic acidosis
  - Encephalopathy

 TREATMENT

- Oral activated charcoal 60–100 g mixed in aqueous slurry (if given within 1–2 h of acute ingestion)
- Oral *N*-acetylcysteine (NAC), 140 mg/kg oral loading dose, followed by 70 mg/kg q4h
- Traditional US oral regimen 72 h (17 doses), although many stop at 36 h (9 doses) if transaminases normal
- Newly approved IV NAC (Acetadote), 150 mg/kg IV × 1 over 60 min, then 50 mg/k IV × 1 over 4h, then 100 mg/kg IV × 1 over 16h (21 h infusion)
- Fulminant liver failure may require emergency liver transplantation

Achalasia

 KEY FEATURES

ESSENTIALS OF DIAGNOSIS

- Gradual, progressive dysphagia for solids and liquids
- Regurgitation of undigested food
- Barium esophagogram shows "bird's beak" distal esophagus
- Esophageal manometry confirms diagnosis

GENERAL CONSIDERATIONS

- Idiopathic motility disorder characterized by loss of peristalsis in the distal two-thirds (smooth muscle) of the esophagus and impaired relaxation of the lower esophageal sphincter
- Cause unknown

DEMOGRAPHICS

- Increased incidence with advancing age

 CLINICAL FINDINGS

SYMPTOMS AND SIGNS

- Gradual onset of dysphagia for solid foods and, in the majority, liquids also
- Symptoms persist for months to years
- Substernal chest pain, discomfort, or fullness
- Regurgitation of undigested food
- Nocturnal regurgitation
- Coughing or aspiration
- Weight loss is common
- Physical examination unhelpful

DIFFERENTIAL DIAGNOSIS

- Chagas' disease
- Primary or metastatic tumors at the gastroesophageal junction
- Diffuse esophageal spasm
- Scleroderma esophagus
- Peptic stricture

 DIAGNOSIS

IMAGING STUDIES

- Chest x-ray: air-fluid level in an enlarged, fluid-filled esophagus
- Barium esophagography
  - Esophageal dilation
  - Loss of esophageal peristalsis
  - Poor esophageal emptying
  - A smooth, symmetric "bird's beak" tapering of the distal esophagus

DIAGNOSTIC PROCEDURES

- Endoscopy to exclude a distal stricture or carcinoma
- Esophageal manometry confirms the diagnosis; characteristic features include
  - Complete absence of peristalsis

– Elevated lower esophageal sphincter pressure with incomplete relaxation during swallowing

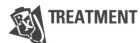 **TREATMENT**

MEDICATIONS

- Calcium channel blockers (nifedipine) may provide temporary symptomatic improvement

SURGERY

- Surgical myotomy
  – Modified Heller cardiomyotomy of the lower esophageal sphincter and cardia plus an antireflux procedure (fundoplication) results in improvement in > 85%; now routinely performed laparoscopically

THERAPEUTIC PROCEDURES

- Botulinum toxin injection
  – Endoscopically guided injection of botulinum toxin directly into the lower esophageal sphincter results in improvement in 85%
  – Symptom relapse occurs in > 50% within 6–9 months
  – May cause submucosal scarring that may make subsequent surgical myotomy more difficult
- 75% of initial responders to botulinum toxin injection who relapse improve with repeated injections
- Pneumatic dilation; goal is to disrupt lower esophageal sphincter
  – Over 75–85% of patients experience good to excellent relief of dysphagia after 1–3 sessions
  – > 50–70% achieve long-term relief

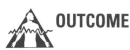 **OUTCOME**

FOLLOW-UP

- No follow-up necessary unless symptoms recur

COMPLICATIONS

- Perforations occur in < 3% of pneumatic dilations, may require operative repair
- Increased risk of squamous cell esophageal cancer

PROGNOSIS

- After successful dilation or myotomy, patients have near-normal swallowing, although esophageal peristalsis is absent

WHEN TO REFER

- Patients with achalasia should be evaluated by a gastrointestinal specialist

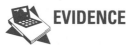 **EVIDENCE**

PRACTICE GUIDELINES

- National Guideline Clearinghouse
- Patient Care Committee; Society for Surgery of the Alimentary Tract: Esophageal achalasia. SSAT patient care guidelines. J Gastrointest Surg. 2004;8:367. [PMID: 15115006]
- Society for Surgery of the Alimentary Tract

INFORMATION FOR PATIENTS

- MedlinePlus
- Society of Thoracic Surgeons

REFERENCES

- Karamanolis G et al. Long-term outcome of pneumatic dilation in the treatment of achalasia. Am J Gastroenterol. 2005 Feb;100(2):270–4. [PMID: 15667481]
- Lake JM et al. Review article: the management of achalasia—a comparison of different treatment modalities. Aliment Pharmacol Ther. 2006 Sep 15; 24(6):909–18. [PMID: 16948803]
- Park W et al. Etiology and pathogenesis of achalasia: the current understanding. Am J Gastroenterol. 2005 Jun; 100(6):1404–14. [PMID: 15929777]
- Vela MF et al. The long-term efficacy of pnematic dilation and Heller myotomy for the treatment of achalasia. Clin Gastroenterol Hepatol. 2006 May; 4(5):580–7. [PMID: 16630776]

Acidosis, Lactic

 KEY FEATURES

ESSENTIALS OF DIAGNOSIS

- Severe acidosis with hyperventilation
- Blood pH below 7.30
- Serum bicarbonate < 15 mEq/L
- Anion gap > 15 mEq/L
- Absent serum ketones
- Serum lactate > 5 mmol/L

GENERAL CONSIDERATIONS

- Characterized by overproduction of lactic acid (tissue hypoxia), deficient removal (hepatic failure), or both (circulatory collapse)
- Occurs often in severely ill patients suffering from
  – Cardiac decompensation
  – Respiratory or hepatic failure
  – Septicemia
  – Infarction of bowel or extremities
- With the discontinuance of phenformin therapy in the United States, lactic acidosis in diabetics is uncommon but occasionally occurs with use of metformin. It must be considered in the acidotic diabetic, especially if the patient is seriously ill

Etiology

- Tissue hypoxia, eg, cardiogenic, septic, or hemorrhagic shock; seizure; carbon monoxide or cyanide poisoning
- Hepatic failure
- Ischemic bowel
- Infarction of extremities
- Diabetes, especially with metformin use
- Ketoacidosis
- Renal failure
- Infection
- Leukemia or lymphoma
- Drugs: ethanol, methanol, salicylates, isoniazid
- AIDS
- Idiopathic

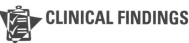 **CLINICAL FINDINGS**

SYMPTOMS AND SIGNS

- Main clinical feature is marked hyperventilation
- When lactic acidosis is secondary to tissue hypoxia or vascular collapse, the clinical presentation is variable, being that of the prevailing catastrophic illness
- In idiopathic, or spontaneous, lactic acidosis
  – Onset is rapid (usually over a few hours)
  – Blood pressure is normal
  – Peripheral circulation is good
  – No cyanosis

DIFFERENTIAL DIAGNOSIS

Other causes of metabolic acidosis

- Diabetic ketoacidosis
- Starvation ketoacidosis
- Alcoholic ketoacidosis

- Renal failure (acute or chronic)
- Ethylene glycol toxicity
- Methanol toxicity
- Salicylate toxicity
- Other: paraldehyde, metformin, isoniazid, iron, rhabdomyolysis

DIAGNOSIS

LABORATORY TESTS

- High anion gap (serum sodium minus the sum of chloride and bicarbonate anions [in mEq/L] should be no greater than 15). A higher value indicates the existence of an abnormal compartment of anions
- Plasma bicarbonate and blood pH are quite low, indicating the presence of severe metabolic acidosis
- Ketones are usually absent from plasma and urine, or at least not prominent
- In the absence of azotemia, hyperphosphatemia occurs in lactic acidosis for reasons that are not clear
- The diagnosis is confirmed by demonstrating, in a sample of blood that is promptly chilled and separated, a plasma lactic acid concentration of 5 mmol/L or higher (values as high as 30 mmol/L have been reported)
- Normal plasma values average 1 mmol/L, with a normal lactate–pyruvate ratio of 10:1. This ratio is greatly exceeded in lactic acidosis

TREATMENT

- Empiric antibiotic coverage for sepsis should be given after culture samples are obtained if the cause of lactic acidosis is unknown
- Alkalinization with IV sodium bicarbonate to keep the pH above 7.2 in the emergency treatment of lactic acidosis is controversial; as much as 2000 mEq in 24 h has been used. However, there is no evidence that the mortality rate is favorably affected by administering bicarbonate

THERAPEUTIC PROCEDURES

- Aggressive treatment of the precipitating cause is the main component of therapy, such as ensuring adequate oxygenation and vascular perfusion of tissues
- Hemodialysis may be useful when large sodium loads are poorly tolerated

OUTCOME

PROGNOSIS

- Mortality rate of spontaneous lactic acidosis is high
- Early and aggressive treatment of metformin-induced lactic acidosis with hemofiltration improves outcome
- Prognosis in most cases is that of the primary disorder that produced the lactic acidosis

WHEN TO ADMIT

- All patients because of the high mortality rate

EVIDENCE

PRACTICE GUIDELINES

- National Guideline Clearinghouse: Surviving Sepsis Campaign Guidelines for Management of Severe Sepsis and Septic Shock

REFERENCES

- Forsythe SM et al. Sodium bicarbonate for the treatment of lactic acidosis. Chest. 2000 Jan;117(1):260–7. [PMID: 10631227]
- Salpeter S et al. Risk of fatal and nonfatal lactic acidosis with metformin use in type 2 diabetes mellitus. Cochrane Database Syst Rev. 2006 Jan 25;(1):CD002967. [PMID: 16437448]

Acidosis, Metabolic, Decreased or Normal Anion Gap

KEY FEATURES

ESSENTIALS OF DIAGNOSIS

- The hallmark of this disorder is that the low HCO_3^- of metabolic acidosis is associated with hyperchloremia, so that the anion gap remains normal
- Decreased HCO_3^- is seen also in respiratory alkalosis, but the pH distinguishes between the two disorders

GENERAL CONSIDERATIONS

- Most common causes
  - Gastrointestinal (GI) HCO_3^- loss
  - Defects in renal acidification (renal tubular acidoses)
- The urinary anion gap can differentiate between these two causes

Renal tubular acidosis (RTA)

- Hyperchloremic acidosis with a normal anion gap and normal or near normal glomerular filtration rate, in the absence of diarrhea
- Three major types of RTA can be differentiated by the clinical setting: urinary pH, urinary anion gap (see below), serum K^+ level

HCO_3^- loss

- **Normal anion gap (6–12 mEq)**
  - GI loss of HCO_3^-, eg, diarrhea, pancreatic ileostomy, or ileal loop bladder
  - RTA
  - Recovery from diabetic ketoacidosis
  - Dilutional acidosis from rapid administration of 0.9% NaCl
  - Carbonic anhydrase inhibitors
  - Chloride retention or administration of HCl equivalent or NH_4Cl
- **Decreased anion gap (< 6 mEq)**
  - Plasma cell dyscrasias, eg, multiple myeloma (cationic paraproteins accompanied by chloride and bicarbonate)
  - Bromide or lithium intoxication
- **Decreased anion gap without acidosis**
  - Hypoalbuminemia (decreased unmeasured anion)
  - Severe hyperlipidemia

Renal tubular acidoses

- **Type I (distal H^+ secretion defect)**
  - Due to selective deficiency in H^+ secretion in the distal nephron
  - Low serum K^+
  - Despite acidosis, urinary pH cannot be acidified (urine pH > 5.5)
  - Associated with autoimmune disease, hypercalcemia
- **Type II (proximal HCO_3^- reabsorption defect)**
  - Due to a selective defect in the proximal tubule's ability to adequately reabsorb filtered HCO_3^-
  - Low serum K^+
  - Urine pH < 5.5
  - Associated with multiple myeloma and drugs, eg, sulfa, carbonic anhydrase inhibitors (acetazolamide)
- **Type IV (hyporeninemic hypoaldosteronism)**
  - Only RTA characterized by hyperkalemic, hyperchloremic acidosis
  - Defect is aldosterone deficiency or antagonism, which impairs distal

nephron Na^+ reabsorption and K^+ and H^+ excretion

– Urine pH < 5.5

– Renal salt wasting is frequently present

– Most common in diabetic nephropathy, tubulointerstitial renal diseases, AIDS, and hypertensive nephrosclerosis

 CLINICAL FINDINGS

SYMPTOMS AND SIGNS

• Symptoms are mainly those of the underlying disorder

• Compensatory hyperventilation may be misinterpreted as a primary respiratory disorder

• When acidosis is severe, Kussmaul respirations (deep, regular, sighing respirations) occur and are indicative of intense stimulation of the respiratory center

 DIAGNOSIS

LABORATORY TESTS

• See Table 32

• Blood pH, serum HCO_3^-, and PCO_2 are decreased

• Anion gap is normal (hyperchloremic) or decreased

• Hyperkalemia may be seen

• Urinary anion gap from a random urine sample ($[Na^+ + K^+] - Cl^-$) reflects the ability of the kidney to excrete NH_4Cl as in the following equation:

$$Na^+ + K^+ + NH_3^+ = Cl^- + 80$$

where 80 is the average value for the difference in the urinary anions and cations other than Na^+, K^+, NH_3^+, and Cl^-

• Urinary anion gap is equal to $80 - NH_3^+$; this gap aids in the distinction between GI and renal causes of hyperchloremic acidosis:

– If the cause of the metabolic acidosis is GI

▫ HCO_3^- loss (diarrhea), renal acidification ability remains normal

▫ NH_4Cl excretion increases in response to the acidosis

▫ Urinary anion gap is negative (eg, –30 mEq/L)

– If the cause is distal RTA

▫ The kidney is unable to excrete H^+ and thus unable to increase NH_4Cl excretion

▫ Therefore, urinary anion gap is positive (eg, +25 mEq/L)

– In type II (proximal) RTA

▫ The kidney has defective HCO_3^- reabsorption, leading to increased

HCO_3^- excretion rather than decreased NH_4Cl excretion

▫ Thus, the urinary anion gap is often negative

• Urinary pH may not as readily differentiate between renal and GI etiologies

 TREATMENT

MEDICATIONS

• See Table 32

• Treatment of RTA is mainly achieved by administration of alkali (either as bicarbonate or citrate) to correct metabolic abnormalities and prevent nephrocalcinosis and renal failure

• Type I distal RTA

– Supplementation of bicarbonate is necessary since acid accumulates systemically

• Type II proximal RTA

– Correction of low serum bicarbonate is not indicated except in severe cases

– Large amounts of alkali (10–15 mEq/kg/day) may be required because much of the alkali is secreted into the urine, which exacerbates hypokalemia

– A mixture of sodium and potassium salts, such as K-Shohl, is preferred

 OUTCOME

COMPLICATIONS

• The hyperkalemia can be exacerbated by drugs, including

– Angiotensin-converting enzyme inhibitors

– Aldosterone receptor blockers, such as spironolactone

– Nonsteroidal anti-inflammatory drugs

WHEN TO REFER

• If expertise is needed in determining the etiology of the metabolic acidosis

• If consultation is needed on whether bicarbonate should be administered

WHEN TO ADMIT

• Respiratory muscle weakness from severe hypokalemia

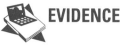 **EVIDENCE**

WEB SITE

• National Kidney Foundation

INFORMATION FOR PATIENTS

• MedlinePlus: Metabolic Acidosis

• MedlinePlus: Distal Renal Tubular Acidosis

• MedlinePlus: Proximal Renal Tubular Acidosis

• National Kidney and Urologic Diseases Information Clearinghouse: Renal Tubular Acidosis

REFERENCES

• Casaletto JJ. Differential diagnosis of metabolic acidosis. Emerg Med Clin North Am. 2005;23:771. [PMID: 15982545]

• Eledrisi MS et al. Overview of the diagnosis and management of diabetic ketoacidosis. Am J Med Sci. 2006 May; 331(5):243–51. [PMID: 16702793]

• Forni LG et al. Circulating anions usually associated with the Krebs cycle in patients with metabolic acidosis. Crit Care. 2005 Oct 5;9(5):R591–5. [PMID: 16277723]

• Matin MJ et al. Use of serum bicarbonate measurement in place of arterial base deficit in the surgical intensive care unit. Arch Surg. 2005 Aug;140(8):745–51. [PMID: 16103283]

• Moe OW et al. Clinical acid-base pathophysiology: disorders of plasma anion gap. Best Pract Res Clin Endocrinol Metab. 2003 Dec;17(4):559–74. [PMID: 14687589]

• Rosival V. Metabolic acidosis. Crit Care Med. 2004 Dec;32(12):2563–4. [PMID: 15599180]

Acidosis, Metabolic, Increased Anion Gap

 KEY FEATURES

ESSENTIALS OF DIAGNOSIS

• Hallmark of this disorder is that metabolic acidosis (thus low HCO_3^-) is associated with normal serum Cl^-, so that the anion gap increases

• Decreased HCO_3^- is also seen also in respiratory alkalosis, but pH distinguishes between the two disorders

GENERAL CONSIDERATIONS

- Calculation of the anion gap is useful in determining the cause of the metabolic acidosis
- Normochloremic (increased anion gap) metabolic acidosis
  - Generally results from addition to the blood of nonchloride acids such as lactate, acetoacetate, β-hydroxybutyrate, and exogenous toxins (exception: uremia, with underexcretion of organic acids and anions)

Etiology

- Lactic acidosis
  - Type A (tissue hypoxia): cardiogenic, septic, or hemorrhagic shock; seizure; carbon monoxide or cyanide poisoning
  - Type B (nonhypoxic): hepatic or renal failure, ischemic bowel, diabetes mellitus (especially with metformin use), ketoacidosis, infection, leukemia or lymphoma, drugs (ethanol, methanol, salicylates, isoniazid), AIDS, idiopathic (usually in debilitated patients)
- Diabetic ketoacidosis
- Starvation ketoacidosis
- Alcoholic ketoacidosis
  - Acid-base disorders in alcoholism are frequently mixed (10% have triple acid-base disorder)
  - Three types of metabolic acidoses: ketoacidosis, lactic acidosis, and hyperchloremic acidosis from bicarbonate loss in urine from ketonuria
  - Metabolic alkalosis from volume contraction and vomiting
  - Respiratory alkalosis from alcohol withdrawal, pain, sepsis, or liver disease
- Uremic acidosis (usually at glomerular filtration rate < 20 mL/min)
- Ethylene glycol toxicity
- Methanol toxicity
- Salicylate toxicity (mixed metabolic acidosis with respiratory alkalosis)
- Other: paraldehyde, isoniazid, iron, rhabdomyolysis

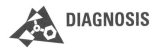 **CLINICAL FINDINGS**

SYMPTOMS AND SIGNS

- Symptoms are mainly those of the underlying disorder
- Compensatory hyperventilation may be misinterpreted as a primary respiratory disorder
- When severe, Kussmaul respirations (deep, regular, sighing respirations indi-

cating intense stimulation of the respiratory center) occur

 DIAGNOSIS

LABORATORY TESTS

- See Table 31
- Blood pH, serum HCO_3^-, and PCO_2 are decreased
- Anion gap is increased (normochloremic)
- Hyperkalemia may be seen
- In lactic acidosis, lactate levels are at least 4–5 mEq/L but commonly 10–30 mEq/L
- The diagnosis of alcoholic ketoacidosis is supported by the absence of a diabetic history and no evidence of glucose intolerance after initial therapy

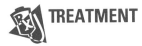 **TREATMENT**

MEDICATIONS

- Supplemental HCO_3^- is indicated for treatment of hyperkalemia but is controversial for treatment of increased anion gap metabolic acidosis
- Administration of large amounts of HCO_3^- may have deleterious effects, including
  - Hypernatremia
  - Hyperosmolality
  - Worsening of intracellular acidosis
- In salicylate intoxication, alkali therapy must be started unless blood pH is already alkalinized by respiratory alkalosis, because the increment in pH converts salicylate to more impermeable salicylic acid and thus prevents CNS damage
- The amount of HCO_3^- deficit can be calculated as follows:

$$\text{Amount of } HCO_3^- \text{ deficit} = 0.5 \times \text{bodyweight} \times (24 - HCO_3^-)$$

- Half of the calculated deficit should be administered within the first 3–4 h to avoid overcorrection and volume overload
- In methanol intoxication, ethanol is administered as a competitive substrate for alcohol dehydrogenase, the enzyme that metabolizes methanol to formaldehyde

THERAPEUTIC PROCEDURES

- Treatment is aimed at the underlying disorder, such as insulin and volume resuscitation to restore tissue perfusion
- Lactate will later be metabolized to produce HCO_3^- and increase pH

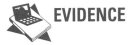 **OUTCOME**

PROGNOSIS

- The mortality rate of lactic acidosis exceeds 50%

WHEN TO ADMIT

- Because of the high mortality rate, all patients with lactic acidosis should be admitted
- Most other patients with significant metabolic acidosis are admitted as well

PREVENTION

- Avoid metformin use if there is tissue hypoxia or renal insufficiency
- Acute renal failure can occur rarely with the use of radiocontrast agents in patients receiving metformin therapy
- Metformin should be temporarily halted on the day of the test and for 2 days after injection of radiocontrast agents to avoid potential lactic acidosis if renal failure occurs

EVIDENCE

PRACTICE GUIDELINES

- American Diabetes Association: Hyperglycemic Crises in Diabetes, 2004

INFORMATION FOR PATIENTS

- MedlinePlus: Metabolic Acidosis
- American Diabetes Association: Ketoacidosis
- MedlinePlus: Alcoholic Ketoacidosis

REFERENCES

- Casaletto JJ. Differential diagnosis of metabolic acidosis. Emerg Med Clin North Am. 2005;23:771. [PMID: 15982545]
- Eledrisi MS et al. Overview of the diagnosis and management of diabetic ketoacidosis. Am J Med Sci. 2006 May; 331(5):243–51. [PMID: 16702793]
- Forni LG et al. Circulating anions usually associated with the Krebs cycle in patients with metabolic acidosis. Crit Care. 2005 Oct 5;9(5):R591–5. [PMID: 16277723]
- Matin MJ et al. Use of serum bicarbonate measurement in place of arterial base deficit in the surgical intensive care unit. Arch Surg. 2005 Aug;140(8):745–51. [PMID: 16103283]

- Moe OW et al. Clinical acid-base pathophysiology: disorders of plasma anion gap. Best Pract Res Clin Endocrinol Metab. 2003 Dec;17(4):559–74. [PMID: 14687589]
- Rosival V. Metabolic acidosis. Crit Care Med. 2004 Dec;32(12):2563–4. [PMID: 15599180]

Acidosis, Respiratory

 KEY FEATURES

- Respiratory acidosis results from decreased alveolar ventilation and subsequent hypercapnia
- Be mindful of readily reversible causes, such as respiratory depression from opioids
- Acid-base compensation
  - Acute respiratory acidosis: an increase in serum HCO_3^- of 1 mEq/L per 10 mm Hg increase in PCO_2
  - Chronic respiratory acidosis (after 6–12 h): an increase in serum HCO_3^- of 3.5 mEq/L per 10 mm Hg increase in PCO_2
- When chronic respiratory acidosis is corrected suddenly, there is a 2- to 3-day lag in renal bicarbonate excretion, resulting in posthypercapnic metabolic alkalosis

 CLINICAL FINDINGS

- Acute respiratory acidosis: somnolence, confusion, myoclonus, asterixis
- Increased intracranial pressure (papilledema, pseudotumor cerebri)
- Coma from CO_2 narcosis

 DIAGNOSIS

- Low arterial pH, increased PCO_2
- Chronic respiratory acidosis: HCO_3^- may be elevated along with hypochloremia from NH_4^+ and Cl^- renal loss (Table 31)

 TREATMENT

- Administer naloxone, 0.04–2.0 mg IV or SQ (or IM) q 2-3 min × 3 doses if needed, for possible opioid overdose
- For all forms of respiratory acidosis, treatment must aim to improve ventilation

Acne Vulgaris

 KEY FEATURES

ESSENTIALS OF DIAGNOSIS

- Occurs at puberty, though onset may be delayed into the third or fourth decade
- Open and closed comedones are the hallmark of acne vulgaris
- The most common of all skin conditions
- Severity varies from purely comedonal to papular or pustular inflammatory acne to cysts or nodules
- Face and upper trunk may be affected
- Scarring may be a sequela of the disease or picking and manipulating by the patient

GENERAL CONSIDERATIONS

- The disease is activated by androgens in those who are genetically predisposed
- The skin lesions parallel sebaceous activity
- Pathogenic events include
  - Plugging of the infundibulum of the follicles
  - Retention of sebum
  - Overgrowth of the acne bacillus (*Propionibacterium acnes*) with resultant release of and irritation by accumulated fatty acids
  - Foreign body reaction to extrafollicular sebum
- When a resistant case of acne is encountered in a woman, hyperandrogenism may be suspected

DEMOGRAPHICS

- Acne vulgaris is more common and more severe in males
- 12% of women and 3% of men over age 25 have acne vulgaris

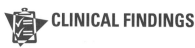 CLINICAL FINDINGS

SYMPTOMS AND SIGNS

- Mild soreness, pain, or itching
- Lesions occur mainly over the face, neck, upper chest, back, and shoulders
- Comedones are the hallmark
- Closed comedones are tiny, flesh-colored, noninflamed bumps that give the skin a rough texture or appearance
- Open comedones typically are a bit larger and have black material in them
- Inflammatory papules, pustules, ectatic pores, acne cysts, and scarring are also seen
- Acne may have different presentations at different ages

DIFFERENTIAL DIAGNOSIS

- Acne rosacea (face)
- Bacterial folliculitis (face or trunk)
- Tinea (face or trunk)
- Topical corticosteroid use (face)
- Perioral dermatitis (face)
- Pseudofolliculitis barbae (ingrown beard hairs)
- Miliaria (heat rash) (trunk)
- Eosinophilic folliculitis (trunk)
- Hyperandrogenic states in women
- Pustules on the face can also be caused by tinea infections

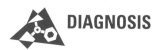 DIAGNOSIS

LABORATORY TESTS

- Culture in refractory cases

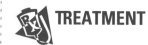 TREATMENT

MEDICATIONS

- See Table 150

Comedonal acne

- Soaps play little part and, if any are used, they should be mild
- Topical retinoids
  - Tretinoin
    - Very effective
    - Start with 0.025% cream (not gel) twice weekly at night
    - Then, build up to as often as nightly
    - Pea-sized amount is sufficient to cover half the entire face
    - Wait 20 min after washing to apply
  - If standard tretinoin preparations cause irritation, other options include
    - Adapalene gel 0.1%

□ Reformulated tretinoin (Renova, Retin A Micro, Avita)

□ Tazarotene gel 0.05% or 0.1%

– Lesions may flare in the first 4 weeks of treatment

– Should not be used during pregnancy

• Benzoyl peroxide is available in many concentrations but 2.5% is as effective as 10% and less irritating

Papular inflammatory acne

• Antibiotics are the mainstay, used topically or orally

• **Mild acne**

– The first choice of topical antibiotics is the combination of erythromycin or clindamycin with benzoyl peroxide topical gel

□ Clindamycin (Cleocin T) lotion (least irritating), gel, or solution or topical erythromycin gel or solution may be used BID and benzoyl peroxide in the morning

□ A combination of erythromycin or clindamycin with benzoyl peroxide is available as a prescription item

– The addition of tretinoin 0.025% cream or 0.01% gel at night enhances efficacy

• **Moderate acne**

– Tetracycline, 500 mg BID, doxycycline, 100 mg BID, and minocycline, 50–100 mg BID, are all effective

– Tetracycline, minocycline, and doxycycline are contraindicated in pregnancy

– If the skin is clear, taper the dose by 250 mg for tetracycline, by 100 mg for doxycycline, every 6–8 weeks—while treating with topicals—to arrive at the lowest systemic dose needed

– Lowering the dose to zero without other therapy usually results in recurrence of the acne

– Oral contraceptives or spironolactone (50–100 mg daily) may be added as an antiandrogen in women with antibiotic-resistant acne or in women in whom relapse occurs after isotretinoin therapy

• **Severe cystic acne**

– Isotretinoin (Accutane) should be used before significant scarring occurs or if symptoms are not promptly controlled by antibiotics

– Informed consent must be obtained before its use in all patients

– Dosage of 0.5–1.0 mg/kg/day for 20 weeks for a cumulative dose of at least 120 mg/kg is usually adequate

– The drug is teratogenic and must not be used in pregnancy

□ Obtain two serum pregnancy tests before starting the drug and every month thereafter

□ Sufficient medication for only 1 month should be dispensed

□ Two forms of effective contraception must be used

– Patient must be registered in iPledge system

– Side effects

□ Dry skin and mucous membranes occur in most patients

□ If headache occurs, consider pseudotumor cerebri

□ At higher dosages, elevation of cholesterol and triglycerides and a lowering of high-density lipoproteins can occur

□ Minor elevations of liver function tests and fasting blood sugar can occur

□ Moderate to severe myalgias necessitate decreasing the dosage or stopping the drug

• Monitor baseline and Q month cholesterol, triglycerides, and liver function studies when using isotretinoin

THERAPEUTIC PROCEDURES

• Comedones may be removed with a comedo extractor but will recur if not prevented by treatment

• In otherwise moderate acne, injection of triamcinolone acetonide (2.5 mg/mL, 0.05 mL per lesion) may hasten resolution of deeper papules and cysts

• Cosmetic improvement of scars may be achieved with surgical procedures

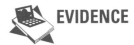 **OUTCOME**

COMPLICATIONS

• Cyst formation

• Pigmentary changes in pigmented patients

• Severe scarring

• Psychological problems may result

PROGNOSIS

• The disease flares intermittently in spite of treatment

• The condition may persist through adulthood and may lead to severe scarring if left untreated

• Antibiotics continue to improve skin for the first 3–6 months of use

• Relapse during treatment may suggest the emergence of resistant *P acnes*

• Remissions following systemic treatment with isotretinoin may be lasting in up to 60% of cases

• Relapses after isotretinoin usually occur within 3 years and require a second course in up to 20% of patients

WHEN TO REFER

• Failure to respond to standard regimens

• When the diagnosis is in question

• Fulminant scarring disease (acne fulmincans)

PREVENTION

• Foods do not cause or exacerbate acne

• Educate patients not to manipulate lesions

• Avoid topical exposure to oils, cocoa butter, and greases

EVIDENCE

PRACTICE GUIDELINES

• Institute for Clinical Systems Improvement. Acne management. 2003

• Madden WS et al. Treatment of acne vulgaris and prevention of acne scarring: Canadian consensus guidelines. J Cutan Med Surg. 2000;4 (Suppl 1):S2. [PMID: 11749902]

WEB SITE

• American Academy of Dermatology

INFORMATION FOR PATIENTS

• American Academy of Dermatology: What is Acne?

• MedlinePlus: Acne Interactive Tutorial

• National Institute of Arthritis, and Musculoskeletal and Skin Diseases: Acne

• Torpy JM et al. JAMA patient page: Acne. JAMA. 2004;292:764. [PMID: 15304474]

REFERENCES

• Haider A et al. Treatment of acne vulgaris. JAMA. 2004 Aug 11;292(6):726–35. [PMID: 15304471]

• James WD. Clinical practice. Acne. N Engl J Med. 2005 Apr 7;352(14):1463–72. [PMID: 15814882]

• Zane LT. Acne maintenance therapy: expanding the role of topical retinoids? Arch Dermatol. 2006 May;142(5):638–40. [PMID: 16702503]

Acromegaly & Gigantism

KEY FEATURES

ESSENTIALS OF DIAGNOSIS

- Excessive growth of hands, feet, jaw, and internal organs
- Gigantism if growth hormone (GH) excess before closure of epiphyses; acromegaly if after closure
- Amenorrhea, headaches, visual field loss, weakness
- Soft, doughy, sweaty handshake
- Elevated insulin-like growth factor 1 (IGF-1)
- Serum GH not suppressed following oral glucose

GENERAL CONSIDERATIONS

- GH exerts much of its effects by stimulating release of IGF-1
- Nearly always caused by pituitary adenoma, usually macroadenomas (> 1 cm); may be locally invasive but < 1% are malignant
- GH-secreting pituitary tumors usually cause hypogonadism by cosecretion of prolactin or direct pressure on pituitary
- Usually sporadic, rarely familial
- May be associated with endocrine tumors of parathyroids or pancreas (multiple endocrine neoplasia type 1 [MEN-1])
- Acromegaly may be seen in McCune-Albright syndrome and as part of Carney's syndrome (atrial myxoma, acoustic neuroma, lentigines, adrenal hypercortisolism)
- Rarely caused by ectopic secretion of growth hormone-releasing hormone or GH secreted by lymphoma, hypothalamic tumor, bronchial carcinoid, or pancreatic tumor

CLINICAL FINDINGS

SYMPTOMS AND SIGNS

- Tall stature
- Head and neck
  - Facial features coarsen
  - Hat size increases, tooth spacing widens
  - Mandible becomes more prominent
  - Macroglossia and hypertrophy of pharyngeal and laryngeal tissue
    - Deep, coarse voice
    - May cause obstructive sleep apnea
  - Goiter may be noted
- Hands
  - Enlarged
  - Fingers widen and rings no longer fit
  - Carpal tunnel syndrome is common
- Feet grow, particularly in shoe width
- Hypertension (50%) and cardiomegaly
- Weight gain
- Arthralgias, degenerative arthritis, and spinal stenosis may occur
- Colon polyps common
- Skin
  - Hyperhidrosis
  - Thickening
  - Cystic acne
  - Skin tags
  - Acanthosis nigricans
- Symptoms of hypopituitarism
  - Hypogonadism: decreased libido, impotence, irregular menses or amenorrhea common
  - Secondary hypothyroidism sometimes occurs, hypoadrenalism is unusual
  - Headaches and temporal hemianopia

DIFFERENTIAL DIAGNOSIS

- Familial tall stature, coarse features, or large hands and feet
- Physiologic growth spurt
- Pseudoacromegaly (acromegaly features, insulin resistance)
- Inactive ("burned-out") acromegaly (spontaneous remission due to pituitary adenoma infarction)
- Myxedema
- Isolated prognathism (jaw protrusion)
- Aromatase deficiency or estrogen receptor deficiency causing tall stature
- Other causes of increased growth hormone level
  - Exercise or eating prior to test
  - Acute illness or agitation
  - Hepatic or renal failure
  - Malnourishment
  - Diabetes mellitus
  - Drugs (estrogens, β-blockers, clonidine)

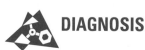

DIAGNOSIS

LABORATORY TESTS

- IGF-1 levels > 5 times normal in most acromegalics
- Glucose tolerance test: glucose syrup 75 g PO
  - GH measured 60 min later
  - Acromegaly excluded if GH < 1 ng/mL (IRMA or chemiluminescent assays) or < 2 ng/mL (older radioimmunoassays) and if IGF-1 is normal
- Prolactin may be elevated (cosecreted by many GH-secreting tumors)
- Insulin resistance usually present, often causing hyperglycemia (common) and diabetes mellitus (30%)
- Thyroid-stimulating hormone and free thyroxine may show secondary hypothyroidism
- Serum phosphorus frequently elevated
- Serum calcium elevated if hyperparathyroidism as in MEN-1

IMAGING STUDIES

- MRI shows pituitary tumor in 90%
- MRI superior to CT, especially postoperatively
- Skull radiographs may show enlarged sella and thickened skull
- Radiographs may show tufting of terminal phalanges of fingers and toes
- Lateral view of foot shows increased thickness of heel pad

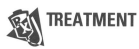

TREATMENT

MEDICATIONS

- Dopamine agonist
  - Use if surgery does not produce clinical remission or normalization of GH
  - Cabergoline 0.25–1.0 mg PO twice weekly; most successful if tumor secretes both prolactin and GH
- Somatostatin analogs
  - Use if acromegaly persists despite pituitary surgery
  - Octreotide
    - Begin with short-acting octreotide 50 mcg SQ TID
    - Switch to long-acting octreotide 20 mg IM every month if short-acting drug is tolerated
  - Adjust dose up to 40 mg IM every month to maintain serum GH between 1 ng/mL and 2.5 ng/mL, keeping IGF-1 levels normal
  - Lanreotide SR 30 mg SQ q7–14d (not available in the United States)
  - Lanreotide Autogel 60–120 mg SQ q28d, better tolerated than lanreotide SR (not available in the United States)
- GH receptor antagonist
  - Pegvisomant 10–30 mg/day SQ, following IGF-1 levels

SURGERY

- Endoscopic transnasal, transsphenoidal resection is treatment of choice for pituitary adenoma; the normal pituitary is often preserved
- GH levels fall immediately
- Infection, cerebrospinal fluid leak, or hypopituitarism develops in about 10% of patients
- Hyponatremia can occur 4–13 days postoperatively; serum sodium must be monitered closely

THERAPEUTIC PROCEDURES

- Pituitary irradiation suggested if not cured by surgical and medical therapy. Stereotactic radiosurgery (cyber knife or gamma knife) preferred
- Heavy particle radiation available in certain centers

 OUTCOME

FOLLOW-UP

- Postoperative normal pituitary function usually preserved
- Postoperative GH levels > 5 ng/mL and rising IGF-1 levels usually indicate recurrent tumor
- Soft tissue swelling regresses but bone enlargement is permanent
- Hypertension frequently persists
- Carpal tunnel syndrome and diaphoresis often improve within a day of surgery

COMPLICATIONS

- Hypopituitarism
- Hypertension
- Diabetes mellitus
- Cardiomegaly and cardiac failure
- Carpal tunnel syndrome
- Arthritis of hips, knees, and spine
- Spinal cord compression may be seen
- Visual field defects may be severe and progressive
- Tumor may be locally invasive, particularly into the cavernous sinus
- Acute loss of vision or cranial nerve palsy if tumor undergoes spontaneous hemorrhage and necrosis (pituitary apoplexy)
- Intubation may be difficult due to macroglossia and hypertrophy of pharyngeal and laryngeal tissue

PROGNOSIS

- Persistent acromegaly usually causes premature cardiovascular disease and progressive acromegalic symptoms
- Transsphenoidal pituitary surgery successful in 80–90% if tumor < 2 cm and GH < 50 ng/mL
- Conventional radiation therapy (alone) produces remission in 40% by 2 years and 75% by 5 years
- Gamma knife radiation reduces GH levels an average of 77%, with 20% in remission at 12 months
- Heavy particle pituitary radiation produces remission in 70% by 2 years and 80% by 5 years
- Radiation therapy usually produces some degree of hypopituitarism
- Conventional radiation therapy may cause some degree of organic brain syndrome and predisposes to small strokes

 EVIDENCE

PRACTICE GUIDELINES

- AACE Practice Guidelines
- Melmed S et al. Guidelines for acromegaly management. J Clin Endocrinol Metab. 2002;87:4054. [PMID: 12213843]
- Scandinavian Workshop on the Treatment of Acromegaly. Treatment guidelines for acromegaly. Report from a Scandinavian workshop: first Scandinavian Workshop on the Treatment of Acromegaly. Growth Horm IGF Res. 2001;11:72. [PMID: 11472072]

WEB SITE

- National Institute of Diabetes and Digestive and Kidney Diseases (NIDDK)—Endocrine and metabolic diseases

INFORMATION FOR PATIENTS

- Acromegaly.org
- Mayo Clinic—Acromegaly

REFERENCES

- Castinetti F et al. Outcome of gamma knife radiosurgery in 82 patients with acromegaly: correlation with initial hypersecretion. J Clin Endocrinol Metab. 2005 Aug;90(8):4483–8. [PMID: 15899958]
- Feenstra J et al. Combined therapy with somatostatin analogues and weekly pegvisomant in active acromegaly. Lan-

cet. 2005 May 7–13;365(9471):1644–6. [PMID: 15885297]
- Galland F et al. McCune-Albright syndrome and acromegaly: Effects of hypothalamopituitary radiotherapy and/or pegvisomant in somatostatin analog-resistant patients. J Clin Endocrinol Metab. 2006 Dec;91(12):4957–61. [PMID: 16984995]
- Melmed S. Acromegaly. N Engl J Med. 2006 Dec 14;355(24):2558–73. [PMID: 17167139]

Actinic Keratosis

 KEY FEATURES

- Actinic keratoses are considered premalignant, but only 1:1000 lesions/year progresses to become squamous cell carcinoma

 CLINICAL FINDINGS

- Actinic keratoses are small (0.2–1.0 cm) papules—flesh-colored, pink, or slightly hyperpigmented—that feel like sandpaper and are tender when the finger is drawn over them
- They occur on sun-exposed parts of the body in persons of fair complexion

 DIAGNOSIS

- Clinical
- Differential diagnosis
  - Squamous cell carcinoma
  - Bowen's disease (squamous cell carcinoma in situ)
  - Nonpigmented seborrheic keratosis
  - Psoriasis
  - Seborrheic dermatitis
  - Seborrheic keratosis
  - Paget's disease

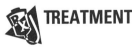 **TREATMENT**

- Liquid nitrogen is a rapid, effective method of eradication. The lesions crust and disappear in 10–14 days
- An alternative treatment is the use of 1–5% fluorouracil cream

– This agent may be rubbed into the lesions morning and night until they become red and sore, crusted, and eroded (usually 2–3 weeks)

– Alternatively, 5-fluorouracil 0.5% cream once daily for 4–6 weeks

– Imiquimod 5% cream applied once daily 3–5 times per week can be used instead of 5-fluorouracil

Actinomycosis

 KEY FEATURES

ESSENTIALS OF DIAGNOSIS

- History of recent dental infection or abdominal trauma
- Chronic pneumonia or indolent intra-abdominal or cervicofacial abscess
- Sinus tract formation

GENERAL CONSIDERATIONS

- Organisms are anaerobic, gram-positive, branching filamentous bacteria (1 mcm in diameter) that may fragment into bacillary forms
- Occur in the normal flora of the mouth and tonsillar crypts
- When introduced into traumatized tissue and associated with other anaerobic bacteria, actinomycetes become pathogens
- Most common site of infection is cervicofacial area (about 60% of cases)
- Infection typically follows extraction of a tooth or other trauma
- Lesions may develop in the gastrointestinal tract or lungs following ingestion or aspiration of the organism from its endogenous source in the mouth

 CLINICAL FINDINGS

SYMPTOMS AND SIGNS

Cervicofacial actinomycosis

- Develops slowly, becomes markedly indurated, and the overlying skin becomes reddish or cyanotic
- Abscesses eventually drain to the surface
- Persist for long periods
- Sulfur granules—masses of filamentous organisms—may be found in the pus
- There is usually little pain unless there is secondary infection

Thoracic actinomycosis

- Fever, cough, sputum production
- Night sweats, weight loss
- Pleuritic pain
- Multiple sinuses may extend through the chest wall to the heart or abdomen

Abdominal actinomycosis

- Pain in the ileocecal region
- Spiking fever and chills
- Vomiting
- Weight loss
- Irregular abdominal masses may be palpated
- Pelvic inflammatory disease caused by actinomycetes has been associated with prolonged use of an intrauterine contraceptive device
- Sinuses draining to the exterior may develop

DIFFERENTIAL DIAGNOSIS

- Lung cancer
- Tuberculous lymphadenitis (scrofula)
- Other cause of cervical lymphadenopathy
- Nocardiosis
- Crohn's disease
- Pelvic inflammatory disease from another cause

 DIAGNOSIS

LABORATORY TESTS

- Organisms may be demonstrated as a granule or as scattered branching gram-positive filaments in the pus
- Anaerobic culture is necessary to distinguish from *Nocardia*

IMAGING STUDIES

- Chest radiograph shows areas of consolidation and, in many cases, pleural effusion
- Abdominal pelvic CT scanning reveals an inflammatory mass that may extend to involve bone

 TREATMENT

MEDICATIONS

- Penicillin G
  - Drug of choice
  - 10 to 20 million units IV for 4–6 weeks followed by penicillin V, 500 mg PO QID
- Alternatives include: ampicillin, 12 g/d IV for 4–6 weeks, followed by amoxicillin, 500 mg PO TID; or doxycycline, 100 mg BID IV or PO
- Sulfonamides such as sulfamethoxazole may be an alternative regimen at a total daily dosage of 2–4 g
- Therapy should be continued for weeks to months after clinical manifestations have disappeared in order to ensure cure

SURGERY

- Drainage and resection may be beneficial

THERAPEUTIC PROCEDURES

- Therapy should be continued for weeks to months after clinical manifestations have disappeared in order to ensure cure
- Response to therapy is slow

 OUTCOME

PROGNOSIS

- With penicillin and surgery, the prognosis is good
- The difficulties of diagnosis may result in extensive destruction of tissue before therapy is started

WHEN TO REFER

- Refer early to an infectious disease specialist for diagnosis and management

WHEN TO ADMIT

- All patients with thoracic or abdominal actinomycosis
- Patients with cervicofacial actinomycosis if the diagnosis is in question, to control symptoms, or initiate IV antibiotics

EVIDENCE

PRACTICE GUIDELINES

- Cayley J et al. Recommendations for clinical practice: actinomyces like organisms and intrauterine contraceptives. The Clinical and Scientific Committee. Br J Fam Plann. 1998;23:137. [PMID: 9882769]

WEB SITE

- Karolinska Institute: Diseases and Disorders—Links Pertaining to Bacterial Infections and Mycoses

INFORMATION FOR PATIENTS

- National Institutes of Health: Actinomycosis

- National Institutes of Health: Pulmonary Actinomycosis

REFERENCE

- Yildiz O et al. *Actinomycoses* and *Nocardia* pulmonary infections. Curr Opin Pulm Med. 2006 May;12(3):228–34. [PMID: 16582679]

Acute Respiratory Distress Syndrome (ARDS)

KEY FEATURES

ESSENTIALS OF DIAGNOSIS

- Bilateral radiographic pulmonary opacities
- Absence of elevated left atrial pressure; if measured, pulmonary arterial wedge pressure < 18 mm Hg
- Ratio of $Pao_2/FIO_2 < 200$, regardless of the level of peak end-expiratory pressure (PEEP)

GENERAL CONSIDERATIONS

- Acute hypoxemic respiratory failure following a systemic or pulmonary insult without evidence of left-sided heart failure
- Common risk factors (Table 122)
  - Sepsis
  - Aspiration of gastric contents
  - Shock
  - Infection, pulmonary or systemic
  - Lung contusion
  - Trauma
  - Toxic inhalation
  - Near-drowning
  - Multiple blood product transfusions
- Damage to pulmonary capillary endothelial and alveolar epithelial cells is found, regardless of the cause of ARDS

Systemic causes

- Sepsis
- Shock
- Pancreatitis
- Multiple blood-product transfusions
- Trauma
- Burns
- Disseminated intravascular coagulation (DIC) and thrombotic thrombocytopenia purpura (TTP)

- Drugs
  - Opioids
  - Aspirin
  - Phenothiazines
  - Tricyclic antidepressants
  - Amiodarone
  - Chemotherapeutics
  - Nitrofurantoin
  - Protamine
- Cardiopulmonary bypass
- Head injury
- Paraquat exposure

Pulmonary causes

- Aspiration of gastric contents
- Near-drowning
- Pneumonia, bacterial, viral, or fungal
- Miliary tuberculosis
- Toxic gas inhalation
  - Nitrogen dioxide
  - Chlorine
  - Sulfur dioxide
  - Ammonia
  - Smoke inhalation
- Free-base cocaine smoking
- Embolism of thrombus, fat, air, or amniotic fluid
- Lung contusion
- Acute eosinophilic pneumonia
- Bronchiolitis obliterans organizing pneumonia (BOOP) (now more commonly referred to as cryptogenic organizing pneumonia)
- Acute upper airway obstruction
- Lung reexpansion or reperfusion
- Radiation exposure
- High-altitude exposure
- Oxygen toxicity

CLINICAL FINDINGS

SYMPTOMS AND SIGNS

- Rapid onset of profound dyspnea, usually 12–48 hours after the initiating event
- Labored breathing and tachypnea, with rales on examination
- Marked hypoxemia refractory to supplemental oxygen
- Multiple-organ failure is seen in many patients

DIFFERENTIAL DIAGNOSIS

- Because ARDS is a syndrome, the concept of differential diagnosis applies only in considering the precipitating illness or injury
- Cardiogenic (hydrostatic) pulmonary edema
- Neurogenic pulmonary edema

- Pneumonia
- Aspiration
- Diffuse alveolar hemorrhage
- Acute interstitial pneumonitis
- Acute eosinophilic pneumonia
- Acute hypersensitivity pneumonitis
- BOOP
- Pulmonary contusion
- Drug-induced lung disease

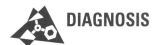

DIAGNOSIS

LABORATORY TESTS

- Tests to identify the systemic or pulmonary causes of ARDS are indicated

IMAGING STUDIES

- Chest radiograph shows diffuse or patchy bilateral opacities that rapidly become confluent
- Air bronchograms are seen in 80% of cases
- Features of congestive heart failure (pleural effusions, cardiomegaly, venous engorgement in upper lung zones, indistinct blood vessels) are absent

DIAGNOSTIC PROCEDURES

- When indicated to exclude cardiogenic pulmonary edema, pulmonary artery catheterization will demonstrate pulmonary arterial wedge pressures < 18 mm Hg

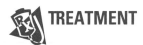

TREATMENT

MEDICATIONS

- Medications directed at the underlying cause of ARDS are indicated
- Intravascular volume should be maintained at the lowest level required to maintain adequate cardiac output
- Diuretics may be needed to reduce pulmonary capillary wedge pressure and improve oxygenation
- Judicious use of inotropes to maintain cardiac output at higher levels of PEEP may be necessary
- Achieving supranormal oxygen delivery through the use of inotropes and blood transfusion is not clinically useful and may be harmful
- Sedatives, analgesics, and antipyretics may be used to decrease oxygen consumption
- Systemic corticosteroids have not been shown to reliably improve outcomes

THERAPEUTIC PROCEDURES

- Intubation and mechanical ventilation are usually required to treat hypoxemia
- Use the lowest levels of PEEP and FiO_2 needed to maintain $Pao_2 > 60$ mm Hg
- Mechanical ventilation with small tidal volumes (6 mL/kg of ideal body weight) and airway plateau pressure limits (< 30 cm H_2O) has been shown to reduce mortality by 10% in a large multicenter trial
- PEEP may be increased as long as cardiac output and oxygen delivery are not impaired and pulmonary pressures are not excessive
- Prone positioning may improve oxygenation in selected patients

 OUTCOME

FOLLOW-UP

- Efforts should be made to decrease FiO_2 below 60% as early as possible
- For patients who recover, no specific follow-up is required

COMPLICATIONS

- Complications are those associated with ICU level care and mechanical ventilation

PROGNOSIS

- Mortality is 30–40% in ARDS, 90% when associated with sepsis
- Median survival is 2 weeks
- Many patients with ARDS die when support is withdrawn
- Survivors of ARDS are left with some pulmonary symptoms, which tend to improve over time
- Mild abnormalities of oxygenation, diffusion capacity, and lung mechanics may persist in some survivors

WHEN TO REFER

- Care of patients with ARDS should involve a clinician who is familiar with the syndrome, typically a pulmonologist or intensivist

WHEN TO ADMIT

- Because of the profound hypoxemia that defines ARDS, all patients need admission and intensive care

PREVENTION

- No measures have been identified to effectively prevent ARDS

- Prophylactic PEEP, methylprednisolone, or other interventions are not helpful in patients at risk

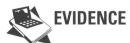 EVIDENCE

INFORMATION FOR PATIENTS

- National Institutes of Health

REFERENCES

- Adhikari N et al. Pharmacologic therapies for adults with acute lung injury and acute respiratory distress syndrome. Cochrane Database Syst Rev. 2004 Oct 18;(4):CD004477. [PMID: 15495113]
- Bernard GR. Acute respiratory distress syndrome: a historical perspective. Am J Respir Crit Care Med. 2005 Oct 1; 172(7):798–806. [PMID: 16020801]
- Hager DN et al. Tidal volume reduction in patients with acute lung injury when plateau pressures are not high. Am J Respir Crit Care Med. 2005 Nov 15; 172(10):1241–5. [PMID: 16081547]
- Matthay MA et al. Acute lung injury and the acute respiratory distress syndrome: four decades of inquiry into pathogenesis and rational management. Am J Respir Cell Mol Biol. 2005 Oct; 33(4):319–27. [PMID: 16172252]
- National Heart, Lung, and Blood Institute Acute Respiratory Distress Syndrome (ARDS) Clinical Trials Network; Wheeler AP et al. Pulmonary-artery versus central venous catheter to guide treatment of acute lung injury. N Engl J Med. 2006 May 25;354(21):2213–24. [PMID: 16714768]
- National Heart, Lung, and Blood Institute Acute Respiratory Distress Syndrome (ARDS) Clinical Trials Network; Wiedemann HP et al. Comparison of two fluid-management strategies in acute lung injury. N Engl J Med. 2006 Jun 15;354(24):2564–75. [PMID: 16714767]
- Rubenfeld GD et al. Incidence and outcomes of acute lung injury. N Engl J Med. 2005 Oct 20;353(16):1685–93. [PMID: 16236739]
- Schwarz MI et al. "Imitators" of the ARDS: implications for diagnosis and treatment. Chest. 2004 Apr; 125(4):1530–5. [PMID: 15078770]
- Steinberg KP et al; National Heart, Lung, and Blood Institute Acute Respiratory Distress Syndrome (ARDS) Clinical Trials Network. Efficacy and safety of corticosteroids for persistent acute respiratory distress syndrome. N Engl J Med. 2006 Apr 20;354(16):1671–84. [PMID: 16625008]
- Ventilation with lower tidal volumes as compared with traditional tidal volumes for acute lung injury and the acute respiratory distress syndrome. The Acute Respiratory Distress Syndrome Network. N Engl J Med. 2000 May 4; 342(18):1301–8. [PMID: 10793162]

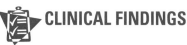

Adenovirus Infections

 KEY FEATURES

- More than 40 types, which produce a variety of clinical syndromes
- Usually self-limited except in immunosuppressed hosts

 CLINICAL FINDINGS

- Common cold
- Nonstreptococcal exudative pharyngitis
- Lower respiratory tract infections
- Epidemic keratoconjunctivitis
- Hemorrhagic cystitis
- Acute gastroenteritis
- Disseminated disease in transplant recipients

 DIAGNOSIS

- Can be cultured from appropriate specimens when definitive diagnosis is desired

TREATMENT

- Disease usually self-limited
- Immunocompromised patients often treated with ribavirin, although efficacy unclear
- Vaccine against certain strains used in military personnel to prevent outbreaks

Adrenocortical Insufficiency, Acute (Adrenal Crisis)

 KEY FEATURES

ESSENTIALS OF DIAGNOSIS

- Weakness, abdominal pain, fever, confusion, vomiting
- Low blood pressure, dehydration
- Skin pigmentation may be increased
- Serum potassium high, sodium low, blood urea nitrogen high
- Cosyntropin ($ACTH_{1-24}$) unable to stimulate a normal increase in serum cortisol

GENERAL CONSIDERATIONS

- An emergency caused by insufficient cortisol
- Causes
  - May occur in patients treated for chronic adrenal insufficiency or as its presenting manifestation
  - More common in primary adrenal insufficiency (adrenal gland disorder; Addison's disease) than secondary adrenocortical hypofunction (pituitary gland disorder)
  - Stress, eg, trauma, surgery, infection, or prolonged fasting in patient with latent insufficiency
  - Withdrawal of adrenocortical hormone replacement in patient with chronic adrenal insufficiency or temporary insufficiency related to withdrawal of exogenous corticosteroids
  - Bilateral adrenalectomy or removal of a functioning adrenal tumor that had suppressed the other adrenal
  - Injury to both adrenals by trauma, hemorrhage, anticoagulant therapy, thrombosis, infection or, rarely, metastatic carcinoma
  - Pituitary necrosis, or when thyroid hormone replacement is given to a patient with adrenal insufficiency

 CLINICAL FINDINGS

SYMPTOMS AND SIGNS

- Headache, lassitude, nausea and vomiting, abdominal pain, and diarrhea
- Confusion or coma
- Fever, as high as 40.6°C or more
- Low blood pressure
- Recurrent hypoglycemia and reduced insulin requirements in patients with preexisting type 1 diabetes mellitus
- Cyanosis, dehydration, skin hyperpigmentation, and sparse axillary hair (if hypogonadism also present)
- Meningococcemia may cause purpura and adrenal insufficiency secondary to adrenal infarction (Waterhouse-Friderichsen syndrome)

DIFFERENTIAL DIAGNOSIS

- Other cause of shock
  - Sepsis
  - Cardiogenic
  - Hypovolemic
  - Anaphylaxis
- Hyperkalemia due to other cause
  - Renal failure
  - Rhabdomyolysis
  - Angiotensin-converting enzyme inhibitors
  - Angiotensin receptor blockers
  - Spironolactone
- Hyponatremia due to other cause
  - Syndrome of inappropriate antidiuretic hormone
  - Cirrhosis
  - Vomiting
- Abdominal pain due to other cause
- Low serum cortisol-binding globulin in critical illness, causing low total serum cortisol; serum free cortisol levels normal

 DIAGNOSIS

LABORATORY TESTS

- Eosinophil count may be high
- Hyponatremia or hyperkalemia (or both) usually present
- Hypoglycemia common
- Hypercalcemia may be present
- Blood, sputum, or urine culture may be positive if bacterial infection is precipitating cause
- Cosyntropin stimulation test
  - Synthetic $ACTH_{1-24}$ (cosyntropin), 0.25 mg, given SQ, IM, or IV
  - Serum cortisol obtained 45 min later
  - Normally, cortisol rises to ≥ 20 mcg/dL
  - For patients taking corticosteroids, hydrocortisone must not be given for at least 8 h before test
  - Other corticosteroids (eg, prednisone, dexamethasone) do not interfere with specific assays for cortisol
- Plasma ACTH markedly elevated if patient has primary adrenal disease (generally > 200 pg/mL)

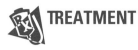 **TREATMENT**

MEDICATIONS

- If diagnosis is suspected
  - Draw blood sample for electrolytes, cortisol, and ACTH determinations
  - Without waiting for results, treat *immediately* with hydrocortisone 100–300 mg IV and saline
- Then, continue hydrocortisone 50–100 mg IV q6h for first day, q8h the second day, and taper as clinically appropriate
- Broad-spectrum antibiotics given empirically while waiting for initial culture results
- $D_{50}W$ to treat hypoglycemia with careful monitoring of serum electrolytes, blood urea nitrogen, and creatinine
- When patient is able to take oral medication
  - Give hydrocortisone, 10–20 mg PO q6h, and taper to maintenance levels
  - Most require hydrocortisone twice daily: 10–20 mg every morning, 5–10 mg every night
- Mineralocorticoid therapy
  - Not needed when large amounts of hydrocortisone are being given
  - However, as the dose is reduced, may need to add fludrocortisone, 0.05–0.2 mg PO once daily
  - Some patients never require fludrocortisone or become edematous at doses > 0.05 mg once or twice weekly

THERAPEUTIC PROCEDURES

- Once the crisis is over, must assess degree of permanent adrenal insufficiency and establish cause if possible

OUTCOME

FOLLOW-UP

- Repeat cosyntropin stimulation test

COMPLICATIONS

- Shock and death if untreated
- Sequelae of infection that commonly precipitate adrenal crisis

PROGNOSIS

- Rapid treatment usually lifesaving

- Frequently unrecognized and untreated since manifestations mimic more common conditions
- Lack of treatment leads to shock that is unresponsive to volume replacement and vasopressors, resulting in death

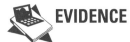 **EVIDENCE**

PRACTICE GUIDELINES

- Arlt W et al. Adrenal insufficiency. Lancet. 2003;361:1881. [PMID: 12788587]
- Clinical practice parameters for hemodynamic support of pediatric and neonatal patients in septic shock. American College of Critical Care Medicine, 2002
- Cooper MS et al. Corticosteroid insufficiency in acutely ill patients. N Engl J Med. 2003;348:727. [PMID: 12594318]
- Oelkers W et al. Therapeutic strategies in adrenal insufficiency. Ann Endocrinol (Paris). 2001;62:212. [PMID: 11353897]

WEB SITE

- National Adrenal Disease Foundation

INFORMATION FOR PATIENTS

- MedlinePlus–Acute adrenal crisis

REFERENCES

- Hamrahian AH et al. Measurements of serum free cortisol in critically ill patients. N Engl J Med. 2004 Apr 15; 350(16):1629–38. [PMID: 15084695]
- Jahangir-Hekmat M et al. Adrenal insufficiency attributable to adrenal hemorrhage: long-term follow-up with reference to glucocorticoid and mineralocorticoid function and replacement. Endocr Pract. 2004 Jan–Feb;10(1):55–61. [PMID: 15251623]

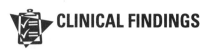

Adrenocortical Insufficiency, Chronic (Addison's Disease)

 KEY FEATURES

ESSENTIALS OF DIAGNOSIS

- Weakness, anorexia, weight loss
- Increased skin pigmentation
- Hypotension, small heart
- Serum sodium may be low; potassium, calcium, and urea nitrogen may be elevated
- Neutropenia, mild anemia, eosinophilia, and relative lymphocytosis may be present
- Plasma cortisol levels low or fail to rise after administration of cosyntropin
- Plasma ACTH level elevated

GENERAL CONSIDERATIONS

- Causes
  - Autoimmune adrenal destruction of adrenal glands is most common cause in the United States
  - May be associated with
    - Autoimmune thyroid disease
    - Hypoparathyroidism
    - Type 1 diabetes mellitus
    - Vitiligo
    - Alopecia areata
    - Celiac sprue
    - Primary ovarian failure
    - Testicular failure
    - Pernicious anemia
  - Combination of Addison's disease and hypothyroidism is Schmidt's syndrome
  - May occur in polyglandular autoimmunity (PGA-1 and PGA-2)
  - Tuberculosis in areas of high prevalence; now rare
  - Bilateral adrenal hemorrhage may occur spontaneously or with
    - Sepsis
    - Heparin-associated thrombocytopenia or anticoagulation
    - Antiphospholipid antibody syndrome
    - Surgery (postoperatively) or trauma
- Rare causes
  - Lymphoma
  - Metastatic carcinoma
  - Coccidioidomycosis
  - Histoplasmosis
  - Cytomegalovirus (more frequent in AIDS)
  - Syphilitic gummas
  - Scleroderma
  - Amyloid disease
  - Hemochromatosis
  - Familial glucocorticoid deficiency
  - Allgrove syndrome (associated with achalasia, alacrima, and neurologic disease)
  - X-linked adrenal leukodystrophy
  - Congenital adrenal hypoplasia or hyperplasia

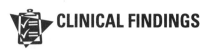 **CLINICAL FINDINGS**

SYMPTOMS AND SIGNS

- Weakness and fatigability, weight loss, myalgias, arthralgias
- Fever
- Anorexia, nausea and vomiting
- Anxiety, mental irritability, and emotional changes common
- Skin
  - Diffuse tanning over nonexposed and exposed skin or multiple freckles
  - Hyperpigmentation, especially knuckles, elbows, knees, posterior neck, palmar creases, nail beds, pressure areas, and new scars
  - Vitiligo (10%)
- Hypoglycemia, when present, may worsen weakness and mental functioning, rarely leading to coma
- Other autoimmune disease manifestations
- In diabetics, increased insulin sensitivity and hypoglycemic reactions
- Hypotension and orthostasis usual
  - 90% have systolic blood pressure (SBP) < 110 mm Hg
  - SBP > 130 mm Hg is rare
- Small heart
- Scant axillary and pubic hair (especially in women)
- Neuropsychiatric symptoms, sometimes without adrenal insufficiency, in adult-onset adrenoleukodystrophy

DIFFERENTIAL DIAGNOSIS

- Hypotension due to other cause, eg, medications
- Hyperkalemia due to other cause, eg, renal failure
- Gastroenteritis
- Occult cancer
- Anorexia nervosa
- Hyperpigmentation due to other cause, eg, hemochromatosis
- Isolated hypoaldosteronism

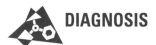 **DIAGNOSIS**

LABORATORY TESTS

- Moderate neutropenia, lymphocytosis, and total eosinophil count > 300/mcL
- Hyponatremia (90%), hyperkalemia (65%). (Patients with diarrhea may not be hyperkalemic.)
- Fasting blood glucose may be low
- Hypercalcemia may be present
- Plasma very-long-chain fatty acid levels to screen for adrenoleukodystrophy in young men with idiopathic Addison's disease
- Plasma cortisol level low (< 5 mg/dL) at 8 AM is diagnostic, especially if accompanied by simultaneous elevated ACTH (usually > 200 pg/mL)
- Cosyntropin stimulation test
  - Synthetic $ACTH_{1-24}$ (cosyntropin), 0.25 mg, given parenterally
  - Serum cortisol obtained 45 min later
  - Normally, cortisol rises to ≥ 20 mcg/dL
  - For patients taking corticosteroids, hydrocortisone must not be given for at least 8 h before the test
  - Other corticosteroids do not interfere with specific assays for cortisol
- Plasma ACTH markedly elevated (generally > 200 pg/mL) if patient has primary adrenal disease
- Serum DHEA > 1000 ng/mL excludes the diagnosis
- Antiadrenal antibodies detected in 50% of autoimmune Addison's disease
- Antithyroid antibodies (45%) and other autoantibodies may be present
- Elevated plasma renin activity indicates
  - Depleted intravascular volume
  - The need for higher doses of fludrocortisone replacement
- Plasma epinephrine levels low
- Serum transferrin saturation elevated in cases of hemochromatosis (rare)

IMAGING STUDIES

- Chest radiograph for tuberculosis, fungal infection, or cancer
- Abdominal CT shows small noncalcified adrenals in autoimmune Addison's disease
  - Adrenals enlarged in about 85% of cases of metastatic or granulomatous disease
  - Calcification noted in cases of tuberculosis (~50%), hemorrhage, fungal infection, and melanoma

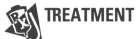 **TREATMENT**

MEDICATIONS

- Corticosteroid and mineralocorticoid replacement required in most cases; hydrocortisone alone may be adequate in mild cases
- Hydrocortisone
  - Drug of choice
  - Usually 15–25 mg PO in two divided doses: two-thirds in morning and one-third in late night or early evening
- Prednisone 2–3 mg PO every morning and 1–2 mg PO every night or evening is an alternative
- Dose adjusted according to clinical response; proper dose usually results in normal WBC differential
- Corticosteroid dose raised in case of infection, trauma, surgery, diagnostic procedures, or other stress
  - Maximum hydrocortisone dose for severe stress is 50 mg IV or IM q6h
  - Lower doses, oral or parenteral, for lesser stress
  - Dose tapered to normal as stress subsides
- Fludrocortisone, 0.05–0.3 mg PO once daily or once every other day, required by many patients
  - Dosage *increased* for
    - Postural hypotension
    - Hyponatremia
    - Hyperkalemia
    - Fatigue
    - Elevated plasma renin activity
  - Dosage *decreased* for
    - Edema
    - Hypokalemia
    - Hypertension
- Treat all infections immediately
- In some women with adrenal insufficiency, dehydroepiandrosterone (DHEA), 50 mg PO every morning, improves sense of well-being, mood, and sexual performance

THERAPEUTIC PROCEDURES

- "Lorenzo's oil" for adrenoleukodystrophy normalizes serum very-long-chain fatty acid concentrations but is ineffective clinically
- Hematopoietic stem cell transplantation from normal donors may improve neurologic manifestations

 OUTCOME

FOLLOW-UP

- Follow clinically and adjust corticosteroid and (if required) mineralocorticoid doses
- Fatigue in treated patients may indicate
  - Suboptimal dosing of medication
  - Electrolyte imbalance
  - Concurrent problems, such as hypothyroidism or diabetes mellitus
- Corticosteroid dose must be increased in case of physiologic stress (see above)

COMPLICATIONS

- Complications of underlying disease (eg, tuberculosis) are more likely
- Adrenal crisis may be precipitated by intercurrent infections
- Associated autoimmune diseases are common (see above)
- Fatigue often persists despite treatment
- Excessive corticosteroid replacement can cause Cushing's syndrome

PROGNOSIS

- Most patients able to live fully active lives
- Life expectancy is normal if adrenal insufficiency is diagnosed and treated with appropriate doses of corticosteroids and (if required) mineralocorticoids
- However, associated conditions can pose additional health risks, eg, patients with adrenal tuberculosis may have serious systemic infection
- Corticosteroid and mineralocorticoid replacement must not be stopped
- Patients should wear medical alert bracelet or medal reading "Adrenal insufficiency—takes hydrocortisone"
- Higher doses of corticosteroids must be administered to patients with infection, trauma, or surgery to prevent adrenal crisis

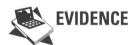 **EVIDENCE**

PRACTICE GUIDELINES

- Arlt W et al. Adrenal insufficiency. Lancet. 2003;361:1881. [PMID: 12788587]
- Don-Wauchope AC et al. Diagnosis and management of Addison's disease. Practitioner. 2000;244:794. [PMID: 11048377]

WEB SITES

- Australian Addison's Disease Association
- National Adrenal Disease Foundation

INFORMATION FOR PATIENTS

- Cleveland Clinic—Addison's disease

REFERENCES

- Alonso N et al. Evaluation of two replacement regimens in primary adrenal insufficiency patients. Effect on clinical symptoms, health-related quality of life and biochemical parameters. J Endocrinol Invest. 2004 May; 27(5):449–54. [PMID: 15279078]
- Betterle C et al. Autoimmune polyglandular syndrome Type 2: the tip of an iceberg? Clin Exp Immunol. 2004 Aug; 137(2):225–33. [PMID: 15270837]
- Libe R et al. Effects of dehydroepiandrosterone (DHEA) supplementation on hormonal, metabolic and behavioral status in patients with hypoadrenalism. J Endocrinol Invest. 2004 Sep;27(8):736–41. [PMID: 15636426]

Alcoholism

 KEY FEATURES

ESSENTIALS OF DIAGNOSIS

- Major criteria
  - Physiologic dependence as evidenced by withdrawal when intake is interrupted
  - Tolerance to the effects of alcohol
  - Evidence of alcohol-associated illnesses, such as alcoholic liver disease
  - Continued drinking despite strong medical and social contraindications
  - Impairment in social and occupational functioning
  - Depression
  - Blackouts
- Other signs
  - Alcohol odor on breath
  - Alcoholic facies
  - Flushed face
  - Scleral injection
  - Tremor
  - Ecchymoses
  - Peripheral neuropathy
  - Surreptitious drinking
  - Unexplained work absences
  - Frequent accidents, falls, or injuries
  - In smokers, cigarette burns on hands or chest

GENERAL CONSIDERATIONS

- The two-phase syndrome includes problem drinking and alcohol addiction

- Problem drinking is the repetitive use of alcohol, often to alleviate anxiety or solve other emotional problems
- Alcohol addiction is a true addiction
- Alcoholism is associated with a high prevalence of lifetime psychiatric disorders, especially depression

DEMOGRAPHICS

- Most suicides and intrafamily homicides involve alcohol
- Major factor in rapes and other assaults
- Male-to-female ratios of 4:1 are converging
- Adoption and twin studies indicate some genetic influence
- Forty percent of Japanese have aldehyde dehydrogenase deficiency, which increases susceptibility to the effects of alcohol

CLINICAL FINDINGS

SYMPTOMS AND SIGNS

Acute intoxication

- Drowsiness, errors of commission, disinhibition, dysarthria, ataxia, and nystagmus
- Ataxia, dysarthria, and vomiting indicate a blood level > 150 mg/dL
- Lethal blood levels: 350–900 mg/dL
- Severe: respiratory depression, stupor, seizures, shock syndrome, coma, and death
- Serious overdoses often include other sedatives combined with alcohol

Withdrawal

- Onset of withdrawal symptoms
  - Usually 8–12 hours
  - Peak intensity 48–72 hours after consumption is stopped
- Anxiety, decreased cognition, tremulousness, increasing irritability, and hyperreactivity to full-blown delirium tremens
- Symptoms of mild withdrawal
  - Tremor, elevated vital signs, anxiety
  - Begin about 8 hours after the last drink and end by day 3
- Generalized seizures
  - Occur within the first 24–38 hours
  - Are more prevalent in patients with previous withdrawal syndromes
- Delirium tremens
  - An acute organic psychosis
  - Usually manifest within 24–72 hours after the last drink but may occur up to 10 days later
  - Mental confusion, tremor

  - Sensory hyperacuity
  - Visual hallucinations
  - Autonomic hyperactivity
  - Cardiac abnormalities
  - Diaphoresis, dehydration
  - Electrolyte disturbances (hypokalemia, hypomagnesemia)
  - Seizures
- Acute withdrawal syndrome often unexpectedly occurs in patients hospitalized for an unrelated reason and presents as a diagnostic problem
- Possible persistence of sleep disturbances, anxiety, depression, excitability, fatigue, and emotional volatility for 3–12 months, becoming chronic in some cases

Alcoholic hallucinosis

- Paranoid psychosis without the tremulousness, confusion, and clouded sensorium seen in withdrawal syndromes
- Occurs during heavy drinking or during withdrawal
- Patient appears normal except for the auditory hallucinations, which are frequently persecutory and may cause the patient to behave aggressively and in a paranoid fashion

Chronic alcoholic brain syndrome characteristics

- Encephalopathies
  - Increasing erratic behavior
  - Memory and recall problems
  - Emotional lability
- Wernicke's encephalopathy
  - Confusion
  - Ataxia
  - Ophthalmoplegia (typically sixth nerve)
- Korsakoff's psychosis is a sequela
  - Anterograde and retrograde amnesia
  - Confabulation early in the course

DIFFERENTIAL DIAGNOSIS

Alcohol dependence

- Alcoholism secondary to psychiatric disease, eg, depression, bipolar disorder, schizophrenia, personality disorder
- Other sedative dependence, eg, benzodiazepines
- Other drug abuse, eg, opioids

Alcohol withdrawal

- Withdrawal from other sedatives, eg, benzodiazepines or opioids
- Drug intoxication, eg, cocaine
- Delirium due to medical illness, eg, hypoxia, hepatic encephalopathy, thiamine deficiency, bacteremia
- Anxiety disorder
- Hallucinosis due to other cause, eg, schizophrenia, amphetamine psychosis
- Seizure due to other cause, eg, hypoglycemia, epilepsy

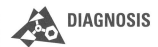

DIAGNOSIS

LABORATORY TESTS

- Blood alcohol levels < 50 mg/dL rarely cause much motor dysfunction
- Carbohydrate-deficient transferrin (CDT) can detect heavy use over a 2-week period with high specificity
- Serious drinking problem likely if
  - Elevation of γ-glutamyl transpeptidase (GGT) (levels > 30 units/L suggest heavy drinking)
  - Mean corpuscular volume (> 95 fL in men and > 100 fL in women)

DIAGNOSTIC PROCEDURES

- Suspect the problem early
- CAGE questionnaire (Table 144)
- Before treating for withdrawal or hallucinosis, meticulous examination for other medical problems is necessary

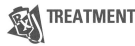

TREATMENT

MEDICATIONS

Alcoholic addiction and withdrawal

- Disulfiram (250–500 mg/day PO); compliance depends on motivation
- Naltrexone (50 mg/day PO) lowers 3–6 month relapse rates
- Acamprosate (333–666 mg PO TID)
  - Reduces craving
  - Maintains abstinence
  - Can be continued during relapse
- Antipsychotic drugs should not be used
- A short course of oral tapering benzodiazepines, eg, 20 mg/day of diazepam initially, decreasing by 5 mg daily, may be a useful adjunct
- In moderate to severe withdrawal, use diazepam (5–10 mg PO hourly depending on severity of withdrawal symptoms)
  - In very severe withdrawal, IV diazepam
  - After stabilization, diazepam (enough to maintain a sedated state) may be given orally q8–12h
  - If withdrawal signs persist (eg, tremulousness), the dosage is increased until moderate sedation occurs
  - Dosage is then gradually reduced by 20% q24h until withdrawal is complete, which usually requires ≥ 1 week of treatment
- Clonidine, 5 mcg/kg PO q2h, or the patch formulation, suppresses cardiovascular signs of withdrawal

- Carbamazepine, 400–800 mg/day PO, compares favorably with benzodiazepines for alcohol withdrawal
- Atenolol, as an adjunct to benzodiazepines, can reduce symptoms of alcohol withdrawal but should not be used when bradycardia is present
  - 100 mg/day PO when the heart rate is above 80 beats per minute
  - 50 mg/day for a heart rate between 50 and 80 beats per minute
- Phenytoin is not useful for alcohol withdrawal seizures unless there is a preexisting seizure disorder
- A general diet should be accompanied by vitamins in high doses
  - Thiamine, 50 mg IV initially (IV glucose given prior to thiamine may precipitate Wernicke's syndrome; concurrent administration is satisfactory)
  - Pyridoxine, 100 mg/day
  - Folic acid, 1 mg/day
  - Ascorbic acid, 100 mg BID

THERAPEUTIC PROCEDURES

- Maintain a nonjudgmental attitude
- Denial is best faced at the first meeting, preferably with family members
- Aversion behavioral therapy has been successful in some patients

OUTCOME

FOLLOW-UP

- Monitoring of vital signs and fluid and electrolyte levels is essential for the severely ill patient with withdrawal
- Patients with alcoholic chronic brain syndrome require careful attention to their social and environmental care

COMPLICATIONS

- Nervous system complications
  - Chronic brain syndromes
  - Cerebellar degeneration
  - Cardiomyopathy
  - Peripheral neuropathies
- Direct liver effects
  - Cirrhosis
  - Eventual hepatic failure
- Indirect effects
  - Protein abnormalities
  - Coagulation defects
  - Hormone deficiencies
  - Increased incidence of liver neoplasms
- Alcoholic hypoglycemia can occur even with low blood alcohol levels

- Traumatic subdural hematoma with liver-induced hypocoagulability
- Fetal alcohol syndrome

PROGNOSIS

- The mortality rate from delirium tremens has steadily decreased with early diagnosis and improved treatment

WHEN TO REFER

- Alcoholics Anonymous (AA)
- Al-Anon for the spouse

WHEN TO ADMIT

- Hallucinosis or severe withdrawal symptoms
- Comorbid conditions (eg, advanced liver disease) that may decompensate during alcohol withdrawal
- Hospitalization is usually not necessary

EVIDENCE

PRACTICE GUIDELINES

- National Guideline Clearinghouse: Screening and counseling. U.S. Preventive Services Task Force, 2004

WEB SITE

- National Institutes of Health: National Institute on Alcohol Abuse and Alcoholism

INFORMATION FOR PATIENTS

- JAMA patient page. Alcohol abuse and alcoholism. JAMA. 2005;293:1694. [PMID: 15811988]
- JAMA patient page. Alcohol and driving. JAMA. 2000;283:2340. [PMID: 10807396]
- JAMA patient page. Alcohol use and heart disease. JAMA. 2001;285:2040. [PMID: 11336048]
- National Institute on Alcohol Abuse and Alcoholism

REFERENCES

- Anton RF et al; COMBINE Study Research Group. Combined pharmacotherapies and behavioral interventions for alcohol dependence: the COMBINE study: a randomized controlled trial. JAMA. 2006 May 3; 295(17):2003–17. [PMID: 16670409]
- Dongier M. What are the treatment options for comorbid alcohol abuse and depressive disorders? J Psychiatry Neu-

rosci. 2005 May;30(3):224. [PMID: 15944746]

- Mayo-Smith MF et al. Management of alcohol withdrawal delirium. An evidence-based practice guideline. Arch Intern Med. 2004 Jul 12; 164(13):1405–12. Erratum in: Arch Intern Med. 2004 Oct 11; 164(18):2068. dosage error in text. [PMID: 15249349]
- Williams SH. Medications for treating alcohol dependence. Am Fam Physician. 2005 Nov 1;72(9):1775–80. [PMID: 16300039]

Alkalosis, Metabolic

 KEY FEATURES

ESSENTIALS OF DIAGNOSIS

- Characterized by high HCO_3^-, which is also seen in chronic respiratory acidosis, but pH differentiates the two disorders
- Compensatory increase in PCO_2, rarely to 55 mm Hg. A higher value implies a superimposed respiratory acidosis
- Distinguish saline-responsive from saline-unresponsive metabolic alkalosis using effective circulating volume status and urinary chloride concentration

GENERAL CONSIDERATIONS

- Etiology can be classified into saline responsive or saline unresponsive (Table 33)
- **Saline responsive**
  - By far the more common disorder
  - Characterized by normotensive extracellular volume contraction
  - Less frequently, hypotension or orthostatic hypotension are seen
  - Generally associated with hypokalemia, due partly to the direct effect of alkalosis on renal potassium excretion and partly to secondary hyperaldosteronism from volume contraction
- **Saline unresponsive**
  - Implies a volume-expanded state as from hyperaldosteronism with accompanying hypokalemia from the renal mineralocorticoid effect

Etiology

- **Saline responsive (UCl < 10 mEq/ day)**

- Excessive body bicarbonate content
  - Renal alkalosis
    - Diuretic therapy
    - Poorly reabsorbable anion therapy (carbenicillin, penicillin, sulfate, phosphate)
    - Posthypercapnia
  - Gastrointestinal alkalosis
    - Loss of HCl from vomiting or nasogastric suction
    - Intestinal alkalosis: chloride diarrhea
  - Exogenous alkali
    - $NaHCO_3$ (baking soda)
    - Sodium citrate, lactate, gluconate, acetate
    - Transfusions
    - Antacids
- Normal body bicarbonate content: Contraction alkalosis
- **Saline unresponsive (UCl >10 mEq/ day)**
- Excessive body bicarbonate content
  - Renal alkalosis, normotensive
    - Bartter's syndrome (renal salt wasting and secondary hyperaldosteronism)
    - Severe potassium depletion
    - Refeeding alkalosis
    - Hypercalcemia and hypoparathyroidism
  - Renal alkalosis, hypertensive
    - Endogenous mineralocorticoids (primary hyperaldosteronism, hyperreninism, adrenal enzyme deficiency: 11- and 17-hydroxylase, Liddle's syndrome)
    - Exogenous mineralocorticoids (licorice)

 CLINICAL FINDINGS

SYMPTOMS AND SIGNS

- No characteristic symptoms or signs
- Orthostatic hypotension may occur
- Weakness and hyporeflexia occur if serum K^+ is markedly low
- Tetany and neuromuscular irritability occur rarely

 DIAGNOSIS

LABORATORY TESTS

- Elevated arterial blood pH and bicarbonate
- Arterial PCO_2 is increased
- Serum potassium and chloride are decreased
- There may be an increased anion gap

- Urinary chloride is lower (< 10 mEq/ day) in saline-responsive disorders
- Urinary chloride is higher (> 10 mEq/ day) in saline-unresponsive disorders

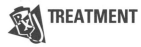 **TREATMENT**

MEDICATIONS

Saline-responsive

- Correct the extracellular volume deficit with adequate amounts of 0.9% NaCl and KCl
- For alkalosis due to nasogastric suction, discontinuation of diuretics and administration of H_2-blockers can be useful
- Acetazolamide can be used if cardiovascular status prohibits adequate volume repletion
  - Give 250–500 mg IV q4–6h
  - Monitor for the development of hypokalemia
- Administration of acid can be used as emergency therapy
  - HCl, 0.1 mol/L, is infused via a central vein (the solution is sclerosing)
  - Dosage is calculated to decrease the HCO_3^- level by one-half over 2–4 h, assuming a HCO_3^- volume of distribution (L) of 0.5 × body weight (kg)

Saline-unresponsive

- Block aldosterone effect with an angiotensin-converting enzyme inhibitor or with an aldosterone receptor antagonist (eg, spironolactone)
- Metabolic alkalosis in primary hyperaldosteronism can be treated only with potassium repletion

THERAPEUTIC PROCEDURES

- Mild alkalosis is generally well tolerated
- Severe or symptomatic alkalosis (pH > 7.60) requires urgent treatment
- Patients with marked renal failure may require dialysis

SURGERY

- Therapy for saline-unresponsive metabolic alkalosis includes surgical removal of a mineralocorticoid-producing tumor

 OUTCOME

WHEN TO REFER

- If expertise is needed for the work-up
- For treatment of saline-unresponsive metabolic alkalosis

WHEN TO ADMIT

- For persistent metabolic alkalosis in the absence of hypovolemia or associated with severe hypokalemia
- If administration of acid is needed for emergency therapy

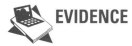 **EVIDENCE**

WEB SITE

- National Kidney Foundation

INFORMATION FOR PATIENTS

- MedlinePlus: Alkalosis
- MedlinePlus: Bartter's Syndrome
- MedlinePlus: Milk-Alkali Syndrome

REFERENCE

- Khanna A et al. Metabolic alkalosis. J Nephrol. 2006 Mar–Apr;19 Suppl 9:S86–96. [PMID: 16736446]

Alkalosis, Respiratory

 KEY FEATURES

- Acute respiratory alkalosis symptoms are related to decreased cerebral blood flow
- Causes
  - Hyperventilation syndrome
  - Hypoxia, severe anemia
  - CNS-mediated disorders (anxiety-related hyperventilation, cerebrovascular accident, infection, trauma, tumor, pharmacologic and hormonal stimulation [salicylates, nicotine, xanthines], pregnancy [progesterone], hepatic failure, septicemia, recovery from metabolic acidosis, heat exposure)
  - Pulmonary disease
  - Mechanical overventilation

 CLINICAL FINDINGS

- Acute respiratory alkalosis
  - Light-headedness
  - Anxiety
  - Paresthesias
  - Numbness about the mouth

- Tingling sensation in the hands and feet
  - Tetany in severe alkalosis from a fall in ionized calcium
- Chronic respiratory alkalosis: findings are those of the responsible condition

 DIAGNOSIS

- Elevated arterial blood pH, low P_{CO_2}
- Serum HCO_3^- is decreased in chronic respiratory alkalosis
- Although serum HCO_3^- is frequently below 15 mEq/L in metabolic acidosis, it is unusual to see such a low level in respiratory alkalosis, and its presence implies a superimposed (noncompensatory) metabolic acidosis

 TREATMENT

- Rapid correction of chronic respiratory alkalosis may result in metabolic acidosis as P_{CO_2} is increased in the setting of previous compensatory decrease in HCO_3^-
- Treatment is directed toward the underlying cause
- In acute hyperventilation syndrome from anxiety, rebreathing into a paper bag increases P_{CO_2}. Sedation may be necessary if the process persists

Alkaptonuria

 KEY FEATURES

- Alkaptonuria is caused by a recessively inherited deficiency of the enzyme homogentisic acid oxidase
- Homogentisic acid accumulates slowly in cartilage throughout the body, leading to degenerative joint disease of the spine and peripheral joints

 CLINICAL FINDINGS

- Back pain; difficult to distinguish from ankylosing spondylitis
- On radiograph, sacroiliac joints are not fused

- Ochronosis (gray-black discoloration of connective tissue, including sclerae, ears, and cartilage)
- Accumulation of metabolites in heart valves can lead to aortic or mitral stenosis
- Predisposition to coronary artery disease and nephrolithiasis

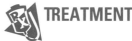 **DIAGNOSIS**

- Homogentisic acid is present in large amounts in the urine, which turns black spontaneously on exposure to air

 TREATMENT

- Nonsteroidal anti-inflammatory drugs for arthritis
- Replacement of defective heart valves and joints
- Although the syndrome causes considerable morbidity, life expectancy is reduced only modestly

Allergic Bronchopulmonary Aspergillosis (ABPA)

 KEY FEATURES

- Also known as allergic bronchopulmonary mycosis
- A bronchopulmonary hypersensitivity disorder caused by allergy to fungal antigens
- Seen in atopic asthmatic persons aged 20–40 years, usually in response to *Aspergillus* species

 CLINICAL FINDINGS

- Symptoms
  - Dyspnea
  - Wheezing
  - Cough
  - Brown-flecked sputum
- Relapses after therapy are common

- Complications
  - Bronchiectasis
  - Hemoptysis
  - Pulmonary fibrosis

DIAGNOSIS

- Primary criteria
  - History of asthma
  - Peripheral eosinophilia
  - Immediate skin reactivity to *Aspergillus* antigen
  - Precipitating antibodies to *Aspergillus* antigen
  - Elevated serum IgE
  - Pulmonary infiltrates
  - Central bronchiectasis
- Secondary criteria
  - *Aspergillus* in sputum
  - History of brown-flecked sputum
  - Delayed skin reactivity to *Aspergillus* antigen
- Presence of primary criteria 1–6 makes diagnosis almost certain

TREATMENT

- Prednisone, 0.5–1.0 mg/kg/day for at least 2 months, then careful tapering
- Itraconazole, 200 mg once daily to BID, may be added for steroid-dependent patients
- Bronchodilators are helpful

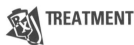

Allergy, Drug & Food

KEY FEATURES

ESSENTIALS OF DIAGNOSIS

- An immunologically mediated reaction to a food or drug
- Many drugs have toxicities or idiosyncratic reactions that are not immune-mediated and therefore are not drug allergies
- 90% of food allergies are caused by peanuts, tree nuts, fish, and shellfish

GENERAL CONSIDERATIONS

- Immediate hypersensitivity
  - IgE-mediated
  - Previously sensitized individuals

- Rapid development of urticaria, angioedema, or anaphylaxis
- Immune complex-mediated disorder
  - Serum-sickness, IgG-mediated
  - Delayed onset of urticaria accompanied by fever, arthralgias, and nephritis
- Immune hypersensitivity mechanisms
  - Drug fever
  - Stevens-Johnson syndrome
- Some drugs are clearly more immunogenic than others, and this can be reflected in the incidence of drug hypersensitivity
- Partial list of drugs frequently implicated in drug reactions
  - β-Lactam antibiotics, sulfonamides
  - Phenytoin, carbamazepine
  - Allopurinol
  - Muscle relaxants used for general anesthesia
  - Nonsteroidal anti-inflammatory drugs
  - Antisera
  - Antiarrhythmic agents
- Drug toxicities, drug interactions, or idiosyncratic reactions must be distinguished from true hypersensitivity reactions because the prognosis and management differ
- Food hypersensitivity must be distinguished from more common food intolerance (eg, lactose intolerance)

DEMOGRAPHICS

- Some estimate that 10% or less of adverse reactions to drugs are true hypersensitivity reactions

CLINICAL FINDINGS

SYMPTOMS AND SIGNS

- Urticaria
- Angioedema
- Anaphylaxis
- Fever, arthralgias, nephritis
- Stevens-Johnson syndrome
- Morbilliform eruptions, lupus-like skin syndromes, cutaneous vasculitides
- Symptoms of IgE-mediated immediate hypersensitivity/anaphylaxis; may be accompanied by abdominal pain, nausea, vomiting, and diarrhea
- Atopic dermatitis (more rare than hypersensitivity)
- Oral allergy syndrome
  - Pruritus of lips, tongue, palate
  - Typically without other signs of systemic anaphylaxis

DIFFERENTIAL DIAGNOSIS

- Vasculitis
- Erythema multiforme
- Contact dermatitis (eg, poison oak or ivy)
- Erythema migrans (Lyme disease)
- Arthropod bites (insect bites)
- Physical factors: heat, cold, solar, pressure, water, vibratory
- Cholinergic urticaria: exercise, excitement, hot showers
- Other allergic causes: feathers, dander, shellfish, tomatoes, strawberries, vaccines, chemicals, cosmetics
- Infection (eg, otitis media, sinusitis, hepatitis)
- Serum sickness
- Angioedema: hereditary or acquired complement-mediated, angiotensin-converting enzyme inhibitors
- Food intolerance

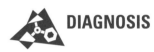

DIAGNOSIS

LABORATORY TESTS

- **Allergy testing**
  - Observed allergic reaction in the setting of a new or old drug
  - Skin testing (available for very few drugs, eg, penicillin)
  - A negative penicillin skin test makes penicillin allergy unlikely
  - Consider judicious test dose challenges in a monitored setting (performed only by a practitioner skilled and experienced with these procedures)
    □ If the likelihood of immunologic reaction is low—based on the history and the likely offending agent
    □ If no allergy testing is available
    □ If the likelihood of an IgE-mediated reaction is significant, these challenges are risky and rapid drug desensitization is indicated instead
  - The gold standard for allergy food testing is skin-prick testing with actual food items
  - However, due to the potential risk for systemic reactions, testing is usually preceded by IgE RAST testing or skin-prick testing with commercially available extracts
  - May be helpful in some cases of occupational asthma
- **Oral provocation tests**
  - Placebo-controlled oral challenge is definitive test in most cases of suspected food or drug allergy
  - Freeze-dried foods in large opaque capsules provide a sufficient dose of allergen for testing

– Should be conducted in a monitored setting
– Should not be administered to patients with suspected food-induced anaphylaxis

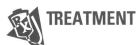 TREATMENT

MEDICATIONS

- Same as for other allergic reactions (antihistamines, corticosteroids, or subcutaneous epinephrine)
- Acute rapid desensitization can be done if the drug (eg, penicillin or insulin) must be administered
  - Rapid escalation of miniscule doses of the drug is followed by full-dose administration
  - Administer a course of oral or parenteral doses starting with extremely low doses (dilutions of 1×10^{-6} or 1×10^{-5} units) and increasing to the full dose over a period of hours
- Slow desensitization protocols are available for patients with late-appearing morbilliform eruptions (sulfamethoxazole-induced dermatitis in AIDS patients, aspirin, NSAIDs, allopurinol)
- Any history of toxic epidermal necrolysis or Stevens-Johnson syndrome is an absolute contraindication to drug readministration
- Epi-Pen, as indicated

 OUTCOME

WHEN TO REFER

- Refer to an allergist for specialized diagnostic or therapeutic interventions, such as oral provocation or rapid desensitization

WHEN TO ADMIT

- For rapid desensitization procedures, especially when there is a history of possible or probable anaphylaxis
- Rapid desensitization carries significant risk and should be undertaken in an intensively monitored setting

PREVENTION

- Avoid the drug and all chemically related compounds in the future
- Many antigens involved in food allergies denature during cooking

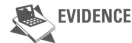 EVIDENCE

PRACTICE GUIDELINES

- Joint Task Force on Practice Parameters, the American Academy of Allergy, Asthma and Immunology, and the Joint Council of Allergy, Asthma and Immunology. Executive summary of disease management of drug hypersensitivity: a practice parameter. Ann Allergy Asthma Immunol. 1999;83(6 Pt 3):665. [PMID: 10616910]

WEB SITES

- American Academy of Allergy, Asthma, and Immunology
- MedlinePlus: Allergy

INFORMATION FOR PATIENTS

- JAMA patient page. Understanding allergies. JAMA. 2000;283:424. [PMID: 10647806]
- American College of Allergy, Asthma and Immunology: Drug Reactions
- MedlinePlus: Drug Allergies

REFERENCES

- Grammer LC et al. Drug allergy and protocols for management of drug allergies, 3rd edition. Part II. General principles of prevention of allergic drug reactions. Allergy Asthma Proc. 2004 July–August; 25(4):267–272.
- Nowak-Wegrzyn A et al. Adverse reactions to foods. Med Clin North Am. 2006 Jan;90(1):97–127. [PMID: 16310526]
- Sicherer SH et al. An expanding evidence base provides food for thought to avoid indigestion in managing difficult dilemmas in food allergy. J Clin Allergy Immunol. 2006 Jun;117(6):1419–22. [PMID: 16751007]

Amebiasis

 KEY FEATURES

ESSENTIALS OF DIAGNOSIS

- Mild to severe colitis
- Amebas or antigen in stools or abscess aspirate
- Serologic tests positive with colitis but may represent prior infections

GENERAL CONSIDERATIONS

- The *Entamoeba* complex contains two morphologically identical species
  - *E dispar*, which is avirulent
  - *E histolytica*, which may be an avirulent intestinal commensal or lead to serious disease
- Humans are the only established host for *E histolytica*
- Transmission occurs through ingestion of cysts from fecally contaminated food or water
- Infection can be transmitted person-to-person
- Flies and other arthropods also serve as mechanical vectors
- Disease follows penetration of the intestinal wall, resulting in diarrhea, dysentery, and extraintestinal disease (see Amebic Liver Disease)

DEMOGRAPHICS

- *E histolytica* infections are present worldwide but are most prevalent in subtropical and tropical areas with crowded conditions, poor sanitation, and poor nutrition
- Urban outbreaks have occurred because of common-source water contamination
- Of 500 million persons worldwide infected with *Entamoeba*, most are infected with *E dispar* and an estimated 10% (50 million) are infected with *E histolytica*
- Mortality from invasive *E histolytica* is about 100,000 per year
- Severe disease is more common in
  - Young children
  - Pregnant women
  - Persons who are malnourished
  - Persons receiving corticosteroids

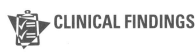 CLINICAL FINDINGS

SYMPTOMS AND SIGNS

- In most infected persons, the organism lives as a commensal, and the carrier is without symptoms

Mild disease

- Diarrhea may begin within a week of infection, although an incubation period of 2–4 weeks is more common
- Onset of abdominal pain and diarrhea is gradual
- Fever is uncommon
- Periods of remission and recurrence may last days to weeks or longer

- Abdominal examination may show
  - Distention
  - Tenderness
  - Hyperperistalsis
  - Hepatomegaly

Severe disease

- Includes colitis and dysentery, with more extensive diarrhea (10–20 stools per day) and the appearance of bloody stools
- Physical findings of dysentery
  - High fevers
  - Prostration
  - Vomiting
  - Abdominal pain and tenderness
  - Hepatic enlargement
  - Hypotension
- Fulminant amebic colitis can progress to
  - Necrotizing colitis
  - Intestinal perforation
  - Mucosal sloughing
  - Severe hemorrhage
- Localized granulomatous lesions (amebomas)
  - Can present after either dysentery or chronic intestinal infection
  - Clinical findings include pain, obstructive symptoms, and hemorrhage and may suggest intestinal carcinoma

DIFFERENTIAL DIAGNOSIS

- Inflammatory bowel disease
- Giardiasis, *Shigella*, *Salmonella*, *Campylobacter*
- Irritable bowel syndrome
- Lactase deficiency
- Cryptosporidiosis, cyclosporiasis
- Annular colonic carcinoma, tuberculosis, or lymphogranuloma venereum

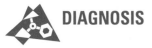 **DIAGNOSIS**

LABORATORY TESTS

- Diagnosis is most commonly made by identifying organisms in the stool
- *E histolytica* and *E dispar* cannot be distinguished, but identification of amebic trophozoites or cysts in a symptomatic patient is highly suggestive of amebiasis
- Stool evaluation for organisms
  - Not highly sensitive (~30–50% for amebic colitis)
  - At least three stool specimens should be evaluated after concentration and staining
- A commercially available stool antigen test (TechLab)
  - Offers improved sensitivity (> 90% for colitis)

- Requires fresh or frozen (not preserved) stool specimens
- Multiple serologic assays are available
  - These tests are fairly sensitive, although sensitivity is lower (~70% in colitis) early in illness
  - They cannot distinguish recent and old disease
- Examination of fresh ulcer exudate for motile trophozoites and for *E histolytica* antigen may yield a diagnosis
- In mild disease, microscopic hematochezia is common
- In severe disease, leukocytosis and hematochezia, with fecal leukocytes not present in all cases

DIAGNOSTIC PROCEDURES

- Colonoscopy of uncleansed bowel
  - In mild intestinal disease, shows no specific findings
  - In severe disease, ulcers may be found with intact intervening friable mucosa, resembling inflammatory bowel disease

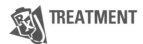 **TREATMENT**

MEDICATIONS

- See Table 79
- Asymptomatic infection with *E dispar* does not require therapy
- Colonization with *E histolytica* generally treated with luminal agent
- Luminal agents
  - Diloxanide furoate (500 mg TID with meals for 10 days)
  - Iodoquinol (diiodohydroxyquin; 650 mg TID for 21 days)
  - Paromomycin (30 mg/kg base, maximum 3 g, in three divided doses after meals daily for 7 days)
  - Side effects
    □ Flatulence with diloxanide furoate
    □ Mild diarrhea with iodoquinol
    □ Gastrointestinal symptoms with paromomycin
  - Relative contraindications
    □ Thyroid disease for iodoquinol
    □ Renal disease for iodoquinol or paromomycin
- Metronidazole (750 mg TID for 10 days) or tinidazole (2 g once daily for 3 days for mild disease and 5 days for serious disease) plus a luminal agent is treatment of choice
- Metronidazole
  - Most commonly used in the United States

- However, tinidazole offers simpler dosing and fewer side effects
- Often induces transient nausea, vomiting, epigastric discomfort, headache, or a metallic taste
- A disulfram-like reaction may occur if alcohol is coingested
- Drug interactions with cimetidine, some anticoagulants, phenytoin, phenobarbital, lithium, and other drugs have been reported
- Should be avoided in pregnant or nursing mothers if possible
- Tetracycline (250–500 mg QID for 10 days) plus chloroquine (500 mg/d for 7 days)
  - Alternative therapy
  - Tetracycline should be avoided in children and pregnant women
- Emetine or dehydroemetine can be given SQ (preferred) or IV in a dose of 1–1.5 mg/kg/d
  - Maximum daily doses
    □ For emetine, 65 mg
    □ For dehydroemetine, 90 mg
  - These agents only used until severe disease is controlled because they are cardiotoxic with a narrow therapeutic range
  - Side effects include nausea, vomiting, pain at injection site
  - Emetine is not available in the United States; dehydroemetine only available from the CDC Drug Service

SURGERY

- Surgical management of acute complications of intestinal amebiasis is best avoided whenever possible

THERAPEUTIC PROCEDURES

- Fluid and electrolyte replacement is important for patients with significant diarrhea

 OUTCOME

FOLLOW-UP

- Examine at least three stools at 2- to 3-day intervals, starting 2–4 weeks after the end of treatment
- Colonoscopy and reexamination of stools within 3 months may be indicated

COMPLICATIONS

- See Amebic Liver Disease
- Successful therapy of severe amebic colitis may be followed by postdysenteric colitis, with continued diarrhea without persistent infection

- More chronic complications of intestinal amebiasis include
  - Chronic diarrhea with weight loss, which may last for months to years
  - Bowel ulcerations
  - Amebic appendicitis

PROGNOSIS

- Postdysenteric colitis generally resolves in weeks to months
- Mortality rate of fulminant amebic colitis is > 40%

WHEN TO REFER

- Progressive colitis despite therapy

WHEN TO ADMIT

- Severe colitis or hepatic abscess

PREVENTION

- Safe water supplies; water can be
  - Boiled
  - Treated with iodine (0.5 mL tincture of iodine per liter for 20 min; cysts are resistant to standard concentrations of chlorine)
  - Filtered
- Sanitary disposal of human feces
- Adequate cooking of foods
- Protection of foods from fly contamination
- Handwashing
- In endemic areas, avoidance of foods that cannot be cooked or peeled

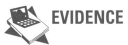 **EVIDENCE**

PRACTICE GUIDELINES

- National Guideline Clearinghouse

WEB SITE

- Centers for Disease Control and Prevention—Division of Parasitic Diseases

INFORMATION FOR PATIENTS

- Centers for Disease Control and Prevention
- Nemours Foundation
- National Institutes of Health

REFERENCES

- Blessman J et al. Ultrasound patterns and frequency of focal liver lesions after successful treatment of amoebic liver abscess. Trop Med Int Health. 2006 Apr;11(4):504–8. [PMID: 16553933]
- Haque R et al. Amebiasis. N Engl J Med. 2003 Apr 17;348(16):1565–73. [PMID: 12700377]
- Stanley SL Jr. Amoebiasis. Lancet. 2003 Mar 22;361(9362):1025–34. [PMID: 12660071]
- Tinidazole (Tindamax)—a new antiprotozoal drug. Med Lett Drugs Ther. 2004 Aug 30;46(1190):70–2. [PMID: 15375353]

Amebic Liver Disease

 KEY FEATURES

ESSENTIALS OF DIAGNOSIS

- Fever, abdominal pain
- Amebas or antigen in stool or abscess aspirate
- Positive serologic tests but may represent prior infections
- Hepatomegaly, hepatic abscess on imaging studies

GENERAL CONSIDERATIONS

- The *Entamoeba* complex contains two morphologically identical species
  - *E dispar,* which is avirulent
  - *E histolytica,* which may be an avirulent intestinal commensal or lead to serious disease
- Humans are the only established host for *E histolytica*
- Transmission occurs through ingestion of cysts from fecally contaminated food or water
- Infection can be transmitted person-to-person
- Flies and other arthropods also serve as mechanical vectors
- Disease follows penetration of the intestinal wall, resulting in
  - Diarrhea
  - Dysentery
  - Extraintestinal disease, most commonly liver abscess

DEMOGRAPHICS

- *E histolytica* infections are present worldwide but are most prevalent in subtropical and tropical areas under conditions of crowding, poor sanitation, and poor nutrition
- Of 500 million persons worldwide infected with *Entamoeba,* most are infected with *E dispar* and an estimated 10% (50 million) are infected with *E histolytica*
- Mortality from invasive *E histolytica* is about 100,000 per year
- Severe disease is more common in
  - Young children
  - Pregnant women
  - Persons who are malnourished
  - Persons receiving corticosteroids
- Hepatic abscesses more common in men

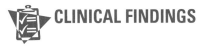 **CLINICAL FINDINGS**

SYMPTOMS AND SIGNS

- Many patients do not have current or a past history of intestinal symptoms
- Acute or gradual onset of abdominal pain
- Fever
- Enlarged and tender liver
- Anorexia
- Weight loss
- Intercostal tenderness
- Diarrhea is present in a small number of patients
- Abscesses are most commonly single and in the right lobe of the liver
- Amebic infections may rarely occur throughout the body, including the lungs, brain, and genitourinary system

DIFFERENTIAL DIAGNOSIS

- Pyogenic liver abscess
- Echinococcosis (hydatid disease)
- Cholecystitis or cholangitis
- Right lower lobe pneumonia
- Pancreatitis
- Hepatocellular carcinoma

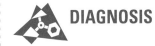 **DIAGNOSIS**

LABORATORY TESTS

- Leukocytosis and elevated liver function studies
- Serologic tests for anti-amebic antibodies are almost always positive, except very early in the infection
- Thus, a negative test in a suspicious case should be repeated in about a week
- The stool *E histolytica* antigen test is positive in ~40% of cases; a serum antigen test is under development
- Examination of stools for the organisms or antigen is frequently negative

IMAGING STUDIES

- Ultrasonography, CT, or MRI show abscesses as round or oval low-density nonhomogeneous lesions with abrupt transition from normal liver to the lesion and hypoechoic centers

DIAGNOSTIC PROCEDURES

- Percutaneous aspiration
  - May be needed to distinguish between amebic and pyogenic abscesses
  - Best done by an image-guided needle
  - Typically yields brown or yellow fluid
  - Detection of organisms in the aspirate is uncommon, but detection of *E histolytica* antigen is very sensitive and diagnostic
  - The key risk is peritoneal spillage leading to peritonitis from amebas or other (pyogenic or echinococcal) organisms

 TREATMENT

MEDICATIONS

- See Table 79
- Treatment is metronidazole or tinidazole plus a luminal agent
- IV metronidazole can be used when necessary
- If initial treatment with metronidazole or tinidazole fails, add chloroquine, emetine, or dehydroemetine

THERAPEUTIC PROCEDURES

- Needle aspiration may be helpful for large abscesses (over 5–10 cm), in particular if
  - The diagnosis remains uncertain
  - There is an initial lack of response
  - Patient is very ill, suggesting imminent abscess rupture

 OUTCOME

COMPLICATIONS

- Without prompt treatment, amebic abscesses may rupture into the pleural, peritoneal, or pericardial space, which is often fatal

PROGNOSIS

- With successful therapy, abscesses disappear slowly (over months)

WHEN TO ADMIT

- All patients should be admitted

PREVENTION

- Safe water supplies; water can be
  - Boiled
  - Treated with iodine (0.5 mL tincture of iodine per liter for 20 min; cysts are resistant to standard concentration of chlorine)
  - Filtered
- Sanitary disposal of human feces
- Adequate cooking of foods
- Protection of foods from fly contamination
- Handwashing
- In endemic areas, avoidance of foods that cannot be cooked or peeled

 EVIDENCE

INFORMATION FOR PATIENTS

- Centers for Disease Control and Prevention
- National Institutes of Health

REFERENCES

- Blessman J et al. Ultrasound patterns and frequency of focal liver lesions after successful treatment of amoebic liver abscess. Trop Med Int Health. 2006 Apr;11(4):504–8. [PMID: 16553933]
- Haque R et al. Amebiasis. N Engl J Med. 2003 Apr 17;348(16):1565–73. [PMID: 12700377]
- Stanley SL Jr. Amoebiasis. Lancet. 2003 Mar 22;361(9362):1025–34. [PMID: 12660071]
- Tinidazole (Tindamax)—a new antiprotozoal drug. Med Lett Drugs Ther. 2004 Aug 30;46(1190):70–2. [PMID: 15375353]

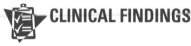

Amebic Meningoencephalitis, Primary

 KEY FEATURES

ESSENTIALS OF DIAGNOSIS

- A fulminating, hemorrhagic, necrotizing meningoencephalitis
- Occurs in healthy children and young adults and is rapidly fatal

GENERAL CONSIDERATIONS

- Caused by free-living amebas
  - *Naegleria fowleri* (most commonly)
  - *Balamuthia mandrillaris*
  - *Acanthamoeba* species
- The incubation period varies from 2 to 15 days

DEMOGRAPHICS

- *N fowleri* is a thermophilic organism found in
  - Fresh and polluted warm lake water
  - Domestic water supplies
  - Swimming pools
  - Thermal water
  - Sewers
- Most patients give a history of exposure to fresh water

 CLINICAL FINDINGS

SYMPTOMS AND SIGNS

- Early symptoms include headache, fever, stiff neck, and lethargy, often associated with rhinitis and pharyngitis
- Vomiting, disorientation, and other signs of meningoencephalitis develop within 1 or 2 days, followed by coma and then death within 7–10 days

DIFFERENTIAL DIAGNOSIS

- No distinctive clinical features distinguish the infection from acute bacterial meningoencephalitis

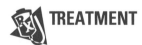 **DIAGNOSIS**

LABORATORY TESTS

- Cerebrospinal fluid (CSF) shows hundred to thousands of leukocytes and erythrocytes per cubic millimeter
- Protein is usually elevated, and glucose is normal or moderately reduced
- A fresh wet mount of the CSF may show motile trophozoites
- Staining with Giemsa or Wright stain will identify trophozoites
- Species identification is based on morphology and immunologic methods

TREATMENT

MEDICATIONS

- Amphotericin B is drug of choice

- One survivor of this disease was treated with intravenous and intrathecal amphotericin B, intravenous miconazole, and oral rifampin

OUTCOME

PROGNOSIS
- Nearly always fatal

WHEN TO ADMIT
- All patients with confirmed or suspected disease

EVIDENCE

WEB SITE
- Centers for Disease Control and Prevention—Division of Parasitic Diseases

INFORMATION FOR PATIENTS
- Centers for Disease Control and Prevention

REFERENCES
- Driebe WT Jr. Present status of contact lens-induced corneal infections. Ophthalmol Clin North Am. 2003 Sep;16(3):485–94. [PMID: 14564769]
- Marciano-Cabral F et al. *Acanthamoeba* spp. as agents of disease in humans. Clin Microbiol Rev. 2003 Apr;16(2):273–307. [PMID: 12692099]
- Vargas-Zepeda J et al. Successful treatment of *Naegleria fowleri* meningoencephalitis by using intravenous amphotericin B, fluconazole and rifampicin. Arch Med Res. 2005 Jan–Feb;36(1):83–6. [PMID: 15900627]

Amenorrhea, Primary

KEY FEATURES

- Menarche ordinarily occurs between 11 and 15 years (average in US, 12.7 years)
- Primary amenorrhea is failure of any menses to appear

- Evaluate at age 14 if no menarche or breast development or if height in lowest 3%, or at age 16 if no menarche
- Causes
  – Hypothalamic-pituitary (low-normal FSH)
    □ Idiopathic delayed puberty
    □ Pituitary tumor
    □ Hypothalamic amenorrhea (eg, stress, weight change, exercise)
    □ Anorexia nervosa
    □ Hypothyroidism
    □ Cushing's syndrome
    □ GnRH or gonadotropin deficiency
  – Hyperandrogenism (low-normal FSH)
    □ Adrenal tumor or adrenal hyperplasia
    □ Polycystic ovary syndrome
    □ Ovarian tumor
    □ Exogenous androgenic steroids
  – Ovarian causes (high FSH)
    □ Turner's syndrome
    □ Autoimmune ovarian failure
  – Pseudohermaphroditism (high LH)
    □ Testosterone synthesis defect
    □ Complete androgen resistance
  – Anatomic defect (normal FSH)
    □ Absent uterus
    □ Imperforate hymen
  – Pregnancy (high hCG)

CLINICAL FINDINGS

- Nausea, breast engorgement suggest pregnancy
- Headaches or visual field abnormalities suggest pituitary tumor
- Obesity suggests Cushing's syndrome
- Hirsutism, virilization, and acne suggest excessive testosterone
- Short stature suggests growth hormone or thyroid hormone deficiency
- Short stature and gonadal dysgenesis indicate Turner's syndrome
- Tall stature suggests eunuchoidism or gigantism
- Anosmia suggests Kallmann's syndrome
- Perform pelvic examination to assess for hymenal patency and presence of a uterus

DIAGNOSIS

- Serum FSH, LH, prolactin, testosterone, TSH, free T_4, and pregnancy test
- Serum electrolytes
- Further hormone evaluation if patient is virilized or hypertensive

- Obtain MRI of hypothalamus and pituitary if low-normal FSH and LH, especially if high prolactin
- Karyotyping

TREATMENT

- Treatment directed at underlying cause
- Hormone replacement therapy for females with permanent hypogonadism
- See Amenorrhea, Secondary & Menopause

Amenorrhea, Secondary & Menopause

KEY FEATURES

ESSENTIALS OF DIAGNOSIS
- Secondary amenorrhea: absence of menses for 3 consecutive months in women who have passed menarche
- Menopause: termination of naturally occurring menses; usually diagnosed after 6 months of amenorrhea

GENERAL CONSIDERATIONS
Causes of secondary amenorrhea
- High human chorionic gonadotropin (hCG)
  – Pregnancy most common cause
  – Rarely caused by ectopic secretion of hCG by choriocarcinoma or bronchogenic carcinoma
- Hypothalamic-pituitary causes (low-normal follicle-stimulating hormone [FSH])
- "Hypothalamic amenorrhea"
  – Idiopathic
  – Stress
  – Strict dieting
  – Vigorous exercise
  – Organic illness
  – Anorexia nervosa
- Hyperprolactinemia, pituitary tumors, and corticosteroid excess can suppress gonadotropins
- Hyperandrogenism (low-normal FSH)
  – Polycystic ovarian syndrome
  – Use of anabolic steroids
  – Rarely caused by
    □ Adrenal P-450c21 deficiency

- □ Ovarian or adrenal malignancy
- □ Ectopic ACTH from malignancy
- □ Cushing's disease
- Endometritis (normal FSH)
  - Scarring (Asherman's syndrome) occurring spontaneously
  - Following delivery or D&C
  - Tuberculosis or schistosomiasis in endemic areas
- Premature ovarian failure (high FSH) (primary hypogonadism before age 40)
  - Autoimmune
  - XO/XX chromosome mosaicism
  - Bilateral oophorectomy
  - Pelvic radiation therapy
  - Chemotherapy
  - Rarely caused by
    - □ Myotonic dystrophy
    - □ Galactosemia
    - □ Mumps oophoritis
    - □ Familial or idiopathic
- Menopause (high FSH)

DEMOGRAPHICS

- Normal age of menopause in the United States is 48–55 years (average 51.5 years)

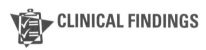 **CLINICAL FINDINGS**

SYMPTOMS AND SIGNS

- Nausea and breast engorgement suggest pregnancy
- Headache or visual field abnormalities suggest pituitary tumor
- Thirst and polyuria with diabetes insipidus indicate hypothalamic or pituitary lesion
- Acromegaly or gigantism indicate pituitary tumor
- Goiter suggests hyperthyroidism
- Weight loss, diarrhea, or skin darkening suggests adrenal insufficiency
- Weight loss with distorted body image suggests anorexia nervosa
- Galactorrhea suggests hyperprolactinemia due to pituitary tumor or various drugs
- Hirsutism or virilization occurs with hyperandrogenism
- Weakness, psychiatric changes, hypertension, central obesity, hirsutism, thin skin, ecchymoses suggest Cushing's syndrome or alcoholism
- Perform pelvic examination to check for uterine or adnexal enlargement
- Vasomotor instability (hot flushes), depression, irritability, fatigue, insomnia, headache, diminished libido, or rheumatologic symptoms suggest menopause

- Vasomotor instability in 80%, lasts seconds to many minutes; may be most severe at night or triggered by emotional stress, may persist for > 5 years in 35%
- Urogenital atrophy, vaginal dryness, and dyspareunia; dysuria, frequency, and incontinence; osteoporotic fractures are late manifestations of estrogen deficiency

DIFFERENTIAL DIAGNOSIS

- Pregnancy
- Menopause or perimenopause
- Polycystic ovary syndrome
- Hypothalamic amenorrhea, eg, stress, weight change, exercise
- Hyperprolactinemia
- Hypothyroidism or hyperthyroidism
- Diabetes mellitus
- Premature ovarian failure
- Anorexia nervosa

 DIAGNOSIS

LABORATORY TESTS

- Serum pregnancy test
  - For all women of childbearing age
  - False-positive tests may occur rarely with ectopic hCG secretion (eg, choriocarcinoma or bronchogenic carcinoma)
- If not pregnant, check serum levels of
  - Prolactin
  - FSH
  - Luteinizing hormone
  - Thyroid-stimulating hormone
  - Potassium
  - Creatinine
  - Liver enzymes
- Check serum testosterone in hirsute or virilized women
- Perform 1-mg overnight dexamethasone suppression test (see Cushing's syndrome) if signs of hypercortisolism
- Perform Papanicolaou smear and vaginal smear to assess estrogen effect
- Progestin withdrawal test
  - Nonpregnant women with normal pelvic examination and laboratory tests are given a 10-day course of progestin (eg, medroxyprogesterone acetate 10 mg PO once daily)
    - □ Absence of withdrawal menses indicates possible pregnancy, uterine abnormality, or estrogen deficiency
    - □ Occurrence of withdrawal bleeding indicates anovulation likely due to noncyclic gonadotropin secretion (eg, polycystic ovaries, idiopathic anovulation)

IMAGING STUDIES

- Hyperprolactinemia or hypopituitarism without obvious cause should prompt pituitary MRI (see Hypopituitarism)

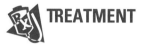 **TREATMENT**

MEDICATIONS

Guidelines

- Hormone replacement therapy (HRT) recommended for
  - Women with premature ovarian failure (< 40 years of age)
  - Older women on a case-by-case basis
- Estrogens
  - Lower-dose estrogen is favored
  - Transdermal estradiol and vaginal estrogen are favored over oral estrogen
  - Transdermal estradiol: do not apply to the breasts
  - Vaginal estrogen creams, tablets, and rings
    - □ Relieve vaginal dryness and discomfort, dyspareunia, urinary urgency, and dysuria
    - □ Can cause endometrial proliferation with prolonged use
- Progestins
  - Added to conventional-dose estrogen for women with a uterus to avoid endometrial hyperplasia
  - Exposure can be minimized by using lower-dose estrogen or progestin-eluting intrauterine devices (IUDs)
  - Progestin-eluting IUDs
    - □ Available as levonorgestrel (eg, Norplant); replaced every 5 years
    - □ Best tolerated by parous women
- Selective estrogen receptor modulators (SERMs; eg, raloxifene)
  - Alternative to estrogen replacement for osteoporosis prevention; does not increase risk of breast or uterine cancer

Benefits and risks

- **HRT: Benefits**
  - Improvement in hot flushes, vaginal moisture, sleep, rheumatic complaints
  - Improved bone density; fewer fractures
  - Improved skin moisture and thickness
- **HRT: Risks**
  - Dose-dependent
  - Oral estrogens
    - □ Increase risk of deep venous thrombosis and stroke
    - □ Can cause hypertriglyceridemia, particularly in women with preexistent hyperlipidemia, rarely resulting in pancreatitis

▫ These can be reduced by using non-oral estrogen replacement

- **Estrogen replacement without progestin: Benefits**
  - Improvement in menopause-related depression
  - Better control of type 2 diabetes mellitus
  - Slightly reduced risk of breast cancer
- **Estrogen replacement without progestin: Risks**
  - Increased risk of stroke among women taking conjugated equine estrogens
  - Endometrial hyperplasia and dysfunctional uterine bleeding (DUB)
  - Endometrial carcinoma, low absolute risk
  - Mortality from ovarian cancer, low absolute risk
- **Estrogen replacement with progestin: Benefits**
  - 0.7% lower risk for developing diabetes
  - Reduced risk for DUB and endometrial carcinoma
- **Estrogen replacement with progestin: Risks**
  - Conventional-dose oral combined HRT results in an increased risk for myocardial infarction (6 additional heart attacks per 10,000 women), mostly in preexistent coronary disease in the first year of therapy

THERAPEUTIC PROCEDURES

- Postmenopausal women should be evaluated for osteoporosis and treated if appropriate (see Osteoporosis)

 ## OUTCOME

FOLLOW-UP

- Hypothalamic amenorrhea
  - Patients typically recover spontaneously
  - However, they should have regular evaluations and a progestin withdrawal test about every 3 months to detect loss of estrogen effect

PROGNOSIS

- Ovarian failure (premature or menopausal) is usually irreversible

COMPLICATIONS

- Menopause
  - Osteoporosis and fractures
  - Increased LDL/HDL cholesterol ratio causes increased risk of atherosclerosis

PREVENTION

- Diet adequate in protein, calories, calcium, and vitamins; calcium and vitamin D supplements and exercise for those at risk for osteoporosis
- Consider bisphosphonate for osteoporosis
- Mammography recommended yearly for menopausal women receiving HRT
- Tamoxifen and raloxifene offer protection against osteoporosis but aggravate hot flushes

 ## EVIDENCE

PRACTICE GUIDELINES

- Practice Committee of the American Society for Reproductive Medicine. Current evaluation of amenorrhea. Fertil Steril. 2004;82:266. [PMID: 15237040]

INFORMATION FOR PATIENTS

- Mayo Clinic: Amenorrhea
- MedlinePlus: Secondary Amenorrhea
- National Women's Health Information Center: Menopause

REFERENCES

- Anderson GL et al. Effects of conjugated equine estrogen in postmenopausal women with hysterectomy: the Women's Health Initiative randomized controlled trial. JAMA. 2004 Apr 14; 291(14):1701–12. [PMID: 15082697]
- Barnabei VM et al; Women's Health Initiative Investigators. Menopausal symptoms and treatment-related effects of estrogen and progestin in the Women's Health Initiative. Obstet Gynecol. 2005 May;105(5 Pt 1):1063–73. [PMID: 15863546]
- Basaria S et al. Clinical review: Controversies regarding transdermal androgen therapy in postmenopausal women. J Clin Endocrinol Metab. 2006 Dec; 91(12):4743–52. [PMID: 16984993]
- Evans ML et al. Management of postmenopausal hot flushes with venlafaxine hydrochloride: a randomized, controlled trial. Obstet Gynecol. 2005 Jan; 105(1):161–6. [PMID: 15625158]
- Nair KS et al. DHEA in elderly women and DHEA or testosterone in elderly men. N Engl J Med. 2006 Oct 19; 355(16):1647–59. [PMID: 17050889]
- Reddy SY et al. Gabapentin, estrogen, and placebo for treating hot flushes: A randomized controlled trial. Obstet Gynecol. 2006 Jul;108(1):41–8. [PMID: 16816054]

Amphetamine & Cocaine Overdose

 ## KEY FEATURES

ESSENTIALS OF DIAGNOSIS

- Agitation, paranoia, psychosis
- Seizures, hyperthermia
- Hypertension, tachycardia
- Hyponatremia may occur with methylenedioxymethamphetamine (MDMA, "ecstasy")

GENERAL CONSIDERATIONS

- Amphetamines and cocaine are widely abused for their euphorigenic and stimulant properties
- Both drugs may be smoked, snorted, ingested, or injected
- The toxic dose of each drug is highly variable and depends on the route of administration and individual tolerance
- Amphetamine derivatives and related drugs include
  - Methamphetamine ("crystal meth," "crank")
  - MDMA
  - Ephedrine
  - Methcathinone ("cat")
- Nonprescription medications and nutritional supplements may contain stimulant or sympathomimetic drugs, such as
  - Ephedrine
  - Yohimbine
  - Caffeine

CLINICAL FINDINGS

SYMPTOMS AND SIGNS

- CNS stimulation and a generalized increase in central and peripheral sympathetic activity
- The onset of effects is most rapid after IV injection or smoking
- Anxiety
- Tremulousness
- Tachycardia
- Hypertension
- Diaphoresis
- Dilated pupils
- Agitation
- Muscular hyperactivity
- Psychosis

- In severe intoxication, seizures and hyperthermia may occur

DIFFERENTIAL DIAGNOSIS

- Pseudoephedrine, caffeine
- Anticholinergic poisoning
- Psychosis
- Heat stroke
- Alcohol or sedative-hypnotic withdrawal
- Serotonin syndrome

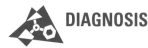 DIAGNOSIS

LABORATORY TESTS

- Urine screening usually tests for amphetamines, cocaine metabolite benzoylecgonine
- Blood screening is generally not sensitive enough to detect these drugs
- Elevated serum creatine kinase (CK) suggests rhabdomyolysis
- Hyponatremia has been reported after MDMA use
- Massive cocaine intoxication can cause QRS interval prolongation similar to tricyclic antidepressant overdose

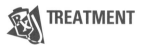 TREATMENT

MEDICATIONS

Emergency and supportive measures
- Rapidly lower the body temperature (see Hyperthermia) in patients who are hyperthermic (40°C)
- Treat agitation or psychosis with a benzodiazepine
  - Lorazepam, 2–3 mg IV repeated PRN up to 8–10 mg
  - Midazolam, 0.1–0.2 mg/kg IM

Specific treatment
- Treat agitation with a sedative such as lorazepam, 2–3 mg IV
- Treat seizures with lorazepam (2–3 mg IV) or phenobarbital (15 mg/kg IV)
- Treat hypertension with a
  - Vasodilator drug, such as phentolamine, 1–5 mg IV, or nitroprusside 0.5–10 mcg/kg/min
  - Combined α- and β-adrenergic blocker such as labetalol, 10–20 mg IV
  - Do *not* administer a pure β-blocker, such as propranolol alone, because this may result in paradoxic worsening of the hypertension as a result of unopposed α-adrenergic effects

- Treat tachycardia or tachyarrhythmias with a short-acting β-blocker such as esmolol, 25–100 mcg/kg/min by IV infusion
- Treat hyponatremia (see Hyponatremia)
- Treat hyperthermia (see Hyperthermia)

 OUTCOME

COMPLICATIONS

- Sustained or severe hypertension may result in
  - Intracranial hemorrhage
  - Aortic dissection
  - Myocardial infarction
- Hyperthermia may cause
  - Multiorgan failure
  - Permanent brain damage
- Muscle hyperactivity may lead to metabolic acidosis and rhabdomyolysis

PROGNOSIS

- Good if only a single brief seizure or mild-moderate agitation or cardiovascular effects
- Poor after severe hyperthermia (eg, temperature > 40°C) or intracranial hemorrhage

WHEN TO ADMIT

- Persistent hypertension, tachycardia
- Hyperthermia
- Hyponatremia
- Multiple or prolonged seizures

 EVIDENCE

PRACTICE GUIDELINES

- National Guideline Clearinghouse: VHA/DoD Clinical Practice Guideline for the Management of Substance Abuse Disorders

WEB SITES

- eMedicine: Toxicology Articles
- National Institute on Drug Abuse: Info-Facts: Crack and Cocaine

INFORMATION FOR PATIENTS

- JAMA patient page. Cocaine addiction. JAMA. 2002 Jan 2;287(1):146. [PMID: 11797622]
- JAMA patient page. Drug abuse. JAMA. 2000 Mar 8;283(10):1378. [PMID: 10714739]

REFERENCES

- El-Mallakh RS et al. MDMA (Ecstasy). Ann Clin Psychiatry. 2007 Jan–Mar; 19(1):45–52. [PMID: 17453661]
- Kleber HD et al; Work Group on Substance Use Disorders; American Psychiatric Association Steering Committee on Practice Guidelines. Treatment of patients with substance use disorders, second edition. American Psychiatric Association. Am J Psychiatry. 2007 Apr;164(4 Suppl):5–123. [PMID: 17569411]
- McGuinness T. Methamphetamine abuse. Am J Nurs. 2006 Dec; 106(12):54–9. [PMID: 17133009]
- Preti A. New developments in the pharmacotherapy of cocaine abuse. Addict Biol. 2007 Jun;12(2):133–51. [PMID: 17508985]
- Romanelli F et al. Clinical effects and management of methamphetamine abuse. Pharmacotherapy. 2006 Aug; 26(8):1148–56. [PMID: 16863490]
- Treadwell SD et al. Cocaine use and stroke. Postgrad Med J. 2007 Jun; 83(980):389–94. [PMID: 17551070]

Amyloidosis

 KEY FEATURES

ESSENTIALS OF DIAGNOSIS

- The diagnosis is based on clinical suspicion, family history, and preexisting long-standing infection or debilitating illness
- Microscopic examination of biopsy (eg, gingival, renal, rectal) or surgical specimens is diagnostic
- Fine-needle biopsy of subcutaneous abdominal fat is a simple and reliable method for diagnosing secondary systemic amyloidosis

GENERAL CONSIDERATIONS

- A group of disorders characterized by impaired organ function due to infiltration with insoluble protein fibrils
- Different fibrils are correlated with the clinical syndromes
- In **primary amyloidosis** (AL), the protein fibrils are monoclonal immunoglobulin light chains
- **Secondary amyloid** (AA) proteins are derived from acute-phase reactant apolipoprotein precursors

- Familial syndromes commonly cause infiltrative neuropathies
- Other types of amyloidosis may also be hereditary
- Over 20 types of fibrils have been identified in amyloid deposits
- Amyloidosis due to deposition of β_2-microglobulin in carpal ligaments occurs in chronic hemodialysis patients

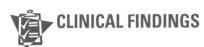

CLINICAL FINDINGS

SYMPTOMS AND SIGNS

- Related to malfunction of the infiltrated organ
- The hereditary amyloidoses usually cause neuropathies

Primary amyloidosis

- Causes widespread disease
- Nephrotic syndrome and renal failure
- Cardiomyopathy and cardiac conduction defects
- Intestinal malabsorption and pseudoobstruction
- Alzheimer's disease
- Carpal tunnel syndrome
- Macroglossia
- Peripheral neuropathy
- End-organ insufficiency of endocrine glands
- Respiratory failure
- Capillary damage with ecchymosis

Secondary amyloidosis

- Usually limited to the liver, spleen, and adrenals

DIFFERENTIAL DIAGNOSIS

- Multiple myeloma
- Hemochromatosis
- Sarcoidosis
- Waldenström's macroglobulinemia
- Metastatic cancer
- Other causes of nephrotic syndrome, eg, lupus nephritis

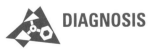

DIAGNOSIS

LABORATORY TESTS

- Monoclonal gammopathy on serum protein electrophoresis (in primary amyloidosis)

DIAGNOSTIC PROCEDURES

- Abdominal fat pad, rectal, or gingival biopsy with microscopic examination

revealing amyloid protein (green birefringence under polarizing microscope after Congo red staining)

- In systemic disease, rectal or gingival biopsies show a sensitivity of about 80%, bone marrow biopsy about 50%, and abdominal fat aspiration between 70% and 80%

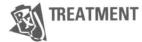

TREATMENT

MEDICATIONS

- Myeloma-associated amyloid can be treated with melphalan and prednisone

SURGERY

- Treatment of localized amyloid tumors is by surgical excision
- Some hereditary forms of amyloid are being treated with liver transplantation

THERAPEUTIC PROCEDURES

Systemic amyloidosis

- There is no effective treatment
- Supportive care/specific care pertinent to involved organs
- Hemodialysis and immunosuppressive therapy may be useful

Secondary disease

- Usually approached by aggressively treating the predisposing disease, but remission of fibril deposition does not occur
- Bone marrow transplant after chemotherapy has been used in selected patients

OUTCOME

PROGNOSIS

- Death usually occurs within 1–3 years of diagnosis with systemic amyloidosis

WHEN TO REFER

- Refer to a hematologist to confirm the diagnosis and for management
- Refer to a specialist on the organ(s) involved (eg, cardiologist, nephrologist)

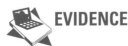

EVIDENCE

PRACTICE GUIDELINES

- Guidelines Working Group of UK Myeloma Forum; British Committee for Standards in Haematology, British

Society for Haematology. Guidelines on the diagnosis and management of AL amyloidosis. Br J Haematol. 2004; 125:681. [PMID: 15180858]

WEB SITE

- Amyloidosis Support Network

INFORMATION FOR PATIENTS

- Mayo Clinic: Amyloidosis

REFERENCES

- Gertz MA et al. Amyloidosis: diagnosis and management. Clin Lymphoma Myeloma. 2005 Nov;6(3):208–19. [PMID: 16354326]
- Gertz MA et al. Amyloidosis. Best Pract Res Clin Haematol. 2005;18(4):709–27. [PMID: 16026746]
- Merlini G et al. Molecular mechanisms of amyloidosis. N Engl J Med. 2003 Aug 7;349(6):583–96. [PMID: 12904524]
- Vesole DH et al; Plasma Cell Disorders Working Committee of the Center for International Blood and Marrow Transplant Research. High-dose therapy and autologous hematopoietic stem cell transplantation for patients with primary systemic amyloidosis: a Center for International Blood and Marrow Transplant Research Study. Mayo Clin Proc. 2006 Jul;81(7):880–8. [PMID: 16835967]

Anaerobic Infections, Bacteremia & Endocarditis

KEY FEATURES

- Anaerobic bacteremia usually originates from the
  - Gastrointestinal tract
  - Oropharynx
  - Decubitus ulcers
  - Female genital tract
- Endocarditis resulting from anaerobic and microaerophilic streptococci and bacteroides (rare) originates from the same sites

CLINICAL FINDINGS

- Related to site of original and metastatic infection

DIAGNOSIS

- Culture of blood and affected tissues

TREATMENT

- Most cases of anaerobic or microaerophilic streptococcal endocarditis can be effectively treated with 12–20 million units of penicillin G daily for 4–6 weeks
- However, optimal therapy for other types of anaerobic bacterial endocarditis must rely on laboratory guidance
- Metronidazole, 500 mg IV q8h, should be used if *Bacteroides* species is identified

Anaerobic Infections, Central Nervous System

KEY FEATURES

- Common cause of brain abscess, subdural empyema, or septic CNS thrombophlebitis
- The organisms reach CNS by direct extension from sinusitis, otitis, or mastoiditis or by hematogenous spread from chronic lung infections

CLINICAL FINDINGS

- Various neurologic deficits

DIAGNOSIS

- MRI scan (most sensitive) or CT scan
- Culture of infected tissue

TREATMENT

- Antimicrobial therapy is an important adjunct to surgical drainage
  - Ceftriaxone, 2 g IV q12h, plus metronidazole, 750 mg IV q8h
- Duration of antibiotic therapy is 6–8 weeks
- Some small multiple brain abscesses can be treated with antibiotics alone without surgical drainage

Anaerobic Infections, Chest

KEY FEATURES

- Frequently occur in the setting of poor oral hygiene and periodontal disease, aspiration of saliva (which contains 10^8 anaerobic organisms per milliliter in addition to aerobes)
- May lead to necrotizing pneumonia, lung abscess, and empyema
- Polymicrobial infection is the rule
- Anaerobes are frequently isolated etiologic agents, particularly
  - *Prevotella melaninogenica*
  - Fusobacteria
  - Peptostreptococci
- Septic internal jugular thrombophlebitis (Lemierre's syndrome)
  - May originate from mouth anaerobes, classically *Fusobacterium necrophorum*
  - May cause septic pulmonary embolization
  - Severe sore throat is concomitant

CLINICAL FINDINGS

- Fever
- Productive cough
- Night sweats
- Weight loss
- Chronic course of illness
- Poor dentition (frequently)

DIAGNOSIS

- Pleural fluid culture
- Chest radiograph
- CT scan

TREATMENT

- Clindamycin, 600 mg IV once, followed by 300 mg PO q6–8h, is the treatment of choice
- Metronidazole is an alternative
  - But does not cover facultative streptococci, which are often present
  - So, if used, a second agent active against streptococci, such as ceftriaxone, 1 g/day IV or IM should be added
- Penicillin, 2 million units IV q4h, followed by amoxicillin, 750–1000 mg PO q12h, is an alternative, although increasing prevalence of β-lactamase producing organisms is common
- Moxifloxacin, 400 mg PO or IV, once daily may be used
- Because these infections respond slowly, a prolonged course of therapy (eg, 4–6 weeks) is generally recommended

Anaerobic Infections, Head & Neck

KEY FEATURES

- *Prevotella melaninogenica* and anaerobic spirochetes are commonly involved in periodontal infections
- These organisms, fusobacteria, and peptostreptococci may cause
  - Chronic sinusitis
  - Peritonsillar abscess
  - Chronic otitis media
  - Mastoiditis
  - Venous thrombosis

CLINICAL FINDINGS

- Related to infected organ

DIAGNOSIS

- Culture
- CT scan

TREATMENT

- Tables 62 and 63
- Oral anaerobic organisms have been uniformly susceptible to penicillin
- However, there has been a trend of increasing penicillin resistance, usually resulting from β-lactamase production
- Penicillin
  - 1–2 million units IV q4h (if parenteral therapy is required) **or**
  - 500 mg PO QID for less severe infections
- Clindamycin is alternative
  - 600 mg IV q8h **or**
  - 300 mg PO q6h
- Indolent, established infections (eg, mastoiditis or osteomyelitis) may require prolonged courses of therapy (eg, 4–6 weeks or longer)

Anaerobic Infections, Intra-Abdominal

KEY FEATURES

- Each gram of stool contains up to 10^{11} anaerobes, predominantly
  - *Bacteroides fragilis*
  - Clostridia
  - Peptostreptococci
- These organisms play a central role in most intra-abdominal abscesses
  - Diverticulitis
  - Appendicitis
  - Perirectal abscess
- They may also participate in hepatic abscess and cholecystitis
- The bacteriology of these infections includes anaerobes as well as enteric gram-negative rods and, on occasion, enterococci

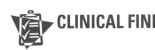

CLINICAL FINDINGS

- Related to infected organ

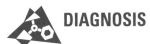

DIAGNOSIS

- Examination, laboratory tests, cultures, and CT scan

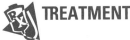

TREATMENT

- Therapy should be directed both against anaerobes and gram-negative aerobes
- Antibiotics that are reliably active against *B fragilis* include
  - Metronidazole
  - Chloramphenicol
  - Carbapenems
  - Ampicillin-sulbactam
  - Ticarcillin-clavulanic acid
  - Piperacillin-tazobactam
- Table 76 summarizes the antibiotic regimens for management of
  - Moderate to moderately severe infections (eg, patient hemodynamically stable, good surgical drainage possible or established, low APACHE score, no multiple-organ failure)
  - Severe infections (eg, major peritoneal soilage, large or multiple abscesses, patient hemodynamically unstable), particularly if drug-resistant organisms are suspected

Anaerobic Infections, Skin & Soft Tissue

KEY FEATURES

- Several terms have been used to classify these infections
  - Bacterial synergistic gangrene
  - Synergistic necrotizing cellulitis
  - Necrotizing fasciitis
  - Nonclostridial crepitant cellulitis
- Usually occur
  - After trauma or surgery
  - With inadequate blood supply
  - In association with diabetes mellitus
- Most common in areas contaminated by oral or fecal flora
- All are mixed infections caused by aerobic and anaerobic organisms
- Although there are some differences in microbiology among these infections, their differentiation on clinical grounds alone is difficult

CLINICAL FINDINGS

- There may be progressive tissue necrosis, evidence of gas in the tissues (crepitance) and a putrid odor
- Pain out of proportion to the clinical findings
- Hemodynamic instability and systemic toxicity may be present

DIAGNOSIS

- Surgical exploration

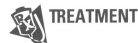

TREATMENT

- Broad-spectrum antibiotics active against both anaerobes and gram-positive and gram-negative aerobes should be instituted empirically and modified by culture results (Tables 62, 63, and 76)
  - Piperacillin-tazobactam
  - A carbapenem (eg, imipenem, meropenem)
  - Vancomycin plus metronidazole plus a fluoroquinolone or gentamicin or tobramycin
- Require aggressive surgical débridement of necrotic tissue for cure

Anal Cancer

KEY FEATURES

- Carcinoma of the anus is relatively rare: only 1–2% of all cancers of the large intestine and anus
- Squamous cancers (keratinizing, transitional cell, and cloacogenic), 80%; adenocarcinomas, 20%
- Increased incidence among
  - People practicing receptive anal intercourse
  - Those with a history of other sexually transmitted diseases
  - Those with HIV infection
- Human papillomavirus (HPV) infection in > 80%
- Increased risk in combined HIV and HPV infection

CLINICAL FINDINGS

- Anal bleeding
- Pain
- Local tumor

DIAGNOSIS

- Anoscopy and biopsy for diagnosis
- MRI and endoluminal ultrasonogram for staging

TREATMENT

- Local excision for small superficial lesions of the perianal skin
- Combined-modality therapy for tumors invading the sphincter or rectum: external radiation with simultaneous chemotherapy (fluorouracil and either mitomycin or cisplatin)
- Local control achieved in 80% of patients
- Radical surgery (abdominoperineal resection) for patients in whom chemotherapy and radiation therapy fail
- 5-year survival rate
  – 60–70% for localized (stages I–III) disease
  – > 25% for metastatic (stage IV) disease

Anal Fissures

KEY FEATURES

- Linear or rocket-shaped ulcers, usually < 5 mm
- Most commonly occur in the posterior midline; 10% occur anteriorly
- Arise from trauma during defecation

CLINICAL FINDINGS

- Severe, tearing pain during defecation followed by throbbing discomfort
- May lead to constipation because of fear of recurrent pain
- Mild associated hematochezia
- With chronic fissures, there is fibrosis and a skin tag at the outermost edge (sentinel pile)

DIAGNOSIS

- Diagnosis is confirmed by visual inspection of the anal verge while gently separating the buttocks
- Digital and anoscopic examinations may cause severe pain and may not be possible
- Fissures that occur off the midline suggest
  – Crohn's disease
  – Syphilis
  – Tuberculosis
  – HIV/AIDS
  – Anal carcinoma

TREATMENT

- Fiber supplements, stool softeners
- Sitz baths
- Topical anesthetics (EMLA cream) may provide temporary relief
- Chronic fissures may be treated with
  – Topical 0.2–0.4% nitroglycerin or diltiazem 2% ointment (1 cm of ointment) applied just inside anus with tip of finger BID for 4–8 weeks
  – Injection of botulinum toxin (20 units) into anal sphincter
- Internal sphincterotomy is effective for chronic or recurrent fissures but may be complicated by minor fecal incontinence

Anaphylaxis

KEY FEATURES

ESSENTIALS OF DIAGNOSIS

- **Anaphylaxis**
  – Systemic reaction with cutaneous symptoms
  – Dyspnea, visceral edema, and hypotension
- **Urticaria**
  – Large, irregularly shaped, pruritic, erythematous wheals
- **Angioedema**
  – Painless subcutaneous swelling, often involving periorbital, circumoral, and facial regions
- These disorders may be diagnosed clinically, especially in the context of allergen exposure; detection of specific IgE or elevated serum tryptase can confirm diagnosis

GENERAL CONSIDERATIONS

- The most common allergens that induce this IgE antibody-mediated response are drugs, insect venoms, and foods
- A generalized release of mediators from mast cells can result in systemic anaphylaxis
- Can affect both nonatopic and atopic persons
- Isolated urticaria and angioedema are more common cutaneous forms of anaphylaxis with a better prognosis
- Chronic relapsing urticaria, angioedema, and anaphylaxis are not always due to IgE-mediated hypersensitivity; consider underlying systemic disorders such as systemic mastocytosis or subclinical infection or inflammatory disorders
- Idiopathic autoimmune processes include the production of histamine-liberating autoantibodies directed against Fcε mast cell membrane receptors

DEMOGRAPHICS

In the United States

- Approximately 34,000 patients have idiopathic anaphylaxis
- Food allergies cause an estimated 150 fatalities per year
- Most food allergy fatalities are due to peanuts, tree nuts, shellfish, and fish
- β-Lactam antibiotics may be involved in 400–800 fatalities per year
- Stinging insect venom causes about 50 fatalities per year
- 20% of the population will experience urticaria or angioedema during their lifetime

CLINICAL FINDINGS

SYMPTOMS AND SIGNS

- Hypotension/shock from widespread vasodilation
- Respiratory distress from bronchospasm or laryngeal edema
- Gastrointestinal or uterine smooth muscle contraction
- Flushing, pruritus, urticaria, and angioedema

DIFFERENTIAL DIAGNOSIS

- Other causes of shock
  – Sepsis
  – Cardiogenic
  – Hypovolemic
  – Neurogenic

- Asthma
- Adrenal insufficiency
- Vasovagal reaction

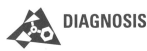 **DIAGNOSIS**

LABORATORY TESTS

- Based on the clinical presentation and a history of allergen exposure
- An elevated serum tryptase (a mast cell protease) measured during the episode can confirm the diagnosis
- Detection of a specific IgE, skin testing, or radioallergosorbent test (RAST) against the suspected antigen can confirm the allergic diathesis
- A serum C4 level
  - Adequate screening test in CI-esterase inhibitor deficiency/hereditary angioedema in patients with recurrent angioedema
  - Usually low when there is CI-esterase inhibitor deficiency

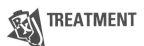 **TREATMENT**

MEDICATIONS

Anaphylaxis

- Epinephrine 1:1000 in a dose of 0.2–0.5 mL (0.2–0.5 mg) injected IM in the anterolateral thigh (more predictable and rapidly absorbed than SQ administration); repeated injections can be given every 5–15 min if necessary
- Rapid infusions of normal saline
- Inhaled β_2-adrenergic agonists, or IV aminophylline (0.5 mg/kg/h with 6-mg/kg loading dose over 30 min) for bronchospasm
- Antihistamines (H_1- and H_2-receptor antagonists) such as diphenhydramine (25–50 mg PO, IM, or IV q4–6h) and ranitidine (150 mg PO q12h or 50 mg IM or IV q6–8h)
- Anaphylaxis from β-adrenergic blocker drugs can be particularly problematic because of refractoriness to epinephrine and selective β-adrenergic agonists
- Higher-dose adrenergic drugs are required: glucagon (0.5–1.0 mg IV, IM, or SQ; may be repeated after 30 min) may be beneficial
- IV corticosteroids (which may mitigate the late-phase response that occurs 24 h after onset)
- 12–24 h of observation
- See Urticaria & Angioedema

THERAPEUTIC PROCEDURES

- Endotracheal intubation for laryngeal edema or severe bronchospasm

 OUTCOME

FOLLOW-UP

- Follow up with an allergist and receive a subcutaneous epinephrine self-injection kit; further management may involve antihistamines or immunotherapy

WHEN TO REFER

- Early referral to an allergist may help with management
- Refer for desensitization and immunotherapy

WHEN TO ADMIT

- Patients with anaphylaxis should be admitted for 12–24 h of observation for recurrence of symptoms

PREVENTION

- Long-term combined oral antihistamine and prednisone therapy reduces the number and severity of attacks of life-threatening idiopathic anaphylaxis
- Medical therapy does not reliably prevent true IgE-mediated hypersensitivity reactions

Venom immunotherapy

- Patients with immediate hypersensitivity reactions to stinging insects and documented venom-specific IgE on allergy testing should receive a 5-year course of venom immunotherapy for prevention of anaphylaxis. Large, isolated, local reactions to insect stings are not a predisposing factor for systemic anaphylaxis
- Untreated individuals have a 50–60% risk of anaphylactic response to subsequent stings
- Venom immunotherapy provides 98% protection from life-threatening reactions on rechallenge

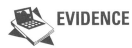 **EVIDENCE**

PRACTICE GUIDELINES

- The diagnosis and management of anaphylaxis: Updated. Joint Task Force on Practice Parameters, Work Group on Diagnosis and Management of Anaphylaxis.
- Joint Task Force on Practice Parameters; American Academy of Allergy, Asthma and Immunology; American College of Allergy, Asthma and Immunology; Joint Council of Allergy, Asthma and Immunology. The diagnosis and management of anaphylaxis: an updated practice parameter. J Allergy Clin Immunol. 2005 Mar;115(3 Suppl 2):S483–523. [PMID: 15753926]

WEB SITES

- American Academy of Allergy, Asthma, and Immunology
- Food Allergy & Anaphylaxis Network

INFORMATION FOR PATIENTS

- American Academy of Allergy, Asthma & Immunology: Anaphylaxis
- American Academy of Allergy, Asthma & Immunology: What Is Anaphylaxis?
- FamilyDoctor.org: Anaphylaxis
- MedlinePlus: Anaphylaxis

REFERENCES

- Dibbern DA Jr. Urticaria: selected highlights and recent advances. Med Clin North Am. 2006 Jan;90(1):187–209. [PMID: 16310530]
- Kemp SF. Office approach to anaphylaxis: sooner better than later. Am J Med. 2007 Aug;120(8):664–8. [PMID: 17679121]
- Moffitt JE et al. Stinging insect hypersensitivity: A practice parameter update. J Allergy Clin Immunol. 2004 Oct; 114(4):869–86. [PMID: 15480329]
- Oswalt ML et al. Anaphylaxis: office management and prevention. Immunol Allergy Clin North Am. 2007 May; 27(2):177–91, vi. [PMID: 17493497]
- Simons FE. Anaphylaxis, killer allergy: long-term management in the community. J Allergy Clin Immunol. 2006 Feb; 117(2):367–77. [PMID: 16461138]
- Weiler CR et al. Genetic test indications and interpretations in patients with hereditary angioedema. Mayo Clin Proc. 2006 Jul;81(7):958–72. [PMID: 16835976]

Anemia of Chronic Disease

 KEY FEATURES

- Many chronic systemic diseases associated with mild or moderate anemia (eg, chronic infection or inflammation, cancer, liver disease)
- Anemia of chronic renal failure has different pathophysiology (reduced erythropoietin); is usually more severe
- Largely caused by sequestration of iron within reticuloendothelial system
- Decreased dietary intake of folate or iron common in ill patients, causing coexistent folate or iron deficiency
- Many also have ongoing GI bleeding
- Hemodialysis patients regularly lose iron and folate during dialysis

 CLINICAL FINDINGS

- Symptoms of anemia, which is usually modest
- Suspect diagnosis in patients with known chronic diseases

 DIAGNOSIS

- Hematocrit usually > 25% (except in renal failure); if < 25%, evaluate for coexistent iron deficiency or folic acid deficiency
- Mean corpuscular volume usually normal or slightly low
- Red blood cell morphology nondiagnostic; reticulocyte count neither strikingly reduced nor increased
- Low serum iron, low transferrin saturation
- Normal or increased serum ferritin; serum ferritin < 30 mcg/L suggests coexistent iron deficiency
- Normal or increased bone marrow iron stores

 TREATMENT

- In most cases, no treatment necessary
- Purified recombinant erythropoietin (eg, 30,000 units SQ every week) effective for anemia of renal failure, AIDS, cancer, rheumatoid arthritis
- In renal failure, optimal response to erythropoietin requires adequate dialysis
- Erythropoietin very expensive; used only when patient is transfusion-dependent or when quality of life clearly improved by hematologic response

Anemia, Aplastic

 KEY FEATURES

ESSENTIALS OF DIAGNOSIS

- Pancytopenia
- No abnormal cells seen
- Hypocellular bone marrow

GENERAL CONSIDERATIONS

- In aplastic anemia, bone marrow failure and pancytopenia arise from injury to or abnormal expression of the hematopoietic stem cell

Causes of aplastic anemia
- "Idiopathic" (probably autoimmune)
- Drugs
  – Chloramphenicol
  – Phenylbutazone
  – Gold salts
  – Sulfonamides
  – Phenytoin
  – Carbamazepine
  – Quinacrine
  – Tolbutamide
- Systemic lupus erythematosus
- Toxins: benzene, toluene, insecticides
- Posthepatitis
- Pregnancy
- Paroxysmal nocturnal hemoglobinuria
- Congenital (rare)

 CLINICAL FINDINGS

SYMPTOMS AND SIGNS

- Weakness and fatigue from anemia
- Vulnerability to bacterial infections from neutropenia
- Mucosal and skin bleeding from thrombocytopenia
- Pallor, purpura, and petechiae
- Hepatosplenomegaly, lymphadenopathy, or bone tenderness should *not* be present

DIFFERENTIAL DIAGNOSIS

- Acute leukemia
- Hairy cell leukemia
- Myelodysplastic syndrome
- Bone marrow infiltrative process (eg, tumor, infection, granulomatous disease)
- Hypersplenism
- Systemic lupus erythematosus

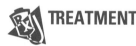 **DIAGNOSIS**

LABORATORY TESTS

- Pancytopenia, although in early disease only one or two cell lines may be reduced
- Anemia may be severe
- Reticulocytes always decreased
- Red blood cell morphology unremarkable
- Neutrophils and platelets reduced in number, no immature or abnormal forms seen
- Severe aplastic anemia defined by neutrophils < 500/mcL, platelets < 20,000/mcL, reticulocytes < 1%, and bone marrow cellularity < 20%

DIAGNOSTIC PROCEDURES

- Bone marrow aspirate and bone marrow biopsy appear hypocellular, with scant amounts of normal hematopoietic progenitors; no abnormal cells are seen

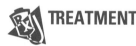 **TREATMENT**

MEDICATIONS

- Antibiotics to treat infections
- Immunosuppression with antithymocyte globulin (ATG) plus cyclosporine (or tacrolimus) for severe aplastic anemia in adults aged > 60 or those without HLA-matched siblings
- Useful regimen is equine ATG, 40 mg/kg/day IV for 4 days, in combination with cyclosporine, 6 mg/kg PO BID, given in hospital in conjunction with corticosteroids, and transfusion and antibiotic support
- Corticosteroids are given with ATG (prednisone 1–2 mg/kg/day initially followed by taper over 2–3 weeks) to avoid complications of serum sickness
- Rabbit ATG is more immunosuppressive than equine ATG and may also be used
- Antibiotics and transfusion often required for prolonged pancytopenia
- Androgens (eg, oxymetholone, 2–3 mg/kg PO once daily) used commonly in past

- Despite low response rate, some patients can be maintained successfully with androgens

THERAPEUTIC PROCEDURES

- Supportive measures only for mild cases
- Allogeneic bone marrow transplantation is treatment of choice for severe aplastic anemia in adults aged < 50 with HLA-matched siblings
- Allogeneic transplantation using unrelated donor if immunosuppression is not effective
- Red blood cell and platelet transfusions as necessary

OUTCOME

COMPLICATIONS

- Infections
- Bleeding

PROGNOSIS

- Median survival in severe aplastic anemia without treatment is ~3 months, and 1-year survival is only 20%
- Allogeneic bone marrow transplantation is highly successful in children and young adults with HLA-matched siblings, with durable complete response rate > 80%
- ATG treatment produces partial response in ~60% of adults, usually in 4–12 weeks; long-term prognosis of responders is good
- Paroxysmal nocturnal hemoglobinuria or myelodysplasia or other clonal hematologic disorders develop in < 25% of nontransplanted patients after many years of follow-up

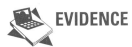

EVIDENCE

PRACTICE GUIDELINES

- Marsh JC et al. Guidelines for the diagnosis and management of acquired aplastic anaemia. Br J Haematol. 2003; 123:782. Erratum in: Br J Haematol. 2004;126:625. [PMID: 14632769]

INFORMATION FOR PATIENTS

- American Cancer Society: Detailed Guide: Aplastic Anemia
- Aplastic Anemia & MDS International Foundation
- MedlinePlus: Idiopathic Aplastic Anemia
- MedlinePlus: Secondary Aplastic Anemia

REFERENCES

- Ades L et al. Long-term outcome after bone marrow transplantation for severe aplastic anemia. Blood. 2004 Apr 1; 103(7):2490–7. [PMID: 14656884]
- Marsh J. Making therapeutic decisions in adults with aplastic anemia. Hematology Am Soc Hematol Educ Program. 2006:78–85. [PMID: 17124044]
- Yamaguchi H et al. Mutations in TERT, the gene for telomerase reverse transcriptase, in aplastic anemia. N Engl J Med. 2005 Apr 7;352(14):1413–24. [PMID: 15814878]

Anemia, Autoimmune Hemolytic

KEY FEATURES

ESSENTIALS OF DIAGNOSIS

- Acquired anemia caused by immunoglobulin G (IgG) autoantibody
- Spherocytes and reticulocytosis on peripheral blood smear
- Positive direct Coombs test

GENERAL CONSIDERATIONS

- Acquired disorder in which IgG autoantibody binds to red blood cell (RBC) membrane
  - Macrophages in spleen and other portions of reticuloendothelial system then remove portion of RBC membrane, forming a spherocyte because of decreased surface-to-volume ratio of RBC
  - Spherocytes less deformable and become trapped in spleen
- Causes include
  - Idiopathic (~50% of cases)
  - Systemic lupus erythematosus
  - Chronic lymphocytic leukemia
  - Lymphomas
- Must be distinguished from drug-induced hemolytic anemia (eg, penicillin and other drugs), which coats RBC membrane; antibody is directed against membrane–drug complex
- Typically produces anemia of rapid onset that may be life-threatening

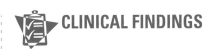

CLINICAL FINDINGS

SYMPTOMS AND SIGNS

- Fatigue, angina pectoris, symptoms of congestive heart failure
- Jaundice and splenomegaly may be present

DIFFERENTIAL DIAGNOSIS

- Hereditary spherocytosis
- Alloimmune transfusion reaction
- Glucose-6-phosphate dehydrogenase deficiency
- Microangiopathic hemolytic anemia
  - Thrombotic thrombocytopenic purpura
  - Hemolytic-uremic syndrome
  - Disseminated intravascular coagulation
- Splenic sequestration

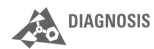

DIAGNOSIS

LABORATORY TESTS

- Anemia of variable severity, although hematocrit may be < 10%
- Reticulocytosis usually present
- Spherocytes on peripheral blood smear
- Indirect bilirubin increased
- Coincident immune thrombocytopenia (Evans syndrome) in ~10%
- Coombs antiglobulin test is basis for diagnosis; reagent is rabbit IgM antibody against human IgG or human complement
- Direct Coombs test positive: patient's RBCs mixed with Coombs reagent; agglutination indicates antibody on RBC surface
- Indirect Coombs test may or may not be positive: patient's serum mixed with panel of type O RBCs, then Coombs reagent added; agglutination indicates presence of large amount of autoantibody that has saturated binding sites on RBC and consequently appears in serum
- Micro-Coombs test is more sensitive and is necessary to make diagnosis in ~10% of cases; test indicated in patient with acquired spherocytic hemolytic anemia that may be autoimmune who has a negative direct Coombs test

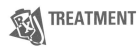

TREATMENT

MEDICATIONS

- Prednisone, 1–2 mg/kg/day in divided doses, is initial therapy

- Splenectomy if prednisone ineffective or if disease recurs on tapering dose
- Danazol, 600–800 mg/day, is less effective than in immune thrombocytopenia
- Rituximab, 375 mg/m^2 IV every week for 4 weeks, is effective and has low toxicity
- Immunosuppressive agents (eg, cyclosporine, mycophenolate mofetil) may be effective
- Cytotoxic immunosuppressive agents (eg, cyclophosphamide, azathioprine) may be effective, but with toxicity
- High-dose IVIG, 1 g daily for 1 or 2 days
  – May be highly effective in controlling hemolysis
  – Benefit is short lived (1–3 weeks)
  – It is expensive

SURGERY

- Splenectomy is often successful

THERAPEUTIC PROCEDURES

- Transfusion may be problematic because of difficulty in performing cross-match; thus, incompatible blood may be given
- If compatible, most transfused blood survives similarly to patient's own RBCs

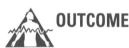 **OUTCOME**

COMPLICATIONS

- Possible transfusion reactions
- Drops in hematocrit may be sudden and severe

PROGNOSIS

- Long-term prognosis is good, especially if there is no underlying autoimmune disorder or lymphoma

WHEN TO REFER

- Decisions regarding transfusions should be made in consultation with a hematologist

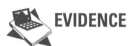 **EVIDENCE**

WEB SITES

- American Academy of Family Physicians: Hemolytic Anemia

INFORMATION FOR PATIENTS

- MedlinePlus: Idiopathic Autoimmune Hemolytic Anemia

- National Institutes of Health: Questions and Answers About Autoimmunity
- The Regional Cancer Center: Autoimmune Hemolytic Anemia

REFERENCES

- Petz LD. A physician's guide to transfusion in autoimmune haemolytic anaemia. Br J Haematol. 2004 Mar; 124(6):712–6. [PMID: 15009058]
- Robak T. Monoclonal antibodies in the treatment of autoimmune cytopenias. Eur J Haematol. 2004 Feb;72(2):79–88. [PMID: 14962245]

Anemia, Hemolytic

 KEY FEATURES

- **Coombs positive hemolytic anemia** may be autoimmune or related to drugs, infection, lymphoproliferative disease, Rh or ABO incompatibility
- **Coombs negative hemolytic anemia** may be intrinsic RBC disease
  – Abnormal hemoglobin: sickle cell disease, thalassemia, methemoglobinemia
  – Membrane defect: hereditary spherocytosis, hereditary elliptocytosis, paroxysmal nocturnal hemoglobinuria
  – Enzyme defect: G6PD deficiency, pyruvate kinase deficiency
- **Coombs negative hemolytic anemia** may be extrinsic
  – Microangiopathic hemolytic anemia
    ▫ TTP
    ▫ Hemolytic-uremic syndrome
    ▫ DIC
    ▫ Prosthetic valve hemolysis
    ▫ Metastatic adenocarcinoma
    ▫ Vasculitis
    ▫ Malignant hypertension
    ▫ HELLP syndrome
  – Splenic sequestration
  – *Plasmodium, Clostridium, Borrelia* infection
  – Burns

 CLINICAL FINDINGS

- Symptoms of anemia
- Jaundice, pigment gallstones, cholecystitis in chronic cases
- Palpable spleen

 DIAGNOSIS

- Serum haptoglobin may be low but is neither specific nor sensitive
- Reticulocytosis present unless second disorder (infection, folate deficiency) superimposed on hemolysis
- Transient hemoglobinemia with intravascular hemolysis
- Hemoglobinuria when capacity for reabsorption of hemoglobin by renal tubular cells exceeded
- Urine hemosiderin test positive; indicates prior intravascular hemolysis
- Hemoglobinemia and methemalbuminemia if severe intravascular hemolysis
- Indirect bilirubin elevated, total bilirubin elevated to ≥ 4 mg/dL
- Serum LDH elevated in microangiopathic hemolysis; may be elevated in other hemolytic anemias

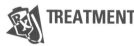 **TREATMENT**

- Treat underlying cause
- Folic acid, 1 mg PO once daily
- Transfusions possible

Anemia, Iron Deficiency

 KEY FEATURES

ESSENTIALS OF DIAGNOSIS

- Absent bone marrow iron stores or serum ferritin < 12 mcg/L are both pathognomonic
- Caused by bleeding in adults unless proved otherwise
- Response to iron therapy

GENERAL CONSIDERATIONS

- Most common cause of anemia worldwide
- Causes
  – Blood loss (gastrointestinal [GI], menstrual, repeated blood donation)
  – Deficient diet
  – Increased requirements (pregnancy, lactation)
  – Hemoglobinuria (eg, paroxysmal nocturnal hemoglobinuria)

- Malabsorption (eg, gastric surgery, celiac disease)
- Intravascular hemolysis
- Pulmonary hemosiderosis (iron sequestration)
- Women with heavy menstrual losses may require more iron than can reasonably be absorbed; thus, they often become iron deficient
- Pregnancy and lactation also increase requirement for iron, necessitating medicinal iron supplementation
- Long-term aspirin use may cause blood loss even without documented structural lesion
- Search for source of GI bleeding if other sites of blood loss (menorrhagia, other uterine bleeding, and repeated blood donations) are excluded

DEMOGRAPHICS

- More common in women as a result of menstrual losses

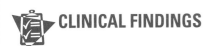 CLINICAL FINDINGS

SYMPTOMS AND SIGNS

- Symptoms of anemia (eg, easy fatigability, tachycardia, palpitations and tachypnea on exertion)
- Skin and mucosal changes (eg, smooth tongue, brittle nails, and cheilosis) in severe iron deficiency
- Dysphagia resulting from esophageal webs (Plummer-Vinson syndrome)
- Pica (ie, craving for specific foods [eg, ice chips, lettuce] often not rich in iron) is frequent

DIFFERENTIAL DIAGNOSIS

- Microcytic anemia resulting from other causes
  - Thalassemia
  - Anemia of chronic disease
  - Sideroblastic anemia
  - Lead poisoning

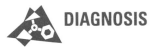 DIAGNOSIS

LABORATORY TESTS

- Diagnosis can be made by
  - Laboratory confirmation of an iron-deficient state
  - Evaluation of response to a therapeutic trial of iron replacement
- Hematocrit low, but mean corpuscular hemoglobin (MCV) initially normal; later MCV low

- Platelet count may be increased
- Serum ferritin low; value < 30 mcg/L highly reliable indicator of iron deficiency
- Serum total iron-binding capacity (TIBC) rises, serum iron < 30 mcg/dL, and transferrin saturation < 15% after iron stores depleted
- Blood smear becomes abnormal in moderate to severe cases, showing hypochromic microcytic cells, anisocytosis (variation in red blood cell [RBC] size), and poikilocytosis (variation in RBC shape)
- Severely hypochromic cells, target cells, hypochromic pencil-shaped cells, and occasionally small numbers of nucleated RBCs in severe iron deficiency
- Fecal occult blood testing often positive with GI bleeding

DIAGNOSTIC PROCEDURES

- Colonoscopy or flexible sigmoidoscopy may be required in evaluation of suspected GI bleeding

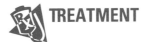 TREATMENT

MEDICATIONS

- Ferrous sulfate, 325 mg PO TID
  - Treatment of choice
  - May cause GI side effects
- Compliance improved by starting 325 mg PO once daily with food, then gradually escalating dose
- Preferable to prescribe a lower dose of iron or to allow ingestion concurrent with food rather than insist on a regimen that will not be followed
- Continue iron therapy for 3–6 months after restoration of normal hematologic values to replenish iron stores
- Failure of response to iron therapy
  - Usually due to noncompliance
  - Occasional patients absorb iron poorly
  - Other reasons include incorrect diagnosis (anemia of chronic disease, thalassemia) and ongoing GI blood loss
- Indications for parenteral iron
  - Intolerance of oral iron
  - Refractoriness to oral iron
  - GI disease (usually inflammatory bowel disease) precluding use of oral iron
  - Continued blood loss that cannot be corrected
- Because of risk of anaphylaxis, parenteral iron used only for persistent anemia after reasonable trial of oral therapy
- Dose of IV iron (total 1.5–2.0 g) is calculated by estimating decrease in vol-

ume of RBC mass and supplying 1 mg of iron for each milliliter of volume below normal
  - Then add approximately 1 g for storage iron
  - Entire dose may be given as IV infusion over 4–6 h
  - Test dose of dilute solution given first; observe patient during entire infusion for anaphylaxis

THERAPEUTIC PROCEDURES

- Treat underlying cause such as source of GI bleeding

OUTCOME

FOLLOW-UP

- Recheck complete blood cell count to observe for response to iron replacement by return of hematocrit to halfway toward normal within 3 weeks and fully to baseline after 2 months
- Iron supplementation during pregnancy and lactation: included in prenatal vitamins

EVIDENCE

PRACTICE GUIDELINES

- Goddard AF et al. Guidelines for the management of iron deficiency anaemia. British Society of Gastroenterology. Gut. 2000;46(Suppl 3–4):IV1. [PMID: 10862605]
- CDC Recommendations to Prevent and Control Iron Deficiency in the United States. MMWR Recomm Rep 1998;47:1

WEB SITES

- National Heart, Lung, and Blood Institute
- NIH Office of Dietary Supplements: Iron Fact Sheet

INFORMATION FOR PATIENTS

- American Academy of Family Physicians: Anemia: When Low Iron Is the Cause
- National Women's Health Information Center: Anemia
- Mayo Clinic: Iron Deficiency Anemia

REFERENCES

- Capurso G et al. Can patient characteristics predict the outcome of endoscopic evaluation of iron deficiency anemia: a multiple logistic regression analysis.

Gastrointest Endosc. 2004 Jun; 59(7):766–71. [PMID: 15173787]

- Cook JD et al. The quantitative assessment of body iron. Blood. 2003 May 1; 101(9):3359–64. [PMID: 12521995]
- Eichbaum Q et al. Is iron gluconate really safer than iron dextran? Blood. 2003 May 1;101(9):3756–7. [PMID: 12707229]
- Makrides M et al. Efficacy and tolerability of low-dose iron supplements during pregnancy: a randomized controlled trial. Am J Clin Nutr. 2003 Jul; 78(1):145–53. [PMID: 12816784]
- Yates JM et al. Iron deficiency anaemia in general practice: clinical outcomes over three years and factors influencing diagnostic investigations. Postgrad Med J. 2004 Jul;80(945):405–10. [PMID: 15254305]

- Peripheral blood smear characteristically shows dimorphic population of RBCs: 1 normal and 1 hypochromic
- Coarse basophilic stippling of RBCs and serum lead level elevated in lead poisoning
- Bone marrow iron stain shows generalized increase in iron stores and ringed sideroblasts (RBCs with iron deposits encircling the nucleus) and marked erythroid hyperplasia (resulting from ineffective erythropoiesis)
- Serum iron and transferrin saturation high

TREATMENT

- Occasionally, transfusion required for severe anemia
- Erythropoietin therapy not usually effective

Anemia, Sideroblastic

KEY FEATURES

- Heterogeneous group of disorders in which reduced hemoglobin synthesis occurs because of failure to incorporate heme into protoporphyrin to form hemoglobin
- Iron accumulates, particularly in mitochondria
- Sometimes represents stage in evolution of a generalized bone marrow disorder (myelodysplasia)
- Other causes include chronic alcoholism and lead poisoning

CLINICAL FINDINGS

- Symptoms of anemia; no other specific clinical features

DIAGNOSIS

- Anemia usually moderate, hematocrit 20–30%
- Mean corpuscular volume usually normal or slightly increased, but occasionally low, leading to confusion with iron deficiency

Aneurysm, Intracranial

KEY FEATURES

ESSENTIALS OF DIAGNOSIS

- Subarachnoid hemorrhage or focal deficit
- "Warning leak" may precede the major hemorrhage
- Abnormal imaging studies

GENERAL CONSIDERATIONS

- Most aneurysms are located
  - On the anterior part of the circle of Willis, particularly on the anterior or posterior communicating arteries
  - At the bifurcation of the middle cerebral artery
  - At the bifurcation of the internal carotid artery
- Saccular aneurysms ("berry" aneurysms)
  - Occur at arterial bifurcations
  - Are more common in adults than in children
  - Are frequently multiple (20% of cases)
  - Are usually asymptomatic
  - May be associated with polycystic kidney disease and coarctation of the aorta

DEMOGRAPHICS

- Risk factors for aneurysm formation include smoking, hypertension, and hypercholesterolemia

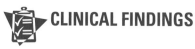

SYMPTOMS AND SIGNS

- May cause a focal neurologic deficit by compressing adjacent structures
- Most are asymptomatic or produce only nonspecific symptoms until they rupture, causing a subarachnoid hemorrhage
- "Warning leaks" of a small amount of blood from the aneurysm sometimes precede the major hemorrhage by a few hours or days, leading to headaches, nausea, and neck stiffness
- Focal neurologic signs may be absent in subarachnoid hemorrhage and secondary to a focal hematoma or ischemia in the territory of the vessel with the ruptured aneurysm
- Focal arterial spasm in the area of the ruptured aneurysm may occur after 1–14 days, causing hemiplegia or other focal deficits
- Cause of vasospasm is unknown and likely multifactorial
- Vasospasm may lead to significant cerebral ischemia or infarction and increase in intracranial pressure
- Subacute hydrocephalus due to interference with the flow of cerebrospinal fluid may occur after 2 or more weeks; leads to delayed clinical deterioration and is relieved by shunting

DIFFERENTIAL DIAGNOSIS

- Meningitis or meningoencephalitis
- Ischemic stroke
- Space-occupying lesion, eg, brain tumor
- Subdural hemorrhage
- Epidural hemorrhage
- Migraine

DIAGNOSIS

LABORATORY TESTS

- Cerebrospinal fluid is bloodstained if subarachnoid hemorrhage has occurred
- ECG evidence of arrhythmias or myocardial ischemia may occur and probably relates to excessive sympathetic activity
- Peripheral leukocytosis and transient glycosuria also common

IMAGING STUDIES

- CT scan generally confirms that sub-arachnoid hemorrhage has occurred but may be normal
- Angiography (bilateral carotid and vertebral studies) indicates the size and site of the lesion, sometimes reveals multiple aneurysms, and may show arterial spasm
- If subarachnoid hemorrhage is confirmed by lumbar puncture or CT scanning but arteriogram is normal, then the examination should be repeated after 2 weeks because vasospasm may prevent detection of an aneurysm during the initial study

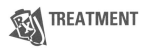 TREATMENT

MEDICATIONS

- Phenytoin to prevent seizures
- Calcium channel blockers reduce or reverse experimental vasospasm, and nimodipine reduces ischemic deficits from arterial spasm without any side effects (60 mg q4h for 21 days)

SURGERY

- Definitive treatment requires surgery and clipping of the aneurysm base, or endovascular treatment by interventional radiology

THERAPEUTIC PROCEDURES

- Major aim is to prevent further hemorrhages
- Conscious patients are
  - Confined to bed
  - Advised against exertion or straining
  - Treated symptomatically for headache and anxiety
  - Given laxatives or stool softeners
- If severe hypertension, lower blood pressure gradually but not below a diastolic level of 90 mm Hg
- Medical management as outlined for subarachnoid hemorrhage is continued for about 6 weeks and followed by gradual mobilization

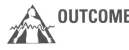 OUTCOME

FOLLOW-UP

- After surgical obliteration of aneurysms, symptomatic vasospasm may be treated by
  - Intravascular volume expansion
  - Induced hypertension
  - Transluminal balloon angioplasty of involved intracranial vessels

PROGNOSIS

- Unruptured aneurysms that are symptomatic merit prompt treatment
- However, small asymptomatic aneurysms discovered incidentally are often monitored arteriographically and corrected surgically only if > 10 mm
- Greatest risk of further hemorrhage is within a few days of initial bleed; thus, early obliteration (within 2 days) is preferred
- Approximately 20% of patients will have further bleeding within 2 weeks and 40% within 6 months

WHEN TO ADMIT

- All patients need admission and referral to specialized care

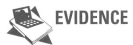 EVIDENCE

PRACTICE GUIDELINES

- American Society of Interventional and Therapeutic Neuroradiology. Aneurysm endovascular therapy. AJNR Am J Neuroradiol. 2001;22(8 Suppl):S4. [PMID: 11686074]
- National Guideline Clearinghouse

WEB SITES

- 3-D Visualization of brain aneurysms
- CNS Pathology Index

INFORMATION FOR PATIENTS

- National Institute of Neurological Disorders and Stroke
- UCSF Neurocritical Care and Stroke Patient Information

REFERENCES

- Doerfler A et al. Endovascular treatment of cerebrovascular disease. Curr Opin Neurol. 2004 Aug;17(4):481–7. [PMID: 15247546]
- Molyneux AJ et al. International Subarachnoid Aneurysm Trial (ISAT) of neurosurgical clipping versus endovascular coiling in 2143 patients with ruptured intracranial aneurysms: a randomised comparison of effects on survival, dependency, seizures, rebleeding, subgroups, and aneurysm occlusion. Lancet. 2005 Sep 3–9;366(9488):809–17. [PMID: 16139655]
- Nieuwkamp DJ et al. Subarachnoid haemorrhage in patients ≥ 75 years: clinical course, treatment and outcome. J Neurol Neurosurg Psychiatry. 2006 Aug;77(8):933-7. [PMID: 16638789]

- Pouratian N et al. Endovascular management of unruptured intracranial aneurysms. J Neurol Neurosurg Psychiatry. 2006 May;77(5):572–8. [PMID: 16614015]

Angiitis of the CNS, Primary

 KEY FEATURES

- Small and medium-sized vasculitis limited to the brain and spinal cord

 CLINICAL FINDINGS

- Biopsy-proved cases have predominated in men who present with a history of weeks to months of headaches, encephalopathy, and multifocal strokes
- Systemic symptoms and signs are absent

 DIAGNOSIS

- MRI of the brain is almost always abnormal
- Spinal fluid often reveals a mild lymphocytosis and a modest increase in protein level
- Angiograms classically reveal a "string of beads" pattern produced by alternating segments of arterial narrowing and dilation
- However, neither MRI nor angiogram appearance is specific for vasculitis
- Definitive diagnosis requires
  - A compatible clinical picture
  - Exclusion of infection, neoplasm, or metabolic disorder or drug exposure (eg, cocaine) that can mimic primary angiitis of the CNS
  - A positive brain biopsy
- Many patients who fit the clinical profile of stroke, headache, but no encephalopathy may have reversible cerebral vasoconstriction rather than true vasculitis
- Routine laboratory tests are usually normal

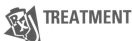 TREATMENT

- Usually improve with prednisone therapy
- May require cyclophosphamide

- Reversible cerebral vasoconstriction may be best treated with calcium channel blockers (eg, nimodipine or verapamil) and possibly a short course of corticosteroids

Angina Pectoris

 KEY FEATURES

ESSENTIALS OF DIAGNOSIS

- Precordial chest pain, usually precipitated by stress or exertion, and rapidly relieved by resting or nitrates
- Pain
  - Usually pressure-like and not sharp
  - Radiation common, especially to jaws, neck, or arm
  - May be associated with systemic symptoms, such as nausea, diaphoresis, dyspnea, palpitations
- ECG, echocardiographic, or scintigraphic evidence of ischemia during pain or stress testing
- Angiographic evidence of significant obstruction of major coronary arteries

GENERAL CONSIDERATIONS

- Usually due to atherosclerotic coronary artery disease
- Less common causes
  - Coronary vasospasm
  - Congenital anomalies
  - Emboli
  - Arteritis
  - Dissection
  - Severe ventricular hypertrophy
  - Severe aortic stenosis or regurgitation
- Commonly exacerbated by increased metabolic demands (eg, hyperthyroidism, anemia, tachycardias)
- Coronary vasospasm may occur spontaneously, or by exposure to cold, emotional stress, vasoconstricting medications, or cocaine

DEMOGRAPHICS

- Underdiagnosed in postmenopausal women

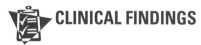 **CLINICAL FINDINGS**

SYMPTOMS AND SIGNS

- Diagnosis depends primarily on the history

- Angina most commonly arises during activity and is relieved by rest
- Patient often prefers to remain upright rather than lie down
- Rather than "pain," patient may describe tightness, squeezing, burning, pressure, choking, aching
- Discomfort behind or slightly to the left of the mid-sternum (in 80–90%)
- May radiate to
  - Left shoulder and upper arm
  - Medial aspect of arm, elbow, forearm, wrist, and fourth and fifth fingers
  - Lower jaw
  - Nape of neck
  - Interscapular area
- Diagnosis strongly supported if sublingual nitroglycerin aborts or attenuates length of attack
- Physical examination during an attack often reveals a significant elevation in systolic and diastolic blood pressure
- Hypotension is a more ominous sign
- An S_3 or arrhythmia may occur (bradycardia more common with involvement of the right coronary artery)

DIFFERENTIAL DIAGNOSIS

- **Cardiovascular**
  - Myocardial infarction (MI)
  - Pericarditis
  - Aortic stenosis
  - Aortic dissection
  - Cardiomyopathy
  - Myocarditis
  - Mitral valve prolapse
  - Pulmonary hypertension
  - Hypertrophic cardiomyopathy
  - Carditis in acute rheumatic fever
  - Aortic insufficiency
  - Right ventricular hypertrophy
- **Pulmonary**
  - Pneumonia
  - Pleuritis
  - Bronchitis
  - Pneumothorax
  - Tumor
  - Mediastinitis
- **Gastrointestinal**
  - Esophageal rupture
  - Gastroesophageal reflux disease
  - Esophageal spasm
  - Mallory-Weiss tear
  - Peptic ulcer disease
  - Biliary disease
  - Pancreatitis
  - Functional gastrointestinal pain
- **Musculoskeletal**
  - Cervical or thoracic disk disease or arthritis
  - Shoulder arthritis

  - Costochondritis or Tietze's syndrome
  - Subacromial bursitis
- **Other**
  - Anxiety
  - Herpes zoster
  - Breast disorders
  - Chest wall tumors
  - Thoracic outlet syndrome

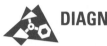 **DIAGNOSIS**

LABORATORY TESTS

- Obtain a fasting lipid profile
- Rule out diabetes mellitus and anemia
- Exercise testing (treadmill or bicycle) is the least expensive and most useful noninvasive procedure to
  - Confirm the diagnosis of angina
  - Determine the severity of limitation of activity
  - Assess prognosis
  - Evaluate responses to therapy

IMAGING STUDIES

- Indications for myocardial stress imaging (scintigraphy, echocardiography, MRI)
  - Patients are physically unable to exercise
  - ECG is difficult to interpret (eg, LBBB)
  - Results of exercise testing contradict the clinical impression
  - Need to localize the ischemia more precisely
  - Assess the completeness of revascularization
  - Prognostic indicator
- Scintigraphy can provide more information about the presence, location, and extent of coronary artery disease than exercise testing
- Scintigraphy is performed both at rest and during stress (exercise or pharmacologic stimulation)

DIAGNOSTIC PROCEDURES

- Obtain an ECG in all patients and, if possible, compare ECGs when pain is and is not present
- During anginal episodes as well as asymptomatic ischemia, the ECG may reveal horizontal or downsloping ST-segment depression, or T wave flattening or inversion that reverses after ischemia disappears or, less commonly, ST-segment elevation
- ECG is normal in ~25% of patients with angina
- Coronary arteriography is the definitive diagnostic procedure

- Arteriography has a mortality rate of ~0.1% and morbidity of ~1–5%, and it is expensive
- Left ventricular angiography performed at the same time assesses left ventricular function and mitral regurgitation

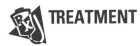 **TREATMENT**

MEDICATIONS

- Nitroglycerin, 0.3–0.6 mg sublingual or 0.4–0.8 mg by spray, with onset of symptoms or prophylactically 5 min before activity
- Long-acting nitrates (isosorbide dinitrate or mononitrate) for symptom management: avoid use for 8–10 h each day to avoid tolerance
- Nitrates relieve symptoms but do not benefit mortality
- β-Blockers reduce myocardial oxygen demand and benefit mortality
- Calcium channel blockers are generally not indicated except to treat coronary vasospasm
- Platelet inhibitors reduce the risk of coronary thromboembolism: aspirin (81–325 mg/day), or clopidogrel (75 mg/day) in aspirin-intolerant patients, benefits mortality
- Ranolazine, 500 mg PO BID, for chronic angina
  - Contraindicated in significant liver and renal disease
  - Can cause QT prolongation

SURGERY

- Revascularization (coronary bypass grafting or angioplasty) is indicated when
  - Symptoms are unacceptable despite maximal medical therapy
  - There is > 50% stenosis of the left main coronary artery with or without symptoms
  - Triple-vessel disease coexists with either an ejection fraction < 50% or a prior MI
  - Unstable angina is present
  - Angina or severe ischemia persists on noninvasive testing after MI
- Coronary bypass grafting is generally reserved for left main and triple-vessel disease

THERAPEUTIC PROCEDURES

- Angioplasty or stenting performed during angiography
  - The procedure of choice for single-vessel disease in the setting of refractory symptoms

  - Superior to medical therapy for symptom relief, but not in preventing infarction or death
  - A high rate (~40%) of restenosis may be reduced with newer stents

 OUTCOME

WHEN TO ADMIT

- Admit patients with unremitting or unstable angina (see Angina pectoris, unstable) for cardiac evaluation, to rule out MI, and to maximize therapy, including possible emergent revascularization

PREVENTION

- Smoking cessation
- β-Blockers, nitrates, and aspirin
- Vigorous treatment of hyperlipidemia (goal LDL < 100 mg/dL, HDL > 45 mg/dL)
- Tight control of diabetes mellitus
- Goal blood pressure (< 140/90 mm Hg)
- Avoiding aggravating factors: strenuous activity, cold temperatures, strong emotion

 EVIDENCE

PRACTICE GUIDELINES

- ACC/AHA 2002 guideline update for the management of patients with unstable angina and non-ST-segment elevation myocardial infarction. A report of the American College of Cardiology/American Heart Association Task Force on Practice Guidelines
- Snow V et al; American College of Physicians; American College of Cardiology Chronic Stable Angina Panel. Primary care management of chronic stable angina and asymptomatic suspected or known coronary artery disease: a clinical practice guideline from the American College of Physicians. Ann Intern Med. 2004;141:562. [PMID: 15466774]

WEB SITES

- American College of Cardiology
- National Heart, Lung, and Blood Institute

INFORMATION FOR PATIENTS

- American Academy of Family Physicians: Angina and Heart Disease
- American Heart Association: Angina Pectoris

- MedlinePlus: Angina Interactive Tutorial
- National Heart, Lung, and Blood Institute: Angina

REFERENCES

- Chaitman BR et al; Combination Assessment of Ranolazine In Stable Angina (CARISA) Investigators. Effects of ranolazine with atenolol, amlodipine, or diltiazem on exercise tolerance and angina frequency in patients with severe chronic angina: a randomized controlled trial. JAMA. 2004 Jan 21; 291(3):309–16. [PMID: 14734593]
- Paetsch I et al. Comparison of dobutamine stress magnetic resonance, adenosine stress magnetic resonance, and adenosine stress magnetic resonance perfusion. Circulation. 2004 Aug 17; 110(7):835–42. [PMID: 15289384]

Angina Pectoris, Unstable

 KEY FEATURES

- Accelerating or "crescendo" pattern of angina pectoris (see Angina Pectoris)
- Worse prognosis than stable angina because more likely to progress to myocardial infarction (MI)
- Unstable new-onset angina, if exertional and responsive to rest and medication, is not associated with poor prognosis

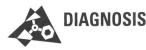 **CLINICAL FINDINGS**

- Angina occurs at rest or with less exertion than previously
- Lasts longer
- Is less responsive to medication

DIAGNOSIS

- Most patients with unstable angina manifest ECG changes during pain: ST-segment depression, T wave flattening or inversion
- ST-segment elevation is more ominous and has to be considered and treated as MI until proved otherwise

- Possible left ventricular dysfunction during pain and for a period afterward
- See Angina Pectoris for other symptoms and signs

 TREATMENT

- Hospitalization, bed rest, telemetry, and supplemental oxygen
- Rule out MI with three serial cardiac enzymes (troponin I or troponin T, and CK-MB) q6–8h and follow-up ECGs
- Cardiology consultation
- Benzodiazepine sedation if anxiety is present
- **Aspirin** (first-line therapy): 325 mg PO immediately and then once daily
- **Heparin** (first-line therapy): if symptoms onset within the past 24 hours, stuttering, or unremitting
- **Low-molecular-weight heparin**: eg, enoxaparin 1 mg/kg SQ q12h, slightly superior to IV heparin
- **Clopidogrel**: 300 mg PO loading dose, then 75 mg/day, sometimes added
- **Nitroglycerin** (first-line therapy): sublingual, oral, or topical initially, but continuous drip if pain persists or recurs
  - Start at 10 mcg/min, titrate up to 1 mcg/kg/min over 30–60 minutes, increasing to higher doses if needed
  - Continuous BP monitoring required
- **Opioids**, for unrelieved pain or pulmonary congestion
- **β-Blockers** (first-line therapy): PO or IV for more rapid effect
  - For example, metoprolol 5-mg IV doses × 3 at 5-min intervals, unless overt heart failure
  - Titrate up for goal heart rate of 60/min as tolerated by BP
- Reduce systolic BP to 100–120 mm Hg with nitroglycerin and β-blockers, except in patients with history of severe hypertension
- Early exercise or pharmacologic stress testing or coronary arteriography
- If continued pain despite above medications, fluctuating ST-segment depression, or positive cardiac enzymes, consider glycoprotein IIb/IIIa receptor blockers (eg, tirofiban, 0.4 mcg/kg/min for 30 min, then 0.1 mcg/kg/min) pending emergent arteriography
- Thrombolytics have no role in unstable angina without ST-segment elevation

Angiostrongyliasis Cantonensis

 KEY FEATURES

ESSENTIALS OF DIAGNOSIS

- Meningoencephalitis
- Transient cranial neuropathies

GENERAL CONSIDERATIONS

- Nematodes of rats of the genus *Angiostrongylus* cause two distinct syndromes in humans
  - *Angiostrongylus cantonensis,* the rat lungworm, causes eosinophilic meningoencephalitis
  - *Angiostrongylus costaricensis* causes gastrointestinal inflammation
- In both diseases, human infection follows ingestion of larvae within slugs or snails (and also crabs or prawns for *A cantonensis*) or on material contaminated by these organisms
- Since the parasites are not in their natural hosts, they cannot complete their life cycles, but they can cause disease after migrating to the brain or gastrointestinal tract
- In *A cantonensis* infection, disease is caused primarily by worm larvae migrating through the CNS and an inflammatory response to dying worms

DEMOGRAPHICS

- *A cantonensis* is seen primarily in southeast Asia and some Pacific islands

 CLINICAL FINDINGS

SYMPTOMS AND SIGNS

- After an incubation period of 1 day to 2 weeks, presenting symptoms and signs include
  - Headache
  - Stiff neck
  - Nausea, vomiting
  - Cranial nerve abnormalities
  - Paresthesias

DIFFERENTIAL DIAGNOSIS

- Tuberculous, coccidioidal, or aseptic meningitis
- Neurocysticercosis
- Neurosyphilis
- Lymphoma
- Paragonimiasis
- Echinococcosis
- Gnathostomiasis

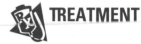 **DIAGNOSIS**

LABORATORY TESTS

- Diagnosis strongly suggested by finding eosinophilic CSF pleocytosis (leukocytosis with over 10% eosinophils) in a patients with a history of travel to endemic area
- Peripheral eosinophilia may not be present
- *A cantonensis* larvae have rarely been recovered from the CSF and the eyes

 TREATMENT

MEDICATIONS

- No specific treatment is available
- Antihelminthic therapy is probably not indicated, since responses to dying worms may worsen with therapy
- Corticosteroids have been used in severe cases

OUTCOME

COMPLICATIONS

- Parasite deaths may exacerbate CNS inflammatory lesions

PROGNOSIS

- Most cases resolve spontaneously after 2–8 weeks
- However, serious sequelae and death have been reported

WHEN TO ADMIT

- All patients

PREVENTION

- Controlling rat population
- Cooking snails, prawns, fish, and crabs for 3–5 min or by freezing them (–15°C for 24 h)
- Examining vegetables for mollusks before eating
- Washing contaminated vegetables to eliminate larvae contained in mollusk mucus is not always successful

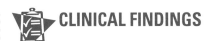 **CLINICAL FINDINGS**

SYMPTOMS AND SIGNS

- Gradual onset before age 40, with intermittent bouts of back pain that may radiate down the thighs
- Symptoms progress in a cephalad direction
- Motion becomes limited, with the normal lumbar curve flattened and the thoracic curvature exaggerated
- Chest expansion is often limited as a consequence of costovertebral joint involvement
- In advanced cases, the entire spine becomes fused, allowing no motion in any direction
- Transient acute arthritis of the peripheral joints occurs in about 50% of cases, and permanent changes—most commonly the hips, shoulders, and knees—are seen in about 25%
- Anterior uveitis in up to 25% of cases
- Constitutional symptoms similar to those of rheumatoid arthritis are absent in most patients

DIFFERENTIAL DIAGNOSIS

- Rheumatoid arthritis
  - Predominantly affects multiple, small, peripheral joints of the hands and feet
  - Usually spares the sacroiliac joints with little effect on the rest of the spine except for C1–C2
- Ankylosing hyperostosis (diffuse idiopathic skeletal hyperostosis [DISH], Forestier's disease)
  - Exuberant osteophyte formation
  - The osteophytes are thicker and more anterior than the syndesmophytes of ankylosing spondylitis
  - Sacroiliac joints are not affected
- Reactive arthritis (Reiter's syndrome)
- Psoriatic arthritis
- Inflammatory bowel disease
- Osteitis condensans ilii
- Hyperparathyroidism
- Whipple's disease
- Synovitis-acne-pustulosis-hyperostosis-osteitis (SAPHO) syndrome
- Sciatica
- Lumbar disk herniation, spinal stenosis, or facet joint degenerative arthritis

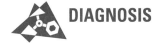 **DIAGNOSIS**

LABORATORY TESTS

- The erythrocyte sedimentation rate is elevated in 85% of cases
- Serologic tests for rheumatoid factor are characteristically negative
- HLA-B27 is found in 90% of white patients and 50% of black patients with ankylosing spondylitis
  - Because this antigen occurs in 8% of the healthy white population (and 2% of healthy blacks), it is not a specific diagnostic test

IMAGING STUDIES

- The earliest radiographic changes of sclerosis and erosion are usually in the sacroiliac joints (early on may be detectable only by MRI)
- Involvement of the apophysial joints of the spine, ossification of the annulus fibrosus, calcification of the anterior and lateral spinal ligaments, and squaring and generalized demineralization of the vertebral bodies may occur in more advanced stages
- "Bamboo spine" describes the late radiographic appearance of the spinal column

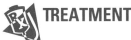 **TREATMENT**

MEDICATIONS

- Postural and breathing exercises
- Nonsteroidal anti-inflammatory drugs (NSAIDs)
- Sulfasalazine (1000 mg PO BID) is sometimes useful for the peripheral arthritis but has little symptomatic effect on spinal and sacroiliac joint disease
- Tumor necrosis factor inhibitors are highly effective in both the spinal and peripheral arthritis. Either etanercept (25 mg SQ twice a week) or infliximab (5 mg/kg every other month) is reasonable for patients whose symptoms are refractory to physical therapy and other interventions

SURGERY

- Total hip replacement benefits those with severe hip involvement

 OUTCOME

COMPLICATIONS

- Spondylitic heart disease, characterized chiefly by atrioventricular conduction defects and aortic insufficiency, occurs in 3–5% of patients with long-standing severe disease
- Pulmonary fibrosis of the upper lobes, with progression to cavitation and bronchiectasis mimicking tuberculosis, may occur

PROGNOSIS

- Almost all patients have persistent symptoms over decades
- The severity of disease varies greatly, with about 10% of patients having work disability after 10 years
- Absence of severe hip disease after the first 5 years is an excellent prognostic sign

WHEN TO REFER

- Refer to a rheumatologist when diagnosis is in doubt or when the patient fails to improve while taking NSAIDs
- Refer to an ophthalmologist for symptoms of uveitis
- Refer for hip replacement

PREVENTION

- Avoid cigarette smoking, since patients are already at risk for restrictive lung disease
- Use a small pillow at night to avoid accelerating flexion deformities of the spine

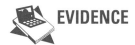 **EVIDENCE**

WEB SITES

- National Institutes of Health
- Spondylitis Association of America

INFORMATION FOR PATIENTS

- Ankylosing Spondylitis International Federation
- Arthritis Foundation
- Mayo Clinic

REFERENCES

- Baraliakos X et al. Magnetic resonance imaging examinations of the spine in patients with ankylosing spondylitis before and after therapy with the tumor necrosis factor alpha receptor fusion protein etanercept. Arthritis Rheum. 2005 Apr;52(4):1216–23. [PMID: 15818694]

- Braun J et al. Persistent clinical response to the anti-TNF-alpha antibody infliximab in patients with ankylosing spondylitis over 3 years. Rheumatology (Oxford). 2005 May;44(5):670–6. [PMID: 15757965]
- van der Heijde D et al. Infliximab improves productivity and reduces workday loss in patients with ankylosing spondylitis: results from a randomized, placebo-controlled trial. Arthritis Rheum. 2006 Aug 15;55(4):569–74. [PMID: 16874778]
- Wanders A et al. Nonsteroidal antiinflammatory drugs reduce radiographic progression in patients with ankylosing spondylitis: A randomized clinical trial. Arthritis Rheum. 2005 Jun; 52(6):1756–65. [PMID: 15934081]

Anorectal Infections

KEY FEATURES

- Proctitis
  - Inflammation of the distal 15 cm of rectum
  - Most cases are sexually transmitted, especially by anal-receptive intercourse
  - Causes include
    - *Neisseria gonorrhoeae*
    - *Treponema pallidum* (syphilis)
    - *Chlamydia trachomatis*, herpes simplex virus type 2 (HSV-2)
    - Human papillomavirus (HPV)
- Venereal warts (condylomata acuminata)
  - Caused by HPV
  - Occur in up to 50% of homosexual men
- Proctocolitis
  - Inflammation that extends above the rectum to the sigmoid colon or more proximally
  - Causes include
    - *Campylobacter*
    - *Entamoeba histolytica*
    - *Shigella*
    - Enteroinvasive *Escherichia coli*

CLINICAL FINDINGS

- Proctitis
  - Anorectal discomfort
  - Tenesmus
  - Constipation
  - Discharge
- Gonorrhea proctitis
  - Itching
  - Burning
  - Tenesmus
  - Mucopurulent discharge
- Complications of untreated gonorrheal infections
  - Strictures
  - Fissures
  - Fistulas
  - Perirectal abscesses
- Anal syphilis
  - Asymptomatic
  - Chancre
  - Proctitis
- In primary syphilis, chancre may mimic a fissure, fistula, or ulcer
- Secondary syphilis causes condylomata lata, foul-smelling mucus discharge, and inguinal lymphadenopathy
- *C trachomatis* causes proctitis similar to gonorrhea or lymphogranuloma venereum, proctocolitis with fever and bloody diarrhea, painful perianal ulcerations, anorectal strictures and fistulas, and inguinal lymphadenopathy (buboes)
- HSV-2 proctitis
  - Severe pain, itching, constipation, tenesmus, urinary retention, and radicular pain
  - Small vesicles or ulcers in the perianal area or anal canal
- Venereal warts are noted on examination of the perianal skin and within the anal canal; otherwise asymptomatic
- Higher rate of HPV progression to high-grade dysplasia or anal cancer in HIV-positive persons

DIAGNOSIS

- Gonorrhea proctitis
  - Blind swab of the anal canal has sensitivity of < 60%
  - Gram's stain and culture from the rectum during anoscopy, cultures from the urethra and pharynx in men, and cultures from the cervix in women
- Anal syphilis
  - Dark-field microscopy of scrapings from the chancre or condylomata
  - Serum VDRL positive in 75% of primary and 99% of secondary syphilis
- Culture of rectal discharge or rectal biopsy for *C trachomatis* has sensitivity of > 80%
- HSV-2
  - Sigmoidoscopy shows vesicular or ulcerative lesions in the distal rectum
  - Diagnosis by viral culture or HSV-2 antigen detection assays of vesicular fluid

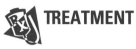 TREATMENT

- For *N gonorrhoeae*
  - Cefixime or cefpodoxime, 400 mg PO once
  - Ceftriaxone, 250 mg IM once
  - Ciprofloxacin, 500 mg PO once
- For *C trachomatis*
  - Doxycycline, 100 mg PO BID for 10 days
  - Ofloxacin, 300 mg PO BID for 21 days
- For *T pallidum*
  - Benzathine penicillin G, 2.4 million units IM once
  - Doxycycline, 100 mg PO BID for 2 weeks
- For HSV-2
  - Acyclovir, 400 mg PO TID for 7–10 days
  - Famciclovir, 250 mg PO TID for 7–10 days
  - Long-term acyclovir suppressive therapy for patients with AIDS and recurrent relapses
- For condylomata acuminata
  - Podophyllum resin applied topically for small perianal warts from HPV
  - CO_2 laser surgery or cryosurgery for anal lesions
  - Higher relapse rate after therapy in HIV-positive persons
- Examine and treat patient's sexual partners
- Surveillance anoscopy every 3–6 months in HIV-positive persons

Anorexia Nervosa

KEY FEATURES

ESSENTIALS OF DIAGNOSIS

- Disturbance of body image and intense fear of becoming fat
- Weight loss, leading to body weight 15% below expected
- In females, absence of three consecutive menstrual cycles

GENERAL CONSIDERATIONS

- Begins in the years between adolescence and young adulthood
- Cause not known, probably of primary psychiatric origin
- Medical or psychiatric illnesses that can account for anorexia and weight loss must be excluded

DEMOGRAPHICS

- Occurs most commonly in females (90%), predominantly middle and upper income
- Estimated prevalence
  - 270 cases per 100,000 population for females
  - 22 cases per 100,000 population for males

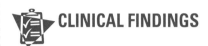 CLINICAL FINDINGS

SYMPTOMS AND SIGNS

- Loss of body fat with severe emaciation
- Dry and scaly skin
- Increased lanugo body hair
- Parotid enlargement and edema
- In severe cases, bradycardia, hypotension, and hypothermia
- Cold intolerance
- Constipation
- Amenorrhea

DIFFERENTIAL DIAGNOSIS

- Endocrine and metabolic disorders
  - Panhypopituitarism
  - Addison's disease
  - Hyperthyroidism
  - Diabetes mellitus
- Gastrointestinal disorders
  - Malabsorption
  - Pancreatic insufficiency
  - Crohn's disease
  - Celiac sprue
- Chronic infections, eg, tuberculosis
- Cancer, eg, lymphoma
- Rare CNS disorders such as hypothalamic tumors
- Severe malnutrition
- Depression
- Obsessive-compulsive disorder
- Body dysmorphic disorder
- Malignancy
- AIDS
- Substance abuse

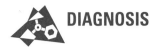 DIAGNOSIS

LABORATORY TESTS

- Check for anemia, leukopenia, electrolyte abnormalities, and elevations of blood urea nitrogen and serum creatinine
- Serum cholesterol level often increased
- Luteinizing hormone level depressed and impaired response to luteinizing hormone-releasing hormone

 TREATMENT

MEDICATIONS

- Tricyclic antidepressants, selective serotonin reuptake inhibitors, and lithium carbonate are effective in some cases

THERAPEUTIC PROCEDURES

- Treatment goal: restoration of normal body weight and resolution of psychological difficulties
- Supportive care
- Structured behavioral therapy
- Intensive psychotherapy
- Family therapy
- Hospitalization may be necessary
- Treatment by experienced teams successful in about two-thirds of cases

 OUTCOME

COMPLICATIONS

- Poor dentition
- Pharyngitis
- Esophagitis
- Aspiration
- Gastric dilatation
- Pancreatitis
- Constipation
- Hemorrhoids
- Dehydration
- Electrolyte abnormalities

PROGNOSIS

- 50% of patients continue to experience difficulties with eating behavior and psychiatric problems
- 2–6% of patients die of the complications of the disorder or from suicide

EVIDENCE

PRACTICE GUIDELINES

- American Dietetic Association
- Ebeling H et al. A practice guideline for treatment of eating disorders in children and adolescents. Ann Med. 2003; 35:488. [PMID: 14649331]
- Wilson GT et al. Eating disorders guidelines from NICE. Lancet. 2005 Jan 1–7;365(9453):79–81. [PMID: 15639682]

WEB SITE

- American Dietetic Association. Position of the American Dietetic Association: Nutrition intervention in the treatment of anorexia nervosa, bulimia nervosa, and eating disorder not otherwise specified (EDNOS).

INFORMATION FOR PATIENTS

- American Academy of Family Physicians
- MedlinePlus—Anorexia nervosa
- National Association of Anorexia Nervosa and Associated Disorders
- National Eating Disorders Association

REFERENCES

- Claudino A et al. Antidepressants for anorexia nervosa. Cochrane Database Syst Rev. 2006 Jan 25;(1):CD004365. [PMID: 16437485]
- McIntosh VV et al. Three psychotherapies for anorexia nervosa: a randomized, controlled trial. Am J Psychiatry. 2005 Apr;162(4):741–7. [PMID: 15800147]
- Pompili M et al. Suicide in anorexia nervosa: a meta-analysis. Int J Eat Disord. 2004 Jul;36(1):99–103. [PMID: 15185278]
- Taylor CB et al. Prevention of eating disorders in at-risk college-age women. Arch Gen Psychiatry. 2006 Aug; 63(8):881–8. [PMID: 16894064]
- Wadden TA et al. Dieting and the development of eating disorders in obese women: results of a randomized controlled trial. Am J Clin Nutr. 2004 Sep; 80(3):560–8. [PMID: 15321793]
- Walsh BT et al. Fluoxetine after weight restoration in anorexia nervosa: a randomized controlled trial. JAMA. 2006 Jun 14;295(22):2605–12. [PMID: 16772623]
- Yager J et al. Clinical practice. Anorexia nervosa. N Engl J Med. 2005 Oct 6; 353(14):1481–8. [PMID: 16207850]

Anthrax

KEY FEATURES

ESSENTIALS OF DIAGNOSIS

- Appropriate epidemiologic setting
  - Exposure to animals or animal hides
  - Exposure resulting from an act of bioterrorism
- Cutaneous anthrax
  - Black eschar on exposed areas of the skin
  - Marked surrounding edema and vesicles
  - Typically painless
- Inhalational anthrax
  - Nonspecific flu-like symptoms
  - Rapidly progresses to extreme dyspnea and shock
  - Chest radiograph shows mediastinal widening and pleural effusions

GENERAL CONSIDERATIONS

- Naturally occurring anthrax is a disease of sheep, cattle, horses, goats, and swine
- *Bacillus anthracis*
  - A gram-positive spore-forming aerobic rod
  - Spores—not vegetative bacteria—are the infectious form of the organism
- Transmitted to humans from contaminated animals, animal products, or soil by inoculation of broken skin or mucous membranes, by inhalation of aerosolized spores or, rarely, by ingestion, resulting in cutaneous, inhalational, or gastrointestinal forms of anthrax, respectively
- Spores entering the lungs are ingested by macrophages and carried via lymphatics to regional lymph nodes, where they germinate
  - The bacteria rapidly multiply within the lymphatics, causing a hemorrhagic lymphadenitis
  - Invasion of the bloodstream leads to overwhelming sepsis, killing the host

CLINICAL FINDINGS

SYMPTOMS AND SIGNS

Cutaneous anthrax

- Onset occurs within 2 weeks of exposure
- Initial lesion is erythematous papule, often on exposed area of skin, that vesiculates, ulcerates, and undergoes necrosis, ultimately progressing to a purple-to-black eschar
- Surrounding area is edematous and vesicular but not purulent
- Infection is usually self-limited

Inhalational anthrax

- Nonspecific viral-like symptoms
- Anterior chest pain is an early symptom of mediastinitis
- Within hours to days, patient progresses to fulminant stage of infection, in which symptoms and signs of overwhelming sepsis predominate
- Dissemination may occur, resulting in meningitis

Gastrointestinal anthrax

- Symptoms begin 2–5 days after ingestion of meat contaminated with anthrax spores
- Fever, diffuse abdominal pain, rebound abdominal tenderness, vomiting, constipation, and diarrhea occur
- Because the primary lesion is ulcerative, emesis is blood tinged or has coffee-ground appearance; stool may be blood tinged or melenic
- Bowel perforation can occur

DIFFERENTIAL DIAGNOSIS

Cutaneous anthrax

- Ecthyma gangrenosum (neutropenic, *Pseudomonas*)
- Tularemia
- Plague
- Brown recluse spider bite
- Aspergillosis or mucormycosis
- Antiphospholipid antibody syndrome
- Warfarin necrosis
- Rat-bite fever
- Rickettsialpox
- Orf (parapoxvirus infection)
- Cutaneous mycobacterial infection
- Cutaneous leishmaniasis

Inhalational anthrax

- Influenza
- Bacterial mediastinitis
- Fibrous mediastinitis from
  - Histoplasmosis
  - Coccidioidomycosis
  - Atypical or viral pneumonia
  - Silicosis
  - Sarcoidosis
- Other causes of mediastinal widening
  - Ruptured aortic aneurysm
  - Lymphoma
  - Superior vena cava syndrome
- Tuberculosis

Gastrointestinal anthrax

- Bowel obstruction
- Perforated viscus
- Peritonitis
- Gastroenteritis
- Peptic ulcer disease

DIAGNOSIS

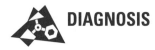

LABORATORY TESTS

- Pleural fluid in inhalational anthrax is hemorrhagic with few white blood cells
- Cerebrospinal fluid from meningitis cases is hemorrhagic
- Gram stain of fluid from a cutaneous lesion, pleural fluid, cerebrospinal fluid, unspun blood, or blood culture may show the characteristic boxcar-shaped encapsulated rods in chains
- The diagnosis is established by isolation of the organism from culture of the skin lesion (or fluid expressed from it), blood, or pleural fluid or cerebrospinal fluid (in cases of meningitis)
- In the absence of prior antimicrobial therapy, cultures are invariably positive

IMAGING STUDIES

- Chest radiograph is most sensitive test for inhalational disease, eg, being abnormal initially in every case of bioterrorism-associated inhalational anthrax
- Mediastinal widening from hemorrhagic lymphadenitis in 70% of the bioterrorism-related cases
- Pleural effusions were present initially or occurred over the course of illness in all cases, and approximately three-fourths had pulmonary infiltrates or signs of consolidation

TREATMENT

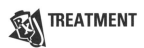

MEDICATIONS

- Ciprofloxacin is the drug of choice
- Other fluoroquinolones are probably as effective
- Doxycycline is an alternative first-line agent
- Ciprofloxacin is used in combination with other agents (Table 71) for inhalational anthrax, disseminated disease, cutaneous infections of the head, face or neck, or when associated with extensive local edema or signs of systemic infection
- *B anthracis*
  - May express β-lactamases that confer resistance to cephalosporins and penicillins

– For this reason, penicillin and amoxicillin are no longer recommended for use as single agents in the treatment of disseminated disease

OUTCOME

PROGNOSIS

- The prognosis for cutaneous infection is excellent; death is unlikely if the infection has remained localized and lesions heal without complications in most cases
- The reported mortality rate for gastrointestinal and inhalational infections is up to 85%

WHEN TO REFER

- Any suspected case of anthrax should be immediately reported to the Centers for Disease Control and Prevention so that a complete investigation can be conducted

PREVENTION

- Ciprofloxacin is considered the drug of choice (Table 71) for prophylaxis following exposure to anthrax spores
- There is an FDA-approved vaccine for persons at high risk for exposure to anthrax spores

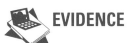

EVIDENCE

PRACTICE GUIDELINES

- National Guideline Clearinghouse

WEB SITES

- Centers for Disease Control and Prevention: Anthrax and Other Bioterrorism-Related Issues
- MedlinePlus: Anthrax

INFORMATION FOR PATIENTS

- Centers for Disease Control: Anthrax
- JAMA patient page. Anthrax. JAMA. 2001;286:2626. [PMID: 11763849]

REFERENCE

- Holty JE et al. Systematic review: A century of inhalational anthrax cases from 1900 to 2005. Ann Intern Med. 2006 Feb 21;144(4):270–80. [PMID: 16490913]

Antiarrhythmic Agent Overdose

KEY FEATURES

- Class Ia antiarrhythmic agents
  - Quinidine
  - Disopyramide
  - Procainamide
- Class Ic antiarrhythmic agent: flecainide

CLINICAL FINDINGS

- Arrhythmias
- Syncope
- Hypotension

DIAGNOSIS

- Blood levels of quinidine and procainamide (and active metabolite NAPA) are generally available from hospital laboratory
- ECG monitoring for QRS and QT interval prolongation
  - Widening of the QRS complex (> 100–120 ms)
  - With type Ia drugs, a lengthened QT interval and atypical or polymorphous ventricular tachycardia (torsades de pointes) may occur

TREATMENT

- Activated charcoal
  - Administer 60–100 g PO or via gastric tube, mixed in aqueous slurry for ingestions within 1 h
  - Do not use for comatose or convulsing patients unless they are endotracheally intubated
- Consider gastric lavage for recent (1 h) large ingestions
- Consider whole bowel irrigation for ingestion of sustained-release formulations
- Perform continuous cardiac monitoring
- Treat cardiotoxicity (hypotension, QRS interval widening) with IV boluses of sodium bicarbonate, 50–100 mEq
- Torsades de pointes ventricular tachycardia may be treated with IV magnesium or overdrive pacing

Anticoagulant Overdose

KEY FEATURES

ESSENTIALS OF DIAGNOSIS

- Prolonged prothrombin time (PT)

GENERAL CONSIDERATIONS

- Warfarin and related compounds (including ingredients of many commercial rodenticides) inhibit the clotting mechanism by blocking hepatic synthesis of vitamin K–dependent clotting factors
- Half-life of the "superwarfarins" used as rodenticides can be weeks or longer

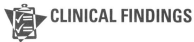

CLINICAL FINDINGS

SYMPTOMS AND SIGNS

- Initially asymptomatic, as evidence of anticoagulant affect usually delayed for 12–24 h
- Hemoptysis
- Gross hematuria
- Bloody stools
- Hemorrhages into organs
- Widespread bruising
- Bleeding into joint spaces

DIFFERENTIAL DIAGNOSIS

- Liver disease
- Hemophilia
- Aspirin overdose

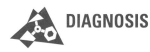

DIAGNOSIS

LABORATORY TESTS

- The PT is increased within 12–24 h (peak 36–48 h) after a single overdose
- After ingestion of brodifacoum and indanedione rodenticides (so-called superwarfarins), inhibition of clotting factor synthesis may persist for several weeks or even months after a single dose

DIAGNOSTIC PROCEDURES

- Obtain daily PT/INR for at least 2 days after ingestion to rule out excessive anticoagulation

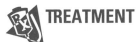 **TREATMENT**

MEDICATIONS

Emergency and supportive measures

- Discontinue the drug at the first sign of gross bleeding
- Determine the PT

Activated charcoal

- Administer activated charcoal, 60–100 g PO or via gastric tube, mixed in aqueous slurry if the patient has ingested an acute overdose

Specific treatment

- If the PT is elevated, give phytonadione (vitamin K_1), 10–25 mg PO, and additional doses as needed to restore the PT to normal
- Do not treat prophylactically—wait for the evidence of anticoagulation (elevated PT)
- Give fresh-frozen plasma or activated Factor VII, or both, as needed to rapidly correct the coagulation factor deficit if there is serious bleeding
- If the patient has been receiving anticoagulation therapy long-term for a medical indication (eg, prosthetic heart valve), give much smaller doses of vitamin K (1 mg) and fresh-frozen plasma (or both) to titrate to the desired PT
- If the patient has ingested brodifacoum or a related superwarfarin, prolonged observation (over weeks) and repeated administration of large doses of vitamin K may be required

 OUTCOME

FOLLOW-UP

- Serial evaluation of PT

COMPLICATIONS

- Bleeding

WHEN TO ADMIT

- All patients with a history of superwarfarin ingestion for 2-day observation of the PT
- All patients with active bleeding

PROGNOSIS

- Very good if no active bleeding and if close outpatient follow-up (and vitamin K treatment, if needed) is maintained (for several weeks or longer after brodifacoum overdose)

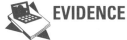 **EVIDENCE**

WEB SITES

- eMedicine: Toxicology Articles
- National Pesticide Information Center: Pesticide Poisonings

INFORMATION FOR PATIENTS

- National Institutes of Health: Anticoagulants (Systemic)

REFERENCES

- Dolin EK et al. A 44-year-old woman with hematemesis and cutaneous hemorrhages as a result of superwarfarin poisoning. J Am Osteopath Assoc. 2006 May;106(5):280–4. [PMID: 16717370]
- Watt BE et al. Anticoagulant rodenticides. Toxicol Rev. 2005;24(4):259–69. [PMID: 16499407]

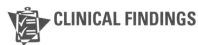
Anticonvulsant Overdose

 KEY FEATURES

ESSENTIALS OF DIAGNOSIS

- Drowsiness, somnolence with all
- Phenytoin: ataxia, slurred speech
- Carbamazepine: coma, seizures, dilated pupils, tachycardia
- Valproic acid: encephalopathy, hypernatremia, metabolic acidosis, hyperammonemia

GENERAL CONSIDERATIONS

- Rapid IV injection of phenytoin can cause acute myocardial depression and cardiac arrest owing to the solvent propylene glycol (does not occur with fosphenytoin injection)
- Phenytoin intoxication can occur with only slightly increased doses because of the small toxic-therapeutic window and zero-order kinetics

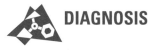 **CLINICAL FINDINGS**

SYMPTOMS AND SIGNS

Phenytoin

- In overdose, often only mild symptoms even with high serum levels

- Most common manifestations
  - Ataxia
  - Nystagmus
  - Drowsiness
- Occasionally, choreoathetoid movements

Carbamazepine

- Most common manifestations
  - Drowsiness, stupor
  - Coma and seizures (with high levels)
  - Dilated pupils
  - Tachycardia

Valproic acid

- Most common manifestations
  - Encephalopathy
  - Hyperammonemia
  - Metabolic acidosis
  - Hypernatremia (from the sodium component of the salt)
  - Hypocalcemia
  - Mild liver aminotransferase elevations
  - Cerebral edema
- Hypoglycemia, as a result of hepatic metabolic dysfunction
- Coma with small pupils, can mimic opioid poisoning

Tiagabine, lamotrigine, topiramate

- Drowsiness, lethargy with all
- Seizures with lamotrigine and tiagabine
- Widened QRS interval with lamotrigine

DIFFERENTIAL DIAGNOSIS

- Opioid intoxication
- Sedative-hypnotic overdose

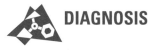 **DIAGNOSIS**

LABORATORY TESTS

- **Phenytoin** toxicity
  - Levels > 20 mg/L associated with ataxia, nystagmus, drowsiness
- **Carbamazepine** toxicity
  - May be seen with serum levels > 20 mg/L, though severe poisoning is usually associated with concentrations > 30–40 mg/L
  - Because of erratic and slow absorption, intoxication may progress over several hours to day
- **Valproic acid** toxicity
  - Obtain frequent repeated levels to rule out delayed absorption from sustained-release formulations (eg, Depakote, Depakote ER)

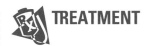

TREATMENT

MEDICATIONS

Activated charcoal

- Repeated doses of activated charcoal, 20–30 g q3–4h, are indicated for massive ingestions of valproic acid or carbamazepine
- Sorbitol or other cathartics should *not* be used with each dose, or resulting large stool volumes may lead to dehydration or hypernatremia

Whole-bowel irrigation

- Indicated for large ingestions of carbamazepine or valproic acid, especially of sustained-release formulations
- Administer the balanced polyethylene glycol-electrolyte solution (CoLyte, GoLYTELY) into the stomach via gastric tube at a rate of 1–2 L/h until the rectal effluent is clear

Specific treatment

- There are no specific antidotes
- Naloxone has been reported to reverse valproic acid overdose in a few anecdotal case reports

THERAPEUTIC PROCEDURES

- Consider hemodialysis for massive intoxication (eg, carbamazepine levels > 60 mg/L or valproic acid levels > 800 mg/L)

OUTCOME

WHEN TO ADMIT

- For phenytoin-induced ataxia if adequate home care is not available
- After symptomatic overdose of any anticonvulsant

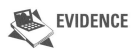

EVIDENCE

PRACTICE GUIDELINES

- Guidelines from the Royal Children's Hospital, Melbourne, Australia: Anticonvulsant Poisoning

WEB SITE

- eMedicine: Toxicology Articles

INFORMATION FOR PATIENTS

- Epilepsy Foundation: Special Concerns About Seizure Medications
- National Institutes of Health: Anticonvulsants: Hydantoin (Systemic)

- National Institutes of Health: Anticonvulsants: Succinimide (Systemic)
- National Institutes of Health: Anticonvulsants: Dione (Systemic)

REFERENCES

- Brahmi N et al. Influence of activated charcoal on the pharmacokinetics and the clinical features of carbamazepine poisoning. Am J Emerg Med. 2006 Jul; 24(4):440–3. [PMID: 16787802]
- Craig S. Phenytoin poisoning. Neurocrit Care. 2005;3(2):161–70. [PMID: 16174888]
- Spiller HA et al. Retrospective evaluation of tiagabine overdose. Clin Toxicol (Phila). 2005;43(7):855–9. [PMID: 16440513]

Antipsychotic Agent Overdose

KEY FEATURES

- Antipsychotic drugs
  - Phenothiazines (chlorpromazine, prochlorperazine, promethazine)
  - Butyrophenones (haloperidol, droperidol)
  - New "atypical" drugs (aripiprazole, olanzapine, quetiapine, ziprasidone)

CLINICAL FINDINGS

- Drowsiness, orthostatic hypotension, especially with α-blocking agents
- Large overdose
  - Miosis
  - Severe hypotension
  - Tachycardia
  - Convulsions
  - Obtundation or coma
- Prolongation of QRS interval (thioridazine) or QT interval (with possible torsades de pointes)
- An acute extrapyramidal dystonic reaction may occur with therapeutic or toxic doses
  - Spasmodic contractions of the face and neck muscles, extensor rigidity of the back muscles, carpopedal spasm, and motor restlessness

- More common with butyrophenones, less common with atypical drugs
- Severe rigidity, hyperthermia, and metabolic acidosis (neuroleptic malignant syndrome) may occasionally occur and are life-threatening

DIAGNOSIS

- Largely based on history of exposure
- Most agents are not detected in routine rapid toxicology screens
- Serum levels not helpful
- ECG monitoring for QRS, QT prolongation

TREATMENT

- Activated charcoal
  - Give 60–100 g (in aqueous slurry) PO or via gastric tube
  - Do not use for comatose or convulsing patients unless they are endotracheally intubated
- Consider gastric lavage for large recent ingestions
- Treat hypotension with fluids and pressor agents
- Widened QRS interval
  - Seen in thioridazine poisoning
  - May respond to IV NaHCO$_3$ as used for tricyclic antidepressants
- Prolonged QT interval or torsades de pointes, or both
  - Magnesium 1–2 g IV
  - Consider overdrive pacing
- Treat hyperthermia, maintain cardiac monitoring
- For extrapyramidal signs
  - Diphenhydramine, 0.5–1.0 mg/kg IV, or benztropine mesylate, 0.01–0.02 mg/kg IM
  - Continue with PO doses for 1–2 days

Anxiety & Dissociative Disorders

 KEY FEATURES

ESSENTIALS OF DIAGNOSIS

- Overt anxiety or an overt manifestation of a coping mechanism (eg, a phobia), or both
- Not limited to an adjustment disorder
- Somatic symptoms referable to the autonomic nervous system or to a specific organ system (eg, dyspnea, palpitations, paresthesias)
- Not a result of physical disorders, psychiatric conditions (eg, schizophrenia), or drug abuse

GENERAL CONSIDERATIONS

- Group of disorders
  - Generalized anxiety disorder (GAD)
  - Panic disorder
  - Obsessive-compulsive disorder (OCD)
  - Phobic disorder
  - Dissociative disorder
- GAD
  - Everyday activities trigger symptoms
  - Symptoms present on most days for at least 6 months
- Panic disorder
  - Symptoms occur in recurrent, short-lived episodes with unpredictable triggers
  - Somatic symptoms are often marked
- OCD
  - Patients experience recurrent intrusive thoughts or obsessions
  - They engage in compulsive actions or rituals to maintain control
- Phobic disorder
  - Symptoms occur predictably
  - Follows exposure to certain objects or situations
- Dissociative disorder
  - Reaction is precipitated by emotional crisis
  - Symptom produces anxiety reduction and a temporary solution of the crisis
  - Mechanisms include repression and isolation as well as particularly limited scope of attention, as seen in hypnotic states

DEMOGRAPHICS

- Incidence of OCD: 2–5%
- Prevalence of panic disorder: 3–5%, 25% with coincident OCD
- Age
  - Panic disorder: onset < 25 years
  - OCD: onset 20–35 years
- Risk factors for OCD: divorce or separation, unemployment

 CLINICAL FINDINGS

SYMPTOMS AND SIGNS

- Anxiety or fear
- Apprehension or worry
- Difficulty concentrating
- Insomnia and fatigue
- Irritability
- Feelings of impending doom
- Recurrent thoughts or fears
- Repetitive actions and rituals
- Avoidant behaviors
- Sympathomimetic symptoms
  - Tachycardia
  - Hyperventilation
  - Tremor
  - Sweating
- Somatic symptoms
  - Headache
  - Paresthesias
  - Dizziness
  - Nausea
  - Bloating
  - Chest pain
  - Palpitations
- Examples of dissociative states
  - Fugue (the sudden, unexpected travel away from one's home with inability to recall one's past)
  - Amnesia
  - Somnambulism
  - Dissociative identity disorder (multiple personality disorder)
  - Depersonalization

DIFFERENTIAL DIAGNOSIS

- Hyperthyroidism
- Pheochromocytoma
- Sympathomimetic drug use
- Myocardial infarction
- Hypoglycemia
- Adjustment disorders
- Dissociative symptoms are similar to symptoms of temporal lobe dysfunction

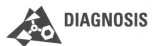 **DIAGNOSIS**

LABORATORY TESTS

- Thyroid-stimulating hormone
- Complete blood cell count
- Toxicology screen (if suspected)
- Glucose (as appropriate to rule out medical disorders)

IMAGING STUDIES

- Chest radiograph may be indicated
- Head CT may be useful in dissociative symptoms to rule out temporal lobe dysfunction

DIAGNOSTIC PROCEDURES

- ECG
- Electroencephalogram may be useful in dissociative symptoms to rule out temporal lobe dysfunction

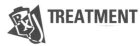 **TREATMENT**

MEDICATIONS

- See Table 145
- GAD
  - Benzodiazepines initially (diazepam 5–10 mg PO BID [or equivalent])
  - Buspirone (total dosage 15–60 mg PO divided TID)
  - Venlafaxine (start 37.5–75.0 mg PO once daily)
  - Possibly selective serotonin reuptake inhibitors (SSRIs), paroxetine
- Panic disorder
  - Lorazepam (0.5–2.0 mg PO) or alprazolam SL (0.5–1.0 mg) as acute treatment
  - SSRIs (eg, sertraline 25 mg PO once daily, titrate upward after 1 week) for ongoing treatment
- OCD
  - SSRIs, usually in doses higher than for depression (eg, fluoxetine, up to 60–80 mg PO once daily)
  - Clomipramine
  - In refractory cases, antipsychotics may be helpful as adjuncts to antidepressants
- Phobic disorder
  - SSRIs (paroxetine, sertraline, fluvoxamine)
  - Monoamine oxidase inhibitors
  - Gabapentin (900–3600 mg PO divided TID) for global social phobia
  - Propranolol 20–40 mg PO 1 hour before exposure for specific phobias (eg, performance)

SURGERY

- Stereotactic modified cingulotomy of limited use in severe, unremitting OCD

THERAPEUTIC PROCEDURES

- Behavioral/cognitive
  - Frequently used in conjunction with medical therapies
  - Relaxation techniques (particularly effective for physiologic symptoms in panic disorder)
  - Desensitization, via graded exposure to a phobic object
  - Emotive imagery (imagining anxiety-provoking situation while using relaxation techniques)
  - Cognitive therapy
- Social
  - Support groups
  - Family counseling
  - School, vocational counseling

 OUTCOME

FOLLOW-UP

- Every 1–2 weeks until stabilized, then as agreed upon with patient

COMPLICATIONS

- Alcohol and substance abuse

WHEN TO REFER

- Refer to a psychiatrist
  - If the diagnosis is in question
  - To receive recommendations on therapy
  - If first-line therapy has failed
  - If patient presents with management problems

PROGNOSIS

- Usually long-standing and difficult to treat
- All disorders relieved to varying degrees by medication and behavioral techniques (eg, 60% response rate to SSRIs for OCD)

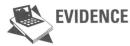 **EVIDENCE**

PRACTICE GUIDELINES

- Bandelow B et al. World Federation of Societies of Biological Psychiatry (WFSBP) guidelines for the pharmacological treatment of anxiety, obsessive-compulsive and posttraumatic stress dis-orders. World J Biol Psychiatry. 2002; 3:171. [PMID: 12516310]
- National Guideline Clearinghouse: Anxiety Disorders. Singapore Ministry of Health, 2003

WEB SITES

- American Psychiatric Association
- Anxiety Disorders Association of America
- Internet Mental Health

INFORMATION FOR PATIENTS

- American Psychiatric Association
- JAMA patient page. Obsessive-compulsive disorder. JAMA. 1998;280:1806. [PMID: 9842960]
- National Institute of Mental Health

REFERENCES

- Leopola U et al. Sertraline versus imipramine treatment of comorbid panic disorder and major depressive disorder. J Clin Psychiatry. 2003 Jun;64(6):654–62. [PMID: 12823079]
- Rickels K et al. Paroxetine treatment of generalized anxiety disorder: a double blind, placebo controlled study. Am J Psychiatry. 2003 Apr;160(4):749–56. [PMID: 12668365]

Aortic Dissection

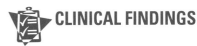 **KEY FEATURES**

ESSENTIALS OF DIAGNOSIS

- Sudden searing chest pain with radiation to back, abdomen, or neck in a hypertensive patient
- Widened mediastinum on chest radiograph
- Pulse discrepancy in the extremities
- Acute aortic regurgitation may develop

GENERAL CONSIDERATIONS

- Occurs when a spontaneous intimal tear develops and blood dissects into the media of the aorta
- Tear probably results from repetitive torque applied to ascending and proximal descending aorta during the cardiac cycle
- Blood entering the intimal tear may extend the dissection into the
  - Abdominal aorta
  - Lower extremities
  - Carotid arteries
  - Subclavian arteries (less commonly)
- Hypertension is important component
- Abnormalities of smooth muscle, elastic tissue, or collagen are more common in patients without hypertension
- Both absolute pressure levels and the pulse pressure are important in propagation of dissection
- **Type A dissection**
  - Involves the arch proximal to the left subclavian artery
  - Death may occur within hours, usually due to rupture of aorta into pericardial sac
  - Rupture into plural cavity also possible
  - Flap of aortic wall created by the dissection may occlude major vessels that branch off aorta, resulting in ischemia of brain, intestines, kidney, or lower extremities
- **Type B dissection** typically occurs in the proximal descending thoracic aorta just beyond the left subclavian artery
- Conditions associated with increased risk of dissection
  - Pregnancy
  - Bicuspid aortic valve
  - Coarctation

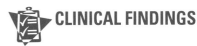 **CLINICAL FINDINGS**

SYMPTOMS AND SIGNS

- Sudden onset of severe persistent chest pain
  - Characteristically radiates down the back or possibly into the anterior chest
  - May also radiate into the neck
- Dissections may occur with minimal pain
- Hypertension
- Syncope
- Hemiplegia
- Paralysis of lower extremities
- Intestinal ischemia or renal insufficiency
- Peripheral pulses may be diminished or unequal
- A diastolic murmur may develop as a result of a dissection in the ascending aorta close to the aortic valve, causing valvular regurgitation, heart failure, and cardiac tamponade

DIFFERENTIAL DIAGNOSIS

- Myocardial infarction
- Pulmonary embolism
- Arterial embolism

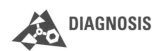

DIAGNOSIS

IMAGING STUDIES

- CT scanning
  - Immediate diagnostic imaging modality of choice
  - Should be obtained in any hypertensive patient with chest pain and equivocal findings on ECG
  - Should include both the chest and abdomen to fully delineate the extent of the dissected aorta
- MRI
  - Excellent imaging modality for chronic dissections
  - The longer imaging time and the difficulty of monitoring patients in the scanner make CT scanning preferable in acute situations
- Chest radiographs may reveal
  - An abnormal aortic contour
  - Widened superior mediastinum
- Transesophageal echocardiography
  - An excellent diagnostic imaging method
  - However, it is not readily available in the acute setting

DIAGNOSTIC PROCEDURES

- ECG findings
  - May be normal in some patients
  - Left ventricular hypertrophy from long-standing hypertension often present
  - Acute changes suggesting myocardial ischemia do not develop unless dissection involves the coronary artery ostium
  - Classically, inferior wall abnormalities predominate since dissection leads to compromise of the right rather than the left coronary artery

TREATMENT

- Aortic dissection is a true emergency; requires immediate control of blood pressure to limit extent
- Use aggressive measures to lower blood pressure when dissection is suspected, even before diagnostic studies have been completed
- Treatment requires a simultaneous reduction of the systolic blood pressure to 100–120 mm Hg and the pulsatile aortic flow

MEDICATIONS

- β-Blockers
  - Have the most desirable effect of reducing the left ventricular ejection force that continues to weaken the arterial wall
  - Should be used with antihypertensive regimen in long-term medical care of patients
- Labetalol
  - Both an α- and β-blocker
  - Lowers pulse pressure and achieves rapid blood pressure control
  - Give 20 mg over 2 minutes by IV injection
  - Additional doses of 40–80 mg IV can be given every 10 minutes (maximum dose 300 mg) until the desired blood pressure has been reached
  - Alternatively, 2 mg/min may be given by IV infusion, titrated to desired effect
- Esmolol
  - Has short half-life
  - Reasonable choice in patients who have asthma, bradycardia, or other conditions that require the patient's reaction to β-blockers be tested
  - Give loading dose of 0.5 mg/kg over 1 minute followed by an infusion of 0.0025–0.02 mg/kg/min
  - Titrate the infusion to a goal heart rate of 60–70 beats/min
- Nitroprusside may be added if β-blockade alone does not control the hypertension
  - 50 mg in 1000 mL of 5% dextrose water, infused at a rate of 0.5 mL/min
  - Infusion rate is increased by 0.5 mL every 5 minutes until adequate control of the pressure has been achieved
- Calcium-channel antagonists
  - No data supporting use in patients with bronchial asthma
  - However, diltiazem and verapamil are potential alternatives to β-blockers
- Morphine sulfate is appropriate for pain relief

SURGERY

- Type A aneurysms
  - Urgent intervention is required
  - Procedure involves grafting and replacing the diseased portion of the arch and brachiocephalic vessels as necessary
  - Replacement of the aortic valve may be required with reattachment of the coronary arteries
- Type B aneurysms
  - Urgent surgery is required if dissection is continuing or there is aortic branch compromise
  - Endovascular repair is treatment of choice, if anatomically feasible

OUTCOME

FOLLOW-UP

- Yearly CT scans are required to monitor the size of the dissecting aneurysm

PROGNOSIS

- Mortality rate for untreated type A dissections
  - Approximately 1% per hour for 72 hours
  - Over 90% at 3 months
- Untreated complicated type B dissections
  - Mortality rate is extremely high
  - Surgical and endovascular options are technically demanding and require an experienced team to achieve perioperative mortalities of < 10%
  - Patients whose blood pressure is controlled and who survive the acute episode without complications may have long-term survival without surgical treatment
  - Aneurysmal enlargement of the false lumen may develop in these patients despite adequate antihypertensive therapy

EVIDENCE

INFORMATION FOR PATIENTS

- American Heart Association: Aortic Dissection
- Mayo Clinic: Aortic Dissection
- MedlinePlus: Aortic Dissection

REFERENCES

- Bortone AS et al. Endovascular treatment of thoracic aortic disease: four years of experience. Circulation. 2004 Sep 14;110(11 Suppl 1):II262–7. [PMID: 15364873]
- Ince H et al. Diagnosis and management of patients with aortic dissection. Heart. 2007 Feb;93(2):266–70. [PMID: 17228080]
- Shiga T et al. Diagnostic accuracy of transesophageal echocardiography, helical computed tomography, and magnetic resonance imaging for suspected thoracic aortic dissection: systematic review and meta-analysis. Arch Intern Med. 2006 Jul 10;166(13):1350–6. [PMID: 16831999]

Aortic Regurgitation

 KEY FEATURES

- Rheumatic causes less common since advent of antibiotics
- Nonrheumatic causes predominate
  - Congenitally bicuspid valve
  - Infective endocarditis
  - Hypertension
  - Cystic medial necrosis
  - Marfan syndrome
  - Aortic dissection
  - Ankylosing spondylitis
  - Reiter's syndrome
- Rarely atherosclerotic in nature

 CLINICAL FINDINGS

- High-pitched, decrescendo diastolic murmur along the left sternal border; no change with respiration
- Hyperactive, enlarged left ventricle (LV)
- Wide pulse pressure with peripheral signs
  - Quincke's pulses: pulsatile nail beds
  - Duroziez's sign: to and fro bruit in femoral artery when systolic bruit created by compression with edge of stethoscope
  - Hill's sign: leg systolic pressure > 40 mm Hg higher than arm
- Usually slowly progressive and asymptomatic until middle age, although onset may sometimes be rapid, as in infective endocarditis or aortic dissection
- Exertional dyspnea and fatigue are the most frequent symptoms, but paroxysmal nocturnal dyspnea and pulmonary edema may also occur
- May present with left-sided failure; chest pain rare
- Need to operate before symptoms emerge

 DIAGNOSIS

- ECG: LV hypertrophy
- Chest radiograph: LV and often aortic dilation
- Doppler echocardiography
  - Confirms the diagnosis
  - Estimates severity
- Serial echocardiographic assessments of LV size and function are critical in determining the timing of valve replacement
- CT or MRI
  - Can estimate aortic root size
  - Can exclude ascending aneurysm
- Cardiac catheterization
  - Can help quantify severity
  - Can evaluate the coronary and aortic root anatomy preoperatively

 TREATMENT

- Surgery may be urgent in acute aortic regurgitation (usually due to endocarditis or dissection)
- Current recommendations advocate afterload reduction though data are derived from very few patients and its use remains controversial
  - Most providers prescribe ACE inhibitors
  - β-Blocker therapy may slow rate of aortic dilation in Marfan syndrome
- Surgery is indicated once aortic regurgitation causes symptoms
- Surgery is also indicated for those who have an ejection fraction < 55% or increasing end-systolic LV volume
- Surgery for asymptomatic ascending aneurysm indicated when maximal dimension > 55 mm (> 50 mm in patients with Marfan syndrome)
- Operative mortality is usually 3–5%

Aortic Stenosis

 KEY FEATURES

- In middle-aged persons: congenital bicuspid valve
- In the elderly: valvular degeneration caused by progressive valvular calcification (sclerosis precedes stenosis)
- Increasingly common with age; 1–3% over age 65 have aortic stenosis (AS)
- In developed countries, AS is most common valve lesion requiring surgery
- Much more frequent in men, smokers, and patients with hypercholesterolemia and hypertension
- Pathologically, calcific AS likely contributed to by same process as atherosclerosis

 CLINICAL FINDINGS

- Delayed and diminished carotid pulses; delay less common in the elderly
- If AS is severe, soft, absent, or paradoxically split S_2
- Harsh systolic murmur
  - Sometimes with thrill along left sternal border, often radiating to the neck
  - May be louder at apex in older patients and resemble mitral regurgitation (Gallavardin phenomenon)
- With bicuspid valve, usually asymptomatic until middle or old age
  - Always check for an associated coarctation of the aorta
  - Many persons have a dilated root due to intrinsic root disease (cystic medial necrosis)
- Left ventricular (LV) hypertrophy progresses over time
- Patients may present with LV failure, angina pectoris, or syncope, all with exertion
- Sudden death is rare without premonitory symptoms
- Syncope
  - Occurs with exertion as the LV pressures rises, stimulating the LV baroreceptors to cause peripherally vasodilation
  - This vasodilation results in need for increased stroke volume, which increases the LV systolic pressure again, creating a cycle of vasodilation and stimulation of the baroreceptors that eventually results in a drop in blood pressure, as the stenotic valve prevents further increase in stroke volume

 DIAGNOSIS

- ECG: usually shows LV hypertrophy
- Chest radiograph fluoroscopy: calcified valve and/or dilated aorta
- Doppler echocardiography
  - Usually diagnostic
  - Can estimate the aortic valve gradient
- Cardiac catheterization
  - Provides confirmatory data
  - Assesses hemodynamics
  - Excludes concomitant coronary artery disease
- Stenosis must be distinguished from supravalvular and outflow obstruction of the LV infundibulum

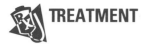 TREATMENT

- After onset of heart failure, angina, or syncope, the mortality rate without surgery is 50% within 3 yr
- Aortic valve replacement (in middle age or older) or Ross procedure (in younger age) is indicated for all symptomatic patients, and those with LV dysfunction or peak gradient > 64 mm Hg by echo/Doppler
- Coronary artery disease is present in over one-third
- Surgical mortality rate is low (2–5%) even in the elderly
- Balloon valvuloplasty is palliative in adolescents, but ineffective long-term in adults
- Type of prosthetic valve depends on patient age and risk of anticoagulation with warfarin
- Pericardial valves appear to last longer than porcine valves; neither require warfarin
- Mechanical valves have longest life, but require warfarin therapy

Aphthous Ulcer

KEY FEATURES

- Canker sore or ulcerative stomatitis
- Large or persistent areas of ulcerative stomatitis may be secondary to
  - Erythema multiforme or drug allergies
  - Acute herpes simplex
  - Pemphigus
  - Pemphigoid
  - Epidermolysis bullosa acquisita
  - Bullous lichen planus
  - Behçet's disease
  - Inflammatory bowel disease
- Cause remains uncertain, although an association with human herpesvirus 6 has been suggested

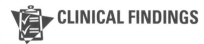 CLINICAL FINDINGS

- Very common and easy to recognize
- Found on nonkeratinized mucosa (eg, buccal and labial mucosa and not attached gingiva or palate)
- May be single or multiple, are usually recurrent, and appear as small (usually 1–2 mm but sometimes 1–2 cm), round

painful ulcerations with yellow-gray fibrinoid centers surrounded by red halos
- The painful stage lasts 7–10 days; healing is completed in 1–3 weeks

DIAGNOSIS

- Based on clinical appearance
- Squamous cell carcinoma may occasionally present in this fashion. When the diagnosis is not clear, incisional biopsy is indicated

TREATMENT

- Topical corticosteroids (triamcinolone acetonide, 0.1%, or fluocinonide ointment, 0.05%) in an adhesive base (Orabase-Plain) provide symptomatic relief
- Other topical therapies are diclofenac 3% in hyaluronan 2.5%, doxymycine-cyanoacrylate, mouthwashes containing the enzymes amyloglucosidase and glucose oxidase, and amlexanox 5% oral paste
- A 1-week tapering course of prednisone (40–60 mg PO daily) can be used
- For recurrent ulcers
  - Cimetidine maintenance therapy
  - Thalidomide has been used selectively in those who are also HIV-positive

Appendicitis

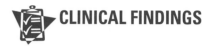 KEY FEATURES

ESSENTIALS OF DIAGNOSIS

- Early: periumbilical pain
- Later: right lower quadrant pain and tenderness
- Anorexia, nausea and vomiting, obstipation
- Tenderness or localized rigidity at McBurney's point
- Additional points for the compare
- Low-grade fever and leukocytosis

GENERAL CONSIDERATIONS

- The most common abdominal surgical emergency, affecting ~10% of the population
- Occurs most commonly between the ages of 10 and 30 years

- Caused by obstruction of the appendix by a fecalith, inflammation, foreign body, or neoplasm
- If untreated, gangrene and perforation develop within 36 hours

CLINICAL FINDINGS

SYMPTOMS AND SIGNS

- Vague, often colicky, periumbilical or epigastric pain
- Within 12 hours, pain shifts to right lower quadrant, with steady ache worsened by walking or coughing
- Nausea and one or two episodes of vomiting in almost all
- Constipation
- Low-grade fever (< 38°C)
- Localized tenderness with guarding in the right lower quadrant
- Rebound tenderness
- Psoas sign (pain on passive extension of the right hip)
- Obturator sign (pain with passive flexion and internal rotation of the right hip)
- Atypical presentations include
  - Pain less intense and poorly localized; tenderness minimal in the right flank
  - Pain in the lower abdomen, often on the left; urge to urinate or defecate
  - Abdominal tenderness absent, but tenderness on pelvic or rectal examination

DIFFERENTIAL DIAGNOSIS

- Gastroenteritis or colitis
- Gynecologic
  - Pelvic inflammatory disease
  - Tuboovarian abscess
  - Ovarian torsion
  - Ruptured ectopic pregnancy or ovarian cyst
  - Mittelschmerz
  - Endometriosis
- Urologic
  - Testicular torsion
  - Acute epididymitis
- Urinary calculus
- Pyelonephritis
- Diverticulitis
- Meckel's diverticulitis
- Carcinoid of the appendix
- Perforated colon cancer
- Crohn's ileitis
- Perforated peptic ulcer
- Cholecystitis
- Mesenteric adenitis

- Typhlitis (neutropenic colitis)
- Mesenteric ischemia

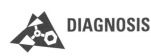

DIAGNOSIS

LABORATORY TESTS

- Moderate leukocytosis (10,000–20,000/mcL) with neutrophilia
- Microscopic hematuria and pyuria in 25%

IMAGING STUDIES

- No imaging necessary in typical appendicitis
  - Imaging may be useful in patients in whom the diagnosis is uncertain
  - Imaging studies (US or CT) suggest alternative diagnosis in up to 15%
- Abdominal or transvaginal ultrasound
  - Diagnostic accuracy of > 85%
  - Useful in the exclusion of adnexal disease in younger women
- Abdominal CT
  - Most accurate test for diagnosis (sensitivity and specific 95%)
  - Useful in suspected appendiceal perforation to diagnose a periappendiceal abscess

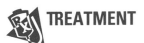

TREATMENT

MEDICATIONS

- Systemic antibiotics reduce the incidence of postoperative wound infections

SURGERY

- Surgical appendectomy by laparotomy or by laparoscopy in patients with uncomplicated appendicitis
- Emergency appendectomy in patients with perforated appendicitis with generalized peritonitis

THERAPEUTIC PROCEDURES

- Percutaneous CT-guided drainage of periappendiceal abscess, intravenous fluids and antibiotics, and interval appendectomy after 6 weeks in stable patients with perforated appendicitis

OUTCOME

COMPLICATIONS

- Perforation in 20%
- Periappendiceal abscess
- Suppurative peritonitis

- Septic thrombophlebitis (pylephlebitis) of the portal venous system

PROGNOSIS

- Mortality rate of uncomplicated appendicitis is extremely low
- Mortality rate of perforated appendicitis is 0.2%, but 15% in the elderly

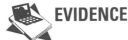

EVIDENCE

PRACTICE GUIDELINES

- National Guideline Clearinghouse

WEB SITE

- Gastrointestinal Pathology Index

INFORMATION FOR PATIENTS

- Mayo Clinic
- NDDIC–NIH

REFERENCE

- Dominguez EP et al. Diagnosis and management of diverticulitis and appendicitis. Gastroenterol Clin North Am. 2006 Jun;35(2):367–91. [PMID: 16880071]

Arbovirus Encephalitides

KEY FEATURES

- Caused by arthropod-borne viruses
- St. Louis and California encephalitides common in United States
- West Nile encephalitis identified in 1999; now present in much of United States
- Disease in United States tends to occur in outbreaks during periods of mosquito proliferation

CLINICAL FINDINGS

- Age-dependent; residual neurologic deficits more likely in the elderly
- Fevers, sore throat, stiff neck, nausea, vomiting, lethargy, coma

- Signs of meningeal irritation, tremors, cranial nerve palsies are common
- CSF
  - Elevated protein
  - Elevated opening pressure
  - Lymphocytosis
- West Nile virus infections show age-related neurologic manifestations
  - Headaches in the young
  - Poliomyelitis-like syndromes in middle age
  - Encephalitis in the elderly

DIAGNOSIS

- Clinical symptoms, with history of mosquito or other vector exposure
- Lymphocytopenia
- Polymerase chain reaction assays may be diagnostic
- West Nile: serum and CSF IgM ELISA confirm the diagnosis

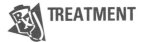

TREATMENT

- Vigorous supportive measures
- Prevention: mosquito control measures
- Ribavirin may be of some use in West Nile encephalitis

Arsenic Poisoning

KEY FEATURES

- Found in some pesticides and industrial chemicals

CLINICAL FINDINGS

- Symptoms usually appear within 1 h after ingestion but may be delayed as long as 12 h
- Abdominal pain, vomiting, watery diarrhea, and skeletal muscle cramps
- Profound dehydration and shock may occur
- In chronic poisoning, symptoms can be vague but often include those of peripheral sensory neuropathy

DIAGNOSIS

- Urinary arsenic levels may be falsely elevated after certain meals (eg, seafood) that contain large quantities of relatively nontoxic organic arsenic

 TREATMENT

Emergency measures

- Perform gastric lavage and administer 60–100 g of activated charcoal mixed in aqueous slurry

Antidote

- For symptomatic patients or those with massive overdose
  - Give dimercaprol injection (British Anti-Lewisite, BAL), 10% solution in oil, 3–5 mg/kg IM q4–6h for 2 days
  - Side effects include nausea, vomiting, headache, and hypertension
- Follow dimercaprol with oral penicillamine, 100 mg/kg/day in 4 divided doses (maximum, 2 g/day), or succimer (DMSA), 10 mg/kg q8h for 1 week
- Consult a medical toxicologist or regional poison control center for advice regarding chelation

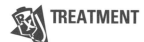
Arteriovenous Malformations, Intracranial

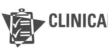 **KEY FEATURES**

ESSENTIALS OF DIAGNOSIS

- Sudden onset of subarachnoid or intracerebral hemorrhage
- Distinctive neurologic signs reflect the region of the brain involved
- Signs of meningeal irritation in patients presenting with subarachnoid hemorrhage
- Seizures or focal deficits may occur

GENERAL CONSIDERATIONS

- See Table 131
- Congenital vascular malformations
  - Result from a localized maldevelopment of part of the primitive vascular plexus

- Vary in size, ranging from massive lesions fed by multiple vessels to small lesions that are hard to identify at arteriography, surgery, or autopsy
- Symptoms may relate to hemorrhage or to cerebral ischemia due to diversion of blood by the anomalous arteriovenous shunt or venous stagnation
- Most cerebral arteriovenous malformations (AVMs) are **supratentorial** and in the middle cerebral artery territory
- **Infratentorial** lesions include brainstem or cerebellar AVMs
- Small AVMs are more likely to bleed than large ones
- AVM that have bled once are more likely to bleed again
- Bleeding is unrelated to sex or lesion site
- Hemorrhage is intracerebral and subarachnoid (with 10% of cases fatal)

DEMOGRAPHICS

- Up to 70% of AVMs bleed, most commonly before the age of 40
- Approximately 10% of cases are associated with arterial aneurysms, while 1–2% of patients with aneurysms have AVMs

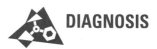 **CLINICAL FINDINGS**

SYMPTOMS AND SIGNS

Supratentorial lesions

- Initial symptoms
  - Hemorrhage in 30–60% of cases
  - Recurrent seizures in 20–40%
  - Headache in 5–25%
  - Miscellaneous complaints (including focal deficits) in 10–15%
- Focal or generalized seizures may accompany or follow hemorrhage or may be the initial presentation, especially with frontal or parietal AVMs
- Headaches, especially when the external carotid arteries are involved (sometimes simulate migraine but usually are nonspecific in character)
- In patients with subarachnoid hemorrhage, examination may reveal an abnormal mental status and signs of meningeal irritation
- Symptoms of increased intracranial pressure may be present
  - Headache
  - Visual obscurations
  - Obtundation
- A cranial bruit may be present but may also be found with
  - Aneurysms
  - Meningiomas

- Acquired arteriovenous fistulas
- AVMs involving the scalp, calvarium, or orbit
- Bruits are best heard over the ipsilateral eye or mastoid region and help in lateralization but not localization
- Absence of a bruit does not exclude an AVM

Infratentorial lesions

- Brainstem AVMs are often clinically silent but
  - May hemorrhage
  - Cause obstructive hydrocephalus
  - Lead to progressive or relapsing brainstem deficits
- Cerebellar AVMs
  - May also be clinically inconspicuous
  - Sometimes lead to cerebellar hemorrhage

DIFFERENTIAL DIAGNOSIS

- Aneurysmal hemorrhage
- Intracerebral hemorrhage from other causes
- Space-occupying lesion, eg, brain tumor

 DIAGNOSIS

IMAGING STUDIES

- CT scanning
  - Indicates whether subarachnoid or intracerebral bleeding has recently occurred
  - Helps localize source of bleeding
  - May reveal the AVM
- Arteriography
  - If the source of hemorrhage is not evident on the CT scan, arteriography is necessary to exclude aneurysm or AVM. MR angiography is not always sensitive enough for this purpose
  - Even if the findings on CT scan suggest AVM, bilateral arteriography of the internal and external carotid and vertebral arteries is required to establish the nature of the lesion
  - AVMs typically appear as a tangled vascular mass with distended tortuous afferent and efferent vessels, a rapid circulation time, and arteriovenous shunting
- MRI typically reveals the lesion but does not define its blood supply
- Plain radiographs of the skull are often normal unless an intracerebral hematoma is present, in which case there may be changes suggestive of raised intracranial pressure, such as displacement of a calcified pineal gland

DIAGNOSTIC PROCEDURES

- If the CT scan shows no evidence of bleeding but subarachnoid hemorrhage is diagnosed clinically, the cerebrospinal fluid should be examined
- Electroencephalography
  - Indicated in patients with seizures
  - May show consistently focal or lateralized abnormalities resulting from the underlying cerebral AVM

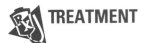 TREATMENT

MEDICATIONS

- In patients presenting solely with seizures, anticonvulsant drug treatment is usually sufficient, and surgery is unnecessary

SURGERY

- Surgical treatment is justified to prevent further hemorrhage when AVMs have bled, provided that the lesion is accessible and the patient has a reasonable life expectancy
- Surgical treatment is appropriate if intracranial pressure is increased and if a focal neurologic deficit to prevent further progression
- Definitive operative treatment consists of excision of the AVM if it is surgically accessible

THERAPEUTIC PROCEDURES

- Inoperable AVMs are sometimes treated solely by embolization; although the risk of hemorrhage is not reduced, neurologic deficits may be stabilized or even reversed by this procedure
- Other techniques
  - Injection of a vascular occlusive polymer through a flow-guided microcatheter
  - Permanent occlusion of feeding vessels by positioning detachable balloon catheters in the desired sites and then inflating them with quickly solidifying contrast material
- Stereotactic radiosurgery with the gamma knife is also useful in the management of inoperable cerebral AVMs

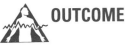 OUTCOME

FOLLOW-UP

- Serial MRIs help monitor malformations that are not treated surgically

COMPLICATIONS

- Communicating or obstructive hydrocephalus may occur and lead to symptoms

PROGNOSIS

- Depends on site of malformation and whether it has bled

WHEN TO REFER

- All patients

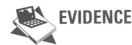 EVIDENCE

PRACTICE GUIDELINES

- American Society of Interventional and Therapeutic Neuroradiology. Embolization of spinal arteriovenous fistulae, spinal arteriovenous malformations, and tumors of the spinal axis. AJNR Am J Neuroradiol. 2001;22(8 Suppl):S28. [PMID: 11686072]
- Ogilvy CS et al. AHA Scientific Statement: recommendations for the management of intracranial arteriovenous malformations. Stroke. 2001;32:1458. [PMID: 11387517]

WEB SITE

- The Whole Brain Atlas

INFORMATION FOR PATIENTS

- Columbia University College of Physicians and Surgeons Cerebrovascular Center
- National Institute of Neurological Disorders and Stroke
- UCSF Neurocritical Care and Stroke Patient Information

REFERENCES

- Choi JH et al. Brain arteriovenous malformations in adults. Lancet Neurol. 2005 May;4(5):299–308. [PMID: 15847843]
- Hartmann A et al. Treatment of arteriovenous malformations of the brain. Curr Neurol Neurosci Rep. 2007 Jan; 7(1):28–34. [PMID: 17217851]

Arthritis & Inflammatory Bowel Diseases

 KEY FEATURES

- 20% of patients with inflammatory bowel disease have arthritis
- Second most common extraintestinal manifestation (after anemia)

 CLINICAL FINDINGS

- Two distinct forms of arthritis occur
  - Peripheral arthritis—usually a nondeforming asymmetric oligoarthritis of large joints—in which the activity of the joint disease parallels that of the bowel disease
  - Spondylitis that is indistinguishable by symptoms or radiograph from ankylosing spondylitis and follows a course independent of the bowel disease. About 50% of these patients are HLA-B27–positive
- About two-thirds of patients with Whipple's disease experience arthralgia or arthritis, most often an episodic, large-joint polyarthritis. The arthritis usually precedes gastrointestinal manifestations by years and resolves as the diarrhea develops

 DIAGNOSIS

- Clinical
- Differential diagnosis
  - Reactive arthritis (Reiter's syndrome)
  - Ankylosing spondylitis
  - Psoriatic arthritis
  - Whipple's disease

 TREATMENT

- Controlling the intestinal inflammation usually eliminates the peripheral arthritis
- Spondylitis often requires NSAIDs, which need to be used cautiously because they may activate the bowel disease in a few patients

Arthritis in Sarcoidosis

 KEY FEATURES

- May occur early (within 6 months of onset of symptoms) or late
- Often associated with erythema nodosum
- Rarely deforming

 CLINICAL FINDINGS

- **Early arthritis**
  - Usually begins in one or both ankles and can additively involve knees, wrists, and hands
  - Strongly associated with erythema nodosum and often produces more periarticular swelling than frank joint swelling
  - Axial skeleton spared
  - Commonly self-limited, resolving after several weeks or months and rarely resulting in chronic arthritis, joint destruction, or significant deformity
- **Late arthritis** is less severe and less widespread
- Dactylitis (sausage digit) may occur in association with overlying cutaneous sarcoidosis
- Often associated with erythema nodosum

 DIAGNOSIS

- Contingent on demonstration of other extra-articular manifestations of sarcoidosis and biopsy evidence of noncaseating granulomas
- In chronic arthritis, radiographs show typical changes in the bones of the extremities with intact cortex and cystic changes

 TREATMENT

- Usually symptomatic and supportive
- A short course of corticosteroids may be effective in severe and progressive joint disease
- Colchicine may be of value

Arthritis, Gonococcal

 KEY FEATURES

ESSENTIALS OF DIAGNOSIS

- Prodromal migratory polyarthralgias
- Tenosynovitis most common sign
- Purulent monarthritis in 50%
- Characteristic skin rash
- Most common in young women during menses or pregnancy
- Symptoms of urethritis frequently absent
- Dramatic response to antibiotics

GENERAL CONSIDERATIONS

- Usually occurs in otherwise healthy individuals
- Most common cause of infectious arthritis in large urban areas
- Recurrent disseminated gonococcal infection occurs when there is a congenital deficiency of terminal complement components, especially C7 and C8

DEMOGRAPHICS

- Two to three times more common in women than in men and is especially common during menses and pregnancy
- Gonococcal arthritis is also common in male homosexuals
- Rare after age 40

 CLINICAL FINDINGS

SYMPTOMS AND SIGNS

- One to 4 days of migratory polyarthralgias involving the wrist, knee, ankle, or elbow
- Thereafter, two patterns emerge
  - 60% of patients characterized by tenosynovitis (most often affecting wrists, fingers, ankles, or toes)
  - 40% of patients characterized by purulent monarthritis (most frequently involving the knee, wrist, ankle or elbow)
- Less than half of patients have fever
- Less than one-fourth have genitourinary symptoms
- Most patients will have asymptomatic but highly characteristic skin lesions: two to ten small necrotic pustules distributed over the extremities, especially the palms and soles

DIFFERENTIAL DIAGNOSIS

- Reactive arthritis (Reiter's syndrome)
  - Can produce acute monarthritis in a young person
  - However, it is distinguished by negative cultures, sacroiliitis, and failure to respond to antibiotics
- Lyme disease involving the knee
  - Less acute
  - Does not show positive cultures
  - May be preceded by known tick exposure and characteristic rash
- Infective endocarditis with septic arthritis
- Nongonococcal septic arthritis
- Gout or pseudogout
- Rheumatic fever
- Sarcoidosis
- Meningococcemia

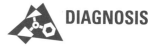 **DIAGNOSIS**

LABORATORY TESTS

- Synovial fluid
  - White blood cell count is typically over 50,000 cells/mcL
  - Gram stain is positive in one-fourth of cases and culture in less than half
- Positive blood cultures are seen in 40% of patients with tenosynovitis and virtually never in patients with suppurative arthritis
- Urethral, throat, and rectal cultures should be done in all patients, since they are often positive in the absence of local symptoms
- The peripheral blood leukocyte count averages 10,000 cells/mcL and is elevated in less than one-third of patients

IMAGING STUDIES

- Radiographs are usually normal or show only soft tissue swelling

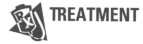 **TREATMENT**

MEDICATIONS

- Approximately 25% of patients have absolute or relative resistance to penicillin
- The recommended initial treatment is ceftriaxone, 1 g IV daily **or**
  - Cefotaxime, 1 g IV q8h **or**
  - Ceftizoxime, 1 g IV q8h **or**

– Ciprofloxacin, 400 mg IV q12h **or**
– Ofloxacin, 400 mg IV q12h **or**
– Levofloxacin, 250 mg/day IV
• Spectinomycin, 2 g IM q12h, can be given to patients with β-lactam allergy
• Once improvement from parenteral antibiotics has been achieved for 24–48 h, patients can be switched to an oral regimen to complete a 7- to 10-day course
– Oral cefixime, 400 mg BID
– Levofloxacin, 500 mg daily, or ciprofloxacin, 500 mg BID (in regions with low rates of quinolone resistance)

THERAPEUTIC PROCEDURES

• Generally responds dramatically in 24–48 h after initiation of antibiotics so that daily joint aspirations are rarely needed

 OUTCOME

PROGNOSIS

• Complete recovery is the rule

WHEN TO REFER

• When diagnosis is in doubt
• Report to the public health department for tracing contacts

WHEN TO ADMIT

• While outpatient treatment has been recommended in the past, the rapid rise in gonococci resistant to penicillin makes initial inpatient treatment advisable
• Patients in whom gonococcal arthritis is suspected should be admitted to the hospital to
– Confirm the diagnosis
– Exclude endocarditis
– Start treatment

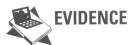 **EVIDENCE**

REFERENCE

• Rice PA. Gonococcal arthritis (disseminated gonococcal infection). Infect Dis Clin North Am. 2005 Dec;19(4):853–61. [PMID: 16297736]

Arthritis, Nongonococcal Acute Bacterial (Septic)

 KEY FEATURES

ESSENTIALS OF DIAGNOSIS

• Sudden onset of acute monarticular arthritis, most often in large weight-bearing joints and wrists
• Previous joint damage or injection drug use are common risk factors
• Infection with causative organisms commonly found elsewhere in body
• Joint effusions are usually large, with white blood cell counts commonly > 50,000/mcL

GENERAL CONSIDERATIONS

• A disease of an abnormal host
• Key risk factors are
– Persistent bacteremia (eg, injection drug use, endocarditis)
– Damaged joints (eg, rheumatoid arthritis)
– Compromised immunity (eg, diabetes, renal failure, alcoholism, cirrhosis, and immunosuppressive therapy)
– Loss of skin integrity (eg, psoriasis)
• *Staphylococcus aureus* is the most common cause of nongonococcal septic arthritis, accounting for about 50% of all cases
• Methicillin-resistant *S aureus* (MRSA) and group B streptococcus have become increasing frequent and important causes of septic arthritis
• Gram-negative septic arthritis is seen in injection drug users and in other immunocompromised patients
• *Staphylococcus epidermidis* is the usual organism in prosthetic joint arthritis

 CLINICAL FINDINGS

SYMPTOMS AND SIGNS

• Sudden onset, with pain, swelling, and heat of one joint—most frequently the knee
• Unusual sites, such as the sternoclavicular or sacroiliac joint, can be involved in injection drug users

• Chills and fever are common but are absent in up to 20% of patients
• Infection of the hip usually does not produce apparent swelling but results in groin pain greatly aggravated by walking
• Polyarticular septic arthritis is uncommon except in patients with rheumatoid arthritis or with group B streptococcal infections

DIFFERENTIAL DIAGNOSIS

• Gout and pseudogout are excluded by the failure to find crystals on synovial fluid analysis
• Acute rheumatic fever and rheumatoid arthritis commonly involve many joints
• Still's disease may mimic septic arthritis, but laboratory evidence of infection is absent

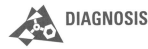 **DIAGNOSIS**

LABORATORY TESTS

• Blood cultures are positive in approximately 50% of patients
• The leukocyte count of the synovial fluid exceeds 50,000/mcL and often 100,000/mcL, with 90% or more polymorphonuclear cells
• Gram stain of the synovial fluid is positive in 75% of staphylococcal infections and in 50% of gram-negative infections

IMAGING STUDIES

• Radiographs are usually normal early in the disease, but evidence of demineralization may be present within days of onset
• MRI and CT are more sensitive in detecting fluid in joints that are not accessible to physical examination (eg, the hip)
• Bony erosions and narrowing of the joint space followed by osteomyelitis and periostitis may be seen within 2 weeks

DIAGNOSTIC PROCEDURES

• Joint aspiration is required to establish the diagnosis

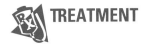 **TREATMENT**

MEDICATIONS

• Prompt systemic antibiotic therapy of any septic arthritis should be based on the best clinical judgment of the causative organism
• If the organism cannot be determined clinically, treatment should be started

with bactericidal antibiotics effective against staphylococci, streptococci, and gram-negative organisms
• Vancomycin should be used whenever MRSA is reasonably likely

SURGERY

• Immediate surgical drainage is reserved for septic arthritis of the hip, because that site is inaccessible to repeated aspiration
• For most other joints, surgical drainage is used only if medical therapy fails over 2–4 days to improve the fever and the synovial fluid volume, white blood cell count, and culture results

THERAPEUTIC PROCEDURES

• Rest, immobilization, and elevation are used at the onset of treatment. Early active motion exercises within the limits of tolerance will hasten recovery
• Frequent (even daily) local aspiration is indicated to complement antibiotic therapy when synovial fluid rapidly reaccumulates and causes symptoms

 OUTCOME

COMPLICATIONS

• Bony ankylosis and articular destruction occur if treatment is delayed or inadequate

PROGNOSIS

• With prompt antibiotic therapy and no serious underlying disease, functional recovery is usually good
• Five to 10% of patients with an infected joint die, chiefly from respiratory complications of sepsis
• The mortality rate is 30% for patients with polyarticular sepsis

WHEN TO REFER

• Refer to an orthopedist if the infected joint is not easy to aspirate repeatedly (eg, hip)

WHEN TO ADMIT

• Admit for presumed or confirmed septic arthritis

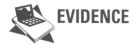 **EVIDENCE**

INFORMATION FOR PATIENTS

• American Association for Clinical Chemistry

REFERENCES

• Ross JJ et al. Septic arthritis. Infect Dis Clin North Am. 2005 Dec;19(4):799–817. [PMID: 16297733]
• Zimmerli W et al. Prosthetic-joint infections. N Engl J Med. 2004 Oct 14; 351(16):1645–54. [PMID: 15483283]

Arthritis, Reactive (Reiter's Syndrome)

 KEY FEATURES

ESSENTIALS OF DIAGNOSIS

• Oligoarthritis, conjunctivitis, urethritis, and mouth ulcers most common features
• Usually follows dysentery or a sexually transmitted infection
• Fifty to 80% of patients are HLA-B27 positive

GENERAL CONSIDERATIONS

• Reiter's syndrome (also called reactive arthritis) is a clinical tetrad
  – Urethritis
  – Conjunctivitis (or, less commonly, uveitis)
  – Mucocutaneous lesions
  – Aseptic arthritis
• Most cases develop within days or weeks after definite or implicated triggers
  – Dysentery: *Shigella, Salmonella, Yersinia, Campylobacter*
  – Sexually transmitted disease: *Chlamydia trachomatis, Ureaplasma urealyticum*, gonorrhea
  – Other: *Chlamydophila pneumoniae, Clostridium difficile*
• Gonococcal arthritis can initially mimic Reiter's syndrome, but the marked improvement after 24–48 h of antibiotic administration and the culture results distinguish the two disorders

DEMOGRAPHICS

• Most commonly in young men
• The gender ratio: 1:1 after enteric infections but 9:1 with male predominance after sexually transmitted infections
• Associated with HLA-B27 in 80% of white patients and 50–60% of blacks

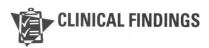 **CLINICAL FINDINGS**

SYMPTOMS AND SIGNS

• The arthritis is most commonly asymmetric and frequently involves the large weight-bearing joints (chiefly the knee and ankle)
• Sacroiliitis or ankylosing spondylitis is observed in at least 20% of patients
• Systemic symptoms including fever and weight loss are common at the onset of disease
• The mucocutaneous lesions may include circinate balanitis, stomatitis, and keratoderma blenorrhagicum, indistinguishable from pustular psoriasis
• Carditis and aortic regurgitation may occur

DIFFERENTIAL DIAGNOSIS

• Gonococcal arthritis
• Psoriatic arthritis
• Ankylosing spondylitis
• Rheumatoid arthritis
• Arthritis associated with inflammatory bowel disease

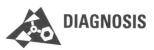 **DIAGNOSIS**

LABORATORY TESTS

• HLA B-27 test is useful in the diagnosis

IMAGING STUDIES

• Radiographic signs of permanent or progressive joint disease may be seen in the sacroiliac as well as the peripheral joints

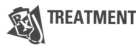 **TREATMENT**

MEDICATIONS

• Nonsteroidal anti-inflammatory drugs (NSAIDs) have been the mainstay of therapy
• Corticosteroids are typically not helpful
• Tetracycline (250 mg PO QID) given for 3 months to patients with Reiter's syndrome associated with *C trachomatis* reduces the duration of symptoms
• Patients who do not respond to NSAIDs and tetracycline may respond to sulfasalazine, 1000 mg PO BID
• Antitumor necrosing factor agents (etanercept, infliximab, adalimumab) may be helpful for patients with refractory disease

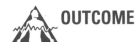

OUTCOME

PROGNOSIS

- While most signs of the disease disappear within days or weeks, the arthritis may persist for several months or even years
- Recurrences involving any combination of the clinical manifestations are common and are sometimes followed by permanent sequelae, especially in the joints

WHEN TO REFER

- Refer to a rheumatologist for progressive symptoms despite therapy

PREVENTION

- Antibiotics given at the time of a non-gonococcal sexually transmitted infection reduce the chance that Reiter's syndrome will develop

EVIDENCE

INFORMATION FOR PATIENTS

- American Academy of Family Physicians
- National Institute of Arthritis and Musculoskeletal and Skin Diseases

REFERENCE

- Putschy N et al. Comparing 10-day and 4-month doxycycline courses for treatment of *Chlamydia trachomatis*-reactive arthritis: a prospective, double-blind trial. Ann Rheum Dis. 2006 Nov; 65(11):1521–4. [PMID: 17038453]

Arthritis, Viral
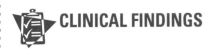

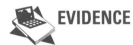

KEY FEATURES

- Arthritis may be a manifestation of many viral infections
- Generally mild and of short duration, terminating without lasting ill effects

CLINICAL FINDINGS

- **Mumps arthritis** may occur in the absence of parotitis

- **Rubella arthritis**
  - Occurs more commonly in adults than in children
  - May appear immediately before, during, or soon after the disappearance of the rash
  - Its usual polyarticular and symmetric distribution mimics that of rheumatoid arthritis
- **Human parvovirus B19:** In adults, polyarthritis may follow infection with the virus
- **Hepatitis B**
  - Transient polyarthritis may be associated with type B hepatitis
  - Typically occurs before the onset of jaundice; it may occur in anicteric hepatitis as well
- **Hepatitis C:** Infection may be associated with chronic polyarthralgia or polyarthritis that mimics rheumatoid arthritis

DIAGNOSIS

- Viral serologies

TREATMENT

- NSAIDs are the mainstay of treatment for most forms of viral arthritis
- Symptoms secondary to hepatitis C virus may respond to interferon-α if the virologic response is good

Asbestosis

KEY FEATURES

- A nodular interstitial fibrosis occurring in workers who are exposed to asbestos fibers long-term
- Cigarette smoking increases the prevalence of pleural and parenchymal changes and markedly increases the incidence of lung carcinoma

CLINICAL FINDINGS

- Inexorably progressive dyspnea, inspiratory crackles
- Clubbing and cyanosis present in some patients

- Lower lung zones involved more than upper lung zones
- Pulmonary function tests typically show a restrictive defect and reduced diffusing capacity

DIAGNOSIS

- Radiographic features
  - Interstitial fibrosis
  - Thickened pleura
  - Calcified pleural plaques on lateral chest walls and diaphragm
- High-resolution CT— the best imaging method

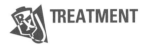

TREATMENT

- No specific treatment

Ascariasis

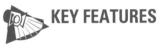

KEY FEATURES

ESSENTIALS OF DIAGNOSIS

- Transient cough, urticaria, pulmonary infiltrates
- Eosinophilia
- Nonspecific abdominal symptoms
- Eggs in stools; adult worms occasionally passed

GENERAL CONSIDERATIONS

- *Ascaris lumbricoides* is the most common intestinal helminth
- Infection follows ingestion of eggs in contaminated food
- Larvae hatch in the small intestine, penetrate into the bloodstream, migrate to lungs, and then back to the gastrointestinal tract where they develop into adult worms
- Adult worms can be up to 40 cm long and live for 1–2 years

DEMOGRAPHICS

- About one-quarter of the world's population is infected, with 12 million acute cases and 10,000 or more deaths annually
- Prevalence is high wherever there is poor hygiene and sanitation or where human feces are used as fertilizer

• Heavy infections are most common in children

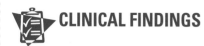

CLINICAL FINDINGS

SYMPTOMS AND SIGNS

• Most infected persons are asymptomatic
• The following symptoms develop in a small number of patients during migration of worms through the lungs
  – Fever
  – Nonproductive cough
  – Chest pain
  – Dyspnea
  – Eosinophilia
  – Eosinophilic pneumonia (occasionally)
• Rarely, larvae lodge ectopically in the brain, kidney, eye, spinal cord, and other sites and may cause local symptoms
• With heavy infection, abdominal discomfort may be seen
• Adult worms may migrate and be coughed up, vomited, or may emerge through the nose or anus
• They may also migrate into the common bile duct, pancreatic duct, appendix, and other sites, which may lead to
  – Cholangitis
  – Cholecystitis
  – Pyogenic liver abscess
  – Pancreatitis
  – Obstructive jaundice
  – Appendicitis
• With very heavy infestations, masses of worms may cause
  – Intestinal obstruction
  – Volvulus
  – Intussusception
  – Death
• Moderate to high worm loads in children are also associated with nutritional abnormalities

DIFFERENTIAL DIAGNOSIS

• Asthma
• Allergic bronchopulmonary aspergillosis (ABPA)
• Acute eosinophilic pneumonia (Löffler's syndrome)
• Paragonimiasis
• Tropical pulmonary eosinophilia (*Wuchereria bancrofti, Brugia malayi*)
• Hookworm disease
• Strongyloidiasis
• Toxocariasis (visceral larva migrans)
• Peptic ulcer disease
• Other causes of cholangitis, cholecystitis, pancreatitis, appendicitis, diverticulitis

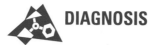

DIAGNOSIS

LABORATORY TESTS

• Diagnosis is made after adult worms emerge from the mouth, nose, or anus or by identifying characteristic eggs in the feces
• Due to the very high egg burden, concentration techniques are generally not needed
• Eosinophilia is marked during worm migration but may be absent during intestinal infection

IMAGING STUDIES

• Chest radiographs show pulmonary infiltrates
• Plain abdominal films and ultrasonography can demonstrate worms, with filling defects in contrast studies and at times evidence of intestinal or biliary obstruction

TREATMENT

MEDICATIONS

• All infections should be treated
• Treatments of choice
  – Albendazole (400 mg single dose)
  – Mebendazole (500 mg single dose or 100 mg BID for 3 days)
  – Pyrantel pamoate (11 mg/kg single dose, maximum 1 g)
• All three of these drugs are
  – Well tolerated but may cause mild gastrointestinal toxicity
  – Considered safe for children older than 1 year and in pregnancy, although use in the first trimester is best avoided
• Intestinal obstruction usually responds to conservative management and antihelminthic therapy

SURGERY

• May be required for appendicitis and other gastrointestinal complications

OUTCOME

FOLLOW-UP

• Stools should be rechecked at 2 weeks after treatment and patients retreated until all ascarids are removed
• Because anesthesia stimulates worms to hypermotility, they should be removed

in advance in infected patients undergoing elective surgery
• The complications caused by wandering adult worms require that all *Ascaris* infections be treated and eradicated

WHEN TO REFER

• If there is difficulty in making the diagnosis or progressive symptoms despite therapy

WHEN TO ADMIT

• Intestinal obstruction or biliary ascariasis

EVIDENCE

WEB SITE

• Centers for Disease Control and Prevention—Division of Parasitic Diseases

INFORMATION FOR PATIENTS

• Centers for Disease Control and Prevention—Division of Parasitic Diseases
• National Institute of Allergy and Infectious Disease
• Nemours Foundation

REFERENCES

• Asdamongkol N et al. Risk factors for strongyloidiasis hyperinfection and clinical outcomes. Southeast Asian J Trop Med Public Health. 2006 Sep; 37(5):875–84. [PMID: 17333728]
• Bethony J et al. Soil-transmitted helminth infections: ascariasis, trichuriasis, and hookworm. Lancet. 2006 May 6; 367(9521):1521–32. [PMID: 16679166]
• Burkhart CN et al. Assessment of frequency, transmission, and genitourinary complications of enterobiasis (pinworms). Int J Dermatol. 2005 Oct; 44(10):837–40. [PMID: 16207185]
• Hotez PJ et al. Hookworm infection. N Engl J Med. 2004 Aug 19;351(8):799–807. [PMID: 15317893]
• Lim S et al. Complicated and fatal *Strongyloides* infection in Canadians: risk factors, diagnosis and management. CMAJ. 2004 Aug 31;171(5):479–84. [PMID: 15337730]
• Petro M et al. Unusual endoscopic and microscopic view of *Enterobius vermicularis*: a case report with a review of the literature. South Med J. 2005 Sep; 98(9):927–9. [PMID: 16217987]

Ascites

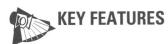 **KEY FEATURES**

ESSENTIALS OF DIAGNOSIS

- Pathologic accumulation of fluid in the peritoneal cavity

GENERAL CONSIDERATIONS

- Two broad categories of ascites
  - Associated with a normal peritoneum
  - Due to a diseased peritoneum (Table 38)
- Most common cause is portal hypertension secondary to chronic liver disease (> 80% of cases)
- Other causes
  - Infections (tuberculous peritonitis)
  - Intra-abdominal malignancy
  - Inflammatory disorders of the peritoneum
  - Ductal disruptions (chylous, pancreatic, biliary)
- Risk factors for ascites include causes of liver disease
  - Ethanol consumption
  - Transfusions
  - Tattoos
  - Injection drug use
  - History of viral hepatitis or jaundice
  - Birth in an area endemic for hepatitis
- History of cancer or marked weight loss suggests malignancy
- Fevers suggest infected peritoneal fluid, including bacterial peritonitis (spontaneous or secondary)

DEMOGRAPHICS

- Tuberculous peritonitis occurs in
  - Immigrants
  - HIV-infected
  - Urban poor, alcoholics
- Cirrhosis with portal hypertensive ascites most commonly caused by chronic alcoholism or chronic viral infection (hepatitis B or C)

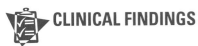 **CLINICAL FINDINGS**

SYMPTOMS AND SIGNS

- Increasing abdominal girth
- Abdominal pain
- In portal hypertension: large abdominal wall veins with cephalad flow; inferiorly directed flow implies hepatic vein obstruction
- In portal hypertension and chronic liver disease
  - Palmar erythema
  - Cutaneous spider angiomas
  - Gynecomastia
  - Asterixis
- In right-sided congestive heart failure or constrictive pericarditis: elevated jugular venous pressure
- In acute alcoholic hepatitis or Budd-Chiari syndrome: large tender liver
- In congestive heart failure or nephrotic syndrome: anasarca
- In malignancy: firm lymph nodes in the left supraclavicular region or umbilicus

DIFFERENTIAL DIAGNOSIS

- See Table 38
- Cirrhosis (80–85%)
- Malignancy (10%)
- Congestive heart failure (3%)
- Tuberculous peritonitis
- Dialysis-related
- Bile or pancreatic ascites
- Lymphatic tear (chylous ascites)
- Nephrotic syndrome

 DIAGNOSIS

LABORATORY TESTS

- Ascitic fluid cell count: normal cell count is < 500 leukocytes/mcL and < 250 polymorphonuclear neutrophils (PMNs)/mcL
- PMN count of > 250/mcL (neutrocytic ascites), with > 75% of all white blood cells (WBCs) being PMNs usually indicates bacterial peritonitis
- Ascitic fluid culture and Gram's stain in suspected peritonitis
- Elevated WBCs with a predominance of lymphocytes occur in tuberculosis or peritoneal carcinomatosis
- Cloudy ascitic fluid suggests infection
- Milky fluid occurs in chylous ascites
- Bloody fluid suggests traumatic paracentesis, malignant ascites
- Serum-ascites albumin gradient (SAAG) classifies ascites into portal hypertensive and nonportal hypertensive causes (Table 38)
- SAAG is calculated by subtracting the ascitic fluid albumin from the serum albumin
  - SAAG > 1.1 g/dL suggests underlying portal hypertension
  - SAAG < 1.1 g/dL implicates nonportal hypertensive causes

- ~4% of patients have "mixed ascites: portal hypertension" (SAAG > 1.1 g/dL) complicated by a second cause for ascites (such as malignancy or tuberculosis)
- SAAG > 1.1 g/dL with a high ascitic fluid total protein (> 2.5 g/dL) occurs in
  - Portal hypertension secondary to cardiac disease or Budd-Chiari syndrome
  - Up to 20% of cases of portal hypertension caused by uncomplicated cirrhosis
- Ascitic fluid amylase is elevated in pancreatic ascites or perforation of the gastrointestinal tract
- Ascitic fluid bilirubin concentration is greater than the serum bilirubin in perforation of the biliary tree
- Ascitic fluid creatinine is elevated in leakage of urine from the bladder or ureters

IMAGING STUDIES

- Ultrasound and CT imaging is useful in
  - Distinguishing between causes of portal and nonportal hypertensive ascites
  - Detecting thrombosis of the hepatic veins (Budd-Chiari syndrome) or portal veins
  - Detecting lymphadenopathy and masses
  - Directing percutaneous needle biopsies of abnormal lymph nodes or solid organic masses

DIAGNOSTIC PROCEDURES

- Physical examination is insensitive for detecting < 1500 mL of ascites fluid
- Abdominal paracentesis is indicated in
  - Patients with new-onset ascites to determine etiology (portal vs. non-portal hypertensive)
  - Patients admitted to the hospital with cirrhosis and ascites to diagnose bacterial peritonitis
  - Patients with known ascites who deteriorate clinically (fever, abdominal pain, rapid worsening of renal function, or worsened hepatic encephalopathy)
- When fluid volume is small or fluid is loculated, abdominal ultrasound confirms presence of ascites and facilitates paracentesis
- Cytologic examination is indicated if peritoneal carcinomatosis is suspected
- Laparoscopy permits direct visualization and biopsy of the peritoneum, liver, and some intra-abdominal lymph nodes in suspected peritoneal tuberculosis or malignancy

TREATMENT

MEDICATIONS

- Portal hypertensive ascites: diuretics such as spironolactone, 100 mg/day, and furosemide, 40 mg/day
- Dose increased every 5–7 days until diuresis achieved, to maximum of 400 mg/day of aldactone and 160 mg/day of furosemide
- Goal is to lose 0.5 kg/day
- Careful monitoring of serum sodium, potassium, and creatinine required

THERAPEUTIC PROCEDURES

- In ascites caused by portal hypertension, dietary sodium restriction to 1–2 g/day; fluid intake restriction if serum Na < 125 mEq/L
- Large-volume paracentesis (4–6 L) is indicated for patients with massive ascites or ascites refractory to diuretics
  - Intravenous albumin should be administered with large-volume paracentesis to reduce acute and long-term complications: 10 g albumin/L of ascites removed
- Transjugular intrahepatic portosystemic shunt (TIPS) effectively controls 75% of carefully selected patients with portal hypertension and refractory ascites

OUTCOME

COMPLICATIONS

- Portal hypertensive ascites: spontaneous bacterial peritonitis occurs in 20–30%; patients with ascites total protein < 1 g/dL are at higher risk (40%)
- Massive ascites
  - Ruptured umbilical hernia
  - Hepatic hydrothorax
  - Respiratory compromise
  - Poor nutritional intake
- TIPS: encephalopathy in 30% and shunt stenosis or occlusion in 30–60% within 1 year, requiring periodic revisions

PROGNOSIS

- In patients with cirrhosis, ascites is a poor prognostic indicator, with 50% survival at 2 years

WHEN TO ADMIT

- Suspected peritonitis

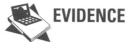

EVIDENCE

PRACTICE GUIDELINES

- National Guideline Clearinghouse
- Runyon BA. AASLD Practice Guideline. Management of adult patients with ascites due to cirrhosis. Hepatology. 2004 Mar;39(3):841–56. [PMID: 14999706]

WEB SITE

- American Association for the Study of Liver Diseases

INFORMATION FOR PATIENTS

- Cancerbacup
- MedlinePlus
- Merck Manual

REFERENCES

- Heidelbaugh JJ et al. Cirrhosis and chronic liver failure: part 1. Diagnosis and evaluation. Am Fam Physician. 2006 Sep 1;74(5):756-62. [PMID: 16970020]
- Heidelbaugh JJ et al. Cirrhosis and chronic liver failure: part 2: Complications and treatment. Am Fam Physician. 2006 Sep 1;74(5):767-76. [PMID: 16970019]

Ascites, Malignant

KEY FEATURES

- Two-thirds of cases are due to peritoneal carcinomatosis from adenocarcinomas of the
  - Ovary
  - Uterus
  - Pancreas
  - Stomach
  - Colon
  - Lung
  - Breast
- One-third of cases are due to lymphatic obstruction or portal hypertension from
  - Hepatocellular carcinoma
  - Diffuse hepatic metastases

CLINICAL FINDINGS

- Nonspecific abdominal discomfort and weight loss
- Increased abdominal girth
- Nausea or vomiting caused by partial or complete intestinal obstruction

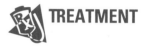

DIAGNOSIS

- Abdominal CT
  - Useful to demonstrate primary malignancy or hepatic metastases
  - Seldom confirms diagnosis of peritoneal carcinomatosis
- Paracentesis demonstrates
  - Low serum ascites–albumin gradient (< 1.1 mg/dL)
  - Increased total protein (> 2.5 g/dL)
  - Elevated WBC (often both neutrophils and mononuclear cells but with a lymphocyte predominance)
- Ascitic fluid cytology is positive in 95%
- Laparoscopy is diagnostic in patients with negative cytology

TREATMENT

- Diuretics not useful in controlling ascites
- Periodic large-volume paracentesis for symptomatic relief
- Intraperitoneal chemotherapy sometimes used
- Prognosis is extremely poor: only 10% survival at 6 months
- Ovarian cancer is an exception; with surgical debulking and intraperitoneal chemotherapy, long-term survival is possible

Atrial Fibrillation

KEY FEATURES

ESSENTIALS OF DIAGNOSIS

- Irregularly irregular heart rhythm
- Tachycardia usually present
- Often associated with palpitations (acute onset) or fatigue (chronic)
- ECG shows erratic atrial activity with irregular ventricular response

GENERAL CONSIDERATIONS

- The most common chronic arrhythmia, affecting nearly 10% of individuals older than 80

- The incidence increases significantly with age starting in the 7th decade of life
- Rarely life-threatening
- If the ventricular rate is rapid enough, it can precipitate hypotension, myocardial ischemia, or myocardial dysfunction
- Approximately 60% of patients with a first episode will revert to sinus rhythm within 24 hours

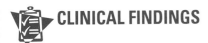

CLINICAL FINDINGS

SYMPTOMS AND SIGNS

- Irregularly irregular pulse (harder to distinguish with more rapid heart rates)
- Often occurs paroxysmally before becoming the established rhythm
- Older or inactive individuals may have relatively few symptoms
- However, some patients are made uncomfortable by the irregular rhythm due to palpitations or fatigue
- In patients with heart disease, rheumatic disease, and other valvular heart disease, attacks can be caused by
  - Dilated cardiomyopathy
  - Atrial septal defect
  - Hypertension
  - Coronary heart disease
  - Thyrotoxicosis
- In patients with normal hearts, attacks can be caused by
  - Pericarditis
  - Chest trauma
  - Thoracic or cardiac surgery
  - Pulmonary disease
  - Electrolyte disturbances
  - Acute alcohol excess or withdrawal
  - Medications, such as theophylline and β-adrenergic agonists

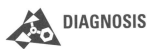

DIAGNOSIS

LABORATORY TESTS

- ECG
  - Lack of normal P waves and an irregular, rapidly fluctuating baseline
  - Irregular ventricular rhythm, with heart rate usually 80–180 bpm
- Echocardiography
  - Visualization of fibrillating atria with irregular ventricular contractions
  - Recommended in patients with newly diagnosed atrial fibrillation to exclude occult valvular or myocardial disease

- Ambulatory ECG monitoring or event recorders are indicated when paroxysmal atrial fibrillation is suspected
- Obtain thyroid-stimulating hormone level to exclude thyrotoxicosis as a potential cause

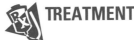

TREATMENT

MEDICATIONS

- If atrial fibrillation persists for > 1 week
  - Spontaneous conversion is unlikely
  - Management consists of rate control and anticoagulation with warfarin (goal INR of 2–3)
- Rate control is defined as ventricular rate of 50–100 bpm with usual daily activities and not exceeding 120 bpm except with moderate to strenuous activity
- Conventional rate-control agents used singly or, in younger adults, often in combination, include
  - β-Blockers
  - Digoxin
  - Calcium channel blockers (Table 12)
- In patients with heart failure, coronary artery disease, or ongoing ischemia, β-blockers or digoxin are preferred
- Amiodarone (among other antiarrhythmic drugs) is useful
  - When rate control with other agents is incomplete or contraindicated
  - When cardioversion is anticipated
- Do not use digoxin, verapamil, or β-blockers if atrial fibrillation is associated with a known or suspected accessory pathway

THERAPEUTIC PROCEDURES

- Urgent electrical cardioversion is recommended in patients who are hemodynamically unstable even if atrial fibrillation has been present for > 48 h
- Elective electrical or pharmacologic cardioversion is recommended in patients
  - With an initial episode of recent onset when there is an identifiable precipitating factor
  - Who remain symptomatic despite aggressive efforts at rate control
- If cardioversion is planned and the duration of atrial fibrillation is unknown
  - Perform a transesophageal echocardiography to exclude an atrial thrombus
  - Attempt electrical cardioversion while the patient remains sedated
- If thrombus is present, delay cardioversion until therapeutic warfarin anticoagulation has been achieved for 4 weeks (goal INR of 2–3)

- Use heparin while awaiting therapeutic warfarin anticoagulation in atrial fibrillation with mitral stenosis, a history of embolic events, or demonstrated thrombus on transesophageal echocardiography
- After cardioversion, maintain therapeutic anticoagulation for at least 1–6 mo
- Patients with atrial fibrillation who fail to convert should receive anticoagulation therapy indefinitely
- However, indefinite anticoagulation therapy is not indicated for those with "lone atrial fibrillation," defined as
  - Age < 65
  - No associated heart disease, hypertension, atherosclerotic vascular disease, or diabetes mellitus
- For drug refractory, symptomatic atrial fibrillation, consider radiofrequency catheter ablation or radiofrequency atrioventricular node ablation and permanent pacing

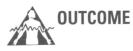

OUTCOME

COMPLICATIONS

- Propensity for stroke from embolization of an atrial thrombus

WHEN TO REFER

- For elective cardioversion, initiation of antiarrhythmic drug therapy, catheter ablation of atrial fibrillation triggers/substrate or radiofrequency ablation of the atrioventricular node and permanent pacemaker implantation

WHEN TO ADMIT

- When the patient is hemodynamically unstable and immediate treatment is required

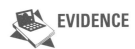

EVIDENCE

PRACTICE GUIDELINES

- McKeown PP et al; American College of Chest Physicians. Executive summary: American College of Chest Physicians guidelines for the prevention and management of postoperative atrial fibrillation after cardiac surgery. Chest. 2005 Aug;128(2 Suppl):1S–5S. [PMID: 16167657]
- Rockson SG et al. Comparing the guidelines: anticoagulation therapy to optimize stroke prevention in patients with atrial fibrillation. J Am Coll Cardiol. 2004 Mar 17;43(6):929–35. [PMID: 15028346]

- Snow V et al. Management of newly detected atrial fibrillation: a clinical practice guideline from the American Academy of Family Physicians and the American College of Physicians. Ann Intern Med. 2003;139:1009. [PMID: 14678921]

WEB SITE

- American College of Cardiology Foundation, Management of Patients with Atrial Fibrillation - Executive Summary

INFORMATION FOR PATIENTS

- American Heart Association
- Parmet S et al. JAMA patient page. Atrial fibrillation. JAMA. 2003; 290:1118. [PMID: 12941685]

REFERENCES

- Corley SD et al; AFFIRM Investigators. Relationships between sinus rhythm, treatment, and survival in the Atrial Fibrillation Follow-Up Investigation of Rhythm Management (AFFIRM) Study. Circulation. 2004 Mar 30; 109(12):1509–13. [PMID: 15007003]
- de Denus S et al. Rate vs rhythm control in patients with atrial fibrillation: a meta-analysis. Arch Intern Med. 2005 Feb 14;165(3):258–62. [PMID: 15710787]
- Gage BF et al. Selecting patients with atrial fibrillation for anticoagulation: stroke risk stratification in patients taking aspirin. Circulation. 2004 Oct 19; 110(16):2287–92. [PMID: 15477396]
- Joglar JA et al. Electrical cardioversion of atrial fibrillation. Cardiol Clin. 2004 Feb;22(1):101–11. [PMID: 14994851]
- Wang TJ et al. A risk score for predicting stroke or death for individuals with new-onset atrial fibrillation in the community: the Framingham Heart Study. JAMA. 2003 Aug 27;290(8):1049–56. [PMID: 12941677]
- Wazni OM et al. Radiofrequency ablation vs antiarrhythmic drugs as first-line treatment of symptomatic atrial fibrillation: a randomized trial. JAMA. 2005 Jun 1;293(21):2634–40. [PMID: 15928285]

Atrial Flutter

 KEY FEATURES

- Reentrant circuit generates atrial rates of 250–350/min, with transmission of every second, third, or fourth impulse to the ventricles
- Atrial flutter is less common than fibrillation
- Occurs most often in chronic obstructive pulmonary disease (COPD)
- Occurs less commonly with
  - Rheumatic or coronary heart disease
  - Congestive heart failure (CHF)
  - Atrial septal defect
  - Surgically repaired congenital heart disease
- Ventricular rate control is attempted as in atrial fibrillation but is much more difficult to achieve
- Risk of systemic embolization is slightly increased

 CLINICAL FINDINGS

- Usually a regular pulse with atrial rate between 250–350 bpm and ventricular rate between 75–150 bpm
- Symptoms include anxiety, shortness of breath, light-headedness
- Physical findings of COPD or CHF

 DIAGNOSIS

- ECG: characteristic atrial flutter waves transmitted in a regular 2:1, 3:1, or 4:1 pattern to the ventricles

 TREATMENT

- Initially, digoxin, a β-blocker, or a calcium channel blocker (Table 12) is used for rate control; conversion to sinus rhythm may result
- If not, ibutilide converts atrial flutter to sinus rhythm in ~50–70% of patients within 15–90 min
- Electrical cardioversion (25–50 J) is effective in ~90% of patients
- Precardioversion anticoagulation is not necessary for atrial flutter of < 48 h duration except in the setting of mitral valve disease

- Anticoagulation is prudent in chronic atrial flutter
- If atrial flutter is recurrent, consider radiofrequency catheter ablation of the reentrant circuit

Atrial Septal Defect

 KEY FEATURES

- Four common forms
  - Ostium secundum defect (midseptum) (80% of cases)
  - Ostium primum defect (low septum)
  - Sinus venosus defect (upper septum), often associated with partial anomalous pulmonary venous connection
  - Coronary sinus defect (unroofed coronary sinus)
- Shunt due to oxygenated blood from higher-pressure LA shunting into RA, increasing RV output and pulmonary blood flow
- Prolonged high flow through pulmonary circulation often leads to elevated pulmonary pressure, but severe pulmonary hypertension with cyanosis (Eisenmenger's physiology) uncommon (10–15%)
- Patent foramen ovale (present in 20–30% of adults) is responsible for most paradoxical emboli especially if associated with redundant septal tissue (septal aneurysm)

 CLINICAL FINDINGS

- Most small or moderate ASDs are asymptomatic for long periods
- Direction of left-to-right at the atrial level depends on respective complicance of atria (which depend on ventricular compliance)
  - Normally, LV compliance worsens with age, and left-to-right shunt increases with age
  - If shunt results in a reduced RV compliance over time, then left-to-right shunt may be lessened and even reverse
  - If it reverses, cyanosis is present
- Large shunts can produce exertional dyspnea

- When RV failure occurs, rather than the jugular venous pressure increasing, a right-to-left shunt may simply be noted
- Moderately loud systolic ejection murmur in the second and third interspaces due to flow across the pulmonary valve; S_2 widely split, does not vary with breathing
- Prominent RV and pulmonary artery pulsations
- Atrial arrhythmias are common

 DIAGNOSIS

- ECG
  - Incomplete or complete right bundle branch block
  - Right axis deviation, RV hypertrophy
  - Negative P waves in limb leads suggestive of a sinus venosus ASD
- Chest radiograph
  - Large pulmonary arteries
  - Increased pulmonary vascularity
  - Enlarged RA and RV
- Echocardiography usually diagnostic
  - Saline bubble contrast demonstrates right-to-left shunting (occurring in essentially all) and Doppler flow can demonstrate shunting in both directions
  - Transesophageal echocardiography has superior sensitivity for small shunts, can separate patent foramen ovale from secundum ASD, and must be done before percutaneous closure
- Cardiac catheterization can
  - Show increase in oxygen saturation between venae cava and RV
  - Quantify shunt
  - Measure pulmonary vascular resistance

 TREATMENT

- Small shunts (< 1.5:1) do not require intervention
- If the RA and RV are enlarged, most clinicians would consider closure
- Percutaneous devices can close most secundum ASDs without surgery
- Ostium primum, sinus venosus ASDs, and coronary sinus ASDs require surgery
- If predominantly a right-to-left shunt, closure probably not effective (consistent with Eisenmenger's physiology)

Atropine and Anticholinergic Poisoning

 KEY FEATURES

- Antimuscarinic agents with variable CNS effects
  - Atropine
  - Scopolamine
  - Belladonna
  - Diphenoxylate with atropine
  - *Datura stramonium*
  - *Hyoscyamus niger*
  - Some mushrooms
  - Tricyclic antidepressants
  - Antihistamines

 CLINICAL FINDINGS

- Anticholinergic syndrome
  - Dryness of the mouth, difficulty swallowing, blurring of vision
  - Dilated pupils, flushed skin, tachycardia, fever, delirium, myoclonus, ileus, flushed appearance
- Dilated pupils, flushed skin, tachycardia, fever, delirium, myoclonus, ileus, flushed appearance
- Antidepressants and antihistamines may induce convulsions
- Diphenhydramine commonly causes delirium, tachycardia, and seizures; massive overdose may mimic tricyclic antidepressant poisoning
- Terfenadine and astemizole cause QT interval prolongation and torsades de pointes and were removed from US market

 DIAGNOSIS

- Based on history of ingestion, typical "anticholinergic syndrome"
- Serum levels not useful
- ECG monitoring for wide QRS, QT prolongation

 TREATMENT

Emergency and supportive measures
- Activated charcoal
  - Administer 60–100 g mixed in aqueous slurry PO or via gastric tube
  - Do not use for comatose or convulsing patients unless they are endotracheally intubated

Specific treatment
- For pure atropine or related anticholinergic syndrome, if symptoms are severe (eg, agitated delirium or excessively rapid tachycardia), give physostigmine salicylate, 0.5–1.0 mg IV slowly over 5 min, with ECG monitoring, until symptoms are controlled
- *Caution:* bradyarrhythmias and convulsions are a hazard with physostigmine administration, and it should **not** be used in patients with tricyclic antidepressant overdose
- Alternate treatment for agitation: lorazepam 1–2 mg IV

Avascular Necrosis of Bone

 KEY FEATURES

- A complication of
  - Corticosteroid use
  - Trauma
  - Systemic lupus erythematosus (SLE)
  - Pancreatitis
  - Alcoholism
  - Gout
  - Sickle cell disease
  - Infiltrative diseases (eg, Gaucher's disease)
- Most commonly affected sites are the proximal and distal femoral heads
- The natural history is usually progression of the bony infarction to cortical collapse, resulting in significant joint dysfunction

 CLINICAL FINDINGS

- Hip or knee pain
- Many patients with hip disease first present with pain referred to the knee; however, internal rotation of the hip—not movement of the knee—is painful

DIAGNOSIS

- Initially, radiographs are often normal
- MRI, CT scan, and bone scan are all more sensitive techniques
- Differential diagnosis
  – Osteoarthritis or rheumatoid arthritis
  – Fracture
  – Joint pain resulting from other cause

 TREATMENT

- Avoidance of weight bearing on the affected joint for at least several weeks
- Surgical core decompression is controversial
- Total hip replacement is the usual outcome for all patients who are suitable candidates

Babesiosis

 KEY FEATURES

ESSENTIALS OF DIAGNOSIS

- History of tick bite or exposure to ticks
- Fever, flu-like symptoms, anemia
- Intraerythrocytic parasites on Giemsa-stained blood smears
- Positive serologic tests

GENERAL CONSIDERATIONS

- Babesiosis is an uncommon intraerythrocytic infection caused mainly by two *Babesia* species and transmitted by *Ixodes* ticks
- Symptoms of *Babesia microti* infections appear 1 week to several weeks after tick bite; parasitemia evident after 2–4 weeks
- Patients usually do not recall the tick bite

DEMOGRAPHICS

- In Europe, infection is caused by *Babesia divergens,* which also infects cattle
- In the United States, infection is caused by *B microti,* which also infects wild mammals
- Most infections in the United States occur in the coastal northeast, with some cases also in the upper midwest
- Rare episodes of illnesses caused by *B microti, B divergens,* and other *Babesia*-like organisms have been reported from other areas

 CLINICAL FINDINGS

SYMPTOMS AND SIGNS

- Fever, fatigue, headache, arthralgia, and myalgia develop gradually and are characteristic
- Other findings
  - Nausea, vomiting
  - Abdominal pain
  - Sore throat
  - Depression, emotional lability
  - Anemia
  - Thrombocytopenia, splenomegaly
- *B divergens* infections in splenectomized patients present with
  - Rapidly progressive high fever
  - Severe hemolytic anemia
  - Jaundice
  - Hemoglobinuria
  - Renal failure

DIFFERENTIAL DIAGNOSIS

- Malaria
- Infectious mononucleosis
- Viral hepatitis
- Ehrlichiosis
- Lyme disease

 DIAGNOSIS

LABORATORY TESTS

- Diagnosis made by identifying the parasite on Giemsa-stained blood smears
- Repeated smears are often necessary because < 1% of erythrocytes may be infected, especially early in infection, although parasitemias can exceed 10%
- An indirect immunofluorescent antibody test for *B microti* is available from the CDC; antibody is detectable within 2–4 weeks after the onset of symptoms and persists for months
- Diagnosis can also be made by polymerase chain reaction or by inoculation of hamsters or gerbils

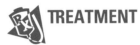 **TREATMENT**

MEDICATIONS

- Most patients have a mild illness and recover without therapy
- Standard therapy is a 7-day course of quinine (650 mg PO TID) plus clindamycin (600 mg PO TID)
- An alternative is a 7-day course of atovaquone (750 mg PO q12h) plus azithromycin (600 mg PO once daily)

THERAPEUTIC PROCEDURE

- Exchange transfusion has been used successfully in severely ill asplenic patients and those with parasitemia > 10%

 OUTCOME

COMPLICATIONS

- Respiratory failure
- Hemolytic anemia
- Disseminated intravascular coagulation
- Congestive heart failure
- Renal failure

PROGNOSIS

- Although parasitemia may continue for months, with or without symptoms, the disease is self-limited

- Older persons and those who have had a splenectomy are most likely to have severe complications
- Mortality rate
  - Among hospitalized patients with *B microti* infections is 6.5%
  - Among splenectomized patients with *B divergens* infection is > 40%

WHEN TO REFER

- Patients not responding to therapy

WHEN TO ADMIT

- All splenectomized or older patients

 EVIDENCE

WEB SITE

- Centers for Disease Control and Prevention—Division of Parasitic Diseases

INFORMATION FOR PATIENTS

- American Academy of Family Physicians
- American College of Emergency Physicians

REFERENCES

- Herwaldt BL et al. *Babesia divergens*-like infection, Washington State. Emerg Infect Dis. 2004 Apr;10(4):622–9. [PMID: 15200851]
- Kogut SJ et al. *Babesia microti,* upstate New York. Emerg Infect Dis. 2005 Mar; 11(3):476–8. [PMID: 15757571]

Baldness

 KEY FEATURES

ESSENTIALS OF DIAGNOSIS

Forms of hair loss
- Baldness due to scarring (cicatricial baldness, irreversible)
- Baldness not due to scarring

GENERAL CONSIDERATIONS

Baldness due to scarring
- Irreversible and permanent, thus it is important to treat the scarring process as early as possible
- May occur following
  - Chemical or physical trauma

– Lichen planopilaris
– Severe bacterial or fungal infections
– Severe herpes zoster
– Chronic discoid lupus erythematosus
– Scleroderma
– Excessive ionizing radiation
• The specific cause is often suggested by
– The history
– The distribution of hair loss
– The appearance of the skin, as in lupus erythematosus

Baldness not due to scarring

• Nonscarring alopecia may occur in association with various systemic diseases such as
– Systemic lupus erythematosus
– Secondary syphilis
– Hyperthyroidism or hypothyroidism
– Iron deficiency anemia
– Pituitary insufficiency

Androgenetic baldness

• Both men and women are affected, often starting in the third decade

Telogen effluvium

• A transitory increase in the number of hairs in the telogen (resting) phase of the hair growth cycle
• Causes
– Spontaneous occurrence
– Iron deficiency
– May appear at the termination of pregnancy
– Precipitated by "crash dieting," high fever, stress from surgery or shock, or malnutrition
– Provoked by hormonal contraceptives
• Latent period of 2–4 months
• The prognosis is generally good

Alopecia areata

• Unknown cause but is believed to be an immunologic process (autoimmune)
• Occasionally associated with Hashimoto's thyroiditis, pernicious anemia, Addison's disease, and vitiligo

Drug-induced alopecia

• Becoming increasingly important
• Incriminated drugs include
– Thallium
– Excessive and prolonged use of vitamin A
– Retinoids
– Antimitotic agents
– Anticoagulants
– Antithyroid drugs
– Oral contraceptives
– Trimethadione
– Allopurinol
– Propranolol
– Indomethacin, salicylates
– Amphetamines
– Gentamicin
– Levodopa

• While chemotherapy-induced alopecia is very distressing, it must be emphasized to the patient before treatment that it is invariably reversible

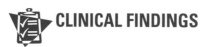

CLINICAL FINDINGS

SYMPTOMS AND SIGNS

Androgenetic baldness

• The earliest changes occur at the anterior portions of the calvarium on either side of the "widow's peak" (in men) and on the crown (vertex) of the skull (in men and women)
• The extent of hair loss is variable and unpredictable
• Occurs in both women and men

Alopecia areata

• Typically, there are patches that are perfectly smooth and without scarring
• Tiny hairs 2–3 mm in length, called "exclamation hairs," may be seen
• Telogen hairs are easily dislodged from the periphery of active lesions
• The beard, brows, and lashes may be involved
• Involvement may extend to all of the scalp hair (alopecia totalis) or to all scalp and body hair (alopecia universalis)

DIFFERENTIAL DIAGNOSIS

• Scarring (cicatricial)
– Chemical or physical trauma
– Lichen planopilaris
– Bacterial or fungal infection (severe)
– Herpes zoster (shingles) (severe)
– Discoid lupus erythematosus
– Scleroderma
– Excessive ionizing radiation
• Nonscarring
– Androgenic (male pattern) baldness
– Telogen effluvium
– Alopecia areata
– Trichotillomania
– Drug-induced alopecia
– Systemic lupus erythematosus
– Secondary syphilis
– Hyperthyroidism
– Hypothyroidism
– Iron deficiency anemia
– Pituitary insufficiency

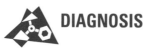

DIAGNOSIS

LABORATORY TESTS

• Serum testosterone, DHEAS, iron, total iron-binding capacity, and thyroid function tests and a complete blood cell count will identify most other causes of hair thinning in premenopausal women

Telogen effluvium

• Diagnosed by the presence of large numbers of hairs with white bulbs coming out upon gentle tugging
• Counts of hairs lost on combing or shampooing often exceed 150 per day, compared with an average of 70–100

DIAGNOSTIC PROCEDURES

• Biopsy is useful in the diagnosis of scarring alopecia, but specimens must be taken from the active border and not from the scarred central zone

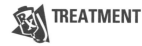

TREATMENT

MEDICATIONS

Androgenetic baldness

• Rogaine extra strength
– Solution containing 50 mg/mL of minoxidil; available over the counter; best results achieved in persons with recent onset (< 5 years) and smaller areas of alopecia
– Approximately 40% of patients treated twice daily for 1 year will have moderate to dense growth
• Finasteride (Propecia): 1 mg PO daily, has similar efficacy to Rogaine and may be additive to minoxidil; used only in males

Hair loss or thinning in women

• May be treated with minoxidil

Alopecia areata

• Intralesional corticosteroids are frequently effective
• Triamcinolone acetonide in a concentration of 2.5–10 mg/mL is injected in aliquots of 0.1 mL at approximately 1- to 2-cm intervals, not exceeding a total dose of 30 mg per month for adults
• Alternatively, anthralin 0.5% ointment used daily, may help some patients

THERAPEUTIC PROCEDURES

Baldness not due to scarring

• The only treatment necessary is prompt and adequate control of the underlying disorder, in which case hair loss may be reversible

Alopecia areata

• Alopecia areata is usually self-limiting, with complete regrowth of hair in 80% of patients, but some mild cases are resistant
• Support groups for patients with extensive alopecia areata are very beneficial

OUTCOME

FOLLOW-UP

- Women who complain of thin hair but show little evidence of alopecia need follow-up, because more than 50% of the scalp hair can be lost before the clinician can perceive it

COMPLICATIONS

- Scarring alopecia can be very disfiguring

WHEN TO REFER

- All scarring alopecias except clearly diagnosed discoid lupus erythematosus and posttraumatic
- Diagnosis and management questions

EVIDENCE

PRACTICE GUIDELINES

- MacDonald Hull SP et al; British Association of Dermatologists. Guidelines for the management of alopecia areata. Br J Dermatol. 2003;149:692. [PMID: 14616359]
- Recommendations to diagnose and treat adult hair loss disorders or alopecia in primary care settings (nonpregnant female and male adults). University of Texas at Austin, 2004

WEB SITES

- American Academy of Dermatology
- National Alopecia Areata Foundation

INFORMATION FOR PATIENTS

- American Academy of Family Physicians: Hair Loss and Its Causes
- American Medical Association: Male Pattern Baldness
- Mayo Clinic: Baldness
- MedlinePlus: Alopecia Interactive Tutorial
- National Institute of Arthritis and Musculoskeletal and Skin Diseases: Alopecia Areata

REFERENCES

- Dombrowski NC et al. Alopecia areata: what to expect from current treatments. Cleve Clin J Med. 2005 Sep;72(9):758, 760–1, 765–6. [PMID: 16193824]
- Han A et al. Clinical approach to the patient with alopecia. Semin Cutan Med Surg. 2006 Mar;25(1):11–23. [PMID: 16616299]

Bartholin's Duct Cyst and Abscess

KEY FEATURES

- Trauma or infection may cause obstruction of the gland; drainage of secretions is prevented, leading to pain, swelling, and abscess formation
- The infection usually resolves and pain disappears, but stenosis of the duct outlet with distention often persists
- Reinfection causes recurrent tenderness and further enlargement of the duct

CLINICAL FINDINGS

- Periodic painful swelling on either side of the introitus and consequent dyspareunia
- A fluctuant swelling 1–4 cm in diameter in the inferior portion of either labium minus is a sign of occlusion of Bartholin's duct
- Tenderness is evidence of active infection

DIAGNOSIS

- Pus or secretions from the gland should be cultured for *Chlamydia* and other pathogens

TREATMENT

- Treat according to culture results
- Frequent warm soaks may be helpful
- If an abscess develops, aspiration or incision and drainage are the simplest forms of therapy, but the problem may recur
- Marsupialization (in the absence of an abscess), incision and drainage with the insertion of an indwelling Word catheter, or laser treatment will establish a new duct opening. Antibiotics are unnecessary unless cellulitis is present
- An asymptomatic cyst does not require therapy

Basal Cell Carcinoma

KEY FEATURES

ESSENTIALS OF DIAGNOSIS

- Slow-growing lesions
- Pearly or translucent appearance
- Telangiectatic vessels easily visible

GENERAL CONSIDERATIONS

- Most common form of cancer
- Basal cell carcinomas occur on sun-exposed skin in otherwise normal fair-skinned individuals
- Clinicians should examine the skin routinely, looking for bumps, patches, and scabbed lesions

CLINICAL FINDINGS

SYMPTOMS AND SIGNS

- Most common presentation is a papule or nodule that may have a scab or erosion
- Occasionally, the nodules have a brown-gray color or have stippled pigment (pigmented basal cell carcinoma)
- Lesions grow slowly, attaining a size of 1–2 cm or more in diameter, often after years of growth
- There is a waxy, "pearly" appearance, with telangiectatic vessels easily visible
- Pearly or translucent quality of the lesions is most diagnostic, a feature best appreciated if the skin is stretched
- On the back and chest and lower legs, basal cell carcinomas appear as reddish, somewhat shiny, scaly plaques
- When examining the face, look at the eyelid margins and medial canthi, the nose and alar folds, the lips, and then around and behind the ears

DIFFERENTIAL DIAGNOSIS

- Squamous cell carcinoma
- Actinic keratosis
- Intradermal nevus
- Fibrous papule of the nose
- Seborrheic keratosis (unpigmented type)
- Sebaceous (epidermal inclusion) cyst
- Sebaceous hyperplasia
- Keratoacanthoma
- Molluscum contagiosum

- Melanoma
- Paget's disease

 DIAGNOSIS

DIAGNOSTIC PROCEDURES

- Lesions suspected to be basal cell carcinomas should be biopsied, by shave or punch biopsy
- Biopsy confirms the diagnosis

 TREATMENT

MEDICATIONS

- Imiquimod cream 5% three to five times a week for 6–10 weeks may be effective for nonfacial, superficial (by biopsy) basal cell cancers

SURGERY

- Therapy is aimed at eradication with minimal cosmetic deformity, often by excision and suturing with recurrence rates of 5% or less
- The technique of three cycles of curettage and electrodesiccation depends on the skill of the operator and is not recommended for head and neck lesions
- After 4–6 weeks of healing, it leaves a broad, hypopigmented, at times hypertrophic scar
- Mohs surgery
  - Involves removal of the tumor followed by immediate frozen section histopathologic examination of margins with subsequent reexcision of tumor-positive areas and final closure of the defect
  - Gives the highest cure rates (98%) and results in least tissue loss

THERAPEUTIC PROCEDURES

- Radiotherapy
  - Effective and sometimes appropriate for older individuals (age > 75)
  - However, recurrent tumors after radiation therapy are more difficult to treat and may be more aggressive
  - Very expensive, so its use should be restricted to cases where other options are not available

 OUTCOME

FOLLOW-UP

- Patients must be monitored for the first 5 years to detect new or recurrent lesions

PROGNOSIS

- Metastases almost never occur
- Most recurrences appear in the first 1–2 years

WHEN TO REFER

- If diagnosis needs to be confirmed or if biopsy is required

PREVENTION

- Sun avoidance, particularly in children, is essential to lower the incidence of new basal cell cancers

 EVIDENCE

PRACTICE GUIDELINES

- Miller SJ et al; NCCN Basal Cell and Squamous Cell Skin Cancer Practice Guidelines Panel. National Comprehensive Cancer Network: Basal Cell and Squamous Cell Skin Cancers v.1.2004
- US Preventive Services Task Force: Counseling to prevent skin cancer, 2003

WEB SITES

- American Academy of Dermatology
- National Cancer Institute: Skin Cancer Information for Patients and Health Professionals

INFORMATION FOR PATIENTS

- American Academy of Family Physicians: Skin Cancer: Saving Your Skin from Sun Damage
- American Cancer Society: Nonmelanoma Skin Cancer
- MedlinePlus: Skin Cancer Interactive Tutorial
- Skin Cancer Foundation: Basal Cell Carcinoma

REFERENCE

- Rubin AI et al. Basal-cell carcinoma. N Engl J Med. 2005 Nov 24; 353(21):2262–9. [PMID: 16306523]

Behçet's Syndrome

 KEY FEATURES

- Causes recurrent attacks of oral aphthous ulcers, genital ulcers, uveitis, and skin lesions
- Onset usually in young adults, aged 25–35 yr
- Blindness, CNS abnormalities, and thrombosis or rupture of large vessels are the most serious complications

 CLINICAL FINDINGS

- Recurrent oral and genital ulcers
- Eye abnormalities include
  - Keratitis
  - Retinal vasculitis
  - Anterior uveitis (often with hypopyon, or pus in the anterior chamber)
- Seronegative arthritis occurs in about two-thirds of patients, most commonly affecting the knees and ankles
- CNS abnormalities include
  - Cranial nerve palsies
  - Convulsions
  - Encephalitis
  - Mental disturbances
  - Spinal cord lesions
- Clinical course may be chronic but is often characterized by remissions and exacerbations

 DIAGNOSIS

- Clinical diagnosis
- CNS lesions may mimic multiple sclerosis radiologically
- Differential diagnosis
  - Inflammatory bowel disease
  - Systemic lupus erythematosus
  - Recurrent aphthous ulcers
  - Herpes simplex infection
  - Ankylosing spondylitis
  - Reactive arthritis (Reiter's syndrome)
  - Syphilis
  - Sarcoidosis
  - HIV infection

 TREATMENT

- Corticosteroids, azathioprine, chlorambucil, pentoxifylline, and cyclosporine have been used with beneficial results

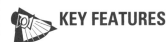

Bell's Palsy

KEY FEATURES

ESSENTIALS OF DIAGNOSIS

- Sudden onset of lower motor neuron facial palsy
- May have hyperacusis or impaired taste
- No other neurologic abnormalities

GENERAL CONSIDERATIONS

- Idiopathic lower motor neuron facial paresis
- Attributed to an inflammatory reaction of the facial nerve near the stylomastoid foramen or in the bony facial canal
- Reactivation of herpes simplex virus has been postulated

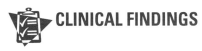

CLINICAL FINDINGS

SYMPTOMS AND SIGNS

- Generally comes on abruptly, but may worsen over 1 or 2 days
- Pain about the ear often precedes or accompanies the weakness but usually lasts for only a few days
- There may be ipsilateral restriction of eye closure and difficulty with eating and fine facial movements
- A disturbance of taste is common, owing to involvement of chorda tympani fibers, and hyperacusis due to involvement of fibers to the stapedius occurs occasionally

DIFFERENTIAL DIAGNOSIS

- HIV-related facial neuropathies
- Lyme disease
- Sarcoidosis
- Ramsay Hunt syndrome (herpes zoster of geniculate ganglion)
- Acoustic neuroma
- Acute or chronic otitis media
- Malignant otitis externa
- Guillain-Barré syndrome
- Tumor, eg, parotid, temporal bone tumor
- Brainstem infarct

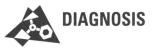

DIAGNOSIS

- Clinical features are characteristic

- Electromyography and nerve excitability or conduction studies provide a guide to prognosis

LABORATORY TESTS

- To exclude other causes of facial neuropathy (see Differential Diagnosis)

TREATMENT

MEDICATIONS

- The only medical treatment that may influence the outcome is administration of corticosteroids, but studies supporting this approach have been criticized
  - Many clinicians prescribe corticosteroids for patients seen within 5 days of onset
  - Others prescribe them only when the palsy is clinically complete or there is severe pain
- Treatment is with prednisone, 60 or 80 mg PO once daily in divided doses for 4 or 5 days, followed by tapering of the dose over the next 7–10 days
- It is helpful to protect the eye with lubricating drops (or lubricating ointment at night) and a patch if eye closure is not possible
- The role of acyclovir or other antiviral agents is unclear

SURGERY

- There is no evidence that surgical procedures to decompress the facial nerve are of benefit

THERAPEUTIC PROCEDURES

- The management is controversial
- Approximately 60% recover completely without treatment
- Considerable improvement occurs in most other cases, and only about 10% of all patients have permanent disfigurement or other long-term sequelae
- Treatment is unnecessary in most cases but is indicated when an unsatisfactory outcome can be predicted
- The best clinical guide to prognosis is the severity of the palsy during the first few days after presentation

OUTCOME

PROGNOSIS

- Patients with clinically complete palsy when first seen are less likely to make a full recovery than those with an incomplete one
- A poor prognosis for recovery is also associated with advanced age, hyperacusis, and severe initial pain

EVIDENCE

PRACTICE GUIDELINES

- Grogan PM et al. Practice parameter: steroids, acyclovir, and surgery for Bell's palsy (an evidenced-based review): report of the Quality Standards Subcommittee of the American Academy of Neurology. Neurology. 2001;56:830. [PMID: 11294918]

INFORMATION FOR PATIENTS

- American Academy of Otolaryngology—Head and Neck Surgery
- National Institute of Neurological Disorders and Stroke

REFERENCES

- Alberton DL et al. Bell's palsy: a review of treatment using antiviral agents. Ann Pharmacother. 2006 Oct;40(10):1838–42. [PMID: 16968821]
- Gilden DH. Clinical practice. Bell's palsy. N Engl J Med. 2004 Sep 23; 351(13):1323–31. [PMID: 15385659]
- Hato N et al. Valacyclovir and prednisolone treatment for Bell's palsy: a multicenter, randomized, placebo-controlled study. Otol Neurotol. 2007 Apr; 28(3):408–13. [PMID: 17414047]
- Salinas RA et al. Corticosteroids for Bell's palsy (idiopathic facial paralysis). Cochrane Database Syst Rev. 2004 Oct 18;(4):CD001942. [PMID: 15495021]

Benign Prostatic Hyperplasia

KEY FEATURES

ESSENTIALS OF DIAGNOSIS

- Obstructive or irritative voiding symptoms
- May have enlarged prostate on rectal examination

- Absence of urinary tract infection, neurologic disorder, urethral stricture disease, prostatic or bladder malignancy

GENERAL CONSIDERATIONS

- Smooth, firm, elastic enlargement of the prostate
  Etiology
- Multifactorial
- Endocrine: dihydrotestosterone (DHT)
- Aging

DEMOGRAPHICS

- The most common benign tumor in men
- Incidence is age related
- Prevalence
  - ~20% in men aged 41–50
  - ~50% in men aged 51–60
  - ~> 90% in men aged 80 and older
- Symptoms are also age related: at age 55, ~25% of men report obstructive voiding symptoms

 CLINICAL FINDINGS

SYMPTOMS AND SIGNS

- Can be divided into obstructive and irritative complaints
- Obstructive symptoms
  - Hesitancy
  - Decreased force and caliber of stream
  - Sensation of incomplete bladder emptying
  - Double voiding (urinating a second time within 2 h)
  - Straining to urinate
  - Postvoid dribbling
- Irritative symptoms
  - Urgency
  - Frequency
  - Nocturia
- American Urological Association (AUA) Symptom Index (Table 153) should be calculated for all patients starting therapy
- Seven questions quantitate the severity of obstructive or irritative complaints on a scale of 0–5. Thus, the score can range from 0 to 35

DIFFERENTIAL DIAGNOSIS

- Prostate cancer
- Urinary tract infection
- Neurogenic bladder
- Urethral stricture

 DIAGNOSIS

DIAGNOSTIC PROCEDURES

- History to exclude other possible causes of symptoms
- Physical examination, digital rectal examination (DRE), and a focused neurologic examination
- DRE: note size and consistency of the prostate
- Examine lower abdomen for a distended bladder
- Renal insufficiency from benign prostatic hyperplasia (BPH)
  - Occurs in only ~2% of patients initially presenting with lower urinary tract symptoms
  - If detected, upper urinary tract imaging is warranted
- If possibility of cancer, further evaluation is needed by serum prostate-specific antigen (PSA), transrectal ultrasound, and biopsy

TREATMENT

MEDICATIONS

- α-Blockers
  - Prazosin, 1 mg PO each night at bedtime for 3 nights, increasing to 1 mg PO BID and then titrating up to 2 mg PO BID if necessary
  - Terazosin, 1 mg PO once daily for 3 days, increasing to 2 mg PO once daily for 11 days, then 5–10 mg PO once daily if necessary
  - Doxazosin, 1 mg PO once daily for 7 days, increasing to 2 mg PO once daily for 7 days, then 4–8 mg PO once daily if necessary
  - Tamsulosin, 0.4 mg PO once daily, increased to 0.8 mg PO once daily if necessary
  - Alfuzosin, 10 mg PO once daily; no dose titration needed
- 5α-Reductase inhibitors
  - Finasteride, 5 mg PO once daily; 6 months of therapy required for maximum effects on prostate size (20% reduction) and symptomatic improvement
  - Dutasteride, 10 mg PO once daily
- Saw palmetto is of no benefit
- Combination therapy
  - α-Blocker and 5α-reductase inhibitor (eg, long-term combination therapy with doxazosin and finasteride)
    □ Safe and reduces risk of overall clinical progression of BPH significantly more than either drug alone

□ Reduces the long-term risk of acute urinary retention and the need for invasive therapy
□ Entails the risks of additional side effects and the cost of two medications

SURGERY

- Indications
  - Refractory urinary retention (failing at least one attempt at catheter removal)
  - Large bladder diverticula
  - Recurrent urinary tract infection
  - Recurrent gross hematuria
  - Bladder stones
  - Renal insufficiency
- Transurethral resection of the prostate (TURP): operative complications
  - Bleeding
  - Urethral stricture or bladder neck contracture
  - Perforation of the prostate capsule with extravasation
  - Transurethral resection syndrome
  - A hypervolemic, hyponatremic state resulting from the absorption of the hypotonic irrigating solution
- TURP: postoperative complications
  - Retrograde ejaculation (75%)
  - Impotence (5–10%)
  - Urinary incontinence (< 1%)
- Transurethral incision of the prostate (TUIP)
  - Removes the zone of the prostate around the urethra leaving the peripheral portion of the prostate and prostate capsule
  - Lower rate of retrograde ejaculation reported (25%)
- Consider open simple prostatectomy when
  - Prostate is too large to remove endoscopically (> 100 g)
  - Concomitant bladder diverticulum
  - Bladder stone is present
  - Dorsal lithotomy positioning is not possible
- Minimally invasive approaches
  - TULIP (transurethral laser-induced prostatectomy) under transrectal ultrasound guidance
  - Visually directed laser techniques under cystoscopic control
  - Interstitial laser therapy usually under cystoscopic control
  - Advantages of laser surgery include
    □ Outpatient surgery
    □ Minimal blood loss
    □ Rare occurrence of transurethral resection syndrome
    □ Ability to treat patients while they are receiving anticoagulation therapy

- Disadvantages of laser surgery include
  □ Lack of tissue for pathologic examination
  □ Longer postoperative catheterization time
  □ More frequent irritative voiding complaints
  □ Expense of laser fibers and generators
- Transurethral needle ablation of the prostate (TUNA)
- Transurethral electrovaporization and KTP laser photovaporization of the prostate
- Hyperthermia—microwave thermotherapy

THERAPEUTIC PROCEDURES

- Watchful waiting: only for patients with mild symptoms (AUA scores 0–7)
- With watchful waiting, ~10% progress to urinary retention, and half demonstrate marked improvement or resolution of symptoms

 OUTCOME

FOLLOW-UP

- Follow AUA Symptom Index for benign prostatic hyperplasia (Table 153)

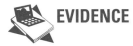 **EVIDENCE**

PRACTICE GUIDELINES

- AUA Practice Guidelines Committee. AUA guideline on management of benign prostatic hyperplasia (2003). Chapter 1: Diagnosis and treatment recommendations. J Urol. 2003 Aug;170(2 Pt 1):530–47. [PMID: 12853821]

WEB SITE

- Male Genital Pathology Index

INFORMATION FOR PATIENTS

- Mayo Clinic
- MedlinePlus—Benign prostatic hyperplasia

REFERENCES

- Bent S et al. Saw palmetto for benign prostatic hyperplasia. N Engl J Med. 2006 Feb 9;354(6):557–66. [PMID: 16467543]
- Djavan B et al. Benign prostatic hyperplasia progression and its impact on treatment. Curr Opin Urol. 2004 Jan; 14(1):45–50. [PMID: 15091050]

- Kaplan SA. Use of alpha-adrenergic inhibitors in treatment of benign prostatic hyperplasia and implications on sexual function. Urology. 2004 Mar; 63(3):428–34. [PMID: 15028431]
- McConnell JD et al; Medical Therapy of Prostatic Symptoms (MTOPS) Research Group. The long-term effect of doxazosin, finasteride, and combination therapy on the clinical progression of benign prostatic hyperplasia. N Engl J Med. 2003 Dec 18;349(25):2387–98. [PMID: 14681504]
- Thorpe A et al. Benign prostatic hyperplasia. Lancet. 2003 Apr 19; 361(9366):1359–67. [PMID: 12711484]
- Wilt TJ et al. Tamsulosin for benign prostatic hyperplasia. Cochrane Database Syst Rev 2003;(1):CD002081. [PMID: 12535426]

Bipolar Disorder

 KEY FEATURES

ESSENTIALS OF DIAGNOSIS

- Episodic mood shifts into mania, major depression, hypomania, and mixed states

GENERAL CONSIDERATIONS

- Manic episodes
  - Begin abruptly and may be triggered by life stresses
  - Last days to months—generally shorter than depressive episodes
  - Most common in spring and summer months
- Cyclothymia
  - Chronic mood disturbances with episodes of depression and hypomania
  - Symptoms are milder than those in a manic or depressive episode, but have at least a 2-year duration
  - Symptoms occasionally escalate to a full-blown manic or depressive episode, warranting a diagnosis of bipolar I or bipolar II disorder

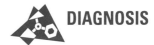 **CLINICAL FINDINGS**

SYMPTOMS AND SIGNS

- Manic episodes
  - Mood ranging from euphoria to irritability

  - Over-involvement in life activities
  - Flight of ideas with distractibility
  - Sleep disruption, little need for sleep
  - Racing thoughts
  - Behaviors may initially attract others
  - Irritability, mood lability, aggression, and grandiosity usually lead to problems in relationships
  - Excessive spending, resignation from a job, a hasty marriage or divorce, sexual acting out, or exhibitionism may occur
  - Atypical episodes involve gross delusions, paranoid ideations, and auditory hallucinations
  - "Rapid cyclers" experience four or more discrete episodes of mood disturbance per year
- Most depressions
  - Lowered mood, varying from mild sadness to intense feelings of guilt, worthlessness, and hopelessness
  - Difficulty in thinking, including inability to concentrate, ruminations, and lack of decisiveness
  - Loss of interest, with diminished involvement in work and recreation
  - Somatic complaints such as
    □ Headache
    □ Disrupted, lessened, or excessive sleep
    □ Loss of energy
    □ Change in appetite
  - Anxiety
- Some severe depressions
  - Psychomotor retardation or agitation
  - Delusions of a hypochondriacal or persecutory nature
  - Withdrawal from activities
  - Physical symptoms of major severity, eg,
    □ Anorexia
    □ Insomnia
    □ Reduced sexual drive
    □ Weight loss
    □ Various somatic complaints
  - Suicidal ideation

DIFFERENTIAL DIAGNOSIS

- Schizophrenia and other psychotic disorders
- Intoxication with stimulants
- Major depressive episode
- Hypothyroidism
- Dysthymia

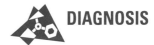 **DIAGNOSIS**

LABORATORY TESTS

- Consider thyroid-stimulating hormone
- Consider toxicology screen

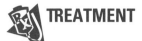

TREATMENT

MEDICATIONS

- Mania
  - Haloperidol (5–10 mg PO or IM q2–3h)
  - Alternatively, atypical neuroleptics (olanzapine 5–20 mg once daily) may be used initially to treat agitation and psychosis
  - Clonazepam (1–2 mg PO q4–6h) may be used instead of or in conjunction with a neuroleptic to control acute behavioral symptoms
  - Lithium (1200–1800 mg PO once daily targeted to therapeutic serum level)
    □ Effective in acute mania or hypomania, but takes several days to take effect
    □ As prophylaxis, can limit the frequency and severity of mood swings in 70% of patients
  - Valproic acid (750 mg/day divided and titrated to therapeutic levels) can be loaded to therapeutic levels in 2–3 days
  - Carbamazepine (800–1600 mg/day)
    □ Used in patients intolerant or unresponsive to lithium
    □ Also more effective than lithium in rapid cyclers
  - Calcium channel blockers (verapamil) have been used in refractory patients
  - Lamotrigine (25–50 mg/day titrated slowly upward) has good efficacy for bipolar depression
  - Topiramate has been found to be effective adjunctive treatment
- Depression
  - See Depression

THERAPEUTIC PROCEDURES

- Electroconvulsive therapy is effective in treatment of manic disorders in pregnant women, in whom medications are contraindicated

OUTCOME

FOLLOW-UP

- Lithium levels should be measured 5–7 days after initiation and dose changes, monthly to bimonthly early in treatment, and every 6–12 months in stable patients
- Thyroid and kidney function should be monitored every 3–4 months in patients taking lithium

- Liver function and blood counts must be monitored in patients taking valproic acid or carbamazepine
- Weight, fasting blood sugar, and lipids must be monitored in patients taking most atypical antipsychotics

COMPLICATIONS

- Suicide (see Depression)
- Drug–drug interactions complicate therapy with all agents—careful review of concomitant medications is needed
- Lithium toxicity occurs at serum levels > 2 mEq/L (see Lithium Toxicity)
- Long-term lithium use can cause cogwheel rigidity and other extrapyramidal signs

PROGNOSIS

- Good prognosis with adequate treatment
- Compliance with lithium is adversely affected by the loss of some hypomanic experiences valued by the patient

WHEN TO REFER

- When diagnosis is in question or when standard management strategies are ineffective
- Any question of suicidiality or irrational behavior

WHEN TO ADMIT

- In a depressive episode, patients who are at risk for suicide or self-harm
- Manic patients whose judgment is sufficiently impaired to make them a risk to themselves or others

EVIDENCE

PRACTICE GUIDELINES

- National Guideline Clearinghouse: American Psychiatric Association

WEB SITES

- American Psychiatric Association
- Internet Mental Health
- National Institute of Mental Health

INFORMATION FOR PATIENTS

- American Psychiatric Association
- National Institute of Mental Health

REFERENCES

- Krishnan KR. Psychiatric and medical comorbidities of bipolar disorder. Psychosom Med. 2005;67:1. [PMID: 15673617]
- Viguera AC et al. Reproductive decisions by women with bipolar disorder after prepregnancy psychiatric consultation. Am J Psychiatry. 2002;159:2102. [PMID: 12450965]

Bites, Animal & Human

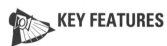

KEY FEATURES

ESSENTIALS OF DIAGNOSIS

- Cat and human bites are more likely to become infected than dog bites
- Bites to the hand are of special concern because of the possiblity of closed-space infection
- Antibiotic prophylaxis indicated for noninfected bites of the hand; hospitalization required for infected hand bites
- All infected wounds need to be cultured to direct therapy

GENERAL CONSIDERATIONS

- Biting animals are usually known by their victims, and most biting incidents are provoked (ie, bites occur while playing with the animal or waking it abruptly from sleep)
- Important determinants of whether bites become infected
  - The animal inflicting the bite
  - The location of the bite
  - Type of injury inflicted
- Bites on the extremities are more likely to become infected than bites on the head, face, and neck
- Failure to elicit a history of provocation is important, because an unprovoked attack raises the possibility of rabies
- **Human bites**
  - Usually inflicted by children while playing or fighting
  - In adults, bites are associated with alcohol use and closed-fist injuries that occur during fights
- Infections following human bites are variable
  - Because bites inflicted by children are superficial, they rarely become infected
  - Bites by adults become infected in 15–30% of cases, with a particularly

high rate of infection in closed-fist injuries
- Self-inflicted "through and through" bites involving the mucosa and skin have an infection rate similar to closed-fist injuries
- **Cat bites**
  - More likely to become infected than human bites
  - 30–50% of cat bites become infected
- **Dog bites,** for unclear reasons, become infected only 5% of the time
- **Puncture wounds** become infected more frequently than lacerations, probably because the latter are easier to irrigate and débride
- The bacteriology of dog and cat bites is polymicrobial
  - Over 50% of infections are caused by aerobes and anaerobes
  - 35% are caused by aerobes alone
  - Pure anaerobic infections are rare
- *Pasteurella* species are the single most common pathogen—75% of cat bites and 50% of dog bites
- Other common aerobes include
  - Streptococci
  - Staphylococci
  - *Moraxella*
  - *Neisseria*
- Common anaerobes include
  - *Fusobacterium*
  - *Bacteroides*
  - *Porphyromonas*
  - *Prevotella*
- Human bites are a mixture of aerobes and anaerobes in over 50% and aerobes alone in 44%
- Staphylococci, streptococci, and *Eikenella corrodens* (isolated in 30% of infections) are the most common aerobes
- *Prevotella* and *Fusobacterium* are the most common anaerobes
- Although the above named organisms are the most common, numerous others have been isolated such as *Capnocytophaga* (dogs and cats), *Pseudomonas,* and *Haemophilus,* emphasizing the need to culture all infected wounds to define bacteriology
- HIV transmission following a bite has been rarely reported; saliva not contaminated with blood is very low risk

DEMOGRAPHICS

- About 1000 dog bite injuries require emergency department attention each day, most often in urban areas
- Dog bites occur most commonly in the summer months

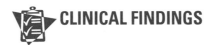

CLINICAL FINDINGS

SYMPTOMS AND SIGNS

Dog and cat bites
- Early infections (within 24 h after the bite) are characterized by
  - Rapid onset and progression
  - Fever
  - Chills
  - Cellulitis
  - Local adenopathy

Human bites
- **Early infections** can produce a rapidly progressive necrotizing infection
- **Late infections** (longer than 24 h after the bite)
  - Present with local swelling and erythema
  - Drainage and systemic symptoms may or may not be present

DIAGNOSIS

LABORATORY TESTS

- Because the bacteriology of the infections is so variable, always culture infected wounds and adjust therapy appropriately, especially if the patient is not responding to initial empiric treatment

IMAGING STUDIES

- Radiographs should be obtained to look for fractures and the presence of foreign bodies

TREATMENT

MEDICATIONS

Prophylactic antibiotics
- Prophylaxis is indicated in high-risk bites, eg, any cat bites and hand bites by any animal or by humans
- The drug of choice is amoxicillin-clavulanate (Augmentin) 500 mg PO TID for 3–5 days
- In the penicillin-allergic patient, clindamycin plus ciprofloxacin or levofloxacin is given
- Moxifloxacin may be suitable monotherapy alternative due to its mixed aerobic and anaerobic activity
- Immunocompromised and asplenic patients are at risk for developing overwhelming bacteremia and sepsis following animal bites and should also receive prophylaxis, even for low-risk bites

Antibiotics
- Infected wounds require antibiotics, either PO or IV, depending on individualized clinical decisions
- *Pasteurella multocida* is best treated with penicillin or a tetracycline
  - Other agents: second- and third-generation cephalosporins, fluoroquinolones, azithromycin or clarithromycin
  - Response to therapy is slow, and therapy should be continued for at least 2–3 weeks
- Human bites frequently require IV therapy with a β-lactam plus a β-lactamase inhibitor combination (Unasyn, Timentin, Zosyn), cefoxitin or, in the penicillin-allergic patient, clindamycin plus a fluoroquinolone

THERAPEUTIC PROCEDURES

- Careful examination to assess the extent of the injury (tendon laceration, joint space penetration) is critical to appropriate care
- Vigorous cleansing and irrigation of the wound as well as débridement of necrotic material are the most important factors in decreasing the incidence of infections
- If wounds require closure for cosmetic or mechanical reasons, suturing can be done
- Never suture an infected wound, and wounds of the hand should generally not be sutured since a closed-space infection of the hand can result in loss of function

OUTCOME

FOLLOW-UP

- Careful follow-up is required every 1–2 days to assess improvement

COMPLICATIONS

- Osteomyelitis
- Tendon rupture
- Abscess

PROGNOSIS

- Generally good, but resolution may be slow, especially with *Pasteurella* infections

WHEN TO REFER

- Bites to the hand
- Failure to improve within 2–3 days

WHEN TO ADMIT

- Human bites to the hand are usually admitted to the hospital

PREVENTION

- All patients must be evaluated for the need for tetanus (Tables 67, 68, and 69) and rabies prophylaxis (see Rabies)

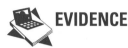

EVIDENCE

PRACTICE GUIDELINES

- Update on emerging infections from the Centers for Disease Control and Prevention. Update rabies postexposure prophylaxis guidelines. Ann Emerg Med. 1999;33:590. [PMID: 10216339]

INFORMATION FOR PATIENTS

- National Institutes of Health
- The Mayo Clinic

REFERENCES

- Brook I. Microbiology and management of human and animal bite wound infections. Prim Care. 2003 Mar;30(1):25–39. [PMID: 12825249]
- Talan DA et al. Clinical presentation and bacteriologic analysis of infected human bites in patients presenting to emergency departments. Clin Infect Dis. 2003 Dec 1;37(11):1481–9. [PMID: 14614671]
- Taplitz RA. Managing bite wounds. Currently recommended antibiotics for treatment and prophylaxis. Postgrad Med. 2004 Aug;116(2):49–52, 55–6, 59. [PMID: 15323154]

Bites, Insect

KEY FEATURES

ESSENTIALS OF DIAGNOSIS

- Localized rash with pruritus
- Furuncle-like lesions containing live arthropods
- Tender erythematous patches that migrate ("larva migrans")
- Generalized urticaria or erythema multiforme in some patients

GENERAL CONSIDERATIONS

- Body lice, fleas, bedbugs, and mosquitoes should be considered
- Arthropods
  - Most persons can readily detect the bites (eg, mosquitoes and biting flies)
  - However, in other persons, the reaction can be delayed for many hours
  - Many persons are allergic
- Spiders
  - Often incorrectly believed to be the source of bites
  - They rarely attack humans
  - However, the brown spider (*Loxosceles laeta, Loxosceles reclusa*) may cause severe necrotic reactions and death due to intravascular hemolysis
  - The black widow spider (*Latrodectus mactans*) may cause severe systemic symptoms and death
- In addition to arthropod bites, the most common lesions are
  - Venomous stings (wasps, hornets, bees, ants, scorpions)
  - Bites (centipedes)
  - Furuncle-like lesions due to fly maggots or sand fleas in the skin
  - Linear creeping eruption due to a migrating larva
- Fleas
  - *Ctenocephalides felis* and *Ctenocephalides canis* are the most common species found on cats and dogs
  - Both species attack humans
  - The human flea is *Pulex irritans*
- Bedbugs are found in crevices of beds or furniture
- Ticks are usually picked up by brushing against low vegetation
- Chiggers or red bugs are larvae of trombiculid mites
- Bird and rodent mites
  - Larger than chiggers
  - Bites are multiple anywhere on the body
- Mites in stored products
  - White and almost invisible
  - Infest products such as vanilla pods, sugar, straw, cottonseeds, cereals
  - Persons who handle these products may be attacked on the hands, forearms and sometimes on the feet
- Caterpillars of moths with urticating hairs
  - Hairs are blown from cocoons or carried by emergent moths, causing severe and often seasonally recurrent outbreaks after mass emergence
  - The gypsy moth is a cause in eastern United States
- Tungiasis
  - Due to the burrowing flea *Tunga penetrans* and found in Africa, the West Indies, South and Central America
  - The female burrows under the skin, sucks blood, swells to 0.5 cm, and then ejects her eggs onto the ground

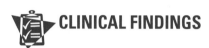

CLINICAL FINDINGS

SYMPTOMS AND SIGNS

- Individual bites are often in clusters and tend to occur either on exposed parts (eg, midges and gnats) or under clothing, especially around the waist or at flexures (eg, small mites or insects in bedding or clothing)
- The reaction is often delayed for 1–24 h or more
- Pruritus is almost always present and may be all but intolerable once the patient starts to scratch
- Secondary infection may follow scratching
- Urticarial wheals are common; papules may become vesicular
- Flea saliva and bedbugs produce papular urticaria in sensitized individuals
- Chiggers or red bugs
  - A few species attack humans, often around the waist, on the ankles, or in flexures, raising intensely itching erythematous papules after a delay of many hours
  - The red chiggers may sometimes be seen in the center of papules that have not yet been scratched
- Tungiasis: ulceration, lymphangitis, gangrene, and septicemia may result, in some cases with lethal effect

DIFFERENTIAL DIAGNOSIS

- Scabies
- Lice
- Fleas
- Bedbugs
- Ticks
- Chiggers or red bugs
- Bird or rodent mites
- Tungiasis (burrowing flea)

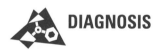

DIAGNOSIS

- Diagnosis is based on the clinical features, but may be aided by searching for exposure to arthropods and by considering the patient's occupation and recent activities

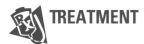

TREATMENT

MEDICATIONS

- Corticosteroid lotions or creams are helpful
- Calamine lotion or a cool wet dressing is always appropriate
- Topical antibiotics may be applied if secondary infection is suspected
- Localized persistent lesions may be treated with intralesional corticosteroids
- Stings produced by many arthropods may be alleviated by applying papain powder (Adolph's Meat Tenderizer) mixed with water, or aluminum chloride hexahydrate (Xerac AC)
- To break the life cycle of the flea, one must repeatedly treat the home and pets, using quick-kill insecticides, residual insecticides, and a growth regulator
- Tungiasis
  - Ethyl chloride spray kills the insect when applied to the lesion
  - Disinfestation may be accomplished with insecticide applied to the terrain
  - Simple surgical excision is usually performed

THERAPEUTIC PROCEDURES

- Living arthropods should be removed carefully with tweezers after application of alcohol and preserved in alcohol for identification

OUTCOME

WHEN TO REFER

- If there is a question about the diagnosis, if recommended therapy is ineffective, or specialized treatment is necessary

PREVENTION

- Avoidance of contaminated areas
- Personal cleanliness
- Disinfection of clothing, bedclothes, and furniture as indicated
- Benzyl benzoate and dimethylphthalate are excellent acaricides
  - Clothing should be impregnated by spray or by dipping in a soapy emulsion

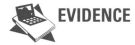

EVIDENCE

PRACTICE GUIDELINES

- Stinging insect hypersensitivity: a practice parameter update. http://www.guideline.gov/summary/summary.aspx?ss=15&doc_id=6888&nbr=4212
- Centers for Disease Control and Prevention

INFORMATION FOR PATIENTS

- American College of Allergy, Asthma & Immunology: Insect Stings
- Centers for Disease Control and Prevention: Protection against Mosquitoes and Other Arthropods
- Mayo Clinic: Insect Bites and Stings
- Nemours Foundation: Bug Bites and Stings (Bedbug, Bee, Black Widow Spider, Brown Recluse Spider, Chigger, Fire Ant, Flea, Gnat, Louse, Mosquito, Scorpion, Tarantula, Tick)

REFERENCES

- Scarupa MD et al. Bedbug bites masquerading as urticaria. J Allergy Clin Immunol. 2006 Jun;117(6):1508–9. [PMID: 16751024]
- Swanson DL et al. Bites of brown recluse spiders and suspected necrotic arachnidism. N Engl J Med. 2005 Feb 17;352(7):700–7. [PMID: 15716564]

Bladder Cancer

KEY FEATURES

ESSENTIALS OF DIAGNOSIS

- Irritative voiding symptoms
- Gross or microscopic hematuria
- Positive urinary cytology in most patients
- Filling defect within bladder noted on imaging

GENERAL CONSIDERATIONS

- Second most common urologic cancer
- More common in men than women (2.7:1)
- Mean age at diagnosis is 65 years
- Risk factors: cigarette smoking, exposure to industrial dyes and solvents

Pathology

- Urothelial cell carcinomas: ~90%
- Squamous cell cancers: ~7%
- Adenocarcinomas: ~2%
- Bladder cancer staging is based on the extent of bladder wall penetration and the presence of either regional or distant metastases
- Natural history is based on tumor recurrence and progression to higher stage disease. Both are related to tumor grade and stage

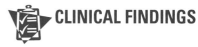

CLINICAL FINDINGS

SYMPTOMS AND SIGNS

- Hematuria is the presenting symptom in 85–90%
- Irritative voiding symptoms in a small percent
- Masses detected on bimanual examination with large-volume or deeply infiltrating cancers
- Lymphedema of the lower extremities with locally advanced cancers or metastases to pelvic lymph nodes
- Hepatomegaly or palpable lymphadenopathy with metastatic disease

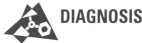

DIAGNOSIS

LABORATORY TESTS

- Urinalysis—hematuria; on occasion, pyuria
- Azotemia
- Anemia

IMAGING STUDIES

- Ultrasound, CT, MRI show filling defects within the bladder

DIAGNOSTIC PROCEDURES

- Cytology useful in detecting disease at initial presentation or recurrence
- Cytology very sensitive (80–90%) in detecting cancers of higher grade and stage
- Imaging done primarily for evaluating the upper urinary tract and staging
- Cystourethroscopy and biopsy
- Diagnosis and staging are by cystoscopy and transurethral resection of bladder tumor (TURBT)
- TURBT can be done under general or regional anesthesia
- Resection down to muscular elements of the bladder
- Random bladder and, on occasion, prostate urethral biopsies

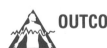

TREATMENT

MEDICATIONS

- Patients with superficial cancers (Ta, T1) are treated with complete TURBT and selective use of intravesical chemotherapy
- Patients with large, high-grade, recurrent Ta lesions, T1 cancers, and carcinoma in situ are treated with TURBT and intravesical chemotherapy
- Patients with more invasive (T2, T3) but still localized cancers require more aggressive surgery (radical cystectomy), or the combination of chemotherapy and selective surgery
- Patients with evidence of lymph node or distant metastases should undergo systemic chemotherapy
- Intravesical chemotherapy
  - Immunotherapeutic or chemotherapeutic agents administered weekly for 6–12 weeks
  - Maintenance therapy after the initial induction regimen includes bacillus Calmette-Guérin, thiotepa, mitomycin, or doxorubicin

SURGERY

- Transurethral resection is diagnostic, allows for proper staging, and controls superficial cancers
- Partial cystectomy is indicated in patients with cancers in a bladder diverticulum
- Radical cystectomy with urinary diversion—a conduit of small or large bowel
- Continent forms of diversion available, improve quality of life

THERAPEUTIC PROCEDURES

- Radiotherapy: external beam therapy over a 6- to 8-week period
- Chemotherapy (systemic)
  - Cisplatin-based combination chemotherapy
  - Combination radiotherapy and systemic chemotherapy or surgery, radiotherapy, and systemic chemotherapy

OUTCOME

COMPLICATIONS

- Intravesical chemotherapy: side effects include irritative voiding symptoms and hemorrhagic cystitis
- Radiotherapy
  - Bladder, bowel, or rectal complications develop in about 10–15% of patients
  - Local recurrence is common (30–70%)

PROGNOSIS

- About 50–80% of bladder cancers are superficial (Ta, Tis, or T1) at initial presentation
  - Lymph node metastases and progression are uncommon in such patients when they are properly treated
  - Survival is excellent at 81%
- 5-year survival of patients with T2 and T3 disease ranges from 50% to 75% after radical cystectomy
- Long-term survival for patients with metastatic disease at presentation is rare

EVIDENCE

PRACTICE GUIDELINES

- Oosterlinck W et al. Guidelines on bladder cancer. Eur Urol. 2002;41:105. [PMID: 12074395]
- Segal R et al; Cancer Care Ontario Practice Guidelines Initiative Genitourinary Cancer Disease Site Group. Adjuvant chemotherapy for deep muscle-invasive transitional cell bladder carcinoma—a practice guideline. Can J Urol. 2002; 9:1625. [PMID: 12431323]

INFORMATION FOR PATIENTS

- American Urological Association
- Cleveland Clinic — Bladder cancer
- Mayo Clinic

REFERENCES

- Carroll PR. Urothelial carcinoma: cancers of the bladder, ureter and renal pelvis. In: *Smith's General Urology,* 16th ed. Tanagho EA, McAninch JW (editors). McGraw-Hill, 2003.
- Droller MJ. Primary care update on kidney and bladder cancer: a urologic perspective. Med Clin North Am. 2004 Mar;88(2):309–28. [PMID: 15049580]
- Habuchi T et al. Prognostic markers for bladder cancer: International consensus panel on bladder tumor markers. Urology. 2005 Dec;66(6 Suppl 1):64–74. [PMID: 16399416]
- Kim HL et al. The current status of bladder preservation in the treatment of muscle invasive bladder cancer. J Urol. 2000 Sep;164(3 Pt 1):627–32. [PMID: 10953112]
- Krejci KG et al. Immunotherapy for urological malignancies. J Urol. 2004 Feb;171(2 Pt 1):870–6. [PMID: 14713844]
- Shelley MD et al. Intravesical bacillus Calmette-Guerin versus mitomycin C for Ta and T1 bladder cancer. Cochrane Database Syst Rev. 2003; (3):CD003231. [PMID: 12917955]
- Sternberg CN et al. Chemotherapy for bladder cancer: treatment guidelines for neoadjuvant chemotherapy, bladder preservation, adjuvant chemotherapy, and metastatic cancer. Urology. 2007 Jan;69(1 Suppl):62–79. [PMID: 17280909]

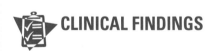

Bone & Joint Mycotic Infections

KEY FEATURES

- **Candidal osteomyelitis**
  - Occurs in malnourished patients undergoing prolonged hospitalization for cancer, neutropenia, trauma, complicated abdominal surgical procedures, or injection drug use
  - Infected IV catheters frequently serve as a hematogenous source
- **Coccidioidomycosis**
  - Usually secondary to a primary pulmonary infection
  - Arthralgia with periarticular swelling, especially in the knees and ankles, occurring as a nonspecific manifestation of systemic coccidioidomycosis, should be distinguished from actual bone or joint infection
  - Osseous lesions commonly occur in cancellous bone of the vertebrae or near the ends of long bones at tendinous insertions; these lesions are initially osteolytic and thus may mimic metastatic tumor or myeloma

CLINICAL FINDINGS

- Joint and bone pain and swelling

DIAGNOSIS

- Culture studies of synovial fluid

- **Coccidioidomycosis**
  - Recovery of *Coccidioides immitis* from the lesion or histologic examination of tissue obtained by open biopsy
  - Rising titers of complement-fixing antibodies also provide evidence of the disseminated nature of the disease

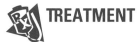 **TREATMENT**

- **Candidal:** fluconazole, 200 mg PO BID, is probably as effective as amphotericin
- **Coccidioidomycosis**
  - Itraconazole, 200 mg BID for 6–12 mo
  - May require operative excision of infected bone and soft tissue
  - Amputation may be the only solution for stubbornly progressive infections

Bone Tumors & Tumor-Like Lesions

 KEY FEATURES

- Persistent pain, swelling, or tenderness of a skeletal part
- Pathologic ("spontaneous") fractures
- Suspicious areas of bony enlargement, deformity, radiodensity, or radiolucency on radiograph
- Histologic evidence of bone neoplasm on biopsy specimen
- Primary tumors of bone are relatively uncommon in comparison with secondary or metastatic neoplasms
- Osteosarcoma, the most common malignancy of bone, typically occurs in adolescents

 CLINICAL FINDINGS

- Osteosarcoma may present as pain or swelling in a bone or joint (especially in or around the knee)
- When the symptoms appear following a sports-related injury, accurate diagnosis may be delayed

 DIAGNOSIS

- Biopsy (which is not always definitive)
- Differential diagnosis
  - Benign developmental skeletal abnormalities
  - Metastatic neoplastic disease
  - Infections (eg, osteomyelitis)
  - Posttraumatic bone lesions
  - Metabolic disease of bone
  - Osteoid osteomas
  - Osteosarcoma
  - Fibrosarcomas
  - Enchondromas
  - Chondromyxoid fibromas
  - Chondrosarcomas
  - Giant cell tumors (osteoclastomas)
  - Chondroblastomas
  - Ewing's sarcoma

 TREATMENT

- Chemotherapy for some
- Osteosarcomas: treated by resection and chemotherapy; 5-year survival rate of 60%
- Osteoid osteomas (seen in children and adolescents) should be surgically removed
- Tumors derived from cartilage treated with appropriate curettement or surgery have good prognosis
- Ewing's sarcoma (affects children, adolescents, and young adults), has a 50% mortality rate in spite of chemotherapy, irradiation, and surgery

Bradycardias

 KEY FEATURES

- Bradycardia most commonly results from impaired sinus node function or from conduction abnormalities, which can occur between sinus node and atrium, within atrioventricular (AV) node or intraventricular conduction pathways
- Sick sinus syndrome (SSS) occurs most commonly in the elderly
- AV block subtypes
  - First-degree and second-degree Mobitz type I block occur with
    □ Heightened vagal tone in normal individuals

    □ Drugs that block the AV node, often in persons with organic heart disease
    □ Ischemia, infarction, inflammatory processes, fibrosis, calcification, or infiltration
  - Second-degree Mobitz type II block occurs with organic heart disease involving the infranodal conduction system
  - Third-degree (complete) block occurs with lesions at or below the His bundle

 CLINICAL FINDINGS

- **SSS, first- and second-degree block**
  - Most patients are asymptomatic
  - Rarely, patients experience syncope, dizziness, confusion, palpitations, heart failure, or angina pectoris
  - Symptoms are nonspecific and thus must coincide temporally with arrhythmias
- **Third-degree block**
  - Patients may be asymptomatic or may complain of weakness, dyspnea, or abrupt syncope if heart rate < 35/min
  - Slow ventricular rate, usually < 50/min, that does not increase with exercise
  - Cannon venous pulsations in the neck

 DIAGNOSIS

- SSS: ECG shows
  - Sinus arrest
  - Sinoatrial exit block (a pause equal to a multiple of the underlying PP interval or progressive shortening of the PP interval before a pause)
  - Persistent sinus bradycardia
- Prolonged ambulatory Holter monitoring or event recorder may be required to document correspondence of bradycardia with symptoms
- AV block
  - First-degree: PR interval > 0.21 s with all atrial impulses conducted
  - Mobitz type I second-degree: progressive lengthening of PR interval and shortening of RR interval before the blocked beat
  - Mobitz type II second-degree: intermittent nonconducted atrial beats are not preceded by a lengthening PR interval
  - Third-degree (complete): ventricular rate usually < 50/min, wide QRS, and no supraventricular impulses being conducted to the ventricles

– Narrow QRS complexes suggest nodal block
– Wide QRS complexes suggest infra-nodal block
• Electrophysiologic studies may be necessary for accurate localization

TREATMENT

• Discontinue offending drugs
• Most symptomatic patients require permanent (preferably dual-chamber) pacemaker implantation
• First-degree and Mobitz type I block
  – Discontinue offending drugs
  – Other therapy is not usually needed
• Mobitz type II block: prophylactic pacemaker implantation is usually required because of risk of progression to third-degree block
• Third-degree block
  – Permanent pacemaker implantation
  – Temporary pacing, if permanent pacing is delayed

Brain Abscess

KEY FEATURES

ESSENTIALS OF DIAGNOSIS

• Symptoms and signs of expanding intracranial mass
• There may be signs of a primary infection or of congenital heart disease
• Fever may be absent

GENERAL CONSIDERATIONS

• Presents as an intracranial space-occupying lesion
• May occur as a sequela of ear or sinus infection, a complication of infection elsewhere in the body, or an infection introduced intracranially by trauma or surgical procedures
• Most common infective organisms
  – Streptococci
  – Staphylococci
  – Anaerobes
• Mixed infections are not uncommon

CLINICAL FINDINGS

SYMPTOMS AND SIGNS

• Early symptoms
  – Headache
  – Drowsiness
  – Inattention
  – Confusion
  – Seizures
• Later signs
  – Increasing intracranial pressure
  – Focal neurologic deficits
• There may be little or no systemic evidence of infection

DIFFERENTIAL DIAGNOSIS

• Other rapidly expanding intracranial space-occupying lesions

DIAGNOSIS

LABORATORY TESTS

• Examination of the cerebrospinal fluid does not help in diagnosis and lumbar puncture may precipitate herniation

IMAGING STUDIES

• CT scan of the head characteristically shows an area of contrast enhancement surrounding a low-density core (similar to metastatic neoplasms)
• MRI permits earlier recognition of focal cerebritis or abscess
• Arteriography indicates the presence of a space-occupying lesion (avascular mass with displacement of normal cerebral vessels) but provides no clue to the nature of the lesion

TREATMENT

MEDICATIONS

• IV antibiotics, combined with surgical drainage (aspiration or excision) if necessary to reduce the mass effect, or to establish the diagnosis
• Broad-spectrum antibiotics are used if the infecting organism is unknown (Table 63)
  – A common regimen is penicillin G (2 million units q2h IV) plus either chloramphenicol (1–2 g IV q6h), metronidazole (750 mg IV q6h), or both
  – Nafcillin is added if *Staphylococcus aureus* is suspected

• Antimicrobial treatment is usually continued parenterally for 6–8 weeks, then orally for another 2–3 weeks
• Dexamethasone (4–25 mg QID, depending on severity, followed by tapering of dose, depending on response) may reduce any associated edema; IV mannitol is sometimes required

THERAPEUTIC PROCEDURES

• Aspiration or excision if necessary to reduce mass effect or to establish the diagnosis

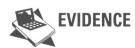

OUTCOME

FOLLOW-UP

• Monitor patient by serial CT scans or MRI every 2 weeks and at deterioration

COMPLICATIONS

• Seizures
• Focal neurologic deficits

PROGNOSIS

• Abscesses smaller than 2 cm can often be cured medically

WHEN TO ADMIT

• When the diagnosis is suspected

EVIDENCE

PRACTICE GUIDELINES

• Evaluation and management of intracranial mass lesions in AIDS. Report of the Quality Standards Subcommittee of the American Academy of Neurology. Neurology. 1998;50:21. [PMID: 9443452]

WEB SITES

• The Whole Brain Atlas
• CNS Pathology Index

INFORMATION FOR PATIENTS

• National Institutes of Health

REFERENCE

• Kastrup O et al. Neuroimaging of infections. NeuroRx. 2005 Apr;2(2):324–32. [PMID: 15897953]

Brain Tumor, Primary

 KEY FEATURES

ESSENTIALS OF DIAGNOSIS

- Personality changes, intellectual decline, emotional lability
- Seizures, headaches, nausea
- Increased intracranial pressure in some patients
- Neuroradiologic evidence of space-occupying lesion

GENERAL CONSIDERATIONS

- Half of all primary intracranial neoplasms (Table 134) are gliomas
- The other half is composed of
  - Meningiomas
  - Pituitary adenomas
  - Neurofibromas
  - Other tumors
- Certain tumors (eg, neurofibromas, hemangioblastomas, and retinoblastomas) have a familial basis
- May lead to a generalized disturbance of cerebral function and symptoms of increased intracranial pressure

DEMOGRAPHICS

- Tumors may occur at any age, but some gliomas are age-specific (Table 134)

 CLINICAL FINDINGS

SYMPTOMS AND SIGNS

Herniation symptoms

- Temporal lobe uncus herniation with compression of the third cranial nerve, midbrain, and posterior cerebral artery
  - Ipsilateral pupillary dilation
  - Followed by stupor, coma, decerebrate posturing, and respiratory arrest
- Cerebellar tonsillar displacement causing medullary compression, apnea, circulatory collapse, and death

Focal deficits

- **Frontal lobe lesions**
  - Progressive intellectual decline, slowing of mental activity, personality changes, and contralateral grasp reflexes
  - Expressive aphasia if the posterior part of the left inferior frontal gyrus is involved
  - Anosmia secondary to pressure on the olfactory nerve
  - Precentral lesions may cause focal motor seizures or contralateral pyramidal deficits
- **Temporal lobe lesions**
  - Seizures with olfactory or gustatory hallucinations, motor automatisms, and impairment of external awareness without actual loss of consciousness
  - Depersonalization, emotional changes, behavioral disturbances, sensations of déjà vu or jamais vu
  - Micropsia or macropsia (objects appear smaller or larger than they are), visual field defects (crossed upper quadrantanopia), and auditory illusions or hallucinations
  - Left-sided lesions may lead to dysnomia and receptive aphasia, while right-sided involvement may disturb the perception of musical notes and melodies
- **Parietal lobe lesions**
  - May cause sensory seizures
  - Contralateral disturbances of sensation, sensory loss or inattention (cortical in type and involves postural sensibility and tactile discrimination, so that the appreciation of shape, size, weight, and texture is impaired)
  - Objects placed in the hand may not be recognized (astereognosis)
  - Extensive lesions may produce contralateral hyperpathia and spontaneous pain (thalamic syndrome)
  - Optic radiation involvement leads to a contralateral homonymous field defect that sometimes consists solely of lower quadrantanopia
  - Left angular gyrus lesions cause Gerstmann's syndrome (alexia, agraphia, acalculia, right-left confusion, and finger agnosia), whereas involvement of the left submarginal gyrus causes ideational apraxia
  - Anosognosia (denial, neglect, or rejection of a paralyzed limb) is seen in patients with lesions of the nondominant (right) hemisphere
  - Constructional apraxia and dressing apraxia may also occur with right-sided lesions
- **Occipital lobe lesions**
  - Crossed homonymous hemianopia or a partial field defect
  - Left-sided or bilateral lesions may cause visual agnosia; irritative lesions on either side can cause unformed visual hallucinations
  - Bilateral occipital lobe involvement causes cortical blindness with preservation of pupillary responses to light and lack of awareness of the defect by the patient
  - Loss of color perception, prosopagnosia (inability to identify a familiar face), simultagnosia (inability to integrate and interpret a composite scene as opposed to its individual elements), and Balint's syndrome (failure to turn the eyes to a particular point in space, despite preservation of spontaneous and reflex eye movements), denial of blindness or a field defect (Anton's syndrome)
- **Brainstem and cerebellar lesions**
  - Brainstem lesions lead to cranial nerve palsies, ataxia, incoordination, nystagmus, and pyramidal and sensory deficits in the limbs
  - Intrinsic brainstem tumors, such as gliomas, cause an increase in intracranial pressure, usually late
  - Marked ataxia of the trunk if the vermis cerebelli is involved
  - Ipsilateral appendicular deficits (ataxia, incoordination and hypotonia of the limbs) if the cerebellar hemispheres are affected
- **False localizing signs**
  - Neurologic signs other than by direct compression or infiltration, leading to errors of clinical localization
  - Include third or sixth nerve palsy and bilateral extensor plantar responses produced by herniation syndromes, and an extensor plantar response occurring ipsilateral to a hemispheric tumor because the opposite cerebral peduncle is compressed against the tentorium

DIFFERENTIAL DIAGNOSIS

- Metastatic intracranial tumors
  - Cerebral metastases
  - Leptomeningeal metastases (carcinomatous meningitis)
- Intracranial mass lesions in AIDS patients

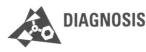 **DIAGNOSIS**

IMAGING STUDIES

- MRI with gadolinium
  - Best for tumors in the posterior fossa
- CT scanning
  - Characteristic appearance of meningiomas is virtually diagnostic
  - Noncontrast CT shows a lesion in the parasagittal and sylvian regions, olfactory groove, sphenoidal ridge, or tuberculum sellae with a homogeneous area of increased density, which enhances uniformly with contrast

- Arteriography
  - May show stretching or displacement of normal cerebral vessels by the tumor and tumor vascularity
  - An avascular mass may be due to tumor, hematoma, abscess, or any space-occupying lesion
  - Used to distinguish between a pituitary adenoma and an arterial aneurysm in patients with normal hormone levels and an intrasellar mass

DIAGNOSTIC PROCEDURES

- Lumbar puncture is rarely necessary
  - Findings are seldom diagnostic
  - Herniation is a risk

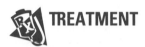 **TREATMENT**

MEDICATIONS

- Corticosteroids help reduce cerebral edema and are usually started before surgery
- Herniation is treated with IV dexamethasone (10–20 mg as a bolus, followed by 4 mg q6h) and IV mannitol (20% solution given in a dose of 1.5 g/kg over about 30 min)
- Anticonvulsants in standard doses (Table 133): controversial whether to start these prophylactically or only after a first seizure

SURGERY

- Complete surgical removal if the tumor is extra-axial (eg, meningioma, acoustic neuroma) or is not in a critical or inaccessible region of the brain (eg, cerebellar hemangioblastoma)
- Surgery may be diagnostic and may relieve intracranial pressure symptoms even if the neoplasm cannot be completely removed
- Simple surgical shunting procedures help in cases with obstructive hydrocephalus

THERAPEUTIC PROCEDURES

- Treatment depends on the type and site of the tumor (Table 134) and the condition of the patient
- Palliative care is important for patients who deteriorate despite treatment
- With malignant gliomas, radiation therapy increases median survival rates regardless of preceding surgery; chemotherapy provides additional benefit
- Indications for irradiation for other primary intracranial neoplasms depend on

tumor type and accessibility and the feasibility of complete surgical removal

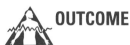 **OUTCOME**

COMPLICATIONS

- Long-term neurocognitive deficits resulting from radiation therapy

WHEN TO REFER

- All patients should be referred to neuro-oncologists or neurosurgeons

WHEN TO ADMIT

- Altered sensorium
- Specialized treatment or surgery

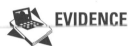 **EVIDENCE**

PRACTICE GUIDELINES

- National Guideline Clearinghouse: Practice parameter: anticonvulsant prophylaxis in patients with newly diagnosed brain tumors. Report of the Quality Standards Subcommittee of the American Academy of Neurology, 2000.

WEB SITES

- Anaplastic Astrocytoma Demonstration Case
- The Whole Brain Atlas
- University of Utah CNS Pathology Index

INFORMATION FOR PATIENTS

- National Cancer Institute
- Patient Education Institute

REFERENCES

- Byrne TN. Cognitive sequelae of brain tumor treatment. Curr Opin Neurol. 2005 Dec;18(6):662–6. [PMID: 16280677]
- Gonzalez J et al. Treatment of astrocytomas. Curr Opin Neurol. 2005 Dec; 18(6):632–8. [PMID: 16280673]
- Henson JW. Treatment of glioblastoma multiforme. Arch Neurol. 2006 Mar; 63(3):337–41. [PMID: 16533960]
- Taillibert S et al. Palliative care in patients with primary brain tumors. Curr Opin Oncol. 2004 Nov; 16(6):587–92. [PMID: 15627022]
- Tam Truong M. Current role of radiation therapy in the management of malignant brain tumors. Hematol Oncol Clin North Am. 2006 Apr; 20(2):431–53. [PMID: 16730301]
- Wen PY et al. Malignant gliomas. Curr Neurol Neurosci Rep. 2004 May; 4(3):218–27. [PMID: 15102348]

Breast Cancer, Female

 KEY FEATURES

ESSENTIALS OF DIAGNOSIS

- Early findings
  - Single, nontender, firm to hard mass with ill-defined margins
  - Mammographic abnormalities
  - No palpable mass
- Later findings
  - Skin or nipple retraction
  - Axillary lymphadenopathy
  - Breast enlargement, redness, edema, pain
  - Fixation of mass to skin or chest wall

GENERAL CONSIDERATIONS

- Second most common cancer in women
- Second most common cause of cancer death in women
- Develops in 1 of 8 American women in her lifetime
- ~178,000 new cases and ~41,000 deaths from breast cancer in US women estimated for 2007

DEMOGRAPHICS

- Mean and median age: 60–61 years
- More common in whites
- 3–4 times increased risk in those whose mother or sister had breast cancer, risk is further increased if family member had premenopausal or bilateral disease
- 1.5 times increased incidence if nulliparous or first full-term pregnancy at age > 35
- Slight increased risk if menarche at age < 12 or natural menopause at age > 50
- Increased incidence in fibrocystic disease with
  - Proliferative changes
  - Papillomatosis
  - Increased breast density on mammogram
  - Atypical ductal epithelial hyperplasia
- Contralateral cancer develops in women with prior breast cancer at a rate of 1–2% per year

- Increased risk with long-term use of hormone replacement therapy
- Increased risk if history of uterine cancer
- 85% lifetime risk in women with *BRCA1* gene mutations
- Increased risk with *BRCA2*, ataxia-telangiectasia, and *p53* gene mutations

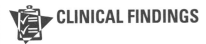

CLINICAL FINDINGS

SYMPTOMS AND SIGNS

- Presenting complaint is a lump (usually painless) in 70%
- Less frequently
  - Breast pain
  - Nipple discharge
  - Erosion, retraction, enlargement, or itching of the nipple
  - Redness, generalized hardness, enlargement, or shrinking of the breast
  - Axillary mass or swelling of the arm (rare)
- With metastatic disease, back or bone pain, jaundice, or weight loss
- Physical examination is done with patient sitting arms at sides and then overhead, and supine with arm abducted
- Findings include
  - Nontender, firm or hard mass with poorly delineated margins
  - Skin or nipple retraction
  - Breast asymmetry
  - Erosions of nipple epithelium
  - Watery, serous or bloody discharge
- Metastatic disease suggested by
  - Firm or hard axillary nodes > 1 cm
  - Axillary nodes that are matted or fixed to skin or deep structures indicate advanced disease (at least stage III)
- Advanced stage (stage IV) cancer suggested by ipsilateral supraclavicular or infraclavicular nodes

DIFFERENTIAL DIAGNOSIS

- Fibrocystic disease or cyst
- Fibroadenoma
- Intraductal papilloma
- Lipoma
- Fat necrosis

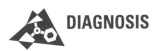

DIAGNOSIS

LABORATORY TESTS

- Alkaline phosphatase increased in liver or bone metastases
- Serum calcium elevated in advanced disease
- Carcinoembryonic antigen (CEA) and CA 15-3 or CA 27-29 are tumor markers for recurrent breast cancer

IMAGING STUDIES

- Mammography
- Breast ultrasound may differentiate cystic from solid masses
- MRI and positron emission tomography (PET) may play a role in imaging atypical lesions but only after diagnostic mammography
- CT scan of chest, abdomen, pelvis, and brain may demonstrate metastases
- Bone scan may show bony metastases in symptomatic patients
- PET scan is under investigation as single test for evaluation of breast, lymphatics, and metastases

DIAGNOSTIC PROCEDURES

- Fine-needle aspiration (FNA) or core biopsy
- Open biopsy under local anesthesia if needle biopsy inconclusive
- Computerized stereotactic or ultrasound guided core needle biopsies for nonpalpable lesions found on mammogram
- TNM staging (I–IV) (Table 48)
- Cytologic examination of breast nipple discharge occasionally helpful

TREATMENT

MEDICATIONS

Potentially curable disease

- Adjuvant chemotherapy improves survival
- Tamoxifen or aromatase inhibitors in hormone receptor-positive patients
- CMF (cyclophosphamide, methotrexate, fluorouracil)
- AC (Adriamycin [doxorubicin], cyclophosphamide) with taxanes (docetaxel or paclitaxel)

Metastatic disease

- Table 50
- For hormone receptor-positive postmenopausal patients, palliative tamoxifen (20 mg PO once daily) or aromatase inhibitors (eg, anastrozole 1 mg PO once daily)
- For patients who initially respond to tamoxifen, but then relapse, consider aromatase inhibitors
- For metastatic disease, chemotherapy should be considered
  - If visceral metastases (especially brain or lung lymphangitic)
  - If hormonal treatment is unsuccessful or disease progresses after initial response to hormonal manipulation
  - If tumor is estrogen receptor-negative
- AC achieves response rate of ~85%
- Combinations of cyclophosphamide, vincristine, methotrexate, fluorouracil, and taxanes achieve response rates of up to 60–70%
- Paclitaxel achieves response rate of 30–40%
- Trastuzumab, a monoclonal antibody that binds to HER-2/*neu* receptors on the cancer cell, is highly effective in HER-2/*neu*-expressive cancers
- High-dose chemotherapy and autologous bone marrow or stem cell transplantation produce no improvement in survival over conventional chemotherapy

SURGERY

- Surgery indicated for stage I and II cancers
- Disease-free survival rates are similar with partial mastectomy plus axillary dissection followed by radiation therapy and with modified radical mastectomy (total mastectomy plus axillary dissection)
- Relative contraindications to breast-conserving therapy
  - Large size and multifocal tumors
  - Fixation to the chest wall
  - Involvement of the nipple or overlying skin
- Axillary dissection generally indicated in women with invasive cancer
- Sentinel node biopsy is an alternative to axillary dissection in selected patients

THERAPEUTIC PROCEDURES

- Radiotherapy after partial mastectomy
  - Improves local control
  - 5–6 weeks of 5 daily fractions to a total dose of 5000–6000 cGy
  - May also improve survival after total mastectomy

OUTCOME

FOLLOW-UP

- Examine patient every 6 months for the first 2 years after diagnosis; thereafter, annually

COMPLICATIONS

- Pleural effusion occurs in almost half of patients with metastatic breast cancer
- Local recurrence occurs in 8%
- Significant edema of the arm occurs in about 10–30%; more commonly if radiotherapy to axilla after surgery

PROGNOSIS

- Stage of breast cancer is the most reliable indicator of prognosis (Table 51)
- Clinical cure rate of localized invasive breast cancer treated with most accepted methods of therapy is 75–90%
- When axillary lymph nodes are involved, the survival rate drops to 50–70% at 5 years and 25–40% at 10 years
- Estrogen and progesterone receptor-positive primary tumors have a more favorable course
- Tumors with marked aneuploidy or high grade have a poor prognosis
- Table 49 lists prognostic factors in node-negative breast cancer

WHEN TO REFER

- Women with exceptional family histories should be referred for genetic counseling and testing

WHEN TO ADMIT

- For definitive therapy by lumpectomy, axillary node dissection or sentinel node biopsy, or mastectomy after diagnosis by FNA or core needle biopsy
- For complications of metastatic disease

PREVENTION

- Screening by combination of clinical examination and mammography: 80–85% detectable only by mammogram; 50% detectable only by examination
- Monthly breast self-examination controversial
- Clinical examination every 2–3 years in women age 20–40, annually in women age > 40
- Mammography every 1–2 years in women 50–79
- For women at high risk for developing breast cancer,
  – Tamoxifen yields a 50% reduction in breast cancer if taken for 5 years
  – Raloxifene also prevents invasive breast cancer in high-risk population

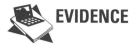

EVIDENCE

PRACTICE GUIDELINES

- Carlson RW et al. NCCN Breast Cancer Practice Guidelines Panel. National Comprehensive Cancer Network: Breast Cancer v.1.2004.

WEB SITE

- National Cancer Institute: Breast Cancer Information for Patients and Health Professionals

INFORMATION FOR PATIENTS

- MedlinePlus: Breast Cancer Interactive Tutorial

REFERENCES

- Albain KS. Adjuvant chemotherapy for lymph node-negative, estrogen receptor-negative breast cancer: a tale of three trials. J Natl Cancer Inst. 2004;96:1801. [PMID: 15601631]
- Giordano SH et al. Breast cancer treatment guidelines in older women. J Clin Oncol. 2005;23:783. [PMID: 15681522]
- Ingle JN et al; North Central Cancer Treatment Group Trial N0032. Fulvestrant in women with advanced breast cancer after progression on prior aromatase inhibitor therapy: North Central Cancer Treatment Group Trial N0032. J Clin Oncol. 2006 Mar 1;24(7):1052–6. [PMID: 16505423]
- Narod SA et al. Prevention and management of hereditary breast cancer. J Clin Oncol. 2005 Mar 10;23(8):1656–63. [PMID: 15755973]
- Smith I. Goals of treatment for patients with metastatic breast cancer. Semin Oncol. 2006;33(1 Suppl 2):2. [PMID: 16472711]

Bronchiectasis

 KEY FEATURES

ESSENTIALS OF DIAGNOSIS

- Chronic productive cough with dyspnea and wheezing
- Recurrent pulmonary infections requiring antibiotics
- A history of recurrent pulmonary infection or inflammation or a predisposing condition
- Radiographic findings of dilated, thickened airways and scattered, irregular opacities

GENERAL CONSIDERATIONS

- A congenital or acquired disorder of large bronchi characterized by abnormal dilation and destruction of bronchial walls
- May be localized or diffuse
- May be caused by recurrent inflammation or infection
- Cystic fibrosis causes 50% of all cases
- Can result from abnormal lung defenses (immunodeficiency states, α_1-antiprotease deficiency, mucociliary clearance disorders, rheumatic disease)
- Airways are often colonized with gram-negative bacilli (especially *Pseudomonas*), *Staphylococcus aureus*, and *Aspergillus* species
- Causes
  – Cystic fibrosis
  – Infection
    □ Tuberculosis
    □ Fungal
    □ Abscess
    □ Pneumonia
  – Abnormal lung defense mechanisms
    □ Hypogammaglobulinemia
    □ Common variable immunodeficiency
    □ Selective IgA, IgM, and IgG subclass deficiency
    □ Acquired immunodeficiency from cytotoxic drugs, AIDS, lymphoma, leukemia, multiple myeloma, chronic renal disease, chronic liver disease
    □ α_1-Antiprotease deficiency with cigarette smoking
    □ Mucociliary clearance disorders (eg, immotile cilia syndrome)
    □ Rheumatic disease (eg, rheumatoid arthritis)
  – Localized airway obstruction

CLINICAL FINDINGS

SYMPTOMS AND SIGNS

- Chronic cough with production of copious, purulent sputum
- Recurrent pneumonia
- Hemoptysis
- Weight loss and anemia common
- Persistent basilar crackles commonly found on examination

- Clubbing
  - Infrequent in mild cases
  - Present in severe disease
- Obstructive pulmonary dysfunction with hypoxemia seen in moderate or severe disease

DIFFERENTIAL DIAGNOSIS

- Chronic obstructive pulmonary disease
- Asthma
- Bronchiolitis
- Allergic bronchopulmonary aspergillosis

 DIAGNOSIS

LABORATORY TESTS

- Sputum smear and culture for bacterial, mycobacterial, and fungal organisms
- Sweat chloride testing
- Quantitative immunoglobulins
- α_1-Antiprotease level
- Excluding patients with humoral immunodeficiencies, most patients have pan-hypergammaglobulinemia, reflecting an immune response to chronic airway infection

IMAGING STUDIES

- Chest radiographs show dilated, thickened central airways and scattered, irregular opacities
- High-resolution CT scanning is the diagnostic test of choice

 TREATMENT

MEDICATIONS

- Antibiotics should be used in acute exacerbations
- Empiric therapy for 10–14 days with amoxicillin or amoxicillin clavulanate, ampicillin or tetracycline, or trimethoprim-sulfamethoxazole
- Sputum smears and cultures should guide therapy where possible
- Preventive or suppressive antibiotics are frequently given to patients with increased purulent sputum, although this practice is not guided by clinical trial data
- Inhaled aerosolized aminoglycosides reduce *Pseudomonas* colonization, but improve FEV_1 and reduce hospitalizations only in cystic fibrosis patients
- Inhaled bronchodilators are commonly used as maintenance therapy and in acute exacerbations

SURGERY

- Resection is reserved for the few patients with localized bronchiectasis and adequate pulmonary function who do not respond to conservative treatment
- Surgical treatment may be necessary to stop bleeding in some cases of massive hemoptysis

THERAPEUTIC PROCEDURES

- Daily chest physiotherapy with postural drainage and chest percussion
- Bronchoscopy may be needed to evaluate hemoptysis, remove retained secretions, and rule out obstructing lesions
- Pulmonary angiography with embolization may be required to control massive hemoptysis

 OUTCOME

FOLLOW-UP

- Monitor serial pulmonary function tests and sputum cultures

COMPLICATIONS

- Hemoptysis
- Hypoxemia
- Cor pulmonale
- Amyloidosis
- Secondary visceral abscesses at distal sites

PROGNOSIS

- Depends on cause and severity

WHEN TO REFER

- Most cases should be referred to a pulmonary, allergy, clinical immunology, or infectious disease specialist to assist in the evaluation and treatment

WHEN TO ADMIT

- Hypoxemia
- Moderate to severe acute airflow obstruction
- Severe infection

PREVENTION

- Influenza vaccine
- Pneumococcal vaccine
- Regular chest physiotherapy

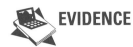 **EVIDENCE**

INFORMATION FOR PATIENTS

- American Lung Association
- National Institutes of Health

REFERENCES

- Barker AF. Bronchiectasis. N Engl J Med. 2002 May 2;346(18):1383–93. [PMID: 11986413]
- Evans DJ et al. Prolonged antibiotics for purulent bronchiectasis. Cochrane Database Syst Rev. 2003; (4):CD001392. [PMID: 14583934]
- Noone PG et al. Primary ciliary dyskinesia: diagnostic and phenotypic features. Am J Respir Crit Care Med. 2004 Feb 15;169(4):459–67. [PMID: 14656747]

Bronchiolitis Obliterans with Organizing Pneumonia

 KEY FEATURES

ESSENTIALS OF DIAGNOSIS

- Dry cough, dyspnea, and constitutional symptoms present for weeks to months prior to presentation
- Patchy, bilateral ground glass or alveolar infiltrates on chest radiograph
- Pulmonary function tests demonstrate restrictive pattern

GENERAL CONSIDERATIONS

- Pathologic classification has two variants
  - Constrictive bronchiolitis (also referred to as obliterative bronchiolitis or bronchiolitis obliterans)
  - Proliferative bronchiolitis
- **Constrictive bronchiolitis**
  - Characterized by chronic inflammation, concentric scarring, and smooth muscle hypertrophy causing luminal obstruction
  - Patients have airflow obstruction on spirometry, minimal radiographic abnormalities, and a progressive, deteriorating clinical course

- **Proliferative bronchiolitis**
  - Occurs when there is an organizing intraluminal exudate, consisting of fibroblasts, foamy macrophages, and other cells that obstruct the lumen
  - When this exudate extends to the alveolar space, the pattern is referred to as bronchiolitis obliterans with organizing pneumonia (BOOP; now more commonly referred to as cryptogenic organizing pneumonitis [COP])
- Disorders associated with bronchiolitis include
  - Organ transplantation
  - Connective tissue diseases
  - Hypersensitivity pneumonitis
- Idiopathic cases are characterized by the insidious onset of dyspnea or cough and include COP

DEMOGRAPHICS

- Affects men and women equally
- Most patients between ages 50 and 70

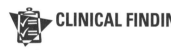 **CLINICAL FINDINGS**

SYMPTOMS AND SIGNS

- Abrupt onset, frequently weeks to a few months after a flu-like illness
- Dyspnea and dry cough are common
- Constitutional symptoms such as fatigue, fever, and weight loss are common
- Crackles are heard in most patients
- Wheezing in approximately one-third of patients
- Clubbing is uncommon

DIFFERENTIAL DIAGNOSIS

- Idiopathic interstitial pneumonias
- Lung disease due to infection (eg, fungal, tuberculosis, *Pneumocystis jiroveci* pneumonia, viral)
- Drug-induced lung disease (eg, amiodarone, bleomycin)
- Sarcoidosis
- Pneumoconiosis
- Hypersensitivity pneumonitis
- Asbestosis

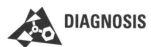 **DIAGNOSIS**

LABORATORY TESTS

- Pulmonary function tests typically show a restrictive ventilatory defect

IMAGING STUDIES

- Chest radiograph typically shows bilateral ground-glass or alveolar infiltrates

 TREATMENT

MEDICATIONS

- Prednisone, 1 mg/kg/day for 1–3 months, tapered slowly to 20–40 mg/day, depending on the response, and weaned over the subsequent 3–6 months as tolerated

 OUTCOME

FOLLOW-UP

- Monitor serial chest radiographs and pulmonary function tests

COMPLICATIONS

- Irreversible scarring or fibrosis of the lung
- Respiratory failure
- Complications of long-term corticosteroid use

PROGNOSIS

- Two-thirds of patients respond rapidly to corticosteroids
- Long-term prognosis is generally good for steroid-responsive patients
- Relapses are common if corticosteroids are stopped prematurely or tapered too quickly

WHEN TO REFER

- Most patients in whom disease is suspected or confirmed should be seen by a pulmonologist

WHEN TO ADMIT

- Respiratory failure
- Signs of acute infection

PREVENTION

- Measures to prevent steroid-induced bone mineral loss

 EVIDENCE

REFERENCES

- Oymak FS et al. Bronchiolitis obliterans organizing pneumonia. Clinical and roentgenological features in 26 cases. Respiration. 2005 May–Jun;72(3):254–62. [PMID: 15942294]
- Ryu JH et al. Bronchiolar disorders. Am J Respir Crit Care Med. 2003 Dec 1; 168(11):1277–92. [PMID: 14644923]
- Schlesinger C et al. The organizing pneumonias: an update and review. Curr Opin Pulm Med. 2005 Sep; 11(5):422–30. [PMID: 16093817]
- Smyth RL et al. Bronchiolitis. Lancet. 2006 Jul 22;368(9532):312–22. [PMID: 16860701]

Bronchogenic Carcinoma

 KEY FEATURES

ESSENTIALS OF DIAGNOSIS

- New cough or change in chronic cough
- Dyspnea, hemoptysis, anorexia
- New or enlarging mass, persistent infiltrate, atelectasis, or pleural effusion on chest radiograph or CT scan
- Cytologic or histologic findings of lung cancer in sputum, pleural fluid, or biopsy specimen

GENERAL CONSIDERATIONS

- Leading cause of cancer deaths
- 90% of lung cancers in men and 79% in women are attributable to smoking
- **Small cell lung cancer** (SCLC)
  - Prone to early hematogenous spread
  - Is rarely amenable to resection
  - Has a very aggressive course
- **Non–small cell lung cancer** (NSCLC)
  - Spreads more slowly
  - Early disease may be cured with resection
  - Histologic types
    - **Squamous cell carcinoma** (25–35%) arises from bronchial epithelium; it is usually centrally located and intraluminal
    - **Adenocarcinoma** (35–40%) arises from mucous glands as a peripheral nodule or mass
    - **Small cell carcinoma** (15–20%) is of bronchial origin, begins centrally, and infiltrates submucosally
    - **Large cell carcinoma** (5–10%) is a heterogeneous group and presents as a central or peripheral mass
    - **Bronchioloalveolar cell carcinoma** (2%) arises from epithelial cells

distal to the terminal bronchiole and spreads intra-alveolarly

DEMOGRAPHICS

- Mean age at diagnosis is 60 years
- Environmental risk factors include
  - Tobacco smoke
  - Radon gas
  - Asbestos
  - Metals
  - Industrial carcinogens
- A familial predisposition is recognized
- Chronic obstructive pulmonary disease, pulmonary fibrosis, and sarcoidosis are associated with an increased risk of lung cancer

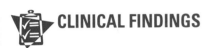 CLINICAL FINDINGS

SYMPTOMS AND SIGNS

- 75–90% are symptomatic at diagnosis
- Presentation depends on
  - Type and location of tumor
  - Extent of spread
  - Presence of paraneoplastic syndromes
- Anorexia, weight loss, and asthenia in 55–90%
- New or changed cough in up to 60%
- Hemoptysis in 5–30%
- Pain, often from bony metastases, in 25–40%
- Local spread may result in endobronchial obstruction and postobstructive pneumonia, effusions, or a change in voice due to recurrent laryngeal nerve involvement
- Superior vena cava (SVC) syndrome
- Horner's syndrome
- Liver metastases are associated with asthenia and weight loss
- Possible presentation of brain metastases
  - Headache
  - Nausea and vomiting
  - Seizures
  - Altered mental status
- **Paraneoplastic syndromes** (Table 10) are not necessarily indicative of metastasis
  - Syndrome of inappropriate antidiuretic hormone secretion occurs in 15% of SCLC patients
  - Hypercalcemia occurs in 10% of SCLC patients

DIFFERENTIAL DIAGNOSIS

- Pneumonia
- Tuberculosis
- Metastatic cancer to lung
- Benign pulmonary nodule or nodules

- Bronchial carcinoid tumor
- Lymphoma
- *Mycobacterium avium* complex infection
- Fungal pneumonia
- Sarcoidosis
- Foreign body aspiration (retained)

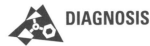 DIAGNOSIS

LABORATORY TESTS

- See Tables 109 and 110
- Tissue or cytology specimen is needed for diagnosis
- Sputum cytology is highly specific, but insensitive; yield is best with lesions in central airways
- Serum tumor markers are neither sensitive nor specific
- Complete blood cell count, renal panel, calcium, liver function tests, and lactate dehydrogenase are a routine part of staging
- Pulmonary function tests are required in all NSCLC patients prior to surgery
  - Preoperative $FEV_1 > 2$ L is adequate to undergo surgery
  - Estimate of postresection FEV_1 is needed if < 2 L preresection
  - Postresection $FEV_1 > 800$ mL or > 40% predicted is associated with a low incidence of perioperative complications

IMAGING STUDIES

- Nearly all patients have abnormal findings on chest radiograph or CT scan
  - Hilar adenopathy and mediastinal thickening (squamous cell)
  - Infiltrates, single or multiple nodules (bronchioloalveolar cell)
  - Central or peripheral masses (large cell)
  - Hilar and mediastinal abnormalities (small cell)
- Chest CT is the most important modality in staging to determine resectability
- For staging, brain MRI, abdominal CT, or radionuclide bone scanning should be targeted to symptoms or signs
- PET imaging can help confirm no metastases in NSCLC patients who are candidates for surgical resection

DIAGNOSTIC PROCEDURES

- Thoracentesis can be diagnostic in the setting of malignant effusions (50–65%)
- If pleural fluid cytology is nondiagnostic after two thoracenteses, thoracoscopy is preferred to blind pleural biopsy

- Fine-needle aspiration of palpable supraclavicular or cervical lymph nodes is frequently diagnostic
- Tissue diagnostic yield from bronchoscopy is 10–90%
- Transthoracic needle biopsy has a sensitivity of 50–90%
- Mediastinoscopy, VATS, or thoracotomy is necessary where less invasive techniques are not diagnostic

Staging
- See Table 109
- NSCLC is staged with the TNM international staging system
  - Stages I and II disease may be cured surgically
  - Stage IIIA disease may benefit from surgery
  - Stage IIIB and IV disease does not benefit from surgery

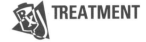 TREATMENT

MEDICATIONS

- See Table 8

Neoadjuvant chemotherapy in NSCLC
- Administration in advance of surgery or radiation therapy
- There is no consensus on the survival impact in stages I and II disease but it is widely used in stage IIIA and IIIB disease

Adjuvant chemotherapy in NSCLC
- Administration of drugs after surgery or radiation therapy
- Multidrug platinum-based therapy shows a trend toward improved survival in stage I and N0 stage II disease (on the order of 3 months at 5 years)
- Data are conflicting for stage IIIA or node-positive stage II disease
- Stage IIIA and IIIB disease, which cannot be treated surgically, has improved survival when treated with combination chemotherapy and radiation therapy
- Performance status and symptom control in stage IIIB and stage IV disease may be improved by chemotherapy

Chemotherapy in SCLC
- 80–100% response to cisplatin/etoposide in limited stage disease (50–70% complete response)
- 60–80% response to cisplatin/etoposide in extensive disease (15–40% complete response)
- Remissions last a median of 6–8 months
- Median survival is 3–4 months after recurrence

SURGERY

- Resection of solitary brain metastases
  - Does not improve survival
  - May improve quality of life in combination with radiation therapy

NSCLC

- Stages I and II are treated with surgical resection where possible
- Stage IIIA disease should be treated with multimodal protocols
- Selected patients with stage IIIB who undergo resection after multimodal therapy have shown long-term survival
- Patients with stage IV disease are treated palliatively

THERAPEUTIC PROCEDURES

- Radiation therapy is used as part of multimodal regimens in NSCLC
- Intraluminal radiation, cryotherapy, and stents are alternative palliative approaches to intraluminal disease
- Palliative care
  - Pain control at the end of life is essential
  - External-beam radiation therapy is used to control
    □ Dyspnea
    □ Hemoptysis
    □ Pain from bony metastases
    □ Obstruction from SVC syndrome
    □ Solitary brain metastases

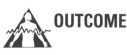 **OUTCOME**

FOLLOW-UP

- Depends on type and stage of cancer as well as the patient's functional status and comorbid conditions

COMPLICATIONS

- SVC syndrome
- Paraneoplastic syndromes
- Venous thrombosis
- Postobstructive pneumonia

PROGNOSIS

- See Table 111
- The overall 5-year survival rate is 15%
- Squamous cell carcinoma may have a better prognosis than adenocarcinoma or large cell carcinoma

WHEN TO REFER

- All patients deserve an evaluation by a multi-disciplinary lung cancer evaluation and treatment program

- A palliative care specialist should be involved in advanced disease care

WHEN TO ADMIT

- Respiratory distress, altered mental status, pain control

PREVENTION

- Smoking cessation
- Screening in high-risk, asymptomatic patients has no proven benefit

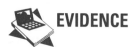 **EVIDENCE**

PRACTICE GUIDELINES

- American College of Chest Physicians; Health and Science Policy Committee. Diagnosis and management of lung cancer. ACCP evidence-based guidelines. Chest. 2003 Jan;123(1 Suppl):D–G, 1S–337S. [PMID: 12527560]
- Rivera MP et al. Diagnosis of lung cancer: the guidelines. Chest 2003;123(1 Suppl):129S. [PMID: 12527572]

INFORMATION FOR PATIENTS

- American Lung Association
- Mayo Clinic
- Parmet S et al. JAMA patient page: Lung cancer. JAMA. 2003;289:380. [PMID: 12532974]

REFERENCES

- Bach PB et al. Computed tomography screening and lung cancer outcomes. JAMA. 2007 Mar 7;297(9):953–61. [PMID: 17341709]
- Black WC et al. CT screening for lung cancer: spiraling into confusion? JAMA. 2007 Mar 7;297(9):995–7. [PMID: 17341714]
- Hamilton W et al. Diagnosis of lung cancer in primary care: a structured review. Fam Pract. 2004 Dec; 21(6):605–11. [PMID: 15520035]
- Henschke CI et al; International Early Lung Cancer Action Program Investigators. Survival of patients with stage I lung cancer detected on CT screening. N Engl J Med. 2006 Oct 26; 355(17):1763–71. [PMID: 17065637]
- Jackman DM et al. Small-cell lung cancer. Lancet. 2005 Oct 15–21; 366(9494):1385–96. [PMID: 16226617]
- Mazzone PJ et al. Lung cancer: Preoperative pulmonary evaluation of the lung resection candidate. Am J Med. 2005 Jun;118(6):578–83. [PMID: 15922686]

- Spira A et al. Multidisciplinary management of lung cancer. N Engl J Med. 2004 Jan 22;350(4):379–92. [PMID: 14736930]
- Spiro SG et al. One hundred years of lung cancer. Am J Respir Crit Care Med. 2005 Sep 1;172(5):523–9. [PMID: 15961694]
- Yang P et al. Clinical features of 5,628 primary lung cancer patients: experience at Mayo Clinic from 1997 to 2003. Chest. 2005 Jul;128(1):452–62. [PMID: 16002972]

Brucellosis

 KEY FEATURES

ESSENTIALS OF DIAGNOSIS

- History of animal exposure, ingestion of unpasteurized milk or cheese
- Insidious onset
  - Easy fatigability
  - Headache
  - Arthralgia
  - Anorexia
  - Sweating
  - Irritability
- Intermittent fever, especially at night, which may become chronic and undulant
- Cervical and axillary lymphadenopathy; hepatosplenomegaly
- Lymphocytosis, positive blood culture, elevated agglutination titer

GENERAL CONSIDERATIONS

- The infection is transmitted from animals to humans. *Brucella abortus* (cattle), *Brucella suis* (hogs), and *Brucella melitensis* (goats) are the main agents
- Transmission to humans occurs by
  - Contact with infected meat (slaughterhouse workers)
  - Placentas of infected animals (farmers, veterinarians)
  - Ingestion of infected unpasteurized milk or cheese
- The incubation period varies from a few days to several weeks
- The disorder may become chronic

DEMOGRAPHICS

- In the United States, brucellosis is very rare except in the midwestern states (*B suis*) and in visitors or immigrants from countries where brucellosis is endemic (eg, Mexico, Spain, South American countries)

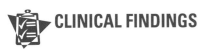

CLINICAL FINDINGS

SYMPTOMS AND SIGNS

- Insidious onset of
  – Weakness
  – Weight loss
  – Low-grade fevers
  – Sweats
  – Exhaustion with minimal activity
- Headache
- Abdominal or back pains with anorexia and constipation
- Arthralgia
- Epididymitis occurs in 10% of cases in men
- 50% of cases have peripheral lymph node enlargement and splenomegaly; hepatomegaly is less common
- Chronic form
  – May assume an undulant nature, with periods of normal temperature between acute attacks
  – Symptoms may persist for years, either continuously or intermittently

DIFFERENTIAL DIAGNOSIS

- Lymphoma
- Tuberculosis
- Infective endocarditis
- Q fever
- Typhoid fever
- Tularemia
- Malaria
- Infectious mononucleosis
- Influenza
- HIV infection
- Disseminated fungal infection, eg, histoplasmosis, coccidioidomycosis

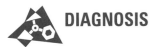

DIAGNOSIS

LABORATORY TESTS

- Early in the course of infection, the organism can be recovered from the blood, cerebrospinal fluid, urine, and bone marrow
- Most modern culture systems can detect growth of the organism in blood by 7 days; cultures are more likely to be negative in chronic cases

- Diagnosis is often made by serologic testing
  – Rising serologic titers or an absolute agglutination titer of > 1:100 supports the diagnosis

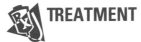

TREATMENT

MEDICATIONS

- Combination regimens of two or three drugs are more effective
- Either doxycycline plus rifampin or streptomycin (or both) *or* doxycycline plus gentamicin *or* trimethoprim-sulfamethoxazole plus rifampin or streptomycin (or both) is effective in doses as follows
  – Doxycycline, 100 mg PO BID for 6 weeks
  – Trimethoprim, 320 mg/day, plus sulfamethoxazole, 1600 mg, PO TID for 6 weeks
  – Rifampin, 600–1200 mg PO once daily for 6 weeks
  – Streptomycin, 500 mg IM BID for 2 weeks
  – Gentamicin 5 mg/kg/d in three divided doses IV for 5–7 days
- Longer courses of therapy (eg, several months) may be required to cure relapses, osteomyelitis, or meningitis

OUTCOME

COMPLICATIONS

Most frequent
- Bone and joint lesions such as spondylitis and suppurative arthritis (usually of a single joint)
- Endocarditis
- Meningoencephalitis

Less common
- Pneumonitis with pleural effusion
- Hepatitis
- Cholecystitis

WHEN TO REFER

- Refer to an infectious disease specialist to confirm the diagnosis or for management of proven cases

WHEN TO ADMIT

- Suspected or known complications such as endocarditis or meningoencephalitis

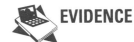

EVIDENCE

WEB SITES

- CDC—Division of Bacterial and Mycotic Diseases
- CDC—Emerging Infectious Diseases
- Karolinska Institute—Directory of bacterial infections and mycoses

REFERENCES

- Hasanjani Roushan MR et al. Efficacy of gentamicin plus doxycycline versus streptomycin plus doxycycline in the treatment of brucellosis in humans. Clin Infect Dis. 2006 Apr 15;42(8):1075–80. [PMID: 16575723]
- Pappas G et al. New approaches to the antibiotic treatment of brucellosis. Int J Antimicrob Agents. 2005 Aug; 26(2):101–5. [PMID: 16039098]

Bullous Pemphigoid

KEY FEATURES

ESSENTIALS OF DIAGNOSIS

- Large, tense blisters that rupture, leaving denuded areas that heal without scarring
- Caused by autoantibodies to specific components of the hemidesmosome

GENERAL CONSIDERATIONS

- Relatively benign pruritic disease characterized by tense blisters in flexural areas, usually remitting in 5 or 6 years, with a course characterized by exacerbations and remissions
- Oral lesions are present in about one-third of affected persons
- The disease may occur in various forms, including localized and urticarial
- There is no statistical association with internal malignant disease

DEMOGRAPHICS

- Most patients are over the age of 60 (often in their 70s and 80s)
- Men are affected twice as frequently as women

CLINICAL FINDINGS

SYMPTOMS AND SIGNS

- Characterized by tense blisters in flexural areas
- Predilection for groin, axillae, flexor forearms, thighs and shins, though may occur anywhere; some have oral involvement
- Appearance of blisters may be preceded by urticarial or edematous lesions for months
- May occur in various forms, including
  – Localized
  – Vesicular
  – Vegetating
  – Erythematous
  – Erythrodermic
  – Nodular
- Course characterized by exacerbations and remissions

DIFFERENTIAL DIAGNOSIS

- Pemphigus
- Drug eruptions
- Erythema multiforme major or toxic epidermal necrolysis
- Bullous impetigo
- Contact dermatitis
- Dermatitis herpetiformis
- Cicatricial pemphigoid
- Paraneoplastic pemphigus
- Linear IgA dermatosis
- Pemphigus foliaceus
- Porphyria cutanea tarda
- Epidermolysis bullosa
- Staphylococcal scalded skin syndrome
- Herpes gestationis
- Graft-versus-host disease

DIAGNOSIS

LABORATORY TESTS

- Circulating anti-basement membrane antibodies can be found in the sera of patients in about 70% of cases

DIAGNOSTIC PROCEDURES

- The diagnosis is made by biopsy and direct immunofluorescence examination
- Light microscopy shows a subepidermal blister
- With direct immunofluorescence, IgG and C3 are found at the dermal–epidermal junction

TREATMENT

MEDICATIONS

- If the patient has only a few blisters, ultrapotent topical corticosteroids may be adequate (Table 150)
- Prednisone at dosages of 60–80 mg/day is often used to achieve rapid control of more widespread disease
- Although slower in onset of action, tetracycline or erythromycin, 1.0–1.5 g/day, alone or combined with nicotinamide—not nicotinic acid or niacin!—(up to 1.5 g/day), if tolerated, may control the disease in patients who cannot use corticosteroids or may allow decreasing or eliminating corticosteroids after control is achieved
- Dapsone is particularly effective in mucous membrane pemphigoid
- If these drugs are not effective, methotrexate, 5–25 mg weekly, or azathioprine, 50 mg QD–TID, may be used as steroid-sparing agents
- Mycophenolate mofetil (1 g BID) or IV immunoglobulin as used for pemphigus vulgaris may be used in refractory cases

OUTCOME

PROGNOSIS

- Usually remitting in 5–6 years

WHEN TO REFER

- If there is a question about the diagnosis, if recommended therapy is ineffective, or specialized treatment is necessary

EVIDENCE

PRACTICE GUIDELINES

- British Association of Dermatologists. Wojnarowska F et al. Guidelines for the management of bullous pemphigoid. Br J Dermatol 2002;147:214. [PMID: 12174090]

WEB SITE

- American Academy of Dermatology

INFORMATION FOR PATIENTS

- American Osteopathic College of Dermatology: Bullous Pemphigoid
- International Pemphigus Foundation: About Pemphigoid
- MedlinePlus: Bullous Pemphigoid

REFERENCES

- Khumalo N et al. Interventions for bullous pemphigoid. Cochrane Database Syst Rev. 2005 Jul 20;(3):CD002292. [PMID: 16034874]
- Mockenhaupt M et al. Daclizumab: a novel therapeutic option in severe bullous pemphigoid. Acta Derm Venereol. 2005;85(1):65–6. [PMID: 15848995]
- Walsh SR et al. Bullous pemphigoid: from bench to bedside. Drugs. 2005; 65(7):905–26. [PMID: 15892587]

Burns

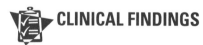

KEY FEATURES

ESSENTIALS OF DIAGNOSIS

- Assess body surface area affected by burns
- Evaluate depth of burn to categorize as first- or second-degree burn
- Consider patient age and associated illness or injury
- Consider hospitalization for hand burns, burns over 10% of total body surface area (TBSA)

GENERAL CONSIDERATIONS

- Only second- and third-degree burns are included in calculating TBSA
- Distinguishing between second- and third-degree burns is not necessary because both are generally treated as full-thickness (third-degree) burns with early excision and grafting

DEMOGRAPHICS

- About 1.25 million burn injuries occur yearly in the United States
- About 51,000 victims of acute burns are hospitalized each year in the United States
- Serious burn injuries occur most frequently in children younger than 5 years old

CLINICAL FINDINGS

SYMPTOMS AND SIGNS

- First-degree burns do not blister initially
- Second-degree burns blister

- In deep second-degree and third-degree burns, hairs are absent or easily extracted, sweat glands become less visible, and the skin appears smoother

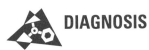 **DIAGNOSIS**

IMAGING STUDIES

- Chest radiographs, usually normal initially, may show acute respiratory distress syndrome in 24–48 h with severe smoke inhalation injury

 TREATMENT

MEDICATIONS

- **Crystalloids:** fluid resuscitation may be instituted simultaneously with initial resuscitation
  - Parkland formula for fluid requirement in first 24 h: lactated Ringer's injection (4 mL/kg body weight per percent TBSA)
  - Deep electrical burns and inhalation injury increase fluid requirement
  - Adequacy of resuscitation determined clinically: urinary output and specific gravity, blood pressure, central venous catheter, or Swan-Ganz catheter readings
  - Half of calculated fluid given in first 8-h period (measured from hour of injury); remaining fluid, split in half, delivered over next 16 h
  - Very large volume of fluid may be needed
- **Colloids:** avoid in routine burn resuscitation because of risk of glomerular filtration decline and association with pulmonary edema

SURGERY

- Because full-thickness circumferential burn may develop ischemia under constricting eschar, escharotomy incisions through anesthetic eschar can save life and limb
- Early excision and grafting of burned areas critical, as soon as 24 h after injury or when patient will hemodynamically tolerate procedure
- Wounds that do not heal in 7–10 days (ie, deep second-degree or third-degree burns) best treated by excision and autograft

THERAPEUTIC PROCEDURES

- Establish airway; evaluate cervical spine, head injuries; stabilize fractures

- Supplemental oxygen
- Intubate if smoke inhalation injury suspected
- **Vascular access**
  - Hypovolemic shock may develop with major burns
  - Remove clothing
  - Establish venous access
    □ Preferably with percutaneous large-bore (14- or 16-gauge) IV line through nonburned skin (eg, femoral lines)
    □ Avoid emergent subclavian lines in volume-depleted patient because of pneumothorax and subclavian vein laceration risk
    □ *Change venous access catheters within 24 h because of high risk of nonsterile placement*
- Protect burn wounds with topical antibiotic (eg, silver sulfadiazine)
- Clean burned areas thoroughly daily

 OUTCOME

FOLLOW-UP

- A Foley catheter is essential for monitoring urinary output
- Monitor smoke inhalation injuries with serial blood gas determination and bronchoscopy

COMPLICATIONS

- Consider comorbid conditions
- Suspect smoke inhalation injury when nasal hairs are singed, mechanism of burn involves closed spaces, sputum is carbonaceous, or carboxyhemoglobin level > 5% in nonsmokers
- Electrical injury that causes burns
  - May also produce cardiac arrhythmias, which require immediate attention, and muscle necrosis
  - Test for elevated creatine kinase levels when rhabdomyolysis is suspected
- Pancreatitis occurs in severe burns along with multiorgan failure
- Nearly all burn patients have one or more septicemic episodes during hospital course; gram-positive infections initially, *Pseudomonas* infections later

PROGNOSIS

- The Baux Score (age + percent burn) predicts mortality after major burn
- Female sex, concomitant nonburn injury, electrical cause of burn, and pediatric age presage poorer outcome
- Physical therapy and psychosocial support are essential

WHEN TO REFER

- Burn units offer the extensive support needed for patients with burns
- Obtain early surgical consultation on burned patients with second- or third-degree burns

PREVENTION

- Maintain normal core body temperature with burns > 20% of TBSA; keep room temperature at 30°C
- Early tube feedings are recommended; begin total parenteral nutrition (TPN) rapidly if patient unable to take tube feedings
- Most patients can be fed adequately with energy equal to 100–120% of estimated basal energy expenditure

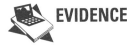 **EVIDENCE**

PRACTICE GUIDELINES

- American Burn Association. Inhalation injury: diagnosis. J Am Coll Surg. 2003; 196:307. [PMID: 12632576]

INFORMATION FOR PATIENTS

- American Academy of Family Physicians: Taking Care of Burns
- Mayo Clinic: Burns
- MedlinePlus: Burns interactive tutorial
- Shriners Hospital

REFERENCES

- Bessey PQ et al. The vulnerabilities of age: burns in children and older adults. Surgery. 2006 Oct;140(4):705–15. [PMID: 17011919]
- Ipaktchi K et al. Advances in burn critical care. Crit Care Med. 2006 Sep;34(9 Suppl):S239–44. [PMID: 16917429]
- Miles JM. Energy expenditure in hospitalized patients: implications for nutritional support. Mayo Clin Proc. 2006 Jun;81(6):809–16. [PMID: 16770981]
- Lee JO et al. Nutrition support strategies for severely burned patients. Nutr Clin Pract. 2005 Jun;20(3):325–30. [PMID: 16207671]
- Oda J et al. Effects of escharotomy as abdominal decompression on cardiopulmonary function and visceral perfusion in abdominal compartment syndrome with burn patients. J Trauma. 2005 Aug;59(2):369–74. [PMID: 16294077]
- Trottier V et al. Survival after prolonged length of stay in a trauma intensive care unit. J Trauma. 2007 Jan;62(1):147-50. [PMID: 17215746]

Bursitis

KEY FEATURES

- Inflammation from trauma, infection, or arthritis (eg, gout, rheumatoid arthritis, or osteoarthritis)
- Subdeltoid, olecranon, ischial, trochanteric, semimembranous-gastrocnemius (Baker's cyst), and prepatellar bursae are common locations

CLINICAL FINDINGS

- More likely than arthritis to begin abruptly and be tender and swollen
- Active and passive range of motion is usually much more limited in arthritis than in bursitis

DIAGNOSIS

- Acute swelling and redness calls for aspiration to rule out infection
- A bursal fluid white blood cell count > 1000/mcL indicates inflammation from infection, rheumatoid arthritis, or gout
- In septic bursitis, the white cell count averages > 50,000/mcL; most cases are caused by *Staphylococcus aureus*
- Chronic, stable olecranon bursa swelling without erythema or other signs of inflammation is unlikely to be infected and does not require aspiration
- A bursa can become symptomatic when it ruptures (eg, Baker's cyst, which, on rupture, can cause calf pain and swelling that mimic thrombophlebitis)
- Treatment of a ruptured cyst includes rest, leg elevation, and injection of triamcinolone, 20–40 mg, into the knee (which communicates with the cyst)

TREATMENT

- Traumatic bursitis responds to local heat, rest, immobilization, NSAIDs, and local corticosteroid injections
- Bursectomy is indicated only when there are repeated infections
- Avoid repetitive minor trauma to the olecranon bursa by not resting the elbow on a hard surface or by wearing an elbow pad

Cancer, Overview
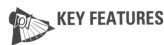

KEY FEATURES

ESSENTIALS OF DIAGNOSIS

- In the United States, second most common cause of death after cardiovascular disease
- In 2006, ~1.4 million new cases of invasive cancer and > 570,000 cancer deaths
- Invasive cancer will develop in one of every two men and one of every three women in their lifetime

GENERAL CONSIDERATIONS

- Cause of most cancers unknown
- DNA mutations in protooncogenes or deletion of tumor suppressor genes (eg, *p53*), or both, cause abnormal cellular proliferation
- Overexpression of *Bcl-2* in breast, colon, prostate, head and neck, and ovarian cancer is one mechanism of resistance to chemotherapy and radiation therapy
- Certain chromosomal abnormalities are associated with specific malignancies and can be used to assess prognosis and determine treatment
- Autoimmune suppression may contribute to development of cancer
- Hereditary predisposition to some cancers, linked to gene mutations, is a relatively rare cause of cancer
- Somatic genetic mutations can be caused by
  - Environmental exposure
  - Genetic susceptibility to environmental toxins
  - Infectious agents
  - Physical agents
  - Drugs, including chemotherapeutic agents such as alkylating agents and topoisomerase II inhibitors

DEMOGRAPHICS

- Risk factors for cancer
  - Age
  - Tobacco use
  - Diet
  - Alcohol consumption
  - Obesity
  - Parity
  - Length of lactation
  - Certain occupations

CLINICAL FINDINGS
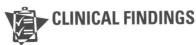

SYMPTOMS AND SIGNS

- Anorexia
- Malaise
- Weight loss
- Fever
- Local effects of tumor growth
- Paraneoplastic syndromes (Table 10)

DIFFERENTIAL DIAGNOSIS

- Depression
- Thyroid disease
- Metabolic disorders (renal, liver disease)
- Chronic infection
- Rheumatologic disease

DIAGNOSIS

LABORATORY TESTS

- Tumor markers primarily used for assessing response to therapy in advanced disease
- Tumor markers should only be used for screening in special circumstances

IMAGING STUDIES

- Radiographs occasionally helpful
- CT, MRI
- PET or PET/CT scan may be more sensitive for certain cancers
- Bone scan to assess for skeletal metastases

DIAGNOSTIC PROCEDURES

- Surgical staging for early-stage disease
- Sentinel lymph node biopsy reduces complications of axillary node dissection in breast cancer
- **Staging**
  - TNM system: used to indicate the extension of cancer before definitive therapy begins
    - Extent of untreated primary tumor (T)
    - Regional lymph node involvement (N)
    - Distant metastases (M)
  - Staging of certain tumors (lymphomas, Hodgkin's disease) differs to reflect their natural history and to better direct treatment decisions
  - Pathologic characteristics of certain tumors add prognostic information (eg, estrogen receptors, tumor grade)
  - Following can have prognostic significance and may direct therapy

- Overexpression or underproduction of oncogene products (HER-2/*neu* in breast cancer)
- Infection of cancer cells with specific viral genomes (HPV subtypes in cervical cancer)
- Certain chromosomal translocations or deletions (alteration of the retinoic acid receptor gene in acute promyelocytic leukemia)

TREATMENT
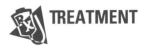

MEDICATIONS

- Systemic chemotherapy
  - As curative therapy for certain malignancies
  - As "neoadjuvant" therapy preoperatively to reduce size and extent of primary tumor, allowing complete excision at surgery
  - As adjuvant therapy to decrease rate of relapse, improve disease-free interval, and improve cure rate
  - As palliative therapy for symptoms and to prolong survival in some patients with incurable malignancies
  - As intensive therapy in combination with bone marrow transplant to improve cure rate in certain cancers, with targeted biological therapy to enhance response
- Regional administration of active chemotherapeutic agents into tumor site can result in palliation and prolonged survival
- Types of cancer responsive to chemotherapy and current treatments of choice: Table 7
- Dosage schedules and toxicities of common chemotherapeutic agents: Table 8
- Hormonal therapy (or ablation) used in treatment and palliation of breast, prostate, endometrial cancers
- Bisphosphonates used to reduce bone pain and fractures in bone metastases
- Other supportive care medications include white and red cell growth factors, pain medications

SURGERY

- Resection is treatment of choice for GI, genitourinary, CNS, breast, thyroid, and skin cancers and sarcomas
- Cryosurgical ablation being evaluated for localized breast and prostate cancer
- Resection of isolated metastases and limited recurrences may result in long-term disease-free survival

THERAPEUTIC PROCEDURES

- Radiation therapy used primarily or in combination with surgery and/or chemotherapy for cancers of the
    - Larynx, oral cavity, pharynx, esophagus
    - Breast
    - Lung
    - Colorectum
    - Uterine cervix, vagina
    - Prostate
    - Skin
    - Brain, spinal cord
    - Hodgkin's and non-Hodgkin's lymphomas

 OUTCOME

FOLLOW-UP

- Monitor for toxicities and need for supportive care (Table 9)
- Evaluate tumor response by examination, radiographic imaging, and tumor markers
    - Partial: ≥ 50% reduction in sum of diameters of original tumor masses
    - Complete: disappearance of tumor
    - Progression: increase in tumor size by ≥ 25% or any new lesions

COMPLICATIONS

Cancer
- Spinal cord compression
- Hypercalcemia
- Hyperuricemia and acute urate nephropathy
- Malignant carcinoid syndrome
- Malignant effusions
- Infection
- Mucositis/esophagitis
- GI symptoms
- Pain
- Anorexia/weight loss
- Paraneoplastic syndromes (Table 10)

Therapy
- Toxicities of common chemotherapeutic agents: Table 8
- **Acute radiation toxicity:** Malaise, anorexia, nausea, vomiting, gastroenteritis, diarrhea, local skin changes, mucosal ulceration of irradiated area, bone marrow suppression, pneumonitis, congestive heart failure
- **Long-term radiation toxicity:** Increased cardiac mortality with chest radiation, secondary leukemias and solid tumors, decreased function of the radiated organ, myelopathy, osteonecrosis, hyperpigmentation and basal cell carcinoma of involved skin

PROGNOSIS

- Functional status at diagnosis (or start of treatment) is major prognostic factor and determinant of outcome with or without tumor-directed therapy
- Depends on stage and tumor biology

WHEN TO REFER

- Patients with strong family histories need referral for genetic screening, counseling

WHEN TO ADMIT

- Oncologic emergencies
- Fever and neutropenia after chemotherapy
- Intractable pain

PREVENTION

Primary
- Smoking cessation
- Diets rich in vegetables and fruit and low in saturated fats
- Reduced exposure to UV light; regular use of sunscreen
- Aspirin and NSAIDs for colon cancer, polyps
- Vitamin E for prostate cancer
- Calcium for colon polyps and selenium for prostate cancer
- Tamoxifen and raloxifene for breast cancer
- Oral contraceptives for ovarian cancer
- Bilateral prophylactic oophorectomy or mastectomy
- Aromatase inhibitors are in clinical trials to determine their effectiveness

Secondary
- Mammography
- Papanicolaou smear and HPV testing
- Fecal occult blood testing, sigmoidoscopy, and colonoscopy
- Prostate-specific antigen in combination with digital rectal examination controversial for prostate cancer screening
- Adjuvant chemotherapy, hormone therapy, and/or radiation therapy to prevent recurrence

 EVIDENCE

PRACTICE GUIDELINES

- National Comprehensive Cancer Network: Clinical Practice Guidelines in Oncology

WEB SITES

- American Cancer Society: Cancer Reference Information
- National Cancer Institute: Statistics, Clinical Trials, Information for Professionals and Patients

INFORMATION FOR PATIENTS

- National Cancer Institute: Cancer: Questions and Answers
- National Cancer Institute: Cancer Information Sources

REFERENCES

- Brenner DE et al. Cancer chemoprevention: lessons learned and future directions. Br J Cancer. 2005;93:735. [PMID: 16160697]
- Domcheck SM et al. Mortality after bilateral salpingo-oophorectomy in *BRCA1* and *BRCA2* mutation carriers. Lancet Oncol. 2006;7:223. [PMID: 16510331]
- Jacobs EJ et al. A large cohort study of aspirin and other nonsteroidal anti-inflammatory drugs and prostate cancer incidence. J Natl Cancer Inst. 2005; 97:975. [PMID: 15998950]
- Kalidas M et al. Aromatase inhibitors for the treatment and prevention of breast cancer. Clin Breast Cancer. 2005; 6:27. [PMID: 15899070]
- Lostumbo L et al. Prophylactic mastectomy for the prevention of breast cancer. Cochrane Database Syst Rev. 2004; (4):CD002748. [PMID: 15495033]

Candidiasis

KEY FEATURES

ESSENTIALS OF DIAGNOSIS

- Common normal flora and opportunistic pathogen
- Mucosal diseases are most common symptomatic infections and include vaginitis, oral thrush, and esophagitis
- Catheter-associated fungemia in hospitalized patients

GENERAL CONSIDERATIONS

- Cutaneous and oral lesions
- Persistent oral or vaginal candidiasis should arouse suspicion of HIV infection

- Fungemia in immunocompromised patients on fluconazole prophylaxis is increasingly due to imidazole-resistant *Candida albicans* or non-*albicans* species

DEMOGRAPHICS

- Mucocutaneous disease occurs with cellular immunodeficiency
- Vulvovaginal candidiasis occurs with
  - Pregnancy
  - Uncontrolled diabetes mellitus
  - Broad-spectrum antibiotics
  - Corticosteroids
  - HIV
- Invasive candidiasis occurs with
  - Prolonged neutropenia
  - Recent surgery
  - Broad-spectrum antibiotics
  - IV catheters (especially for total parenteral nutrition)
  - IV drug use
  - Renal failure
- Candidal endocarditis occurs with repeated inoculation with injection drug use and direct inoculation during valvular heart surgery causing infection of prosthetic valves in first few months following surgery

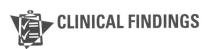 **CLINICAL FINDINGS**

SYMPTOMS AND SIGNS

- Esophageal candidiasis
  - Substernal odynophagia, gastroesophageal reflux, or nausea without substernal pain
  - Oral candidiasis may not be present
- Vulvovaginal candidiasis
  - Acute vulvar pruritus
  - Burning vaginal discharge
  - Dyspareunia
- Disseminated candidiasis
  - Skin, retinal, brain, meningeal, and myocardial involvement
- Hepatosplenic candidiasis: fever and variable abdominal pain weeks after chemotherapy for hematologic cancers, when neutrophil counts have recovered
- Candidal endocarditis
  - Splenomegaly
  - Petechiae
  - Large-vessel embolization

DIFFERENTIAL DIAGNOSIS

- Esophageal
  - Herpes simplex virus (HSV) esophagitis
  - Cytomegalovirus (CMV) esophagitis
  - Varicella-zoster virus esophagitis
  - Pill esophagitis, eg, nonsteroidal anti-inflammatory drugs, bisphosphonates, KCl
  - Gastroesophageal reflux disease
- Vulvovaginal
  - Bacterial vaginosis
  - *Trichomonas* vaginitis
  - Normal vaginal discharge
- Disseminated
  - Histoplasmosis
  - Coccidioidomycosis
  - Tuberculosis
  - Bacterial endocarditis
  - Aspergillosis

 DIAGNOSIS

LABORATORY TESTS

- Disseminated candidiasis
  - Blood cultures are positive in only about 50% of cases
  - While candidemia can be benign, positive blood cultures are sufficient to initiate treatment for disseminated disease
  - Positive mucosal cultures (sputum, urine) may be clue to underlying disseminated candidiasis
  - However, isolated sputum or urine cultures generally represent colonization rather than true infection
  - No current antigens have acceptable sensitivity or specificity for distinguishing colonization from true infection
- Hepatosplenic candidiasis: blood cultures are generally negative, alkaline phosphatase is elevated, and definitive diagnosis is established by tissue biopsy and culture
- Candidal endocarditis: diagnosis requires either positive culture from blood, emboli, or from vegetations found at time of valve replacement

IMAGING STUDIES

- Usually normal in disseminated disease
- Esophageal candidiasis: barium swallow does not allow clear distinction from HSV or CMV esophagitis

DIAGNOSTIC PROCEDURES

- Esophageal candidiasis is best confirmed by endoscopy with biopsy and culture
- For mucosal disease, KOH prep will demonstrate yeast and pseudohyphae
- For invasive disease, definitive proof requires sterile site histologic tests or culture or both
- For suspected fungemia, fundoscopic evaluation may be helpful

 TREATMENT

MEDICATIONS

- Esophageal candidiasis
  - Fluconazole, 100–200 mg PO once daily, or itraconazole solution, 100 mg PO once daily for 10–14 days
  - Voriconazole 200 mg PO BID for refractory cases or cases that develop while on other azoles
  - Caspofungin acetate, 50 mg/day IV, micafungin, 150 mg/day IV, or anidulafungin 50 mg/day IV; all have low toxicity
  - Amphotericin, B 0.3 mg/kg/IV for 10–14 days is reserved for patients who have not responded to other therapies
- Vulvovaginal candidiasis
  - Clotrimazole 100 mg vaginally once daily for 7 days, or miconazole 200 mg vaginally once daily for 3 days
  - Fluconazole 150 mg PO once has equivalent efficacy with better patient acceptance
  - Fluconazole 150 mg PO once weekly helps prevent relapses in patients prone to multiple recurrences
- Candidal funguria
  - Benefit from treatment of asymptomatic candiduria has not been demonstrated
  - Frequently resolves without therapy following discontinuation of antibiotics or removal of bladder catheter
  - Fluconazole, 200 mg PO once daily for 7–14 days, if symptoms persist
- Candidal fungemia
  - Fluconazole 400–800 mg IV once daily with switch to PO therapy when stable; has equivalent efficacy to amphotericin B
  - Amphotericin B, 0.3–0.5 mg/kg/day IV, has excellent efficacy
  - Caspofungin acetate, 70 mg IV for first day then 50 mg/day IV, has equal efficacy to amphotericin B and likely better results versus fluconazole for azole resistant strains
  - Anidulafungin, 200 mg IV for first day then 100 mg/day IV, is also likely better than fluconazole for azole resistant strains
  - Voriconazole, 6 mg/kg IV BID for two doses, then 4 mg/kg IV BID, has increased in vitro activity versus many strains compared with fluconazole
  - Lipid formulations of amphotericin B reduce toxicity allowing for higher doses but are more costly

OUTCOME

COMPLICATIONS

- Candidal funguria: rare ureteral obstruction and dissemination
- Candidal fungemia: endophthalmitis; often no complications if fungemia resolves with removal of IV catheters
- Candidal endocarditis: valve destruction (usually aortic or mitral) is common

PROGNOSIS

- Esophageal candidiasis: relapse common in HIV infection

PREVENTION

- Fluconazole prophylaxis for high-risk patients undergoing induction chemotherapy
- Minimize unnecessary broad-spectrum antibiotics and IV catheters

EVIDENCE

PRACTICE GUIDELINES

- Pappas PG et al. Guidelines for treatment of candidiasis. Clin Infect Dis. 2004;38:161. [PMID: 14699449]

WEB SITE

- Project Inform

INFORMATION FOR PATIENTS

- CDC Disease Information
- JAMA patient page. HIV infection: the basics. JAMA. 2002;288:268. [PMID: 12123237]
- Mayo Clinic
- MedlinePlus

REFERENCES

- Kulberg BJ et al. Voriconazole versus a regimen of amphotericin B followed by fluconazole for candidaemia in non-neutropenic patients: a randomised non-inferiority trial. Lancet. 2005 Oct 22–28;366(9495):1435–42. [PMID: 16243088]
- Pappas PG. Invasive candidiasis. Infect Dis Clin North Am. 2006 Sep; 20(3):485–506. [PMID: 16984866]
- Spellberg BJ et al. Current treatment strategies for disseminated candidiasis. Clin Infect Dis. 2006 Jan 15; 42(2):244–51. [PMID: 16355336]

Candidiasis, Oral

KEY FEATURES

- Risk factors
  - Dentures
  - Debilitated states
  - Diabetes mellitus
  - Anemia
  - Chemotherapy or local irradiation
  - Use of corticosteroids or broad-spectrum antibiotics
- Often the first manifestation of HIV infection
- Angular cheilitis is a symptom, although it can be seen in nutritional deficiencies

CLINICAL FINDINGS

- Painful creamy-white curd-like patches
- White patches can be easily rubbed off by a tongue depressor, unlike leukoplakia or lichen planus, revealing an underlying irregular erythema

DIAGNOSIS

- Clinical
- A wet preparation using potassium hydroxide will reveal spores and may show nonseptate mycelia
- Biopsy will show intraepithelial pseudomycelia of *Candida albicans*

TREATMENT

- Medications
  - Fluconazole (100 mg PO daily for 7–14 days); shorter duration therapy is also effective
  - Ketoconazole (200–400 mg PO with breakfast [requires acidic gastric environment for absorption] for 7–14 days)
  - Clotrimazole troches (10 mg dissolved PO five times daily)
  - Nystatin vaginal troches (100,000 units dissolved PO five times daily) or mouth rinses (500,000 units [5 mL of 100,000 units/mL] held in the mouth before swallowing TID)
- In HIV infection, longer courses may be needed, and itraconazole (200 mg PO daily) may be indicated in fluconazole-refractory cases

- Newer agents, eg, voriconazole, may be needed since many *Candida* species are resistant to first-line azole drugs
- 0.12% chlorhexidine or half-strength hydrogen peroxide mouth rinses may provide local relief
- Nystatin powder (100,000 units/g) applied to dentures TID or QID for several weeks may help denture wearers

Carcinoid Syndrome, Malignant

KEY FEATURES

- Uncommon
- Occurs with tumors of argentaffin cells such as carcinoid tumors of the small bowel metastatic to the liver; less commonly, primary carcinoid tumors of lung or stomach
- Syndrome is caused by release of vasoactive substances
  - Serotonin
  - Histamine
  - Catecholamines
  - Prostaglandins
  - Vasoactive intestinal peptide (VIP)
- A related syndrome occurs in patients with pancreatic tumors that secrete VIP, causing watery diarrhea

CLINICAL FINDINGS

- Facial flushing, telangiectasias
- Abdominal cramps and diarrhea
- Bronchospasm
- Edema of the head and neck (especially with bronchial carcinoid)
- Cardiac valvular lesions (tricuspid or pulmonary stenosis or regurgitation)

DIAGNOSIS

- 24-h urine 5-hydroxyindoleacetic acid (5-HIAA) is increased to > 25 mg/day
- Hold all drugs and serotonin-rich foods such as bananas for several days before the urine collection

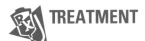 TREATMENT

- Prednisone, 15–30 mg/day
- Hydration and diphenoxylate with atropine for diarrhea
- Octreotide acetate, 100–600 mcg/day SQ in 2–4 divided doses, is the most effective agent for reducing symptoms and levels of urinary 5-HIAA
- Surgical resection of localized carcinoid tumors
- Cyproheptadine, 4 mg PO TID, or methysergide maleate, 2 mg PO TID (up to 16 mg) for severe diarrhea
- Cimetidine and phenothiazines also helpful
- Chemotherapy is moderately effective in metastatic disease
  – Fluorouracil
  – Streptozocin
  – Dacarbazine
  – Cisplatin
  – Doxorubicin
  – Interferon-α

Cardiomyopathy, Dilated

 KEY FEATURES

- Left ventricular (LV) dilation and systolic dysfunction (ejection fraction [EF] < 50%)
- Symptoms and signs of congestive heart failure (most commonly dyspnea)
- Causes
  – Chronic alcohol abuse
  – Unrecognized myocarditis
  – Chronic tachycardia
  – Amyloidosis
  – Sarcoidosis
  – Hemochromatosis
  – Arrhythmogenic right ventricular (RV) dysplasia
  – Uhl's disease (parchment thin RV)
- Often no cause can be identified
- Not associated with ischemic heart disease, hypertension, valvular disease, or congenital defects

 CLINICAL FINDINGS

- Heart failure usually develops gradually, but initial presentation may be severe left or biventricular failure
- Physical examination
  – Low blood pressure
  – Rales
  – Edema
  – Cardiomegaly
  – Elevated jugular venous pressure
  – S_3 and S_4 gallops
  – Murmurs of mitral and tricuspid regurgitation
- Arterial and pulmonary emboli
- Annual mortality rate of 11–13%

 DIAGNOSIS

- ECG
  – Low QRS voltage
  – Sinus tachycardia
  – Left bundle branch block
  – Ventricular or atrial arrhythmias
- Chest radiograph
  – Cardiomegaly
  – Pulmonary venous congestion
  – Pleural effusions
- Doppler echocardiography
  – LV dilatation, thinning, and global dysfunction
  – Can exclude valvular or other lesions
- Exercise or pharmacologic stress myocardial perfusion imaging may suggest underlying coronary disease
- Cardiac MRI helpful in infiltrative diseases

 TREATMENT

- Few cases are amenable to specific therapy
- Discontinue alcohol use
- Treat thyroid dysfunction, acromegaly, pheochromocytoma
- Immunosuppressive therapy is not indicated
- Treat congestive heart failure (see Congestive Heart Failure)
- Long-term anticoagulation for emboli
- Consider biventricular pacing (resynchronization) and implantable cardioverter-defibrillator if EF < 35%
- Persistent symptoms may require consideration for cardiac transplantation

Cardiomyopathy, Hypertrophic

 KEY FEATURES

- Myocardial hypertrophy impinging on the left ventricular (LV) cavity, narrowing the LV outflow tract during systole, can cause dynamic obstruction
- Obstruction is worsened by sympathetic stimulation, digoxin, postextrasystolic beats, Valsalva's maneuver, peripheral vasodilator drugs
- Inherited form has autosomal dominant inheritance and usually presents in early adulthood
- Acquired form presents as diastolic dysfunction in elderly patients with a long history of hypertension
- Atrial fibrillation is a long-term consequence and a poor prognostic sign
- Ventricular arrhythmias are common
- Sudden death may occur, often in athletes after extraordinary exertion

 CLINICAL FINDINGS

- Often presents with dyspnea, chest pain, or syncope (typically postexertional)
- Physical examination
  – Prominent "a" wave in jugular pulse
  – Bisferiens carotid pulse
  – Sustained or triple apical impulse
  – Loud S_4
- Loud systolic murmur along left sternal border that increases with upright posture or Valsalva's maneuver and decreases with squatting
- Mitral regurgitation is frequently present

 DIAGNOSIS

- Chest radiograph: often unimpressive
- ECG: LV hypertrophy and, occasionally, septal Q waves in the absence of myocardial infarction
- Doppler echocardiography
  – Ventricular hypertrophy, which may be asymmetric
  – Usually normal or enhanced contractility and signs of dynamic obstruction
  – Systolic anterior motion of mitral valve if outflow tract obstruction

– Can confirm outflow tract gradient and diastolic filling abnormalities

TREATMENT

- β-Blockers (Table 17) indicated in symptomatic individuals, especially when dynamic outflow obstruction is noted on echocardiogram
- Calcium channel blockers, especially verapamil (Table 19), or disopyramide also effective
- Diuretics (Table 16) for high diastolic and pulmonary capillary wedge pressures
- Nonsurgical septal ablation by injection of alcohol into septal branches of the left coronary artery
- Implantable defibrillator for malignant ventricular arrhythmias or unexplained syncope
- Attempt cardioversion of atrial fibrillation
- Endocarditis prophylaxis

Carpal Tunnel Syndrome

KEY FEATURES

- An entrapment neuropathy from compression of the median nerve in the carpal tunnel, particularly from synovitis of the tendon sheaths or carpal joints and recent or poorly healed fractures
- Most often afflicts those who perform repetitive hand movements
- Associated with
  – Pregnancy
  – Rheumatoid arthritis
  – Myxedema
  – Amyloidosis
  – Sarcoidosis
  – Leukemia (tissue infiltration)
  – Acromegaly
  – Hyperparathyroidism

CLINICAL FINDINGS

- Pain, burning, or tingling in the distribution of the median nerve

- Aching pain may radiate proximally into the forearm and occasionally to the shoulder
- Pain is exacerbated by manual activity, particularly by extremes of volar flexion or dorsiflexion of wrist
- Impairment of sensation in the median nerve distribution may be demonstrable
- Tinel's or Phalen's sign may be positive
  – Tinel's sign is shock-like pain on volar wrist percussion
  – Phalen's sign is pain in the distribution of the median nerve when both wrists are flexed 90 degrees for 1 min
- Muscle weakness or atrophy, especially of the thenar eminence, appears later than sensory disturbances

DIAGNOSIS

- Electromyography and determinations of segmental sensory and motor conduction delay

TREATMENT

- Change of manual activity (or ergonomic improvements); splinting of the hand and forearm at night
- NSAIDs and/or injection of corticosteroid by an experienced operator into the carpal tunnel
- Operative division of the volar carpal ligament gives lasting relief from pain

Cat Scratch Disease

KEY FEATURES

- An acute infection caused by *Bartonella henselae*
- Seen in children and young adults
- It is transmitted from cats to humans as the result of a scratch or bite
- Disseminated forms of the disease occur in HIV-infected persons
  – Bacillary angiomatosis
  – Peliosis hepatis
  – Retinitis
- Endocarditis can occur (usually due to *Bartonella quintana*)

CLINICAL FINDINGS

- A papule or ulcer will develop at the inoculation site within a few days in one-third of patients
- Fever, headache, and malaise occur 1–3 weeks later
- The regional lymph nodes become enlarged, often tender, and may suppurate
- Lymphadenopathy resembles that resulting from neoplasm, tuberculosis, lymphogranuloma venereum, and bacterial lymphadenitis
- Encephalitis occurs rarely

DIAGNOSIS

- Clinical
- Special cultures for *Bartonella,* serology (high antibody titer in an indirect immunofluorescence assay), nucleic acid amplification assay, or excisional biopsy, although rarely necessary, confirm the diagnosis
- Lymph node biopsy revealing necrotizing lymphadenitis is not specific for cat scratch disease

TREATMENT

- Usually self-limited, requiring no specific therapy
- Bacillary angiomatosis responds to treatment with a macrolide (eg, azithromycin, 500 mg PO once daily) or doxycycline, 100 mg PO BID for 4-8 weeks
- For endocarditis, doxycycline 100 mg PO BID for 6 weeks plus gentamicin 3 mg/kg IV in three divided doses for 2 weeks is recommended

Cataract

KEY FEATURES

- Cataract means lens opacity
- Cataracts usually occur bilaterally
- Senile (age-related) cataract is the most common type
- Most persons older than 60 have some degree of lens opacity

- Other causes
  - Congenital infections or inborn errors of metabolism
  - Diabetes mellitus
  - Long-term corticosteroid use
  - Uveitis
  - Ocular trauma

CLINICAL FINDINGS

- Usually gradually progressive visual impairment

DIAGNOSIS

- Ophthalmoscopy, particularly with a dilated pupil, shows opacities in the red reflex
- As the cataract progresses, retinal visualization becomes increasingly difficult

TREATMENT

- When visual impairment significantly affects daily activities, surgical therapy is usually warranted
- Treatment involves surgical removal and insertion of an intraocular lens of appropriate refractive power

Celiac Disease

KEY FEATURES

ESSENTIALS OF DIAGNOSIS

- Typical symptoms
  - Weight loss
  - Chronic diarrhea
  - Abdominal distention
  - Growth retardation
- Atypical symptoms
  - Dermatitis herpetiformis
  - Iron deficiency anemia
  - Osteoporosis
- Abnormal serologic test results
- Abnormal small bowel biopsy
- Clinical improvement on gluten-free diet

GENERAL CONSIDERATIONS

- Caused by an immunologic response to gluten that results in diffuse damage to the proximal small intestinal mucosa with malabsorption of nutrients
- Gluten is a storage protein found in certain grains that is partially digested in the intestinal lumen into glutamine-rich peptides
- Most cases present in childhood or adulthood, although symptoms may manifest between 6 and 24 months of age

DEMOGRAPHICS

- Occurs in 1:100 whites of northern European ancestry but is rare in Africans and Asians
- Clinical diagnosis made in only 1:1000 persons in the United States, so most cases are undiagnosed

CLINICAL FINDINGS

SYMPTOMS AND SIGNS

- "Classic" symptoms of malabsorption more commonly present in infants (< 2 years)
  - Diarrhea
  - Steatorrhea
  - Weight loss
  - Abdominal distention
  - Weakness
  - Muscle wasting
  - Growth retardation
- Older children and adults are less likely to manifest signs of serious malabsorption but may report
  - Chronic diarrhea
  - Dyspepsia
  - Flatulence
  - Variable weight loss
- Many adults have minimal or no gastrointestinal symptoms but present with extraintestinal "atypical" manifestations
  - Fatigue
  - Depression
  - Iron-deficiency anemia
  - Osteoporosis
  - Short stature
  - Delayed puberty
  - Amenorrhea or reduced fertility
- Physical examination
  - In mild cases: may be normal
  - In more severe cases: may reveal signs of malabsorption, loss of muscle mass or subcutaneous fat, pallor, easy bruising, hyperkeratosis, or bone pain
- Abdominal examination may reveal distention with hyperactive bowel sounds
- Dermatitis herpetiformis in < 10%

DIFFERENTIAL DIAGNOSIS

- Irritable bowel syndrome
- Malabsorption due to other causes
- Lactase deficiency
- Viral gastroenteritis, eosinophilic gastroenteritis
- Whipple's disease
- Giardiasis
- Mucosal damage caused by acid hypersecretion associated with gastrinoma

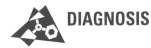

DIAGNOSIS

LABORATORY TESTS

- Obtain complete blood cell count, prothrombin time, serum albumin, iron or ferritin, calcium, alkaline phosphatase, red cell folate, vitamins B_{12}, A, and D levels
- Iron deficiency or megaloblastic anemia occurs because of iron or folate or vitamin B_{12} malabsorption
- Elevation of prothrombin time due to vitamin K deficiency
- Nonanion gap acidosis and hypokalemia in severe diarrhea
- Steatorrhea
  - Detected by a qualitative (Sudan stain) or quantitative 72-hour stool assessment for fecal fat
  - Excretion of more than 10 g/day of fat in patient on a 100-g fat diet is abnormal
- D-Xylose test for malabsorption
- Serologic tests should be performed in all patients with suspected disease
  - IgA endomysial antibody or IgA tissue transglutaminase antibody have > 90% sensitivity and > 95% specificity for diagnosis
  - A negative test result reliably excludes diagnosis whereas a positive test is virtually diagnostic
  - IgG or IgA antigliadin antibodies present in > 85%; however, low specificity (85–90%) limits usefulness as screening test
- Serologic tests become negative (undetectable) 8–12 months after dietary gluten withdrawal

IMAGING

- Dual-energy x-ray densitometry scanning for osteoporosis

DIAGNOSTIC PROCEDURES

- Mucosal biopsy: endoscopic mucosal biopsy of the distal duodenum or proximal jejunum confirms diagnosis

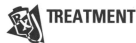

TREATMENT

- Remove all gluten from the diet
- Most patients with celiac disease also have lactose intolerance either temporarily or permanently and should avoid dairy products until the intestinal symptoms have improved on the gluten-free diet

MEDICATIONS

- Nutrient supplements (folate, iron, vitamin B_{12}, calcium, vitamins A and D) in initial stages of therapy, as necessary
- Calcium, vitamin D, and bisphosphonate therapy for osteoporosis

OUTCOME

FOLLOW-UP

- Improvement in symptoms within a few weeks on the gluten-free diet

PROGNOSIS

- Excellent prognosis with appropriate diagnosis and treatment
- Celiac disease that is truly refractory to gluten withdrawal carries a poor prognosis
  - May be caused by enteropathy-associated T-cell lymphoma

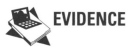

EVIDENCE

PRACTICE GUIDELINES

- American Gastroenterological Association medical position statement: celiac sprue. Gastroenterology 2001; 120:1522. [PMID: 11313323]
- National Institute of Health Consensus Development Conference Statement on Celiac Disease. Gastroenterology 2005; 128:Supplement 1. [PMID: 15825115]
- National Guideline Clearinghouse

WEB SITES

- Celiac Disease Foundation
- Celiac and gluten free support page
- National Institute of Diabetes and Digestive and Kidney Diseases (NIDDK), NIH
- WebPath: Gastrointestinal Pathology Index

INFORMATION FOR PATIENTS

- Mayo Clinic
- National Institute of Diabetes and Digestive and Kidney Diseases (NIDDK), NIH

- Stevens LM. JAMA patient page: Celiac disease. JAMA. 2002;287:1484. [PMID: 11911131]

REFERENCES

- Abrams JA et al. Utility in clinical practice of immunoglobulin A anti-tissue transglutaminase antibody for the diagnosis of celiac disease. Clin Gastroenterol Hepatol. 2006 Jun;4(6):726–30. [PMID: 16630760]
- National Institutes of Health Consensus Development Conference Statement on Celiac Disease, June 28–30, 2004: Gastroenterology. 2005 Apr;128(4 Suppl 1):S1–9. [PMID: 15825115]
- Rostom AA et al. American Gastroenterological Association (AGA) Institute technical review on the diagnosis and management of celiac disease. Gastroenterology. 2006 Dec;131(6):1981–2002. [PMID: 17087937]

Cellulitis & Erysipelas

KEY FEATURES

ESSENTIALS OF DIAGNOSIS

- Diffuse, spreading infection of the skin

GENERAL CONSIDERATIONS

Cellulitis

- Usually due to gram-positive cocci, though gram-negative rods such as *Escherichia coli* may be responsible
- The major portal of entry for lower leg cellulitis is toe web tinea pedis with fissuring of the skin at this site

Erysipelas

- A superficial form of cellulitis that occurs classically on the cheek, caused by β-hemolytic streptococci
- Edematous, spreading, circumscribed, hot, erythematous area, with or without vesicles or bullae
- Pain, chills, fever, and systemic toxicity may be striking
- Erysipeloid, unlike erysipelas, is a benign bacillary infection producing redness of the skin of the fingers or the backs of the hands in fishermen and meat handlers

CLINICAL FINDINGS

SYMPTOMS AND SIGNS

Cellulitis

- The lesion is hot and red
- Pain at the lesion, malaise, chills, and moderate fever
- Usually on the lower leg
- In case of venous stasis, the only clue to cellulitis may be a new localized area of tenderness
- Recurrent attacks may sometimes affect lymphatic vessels, producing a permanent swelling called "solid edema"

Erysipelas

- Central face frequently involved
  - A bright red spot appears first, very often near a fissure at the angle of the nose
  - This spreads to form a tense, sharply demarcated, glistening, smooth, hot area
  - The margin characteristically makes noticeable advances in days or even hours
- The lesion is somewhat edematous and can be pitted slightly with the finger
- Vesicles or bullae occasionally develop on the surface
- The lesion does not usually become pustular or gangrenous and heals without scar formation

DIFFERENTIAL DIAGNOSIS

- Deep venous thrombosis
- Venous stasis
- Candidiasis
- Anthrax
- Erysipeloid
- Contact dermatitis
- Herpes zoster (shingles)
- Scarlet fever
- Angioedema
- Necrotizing fasciitis
- Sclerosing panniculitis
- Underlying osteomyelitis
- Systemic lupus erythematosus

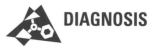

DIAGNOSIS

LABORATORY TESTS

- Attempts to isolate the responsible organism by injecting and then aspirating saline are successful in 20% of cases
- Leukocytosis and an increased sedimentation rate are almost invariably present but are not specific
- Blood cultures may be positive

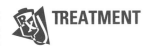 **TREATMENT**

MEDICATIONS

- Intravenous or parenteral antibiotics effective against group A β-hemolytic streptococci and staphylococci may be required for the first 24–48 h
- In mild cases or following the initial parenteral therapy, dicloxacillin or cephalexin, 250–500 mg PO QID for 7–10 days, is usually adequate
- In patients in whom intravenous treatment is not instituted, the first dose of oral antibiotic can be increased to 750–1000 mg to achieve rapid high blood levels

Erysipelas

- Place the patient at bed rest with the head of the bed elevated
- Intravenous antibiotics as above are indicated for the first 48 hours in all but the mildest cases
- A 7-day course is completed with penicillin VK, 250 mg, dicloxacillin, 250 mg, or a first-generation cephalosporin, 250 mg, PO QID
- Either erythromycin, 250 mg PO QID for 7–14 days, or clarithromycin, 250 mg PO BID for 7–14 days, is a good alternative in penicillin-allergic patients

 OUTCOME

COMPLICATIONS

- Unless erysipelas is promptly treated, death may result from extension of the process and systemic toxicity, particularly in the aged

PROGNOSIS

- Erysipelas was at one time a life-threatening infection. It can now usually be quickly controlled with systemic penicillin or erythromycin therapy

WHEN TO REFER

- If there is a question about the diagnosis, if recommended therapy is ineffective, or specialized treatment is necessary

WHEN TO ADMIT

- All but the mildest cases of erysipelas
- Cellulitis with systemic toxicity or in need of IV antibiotics

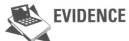 **EVIDENCE**

WEB SITES

- American Academy of Dermatology
- National Institute of Allergy and Infectious Disease

INFORMATION FOR PATIENTS

- MedlinePlus: Erysipelas
- National Institute of Allergy and Infectious Disease: Group A Streptococcal Infections

REFERENCES

- Corwin P et al. Randomized controlled trial of intravenous antibiotic treatment for cellulitis at home compared with hospital. BMJ. 2005 Jan 15; 330(7483):129. [PMID: 15604157]
- Dufel S et al. Simple cellulitis or a more serious infection? J Fam Pract. 2006 May;55(5):396–400. [PMID: 16670034]
- Edwards J et al. A blistering disease: bullous erysipelas. CMAJ. 2006 Aug 1; 175(3):244. [PMID: 16880441]
- Mills AM et al. Are blood cultures necessary in adults with cellulitis? Ann Emerg Med. 2005 May;45(5):548–9. [PMID: 15855955]

Cerebrovascular Disease, Occlusive

 KEY FEATURES

ESSENTIALS OF DIAGNOSIS

- Sudden onset
  - Neurologic deficit consistent with unilateral cortical ischemia
  - Weakness and numbness of an extremity
  - Aphasia
  - Dysarthria
  - Unilateral blindness (amaurosis fugax)
- Bruit heard loudest in the mid neck

GENERAL CONSIDERATIONS

- Unlike the other vascular territories, symptoms of occlusive cerebrovascular disease are predominantly due to emboli

- Symptomatic patients most likely have unstable plaques with ulceration or they have had a recent progression of the stenosis
- Transient ischemic attacks (TIAs) result from small emboli and are the earliest manifestation of carotid stenosis
- These transient symptoms are thought to demonstrate plaque instability, and the risk of additional emboli causing permanent deficits is high
- 25% or more of all strokes may be due to emboli
- In the absence of atrial fibrillation, approximately 90% of these emboli originate from the proximal internal carotid artery
- Lesions in the carotid siphon, the common carotid, and the proximal great vessels are far less common

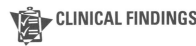 **CLINICAL FINDINGS**

SYMPTOMS AND SIGNS

- Ischemic symptoms of TIAs
  - Generally last only a few minutes
  - May continue for up to 24 hours
- Emboli to the retinal artery cause unilateral blindness which, when transient, is called amaurosis fugax
- Posterior circulation symptoms referable to the brainstem, cerebellum, and visual regions of the brain are
  - Due to atherosclerosis of the vertebral basilar systems
  - Much less common than carotid disease
- Bruits in the mid-cervical area with reduced or absent arm pulses
  - Not specific for narrowing within the vessel
  - Correlation between the degree of stenosis and the presence of the bruit is poor
  - Absence of a bruit does not exclude the possibility of carotid stenosis
- Nonfocal symptoms, such as dizziness and unsteadiness, seldom are related to cerebrovascular atherosclerosis

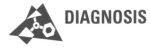 **DIAGNOSIS**

IMAGING STUDIES

- Duplex ultrasonography
  - Imaging modality of choice
  - Has high specificity and sensitivity for detecting and grading degree of stenosis at the carotid bifurcation

- Prospective screening valuable in timing intervention in asymptomatic patients since about 10% will have evidence of plaque progression in a given year
- Magnetic resonance angiography or CT angiography
  - Provides excellent depiction of full anatomy of the cerebrovascular circulation from arch to cranium
  - Each of these modalities may have false-positive or false-negative findings
- Use at least two modalities to confirm degree of stenosis
- Cerebral angiography is reserved for cases that cannot be resolved by these less invasive modalities

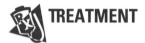

TREATMENT

Asymptomatic patients

- Carotid intervention is likely beneficial in those
  - With no neurologic symptoms but with carotid stenosis on imaging
  - Who are considered to be at low risk and whose expected survival is > 5 years
- Recommendation for intervention also presumes that the stroke rate at the treating institution is acceptable (< 3%)
- Large studies indicate a reduction in stroke from 11.5% to 5.0% over 5 years with surgical treatment of asymptomatic carotid stenoses > 60%
- However, the usual practice is to only treat those patients who have > 80% stenosis

Symptomatic patients

- Patients who have completely or nearly completely recovered from TIAs or stroke
  - Will benefit from carotid intervention if stenosis, ipsilateral to the event, is ≥ 70%
  - Are likely to derive benefit if stenosis is 50–69%
- In these situations, carotid endarterectomy has been shown to have a durable effect in preventing further events

OUTCOME

COMPLICATIONS

- Stroke due to embolization of plaque material during the procedure
- Transient cranial nerve injury (usually vagus or hypoglossal nerve)
- Permanent deficits
- Postoperative neck hematoma, which can compromise the airway

- Myocardial infarction
- Upper limits of acceptable combined morbidity and mortality
  - 3% for asymptomatic
  - 5% for those with TIAs
  - 7% for patients with previous stroke

PROGNOSIS

- Poor for patients with carotid stenosis who have had a TIA or small stroke and no treatment
- 25% of these patients will have a stroke, most occurring in the first year of follow-up
- Patients with carotid stenosis without symptoms have an annual stroke rate of just over 2%
- Concomitant coronary artery disease is common and is an important factor in these patients both for perioperative risk and long-term prognosis

PREVENTION

- Risk factor modification with antiplatelet agents is not nearly as effective in preventing stroke as removing the stenosis

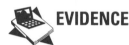

EVIDENCE

PRACTICE GUIDELINES

- Albers GW et al. Antithrombotic and thrombolytic therapy for ischemic stroke: the Seventh ACCP Conference on Antithrombotic and Thrombolytic Therapy. Chest. 2004 Sep;126(3 Suppl):483S–512S. [PMID: 15383482]
- Coull BM et al. Anticoagulants and antiplatelet agents in acute ischemic stroke: report of the Joint Stroke Guideline Development Committee of the American Academy of Neurology and the American Stroke Association (a division of the American Heart Association). Stroke. 2002 Jul;33(7):1934–42. [PMID: 12105379]
- Streefkerk HJ et al. Cerebral revascularization. Adv Tech Stand Neurosurg. 2003;28:145–225. [PMID: 12627810]

WEB SITE

- National Institute of Neurological Disorders and Stroke

INFORMATION FOR PATIENTS

- Cleveland Clinic: Stroke
- Mayo Clinic: Stroke
- MedlinePlus: Stroke Secondary to Atherosclerosis

- National Institute of Neurological Disorders and Stroke: Stroke Information Page

REFERENCES

- Mas JL et al; EVA-3S Investigators. Endarterectomy versus stenting in patients with symptomatic severe carotid stenosis. N Engl J Med. 2006 Oct 19;355(16):1660–71. [PMID: 17050890]
- Safian RD et al; CREATE Pivotal Trial Investigators. Protected carotid stenting in high-risk patients with severe carotid artery stenosis. J Am Coll Cardiol. 2006 Jun 20;47(12):2384–9. [PMID: 16781363]

Cervical Cancer

KEY FEATURES

ESSENTIALS OF DIAGNOSIS

- Abnormal uterine bleeding and vaginal discharge
- Cervical lesion may be visible on inspection as a tumor or ulceration
- Vaginal cytology usually positive; must be confirmed by biopsy

GENERAL CONSIDERATIONS

- Can be considered a sexually transmitted disease
- Both squamous cell and adenocarcinoma of cervix are etiologically related to infection with the human papillomavirus (HPV), especially types 16 and 18
- Smoking and possible dietary factors, such as decreased circulating vitamin A, appear to be cofactors
- Squamous cell carcinoma (SCC) appears first in the intraepithelial layers (the preinvasive stage, or carcinoma in situ)

DEMOGRAPHICS

- Preinvasive cancer (CIN III) is a common diagnosis in women 25–40 years of age
- Incidence of SCC is decreasing while incidence of adenocarcinoma of cervix is increasing

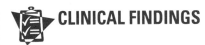 CLINICAL FINDINGS

SYMPTOMS AND SIGNS

- Most common signs
  - Metrorrhagia
  - Postcoital spotting
  - Cervical ulceration
- Bloody or purulent, odorous, nonpruritic discharge may appear after invasion
- Bladder and rectal dysfunction or fistulas and pain are late symptoms

DIFFERENTIAL DIAGNOSIS

- Cervical intraepithelial neoplasia
- Cervical ectropion
- Cervical ectopy (columnar epithelium on face of os, common in adolescence)
- Genital warts (condyloma acuminata)
- Cervical polyp
- Cervicitis
- Nabothian cyst
- Granuloma inguinale

 DIAGNOSIS

LABORATORY TESTS

- Positive Papanicolaou smear

IMAGING STUDIES

- Further staging assessment beyond biopsy may be carried out by abdominal and pelvic CT scanning or MRI

DIAGNOSTIC PROCEDURES

- **Cervical biopsy and endocervical curettage, or conization**
  - These procedures are necessary steps after a positive Papanicolaou smear to determine the extent and depth of invasion of the cancer
  - Even if the smear is positive, treatment is never justified until definitive diagnosis has been established through biopsy
- **"Staging," or estimate of gross spread of cancer of the cervix**
  - The depth of penetration of the malignant cells beyond the basement membrane is a reliable clinical guide to the extent of primary cancer within the cervix and the likelihood of metastases
  - It is customary to stage cancers of the cervix under anesthesia as shown in Table 46

 TREATMENT

- **Carcinoma in situ (stage 0)**
  - In women who have completed childbearing, total hysterectomy is the treatment of choice
  - In women who wish to retain the uterus, acceptable alternatives include cervical conization or ablation of the lesion with cryotherapy or laser
- **Invasive carcinoma**
  - Microinvasive carcinoma (stage IA) is treated with simple, extrafascial hysterectomy
  - Stage IB and stage IIA cancers may be treated with either radical hysterectomy with concomitant radiation and chemotherapy or with radiation plus chemotherapy alone
  - Stage IIB and stage III and IV cancers must be treated with radiation therapy plus cisplatin-based chemotherapy
- **Emergency measures**
  - Vaginal hemorrhage originates from gross ulceration and cavitation in stage II–IV cervical carcinoma
  - Ligation and suturing of the cervix are usually not feasible, but ligation of the uterine or hypogastric arteries may be lifesaving when other measures fail
  - Styptics such as Monsel's solution or acetone are effective, although delayed sloughing may result in further bleeding
  - Wet vaginal packing is helpful
  - Emergency irradiation usually controls bleeding

 OUTCOME

FOLLOW-UP

- Carcinoma in situ
- Close follow-up with Papanicolaou smears every 3 months for 1 year and every 6 months for another year is necessary after cryotherapy or laser

COMPLICATIONS

- Metastases to regional lymph nodes occur with increasing frequency from stage I to stage IV
- The ureters are often obstructed lateral to the cervix, causing hydroureter, hydronephrosis, and renal insufficiency
- Almost two-thirds of untreated patients die of uremia when ureteral obstruction is bilateral
- Pain in the back, in the distribution of the lumbosacral plexus, is often indicative of neurologic involvement
- Gross edema of the legs may be indicative of vascular and lymphatic stasis due to tumor
- Vaginal fistulas to the rectum and urinary tract
- 10–20% of patients with extensive invasive carcinoma die of hemorrhage

PROGNOSIS

- Two to 10 years are required for carcinoma to penetrate the basement membrane and invade the tissues; death usually occurs in 3–5 years in untreated or unresponsive patients
- The overall 5-year relative survival rate is 68% in white women and 55% in black women in the United States
- Survival rates are inversely proportional to the stage of cancer
  - Stage 0, 99–100%
  - Stage IA, > 95%
  - Stage IB–IIA, 80–90%
  - Stage IIB, 65%
  - Stage III, 40%
  - Stage IV, < 20%

WHEN TO REFER

- All patients with invasive cervical cancer should be referred to a gynecologic oncologist

PREVENTION

- Regular Papanicolaou smears (Table 6)
- Smoking cessation

EVIDENCE

PRACTICE GUIDELINES

- Teng N et al; NCCN Cervical Cancer Practice Guidelines Panel. National Comprehensive Cancer Network: Cervical Cancer v.1.2004.
- American College of Obstetricians and Gynecologists. Diagnosis and treatment of cervical carcinomas. ACOG Practice Bulletin 35, 2002.

WEB SITES

- Cervical Cancer Screening: Collection of articles
- National Cancer Institute: Cervical Cancer Information for Patients and Health Professionals

INFORMATION FOR PATIENTS

- American Cancer Society: Cervical Cancer
- CDC: Basic Facts on Cervical Cancer Screening and the Pap Test

- MedlinePlus: Cervical Cancer
- National Cancer Institute

REFERENCES

- Green J et al. Concomitant chemotherapy and radiation therapy for cancer of the uterine cervix. Cochrane Database Syst Rev. 2005;20;(3):CD002225. [PMID: 16034873]
- Tjalma WA et al. Role of human papillomavirus in the carcinogenesis of squamous cell carcinoma and adenocarcinoma of the cervix. Best Pract Res Clin Obstet Gynaecol. 2005 Aug;19(4):469–83. [PMID: 16150388]

Cervical Intraepithelial Neoplasia

KEY FEATURES

ESSENTIALS OF DIAGNOSIS

- The presumptive diagnosis is made by an abnormal Papanicolaou (Pap) smear of an asymptomatic woman with no grossly visible cervical changes
- Diagnose by colposcopically directed biopsy
- Increased in women with HIV

GENERAL CONSIDERATIONS

- Cervical infection with the human papillomavirus (HPV) is associated with a high percentage of all cervical dysplasias and cancers
  - There are over 70 recognized HPV subtypes, of which types 6 and 11 tend to cause mild dysplasia, while types 16, 18, 31, and others cause higher-grade cellular changes
- The varying degrees of dysplasia are defined by the degree of cellular atypia (Table 45)
- The cervical intraepithelial neoplasia (CIN) classification is used along with a description of abnormal cells, including evidence of HPV. The term "squamous intraepithelial lesions (SIL)," low-grade or high-grade, is increasingly used (Table 45)
- HPV testing of cytologic specimens may be useful for triage of atypia (atypical squamous cells of unknown significance; ASCUS)

DEMOGRAPHICS

- Cervical cancer almost never occurs in virginal women
  - It is epidemiologically related to the number of sexual partners a woman has had and the number of other female partners her male partner has had
- Long-term oral contraceptive users, smokers, and women exposed to second-hand smoke are at increased risk
- Women with HIV infection appear to be at increased risk for the disease and of recurrent disease after treatment

CLINICAL FINDINGS

SYMPTOMS AND SIGNS

- There are no specific symptoms or signs of CIN

DIFFERENTIAL DIAGNOSIS

- Cervical cancer
- Cervical ectropion
- Cervical ectopy (columnar epithelium on face of os, common in adolescence)
- Genital warts (condyloma acuminata)
- Cervical polyp
- Cervicitis
- Nabothian cyst
- Granuloma inguinale

DIAGNOSIS

LABORATORY TESTS

Cytologic examination (Pap smear)

- Specimens should be taken from a nonmenstruating patient, spread on a single slide, and fixed or rinsed directly into preservative solution if a thin-layer slide system (ThinPrep) is to be used
- A specimen should be obtained from the squamocolumnar junction with a wooden or plastic spatula and from the endocervix with a cotton swab or nylon brush

DIAGNOSTIC PROCEDURES

Colposcopy

- Viewing the cervix with 10–20× magnification allows for assessment of the size and margins of an abnormal transformation zone and determination of extension into the endocervical canal

- Applying 3–5% acetic acid (vinegar) dissolves mucus, and the acid's desiccating action sharpens the contrast between normal and actively proliferating squamous epithelium
  - Abnormal changes include white patches and vascular atypia, which indicate areas of greatest cellular activity
- Painting the cervix with Lugol's solution (strong iodine solution [Schiller's test]) is also useful
  - Normal squamous epithelium will take the stain
  - Nonstaining squamous epithelium should be biopsied
  - The single-layered, mucus-secreting endocervical tissue will not stain either but can readily be distinguished by its darker pink, shinier appearance

Biopsy

- Both colposcopically-directed punch biopsy and endocervical curettage are office procedures
- If colposcopic examination is not available, the normal-appearing cervix shedding atypical cells can be evaluated by endocervical curettage and by Schiller's test with multiple punch biopsies of nonstaining squamous epithelium or by biopsies from each quadrant of the cervix
- All visibly abnormal cervical lesions should be biopsied

TREATMENT

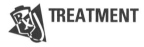

SURGERY

Conization of the cervix

- Conization is surgical removal of the entire transformation zone and endocervical canal
- It should be reserved for cases of severe dysplasia or carcinoma in situ (CIN III), particularly those cases with endocervical extension
- The procedure can be performed by use of the scalpel, the CO_2 laser, the needle electrode, the large-loop excision procedure

THERAPEUTIC PROCEDURES

- Treatment varies depending on the degree and extent of CIN
- Biopsies should always precede treatment

Cauterization or cryosurgery

- The use of either hot cauterization or freezing (cryosurgery) is effective for noninvasive small lesions visible on the cervix without endocervical extension

CO_2 laser

- This well-controlled method minimizes tissue destruction

- It is colposcopically directed and requires special training
- It may be used with large visible lesions
- It involves the vaporization of the transformation zone on the cervix and the distal 5–7 mm of the endocervical canal

Loop excision

- When the CIN is clearly visible in its entirety, a wire loop can be used for excisional biopsy
- Cutting and hemostasis are effected with a low-voltage electrosurgical machine
- This office procedure is done under local anesthesia and is quick and uncomplicated

 OUTCOME

FOLLOW-UP

- All types of dysplasia must be observed and treated if they persist or become more severe
- Because recurrence is possible—especially in the first 2 years after treatment—and because the false-negative rate of a single cervical cytologic test is 20%, close follow-up is imperative
- Cytologic examination
  – Repeat at 4- to 6-month intervals for up to 2 years for CIN II or III
  – Perform at 6 and 12 months for CIN I
- Cytologic specimen HPV DNA testing can be done at 12 months for persistent CIN I
- If repeat testing is normal, then annual cytologic examination can be resumed

PROGNOSIS

- At present, the malignant potential of a specific lesion cannot be predicted. Some lesions remain stable for long periods of time; some regress; and others advance
- Adequately treated CIN very rarely progresses to invasive disease

WHEN TO REFER

- Patients with CIN II/III should be referred to an experienced colposcopist
- Patients requiring conization biopsy should be referred to a gynecologist

PREVENTION

- Preventive measures include the following
  – Regular cytologic screening to detect abnormalities
  – Limiting the number of sexual partners

  – Using a diaphragm or condom for coitus
  – Stopping smoking
  – Avoiding exposure to second-hand smoke
- Women with HIV infection should receive regular cytologic screening and should be monitored closely after treatment for CIN
- HPV (Gardisil) vaccine
  – Prevents cervical cancer caused by HPV types 16 and 18
  – Recommended for girls and women aged 11–26
  – Can be used for girls as young as age 9, if clinically indicated
- A therapeutic vaccine to treat existing HPV infections is in early stages of development
- Because of the very low rate of abnormal Pap smears in women who have undergone hysterectomy for benign disease, routine screening is not justified in this population

 EVIDENCE

PRACTICE GUIDELINES

- Wright TC Jr et al. 2001 Consensus guidelines for the management of women with cervical cytological abnormalities. JAMA. 2002;287:2120. [PMID: 11966387]

WEB SITE

- Colposcopy Atlas

INFORMATION FOR PATIENTS

- American Academy of Family Physicians: Pap Smears: When Yours is Slightly Abnormal
- American Cancer Society: Pap Test
- American Medical Association: Cervical Dysplasia
- JAMA patient page. Papillomavirus. JAMA. 2002;287:2452. [PMID: 12004891]
- National Cancer Institute
- National Cancer Institute: HPV and Cancer

REFERENCES

- American College of Obstetricians-Gynecologists. ACOG Committee Opinion. Evaluation and management of abnormal cervical cytology and histology in the adolescent. Number 330, April 2006. Obstet Gynecol. 2006 Apr; 107(4):963–8. [PMID: 16582143]

- Spitzer M et al. Management of histologic abnormalities of the cervix. Am Fam Physician. 2006 Jan 1;73(1):105–12. [PMID: 16417073]
- Temte JL. HPV vaccine: a cornerstone of female health. Am Fam Physician. 2007 Jan 1;75(1):28, 30. [PMID: 17225700]

Cholangitis & Choledocholithiasis

 KEY FEATURES

ESSENTIALS OF DIAGNOSIS

- Often a history of biliary pain or jaundice
- Sudden onset of severe right upper quadrant or epigastric pain, which may radiate to the right scapula or shoulder
- Occasional patients present with painless jaundice
- Nausea and vomiting
- Acute cholangitis is characterized by fever, which may be followed by hypothermia and gram-negative shock, jaundice, and leukocytosis
- Abdominal films may reveal gallstones

GENERAL CONSIDERATIONS

- Common duct stones usually originate in the gallbladder but may also form spontaneously in the common duct after cholecystectomy
- Symptoms result if there is obstruction
- Biliary pain results from rapid increases in common bile duct pressure due to obstructed bile flow

DEMOGRAPHICS

- About 15% of patients with gallstones have choledocholithiasis (common bile duct stones)
- The percentage rises with age, and the frequency in elderly people with gallstones may be as high as 50%

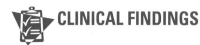 **CLINICAL FINDINGS**

SYMPTOMS AND SIGNS

- See Table 93
- Biliary pain with jaundice in choledocholithiasis

- Frequently recurring attacks of right upper abdominal pain that is severe and persists for hours
- Chills and fever associated with severe pain in acute cholangitis
- **Charcot's triad** (pain, fever [and chills], and jaundice) is characteristic of acute cholangitis
- Altered mental status and septic shock connote acute suppurative cholangitis and constitute an endoscopic or surgical emergency
- Hepatomegaly may be present in calculous biliary obstruction, and tenderness is usually present in the right upper quadrant and epigastrium

DIFFERENTIAL DIAGNOSIS

- Cancer of the pancreas, ampulla of Vater, or common duct
- Acute hepatitis
- Biliary stricture
- Chronic cholestatic liver disease, eg, primary biliary cirrhosis, primary sclerosing cholangitis, drug toxicity
- Pancreatitis
- Sepsis due to other causes
- Underlying *Ascaris* or *Clonorchis*, or hydatid disease

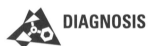 DIAGNOSIS

LABORATORY TESTS

- Bilirubinuria and elevated serum bilirubin
  - Present if the common duct is obstructed
  - Present with cholangitis
  - Levels commonly fluctuate
- Serum alkaline phosphatase levels rise more slowly
- Serum amylase elevations may be present in secondary pancreatitis
- Acute obstruction of the bile duct rarely produces a transient striking increase in serum aminotransferase levels (> 1000 units/L)
- Hypoprothrombinemia can result from obstructed flow of bile to the intestine
- When extrahepatic obstruction persists for more than a few weeks, differentiation of obstruction from chronic cholestatic liver disease becomes progressively more difficult

IMAGING STUDIES

- Ultrasonography and CT scan demonstrate dilated bile ducts
- Radionuclide imaging may show impaired bile flow

- Endoscopic ultrasonography, helical CT, and MR cholangiography can accurately demonstrate common duct stones and, if available, may be used when there is low or intermediate risk for choledocholithiasis

DIAGNOSTIC PROCEDURES

- Endoscopic retrograde cholangiopancreatography (ERCP) or percutaneous transhepatic cholangiography is the best means to determine the cause, location, and extent of obstruction
- If the likelihood that obstruction is caused by a stone is high, ERCP is the procedure of choice because it permits papillotomy or balloon dilation of the papilla with stone extraction or stent placement

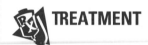 TREATMENT

MEDICATIONS

Hypoprothrombinemia
- Parenteral vitamin K 10 mg or water-soluble oral vitamin K (phytonadione, 5 mg) in 24–36 h

Acute cholangitis
- Ciprofloxacin, 250 mg IV q12h
- Alternatively, in severely ill patients, give mezlocillin, 3 g IV q4h, plus either metronidazole, 500 mg IV q6h (if there has been no prior manipulation of the duct) or gentamicin (2 mg/kg IV as loading dose, plus 1.5 mg/kg every 8 h adjusted for renal function) (or both)
- Aminoglycosides should not be given for more than a few days because the risk of aminoglycoside nephrotoxicity is increased in patients with cholestasis

SURGERY

- At cholecystectomy, operative cholangiography via the cystic duct should be considered
- If stones in the common duct are found, common duct exploration can be performed or a postoperative ERCP and sphincterotomy can be planned
- Following operative choledochostomy, a simple catheter or T tube is placed in the common duct for decompression
  - A properly placed tube should drain bile at the operating table and continuously thereafter; otherwise, it should be considered blocked or dislocated
  - The volume of bile drainage varies from 100 to 1000 mL daily (average, 200–400 mL)
  - Above-average drainage may be due to obstruction at the ampulla (usually by edema)

- Choledocholithiasis discovered at laparoscopic cholecystectomy may be managed via laparoscopic removal or, if necessary, conversion to open surgery or by postoperative endoscopic sphincterotomy
- For the poor-risk patient without cholecystitis, cholecystectomy may be deferred because the risk of subsequent cholecystitis is low

THERAPEUTIC PROCEDURES

- Nutrition should be restored by a high-carbohydrate, high-protein diet and vitamin supplementation
- Common duct stone with cholelithiasis and cholecystitis is usually treated by endoscopic papillotomy and stone extraction followed by laparoscopic cholecystectomy
- ERCP should be performed before cholecystectomy in patients with gallstones and jaundice (serum total bilirubin > 5 mg/dL), a dilated common bile duct (> 7 mm), or stones in the bile duct seen on ultrasound or CT
- Endoscopic balloon dilation of the sphincter of Oddi
  - May be associated with a higher rate of pancreatitis than endoscopic sphincterotomy
  - Is generally reserved for patients with coagulopathy, in whom the risk of bleeding is lower with balloon dilation than with sphincterotomy
- When biliary pancreatitis resolves rapidly, the stone usually passes into the intestine, and ERCP prior to cholecystectomy is not necessary if an intraoperative cholangiogram is done
- In the postcholecystectomy patient with choledocholithiasis, endoscopic papillotomy with stone extraction is preferable to transabdominal surgery
- Lithotripsy (endoscopic or external), direct cholangioscopy, or biliary stenting may be therapeutic for large stones
- For the patient with a T tube and common duct stone, the stone may be extracted via the T tube
- Emergent decompression of the bile duct, generally by ERCP, sphincterotomy, and stone extraction, is generally indicated for patients with acute cholangitis who are septic or do not improve on antibiotics within 12–24 h
- If sphincterotomy cannot be performed, decompression by a biliary stent or nasobiliary catheter can be done
- Once decompressed, antibiotics are generally continued for another 3 days

OUTCOME

FOLLOW-UP

- Postoperative antibiotics are not given routinely after biliary tract surgery; intraoperative bile cultures are taken
- If biliary tract infection was present preoperatively or is apparent at operation, antibiotics are administered postoperatively until the sensitivity tests on culture specimens are available
  - Ampicillin (500 mg IV q6h), gentamicin (1.5 mg/kg q8h), and metronidazole (500 mg q6h) *or*
  - Ciprofloxacin (250 mg IV q12h) *or*
  - A third-generation cephalosporin (eg, cefoperazone, 1–2 g IV q12h)
- A T-tube cholangiogram should be done before the tube is removed, usually about 3 weeks after surgery
- A small amount of bile frequently leaks from the tube site for a few days

COMPLICATIONS

- Common duct obstruction lasting longer than 30 days results in liver damage leading to cirrhosis
- Hepatic failure with portal hypertension occurs in untreated cases

PROGNOSIS

- Medical therapy alone for acute cholangitis is most likely to fail in patients with tachycardia, serum albumin < 3 g/dL, serum bilirubin > 50 mcmol/L, and prothombin time > 14 s on admission

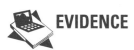 EVIDENCE

PRACTICE GUIDELINES

- Eisen GM et al; American Society for Gastrointestinal Endoscopy. Standards of Practice Committee. An annotated algorithm for the evaluation of choledocholithiasis. Gastrointest Endosc. 2001; 53:864. [PMID: 11375619]
- National Guideline Clearinghouse

WEB SITE

- Choledocholithiasis Demonstration Case

INFORMATION FOR PATIENTS

- Mayo Clinic
- National Institutes of Health

REFERENCES

- Clayton ES et al. Meta-analysis of endoscopy and surgery versus surgery alone for common bile duct stones with the gallbladder in situ. Br J Surg. 2006 Oct; 93(10):1185–91. [PMID: 16964628]
- Drake BB et al. Economical and clinical outcomes of alternative treatment strategies in the management of common bile duct stones in the elderly: wait and see or surgery? Am J Gastroenterol. 2006 Apr;101(4):746–52. [PMID: 16494588]
- Qureshi W. Approach to the patient who has suspected acute bacterial cholangitis. Gastroenterol Clin North Am. 2006 Jun;35(2):409–23. [PMID: 16880073]
- Siddiqui AA et al. Endoscopic sphincterotomy with or without cholecystectomy for choledocholithiasis in high-risk surgical patients: a decision analysis. Aliment Pharmacol Ther. 2006 Oct 1; 24(7):1059–66. [PMID: 16984500]

Cholecystitis, Acute

KEY FEATURES

ESSENTIALS OF DIAGNOSIS

- Steady, severe pain and tenderness in the right hypochondrium or epigastrium
- Nausea and vomiting
- Fever and leukocytosis

GENERAL CONSIDERATIONS

- Associated with gallstones in over 90% of cases
- Occurs when a stone becomes impacted in the cystic duct and inflammation develops behind the obstruction
- Acalculous cholecystitis should be considered when
  - Unexplained fever or right upper quadrant (RUQ) pain occurs within 2–4 weeks of major surgery
  - A critically ill patient has had no oral intake for a prolonged period
- Primarily as a result of ischemic changes secondary to distention, gangrene may develop, resulting in perforation
- Although generalized peritonitis is possible, the leak usually remains localized and forms a chronic, well-circumscribed abscess cavity
- Acute cholecystitis caused by infectious agents (eg, cytomegalovirus, cryptosporidiosis, or microsporidiosis) may occur in patients with AIDS

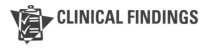 CLINICAL FINDINGS

SYMPTOMS AND SIGNS

- The acute attack is often precipitated by a large or fatty meal
- Relatively sudden, severe, steady pain that is localized to the epigastrium or right hypochondrium and may gradually subside over a period of 12–18 h
- Vomiting occurs in about 75% of patients and affords variable relief in 50%
- RUQ abdominal tenderness
  - Almost always present
  - Usually associated with muscle guarding and rebound pain
- A palpable gallbladder is present in about 15% of cases
- Jaundice
  - Present in about 25% of cases
  - When persistent or severe, suggests the possibility of choledocholithiasis
  - May also result from compression of the common bile or hepatic duct by a cystic duct that is inflamed because of an impacted stone (Mirizzi's syndrome)
- Fever is usually present

DIFFERENTIAL DIAGNOSIS

- Perforated viscus, eg, peptic ulcer, diverticulitis
- Acute pancreatitis
- Appendicitis
- Acute hepatitis or liver abscess
- Right lower lobe pneumonia
- Myocardial infarction
- Radicular pain in T6–T10 dermatome, eg, preeruptive zoster

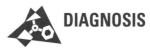 DIAGNOSIS

LABORATORY TESTS

- The white blood cell count is usually high (12,000–15,000/mcL)
- Total serum bilirubin values of 1–4 mg/dL may be seen even in the absence of common duct obstruction
- Serum aminotransferase and alkaline phosphatase are often elevated—the former as high as 300 units/mL, or even higher when associated with ascending cholangitis
- Serum amylase may also be moderately elevated

IMAGING STUDIES

- Plain films of the abdomen may show radiopaque gallstones in 15% of cases
- ^{99m}Tc hepatobiliary imaging (using iminodiacetic acid compounds) (HIDA scan)
  - Useful in demonstrating an obstructed cystic duct, which is the cause of acute cholecystitis in most patients
  - This test is reliable if the bilirubin is under 5 mg/dL (98% sensitivity and 81% specificity for acute cholecystitis)
- RUQ abdominal ultrasound
  - May show the presence of gallstones
  - However, it is not sensitive for acute cholecystitis (67% sensitivity, 82% specificity)

TREATMENT

MEDICATIONS

- Will usually subside on a conservative regimen (withholding of oral feedings, intravenous alimentation, analgesics, and antibiotics, eg, cefoperazone 1–2 g IV q12h)
- Meperidine may be preferable to morphine for pain because of less spasm of the sphincter of Oddi

SURGERY

- Cholecystectomy (generally laparoscopically)
  - Should be performed within 2–3 days after hospitalization because of the high risk of recurrent attacks (up to 10% by 1 month and over 30% by 1 year)
- Surgical treatment of chronic cholecystitis is the same as for acute cholecystitis
  - If indicated, cholangiography can be performed during laparoscopic cholecystectomy
  - Choledocholithiasis can also be excluded by either preoperative or postoperative endoscopic retrograde or magnetic resonance cholangiopancreatography

THERAPEUTIC PROCEDURES

- In high-risk patients, the following may postpone or even avoid the need for surgery:
  - Ultrasound-guided aspiration of the gallbladder
  - Percutaneous cholecystostomy
  - Endoscopic insertion of a stent into the gallbladder
- Cholecystectomy is mandatory when there is evidence of gangrene or perforation

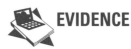 **OUTCOME**

FOLLOW-UP

- If treating nonsurgically, watch the patient (especially if diabetic or elderly) for
  - Recurrent symptoms
  - Evidence of gangrene of the gallbladder
  - Cholangitis

COMPLICATIONS

Gangrene of the gallbladder

- After 24–48 h, the following suggests severe inflammation and possible gangrene of the gallbladder:
  - Continuation or progression of RUQ abdominal pain
  - Tenderness
  - Muscle guarding
  - Fever
  - Leukocytosis
- Necrosis may develop without definite signs in the obese, diabetic, elderly, or immunosuppressed patient
- See Cholangitis & Choledocholithiasis

Chronic cholecystitis and other complications

- Result from repeated episodes of acute cholecystitis or chronic irritation of the gallbladder wall by stones
- Calculi are usually present
- Gallbladder villi undergo polypoid enlargement due to cholesterol deposition ("strawberry gallbladder," cholesterolosis) (5%)
- Marked adenomatous hyperplasia of the gallbladder resembles a myoma (pseudotumor)
- Hydrops of the gallbladder results when acute cholecystitis subsides but cystic duct obstruction persists, producing distention of the gallbladder with a clear mucoid fluid
- A stone in the neck of the gallbladder may compress the bile duct and cause jaundice (Mirizzi's syndrome)
- Cholelithiasis with chronic cholecystitis may be associated with
  - Acute exacerbations of gallbladder inflammation
  - Common duct stone
  - Fistulization to the bowel
  - Pancreatitis
  - Carcinoma of the gallbladder (rarely)
- Calcified (porcelain) gallbladder may have a high association with gallbladder carcinoma (particularly when the calcification is mucosal rather than intramural) and appears to be an indication for cholecystectomy

PROGNOSIS

- The mortality rate of cholecystectomy is less than 0.2%
- Hepatobiliary tract surgery in the elderly has a higher mortality rate
- A successful surgical procedure is generally followed by complete resolution of symptoms

 EVIDENCE

PRACTICE GUIDELINES

- National Guideline Clearinghouse

WEB SITES

- Acute Acalculous Cholecystitis Demonstration Case
- Acute Cholecystitis Demonstration Case

INFORMATION FOR PATIENTS

- Parmet S et al. JAMA patient page: Acute cholecystitis. JAMA. 2003; 289:124. [PMID: 12503995]
- Mayo Clinic
- National Institutes of Health

REFERENCES

- Gurusamy KS et al. Early versus delayed laparoscopic cholecystectomy for acute cholecystitis. Cochrane Database Syst Rev. 2006 Oct 18;(4):CD005440. [PMID: 17054258]
- Lau H et al. Early versus delayed-interval laparoscopic cholecystectomy for acute cholecystitis: a meta-analysis. Surg Endosc. 2006 Jan;20(1):82–7. [PMID: 16247580]

Cholelithiasis (Gallstones)

KEY FEATURES

ESSENTIALS OF DIAGNOSIS

- Biliary pain
- Gallstones in gallbladder on ultrasound
- Patients may be asymptomatic

GENERAL CONSIDERATIONS

- Gallstones are classified according to their predominant composition
  - Cholesterol stones
  - Calcium bilirubinate stones
    □ Comprise < 20% of the stones found in Europe or the United States
    □ Comprise 30–40% of the stones found in Japan

DEMOGRAPHICS

- More common in women than in men
- Incidence increases in both sexes and all races with aging
- In the United States, over 10% of men and 20% of women have gallstones by age 65
- Although cholesterol gallstones are less common in black people, cholelithiasis attributable to hemolysis occurs in over one-third of persons with sickle cell anemia
- Native Americans of both the Northern and Southern Hemispheres have a high rate of cholesterol cholelithiasis, probably because of "thrifty" (*LITH*) genes that promote efficient calorie utilization and fat storage
- As many as 75% of Pima and other American Indian women over the age of 25 years have cholelithiasis
- Risk factors for gallstones
  - Obesity, especially in women
  - Rapid weight loss increases the risk of symptomatic gallstone formation
  - Diabetes and elevated serum insulin levels (insulin resistance) as well as a high intake of carbohydrates and hypertriglyceridemia
  - Pregnancy; also associated with increased risk of symptomatic gallbladder disease
  - Cirrhosis and hepatitis C virus infection (especially in men)
  - Certain drugs (clofibrate, octreotide, ceftriaxone)
  - Crohn's disease
- Prolonged fasting (over 5–10 days) can lead to formation of biliary "sludge" (microlithiasis), which usually resolves with refeeding but can lead to gallstones or biliary symptoms
- Hormone replacement therapy conveys a slight risk for biliary tract surgery

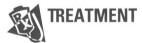 **CLINICAL FINDINGS**

SYMPTOMS AND SIGNS

- See Table 93

- Cholelithiasis is frequently asymptomatic and is discovered incidentally
- "Symptomatic" cholelithiasis usually means characteristic right upper quadrant or epigastric discomfort or pain (biliary pain)
- Small intestinal obstruction due to "gallstone ileus" is the initial manifestation in some patients

DIFFERENTIAL DIAGNOSIS

- Acute cholecystitis
- Acute pancreatitis
- Peptic ulcer disease
- Appendicitis
- Acute hepatitis
- Myocardial infarction
- Radicular pain in T6–T10 dermatome, eg, preeruptive zoster

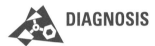 **DIAGNOSIS**

LABORATORY TESTS

- Table 93
- Laboratory tests are normal in persons with asymptomatic gallstones

IMAGING STUDIES

- Ultrasound is the most sensitive imaging modality
- CT is an alternative but usually not necessary

DIAGNOSTIC PROCEDURES

- See Cholecystitis, Acute or Cholangitis & Choledocholithiasis

 TREATMENT

MEDICATIONS

- Cheno- and ursodeoxycholic acids
  - When given orally for up to 2 years dissolve some cholesterol stones
  - May be considered in selected patients who refuse cholecystectomy
  - Dose is 7 mg/kg/day of each or 8–13 mg/kg of ursodeoxycholic acid in divided doses daily
  - They are most effective in patients with a functioning gallbladder, as determined by gallbladder visualization on oral cholecystography, and multiple small "floating" gallstones (representing not more than 15% of patients with gallstones)
  - In 50% of patients, gallstones recur within 5 years after treatment is stopped

SURGERY

- There is generally no need for prophylactic cholecystectomy in an asymptomatic person unless the gallbladder is calcified or gallstones are over 3 cm in diameter
- Laparoscopic cholecystectomy
  - Treatment of choice for symptomatic gallbladder disease
  - The minimal trauma to the abdominal wall makes it possible for patients to go home within 1 day after the procedure and to return to work within 7 days (instead of weeks for those undergoing standard open cholecystectomy)
  - If problems are encountered, the surgery can be converted to a conventional open cholecystectomy
  - See Cholangitis & Choledocholithiasis
- For pregnant patients
  - A conservative approach to biliary pain is advised
  - For those with repeated attacks of biliary pain or acute cholecystitis, cholecystectomy can be performed—even laparoscopically—preferably in the second trimester

THERAPEUTIC PROCEDURES

- Enterolithotomy alone is considered adequate treatment in most patients with gallstone ileus
- Lithotripsy in combination with bile salt therapy for single radiolucent stones < 20 mm in diameter is no longer generally used in the United States

 OUTCOME

COMPLICATIONS

- Cholecystectomy may increase the risk of esophageal, proximal small intestinal, and colonic adenocarcinomas because of increased duodenogastric reflux and changes in intestinal exposure to bile, respectively
- There may be persistence of symptoms after removal of the gallbladder (see Cholecystectomy, Pre- and Post-Syndrome)

PROGNOSIS

- Symptoms (biliary pain) develop in 10–25% of patients with gallstones by 10 years

PREVENTION

- Low-carbohydrate, low-fat, and high-fiber diets and physical activity may help prevent gallstones
- Consumption of caffeinated coffee appears to protect against gallstones in women

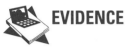

EVIDENCE

PRACTICE GUIDELINES

- National Guideline Clearinghouse
- Patient Care Committee, Society for Surgery of the Alimentary Tract. Treatment of gallstone and gallbladder disease. SSAT patient care guidelines. J Gastrointest Surg. 2004;8:363. [PMID: 15115004]

WEB SITE

- Choledocholithiasis Demonstration Case

INFORMATION FOR PATIENTS

- Mayo Clinic
- National Digestive Diseases Information Clearinghouse
- National Institutes of Health

REFERENCES

- Portincasa P et al. Cholesterol gallstone disease. Lancet. 2006 Jul 15; 368(9531):230–9. [PMID: 16844493]
- Tsai CJ et al. Weight cycling and risk of gallstone disease in men. Arch Intern Med. 2006 Nov 27;166(21):2369–74. [PMID: 17130391]
- Venneman NG et al. Ursodeoxycholic acid exerts no beneficial effect in patients with symptomatic gallstones awaiting cholecystectomy. Hepatology. 2006 Jun; 43(6):1276–83. [PMID: 16729326]

Cholera

KEY FEATURES

ESSENTIALS OF DIAGNOSIS

- History of travel in endemic area or contact with infected person
- Voluminous, watery diarrhea
- Stool is liquid, gray, turbid, and without fecal odor, blood, or pus ("rice water stool")

- Rapid development of marked dehydration
- Positive stool cultures and agglutination of vibrios with specific contaminated food or water

GENERAL CONSIDERATIONS

- An acute diarrheal illness caused by certain serotypes of *Vibrio cholerae*
- The toxin activates adenylyl cyclase in intestinal epithelial cells of the small intestines, producing hypersecretion of water and chloride ion and a massive diarrhea of up to 15 L/day
- Occurs in epidemics under conditions of crowding, war, and famine (eg, in refugee camps) and where sanitation is inadequate
- Infection is acquired by ingestion of contaminated food or water

DEMOGRAPHICS

- Rarely seen in the United States until 1991, when epidemic cholera returned to the Western Hemisphere, originating as an outbreak in coastal cities of Peru
- The epidemic spread to involve several countries in South and Central America as well as Mexico, and cases have been imported into the United States
- A major cause of epidemic diarrhea throughout the developing world

CLINICAL FINDINGS

SYMPTOMS AND SIGNS

- See Table 66
- A sudden onset of severe, frequent watery diarrhea (up to 1 L/h)
- The liquid stool is gray, turbid, and without fecal odor, blood, or pus ("rice water stool")
- Dehydration and hypotension develop rapidly
- The disease is toxin mediated, and fever is unusual

DIFFERENTIAL DIAGNOSIS

- Viral gastroenteritis
- Other small intestinal diarrhea, eg, salmonellosis, enterotoxigenic *Escherichia coli*
- Vasoactive intestinal polypeptide-producing pancreatic tumor (pancreatic cholera)
- Food poisoning, eg, *Staphylococcus aureus*

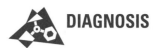

DIAGNOSIS

LABORATORY TESTS

- Stool culture

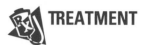

TREATMENT

MEDICATIONS

- Antimicrobial therapy will shorten the course of illness
- Several antimicrobials are active against *V cholerae*, including
  - Tetracycline
  - Ampicillin
  - Chloramphenicol
  - Trimethoprim-sulfamethoxazole
  - Fluoroquinolones
  - Azithromycin
- Multiple drug-resistant strains are increasingly encountered, so susceptibility testing, if available, is advisable
- A single 1 g oral dose of azithromycin was effective for severe cholera caused by strains with reduced susceptibility to fluoroquinolones, but resistance is emerging to this drug as well

THERAPEUTIC PROCEDURES

- Aggressive fluid replacement is essential
- In mild or moderate illness, oral rehydration is usually adequate

OUTCOME

COMPLICATIONS

- Death results from profound hypovolemia

PROGNOSIS

- 25–50% fatality if untreated

WHEN TO ADMIT

- Severe diarrhea
- Moderate to severe dehydration in need of parenteral fluid replacement
- Inability to maintain fluid replacement because there can be rapid development of dehydration

PREVENTION

- A vaccine is available that confers short-lived, limited protection
- Vaccine may be required for entry into or reentry after travel to some countries
- Vaccine is administered in two doses 1–4 weeks apart

- A booster dose every 6 months is recommended for persons remaining in areas where cholera is a hazard
- Vaccination programs are expensive and not particularly effective in managing outbreaks of cholera
- When outbreaks occur, efforts should be directed toward establishing clean water and food sources and proper waste disposal

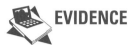 **EVIDENCE**

PRACTICE GUIDELINES

- National Guideline Clearinghouse

WEB SITE

- CDC—Division of Bacterial and Mycotic Diseases

INFORMATION FOR PATIENTS

- JAMA patient page. Preventing dehydration from diarrhea. JAMA. 2001; 285:362. [PMID: 11236756]

REFERENCE

- Saha D et al. Single-dose azithromycin for the treatment of cholera in adults. N Engl J Med. 2006 Jun 8;354(23):2452–62. [PMID: 16760445]

Chronic Fatigue Syndrome

 KEY FEATURES

ESSENTIALS OF DIAGNOSIS

- Weight loss
- Fever
- Sleep-disordered breathing
- Substance use
- Depression

GENERAL CONSIDERATIONS

- Clinically relevant fatigue is composed of three major components
  - Generalized weakness (difficulty in initiating activities)
  - Easy fatigability (difficulty in completing activities)
  - Mental fatigue (difficulty with concentration and memory)
- Fatigue often attributable to
  - Overexertion
  - Poor physical conditioning
  - Sleep disturbance
  - Obesity
  - Undernutrition
  - Emotional problems
- The lifetime prevalence of significant fatigue (present for at least 2 weeks) is about 25%

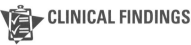 **CLINICAL FINDINGS**

SYMPTOMS AND SIGNS

- Screen for psychiatric disorders
- Evaluation and classification of unexplained chronic fatigue involves
  - History and physical examination
  - Mental status examination (abnormalities require appropriate psychiatric, psychological, or neurologic examination)
  - Screening laboratory tests
- Fatigue is classified as chronic fatigue syndrome if criteria for severity of fatigue are met and four or more of the following symptoms are concurrently present for 6 months or longer
  - Impaired memory or concentration
  - Sore throat
  - Tender cervical or axillary lymph nodes
  - Muscle pain
  - Multijoint pain
  - New headaches
  - Unrefreshing sleep
  - Postexertion malaise
- Fatigue is classified as idiopathic chronic fatigue if criteria for fatigue severity or the symptoms are not met

DIFFERENTIAL DIAGNOSIS

- Hypothyroidism
- Anemia
- Depression
- Obstructive sleep apnea or insufficient sleep
- Infection, eg, tuberculosis, hepatitis, endocarditis, HIV, Lyme disease
- Diabetes mellitus
- Congestive heart failure
- Chronic obstructive pulmonary disease
- Chronic renal failure
- Cancer
- Alcoholism
- Hypercalcemia
- Drugs, eg, sedatives, β-blockers
- Somatoform disorder (somatization)
- Fibromyalgia
- Mononucleosis
- Autoimmune disease

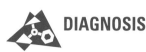 **DIAGNOSIS**

LABORATORY TESTS

- Obtain
  - Complete blood count
  - Erythrocyte sedimentation rate
  - Serum electrolytes
  - Glucose
  - Blood urea nitrogen
  - Creatinine
  - Calcium
  - Liver and thyroid function tests
  - Antinuclear antibody
  - Urinalysis
  - Tuberculin skin test
- Consider, as indicated
  - Serum cortisol
  - Rheumatoid factor
  - Immunoglobulin levels
  - Lyme serology in endemic areas
  - HIV antibody test

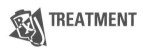 **TREATMENT**

MEDICATIONS

- Treat affective or anxiety disorder only if present
- Treat postural hypotension with fludrocortisone, 0.1 mg/day, and increased dietary sodium
- Psychostimulants, such as methylphenidate, have shown inconsistent results in treatment of cancer-related fatigue

THERAPEUTIC PROCEDURES

- Treatment involves a comprehensive multidisciplinary intervention
  - Optimal medical management of coexisting disorders, eg, depression
  - Cognitive-behavioral therapy
  - Graded exercise program
- Resistance training and aerobic exercise lessens fatigue in a number of chronic conditions, including
  - Congestive heart failure
  - Chronic obstructive pulmonary disease
  - Arthritis
  - Cancer

 OUTCOME

PROGNOSIS

- Although few patients are cured, the treatment effect can be substantial

- Full recovery is eventually possible in many cases

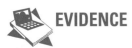 **EVIDENCE**

PRACTICE GUIDELINES

- Veterans Health Administration, Department of Defense: VHA/DoD clinical practice guideline for the management of medically unexplained symptoms: chronic pain and fatigue. 2001.
- Working Group of the Royal Australasian College of Physicians: Chronic fatigue syndrome. Clinical practice guidelines—2002. Med J Aust 2002; 176 (Supp l):S23.

WEB SITE

- Agency for Healthcare Research and Quality: Defining and Managing Chronic Fatigue Syndrome

INFORMATION FOR PATIENTS

- American Academy of Family Physicians: Chronic Fatigue Syndrome
- Mayo Clinic: Chronic Fatigue Syndrome
- National Center for Infectious Diseases: Chronic Fatigue Syndrome
- National Institute of Allergy and Infectious Diseases: Chronic Fatigue Syndrome

REFERENCES

- Chalder T et al. Predictors of outcome in a fatigued population in primary care following a randomized controlled trial. Psychol Med. 2003 Feb;33(2):283–7. [PMID: 12622306]
- Chronic fatigue syndrome. Clinical practice guidelines—2002. Med J Aust. 2002 May 6;176 Suppl:S23–56. [PMID: 12056987]
- Sood A et al. Cancer-related fatigue: an update. Curr Oncol Rep. 2005 Jul; 7(4):277–82. [PMID: 15946587]
- Viner R et al. Fatigue and somatic symptoms. BMJ. 2005 Apr 30; 330(7498):1012–5. [PMID: 15860829]
- Whiting P et al. Interventions for the treatment and management of chronic fatigue syndrome: a systematic review. JAMA. 2001 Sep 19;286(11):1360–8. [PMID: 11560542]

Chronic Obstructive Pulmonary Disease (COPD)

 KEY FEATURES

ESSENTIALS OF DIAGNOSIS

- History of cigarette smoking
- Chronic cough and sputum production (chronic bronchitis) and dyspnea (emphysema)
- Rhonchi, decreased intensity of breath sounds, and prolonged expiration on physical examination
- Airflow limitation on pulmonary function testing

GENERAL CONSIDERATIONS

- Airflow obstruction due to chronic bronchitis or emphysema; most patients have features of both
- Obstruction
  - Is progressive
  - May be accompanied by airway hyperreactivity
  - May be partially reversible
- Chronic bronchitis is characterized by excessive mucous secretions with productive cough for 3 months or more in at least 2 consecutive years
- Emphysema is abnormal enlargement of distal air spaces and destruction of bronchial walls without fibrosis
- Cigarette smoking is the most important cause
  - About 80% of patients have had a significant exposure to tobacco smoke
- Air pollution, airway infection, familial factors, and allergy have been implicated in chronic bronchitis
- α_1-Antiprotease deficiency has been implicated in emphysema

 CLINICAL FINDINGS

SYMPTOMS AND SIGNS

- Presentation
  - Usually at 40–50 years of age
  - Cough
  - Sputum production
  - Shortness of breath

- Dyspnea initially occurs only with heavy exertion, progressing to symptoms at rest in severe disease
- Frequent exacerbations lead to eventual disability
- Viral infections precede exacerbations in most patients
- Late-stage COPD characterized by
  - Hypoxemia
  - Pneumonia
  - Pulmonary hypertension
  - Cor pulmonale
  - Respiratory failure
- Death usually occurs during an exacerbation of COPD in association with respiratory failure
- Clinical findings may be absent early
- Patients are often dichotomized as "pink puffers" or "blue bloaters" depending on whether emphysema or chronic bronchitis predominates (Table 101)

DIFFERENTIAL DIAGNOSIS

- Asthma
- Bronchiectasis, which features recurrent pneumonia and hemoptysis, with distinct radiographic findings
- Severe α_1-antiprotease deficiency
- Cystic fibrosis, which is usually first seen in children and young adults

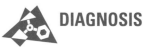 **DIAGNOSIS**

LABORATORY TESTS

- Sputum examination may reveal
  - *Streptococcus pneumoniae*
  - *Haemophilus influenzae*
  - *Moraxella catarrhalis*
  - Cultures correlate poorly with exacerbations
- ECG shows sinus tachycardia, abnormalities consistent with cor pulmonale in severe disease, and/or supraventricular tachycardias and ventricular irritability
- Arterial blood gas values
  - Unnecessary unless hypoxemia or hypercapnia is suspected
  - May show only an increased A–a DO_2 in early disease
  - Hypoxemia in advanced disease
  - Compensated respiratory acidosis with worsening acidemia during exacerbations
- Spirometry
  - Objectively measures pulmonary function and assesses severity
  - Early changes are reductions in mid-expiratory flow and abnormal closing volumes

- FEV_1 and FEV_1/FVC are reduced later in disease
- FVC is reduced in severe disease
- Lung volume measurements show an increase in total lung capacity (TLC), residual volume (RV), and an elevation of RV/TLC indicating air trapping
- α_1-Antiprotease level in young patients with emphysema

IMAGING STUDIES

- Chest radiograph may show hyperinflation, especially when emphysema predominates
- Parenchymal bullae or subpleural blebs are pathognomonic of emphysema
- Nonspecific peribronchial and perivascular markings with chronic bronchitis
- Enlargement of central pulmonary arteries in advanced disease

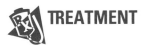 TREATMENT

MEDICATIONS

- Supplemental oxygen
  - In hospitalized patients, oxygen should not be withheld for fear of worsening acidemia
  - Longer survival, reduced hospitalizations, and better quality of life in advanced disease
  - Unless therapy is intended only for night-time or exercise use, 15 hours of nasal oxygen per day is required
  - For most patients, a flow rate of 1–3 L achieves a $PaO_2 > 55$ mm Hg
  - Medicare covers 80% of costs for patients who meet requirements (Table 102)
- Bronchodilators are the most important pharmacologic agents (Tables 99 and 100)
  - **Ipratropium bromide** (2–4 puffs via MDI q6h) is first-line therapy because it is longer-acting and without sympathomimetic side effects
  - Short-acting β-agonists (**albuterol, metaproterenol**) have a shorter onset of action and are less expensive
  - At maximal doses, bronchodilation of β-agonists is equivalent to ipratropium, but with side effects of tremor, tachycardia, and hypokalemia
  - Ipratropium and β-agonists together are more effective than either alone
  - Oral **theophylline** is a third-line agent for patients who do not respond to ipratropium or β-agonists
  - Long-acting β-agonists (**formoterol, salmeterol**) and anticholinergics (**tiotropium**) appear to achieve bronchodilation that is equivalent or superior to what is experienced with ipratropium in addition to similar improvements on health status
- Corticosteroids
  - COPD is generally not steroid responsive; 10–20% of stable outpatients have > a 20% increase in FEV_1 compared with placebo
- Antibiotics improve outcomes slightly when used to treat acute exacerbations
  - Regimens include trimethoprim-sulfamethoxaxole, 160/800 mg PO BID, amoxicillin or amoxicillin-clavulanate 500 mg PO TID, or doxycycline, 100 mg PO BID
- Opioids: severe dyspnea in spite of optimal management may warrant a trial of an opioid
- Sedative-hypnotic drugs (diazepam 5 mg PO TID) may benefit very anxious patients with intractable dyspnea

SURGERY

- Lung transplantation offers substantial improvement in pulmonary function and exercise performance; 1-year survival is 75%
- Lung volume reduction surgery in highly selected patients results in modest improvements in pulmonary function, exercise performance, and dyspnea; surgical mortality rates at experienced centers are 4–10%

THERAPEUTIC PROCEDURES

- Smoking cessation is the single most important goal
- Cough suppressants and sedatives should be avoided as routine measures
- Graded physical exercise programs
- Measure theophylline levels in hospitalized patients
- Noninvasive positive pressure ventilation
  - Reduces the need for intubation
  - Shortens ICU lengths of stay
  - May reduce the risk of nosocomial infection and antibiotic use

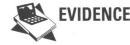 OUTCOME

COMPLICATIONS

- Pulmonary hypertension, cor pulmonale, and chronic respiratory failure are common in advanced disease
- Spontaneous pneumothorax occurs in a small fraction of emphysematous patients
- Hemoptysis may result from chronic bronchitis or bronchogenic carcinoma

PROGNOSIS

- Median survival for severe disease ($FEV_1 < 1$ L) is 4 years
- Degree of dysfunction at presentation is the most important predictor of survival
- A multidimensional index (the BODE index), which includes body mass index (BMI), airway obstruction (FEV_1), dyspnea (Medical Research Council dyspnea score), and exercise capacity, predicts death and hospitalization better than FEV_1 alone

WHEN TO REFER

- Progressive and/or severe airflow obstruction and/or symptoms
- α_1-Antiprotease deficiency
- Large bullae

WHEN TO ADMIT

- Acute exacerbations that fail to respond to measures for ambulatory patients
- Acute respiratory failure
- Cor pulmonale
- Pneumothorax

PREVENTION

- Largely preventable by eliminating chronic exposure to tobacco smoke
- Smoking cessation slows the decline in FEV_1 in middle-aged smokers with mild obstructive disease
- Vaccination against influenza and pneumococcal infection

 EVIDENCE

PRACTICE GUIDELINES

- National Collaborating Centre for Chronic Conditions. Chronic obstructive pulmonary disease. National clinical guideline on management of chronic obstructive pulmonary disease in adults in primary and secondary care. Thorax. 2004;59(Suppl 1):1. [PMID: 15041752]
- Pauwels RA et al. Global strategy for the diagnosis, management, and prevention of chronic obstructive pulmonary disease: National Heart, Lung, and Blood Institute and World Health Organization Global Initiative for Chronic Obstructive Lung Disease (GOLD): executive summary. Respir Care. 2001; 46:798. [PMID: 11463370]
- Sinuff T et al. Clinical practice guideline for the use of noninvasive positive pressure ventilation in COPD patients with acute respiratory failure. J Crit Care. 2004;19:82. [PMID: 15236140]

INFORMATION FOR PATIENTS

- Mayo Clinic
- Parmet S et al. JAMA patient page. Chronic obstructive pulmonary disease. JAMA. 2003;290:2362. [PMID: 14600198]

REFERENCES

- Cote CG et al. New treatment strategies for COPD. Pairing the new with the tried and true. Postgrad Med. 2005 Mar;117(3):27–34. [PMID: 15782671]
- Gluck O et al. Recognizing and treating glucocorticoid-induced osteoporosis in patients with pulmonary diseases. Chest. 2004;125:1859. [PMID: 15136401]
- Hersh CP et al: Predictors of survival in severe, early onset COPD. Chest. 2004 May;126(5):1443–76. [PMID: 15539711]
- Hogg JC et al. The nature of small-airway obstruction in chronic obstructive pulmonary disease. N Engl J Med. 2004 Jun 24;350(26):2645–53. [PMID: 15215480]
- Shapiro SD. COPD unwound. N Engl J Med. 2005 May 12;352(19):2016–9. [PMID: 15888704]

Churg-Strauss Syndrome

 KEY FEATURES

- Idiopathic vasculitis of small- and medium-sized arteries seen in patients with symptoms of asthma
- Affects multiple organ systems, most commonly skin and lung, but heart, gastrointestinal tract, and peripheral nerve involvement may also be affected

 CLINICAL FINDINGS

- Marked peripheral eosinophilia
- Chest radiographic findings range from transient infiltrates to pulmonary nodules

 DIAGNOSIS

- Tissue biopsy demonstrating eosinophilic vasculitis is required to confirm the diagnosis and exclude other causes

 TREATMENT

- Usually requires corticosteroids (prednisone, 1 mg/kg/day, tapering over 3–6 months) and cyclophosphamide (1–2 mg/kg/day, until complete remission is obtained and then tapered slowly)
- Replace cyclophosphamide with methotrexate or azathioprine for maintenance therapy

Cirrhosis

 KEY FEATURES

ESSENTIALS OF DIAGNOSIS

- End result of injury that leads to both fibrosis and nodular regeneration
- The clinical features result from hepatic cell dysfunction, portosystemic shunting, and portal hypertension

GENERAL CONSIDERATIONS

- The most common histologic classification is micronodular, macronodular, and mixed forms cirrhosis
- Each form may be seen at different stages of the disease

Micronodular cirrhosis
- Regenerating nodules are < 1 mm
- Typical of alcoholic liver disease (Laennec's cirrhosis)

Macronodular cirrhosis
- Characterized by larger nodules, up to several centimeters in diameter, and may contain central veins
- Corresponds to postnecrotic (posthepatic) cirrhosis; but may not follow episodes of massive necrosis

Etiology of cirrhosis
- Chronic viral hepatitis
- Alcoholism
- Nonalcoholic fatty liver disease
- Cryptogenic
- Metabolic, eg, hemochromatosis, α_1-antiprotease deficiency, Wilson's disease
- Primary biliary cirrhosis
- Secondary biliary cirrhosis (chronic obstruction due to stone, stricture, neoplasm)
- Congestive heart failure or constrictive pericarditis
- Other
  - Budd-Chiari syndrome
  - Cystic fibrosis
  - Autoimmune hepatitis
  - Glycogen storage disease

DEMOGRAPHICS

- Twelfth leading cause of death in the United States

 CLINICAL FINDINGS

SYMPTOMS AND SIGNS

- Can be asymptomatic for long periods
- Symptoms may be insidious or, less often, abrupt
- Weakness, fatigability, disturbed sleep, muscle cramps, anorexia, and weight loss are common
- Nausea and occasional vomiting
- Jaundice—usually not an initial sign—is mild at first, increasing in severity
- Abdominal pain from hepatic enlargement and stretching of Glisson's capsule or from ascites
- Hematemesis is the presenting symptom in 15–25%
- In women
  - Amenorrhea
- In men
  - Impotence, loss of libido, sterility, and gynecomastia
- In 70% of cases, the liver is enlarged and firm with a sharp or nodular edge; the left lobe may predominate
- Splenomegaly occurs in 35–50%
- Ascites, pleural effusions, peripheral edema, and ecchymoses are late findings
- Fever
  - May be a presenting symptom in up to 35%
  - Usually reflects associated alcoholic hepatitis, spontaneous bacterial peritonitis, or intercurrent infection
- Clubbing and hypoxemia can result from hepatopulmonary syndrome (pulmonary arteriovenous shunting)

Encephalopathy
- Stage 1: day-night reversal, mild confusion
- Stage 2: drowsiness
- Stage 3: stupor
- Stage 4: coma
- Asterixis is characteristic (unless patient is in a coma)
- Coma may be precipitated by an acute hepatocellular insult or GI bleeding

Skin
- Spider nevi on the upper half of the body

- Palmar erythema, Dupuytren's contractures
- Glossitis and cheilosis from vitamin deficiencies are common
- Dilated superficial veins of the abdomen and thorax that fill from below when compressed

 DIAGNOSIS

LABORATORY TESTS

- Laboratory abnormalities are either absent or minimal in early or compensated cirrhosis
- Anemia
  - Usually macrocytic, from suppression of erythropoiesis by alcohol, folate deficiency, hypersplenism, hemolysis, and blood loss from the GI tract
- White blood cell count
  - May be low, reflecting hypersplenism
  - May be high, suggesting infection
- Thrombocytopenia is secondary to
  - Alcoholic marrow suppression
  - Sepsis
  - Folate deficiency
  - Splenic sequestration
- Prolongation of the prothrombin time from reduced levels of clotting factors
- Modest elevations of aspartate aminotransferase (AST) and alkaline phosphatase and progressive elevation of the bilirubin
- Serum albumin is low
- γ-Globulin is increased and may be as high as in autoimmune hepatitis
- Patients with alcoholic cirrhosis may have elevated serum cardiac troponin I levels of uncertain significance
- Combinations of tests (eg, AST and platelet count) are under study for predicting cirrhosis in patients with chronic liver diseases such as chronic hepatitis C
- See Ascites or Peritonitis, Spontaneous Bacterial

IMAGING STUDIES

- Ultrasound
  - Can assess liver size and detect ascites or hepatic nodules, including small hepatocellular carcinomas
  - May establish patency of the splenic, portal, and hepatic veins together with Doppler studies
- Hepatic nodules can be characterized by contrast-enhanced CT scan or MRI
- Nodules suspicious for malignancy may be biopsied under ultrasound or CT guidance

DIAGNOSTIC PROCEDURES

- Perform diagnostic paracentesis for new ascites
- Esophagogastroduodenoscopy confirms the presence of varices and detects specific causes of bleeding
- Liver biopsy

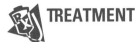 **TREATMENT**

MEDICATIONS

Ascites and edema

- Restrict sodium intake to 400–800 mg/day
- Restrict fluid intake (800–1000 mL/day) for hyponatremia (sodium < 125 mEq/L)
- Ascites may rapidly decrease on bed rest and dietary sodium restriction alone
- Use spironolactone (usually with furosemide) if there is no response to salt restriction
  - The initial dose of spironolactone is 100 mg PO daily
  - May be increased by 100 mg every 3–5 days (up to a maximal conventional daily dose of 400 mg/day, though higher doses have been used) until diuresis is achieved, typically preceded by a rise in the urinary sodium concentration
  - Monitor for hyperkalemia
- Substitute amiloride, 5–10 mg PO daily, if painful gynecomastia develops from spironolactone
- Diuresis can be augmented with the addition of furosemide, 40–160 mg PO daily. Monitor for prerenal azotemia, blood pressure, urinary output, mental status, and serum electrolytes, especially potassium

Anemia

- Iron deficiency anemia: ferrous sulfate, 0.3 g enteric-coated tablets, PO TID after meals
- Macrocytic anemia associated with alcoholism: folic acid, 1 mg/day PO once daily
- Packed red blood cell transfusions may be necessary to replace blood loss

Hemorrhagic tendency

- Treat severe hypoprothrombinemia with vitamin K (eg, phytonadione, 5 mg PO or SQ once daily)
- If this treatment is ineffective, use large volumes of fresh frozen plasma. Because the effect is transient, plasma infusions are indicated only for active bleeding or before an invasive procedure
- Use of recombinant factor VII may be an alternative

SURGERY

- Liver transplantation is indicated in selected cases of irreversible, progressive liver disease
- Absolute contraindications include
  - Malignancy (except small hepatocellular carcinomas in a cirrhotic liver)
  - Sepsis
  - Advanced cardiopulmonary disease (except hepatopulmonary syndrome)

THERAPEUTIC PROCEDURES

- The most important principle is abstinence from alcohol
- Diet
  - Should have adequate calories (25–35 kcal/kg/day) in compensated cirrhosis and 35–40 kcal/kg/day in those with malnutrition
  - Protein should include 1.0–1.2 g/kg/day in compensated cirrhosis and 1.5 g/kg/day in those with malnutrition
  - For hepatic encephalopathy, protein intake should be reduced to 60–80 g/day
- Vitamin supplementation is desirable
- Patients should receive following vaccines
  - HAV, HBV
  - Pneumococcal
  - Influenza (yearly)
- The goal of weight loss with ascites without associated peripheral edema should not exceed 0.5–0.7 kg/day
- Transjugular intrahepatic portosystemic shunt (TIPS)
  - In refractory ascites, reduces ascites recurrence and the risk of hepatorenal syndrome. Preferred to peritoneovenous shunts because of the high rate of complications from the latter
  - Increases the rate of hepatic encephalopathy compared with repeated large-volume paracentesis
  - Survival benefit has not been shown

 OUTCOME

COMPLICATIONS

- Upper GI tract bleeding from varices, portal hypertensive gastropathy, or gastroduodenal ulcer
- Hepatocellular carcinoma
- Spontaneous bacterial peritonitis
- Hepatorenal syndrome
- Hepatopulmonary syndrome and rarely pulmonary hypertension
- Increased risk of systemic infection
- Increased risk of diabetes mellitus

PROGNOSIS

- Factors determining survival include ability to stop alcohol intake and the Child-Turcotte-Pugh class (Table 92)
- The Model for End-Stage Liver Disease (MELD) is used to determine priorities for liver transplantation. Hematemesis, jaundice, and ascites are unfavorable signs
- In patients with a low MELD score (< 21), a low serum sodium concentration (< 130 mEq/L), an elevated hepatic venous pressure gradient, and persistent ascites predict a high mortality rate
- Only 50% of patients with severe hepatic dysfunction (serum albumin < 3 g/dL, bilirubin > 3 mg/dL, ascites, encephalopathy, cachexia, and upper GI bleeding) survive 6 months
- The risk of death is associated with
  - Renal insufficiency
  - Cognitive dysfunction
  - Ventilatory insufficiency
  - Age ≥ 65 years
  - Prothrombin time ≥ 16 s
- Liver transplantation has markedly improved survival, particularly for patients referred for evaluation early

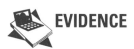

EVIDENCE

PRACTICE GUIDELINES

- Runyon BA. Practice Guidelines Committee, American Association for the Study of Liver Diseases (AASLD). Management of adult patients with ascites due to cirrhosis. Hepatology. 2004; 39:841. [PMID: 14999706]

WEB SITES

- Diseases of the Liver
- Hepatic Pathology Index

INFORMATION FOR PATIENTS

- Mayo Clinic
- Torpy JM et al. JAMA patient page. Hepatitis C. JAMA. 2003;289:2450. [PMID: 12746370]

REFERENCES

- Biggins SW et al. Evidence-based incorporation of serum sodium concentration into MELD. Gastroenterology. 2006 May;130(6):1652–60. [PMID: 16697729]
- Caldwell SH et al. Coagulation disorders and hemostasis in liver disease: pathophysiology and critical assessment of current management. Hepatology. 2006 Oct;44(4):1039–46. [PMID: 17006940]

- Fernández J et al. Adrenal insufficiency in patients with cirrhosis and septic shock: effect of treatment with hydrocortisone on survival. Hepatology. 2006 Nov;44(5):1288–95. [PMID: 17058239]
- Moore KP et al. Guidelines on the management of ascites in cirrhosis. Gut. 2006 Oct;55 Suppl 6:vi1–vi12. [PMID: 16966752]
- Moreau R et al. The use of vasoconstrictors in patients with cirrhosis: type 1 HRS and beyond. Hepatology. 2006 Mar;43(3):385–94. [PMID: 16496352]
- Palma DT et al. The hepatopulmonary syndrome. J Hepatol. 2006 Oct; 45(4):617–25. [PMID: 16899322]

Cirrhosis, Primary Biliary

KEY FEATURES

ESSENTIALS OF DIAGNOSIS

- Middle-aged women
- Often asymptomatic
- Elevated alkaline phosphatase, IgM, cholesterol, antimitochondrial antibodies (+AMA)
- Characteristic liver biopsy
- In later stages, can present with fatigue, jaundice, features of cirrhosis, xanthelasma, xanthomata, steatorrhea

GENERAL CONSIDERATIONS

- Chronic disease of the liver characterized by autoimmune destruction of intrahepatic bile ducts and cholestasis
- Insidious in onset
- Occurs usually in women aged 40–60
- Often detected by the chance finding of elevated alkaline phosphatase levels
- It may be associated with
  - Sjögren's syndrome
  - Autoimmune thyroid disease
  - Raynaud's syndrome
  - Scleroderma
  - Hypothyroidism
  - Celiac disease
- Infection with *Novospingobium aromaticivorans* and *Chlamydophila pneumoniae* may be triggering or causative agents; viral and xenobiotic triggers are also suspected

- Risk factors include
  - History of urinary tract infections
  - Smoking
  - Hormone replacement therapy
- Patients with a clinical and histologic picture of primary biliary cirrhosis but no AMA are said to have "autoimmune cholangitis," which has been associated with
  - Lower serum IgM levels
  - Greater frequency of smooth muscle and antinuclear antibodies

DEMOGRAPHICS

- Estimated incidence and prevalence rates in the United States
  - In women: 4.5 and 65.4 per 100,000, respectively
  - In men: 0.7 and 12.1 per 100,000, respectively

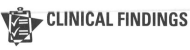 **CLINICAL FINDINGS**

SYMPTOMS AND SIGNS

- Many are asymptomatic for years
- The onset of clinical illness is insidious and is heralded by fatigue and pruritus
- With progression, physical examination reveals hepatosplenomegaly
- Xanthomatous lesions may occur in the skin and tendons and around the eyelids
- Jaundice and signs of portal hypertension are late findings
- The risk of low bone density, osteoporosis, and fractures is increased, as in patients with other forms of chronic liver disease

DIFFERENTIAL DIAGNOSIS

- Chronic biliary tract obstruction (stone or stricture)
- Carcinoma of the bile ducts
- Primary sclerosing cholangitis
- Sarcoidosis
- Cholestatic drug toxicity (eg, chlorpromazine)
- Chronic hepatitis
- Some patients have overlapping features of primary biliary cirrhosis and autoimmune hepatitis

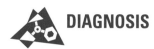 **DIAGNOSIS**

LABORATORY TESTS

- Blood cell counts are normal early in the disease
- Liver biochemical tests reflect cholestasis with elevation of alkaline phosphatase,

- cholesterol (especially high-density lipo-proteins), and, in later stages, bilirubin
- AMA (directed against pyruvate dehydrogenase or other 2-oxo-acid enzymes in mitochondria) are present in 95% of patients, and serum IgM levels are elevated
- Antinuclear antibodies directed against the nuclear pore complex may be detected in specialized laboratories

DIAGNOSTIC PROCEDURES

- Liver biopsy permits histologic staging
  - Stage I: portal inflammation with granulomas
  - Stage II: bile duct proliferation, periportal inflammation
  - Stage III: interlobular fibrous septa
  - Stage IV: cirrhosis

 TREATMENT

MEDICATIONS

- Ursodeoxycholic acid (12–15 mg/kg/day in one or two doses)
  - Preferred medical treatment because lacks toxicity
  - Complete normalization of liver biochemical tests occurs in 25%
- Colchicine (0.6 mg twice daily) and methotrexate (15 mg/week) may improve symptoms and serum levels of alkaline phosphatase and bilirubin
- Methotrexate may also improve liver histology, but overall response rates have been disappointing
- Penicillamine, corticosteroids, and azathioprine are not beneficial
- Budesonide may improve liver histology but worsens osteopenia
- Mycophenolate mofetil is under study
- For pruritus
  - Cholestyramine (4 g) or colestipol (5 g) in water or juice three times daily may be beneficial
  - Rifampin, 150–300 mg orally twice daily, is inconsistently beneficial
  - Opioid antagonists (eg, naloxone, 0.2 μg/kg/min by IV infusion, or naltrexone, 50 mg/day PO) may help
  - The 5-HT$_3$ serotonin receptor antagonist ondansetron may also provide some benefit
  - Plasmapheresis or extracorporeal albumin dialysis may be needed for refractory pruritus
- Deficiencies of vitamins A, K, and D may occur if steatorrhea is present and is aggravated when cholestyramine or colestipol is administered

- Calcium supplementation (500 mg three times daily) may help prevent osteomalacia but is of uncertain benefit in osteoporosis

SURGERY

- For patients with advanced disease, liver transplantation is the treatment of choice

 OUTCOME

PROGNOSIS

- Among asymptomatic patients, at least one-third will become symptomatic within 15 years
- Ursodeoxycholic acid treatment
  - Slows progression of the disease (particularly in early-stage disease)
  - Reduces risk of developing esophageal varices
  - Delays need for liver transplantation
  - Improves long-term survival
- Without liver transplantation, survival averages 7–10 years once symptoms develop
- In advanced disease, adverse prognostic markers are
  - Older age
  - High serum bilirubin
  - Edema
  - Low albumin
  - Prolonged prothrombin time
  - Variceal hemorrhage
- The risk of hepatobiliary malignancies appears to be increased
- Liver transplantation is associated with a 1-year survival rate of 85–90%
- The disease recurs in the graft in 20% of patients by 3 years, but this does not seem to affect survival

 EVIDENCE

WEB SITES

- Diseases of the Liver
- Pathology Index

INFORMATION FOR PATIENTS

- National Digestive Diseases Information Clearinghouse
- National Institutes of Health

REFERENCES

- Kaplan MM et al. Primary biliary cirrhosis. N Engl J Med. 2005 Sep 22; 353(12):1261–73. [PMID: 16177252]
- Shi J et al. Long-term effects of mid-dose ursodeoxycholic acid in primary biliary cirrhosis: a meta-analysis of randomized controlled trials. Am J Gastroenterol. 2006 Jul;101(7):1529–38. [PMID: 16863557]
- Wesierska-Gadek J et al. Correlation of initial autoantibody profile and clinical outcome in primary biliary cirrhosis. Hepatology. 2006 May;43(5):1135–44. [PMID: 16628641]
- Zein CO et al. Smoking and increased severity of hepatic fibrosis in primary biliary cirrhosis: a cross validated retrospective assessment. Hepatology. 2006 Dec; 44(6):1564–71. [PMID: 17133468]

Coarctation of the Aorta

 KEY FEATURES

- Narrowing of the aortic arch distal to the origin of the left subclavian artery
- In most patients, it is due to displaced ductal tissue in the aorta
- Collateral circulation through intercostal arteries and branches of subclavian arteries
- Cause of secondary hypertension
- Bicuspid aortic valve in 50%

 CLINICAL FINDINGS

- Usually no symptoms until hypertension produces left ventricular (LV) failure or cerebral hemorrhage
- Strong arterial pulsations in the neck and suprasternal notch
- Hypertension in the arms, but blood pressure is normal or low in the legs
- Delayed or weak femoral pulsations
- Harsh systolic murmur heard in the back
- Continuous murmurs are heard if collaterals are present around the coarctation
- Blood pressure may not fall after repair of coarctation
- Coarctation can be a major risk in pregnant women

DIAGNOSIS

- ECG: left ventricular hypertrophy (LVH)
- Chest radiograph: scalloping of the ribs as a result of enlarged collateral intercostal arteries
- Doppler echocardiography is diagnostic and can estimate severity of obstruction
- MRI or CT provides excellent visualization of coarctation area
- MRA is diagnostic test of choice
- Cardiac catheterization: measurement of gradient across stenosis

TREATMENT

- Coarctation with peak gradient > 20 mm Hg should be repaired
- Increased collateral flow may reduce gradient seen, even in severe coarctation
- Younger than age 40
  - Surgery advisable if patient has refractory hypertension or significant LVH
  - Surgical mortality rate is 1–4%, and carries risk of spinal cord ischemia
- Older than age 50
  - Surgical mortality rate is considerable
  - Percutaneous stenting is now the procedure of choice if anatomy suitable
- Most untreated patients suffer complications, LV failure, or cerebral hemorrhage
- About 25% of corrected patients remain hypertensive due to resetting of the renin-angiotensin system

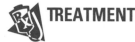

Coccidioidomycosis

KEY FEATURES

ESSENTIALS OF DIAGNOSIS

- Primary infection is an influenza-like illness with malaise, fever, backache, headache, and cough
- Arthralgia and periarticular swelling of knees and ankles
- Erythema nodosum common
- Dissemination may result in meningitis, bone lesions, or skin and soft tissue abscesses
- Chest radiograph varies widely from pneumonitis to cavitation
- Serologic tests useful for diagnosis
- Spherules containing endospores demonstrable in sputum or tissues

GENERAL CONSIDERATIONS

- Consider this diagnosis in any obscure illness in a patient who has been in an endemic area
- Infection results from inhalation of *Coccidioides immitis*, a mold that grows in soil of southwestern United States, Mexico, and Central and South America
- Dissemination occurs in < 1% of immunocompetent hosts, but mortality of disseminated disease is high

DEMOGRAPHICS

- Disseminated coccidioidomycosis occurs in about 0.1% of white and 1% of nonwhite patients. Filipinos and blacks and pregnant women of all races especially susceptible
- In HIV-infected people in endemic areas, coccidioidomycosis is a common opportunistic infection

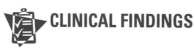

CLINICAL FINDINGS

SYMPTOMS AND SIGNS

Primary coccidioidomycosis
- Incubation period is 10–30 days
- Symptoms, usually respiratory, in 40%
- Nasopharyngitis with fever and chills; bronchitis with dry or slightly productive cough; pleuritic chest pain
- Arthralgias with periarticular swelling of knees and ankles
- Erythema nodosum 2–20 days after symptom onset
- Persistent pulmonary lesions in 5%

Disseminated coccidioidomycosis
- Can involve any organ
- Productive cough
- Enlarged mediastinal lymph nodes
- Lung abscesses, empyema
- Fungemia with diffuse miliary infiltrates on chest radiograph and early death in immunocompromised patients
- Meningitis in 30–50%
- Bone lesions at bony prominences
- Subcutaneous abscesses and verrucous skin lesions
- Lymphadenitis may progress to suppuration
- Mediastinal and retroperitoneal abscesses
- Disseminated in HIV-infected patients more often shows miliary infiltrates, lymphadenopathy, multiple organ involvement and meningitis, but skin lesions are uncommon

DIFFERENTIAL DIAGNOSIS

- Histoplasmosis, cryptococcosis, nocardiosis, blastomycosis
- Sarcoidosis
- Pneumoconiosis, eg, silicosis
- Tuberculosis
- Upper respiratory tract infection
- Atypical pneumonia
- Lymphoma (including lymphocytic interstitial pneumonitis)

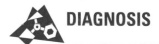

DIAGNOSIS

LABORATORY TESTS

- In primary coccidioidomycosis, moderate leukocytosis and eosinophilia
- IgM antibodies are positive in early disease
- In disseminated coccidioidomycosis, persistent or rising serum complement fixation titer (≥ 1:16); titers can be used to assess treatment adequacy
  - Complement fixation titer may be low in meningitis without other disseminated disease
  - In HIV-infected patients, complement fixation false-negative rate is as high as 30%
- In coccidioidal meningitis, cerebrospinal fluid (CSF) complement-fixing antibodies in > 90%. CSF shows increased cell count, lymphocytosis, and reduced glucose; positive culture in 30%
- Spherules filled with endospores in biopsy specimens, can be cultured
- Blood cultures are rarely positive

IMAGING STUDIES

- Chest radiographic findings vary
  - Nodular infiltrates and thin-walled cavities most common
  - Hilar lymphadenopathy suggests localized disease
  - Mediastinal adenopathy suggests dissemination
  - Pleural effusions
  - Abscesses
  - Bronchiectasis
  - Lytic bone lesions

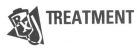

TREATMENT

MEDICATIONS

- For disease limited to the chest with no evidence of progression, symptomatic therapy
- For progressive pulmonary or extrapulmonary disease, IV amphotericin B until favorable clinical response and declining complement fixation titer
- Because of difficulties with intrathecal amphotericin B administration, most meningitis cases are initially treated with high-dose fluconazole, 1000 mg PO once daily, lifelong
- For severe meningitis
  - Lumbar intrathecal amphotericin B daily in increasing doses up to 1–5 mg/day, usually given with IV amphotericin B 0.6 mg/kg/day, until clinically stable
  - Then, taper intrathecal amphotericin to once every 6 weeks, or give oral azole therapy indefinitely
- For chest, bone, and soft-tissue disease, fluconazole, 200–400 mg PO once daily, or itraconazole, 400 mg PO once daily, continued for ≥ 6 months after disease is inactive to prevent relapse

SURGERY

- Thoracic surgery is occasionally indicated for giant, infected, or ruptured cavities
- Surgical drainage useful for soft-tissue abscesses and bone disease
- Following extensive surgical manipulation of infected tissue, give amphotericin B, 1 mg/kg/day IV, until disease is inactive, then change to oral azole therapy
- Ventriculoperitoneal shunting may be needed to control intracranial pressure in meningitis cases

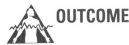

OUTCOME

FOLLOW-UP

- Follow serum complement fixation titers, observe for a decrease during therapy
- Perform serial complement fixation titers after therapy; rising titers indicate relapse and warrant reinstitution of therapy

COMPLICATIONS

- Lung abscesses may rupture into pleural space, producing empyema, and may extend to bones, skin, and occasionally pericardium and myocardium

- Hydrocephalus may complicate chronic meningitis necessitating CSF shunting

PROGNOSIS

- Good for patients with limited disease
- Nodules, cavities, and fibrosis may rarely progress after long periods of stability or regression
- Disseminated and meningeal forms have mortality rates exceeding 50% in the absence of therapy

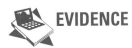

EVIDENCE

PRACTICE GUIDELINES

- 2001 USPHS/IDSA Guidelines for the Prevention of Opportunistic Infections in Persons Infected with Human Immunodeficiency Virus. US Department of Health and Human Services, Public Health Service
- Infectious Diseases Society of America—Practice guidelines for the treatment of coccidioidomycosis

WEB SITE

- AIDS Info by the USDHHS

INFORMATION FOR PATIENTS

- Centers for Disease Control and Prevention—Coccidioidomycosis
- MedlinePlus

REFERENCES

- Johnson RH et al. Coccidioidal meningitis. Clin Infect Dis. 2006 Jan 1; 42(1):103–7. [PMID: 16323099]
- Saubolle MA et al. Epidemiologic, clinical, and diagnostic aspects of coccidioidomycosis. J Clin Microbiol. 2007 Jan; 45(1):26–30. [PMID: 17108067]

Colorectal Cancer

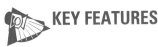

KEY FEATURES

ESSENTIALS OF DIAGNOSIS

- Symptoms or signs depend on tumor location
- Proximal colon: fecal occult blood, anemia
- Distal colon: change in bowel habits, hematochezia

- Characteristic findings on barium enema or CT colonography
- Diagnosis established with colonoscopy and biopsy

GENERAL CONSIDERATIONS

- Almost all colon cancers are adenocarcinomas
- ~50% occur distal to the splenic flexure (descending rectosigmoid) within reach of detection by flexible sigmoidoscopy
- Most colorectal cancers arise from malignant transformation of an adenomatous polyp
- Up to 4% of colorectal cancers are caused by inherited autosomal dominant germline mutations resulting in polyposis syndromes or hereditary nonpolyposis colorectal cancer
- Risk factors
  - Age
  - History of colorectal cancer or adenomatous polyps, breast, uterine, or ovarian cancer
  - Family history of colorectal cancer
  - Inflammatory bowel disease (ulcerative colitis and Crohn's colitis)
  - Diets rich in fats and red meat
  - Race (higher risk in blacks than in whites)

DEMOGRAPHICS

- Second leading cause of death due to malignancy in the United States
- Colorectal cancer will develop in ~6% of Americans and 40% of those will die of the disease
- ~134,000 new cases and 55,000 deaths occur annually in the United States

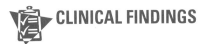

CLINICAL FINDINGS

SYMPTOMS AND SIGNS

- Adenocarcinomas grow slowly and may be asymptomatic
- Right-sided colon cancers cause
  - Iron deficiency anemia
  - Fatigue
  - Weakness from chronic blood loss
- Left-sided colon cancers cause
  - Obstructive symptoms
  - Colicky abdominal pain
  - Change in bowel habits
  - Constipation alternating with loose stools
  - Stool streaked with blood
- Rectal cancers cause
  - Rectal tenesmus
  - Urgency
  - Recurrent hematochezia

- Physical examination usually normal, except in advanced disease: mass may be palpable in the abdomen
- Hepatomegaly suggests metastatic spread

DIFFERENTIAL DIAGNOSIS

- Diverticulosis or diverticulitis
- Hemorrhoids
- Adenomatous polyps
- Ischemic colitis
- Inflammatory bowel disease
- Irritable bowel syndrome
- Infectious colitis
- Iron deficiency due to other cause

 DIAGNOSIS

LABORATORY TESTS

- Complete blood cell count may reveal iron deficiency anemia
- Liver function tests elevated in metastatic disease
- Fecal occult blood tests positive
- Carcinoembryonic antigen (CEA) level elevated in 70%; should normalize after complete surgical resection

IMAGING STUDIES

- Barium enema or CT colonography ("virtual colonoscopy") for initial diagnosis, if colonoscopy not available
- Abdominal and chest CT scan for preoperative staging
- Pelvic MRI and endorectal ultrasonography may guide operative management of rectal cancer

DIAGNOSTIC PROCEDURES

- Colonoscopy is the diagnostic procedure of choice because it visualizes the whole colon and permits biopsy of lesions
- Staging by TNM system correlates with the patient's long-term survival; it is used to determine which patients should receive adjuvant therapy (Table 40)

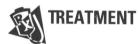 **TREATMENT**

MEDICATIONS

Stage II disease
- Adjuvant chemotherapy beneficial for persons at high risk for recurrence

Stage III disease
- Postoperative adjuvant chemotherapy alternatives include
  - Fluorouracil and leucovorin IV for 6 months improves 5-year disease-free survival rate to 65%
  - Capecitabin
    □ An alternative 5-FU analog, that is given orally, obviating the need for IV infusions
    □ Monotherapy with this drug yields a similar rate of disease-free survival with fewer serious side effects than IV fluorouracil and leucovorin
  - Oxaliplatin
    □ FOLFOX (oxaliplatin, fluorouracil, and leucovorin) is now the preferred postoperative adjuvant chemotherapy regimen
    □ Patients treated with FOLFOX had a higher rate of disease-free survival at 3 4 years (76%) than those treated with fluorouracil and leucovorin alone (69%)
    □ The addition of oxaliplatin was associated with an increased incidence of neutropenia and sensory neuropathy, which generally is reversible

Stage IV (metastatic) disease
- Chemotherapy regimens containing IV fluorouracil and leucovorin or capecitabine prolong median survival to about 11 months
- FOLFOX or FOLFIRI (addition of irinotecan to fluorouracil and leucovorin) further improves tumor response rate (40%) and median survival (15–20 months)
- FOLFOX and FOLFIRI are the preferred first-line treatment regimens
- Patients progressing with one regimen may respond to the alternative regimen, prolonging mean survival to > 20 months
- Biological agents (bevacizumab, cetuximab, and panitumumab) demonstrate further improvement in tumor response rates

SURGERY

- Resection of the primary colonic or rectal cancer
- Regional lymph node removal to determine staging
- For rectal carcinoma, in selected patients, transanal excision
- For all other patients with rectal cancer, low anterior resection with a colorectal anastomosis or an abdominoperineal resection with a colostomy
- For unresectable rectal cancer, diverting colostomy, radiation therapy, laser fulguration, or placement of an expandable wire stent
- For metastatic disease, resection of isolated (one to three) liver or lung metastases

THERAPEUTIC PROCEDURES

- Combined preoperative (or, in some cases, postoperative) adjuvant pelvic radiation and chemotherapy with fluorouracil for both stage II and stage III rectal cancers
- Local ablative techniques (cryosurgery, embolization) for unresectable hepatic metastases

 OUTCOME

FOLLOW-UP

- After resection surgery, patients should be evaluated every 3–6 months for 3–5 years with
  - History
  - Physical examination
  - Fecal occult blood testing
  - Liver function tests
  - Serum CEA levels
- A rise in CEA level that had normalized initially after surgery is suggestive of cancer recurrence
- Obtain colonoscopy
  - 12 months after surgical resection for persons who had complete preoperative colonoscopy
  - 3–6 months postoperatively for persons who did not have complete preoperative colonoscopy
  - Every 3–5 years thereafter
- Change in the patient's clinical picture, abnormal liver function tests, or a rising CEA level warrant chest radiography and abdominal CT

PROGNOSIS

- 5-year survival rates
  - Stage I: 80–100%, even with no adjuvant therapy
  - Stage II (node-negative disease): 50–75%, with no adjuvant therapy, although patients with advanced local stage II disease (T3–T4) should be considered for study protocols of adjuvant chemotherapy or radiotherapy
  - Stage III (node-positive disease): 30–50% without adjuvant chemotherapy; improved by postoperative adjuvant chemotherapy to 65%
- Long-term survival rates
  - Stage I: > 90%
  - Stage II: > 70%

- Stage III with fewer than four positive lymph nodes: 67%
  - Stage III with more than four positive lymph nodes: 33%
  - Stage IV: 5–7%
- For each stage, rectal cancers have a worse prognosis

PREVENTION

- Screening for colorectal neoplasms should be offered to every patient age > 50 (Table 41)
- Chemoprevention
  - Prolonged regular use of aspirin and other nonsteroidal anti-inflammatory drugs may decrease the risk of colorectal neoplasia
  - However, routine use as chemoprevention agents is not recommended currently

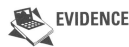

EVIDENCE

PRACTICE GUIDELINES

- National Guideline Clearinghouse
- Practice parameters for colon cancer. Dis Colon Rectum. 2004;47:1269. [PMID: 15484340]
- Screening for colorectal cancer: recommendations and rationale. United States Preventive Services Task Force, 2002
- Winawer S et al. American Gastroenterological Association. Colorectal cancer screening and surveillance: clinical guideline and rationale—update based on new evidence. Gastroenterology. 2003;124:544. [PMID: 12557158]

WEB SITE

- WebPath Gastrointestinal Pathology Index

INFORMATION FOR PATIENTS

- Torpy JM et al. JAMA patient page. Colon cancer screening. JAMA. 2003; 289:1334. [PMID: 12633198]

REFERENCES

- Bernold DM et al. Advances in chemotherapy for colorectal cancer. Clin Gastroenterol Hepatol. 2006 Jul;4(7):808–21. [PMID: 16797250]
- Davila RE et al. ASGE guidelines: colorectal cancer screening and surveillance. Gastrointest Endosc. 2006 Apr; 63(4):546–57. [PMID: 16564851]
- Meyerhardt JA et al. Systematic therapy for colorectal cancer. N Engl J Med. 2005 Feb 3;352(5):476–87. [PMID: 15689586]

- Morikawa T et al. A comparison of the immunochemical fecal occult blood test and total colonoscopy in the asymptomatic population. Gastroenterology. 2005 Aug;129(2):422–8. [PMID: 16083699]
- Rex D et al. Guidelines for colonoscopy surveillance after cancer resection: a consensus update by the American Cancer Society and the US multi-society task force on colorectal cancer. Gastroenterology. 2006 May;130(6):1865–71. [PMID: 16697749]
- Twelves C et al. Capecitabine as adjuvant treatment for stage III colon cancer. N Engl J Med. 2005 Jun 30;352(26):2696–704. [PMID: 15987918]
- Weitz J et al. Colorectal cancer. Lancet. 2005 Jan 8-14;365(9454):153–65. [PMID: 15639298]

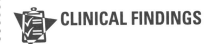

Common Variable Immunodeficiency

KEY FEATURES

ESSENTIALS OF DIAGNOSIS

- Most commonly due to a defect in terminal differentiation of B cells, with absent plasma cells and deficient synthesis of secreted antibody
- Increased susceptibility to pyogenic infections and frequent sinopulmonary infections
- Confirmation by detection of deficient serum immunoglobulin levels and impaired functional antibody responses

GENERAL CONSIDERATIONS

- A heterogeneous immunodeficiency disorder clinically characterized by an increased incidence of recurrent infections, autoimmune phenomena, and neoplastic diseases
- The most common cause of panhypogammaglobulinemia in adults
- The onset is usually during adolescence or early adulthood but can occur at any age
- Paradoxically, there is an increased incidence of autoimmune disease (20%), though patients may not display the usual serologic markers
- Gastrointestinal disorders are commonly associated

DEMOGRAPHICS

- The prevalence is about 1:80,000 in the United States

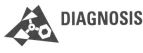

CLINICAL FINDINGS

SYMPTOMS AND SIGNS

- Increased susceptibility to pyogenic infections
- Most patients suffer from recurrent sinusitis
- Bronchitis, otitis, pharyngitis, and pneumonia are also common
- Autoimmune disease
- Sprue-like syndrome, with diarrhea, steatorrhea, malabsorption, protein-losing enteropathy, and hepatosplenomegaly
- Lymphadenopathy
- Increased incidence of cancers—lymphoma, gastric, and skin

DIFFERENTIAL DIAGNOSIS

- Secondary immunodeficiency, eg, AIDS, corticosteroid use, leukemia
- Selective IgA deficiency
- Multiple myeloma
- Cystic fibrosis
- Asplenism
- Celiac sprue
- Systemic lupus erythematosus
- X-linked agammaglobulinemia
- Immunodeficiency with thymoma
- Wegener's granulomatosis

DIAGNOSIS

LABORATORY TESTS

- The pattern of immunoglobulin isotype deficiency is variable
- Typically present with significantly depressed IgG levels (usually < 250 mg/dL), but over time all antibody classes (IgG, IgA, and IgM) may decrease
- Decreased to absent functional antibody responses to protein antigen immunizations establish the diagnosis
- Autoimmune cytopenias are common

DIAGNOSTIC PROCEDURES

- Biopsies of enlarged lymph nodes show marked reduction in plasma cells
- Noncaseating granulomas are frequently found in the spleen, liver, lungs, or skin

TREATMENT

MEDICATIONS

- Antibiotics at the first sign of infection; since antibody deficiency predisposes to high-risk pyogenic infections, antibiotic should cover encapsulated bacteria
- Monthly intravenous immune globulin (IGIV) is effective in decreasing the incidence of potentially life-threatening infections and increasing quality of life

OUTCOME

FOLLOW-UP

- Quarterly until "trough" immunoglobulin levels stabilize within age-adjusted "normal range"; semiannually thereafter for assessment of quantitative immunoglobulin levels and clinical assessment

COMPLICATIONS

- Infections may be of prolonged duration or associated with unusual complications such as meningitis or sepsis
- There is an increased propensity for the development of B cell neoplasms (50- to 400-fold increased risk of lymphoma), gastric carcinomas, and skin cancers

PROGNOSIS

- Good to excellent with monthly replacement immunoglobulin therapy

WHEN TO REFER

- Refer to confirm the need for IGIV
- May need early referral to an infectious disease specialist for severe or prolonged infections
- May need referral to a medical oncologist for staging and treatment of cancer

WHEN TO ADMIT

- For severe or rapidly progressive infections

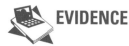

EVIDENCE

WEB SITES

- American Academy of Allergy, Asthma, and Immunology
- Immune Deficiency Foundation

INFORMATION FOR PATIENTS

- National Institutes of Health: Primary Immune Deficiency

- National Primary Immunodeficiency Resource Center: Common Variable Immunodeficiency
- National Primary Immunodeficiency Resource Center: FAQ's

REFERENCES

- Castigli E et al. Molecular basis of common variable immunodeficiency. J Allergy Clin Immunol. 2006 Apr; 117(4):740–6. [PMID: 16630927]
- Cunningham-Rundles C. Immune deficiency: office evaluation and treatment. Allergy Asthma Proc. 2003 Nov–Dec; 24(6):409–15. [PMID: 14763242]
- Weiler CR et al. Common variable immunodeficiency: test indications and interpretations. Mayo Clin Proc. 2005 Sep;80(9):1187–200. [PMID: 16178499]

Complex Regional Pain Syndrome (Reflex Sympathetic Dystrophy)

KEY FEATURES

ESSENTIALS OF DIAGNOSIS

- Rare disorder characterized by autonomic and vasomotor instability
- Intense, burning pain; often greatly worsened by minimal stimuli, such as light touch

GENERAL CONSIDERATIONS

- Most cases are preceded by direct physical trauma, often of relatively minor nature, to the soft tissues, bone, or nerve
- May occur after a knee injury or after arthroscopic knee surgery
- Any extremity can be involved, but the hand is most commonly affected and is associated with ipsilateral restriction of shoulder motion (shoulder-hand syndrome)
- The shoulder-hand variant sometimes complicates myocardial infarction or injuries to the neck or shoulder
- The posttraumatic variant is known as Sudeck's atrophy

CLINICAL FINDINGS

SYMPTOMS AND SIGNS

- No systemic symptoms
- Localized, diffuse pain
- Swelling of involved extremity
- Disturbances of color and temperature in affected limb
- Dystrophic changes in overlying skin and nails
- Limited range of motion

DIFFERENTIAL DIAGNOSIS

- Other cervicobrachial pain syndromes
- Rheumatoid arthritis
- Thoracic outlet obstruction
- Scleroderma

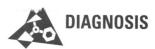

DIAGNOSIS

IMAGING STUDIES

- Bone scans
  - Sensitive in the early phases
  - Show diffuse increased uptake in affected extremity
- Radiographs eventually reveal severe generalized osteopenia

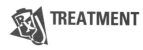

TREATMENT

MEDICATIONS

- Nortriptyline
  - Initial dose: 10 mg PO at bedtime
  - Increase gradually to 40–75 mg at bedtime
- Prednisone, 30–40 mg/d PO for 2 weeks and then tapered over 2 weeks, for resistant cases
- Patients with restricted shoulder motion may benefit from treatment used for scapulohumeral periarthritis

THERAPEUTIC PROCEDURES

- Physical therapy
- Regional nerve blocks and dorsal-column stimulation

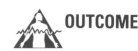

OUTCOME

PROGNOSIS

- Good with early treatment

PREVENTION

- Early mobilization after injury, surgery, or myocardial infarction

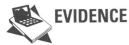

EVIDENCE

PRACTICE GUIDELINES

- Greipp ME. Complex regional pain syndrome—type I: research relevance, practice realities. J Neurosci Nurs. 2003 Feb;35(1):16–20. [PMID: 12789717]
- Turner-Stokes L. Reflex sympathetic dystrophy—a complex regional pain syndrome. Disabil Rehabil. 2002 Dec 15;24(18):939–47. [PMID: 12523947]

INFORMATION FOR PATIENTS

- Mayo Clinic: Complex Regional Pain Syndrome
- MedlinePlus: Complex Regional Pain Syndrome
- National Institute of Neurological Disorders and Stroke: Complex Regional Pain Syndrome Information Page

REFERENCES

- Birklein F. Complex regional pain syndrome. J Neurol. 2005 Feb; 252(2):131–8. [PMID: 15729516]
- Quisel A et al. Complex regional pain syndrome: which treatments show promise? J Fam Pract. 2005 Jul; 54(7):599–603. [PMID: 16009087]
- Teasdall RD et al. Complex regional pain syndrome (reflex sympathetic dystrophy). Clin Sports Med. 2004 Jan; 23(1):145–55. [PMID: 15062588]

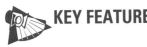

Congestive Heart Failure

KEY FEATURES

ESSENTIALS OF DIAGNOSIS

- Left ventricular (LV) congestive heart failure (CHF)
  - Exertional dyspnea
  - Cough
  - Fatigue
  - Orthopnea
  - Paroxysmal nocturnal dyspnea
  - Cardiac enlargement
  - Rales
  - Gallop rhythm
  - Pulmonary venous congestion
- Right ventricular (RV) CHF
  - Elevated venous pressure
  - Hepatomegaly
  - Dependent edema
  - Usually due to LV failure

GENERAL CONSIDERATIONS

- CHF occurs as a result of depressed contractility with fluid retention and/or impaired cardiac output, or diastolic dysfunction with fluid retention
- Acute exacerbations of chronic CHF are caused by patient nonadherence to or alterations in therapy, excessive salt and fluid intake, arrhythmias, excessive activity, pulmonary emboli, intercurrent infection, progression of the underlying disease
- High-output CHF is caused by thyrotoxicosis, beriberi, severe anemia, arteriovenous shunting, Paget's disease
- Systolic dysfunction is caused by myocardial infarction (MI), ethanol abuse, long-standing hypertension, viral myocarditis (including HIV), Chagas' disease, idiopathic dilated cardiomyopathy
- Diastolic dysfunction is associated with abnormal filling of a ("stiff") LV; caused by chronic hypertension, LV hypertrophy, and diabetes

CLINICAL FINDINGS

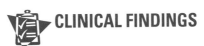

SYMPTOMS AND SIGNS

- Symptoms of diastolic dysfunction are often difficult to distinguish clinically from those of systolic dysfunction
- LV CHF
  - Exertional dyspnea progressing to orthopnea and then dyspnea at rest
  - Paroxysmal nocturnal dyspnea
  - Chronic nonproductive cough (often worse in recumbency)
  - Nocturia
  - Fatigue and exercise intolerance
- RV CHF
  - Anorexia
  - Nausea
  - Right upper quadrant pain due to chronic passive congestion of the liver and gut
- Tachycardia, hypotension, reduced pulse pressure, cold extremities, and diaphoresis
- Long-standing severe CHF: cachexia or cyanosis
- Physical examination findings in LV CHF
  - Crackles at lung bases, pleural effusions and basilar dullness to percussion, expiratory wheezing, and rhonchi
  - Parasternal lift, an enlarged and sustained LV impulse, a diminished first heart sound
  - S_3 gallop
  - S_4 gallop in diastolic dysfunction
- Physical examination findings in RV CHF
  - Elevated jugular venous pressure, abnormal pulsations, such as regurgitant v waves
  - Tender or nontender hepatic enlargement, heptojugular reflux, and ascites
  - Peripheral pitting edema sometimes extending to the thighs and abdominal wall

DIFFERENTIAL DIAGNOSIS

- Chronic obstructive pulmonary disease (COPD)
- Pneumonia
- Cirrhosis
- Peripheral venous insufficiency
- Nephrotic syndrome

DIAGNOSIS

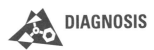

LABORATORY TESTS

- Obtain complete blood cell count, blood urea nitrogen, serum electrolytes, creatinine, thyroid-stimulating hormone
- ECG to look for
  - Arrhythmia
  - MI
  - Nonspecific changes, including low-voltage, intraventricular conduction delay; LV hypertrophy; and repolarization changes
- "B-type" natriuretic peptide (BNP)
  - Elevation is a sensitive indicator of symptomatic (diastolic or systolic) CHF but may be less specific, especially in older patients, women, and patients with COPD
  - Adds to clinical assessment in differentiating dyspnea due to heart failure from noncardiac causes

IMAGING STUDIES

- Chest radiograph shows
  - Cardiomegaly
  - Dilation of the upper lobe veins
  - Perivascular or interstitial edema
  - Alveolar fluid
  - Bilateral or right-sided pleural effusions
- Echocardiography can assess
  - Ventricular size and function
  - Valvular abnormalities

– Pericardial effusions
– Intracardiac shunts
– Segmental wall motion abnormalities
• Radionuclide angiography: measures LV ejection fraction and assesses regional wall motion
• Stress imaging: indicated if ECG abnormalities or suspected myocardial ischemia

DIAGNOSTIC PROCEDURES

• ECG helps to rule out
  – Valvular lesions
  – Myocardial ischemia
  – Arrhythmias
  – Alcohol- or drug-induced myocardial depression
  – Intracardiac shunts
  – High-output states
  – Hyperthyroidism and hypothyroidism
  – Medications
  – Hemochromatosis
  – Sarcoidosis
  – Amyloidosis
• Left heart catheterization
  – To exclude significant valvular disease
  – To delineate presence and extent of coronary artery disease
• Right heart catheterization: to select and monitor therapy in patients not responding to standard therapy

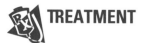 TREATMENT

MEDICATIONS

• Systolic dysfunction: a diuretic and an angiotensin-converting enzyme (ACE) inhibitor (or angiotensin receptor blocker [ARB]) with subsequent addition of a β-blocker
• Diuretics (Table 16)
  – Thiazide
  – Loop
  – Thiazide and loop
  – Thiazide and spironolactone
• Aldosterone blockers (Table 16)
  – Spironolactone, 25 mg PO once daily (may decrease to 12.5 mg or increase to 50 mg depending on renal function, K+, and symptoms)
  – Eplerenone, 25–50 mg PO once daily
• ACE inhibitors (Table 18): start at low doses and titrate to dosages proved effective in clinical trials over 1–3 months; for example
  – Captopril, 50 mg PO TID
  – Enalapril, 10 mg PO BID
  – Lisinopril, 20 mg PO once daily
• ARBs (Table 18) for ACE-intolerant patients

• ARB valsartan (titrated to a dose of 160 mg BID) added to ACE inhibitor therapy reduced composite of death or hospitalization for CHF
• β-Blockers (Table 17): in stable patients, start at low doses and titrate gradually and with great care; for example
  – Carvedilol started at 3.125 mg PO BID, increased to 6.25, 12.5, and 25 mg BID at intervals of ~2 weeks
  – Metoprolol extended-release, started at 12.5 or 25 mg once daily, increased to 50, 75, 100, 150, and 200 mg at intervals of ~2 weeks or longer
• Digoxin
• Positive inotropic agents (eg, dobutamine and milrinone): use is limited to patients
  – With hypoperfusion
  – With rapidly deteriorating renal function
  – Who have not responded to intravenous diuretics
  – Awaiting cardiac transplantation
• Anticoagulation: for patients with LV CHF associated with atrial fibrillation or large recent (within 3–6 months) MI
• Diastolic dysfunction: diuretics, rigorous blood pressure control

SURGERY

• Coronary revascularization may improve symptoms and prevent progression
• Bypass surgery provides more complete revascularization than angioplasty
• Cardiac transplantation for advanced heart failure
• Implantable defibrillators for chronic heart failure and ischemic or nonischemic cardiomyopathy with ejection fraction < 35%
• Biventricular pacing (resynchronization) for patients with moderate to severe systolic CHF and LV dyssynchrony

THERAPEUTIC PROCEDURES

• Moderate salt restriction (2.0–2.5 g sodium or 5–6 g salt per day)
• Temporary restriction of activity

 OUTCOME

FOLLOW-UP

• Monitor patients taking diuretics and ACE inhibitors for hypokalemia, renal failure
• Case management, home monitoring of weight and clinical status, and patient adjustment of diuretics can prevent rehospitalizations

COMPLICATIONS

• Myocardial ischemia in patients with underlying coronary artery disease
• Asymptomatic and symptomatic arrhythmias, especially nonsustained ventricular tachycardia
• Sudden death and unexplained syncope

PROGNOSIS

• Heart failure carries a poor prognosis
• 5-year mortality is approximately 50%
• Mortality rates vary from < 5% per year in those with no or few symptoms to > 30% per year in those with severe and refractory symptoms
• Higher mortality is related to
  – Older age
  – Lower left ventricular ejection fraction
  – More severe symptoms
  – Renal insufficiency
  – Diabetes

PREVENTION

• Antihypertensive therapy
• Antihyperlipidemic therapy
• Treat valvular lesions (aortic stenosis and mitral and aortic regurgitation) early

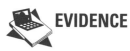 EVIDENCE

PRACTICE GUIDELINES

• Hunt SA et al. ACC/AHA Guidelines for the evaluation and management of chronic heart failure in the adult: executive summary. A report of the American College of Cardiology/American Heart Association Task Force on Practice Guidelines (Committee to Revise the 1995 Guidelines for the Evaluation and Management of Heart Failure). J Am Coll Cardiol. 2001 Dec; 38(7):2101–13. [PMID: 11738322]
• Liu P et al. Canadian Cardiovascular Society. The 2002/3 Canadian Cardiovascular Society consensus guideline update for the diagnosis and management of heart failure. Can J Cardiol. 2003;19:347. [PMID: 12704478]
• Swedberg K et al. Guidelines for the diagnosis and treatment of chronic heart failure: executive summary (update 2005): The Task Force for the Diagnosis and Treatment of Chronic Heart Failure of the European Society of Cardiology. Eur Heart J. 2005 Jun;26(11):1115–40. [PMID: 15901669]

WEB SITES

• American College of Cardiology
• National Heart, Lung, and Blood Institute

INFORMATION FOR PATIENTS

- American Academy of Family Physicians: Heart Failure
- American Heart Association: Heart Failure
- MedlinePlus: Congestive Heart Failure Interactive Tutorial
- National Heart, Lung, and Blood Institute: Heart Failure

REFERENCES

- Angeja BG et al. Evaluation and management of diastolic heart failure. Circulation. 2003 Feb 11;107(5):659–63. [PMID: 12578862]
- Bardy GH; Sudden Cardiac Death in Heart Failure Trial (SCD-HeFT) Investigators. Amiodarone or an implantable cardioverter-defibrillator for congestive heart failure. N Engl J Med. 2005 Jan 20;352(3):225–37. [PMID: 15659722]
- Cleland JG et al. The effect of cardiac resynchronization on morbidity and mortality in heart failure. N Engl J Med. 2005 Apr 14;352(15):1539–49. [PMID: 15753115]
- Mueller C et al. Use of B-type natriuretic peptide in the evaluation and management of acute dyspnea. N Engl J Med. 2004 Feb 12;350(7):647–54. [PMID: 14960741]
- Taylor AL et al; African-American Heart Failure Trial Investigators. Combination of isosorbide dinitrate and hydralazine in blacks with heart failure. N Engl J Med. 2004 Nov 11;351(20):2049–57. [PMID: 15533851]
- Young JB et al; Candesartan in Heart failure Assessment of Reduction in Mortality and morbidity (CHARM) Investigators and Committees. Mortality and morbidity reduction with candesartan in patients with chronic heart failure and left ventricular systolic dysfunction: results of the CHARM low-left ventricular ejection fraction trials. Circulation. 2004 Oct 26; 110(17):2618–26. [PMID: 15492298]

Conjunctivitis

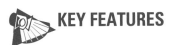 **KEY FEATURES**

ESSENTIALS OF DIAGNOSIS

- The most common eye disease, also known as "pink eye"
- Diffuse redness of the bulbar and tarsal conjunctiva
- Usually mild to moderate ocular irritation and discharge, clear cornea, and normal visual acuity

GENERAL CONSIDERATIONS

- Usually due to bacterial (including gonococcal or chlamydial) or viral infections
- Other common causes include atopy, chemical irritants, and keratoconjunctivitis sicca (dry eyes)
- Mode of transmission of infectious conjunctivitis is usually direct contact via fingers, towels, etc to the other eye, or to other persons
- Clinically important to differentiate conjunctivitis from acute uveitis, acute glaucoma, and corneal disorders

DEMOGRAPHICS

- Precise incidence is unknown, but very common
- Men and women affected equally
- Age group affected depends on the underlying cause
- Trachoma (*Chlamydia trachomatis*) is a major cause of blindness worldwide
- Gonococcal conjunctivitis and inclusion conjunctivitis are caused by the agents involved in the respective genital tract diseases (*Neisseria gonorrhoeae* or *C trachomatis*) and typically occur in sexually active adults
- Viral conjunctivitis is more common in children than adults, with contaminated swimming pools or ophthalmologists' offices often being the source of epidemics
- Keratoconjunctivitis sicca is common in elderly women and sometimes associated with systemic diseases (Sjögren's syndrome)
- Allergic eye disease typically begins in late childhood or young adulthood and usually in people with atopy

CLINICAL FINDINGS

SYMPTOMS AND SIGNS

Bacterial conjunctivitis

- Staphylococci, streptococci, *Haemophilus, Pseudomonas,* and *Moraxella* are the most common organisms isolated
- Purulent discharge
- Usually self-limited, lasting 10–14 days if untreated

Gonococcal conjunctivitis

- Exposure to infected genital secretions is the usual mode of transmission
- Copious purulent discharge
- An ophthalmologic emergency because corneal involvement may rapidly lead to perforation and blindness

Chlamydial conjunctivitis

- Trachoma usually causes recurrent conjunctivitis with scarring during childhood leading to corneal scarring in adulthood
- Inclusion conjunctivitis produces follicular conjunctivitis with redness, discharge, and irritation, and nontender preauricular lymphadenopathy

Viral conjunctivitis

- Adenoviruses are the most common causative pathogens
- Copious watery discharge with severe ocular irritation and possibly visual loss due to keratitis
- Subconjunctival hemorrhages occasionally occur
- There may be pharyngitis, fever, malaise, and preauricular lymphadenopathy

Keratoconjunctivitis sicca

- Due to hypofunction of the lacrimal glands, excessive evaporation of tears, abnormalities of the lipid component of tears, or mucin deficiency
- Ocular dryness, redness, or foreign body sensation
- Marked discomfort, photophobia, and excessive mucus in severe cases
- Corneal ulceration may develop

Allergic eye disease

- Itching is strongly suggestive of allergic eye disease
- Allergic conjunctivitis is a benign disease characterized by conjunctival hyperemia and edema, often of sudden onset, that may be seasonal (hay fever conjunctivitis) or perennial
- Vernal keratoconjunctivitis, characterized by large "cobblestone" papillae on the upper tarsal conjunctiva, and atopic keratoconjunctivitis, characterized by chronic papillary conjunctivitis with fibrosis, are potentially blinding diseases

DIFFERENTIAL DIAGNOSIS

- See Table 23
- Acute anterior uveitis (iritis)
- Acute (angle-closure) glaucoma
- Corneal trauma (eg, foreign body or abrasion)
- Corneal infection or inflammation (eg, corneal ulcer or herpes simplex keratitis)
- Scleritis or episcleritis

DIAGNOSIS

- Diagnosis is usually clinical
- If there is copious purulent discharge, conjunctival swab for Gram stain and bacterial culture to identify gonoccocal infection
- For suspected inclusion conjunctivitis or trachoma, immunologic tests or polymerase chain reaction on conjunctival samples
- For suspected keratoconjunctivitis sicca, Schirmer's test to measure tear production

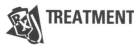

TREATMENT

MEDICATIONS

- See Table 24
- Choice of therapeutic agent should be dictated by underlying cause
- Bacterial conjunctivitis
  – Usually self-limited, lasting about 10–14 days if untreated
  – Topical sulfonamide (eg, sulfacetamide, 10% ophthalmic solution or ointment TID) will usually clear the infection in 2–3 days
  – Povidone-iodine may also be effective
  – Use of topical fluoroquinolones is rarely justified for treatment of a generally self-limiting, benign infection
- Gonococcal conjunctivitis: ceftriaxone 1 g IM but admit to hospital if corneal involvement
- Chlamydial conjunctivitis: single dose therapy with azithromycin or oral tetracycline, erythromycin, doxycyline for 1–4 weeks
- Viral conjunctivitis: if corneal involvement, weak topical corticosteroids under the supervision of an ophthalmologist
- Keratoconjunctivitis sicca
  – Artificial tears (preparations with methylcellulose, polyvinyl alcohol, or polyacrylic acid are longer lasting)
  – Lubricant ointment
- Allergic keratoconjunctivitis
  – Topical antihistamine
  – Nonsteroidal anti-inflammatory or mast cell stabilizing agents
  – If severe, topical corticosteroids under the supervision of an ophthalmologist

SURGERY

- Correction of eyelid deformities and corneal transplantation in the later stages of trachoma

THERAPEUTIC PROCEDURES

- Warm compresses and rest can be helpful and are often the only therapy necessary for mild bacterial or viral conjunctivitis

OUTCOME

FOLLOW-UP

- Most cases of bacterial or viral conjunctivitis do not require follow-up
- Recurrent bacterial conjunctivitis requires ophthalmologic assessment for predisposing factors such as blepharitis
- Gonococcal and inclusion conjunctivitis require follow-up for other sexually transmitted diseases
- Chronic moderate or severe allergic eye disease or keratoconjunctivitis sicca should be managed by an ophthalmologist

COMPLICATIONS

- Corneal ulceration, perforation or scarring, resulting in visual loss, may complicate gonococcal conjunctivitis, trachoma, keratoconjunctivitis sicca, or severe allergic eye disease

PROGNOSIS

- Most cases of conjunctivitis have an excellent prognosis, although long-term treatment may be required in keratoconjunctivitis sicca and chronic allergic eye disease

WHEN TO REFER

- Refer patients with copious purulent discharge, corneal involvement, loss of visual acuity, severe pain, or lack of response to treatment to an ophthalmologist
- Refer patients (or their mothers in the case of neonates) with inclusion conjunctivitis or gonococcal conjunctivitis for identification of genital tract infection and other sexually transmitted diseases to an internist or gynecologist

WHEN TO ADMIT

- Admit patients with gonococcal conjunctivitis involving the cornea

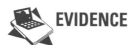

EVIDENCE

PRACTICE GUIDELINES

- American Academy of Ophthalmology
- American Family Physician (Cochrane Interpretation)

WEB SITES

- American Academy of Ophthalmology
- National Eye Institute

INFORMATION FOR PATIENTS

- American Academy of Family Physicians: Allergic Conjunctivitis
- Cleveland Clinic Foundation: Conjunctivitis
- Keratoconjunctivitis sicca

REFERENCE

- Sheikh A et al. Antibiotics versus placebo for acute bacterial conjunctivitis. Cochrane Database Syst Rev. 2006 Apr 19;(2):CD001211. [PMID: 16625540]

Connective Tissue Disease, Mixed

KEY FEATURES

- Features of more than one rheumatic disease; overlap connective tissue disease is the preferred designation for patients having features of different rheumatic diseases
- Patients with overlapping features of systemic lupus erythematosus (SLE), systemic sclerosis, and polymyositis
  – Initially, these patients were thought to have a distinct entity (mixed connective tissue disease [MCTD]) defined by a specific autoantibody to ribonuclear protein (RNP)
  – With time, in many patients, the manifestations evolve to one predominant disease, such as scleroderma, and many patients with antibodies to RNP have clear-cut SLE

CLINICAL FINDINGS

- Characteristics of multiple rheumatic diseases

DIAGNOSIS

- Clinical
- RNP
  – Sensitivity 95–100%, specificity is low

– Negative test essentially excludes MCTD

– Positive test in high titer increases posttest probability of MCTD

• Table 123

• Differential diagnosis
  – SLE
  – Scleroderma
  – Polymyositis
  – Sjögren's syndrome
  – Rheumatoid arthritis
  – Eosinophilic fasciitis
  – Graft-versus-host disease

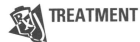 **TREATMENT**

• Symptom directed
• SLE, systemic sclerosis, or polymyositis features are treated the same way as the diseases

Constipation

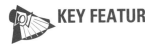 **KEY FEATURES**

ESSENTIALS OF DIAGNOSIS

• Defined as two or fewer bowel movements per week or excessive difficulty and straining at defecation

GENERAL CONSIDERATIONS

Primary constipation

• Most cases cannot be attributed to any structural abnormalities or systemic disease
• Colonic transit time is normal in most patients
• Normal colonic transit time is about 35 hours; > 72 hours is significantly abnormal
• Slow colonic transit
  – Commonly idiopathic but may be part of a generalized gastrointestinal dysmotility syndrome
  – More common in women, some of whom have a history of psychosocial problems (depression, anxiety, eating disorder, childhood trauma) or sexual abuse
• Patients may complain of
  – Infrequent bowel movements and abdominal bloating
  – Excessive straining
  – Sense of incomplete evacuation
  – Need for digital manipulation

Causes of secondary constipation

• Systemic disease
  – Endocrine
    ▫ Hypothyroidism
    ▫ Hyperparathyroidism
    ▫ Diabetes mellitus
  – Metabolic
    ▫ Hypercalcemia
    ▫ Hypokalemia
    ▫ Uremia
    ▫ Porphyria
  – Neurologic
    ▫ Parkinson's diseas
    ▫ Multiple sclerosis
    ▫ Sacral nerve damage (pelvic surgery, tumor)
    ▫ Paraplegia
    ▫ Autonomic neuropathy
  – Rheumatologic
    ▫ Scleroderma
  – Amyloidosis
  – Medications
    ▫ Narcotic
    ▫ Diuretic
    ▫ Calcium channel blocker
    ▫ Anticholinergic
    ▫ Psychotropic
    ▫ Calcium, iron
    ▫ Nonsteroidal anti-inflammatory drugs
    ▫ Clonidine
    ▫ Sucralfate
    ▫ Cholestyramine
  – Infectious: Chagas' disease
• Structural abnormalities
  – Anorectal
    ▫ Rectal prolapse
    ▫ Rectocele
    ▫ Rectal intussusception
    ▫ Anorectal stricture
    ▫ Anal fissure
    ▫ Solitary rectal ulcer syndrome
  – Pelvic floor dysfunction
  – Obstructing colonic mass (cancer)
  – Colonic stricture
    ▫ Radiation
    ▫ Ischemia
    ▫ Diverticulosis
  – Hirschsprung's disease
  – Chagas' disease
• Slow colonic transit
  – Idiopathic: isolated to colon
  – Psychogenic
  – Eating disorders
  – Chronic intestinal pseudo-obstruction

DEMOGRAPHICS

• Occurs in 10–15% of adults
• More common in women
• Elderly are predisposed due to comorbid conditions (eg, medical conditions, decreased mobility, medications, poor eating habits)

 CLINICAL FINDINGS

SYMPTOMS AND SIGNS

• Decreased appetite
• Nausea and vomiting
• Abdominal pain and distention
• Paradoxical "diarrhea"
• Firm feces palpable on digital rectal examination

DIFFERENTIAL DIAGNOSIS

• Inadequate fiber or fluid intake
• Poor bowel habits
• Irritable bowel syndrome

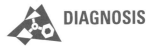 **DIAGNOSIS**

• In healthy patients under age 50 without alarm symptoms, it is reasonable to initiate a trial of empiric treatment without diagnostic tests
• Further diagnostic tests should be performed
  – In patients age > 50 years
  – In patients of any age with
    ▫ Severe constipation
    ▫ Hematochezia
    ▫ Weight loss
    ▫ Positive fecal occult blood
    ▫ Positive family history of colon cancer or inflammatory bowel disease
    ▫ No response to empiric treatment

LABORATORY TESTS

• Complete blood cell count
• Serum electrolytes
• Serum calcium
• Serum thyroid-stimulating hormone
• Fecal occult blood test

IMAGING STUDIES

• Colonoscopy or flexible sigmoidoscopy and barium enema

DIAGNOSTIC PROCEDURES

• Diet, fluid, and medication history
• Physical examination
• Colonic transit and pelvic floor function studies for severe constipation unresponsive to lifestyle changes and laxatives

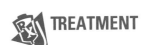 **TREATMENT**

MEDICATIONS

• Fiber supplements
  – Psyllium

– Methylcellulose

– Polycarbophil

• Stool surfactant agents

– Docusate sodium, 100 mg once daily or BID or

– Mineral oil, 15–45 mL/day once daily or BID

• Saline laxatives

– Magnesium-containing saline laxatives (milk of magnesia, magnesium sulfate)

– Sodium phosphate or magnesium citrate

• Osmotic laxatives

– Nonabsorbable carbohydrates: sorbitol (70%) or lactulose, 15–60 mL PO once daily to TID

– Polyethylene glycol powder (MiraLax), 17 g in 8 oz of liquid once daily or BID

• Stimulant agents

– Bisacodyl

– Senna

– Cascara

• Lubiprostone, 24 mcg PO BID

– Avoid in pregnant women

– Reserve for patients who have suboptimal response or side effects with less expensive agents

• Fecal impaction

– Initial treatment: enemas (saline, mineral oil, or diatrizoate) or digital disruption

– Long-term treatment: maintaining soft stools and regular bowel movements

SURGERY

• Subtotal colectomy with ileorectal anastomosis rarely required for severe intractable colonic inertia

• Disimpaction under anesthesia sometimes required for severe impaction

THERAPEUTIC PROCEDURES

• Biofeedback therapy for pelvic floor dysfunction

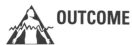 OUTCOME

COMPLICATIONS

• Fecal impaction

• Large bowel obstruction with pain, distention, nausea and vomiting

PROGNOSIS

• Most patients successfully treated with lifestyle changes and intermittent or chronic laxatives

WHEN TO REFER

• Severe constipation unresponsive to laxatives

• Suspected pelvic floor dysfunction (prolonged straining, difficulty with evacuation)

WHEN TO ADMIT

• Severe fecal impaction

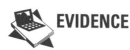 EVIDENCE

PRACTICE GUIDELINES

• American College of Gastroenterology Task Force. An evidence-based approach to the management of chronic constipation in North America. Am J Gastroenterol. 2005;100 Suppl 1:S1–4. [PMID: 16008640]

• American Gastroenterological Association medical position statement: guidelines on constipation. American Gastroenterological Association, 2001

INFORMATION FOR PATIENTS

• American College of Gastroenterology

• Cleveland Clinic

• Mayo Clinic

• National Digestive Diseases Information Clearinghouse—Constipation

REFERENCES

• Chiarioni G et al. Biofeedback is superior to laxatives for normal transit constipation due to pelvic floor dyssynergia. Gastroenterology. 2006 Mar; 130(3):657–64. [PMID: 16530506]

• Hsieh C. Treatment of constipation in older adults. Am Fam Physician. 2005 Dec 1;72(11):2277–84. [PMID: 16342852]

• Kamm MA. Clinical case: chronic constipation. Clin Gastroenterol Hepatol. 2006 Feb;4(2):233–48. [PMID: 16469685]

• McKeage K et al. Lubiprostone. Drugs. 2006;66(6):873–9. [PMID: 16706562]

• Ramkumar D et al. Efficacy and safety of traditional medical therapies for chronic constipation: systematic review. Am J Gastroenterol. 2005 Apr; 100(4):936–71. [PMID: 15784043]

• Rao SS et al. Clinical utility of diagnostic tests for constipation in adults: a systematic review. Am J Gastroenterol. 2005 Jul;100(7):1605–15. [PMID: 15984989]

• Wald A. Constipation in the primary care setting: current concepts and misconceptions. Am J Med. 2006 Sep; 119(9):736–9. [PMID: 16945605]

• Wald A. Severe constipation. Clin Gastroenterol Hepatol. 2005 May; 3(5):432–5. [PMID: 15880311]

Contraception, IUD & Barrier Methods

 KEY FEATURES

GENERAL CONSIDERATIONS

• Contraception should be available to all women and men of reproductive ages

• Education about and access to contraception are especially important for sexually active teenagers and for women following childbirth or abortion

• Intrauterine devices (IUDs) are not abortifacients

Intrauterine devices

• Available IUDs include Mirena (which releases levonorgestrel) and TCu380A (which is copper-bearing)

• The hormone-containing Mirena IUD has the advantage of reducing cramping and menstrual flow

• Nulliparity is not a contraindication to IUD use

• The Mirena IUD may have a protective effect against upper tract infection similar to that of oral contraceptives

• Contraindications to use of IUDs are outlined in Table 54

• A copper-containing IUD can be inserted within 5 days following a single episode of unprotected mid-cycle coitus as a postcoital contraceptive

• An IUD should not be inserted into a pregnant uterus

• If pregnancy occurs as an IUD failure, there is a greater chance of spontaneous abortion if the IUD is left in situ (50%) than if it is removed (25%)

• Spontaneous abortion with an IUD in place is associated with a high risk of severe sepsis, and death can occur rapidly

• Women using an IUD who become pregnant should have the IUD removed if the string is visible

• An IUD can be removed at the time of abortion if this is desired

• If the string is not visible and the patient wants to continue the pregnancy, she should be informed of the serious risk of sepsis and, occasionally, death with such pregnancies

- Such women should be informed that any symptoms of fever, myalgia, headache, or nausea warrant immediate medical attention for possible septic abortion
- Since the ratio of ectopic to intrauterine pregnancies is increased among IUD wearers, clinicians should search for adnexal masses in early pregnancy and should always check the products of conception for placental tissue following abortion

Diaphragm

- The diaphragm (with contraceptive jelly) is safe and effective; the diaphragm stretches from behind the cervix to behind the pubic symphysis
- Its features make it acceptable to some women and not others
- Advantages
  - Has no systemic side effects
  - Gives significant protection against pelvic infection and cervical dysplasia as well as pregnancy
- Disadvantages
  - Must be inserted before and near the time of coitus
  - Pressure from the rim predisposes some women to cystitis after intercourse
- Failure rates range from 6% to 16%, depending on the motivation of the woman and the care with which it is used

Cervical cap

- The cervical cap (with contraceptive jelly) is similar to the diaphragm but fits snugly over the cervix only
- Advantages
  - Can be used by women who cannot be fitted for a diaphragm because of a relaxed anterior vaginal wall
  - Can be used by women who have discomfort or develop repeated bladder infections with the diaphragm
- Disadvantages
  - More difficult to insert and remove than diaphragm
  - Because of the small risk of toxic shock syndrome, a cervical cap or diaphragm should not be left in the vagina for over 12–18 h, nor should these devices be used during the menstrual period (see above)
- Failure rates are 16% (typical use) and 9% (perfect use) in nulliparous women and 32% and 26%, respectively, in parous women

Contraceptive foam, cream, film, sponge, jelly, and suppository

- All contain the spermicide nonoxynol-9, which also has some virucidal and bactericidal activity
  - Nonoxynol-9 does not appear to adversely affect the vaginal colonization of hydrogen peroxide-producing lactobacilli
  - Nonoxynol-9 is not protective against HIV infection, particularly in women who have frequent intercourse
- Advantages
  - Simple to use
  - Easily available without prescription
- Disadvantage is a slightly higher failure rate (2-30%) than the diaphragm or condom

Condom

- The latex or animal membrane **male condom** affords good protection against pregnancy
  - Efficacy is comparable to that of a diaphragm used with spermicidal jelly
  - Latex (but not animal membrane) condoms also offer protection against sexually transmitted disease (STD) and cervical dysplasia
  - For protection against HIV transmission, a latex condom along with spermicide during vaginal or rectal intercourse is advised
  - The failure rate of a condom used with a spermicide, such as vaginal foam, approaches that of oral contraceptives
  - Condoms coated with spermicide are available in the United States
  - Disadvantages of condoms are dulling of sensation and potential for spillage of semen due to tearing, slipping, or leakage with detumescence of the penis
- The polyurethane **female condom** has failure rates of 5% to 21%
  - Efficacy is comparable to that of the diaphragm
  - It is the only female-controlled method that offers significant protection from both pregnancy and STDs

TREATMENT

THERAPEUTIC PROCEDURES

Intrauterine devices

- Insertion can be performed during or after the menses, at midcycle to prevent implantation, or later in the cycle if the patient is not pregnant
- Wait for 6–8 weeks postpartum before inserting an IUD

- When insertion is performed during lactation, there is greater risk of uterine perforation or embedding of the IUD
- Insertion immediately following abortion is acceptable if there is no sepsis and if follow-up insertion a month later will not be possible; otherwise, it is wise to wait until 4 weeks postabortion

OUTCOME

COMPLICATIONS

Intrauterine devices

- **Pelvic infection**
  - Women with a history of recent or recurrent pelvic infection are not good candidates for IUD use
  - At the time of insertion, women with an increased risk of STDs should be screened for gonorrhea and chlamydia
  - There is an increased risk of pelvic infection during the first month following IUD insertion
  - The subsequent risk of pelvic infection appears to be primarily related to the risk of acquiring STDs
- **Infertility** rates do not appear to be increased among women who have previously used the currently available IUDs
- **Menorrhagia or severe dysmenorrhea**
  - The copper IUD can cause heavier menstrual periods, bleeding between periods, and more cramping, so it is generally not suitable for women who already suffer from these problems
  - However, hormone-releasing IUDs can be tried in these cases, as they often cause decreased bleeding and cramping with menses
  - Nonsteroidal anti-inflammatory drugs are also helpful in decreasing bleeding and pain
- **Complete or partial expulsion**
  - Spontaneous expulsion of the IUD occurs in 10–20% of cases during the first year of use
  - Any IUD should be removed if the body of the device can be seen or felt in the cervical os
- **Missing IUD strings**
  - If the transcervical tail cannot be seen, this may signify unnoticed expulsion, perforation of the uterus with abdominal migration of the IUD, or simply retraction of the string into the cervical canal or uterus owing to movement of the IUD or uterine growth with pregnancy
  - Once pregnancy is ruled out, probe for the IUD with a sterile sound or forceps designed for IUD removal,

after administering a paracervical block

- If the IUD cannot be detected, pelvic ultrasound will demonstrate the IUD if it is in the uterus, or anteroposterior and lateral x-rays of the pelvis with another IUD or a sound in the uterus as a marker can confirm an extrauterine IUD
- If the IUD is in the abdominal cavity, remove by laparoscopy or laparotomy
- Open-looped all-plastic IUDs such as the Lippes Loop can be left in the pelvis without danger, but ring-shaped IUDs may strangulate a loop of bowel and copper-bearing IUDs may cause tissue reaction and adhesions

PROGNOSIS

- The IUD is highly effective, with failure rates similar to those achieved with surgical sterilization
- Women who are not in mutually monogamous relationships should use condoms for protection from STDs
- The Mirena IUD is approved for 5 years use and the Tcu380A IUD for 10 years

PREVENTION

- Perforations of the uterus are less likely if insertion is performed slowly, with care taken to follow directions applicable to each type of IUD

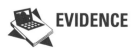 EVIDENCE

PRACTICE GUIDELINES

- Black A et al; Contraception Guidelines Committee. Canadian Contraception Consensus, 2004.

WEB SITE

- Gynecology Handbook

INFORMATION FOR PATIENTS

- American College of Obstetricians and Gynecologists: Birth Control
- Mayo Clinic: IUDs

REFERENCES

- ACOG Committee on Practice Bulletins-Gynecology. ACOG practice bulletin. Clinical Management Guidelines for Obstetrician-Gynecologists. Number 59, January 2005. Intrauterine device. Obstet Gynecol. 2005 Jan; 105(1):223–32. [PMID: 15625179]
- Raymond EG et al. Contraceptive effectiveness and safety of five nonoxynol-9 spermicides: a randomized trial. Obstet Gynecol. 2004 Mar;103(3):430–9. [PMID: 14990402]

Contraception, Oral, Injections, & Implants

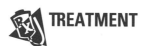 **KEY FEATURES**

GENERAL CONSIDERATIONS

- Contraception should be available to all women and men of reproductive ages
- Education about contraception and access to contraceptive pills or devices are especially important for sexually active teenagers and for women following childbirth or abortion

TREATMENT

MEDICATIONS

Oral contraceptives
- **Combination pills**
  - Have a theoretical failure rate of < 0.3% if taken absolutely on schedule and a typical failure rate of 8%
  - Primary mode of action is suppression of ovulation
  - Pills can be started on the first day of the menstrual cycle, on the first Sunday after the onset of the cycle, or on any day of the cycle
    - If started on any day other than the first day of the cycle, a backup method should be used
    - A pill is taken daily for 21 days, followed by 7 days of placebos or no medication, and this schedule is continued for each cycle
  - There are also pills packaged to be taken continuously for 84 days, followed by 7 days of placebos
    - If an active pill is missed at any time, and no intercourse occurred in the past 5 days, two pills should be taken immediately and a backup method should be used for 7 days
    - If intercourse occurred in the previous 5 days, emergency contraception should be used immediately, and the pills restarted the following day; a backup method should be used for 5 days

- **Benefits**
  - There are many noncontraceptive advantages to oral contraceptives
    - Menstrual flow is lighter
    - Resultant anemia is less common
    - Dysmenorrhea is relieved for most women
  - Functional ovarian cysts generally disappear with oral contraceptive use, and new cysts do not occur
  - Pain with ovulation and postovulatory aching are relieved
  - The risk of ovarian and endometrial cancer is decreased, and the risks of salpingitis and ectopic pregnancy may be diminished
  - Acne is usually improved
  - The frequency of developing myomas is lower in long-term users (> 4 years). There is a beneficial effect on bone mass
- **Selection**
  - Any of the combination oral contraceptives containing 35 mcg or less of estrogen are suitable for most women
  - There is some variation in potency of the various progestins in the pills, but there are essentially no clinically significant differences for most women among the progestins in the low-dose pills
  - Women who have acne or hirsutism may benefit from use of one of the pills containing the third-generation progestins, desogestrel or norgestimate, as they are the least androgenic
  - The low-dose oral contraceptives commonly used in the United States are listed in Table 52
- **Drug interactions**
  - Drugs that interact with oral contraceptives to decrease their efficacy include
    - Phenytoin
    - Phenobarbital (and other barbiturates)
    - Primidone
    - Carbamazepine
    - Rifampin
  - Women taking these drugs should use another means of contraception for maximum safety
- **Contraindications and adverse effects**
  - See Table 53
- **Minor side effects**
  - Nausea and dizziness may occur in the first few months of pill use
- **Efficacy and methods of use**
  - Formulations containing 0.35 mg of norethindrone or 0.075 mg of norgestrel are available in the United States
  - Efficacy is similar to that of combined oral contraceptives, with failure rates of 1–4%

- The minipill is begun on the first day of a menstrual cycle and then taken continuously for as long as contraception is desired

- **Advantages**
  - The low dose and absence of estrogen make the minipill safe during lactation; it may increase the flow of milk
  - It is often tried by women who want minimal doses of hormones and by patients who are over age 35
  - It can be used by women with uterine myomas or sickle cell disease (S/S or S/C)

- **Complications and contraindications**
  - Minipill users often have bleeding irregularities (eg, prolonged flow, spotting, or amenorrhea); such patients may need monthly pregnancy tests
  - Ectopic pregnancies are more frequent, and complaints of abdominal pain should be investigated with this in mind
  - The contraindications listed in Table 53 apply to the minipill
  - Minor side effects of combination oral contraceptives such as weight gain and mild headache may also occur with the minipill

Contraceptive injections and implants

- **Long-acting progestins**
  - Progestin medroxyprogesterone acetate IM, 150 mg every 3 months
  - A new subcutaneous preparation, containing 104 mg of DMPA, is available in the United States
  - Has a contraceptive efficacy of 99.7%
  - Common side effects
    - Irregular bleeding
    - Amenorrhea
    - Weight gain
    - Headache
  - Associated with bone mineral loss
  - Users commonly have irregular bleeding initially and subsequently develop amenorrhea
  - Ovulation may be delayed after the last injection
  - Contraindications are similar to those for the minipill
  - Estradiol cypionate (Lunelle)
    - A monthly injectable that is highly effective, with a first-year pregnancy rate of 0.2%
    - Side effect profile similar to that of oral contraceptives
    - Not being marketed currently
  - Implanon
    - A 40-mm × 2-mm rod containing 68 mg of etonogestrel
    - Insertion and removal much simpler and faster than with Norplant
    - Pregnancy rate was 0.0% in clinical trials

- Side effects similar to minipills, Depo-Provera, and Norplant
- Irregular bleeding most common reason for discontinuation
  - Norplant system
    - A contraceptive implant containing levonorgestrel
    - No longer marketed in the United States

Other hormonal methods

- A transdermal contraceptive patch containing 150 mcg norelgestromin and 20 mcg ethinyl estradiol and measuring 20 cm^2 is available
  - The patch is applied to the lower abdomen, upper torso, or buttock once a week for 3 consecutive weeks, followed by 1 week without the patch
  - The mechanism of action and efficacy are similar to those associated with oral contraceptives, though compliance may be better
  - Because of a higher steady-state serum concentration of estrogen than with low dose oral contraceptives, there may be a higher risk of estrogen-related complications
- A contraceptive vaginal ring that releases 120 mcg of etonogestrel and 15 mcg of ethinyl estradiol daily is available
  - The ring is soft and flexible and is placed in the upper vagina for 3 weeks, removed, and replaced 1 week later
  - The efficacy, mechanism of action, and systemic side effects are similar to those associated with oral contraceptives
  - In addition, users may experience an increased incidence of vaginal discharge

OUTCOME

FOLLOW-UP

- Patients using hormonal contraception are usually seen annually for a review of pertinent history, breast and pelvic examination with Papanicolaou smear

COMPLICATIONS

- Serious complications of combined hormonal contraception include
  - Venous thromboembolism: 10–30/ 100,000 annually
  - Myocardial infarction: 40/100,000 annually in smokers over age 35
  - Hypertension: 1% incidence

EVIDENCE

PRACTICE GUIDELINES

- ACOG Committee on Practice Bulletins—Gynecology. ACOG practice bulletin. No. 73: Use of hormonal contraception in women with coexisting medical conditions. Obstet Gynecol. 2006 Jun;107(6):1453–72. [PMID: 16738183]
- Black A et al; Contraception Guidelines Committee. Canadian Contraception Consensus, 2004.
- FFPRHC Guidance. emergency contraception (April 2003). J Fam Plan Reprod Health Care. 2003;29:9. [PMID: 12681030]

WEB SITES

- Gynecology Handbook for Family Practitioners
- US Food and Drug Administration: Birth Control Guide

INFORMATION FOR PATIENTS

- American College of Obstetricians and Gynecologists
- National Women's Health Information Center: Birth Control Methods
- National Women's Health Information Center: Emergency Contraception
- US Food and Drug Administration: What Kind of Birth Control Is Best for You?

REFERENCES

- Hatcher RA et al. *Contraceptive Technology*, 18th edition. New York, Ardent Media, 2004.
- Kaunitz AM. Beyond the pill: new data and options in hormonal and intrauterine contraception. Am J Obstet Gynecol. 2005 Apr;192(4):998–1004. [PMID: 15846172]
- Reproductive Health and Research; World Health Organization. Medical Eligibilty Criteria for Contraceptive Use. WHO/RHR 2004, Geneva.
- Reproductive Health and Research; World Health Organization. Selected Practice Recommendations for Contraceptive Use. WHO/RHR 2004, Geneva.
- World Health Organization. WHO Statement on Hormonal Contraception and Bone Health 2005 http://www.who.int/reproductive-health/family_planning/docs/hormonal_contraception_bone_health.pdf

Cor Pulmonale

KEY FEATURES

- Right ventricular (RV) hypertrophy and failure from lung disease or pulmonary vascular disease
- Most common cause: chronic obstructive pulmonary disease (COPD) or sleep apnea
- Less common causes
  - Pneumoconiosis
  - Pulmonary fibrosis
  - Kyphoscoliosis
  - Idiopathic pulmonary hypertension
  - Repeated pulmonary embolization
  - Sleep apnea (Pickwickian syndrome)

CLINICAL FINDINGS

- Predominant symptoms—intensified with RV failure—are related to the underlying pulmonary disorder
  - Chronic productive cough
  - Exertional dyspnea
  - Wheezing
  - Easy fatigability
  - Weakness
- Other possible findings
  - Dependent edema
  - Right upper quadrant pain (hepatic congestion)
  - Cyanosis
  - Clubbing
  - Distended neck veins
  - RV heave
  - Gallop
- Polycythemia is often present
- Arterial oxygen saturation often < 85%

DIAGNOSIS

- Symptoms and signs of COPD with elevated jugular venous pressure, parasternal lift, edema, hepatomegaly, ascites
- ECG
  - Tall, peaked P waves (P pulmonale), right axis deviation, and RV hypertrophy
  - Q waves in leads II, III, and aVF may mimic myocardial infarction
  - Frequent, nonspecific supraventricular arrhythmias
- Chest radiograph
  - Enlarged RV and pulmonary artery
  - Possible signs of pulmonary parenchymal disease

- Pulmonary function tests to confirm underlying lung disease
- Echocardiogram or angiography to exclude primary left ventricular failure as a cause of right-sided heart failure
- Multi-slice CT scan to exclude pulmonary emboli

TREATMENT

- Treat underlying lung disease
- Oxygen, salt and fluid restriction, and diuretics, often in combination
- Compensated cor pulmonale has the same prognosis as the underlying lung disease
- Average life expectancy is 2–5 yr when signs of congestive heart failure appear, but survival is significantly longer when uncomplicated emphysema is the cause

Cough

KEY FEATURES

ESSENTIALS OF DIAGNOSIS

- Age
- Duration of cough
- Dyspnea (at rest or with exertion)
- Constitutional symptoms
- Tobacco use history
- Vital signs (temperature, respiratory rate, heart rate)
- Chest examination

GENERAL CONSIDERATIONS

- Cough results from stimulation of mechanical or chemical afferent nerve receptors in the bronchial tree
- Cough illness syndromes are defined as acute (< 3 weeks) or persistent (> 3 weeks)
- Postinfectious cough lasting 3–8 weeks is termed "subacute cough" to distinguish this distinct clinical entity from acute and persistent cough
- The prevalence of pertussis infection in adults with a cough lasting > 3 weeks is 20%
- In about 25% of cases, persistent cough has multiple contributors

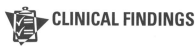

CLINICAL FINDINGS

SYMPTOMS AND SIGNS

- Timing and character of cough are usually not useful in establishing cause
- Acute cough syndromes
  - Most due to viral respiratory tract infections
  - Less common causes include congestive heart failure (CHF), hay fever (allergic rhinitis), and environmental factors
- Search for additional features of infection such as fever, nasal congestion, and sore throat
- Dyspnea (at rest or with exertion) may reflect a more serious condition
- Persistent cough is usually due to
  - Angiotensin-converting enzyme (ACE) inhibitor therapy
  - Postnasal drip
  - Asthma
  - Gastroesophageal reflux disease (GERD)
- Less common causes of persistent cough
  - Bronchogenic carcinoma
  - Chronic bronchitis
  - Bronchiectasis
  - Other chronic lung disease
  - CHF
- Signs of pneumonia
  - Tachycardia
  - Tachypnea
  - Fever
  - Rales
  - Decreased breath sounds
  - Fremitus
  - Egophony
- Signs of acute bronchitis: wheezing and rhonchi
- Signs of chronic sinusitis: postnasal drip
- Signs of chronic obstructive pulmonary disease (COPD)
  - Abnormal match test (inability to blow out a match from 10 inches away)
  - Maximum laryngeal height < 4 cm (measured from the sternal notch to the cricoid cartilage at end expiration)
- Signs of CHF
  - Symmetric basilar rales
  - Abnormal jugular venous pressure
  - Positive hepatojugular reflux

DIFFERENTIAL DIAGNOSIS

Acute cough
- Viral upper respiratory infection or postviral cough (most common)
- Postnasal drip (allergic rhinitis)
- Pneumonia
- Pulmonary edema

- Pulmonary embolism
- Aspiration pneumonia

Persistent cough

- Top three causes: postnasal drip, asthma, GERD
- Pulmonary infection
  - Postviral
  - Pertussis
  - Chronic bronchitis, especially in smokers
  - Bronchiectasis
  - Tuberculosis
  - Cystic fibrosis
  - *Mycobacterium avium* complex
  - *Mycoplasma, Chlamydia,* respiratory syncytial virus (underrecognized in adults)
- Pulmonary noninfectious
  - Asthma (cough-variant asthma)
  - COPD
  - ACE inhibitors
  - Irritant inhalation (eg, smoking)
  - Endobronchial lesion (eg, tumor)
  - Interstitial lung disease
  - Sarcoidosis
  - Chronic microaspiration
  - β-Blockers causing asthma
- Nonpulmonary
  - GERD
  - Postnasal drip (allergic rhinitis)
  - Sinusitis
  - CHF
  - Laryngitis
  - Ear canal or tympanic membrane irritation
  - Psychogenic or habit cough

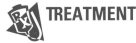 **DIAGNOSIS**

LABORATORY TESTS

- Pulse oximetry or arterial blood gas measurement
- Peak expiratory flow rate or spirometry

IMAGING STUDIES

- Acute cough: obtain chest radiograph if abnormal vital signs or chest examination; higher index of suspicion in elderly and immunocompromised persons
- Persistent cough: obtain chest radiograph if unexplained cough lasts more than 3–6 weeks

DIAGNOSTIC PROCEDURES

- Pertussis detection by culture and polymerase chain reaction of nasopharyngeal swab
- Reserve procedures for patients with persistent cough who do not respond to therapeutic trials

- Sinus CT scan for cough with postnasal drip
- Spirometry (if normal, possible methacholine challenge) for cough with wheezing or possible asthma, though pulmonary function tests are often normal in cough-variant asthma
- Esophageal pH monitoring for cough with GERD symptoms

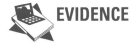 **TREATMENT**

MEDICATIONS

Acute cough

- Treatment should target
  - The underlying cause of the illness
  - The cough reflex itself
  - Any additional factors that exacerbate the cough
- Amantadine, rimantadine, oseltamivir, and zanamivir are equally effective (1 less day of illness) when initiated within 30–48 hours of onset of influenza
- Macrolide or doxycycline are first-line antibiotics for *Chlamydia* or *Mycoplasma*-documented infection
- In patients diagnosed with acute bronchitis, inhaled β₂-agonist therapy reduces severity and duration of cough in some patients
- Dextromethorphan has a modest benefit on the severity of cough due to acute respiratory tract infections
- Treatment of postnasal drip (with antihistamines, decongestants and/or nasal steroids) or gastroesophageal reflux disease (with H_2-blockers or proton-pump inhibitors), when accompanying acute cough illness, can also be helpful
- Vitamin C and echinacea are not effective in reducing the severity of acute cough illness after it develops

Persistent cough

- If due to pertussis, macrolide antibiotic therapy to reduce transmission
- When pertussis infection has lasted more than 7–10 days, antibiotic treatment does not affect the duration of cough—which can last up to 6 months
- Nebulized lidocaine therapy for idiopathic persistent cough

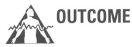 **OUTCOME**

WHEN TO REFER

- When asthma is suspected, refer to pulmonologist

- When due to chronic sinusitis unresponsive to medications, refer to otolaryngologist
- When due to GERD unresponsive to medications, refer to gastroenterologist or surgeon

WHEN TO ADMIT

- Pneumonia, if moderate to severe
- Bronchiectasis exacerbation, if moderate to severe
- COPD exacerbation, if moderate to severe

 EVIDENCE

PRACTICE GUIDELINES

- Gonzales R et al. Principles of appropriate antibiotic use for treatment of uncomplicated acute bronchitis in adults: background. Ann Intern Med. 2001;134:521. [PMID: 11255532]
- Institute for Clinical Systems Improvement (ICSI): Chronic obstructive pulmonary disease, 2004.
- Institute for Clinical Systems Improvement (ICSI): Viral upper respiratory infection (VURI) in adults and children, 2004.

INFORMATION FOR PATIENTS

- American Academy of Family Physicians: Chronic Cough: Causes and Cures
- American College of Chest Physicians: Managing Cough as Defense Mechanism and as a Symptom
- MedlinePlus: Cough

REFERENCES

- Call SA et al. Does this patient have influenza? JAMA. 2005 Feb 23; 293(8):987–97. [PMID: 15728170]
- Hewlett EL et al. Clinical practice. Pertussis—not just for kids. N Engl J Med. 2005 Mar 24;352(12):1215–22. [PMID: 15788498]
- Metlay JP et al. Testing strategies in the initial management of patients with community-acquired pneumonia. Ann Intern Med. 2003 Jan 21;138(2):109–18. [PMID: 12529093]
- Pratter MR et al. An empiric integrative approach to the management of cough: ACCP evidence-based clinical practice guidelines. Chest. 2006 Jan;129(1 Suppl):222S–231S. [PMID: 16428715]
- Schroeder K et al. Over-the-counter medications for acute cough in children and adults in ambulatory settings.

Cochrane Database Syst Rev 2004;
(4):CD001831. [PMID: 15495019]
• Wenzel RP et al. Acute bronchitis. N
Engl J Med. 2006 Nov 16;
355(20):2125–30. [PMID: 17108344]

Crohn's Disease

 KEY FEATURES

ESSENTIALS OF DIAGNOSIS

- Insidious onset
- Intermittent bouts of low-grade fever, diarrhea, and right lower quadrant pain
- Right lower quadrant mass and tenderness
- Perianal disease with abscess, fistulas
- Radiographic evidence of ulceration, stricturing, or fistulas of the small intestine or colon

GENERAL CONSIDERATIONS

- Crohn's disease is a transmural process
- Crohn's may involve
  – Small bowel only, most commonly the terminal ileum (ileitis) in ~33% of cases
  – Small bowel and colon, most often the terminal ileum and adjacent proximal ascending colon (ileocolitis) in ~50%
  – Colon alone in 20%
- Chronic illness with exacerbations and remissions
- Treatment is directed both toward symptomatic improvement and controlling the disease process

DEMOGRAPHICS

- Increased in Europeans, North Americans, and Ashkenazi Jews
- Increased risk among first-degree relatives
- Increased risk in smokers

 CLINICAL FINDINGS

SYMPTOMS AND SIGNS

- Fevers
- Abdominal pain
- Liquid bowel movements
- Abdominal tenderness or abdominal mass

Chronic inflammatory disease
- Malaise, loss of energy
- Diarrhea, nonbloody, intermittent
- Cramping or steady right lower quadrant or periumbilical pain
- Focal tenderness, right lower quadrant
- Palpable, tender mass in the lower abdomen

Intestinal obstruction
- Postprandial bloating, cramping pains, and loud borborygmi
- Small bowel obstruction with distention, cramping abominal pain, nausea, vomiting

Fistulization with or without infection
- Sinus tracts and fistulas can result in intra-abdominal or retroperitoneal abscesses manifested by fevers, chills, and a tender abdominal mass
- Bacterial overgrowth in small bowel may result in diarrhea, weight loss, and malnutrition
- Bladder or vagina recurrent infections
- Cutaneous fistulas
- Perianal disease
  – Anal fissures
  – Perianal abscesses
  – Fistulas

Extraintestinal manifestations
- Oral aphthous lesions
- Gallstones
- Nephrolithiasis with stones

DIFFERENTIAL DIAGNOSIS

- Ulcerative colitis
- Irritable bowel syndrome
- Appendicitis
- *Yersinia enterocolitica* enteritis
- Mesenteric adenitis
- Intestinal lymphoma
- Segmental colitis due to ischemic colitis, tuberculosis, amebiasis, chlamydia
- Diverticulitis with abscess
- Nonsteroidal anti-inflammatory drug–induced colitis
- Perianal fistula due to other cause

 DIAGNOSIS

LABORATORY TESTS

- Obtain complete blood cell count, erythrocyte sedimentation rate or C-reactive protein, serum albumin
- Anemia of chronic inflammation, blood loss, iron deficiency, or vitamin B_{12} malabsorption
- Leukocytosis with abscesses

- Sedimentation rate or C-reactive protein elevated
- Obtain stool for routine pathogens, ova and parasites, and *Clostridium difficile* toxin
- Antibodies to the yeast *Saccharomyces cerevisiae* (ASCA) are found in 60–70%

IMAGING STUDIES

- Barium upper gastrointestinal series with small bowel follow-through
- CT enterography
- Capsuled (video) imaging of small intestine

DIAGNOSTIC PROCEDURES

- Colonoscopy
- Biopsy of intestine reveals granulomas in 25%

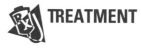 **TREATMENT**

MEDICATIONS

Symptomatic treatment of diarrhea
- Antidiarrheal agents
  – Loperamide (2–4 mg), diphenoxylate with atropine (one tablet), or tincture of opium (5–15 drops) QID PRN
  – Should not be used in patients with active severe colitis
- Broad-spectrum antibiotics if bacterial overgrowth
- Cholestyramine (2–4 g) or colestipol (5 g) PO BID–TID before meals for diarrhea caused by terminal ileal-resection with bile salt malabsorption

Treatment of exacerbations
- 5-Aminosalicylic acid agents
  – Sulfasalazine, 1.5–2 g PO BID
  – Mesalamine (Asacol), 0.8–1.2 g PO QID, or its slow-release form (Pentasa), 1 g PO QID, for mild to moderate colonic disease
  – Limited or no efficacy for small bowel disease
- Antibiotics sometimes used for for ileitis; however, efficacy unproven
  – Metronidazole, 10 mg/kg/day
  – Ciprofloxacin, 500 mg PO BID for perianal disease
- Broad-spectrum antibiotics for abscess
- Ileal-release preparation of topically active compound budesonide, 9 mg PO QD for 8 weeks for mild to moderate disease involving terminal ileal disease or ascending colon, or both
- Corticosteroids
  – Prednisone, 40–60 mg/day for 2–3 weeks

- Taper by 5 mg/week until dosage is 20 mg/day, then by 2.5 mg/week or every other week for acute episodes of moderate to severe disease
- Immunomodulatory drugs
  - Azathioprine (2–2.5 mg/kg) and mercaptopurine (1–1.5 mg/kg) useful for long-term treatment in patients requiring repeated corticosteroids (to help achieve or maintain remission) or infliximab (to reduce formation of antibodies to infliximab)
  - Methotrexate (25 mg IM or SQ weekly for 12 weeks, followed by 12.5–15 mg once weekly) for patients who are intolerant of or who do not respond to azathioprine or mercaptopurine
  - Infliximab, 5 mg/kg given at 0, 2, and 6 weeks is useful in moderate to severe Crohn's, and results in improvement in two-thirds and remission in one-third of patients

Maintenance of remission

- Mesalamine (Asacol), 800 mg PO TID or Pentasa, 500–750 mg PO QID may be of value in disease involving colon
- Corticosteroids should not be used
- Azathioprine, mercaptopurine, and methotrexate help maintain remission
- Long-term infliximab (every 8 weeks) appropriate for some patients with moderate to severe disease

SURGERY

- At least one surgical procedure required by > 50% of patients
- Indications for surgery
  - Intractability to medical therapy
  - Intra-abdominal abscess
  - Massive bleeding
  - Obstruction with fibrous stricture
- Incision and drainage for abscess
- Surgical resection of the stenotic area or stricturoplasty in small bowel obstruction
- Surgical fistulotomy; avoid in active Crohn's disease

THERAPEUTIC PROCEDURES

- Percutaneous drainage for abscess
- Nasogastric suction and IV fluids for small bowel obstruction
- Well-balanced diet
- Avoid lactose-containing foods since lactose intolerance is common
- Fiber supplementation for patients with colonic involvement
- Low-roughage diet for patients with obstructive symptoms
- Low-fat diet for patients with fat malabsorption
- Iron supplement if documented deficiency
- Vitamin B_{12} 100 mcg IM every month if prior terminal ileal resection
- Total parenteral nutrition
  - Used short term in patients with active disease and progressive weight loss or in malnourished patients awaiting surgery
  - Used long term in subset of patients with extensive intestinal resections resulting in short bowel syndrome with malnutrition

OUTCOME

COMPLICATIONS

- Abscess
- Small bowel obstruction
- Fistulas
- Perianal disease
- Hemorrhage (unusual)
- Malabsorption

PROGNOSIS

- With proper medical and surgical treatment, most patients are able to cope with this chronic disease and its complications
- Few patients die of Crohn's disease

WHEN TO ADMIT

- Persisting symptoms despite treatment with oral corticosteroids
- Presence of high fever, persistent vomiting, evidence of intestinal obstruction, severe weight loss, severe abdominal tenderness, or suspicion of an abscess

PREVENTION

- Colonoscopy screening to detect dysplasia or cancer recommended for patients with a history of 8 or more years of Crohn's colitis

EVIDENCE

PRACTICE GUIDELINES

- ACR Appropriateness criteria for imaging recommendations for patients with Crohn's disease. American College of Radiology, 2001
- American Gastroenterological Associates Medical Position Statement. Perianal Crohn's disease. Gastroenterology. 2003;125:1503. [PMID: 14598267]
- Management of Crohn's disease in adults. American College of Gastroenterology, 2001
- National Guideline Clearinghouse

WEB SITE

- WebPath Gastrointestinal Pathology Index

INFORMATION FOR PATIENTS

- Cleveland Clinic—Crohn's disease
- NIH—Patient Education Institute—Crohn's

REFERENCES

- Hanauer SB et al. Human antitumor necrosis factor monoclonal antibody (adalimumab) in Crohn's disease: the CLASSIC-1 trial. Gastroenterology. 2006 Feb;130(2):323–33. [PMID: 16452588]
- Lichtenstein GR. Infliximab: lifetime use for maintenance is appropriate in Crohn's Disease. PRO: maintenance therapy is superior to episodic therapy. Am J Gastroenterol. 2005 Jul;100(7):1433–5. [PMID: 15984959]
- Loftus EV. Infliximab: lifetime use for maintenance is appropriate in Crohn's Disease. CON: "lifetime use" is an awfully long time. Am J Gastroenterol. 2005 Jul;100(7):1435–8. [PMID: 15984960]
- Sandborn WJ et al. Budesonide for maintenance of remission in patients with Crohn's disease in medically induced remission: a predetermined pooled analysis of four randomized, double-blind, placebo-controlled trials. Am J Gastroenterol. 2005 Aug;100(8):1780–7. [PMID: 16086715]
- Sands BE. New therapies for the treatment of inflammatory bowel disease. Surg Clin North Am. 2006 Aug;86(4):1045–64. [PMID: 16905423]
- Wise PE et al. Management of perianal Crohn's disease. Clin Gastroenterol Hepatol. 2006 Apr;4(4):426–30. [PMID: 16616345]

Cushing's Syndrome (Hypercortisolism)

 KEY FEATURES

ESSENTIALS OF DIAGNOSIS

- Central obesity, muscle wasting, psychological changes, hirsutism, purple striae
- Osteoporosis, hypertension
- Hyperglycemia, leukocytosis, lymphocytopenia, hypokalemia
- Elevated serum cortisol and urinary free cortisol. Lack of normal suppression by dexamethasone

GENERAL CONSIDERATIONS

- **Cushing's "syndrome"** refers to manifestations of excessive corticosteroids
  - Commonly due to supraphysiologic doses of corticosteroid drugs
  - Rarely due to excessive spontaneous corticosteroid production
- **Cushing's "disease"**
  - ~45% of cases due to ACTH hypersecretion by a pituitary adenoma, which is usually small and benign
  - ~10% due to nonpituitary neoplasms (eg, small-cell lung carcinoma) that produce excessive ectopic ACTH
  - ~15% due to ACTH from a source that cannot be initially located
  - ~30% due to excessive autonomous secretion of cortisol by the adrenals independent of ACTH (serum ACTH usually low). Usually due to unilateral adrenal tumor of three types
    - □ Benign adrenal adenomas are generally small tumors that produce mostly cortisol
    - □ Adrenal carcinomas usually large and can produce excessive androgens as well as cortisol
    - □ ACTH-independent bilateral adrenal hyperplasia can also produce hypercortisolism
- Impaired glucose tolerance from insulin resistance

DEMOGRAPHICS

- Spontaneous Cushing's syndrome is rare: 2.6 new cases yearly per million population
- ACTH-secreting pituitary adenoma (Cushing's "disease") > 3 times more common in women than men

 CLINICAL FINDINGS

SYMPTOMS AND SIGNS

- Central obesity with plethoric "moon face," "buffalo hump," supraclavicular fat pads, protuberant abdomen, and thin extremities
- Oligomenorrhea or amenorrhea (or impotence in males)
- Weakness, backache, headache
- Hypertension
- Osteoporosis or avascular bone necrosis
- Skin
  - Acne
  - Superficial skin infections
  - Purple striae (especially around the thighs, breasts, and abdomen)
  - Easy bruising, impaired wound healing
- Thirst and polyuria (with or without glycosuria); renal calculi
- Glaucoma
- Mental symptoms range from diminished concentration to increased mood lability to psychosis
- Increased susceptibility to opportunistic infections
- Hirsutism and virilization may occur with adrenal carcinomas

DIFFERENTIAL DIAGNOSIS

- Chronic alcoholism (alcoholic pseudo-Cushing's syndrome)
- Diabetes mellitus
- Depression (may have hypercortisolism)
- Osteoporosis due to other cause
- Obesity due to other cause
- Primary hyperaldosteronism
- Anorexia nervosa (high urine free cortisol)
- Striae distensae ("stress marks") seen in adolescence and in pregnancy
- Lipodystrophy from antiretroviral agents

DIAGNOSIS

LABORATORY TESTS

- Hyperglycemia
- Leukocytosis; relative granulocytosis and lymphopenia
- Hypokalemia (not hypernatremia), particularly with ectopic ACTH secretion
- Easiest screening test involves obtaining a salivary cortisol at 11 PM and then administering 1 mg of dexamethasone orally
  - Collect serum for cortisol determination at about 8 AM next morning

  - Cortisol level < 5 mcg/dL (< 135 nmol/L, fluorometric assay) or < 2 mcg/dL (< 54 nmol/L, high-performance liquid chromatography assay) excludes Cushing's syndrome with 98% certainty
- If hypercortisolism is not excluded, measure 24-hour urine for free cortisol and creatinine
  - High 24-hour urine free cortisol (or free cortisol to creatinine ratio of > 95 mcg cortisol/g creatinine) helps confirm hypercortisolism
  - Misleadingly high urine free cortisol occurs with high fluid intake
- Midnight serum cortisol level > 7.5 mcg/dL is indicative of Cushing's syndrome; patient must be NPO for 3 hours and have IV established in advance for blood draw
- If hypercortisolism is confirmed
  - Plasma ACTH below normal indicates probable adrenal tumor
  - High or normal ACTH indicates pituitary or ectopic tumors
  - Blood for ACTH assay must be collected in a plastic tube, placed on ice, and processed quickly to avoid falsely low results

IMAGING STUDIES

- Pituitary MRI shows adenoma in ~50% of cases of ACTH-dependent Cushing's syndrome
- CT scanning
  - Of chest and abdomen can help locate source of ectopic ACTH in lungs (carcinoid or small-cell carcinomas), thymus, pancreas, or adrenals
  - Of adrenals can localize adrenal tumor in most cases of non-ACTH-dependent Cushing's syndrome
  - However, it fails to detect the source of ACTH in about 40% of patients with ectopic ACTH secretion
- ^{111}In-octreotide scanning is also useful in detecting occult tumors, but [18]FDG-PET scanning is not usually helpful
- Some ectopic ACTH-secreting tumors elude discovery, necessitating bilateral adrenalectomy

DIAGNOSTIC PROCEDURES

- If pituitary MRI is normal or shows incidental irregularity, selective inferior petrosal venous sampling for ACTH is performed (with corticotropin-releasing hormone stimulation) where available to confirm pituitary ACTH source, distinguishing it from an occult nonpituitary tumor secreting ACTH

- In patients with ACTH-dependent Cushing's syndrome
  - Chest masses may be the source of ACTH
  - However, opportunistic infections are common
  - Therefore, it is prudent to biopsy a chest mass to confirm the pathologic diagnosis prior to resection

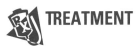 **TREATMENT**

MEDICATIONS

- Hydrocortisone replacement required temporarily after resection of pituitary adenoma or adrenal adenoma (see above)
- Ketoconazole, 200 mg PO q6h, for patients with Cushing's disease who are not surgical candidates; must monitor liver enzymes
- Mitotane for metastatic adrenal carcinomas; ketoconazole or metyrapone may suppress hypercortisolism in unresectable adrenal carcinoma; however, metyrapone may exacerbate female virilization
- Bisphosphonates for patients with osteoporosis

SURGERY

- Selective transsphenoidal resection of pituitary adenoma indicated in Cushing's disease, after which remainder of pituitary usually returns to normal function
  - However, corticotrophs require 6–36 months to recover normal function
  - Thus, hydrocortisone replacement is required temporarily
- Bilateral laparoscopic adrenalectomy if no remission (or recurrence) after pituitary surgery
- Laparoscopic resection for adrenal neoplasms secreting cortisol
- Because contralateral adrenal is suppressed, postoperative hydrocortisone replacement is required until recovery
- Surgical resection of ectopic ACTH-secreting tumors

THERAPEUTIC PROCEDURES

- Stereotactic pituitary radiosurgery (gamma knife) normalizes urine free cortisol in two-thirds of patients within 12 months
- Conventional radiation therapy cures 23%

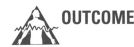 **OUTCOME**

COMPLICATIONS

- Complications of hypertension or diabetes mellitus
- Increased susceptibility to infections
- Nephrolithiasis
- Depression, dementia, psychosis
- Following bilateral adrenalectomy for Cushing's disease, progressive enlargement of pituitary adenoma may cause local effects (eg, visual field impairment) and hyperpigmentation (Nelson's syndrome)
- Steroid withdrawal syndrome after treatment: nausea, myalgias, fatigue, pruritus

PROGNOSIS

- Patients with Cushing's syndrome due to benign adrenal adenoma have
  - 5-year survival rate of 95%
  - 10-year survival rate of 90% following successful adrenalectomy
- Patients with Cushing's disease from pituitary adenoma have similar survival if pituitary surgery is successful
- Transsphenoidal surgery fails in ~10–20%
- Despite complete remission after transsphenoidal surgery, ~15–20% recur over 10 years
- Bilateral laparoscopic adrenalectomy
  - May be required but is often complicated by infection
  - Recurrence of hypercortisolism may occur owing to growth of adrenal remnant stimulated by high ACTH levels
- Prognosis with ectopic ACTH-producing tumors depends on aggressiveness and stage of tumor
- Patients with ACTH of unknown source have
  - 5-year survival rate of 65%
  - 10-year survival rate of 55%
- Patients with adrenal carcinoma have median survival of 7 months

WHEN TO REFER

- If abnormal dexamethasone suppression test

WHEN TO ADMIT

- For transsphenoidal hypophysectomy, adrenalectomy, resection of ectopic ACTH-secreting tumor

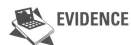 **EVIDENCE**

PRACTICE GUIDELINES

- Morris D et al. The medical management of Cushing's syndrome. Ann NY Acad Sci. 2002;970:119. [PMID: 12381547]
- Nieman LK. Diagnostic tests for Cushing's syndrome. Ann NY Acad Sci. 2002;970:112. [PMID: 12381546]

INFORMATION FOR PATIENTS

- American Academy of Family Physicians—Cushing's syndrome and Cushing's disease
- NIDDK/NIH—Cushing's Syndrome

REFERENCES

- Findling JW et al. Cushing's syndrome: important issues in diagnosis and management. J Clin Endocrinol Metab. 2006 Oct;91(10):3746–53. [PMID: 16868050]
- Ilias I et al. Cushing's syndrome due to ectopic corticotropin secretion: twenty years' experience at the National Institutes of Health. J Clin Endocrinol Metab. 2005 Aug;90(8):4955–62. [PMID: 15914534]
- Viardot A et al. Reproducibility of nighttime salivary cortisol and its use in the diagnosis of hypercortisolism compared with urinary free cortisol and overnight dexamethasone suppression test. J Clin Endocrinol Metab. 2005 Oct; 90(10):5730–6. [PMID: 16014408]

Cystic Fibrosis

 KEY FEATURES

ESSENTIALS OF DIAGNOSIS

- Chronic or recurrent cough, sputum production, dyspnea, and wheezing
- Recurrent infections or chronic colonization of the airways with
  - *Haemophilus influenzae*
  - *Pseudomonas aeruginosa*
  - *Staphylococcus aureus*
  - *Burkholderia cepacia*
  - *Stenotrophomonas maltophilia*
- Bronchiectasis and scarring on chest radiographs
- Airflow obstruction on spirometry

- Pancreatic insufficiency, distal intestinal obstruction syndrome, chronic hepatic disease, nutritional deficiencies, or male urogenital abnormalities
- Sweat chloride concentration above 60 mEq/L on two occasions or mutations in genes known to cause cystic fibrosis

GENERAL CONSIDERATIONS

- Most common fatal hereditary disorder of whites in the United States
- Autosomal recessive disorder due to mutations affecting a membrane chloride channel (the cystic fibrosis transmembrane conductance regulator, or CFTR)
- At least 1000 mutations to the CFTR gene are described, with "ΔF508" accounting for approximately 60% of cases
- Pathophysiology results from production of an abnormal mucous in exocrine glands, which leads to tissue destruction and, in the respiratory tract, impairs mucociliary clearance
- Variety of mutations is reflected in wide range of pulmonary and nonpulmonary manifestations

DEMOGRAPHICS

- Affects 1 in 3200 whites; 1 in 25 is a carrier

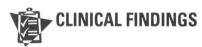 **CLINICAL FINDINGS**

SYMPTOMS AND SIGNS

- Disease should be suspected in young adults with a history of chronic lung disease, pancreatic insufficiency, or infertility
- Productive cough, decreased exercise tolerance, and recurrent hemoptysis are typical
- Sinus pain or pressure with purulent nasal discharge is common
- Pulmonary manifestations
  - Bronchitis
  - Bronchiectasis
  - Pneumonia
  - Atelectasis
  - Peribronchial and parenchymal scarring
- Common extrapulmonary manifestations
  - Steatorrhea
  - Diarrhea
  - Abdominal pain
- Advanced disease manifestations
  - Hypoxemia
  - Hypercapnia
  - Cor pulmonale

- Nearly all male patients have congenital absence of the vas deferens with azoospermia
- Other findings include
  - Digital clubbing
  - Increased anteroposterior chest diameter
  - Apical crackles

DIFFERENTIAL DIAGNOSIS

- Chronic obstructive pulmonary disease
- Asthma
- α_1-Antiprotease deficiency
- Bronchiolitis
- Celiac disease (celiac sprue)
- Chronic sinusitis

 DIAGNOSIS

LABORATORY TESTS

- Arterial blood gases reveal hypoxemia, with compensated respiratory acidosis in advanced disease
- Pulmonary function tests
  - A mixed obstructive and restrictive pattern
  - Reduced FVC, airflow rates, and total lung capacity
  - Air trapping and reduced diffusion capacity are common
- Genotyping, measurement of nasal membrane potential difference, semen analysis, or assessment of pancreatic function can play a role in diagnosis
- Sputum cultures
  - Frequently show *S aureus* and *P aeruginosa*
  - Occasionally show *H influenzae, S maltophilia,* and *B cepacia*

IMAGING STUDIES

- Hyperinflation is seen early on chest radiographs
- Peribronchial cuffing, mucus plugging, bronchiectasis, atelectasis, and increased interstitial markings are sometimes seen
- High-resolution CT is the test of choice to confirm bronchiectasis

DIAGNOSTIC PROCEDURES

- Chloride sweat test reveals elevated sodium and chloride levels; two tests on different days are required for accurate diagnosis
- A normal sweat chloride test does not exclude the diagnosis

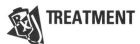 **TREATMENT**

MEDICATIONS

- Inhaled bronchodilators should be considered in patients who demonstrate an increase in FEV_1 of 12% in response to treatment
- rhDNase, 2.5 mg nebulized daily, thins the sputum by cleaving extracellular DNA from neutrophils that accumulate in sputum and increase its viscosity
- Inhalation of hypertonic saline has been associated with small improvements in pulmonary function and fewer exacerbations, perhaps due to improved mucus clearance
- Antibiotics are used to treat airway infection based on results of sputum culture and sensitivity testing
- Aerosolized antibiotics (tobramycin and others) may slow the decline in lung function over time in patients with *P aeruginosa*
- However, there is concern regarding development of resistant organisms and side effects, such as bronchospasm
- Azithromycin (500 mg PO thrice weekly) may slow progression of disease in patients with *P aeruginosa*

SURGERY

- Lung transplantation is the only definitive therapy for advanced disease; double-lung or heart-lung transplantation is required
- 3-year survival rates after transplantation are about 55%

THERAPEUTIC PROCEDURES

- Mechanical interventions to clear lower airway secretions
  - Postural drainage
  - Chest percussion or vibration
  - Positive expiratory pressure valve device
  - Flutter valve breathing devices
  - Directed cough

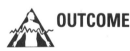 **OUTCOME**

FOLLOW-UP

- Regular assessment of FEV_1
- Regular assessment of nutritional status

COMPLICATIONS

- Pneumothorax and hemoptysis are common
- Cor pulmonale is seen in late disease

- Patients have increased risk of
  - Osteopenia
  - Diabetes mellitus
  - Arthropathies
  - Gastrointestinal malignancies
- Biliary cirrhosis, gallstones, and pancreatitis are seen
- Resistant infections, including methicillin-resistant *S aureus* and *B cepacia*

PROGNOSIS

- Median survival is to age > 30 years
- Death results from pulmonary infections or as a result of chronic respiratory failure and cor pulmonale

WHEN TO REFER

- All patients with suspected or confirmed cystic fibrosis should be referred to a Cystic Fibrosis Center of Excellence for evaluation and treatment recommendations

WHEN TO ADMIT

- Increased cough, sputum production, shortness of breath, decline in FEV_1, weight loss, constitutional symptoms, hemoptysis

PREVENTION

- Vaccination against pneumococcal infection and annual influenza vaccination are recommended
- Screening of family members and genetic counseling are suggested

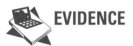 **EVIDENCE**

PRACTICE GUIDELINES

- National Guideline Clearinghouse

INFORMATION FOR PATIENTS

- Cystic Fibrosis Foundation
- Mayo Clinic
- National Institutes of Health

REFERENCES

- Davis PB. Cystic fibrosis since 1938. Am J Respir Crit Care Med. 2006 Mar 1;173(5):475–82. [PMID: 16126935]
- Elkins MR et al; National Hypertonic Saline in Cystic Fibrosis (NHSCF) Study Group. A controlled trial of long-term inhaled hypertonic saline in patients with cystic fibrosis. N Engl J Med. 2006 Jan 19;354(3):229–40. [PMID: 16421364]
- Rowe SM et al. Cystic fibrosis. N Engl J Med. 2005 May 12;352(19):1992–2001. [PMID: 15888700]
- Yankaskas JR et al. Cystic fibrosis adult care: consensus conference report. Chest. 2004 Jan;125(1 Suppl):1S–39S. [PMID: 14734689]

Cysticercosis

 KEY FEATURES

ESSENTIALS OF DIAGNOSIS

- Exposure to *Taenia solium* through fecal contamination of food
- Seizures, headache, and other findings of a focal CNS lesion
- Brain imaging shows cysts; positive serologic tests

GENERAL CONSIDERATIONS

- Caused by tissue infection with cysts of *T solium* that develop after humans ingest food contaminated with eggs from human feces
- Humans are an intermediate host for the parasite
- Infection is one of the most important causes of seizures in the developing world and in immigrants to the United States from endemic countries

DEMOGRAPHICS

- Prevalence is high where parasite is endemic, in particular
  - Mexico
  - Central and South America
  - Philippines
  - Southeast Asia
- Worldwide, an estimated 20 million persons are infected
- Yearly, about 400,000 persons have neurologic symptoms and 50,000 die of the disease
- Antibody prevalence rates to 10% are recognized in some endemic areas

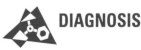 **CLINICAL FINDINGS**

SYMPTOMS AND SIGNS

Neurocysticercosis
- Can cause intracerebral, subarachnoid, and spinal cord lesions and intraventricular cysts

- Single or multiple lesions may be present
- Lesions may persist for years before symptoms develop, generally due to local inflammation or ventricular obstruction
- Presenting symptoms
  - Seizures
  - Focal neurologic deficits
  - Altered cognition
  - Psychiatric disease
- Symptoms develop more quickly with intraventricular cysts, with findings of hydrocephalus and meningeal irritation, including
  - Severe headache
  - Vomiting
  - Papilledema
  - Visual loss
- Racemose cysticercosis
  - Is a particularly aggressive form of the disease
  - Involves proliferation of cysts at the base of the brain
  - Leads to alterations of consciousness and death
- Spinal cord lesions can present with progressive focal findings

Cysticercosis of other organ systems
- Usually clinically benign
- Involvement of muscles
  - Causes discomfort (uncommon)
  - Identified by radiographs of muscle showing multiple calcified lesions
- Subcutaneous involvement presents with multiple painless palpable skin lesions
- Involvement of eyes can present with ptosis due to extraocular muscle involvement or intraocular abnormalities

DIFFERENTIAL DIAGNOSIS

- Epilepsy
- Primary or metastatic cancer
- Tuberculoma
- Echinococcosis (hydatid disease)
- Bacterial or fungal brain abscess
- Toxoplasmosis
- Neurosyphilis

DIAGNOSIS

LABORATORY TESTS

- CSF examination may show
  - Lymphocytic or eosinophilic pleocytosis
  - Decreased glucose
  - Elevated protein
- Serologic tests can indicate prior exposure to *T solium*, but sensitivity and specificity are limited

IMAGING STUDIES

- Neuroimaging by CT or MRI
  - Multiple parenchymal cysts are most typically seen
  - Parenchymal calcification is also common
- MRI is more sensitive than CT for visualizing ventricular cysts

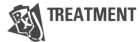 **TREATMENT**

MEDICATIONS

- Benefits of cyst clearance must be weighed against potential harm of an inflammatory response to dying worms
- Antihelminthic therapy
  - Hastens radiologic improvement in parenchymal cysticercosis
  - However, some reports have shown exacerbation of disease after therapy
- Determining when therapy is indicated is difficult
  - Intraventricular cysts may benefit from therapy
  - Inactive calcified lesions probably do not benefit from therapy
- Anticonvulsant therapy is provided if needed

Albendazole
- Treatment of choice
- 10–15 mg/kg/d orally for 8 days
- Increasing dosage to 30 mg/kg/d may improve outcome
- Coadministration of corticosteroids increases circulating levels

Praziquantel
- 50 mg/kg/d orally for 15–30 days
- Coadministration of corticosteroids lowers circulating levels

SURGERY

- Surgical removal of cysts may be helpful for
  - Some difficult cases of neurocysticercosis
  - Symptomatic non-neurologic disease

THERAPEUTIC PROCEDURES

- Shunting is performed if required for elevated intracranial pressure

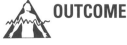 **OUTCOME**

FOLLOW-UP

- Observe patients for evidence of localized inflammatory responses

PROGNOSIS

- The fatality rate for untreated neurocysticercosis is about 50%. Drug treatment has reduced the mortality rate to about 5–15%
- Surgical procedures to relieve intracranial hypertension along with use of corticosteroids to reduce edema improve the prognosis for those not effectively treated with the drugs

WHEN TO REFER

- All patients

WHEN TO ADMIT

- Treatment should be conducted in a hospital

PREVENTION

- All family members should examine their stools over several days for passage of proglottids, and stool specimens should be sent to the laboratory to be examined for proglottids and eggs
- Indiscriminate defecation, free roaming pigs, and ingestion of undercooked pork allow the maintenance of the life cycle and human disease

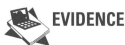 **EVIDENCE**

PRACTICE GUIDELINES

- Garcia HH et al. Current consensus guidelines for treatment of neurocysticercosis. Clin Microbiol Rev. 2002; 15:747. [PMID: 12364377]

WEB SITE

- CDC—Division of Parasitic Diseases

INFORMATION FOR PATIENTS

- Centers for Disease Control
- National Institutes of Health

REFERENCES

- Del Brutto OH et al. Meta-analysis: Cysticidal drugs for neurocysticercosis: albendazole and praziquantel. Ann Intern Med. 2006 Jul 4;145(1):43–51. [PMID: 16818928]
- Garcia HH et al; Cysticercosis Working Group in Peru. Neurocysticercosis: updated concepts about an old disease. Lancet Neurol. 2005 Oct;4(10):653–61. [PMID: 16168934]
- Hawk MW et al. Neurocysticercosis: a review. Surg Neurol. 2005 Feb; 63(2):123–32. [PMID: 15680651]

- Nash TE et al. Treatment of neurocysticercosis: current status and future research needs. Neurology. 2006 Oct 10;67(7):1120–7. [PMID: 17030744]

Cytomegalovirus (CMV) Infection

 KEY FEATURES

- Most CMV infections are asymptomatic
- Age-related rise in seroprevalence
- Acute acquired CMV infection is similar to infectious mononucleosis, except pharyngeal symptoms unusual
- Most CMV-related diseases occur in immunocompromised, especially HIV-infected, persons
  - CMV retinitis
  - Gastrointestinal (GI) and hepatobiliary disease
  - Pulmonary disease
  - Neurologic disease
- CMV is a major pathogen in transplant recipients by both direct infection and reactivation of latent infection, increasing rates of transplant rejection

 CLINICAL FINDINGS

- CMV inclusion disease, with CNS and hepatic malfunction, occurs in infants born to acutely infected mothers
- CMV retinitis, with neovascular and proliferative retinal lesions, occurs primarily in advanced AIDS
- GI and hepatobiliary CMV, with esophagitis, small bowel inflammation, colitis, or cholangiopathy, occurs in AIDS or with high-dose chemotherapy
- Pneumonitis occurs in transplant recipients and AIDS
- Neurologic manifestations include polyneuropathy, transverse myelitis, encephalitis

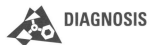

DIAGNOSIS

- Characteristic clinical symptoms in immunosuppressed patients
- Tzanck smear, CMV antibodies, and polymerase chain reaction (PCR) helpful in the proper clinical context
- Tissue biopsy showing characteristic histology is used to document invasive disease

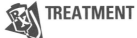

TREATMENT

- Acute, severe infections
  - Ganciclovir IV
  - Valganciclovir
  - Foscarnet
  - Cidofovir
- Improvement of immunosuppression especially important in AIDS and transplant patients
- Prophylactic therapy
  - Ganciclovir IV
  - Valganciclovir PO
  - Valacyclovir (high-dose) PO
- Antigen or PCR tests often used in transplant patients to guide preemptive therapy
- CMV-specific hyperimmune globulin may be used to prevent and treat congenital infection
- Prevention: no vaccine currently available
- Use CMV-negative blood products in immunosuppressed patients

Decubitus Ulcers

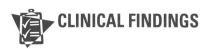

KEY FEATURES

ESSENTIALS OF DIAGNOSIS

- A special type of ulcer caused by impaired blood supply and tissue nutrition
- Results from prolonged pressure over bony or cartilaginous prominences

GENERAL CONSIDERATIONS

- Occur in 3% to 30% of hospitalized patients
- Occur most readily in immobilized (elderly, paralyzed, debilitated, and unconscious) patients
- Staging includes
  - Stage 1: blanchable hyperemia
  - Stage 2: extension through the epidermis
  - Stage 3: full thickness skin loss
  - Stage 4: full thickness wounds with extension into muscle, bone, or supporting structures
- If eschar overlies the wound, staging cannot be done

CLINICAL FINDINGS

SYMPTOMS AND SIGNS

- The skin overlying the sacrum and hips is most commonly involved, but bedsores may also be seen over the occiput, ears, elbows, heels, and ankles

DIFFERENTIAL DIAGNOSIS

- Herpes simplex virus
  - In immunocompromised patients, particularly if there is a scalloped border, representing the erosions of herpetic vesicles
- Skin cancer
  - In the perianal area, a nonhealing ulcer may be cancer
- Pyoderma gangrenosum
  - Rapidly expanding ulcers associated with inflammatory bowel disease
- Ecthyma gangrenosum
  - Ulcerating lesion, commonly due to *Pseudomonas*, observed in neutropenic patients

DIAGNOSIS

LABORATORY TESTS

- Based on clinical appearance
- Suspect an alternative diagnosis if ulcers not healing properly

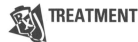

TREATMENT

MEDICATIONS

See Table 44.
- Early lesions
  - Treat with topical antibiotic powders and adhesive absorbent bandage (Gelfoam)
  - Once clean, they may be treated with hydrocolloid dressings such as DuoDerm
- Established lesions
  - Topical antiseptics are not recommended
  - Systemic antibiotics may be required for deep infections if the patient is systemically ill, but should otherwise be avoided because they will promote antibiotic resistance

SURGERY

- Established lesions require surgery for débridement, cleansing, and dressing

THERAPEUTIC PROCEDURES

- For established lesions a spongy foam pad placed under the patient may work best in some cases
- Efforts to promote mobility
- Repositioning of immobile patients every 2–3 h
- Air fluid beds and low air loss beds may be useful

OUTCOME

COMPLICATIONS

- Pain, cellulitis, osteomyelitis, systemic sepsis, and prolonged length of hospital stay

WHEN TO REFER

- If there is a question about the diagnosis, if recommended therapy is ineffective, or if specialized treatment is necessary

PREVENTION

- Good nursing care, good nutrition, and maintenance of skin hygiene are important preventive measures
- The skin and the bed linens should be kept clean and dry
- Bedfast, paralyzed, moribund, listless, or incontinent patients who are candidates for the development of decubiti
  - Must be turned frequently (at least every hour)
  - Must be examined at pressure points for the appearance of small areas of redness and tenderness
- Water-filled mattresses, rubber pillows, alternating-pressure mattresses, and thick papillated foam pads are useful in prevention and in the treatment of lesions
- "Donut" devices should not be used

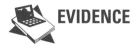

EVIDENCE

WEB SITE

- University of Alabama at Birmingham: Prevention of Pressure Sores Slideshow

INFORMATION FOR PATIENTS

- American Academy of Family Physicians: Pressure Sores
- MedlinePlus: Pressure Ulcer
- Torpy JM et al. JAMA patient page. Pressure ulcers. JAMA. 2003;289:254. [PMID: 12517212]
- University of Alabama at Birmingham: Prevention of Pressure Sores Through Skin Care

REFERENCE

- Grey JE et al. Pressure ulcers. BMJ. 2006 Feb 25;332(7539):472-5. [PMID: 16497764]
- Reddy M et al. Preventing pressure ulcers: a systematic review. JAMA. 2006 Aug 23; 296(8):974-84. [PMID: 16926357]
- Zeller JL et al. JAMA patient page. Pressure ulcers. JAMA. 2006 Aug 23; 296(8):1020. [PMID: 16926361]

Deep Vein Thrombosis

KEY FEATURES

ESSENTIALS OF DIAGNOSIS

- Calf or thigh pain, occasionally associated with swelling

- Alternatively, there may be no symptoms
- Risk factors
  - Recent travel
  - Orthopedic injury
  - Recent abdominal, pelvic, or lower extremity surgery
  - Neoplasia (known or occult)
  - Oral contraceptive use
  - Prolonged inactivity
- Physical signs unreliable
- Duplex ultrasound is diagnostic

GENERAL CONSIDERATIONS

- Thrombosis begins in the deep veins of the calf in about 80% of cases but can arise in femoral or iliac veins
- When thrombosis begins in the calf, propagation into the popliteal and femoral veins takes place in only 10% of cases
- Clinical manifestations
  - Occur in about 3% of patients undergoing major surgical procedures (in the absence of effective prophylaxis)
  - May develop up to 2 weeks postoperatively
- Factors that increase incidence of thromboembolic complications include
  - Certain operations, such as total hip replacement
  - Illnesses that involve periods of bed rest, such as cardiac failure or stroke
- Medications and conditions that contribute to hypercoagulability, which may result in deep vein thrombosis (DVT)
  - Oral contraceptive drugs, especially in women over age 30 and in those who smoke
  - Cancer, particularly adenocarcinoma and tumors of the pancreas, prostate, breast, and ovary
  - Homocystinuria
  - Paroxysmal nocturnal hemoglobinuria
- Consider hereditary factors, such as factor V Leiden, protein C and S deficiencies, and antithrombin III deficiency, in young patients with positive family histories and recurrent venous thrombosis

 CLINICAL FINDINGS

SYMPTOMS AND SIGNS

- Approximately half of patients have no symptoms or signs in the early stages
- Patient may suffer a pulmonary embolism (PE), presumably from the leg veins, without symptoms or demonstrable abnormalities in the extremities

- Ache or pain in the calf or, in more extensive cases, the whole leg, especially when walking
- Typical findings
  - Slight swelling in the involved calf
  - Distention of the superficial venous collaterals
  - Slight fever
  - Tachycardia
- With occlusion of the femoral and iliac veins
  - There may be tenderness over these veins
  - Swelling in the extremity may be marked
  - Skin may be cyanotic if venous obstruction is severe or pale and cool with massive swelling and restriction of blood flow or a reflex arterial spasm is superimposed

DIFFERENTIAL DIAGNOSIS

- Calf muscle strain or contusion
- Cellulitis
- Infection
- Obstruction of the lymphatics or iliac vein in the retroperitoneal area from tumor or irradiation
- Acute arterial occlusion
- Bilateral leg edema due to heart, kidney, or liver disease
- Ruptured Baker cyst

DIAGNOSIS

LABORATORY TESTS

- Evaluate for hereditary and acquired hypercoagulable states (thrombophilia)
  - In young patients
  - If the DVT is not associated with a predisposing event (eg, pregnancy, cancer, limb trauma, surgery, immobility)
- If possible, blood should be drawn for protein C and protein S levels before starting heparin since levels change with anticoagulant therapy
- Genetic tests for factor V Leiden and prothrombin mutations

IMAGING STUDIES

- Doppler ultrasonography
  - Test of choice
  - May be particularly helpful in detecting an extension of small thrombi in the calf veins into the popliteal and femoral veins
- Spiral CT scanning of the chest should be done in patients with respiratory or cardiac symptoms to exclude PE

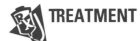 **TREATMENT**

ANTICOAGULANT THERAPY

- Immediate therapy
  - Mandatory in most cases of DVT with the probable exception of thrombosis that is confined to below the knee
  - Reduces clot propagation and risk of PE
- Unfractionated heparin given as a bolus and titrated to keep the partial thromboplastin time (PTT) 1.5 to 2.0 times baseline acts rapidly and effectively but requires hospitalization
- Low-molecular-weight (LMWH)
  - Given subcutaneously
  - Does not require PTT monitoring
  - More expensive than unfractionated heparin
  - Studies show equal efficacy with unfractionated heparin
- After initial anticoagulation with heparin, warfarin should be started
- Once warfarin levels are adequate as reflected by an international normalized ratio (INR) of 2.0–2.5, heparin or LMWH can be stopped
- Duration of therapy
  - First episode: 6 months
  - Second episode: depends on the interval from first episode and the presence of precipitating factors
  - Third episode: lifelong
- Consider permanent anticoagulation if the stimulus to thrombosis is chronic
  - Congestive heart failure
  - Postphlebitic syndrome
  - Presence of a hereditary or acquired hypercoagulable state

THROMBOLYTIC THERAPY

- Catheter-directed therapy with streptokinase, urokinase, or tissue plasminogen activator (TPA) has potential to
  - Rapidly lyse deep venous thrombi
  - Preserve venous valve function
  - Prevent the sequelae of post-thrombotic syndrome
- Indicated in younger patients with large (ileofemoral) thrombi that are detected within 2 weeks of onset
- Risks include bleeding (both at the catheter site and at remote sites), including intracranial hemorrhage

PERCUTANEOUS MECHANICAL THROMBECTOMY

- Nonthrombolytic means of clot removal
- Gaining popularity for rapid treatment of acute symptomatic DVT
- Associated with lower bleeding risk

OUTCOME

COMPLICATIONS

- Pulmonary thromboembolism
- Chronic venous insufficiency with or without secondary varicosities

PROGNOSIS

- Good in most cases once danger of PE has passed
- With adequate treatment, the patient usually returns to normal health and activity with 3–6 weeks
- Occasionally, recurrent episodes of DVT will occur in spite of good local and anticoagulant management
- Such cases may have recurrent PE as well
- Recurrent thrombosis
  - More common in patients with a persistent risk factor for thrombosis (cancer, hereditary or acquired thrombophilia)
  - Less common in patients with an identifiable antecedent risk factor (trauma, pregnancy, surgery) that is no longer present

PREVENTION

- Prophylactic measures may diminish the incidence of venous thrombosis in hospitalized patients (Tables 115 and 116)

Nonpharmacologic measures

- Elevation of the foot of the bed 15–20 degrees
  - Encourages venous flow from the legs, particularly if the head of the bed is kept low or horizontal
  - Slight flexion of the knees is desirable
  - This position is also maintained on the operating table and in the recovery room
  - Sitting in a chair in the early postoperative period should be avoided
- Intermittent pneumatic compression of the legs
  - May be used prophylactically
  - May be the preventive measure of choice in patients in whom all anticoagulants are contraindicated, such as those undergoing neurosurgery
  - Sequential compression devices (SCDs) are not nearly as effective as prophylactic anticoagulation and should not be used as a perioperative substitute in patients at moderate to high risk for DVT
- Elastic antiphlebitic stockings may be used, particularly in patients with varicose veins or a history of phlebitis who will require bed rest for a number of days

- Walking for brief but regular periods postoperatively and during long airplane and automobile trips should be encouraged

Anticoagulation

- May be used in patients considered at high risk for venous thrombosis
- Low-dose heparin
  - 5000 units q8–12h SQ 2 hours preoperatively and during the postoperative period of bed rest and limited ambulation
  - Appears to be effective in reducing the incidence of thromboembolic complications in moderate-risk patients
- LMWH
  - Has lower risk of bleeding complications than unfractionated heparin, although the risk of major bleeding with heparin prophylaxis is generally low (Table 118)
  - Should be used with caution in patients with renal impairment, since it is excreted via the kidneys

EVIDENCE

PRACTICE GUIDELINES

- Abdel-Razeq H et al. Guidelines for diagnosis and treatment of deep venous thrombosis and pulmonary embolism. Methods Mol Med. 2004;93:267–92. [PMID: 14733339]
- American College of Emergency Physicians (ACEP) Clinical Policies Committee; ACEP Clinical Policies Subcommittee on Suspected Lower-Extremity Deep Venous Thrombosis. Clinical policy: critical issues in the evaluation and management of adult patients presenting with suspected lower-extremity deep venous thrombosis. Ann Emerg Med. 2003 Jul; 42(1):124–35. [PMID: 12827132]
- Buller HR et al. Antithrombotic therapy for venous thromboembolic disease: the Seventh ACCP Conference on Antithrombotic and Thrombolytic Therapy. Chest. 2004 Sep;126(3 Suppl):401S–428S. [PMID: 15383479]

INFORMATION FOR PATIENTS

- American Academy of Orthopaedic Surgeons: Deep Vein Thrombosis
- Mayo Clinic: Thrombophlebitis
- MedlinePlus: Deep Venous Thrombosis

REFERENCES

- American College of Physicians and the American Academy of Family Physi-

cians. Ann Intern Med. 2007 Feb 6; 146(3):204–10. [PMID: 17261857]
- Canonico M et al; Estrogen and Thromboembolism Risk (ESTHER) Study Group. Hormone therapy and venous thromboembolism among postmenopausal women: impact of the route of estrogen administration and progestogens: the ESTHER study. Circulation. 2007 Feb 20;115(7):840–5. [PMID: 17309934]
- Dentali F et al. Meta-analysis: anticoagulant prophylaxis to prevent symptomatic venous thromboembolism in hospitalized medical patients. Ann Intern Med. 2007 Feb 20;146(4):278–88. [PMID: 17310052]
- Snow V et al; American College of Physicians; American Academy of Family Physicians Panel on Deep Venous Thrombosis/Pulmonary Embolism. Management of venous thromboembolism: a clinical practice guideline from the American College of Physicians and the American Academy of Family Physicians. Ann Intern Med. 2007 Feb 6; 146(3):204–10. [PMID: 17261857]

Delirium

KEY FEATURES

ESSENTIALS OF DIAGNOSIS

- Acute confusional state
- Transient global disorder of attention, with clouding of consciousness
- Usually a result of systemic problems (eg, drugs, hypoxemia)

GENERAL CONSIDERATIONS

- The organic problem may be a primary brain disease or a secondary manifestation of some general disorder
- The causes of cognitive disorders are listed in Table 149
- Should be considered a syndrome of acute brain dysfunction analogous to acute renal failure
- Delirium can coexist with dementia

DEMOGRAPHICS

- Alcohol or substance withdrawal is the most common cause of delirium in the general hospital

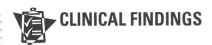 **CLINICAL FINDINGS**

SYMPTOMS AND SIGNS

- Onset is usually rapid
- The mental status fluctuates (impairment is usually least in the morning), with varying inability to concentrate, maintain attention, and sustain purposeful behavior
- "Sundowning"—mild to moderate delirium at night
  - More common in patients with pre-existing dementia
  - May be precipitated by hospitalization, drugs, and sensory deprivation
- There is a marked deficit of memory and recall
- Anxiety and irritability are common
- Amnesia is retrograde (impaired recall of past memories) and anterograde (inability to recall events after the onset of the delirium)
- Orientation problems follow the inability to retain information
- Perceptual disturbances (often visual hallucinations) and psychomotor restlessness with insomnia are common
- Autonomic changes include tachycardia, dilated pupils, and sweating
- Physical findings vary according to the cause

DIFFERENTIAL DIAGNOSIS

- Drugs
  - Opioids
  - Alcohol
  - Sedatives
  - Antipsychotics
- Metabolic
  - Hypoxia
  - Hypoglycemia or hyperglycemia
  - Hypercalcemia
  - Hyponatremia or hypernatremia
  - Uremia
  - Hepatic encephalopathy
  - Hypothyroidism or hyperthyroidism
  - Vitamin B_{12} or thiamine deficiency
  - Carbon monoxide poisoning
  - Wilson's disease
- Infectious
  - Meningitis
  - Encephalitis
  - Bacteremia
  - Urinary tract infections
  - Pneumonia
  - Neurosyphilis
- Structural: space-occupying lesion, eg, brain tumor, subdural hematoma, hydrocephalus
- Vascular
  - Stroke
  - Subarachnoid hemorrhage
  - Hypertensive encephalopathy
  - CNS vasculitis
  - Thrombotic thrombocytopenic purpura
  - Disseminated intravascular coagulation
  - Hyperviscosity
- Psychiatric
  - Schizophrenia
  - Depression
- Other
  - Seizure
  - Hypothermia
  - Heat stroke
  - ICU psychosis

 DIAGNOSIS

LABORATORY TESTS

- Comprehensive physical examination including a search for neurologic abnormalities, infection, or hypoxia
- Routine laboratory tests may include
  - Serum electrolytes
  - Serum glucose
  - Blood urea nitrogen
  - Serum creatinine
  - Liver function tests
  - Thyroid function tests
  - Arterial blood gases
  - Complete blood count
  - Serum calcium, phosphorus, magnesium, vitamin B_{12}, folate
  - Blood cultures
  - Urinalysis
  - Cerebrospinal fluid analysis
- See Table 149

IMAGING STUDIES

- Following may be helpful in diagnosis
  - Electroencephalography (EEG)
  - CT
  - MRI

DIAGNOSTIC PROCEDURES

- EEG usually shows generalized slowing

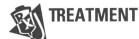 **TREATMENT**

MEDICATIONS

- The first aim of treatment is to identify and correct the etiologic medical problem
- Discontinue drugs that may be contributing to the problem, such as
  - Analgesics
  - Corticosteroids
  - Cimetidine
  - Lidocaine
  - Anticholinergic drugs
  - CNS depressants
  - Mefloquine
- Ideally, the patient should be monitored without further medications while the evaluation is carried out
- Two indications for medication in delirious states
  - Behavioral control (eg, pulling out lines)
  - Subjective distress (eg, pronounced fear due to hallucinations)
  - If these indications are present, medications may be given
- If there is any hint of alcohol or substance withdrawal, a benzodiazepine such as lorazepam (1–2 mg every hour) can be given parenterally
- If there is little likelihood of withdrawal syndrome, haloperidol is often used in doses of 1–10 mg every hour
- Once the underlying condition has been identified and treated, adjunctive medications can be tapered

THERAPEUTIC PROCEDURES

- In addition to the medication, a pleasant, comfortable, nonthreatening, and physically safe environment with adequate nursing or attendant services should be provided

 OUTCOME

PROGNOSIS

- The prognosis is good for recovery of mental functioning in delirium when the underlying condition is reversible
- The average duration is about 1 week, with full recovery in most cases

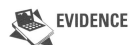 **EVIDENCE**

PRACTICE GUIDELINES

- National Guideline Clearinghouse: American Psychiatric Association, 1999

WEB SITES

- American Academy of Family Physicians
- American Psychiatric Association
- Internet Mental Health

INFORMATION FOR PATIENTS

- National Cancer Institute
- National Institutes of Health

- Torpy JM et al. JAMA patient page: Delirium. JAMA. 2004;291:1794. [PMID: 15082707]

REFERENCES

- McShane R et al. Memantine for dementia. Cochrane Database Syst Rev. 2006 Apr 19;(2):CD003154. [PMID: 16625572]
- Schneider LS et al. Risk of death with atypical antipsychotic drug treatment for dementia: meta-analysis of randomized placebo-controlled trials. JAMA. 2005 Oct 19;294(15):1934–43. [PMID: 16234500]
- Trinh N et al. Efficacy of cholinesterase inhibitors in the treatment of neuropsychiatric symptoms and functional impairment in Alzheimer disease, a meta-analysis. JAMA. 2003 Jan 8; 289(2):210–6. [PMID: 12517232]

Delirium in Elderly

 KEY FEATURES

ESSENTIALS OF DIAGNOSIS

- Rapid onset of acute confusional state
- Fluctuates during the day
- Inability to concentrate, maintain attention, or sustain purposeful behavior
- Altered level of consciousness ranging from hyperalert to drowsy or stuporous
- Increased anxiety and irritability
- The majority of delirium is initiated by problems outside the CNS

GENERAL CONSIDERATIONS

- Delirium is the pathophysiologic consequence of an underlying general medical condition such as
  - Infection
  - Coronary ischemia
  - Hypoxemia
  - Metabolic derangement
- Although the acutely agitated, "sundowning" elderly patient often comes to mind when considering delirium, many episodes are more subtle
- A key component is review of medications
- A large number of drugs, adding a new agent, or discontinuing an agent known to cause withdrawal symptoms is associated with the development of delirium

DEMOGRAPHICS

- Approximately 25% of delirious patients are demented, and 40% of demented hospitalized patients are delirious
- Cognitive impairment is an important risk factor
- Other risk factors
  - Male sex
  - Severe illness
  - Fracture or trauma
  - Fever or hypothermia
  - Functional dependence/immobility
  - Malnutrition/volume depletion
  - Polypharmacy and use of psychoactive medications
  - Sensory impairment
  - Use of restraints
  - Use of IV lines or urinary catheters
  - Metabolic disorders
  - Depression
  - Alcoholism

CLINICAL FINDINGS

SYMPTOMS AND SIGNS

- Acute, fluctuating disturbance of consciousness or mental status
- Inattention, inability to focus on tasks
- Cognitive deficits, disorientation, memory and language impairment
- Irritability
- Hyperactivity or hypoactivity
- Mental slowing
- Hallucinations or illusions

DIFFERENTIAL DIAGNOSIS

- Depression
- Mania
- Once the diagnosis of delirium has been made, an underlying cause should be sought. The underlying causes are wide-ranging
- Dementia, especially Lewy body dementia
- Psychotic disorders
- Seizures

DIAGNOSIS

LABORATORY TESTS

- Laboratory evaluation is aimed at finding an underlying medical condition
- Routine studies include
  - Complete blood cell count
  - Electrolytes
  - Blood urea nitrogen and serum creatinine

  - Glucose, calcium, albumin, liver function studies
  - Urinalysis
  - ECG
- In selected cases, serum magnesium, serum drug levels, arterial blood gas measurements, blood cultures, chest radiographs, urinary toxin screens, head CT scan, and lumbar puncture may be helpful

IMAGING STUDIES

- Consider neuroimaging if evidence of trauma, focal neurologic examination, unable to obtain history

DIAGNOSTIC PROCEDURES

- Electroencephalogram may sometimes be helpful if seizures are in the differential diagnosis

 TREATMENT

MEDICATIONS

- Management entails treating the underlying cause, eliminating unnecessary medications, providing supportive care, and avoidance of restraints
- For refractory cases in which the patient's or others' welfare is at risk, an oral antipsychotic may be necessary
  - Risperidone, 0.25–0.5 mg at bedtime or twice a day
  - Haloperidol, 0.5–1.0 mg at bedtime or twice a day
- In emergency situations, starting haloperidol at 0.5 mg PO or IM and repeating every 30 min until the agitation is controlled may be necessary but is often followed by prolonged sedation or other complications
- In general, benzodiazepines should be avoided unless specifically used to treat alcohol withdrawal

OUTCOME

FOLLOW-UP

- Patients who suffer prolonged episodes of delirium merit closer follow-up for the development of dementia if not already diagnosed

COMPLICATIONS

- May lead to increased number of iatrogenic events

PROGNOSIS

- Delirium is associated with worse clinical outcomes (higher in-hospital and postdischarge mortality, longer lengths of stay, greater probability of placement in a nursing facility), though it is unclear if delirium causes worse outcomes or is simply an ominous marker
- Most episodes clear in a matter of days after correction of the precipitant, but delirium may last for weeks or months

WHEN TO REFER

- Patients in whom restraints are being considered should be referred to a geriatrician or geropsychiatrist
- Refer to a neurologist, geriatrician, or psychiatrist when the etiology is not clear or the patient is not responding to therapy

WHEN TO ADMIT

- Delirium generally signifies an underlying serious medical issue in need of treatment
- Most patients with delirium should be admitted, unless the cause is obvious, treatment is expected to result in rapid response, and they have good social support
- Uncontrollable patients should be admitted

PREVENTION

- Preventive measures include improving
  - Cognition (frequent reorientation, activities)
  - Sleep (massage, noise reduction)
  - Mobility
  - Vision (visual aids and adaptive equipment)
  - Hearing (portable amplifiers, cerumen disimpaction)
  - Hydration status (volume repletion)

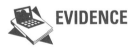

EVIDENCE

PRACTICE GUIDELINES

- American Psychiatric Association

INFORMATION FOR PATIENTS

- American Psychiatric Association
- Torpy JM et al. JAMA patient page: Delirium. JAMA. 2004;291:1794. [PMID: 15082707]

REFERENCE

- Kalisvaart KJ et al. Haloperidol prophylaxis for elderly hip-surgery patients at risk for delirium: a randomized placebo-controlled study. J Am Geriatr Soc. 2005 Oct;53(10):1658–66. [PMID: 16181163]

Dementia in Elderly

KEY FEATURES

ESSENTIALS OF DIAGNOSIS

- Persistent and progressive impairment in intellectual function
- Not due to delirium—diagnosis should not be made during an acute illness
- Primary deficit of short-term memory
- Must have other deficits (executive function, visuospatial function, language) as well

GENERAL CONSIDERATIONS

- A progressive, acquired impairment in multiple cognitive domains, at least one of which is memory
- The deficits must represent a decline in function significant enough to interfere with work or social life
- Frequently coexists with depression and delirium
- Patients have little cognitive reserve and can have acute cognitive or functional decline with a new medical illness

DEMOGRAPHICS

- Alzheimer's disease is the seventh leading cause of death in the United States with a prevalence that doubles every 5 years in the older population, reaching 30–50% at age 85
- Women suffer disproportionately, as patients (even after age adjustment) and as caregivers
- Alzheimer's disease accounts for two-thirds of cases of dementia in the United States, with vascular dementia (either alone or combined with Alzheimer's disease) accounting for much of the rest
- Risk factors
  - Older age
  - Family history
  - Lower education level
  - Female gender

CLINICAL FINDINGS

SYMPTOMS AND SIGNS

- Memory impairment with at least one or more of the following
  - Language impairment (initially just word finding; later, difficulty following a conversation)
  - Apraxia (inability to perform previously learned tasks)
  - Agnosia (inability to recognize objects)
  - Impaired executive function (poor abstraction and judgment)
- Alzheimer's disease
  - Typical earliest deficits are in memory and visuospatial abilities
  - Social graces may be retained despite advanced cognitive decline
  - Personality changes and behavioral difficulties (wandering, inappropriate sexual behavior, agitation) may develop as the disease progresses
  - Hallucinations typically observed only in moderate to severe dementia
  - End-stage disease characterized by
    □ Near-mutism
    □ Inability to sit up
    □ Inability to hold up the head
    □ Inability to track objects with the eyes
    □ Difficulty with eating and swallowing
    □ Weight loss
    □ Bowel or bladder incontinence
    □ Recurrent respiratory or urinary infections
- "Subcortical" dementias
  - Psychomotor slowing
  - Reduced attention
  - Early loss of executive function
  - Personality changes
  - Benefit from cuing in tests of memory
- Dementia with Lewy bodies
  - May be confused with delirium, as fluctuating cognitive impairment is frequently observed
  - Rigidity and bradykinesia are primarily noted; tremor is rare
  - Hallucinations—classically visual and bizarre—may occur
- Frontotemporal dementias
  - Personality change (euphoria, disinhibition, apathy) and compulsive behaviors often predate memory changes
  - In contrast to Alzheimer's disease, visuospatial function is relatively preserved
- Dementia with motor findings: extrapyramidal features or ataxia

DIFFERENTIAL DIAGNOSIS

- Depression
- Mild cognitive impairment
- Delirium
- Medication side effects

 DIAGNOSIS

LABORATORY TESTS

- Recommended tests include
  - Thyroid-stimulating hormone (TSH)
  - Vitamin B$_{12}$
  - Complete blood count
  - Electrolytes
  - Blood urea nitrogen
  - Creatinine
  - Glucose
  - Calcium
- Testing for HIV, neurosyphilis, and heavy metals should not be performed routinely

IMAGING STUDIES

- MRI scanning beneficial for
  - Younger patients
  - Persons who have focal neurologic signs, seizures, gait abnormalities, acute or subacute onset
- Noncontrast CT scanning sufficient in older patients with more classic picture of Alzheimer's disease

DIAGNOSTIC PROCEDURES

- Assess mental status (Figure 1)
- Evaluate for deficits related to cardiovascular accidents, parkinsonism, or peripheral neuropathy
- The combination of the "clock draw" (in which the patient is asked to sketch a clock face, with all the numerals placed properly, the two clock hands positioned at a specified time) and the "three-item recall" is a fairly quick and good test; an abnormally drawn clock markedly increases the probability of dementia
- When patients fail either of these screening tests, further testing with the Mini-Mental State questionnaire, neuropsychological testing, or other instruments is warranted
- Examine for comorbid conditions that may aggravate the disability

 TREATMENT

MEDICATIONS

- Acetylcholinesterase inhibitors (donepezil, galantamine, rivastigmine)
  - Modest improvements in cognitive function in mild to moderate dementia
  - May be modestly beneficial in improving neuropsychiatric symptoms
  - Do not appear to prevent progression of disability or institutionalization
  - Starting dosages
    - Donepezil, 5 mg PO daily (maximum 10 mg daily)
    - Galantamine, 4 mg PO BID (maximum 12 mg BID)
    - Rivastigmine, 1.5 mg PO BID (maximum 6 mg BID)
  - Increase doses gradually as tolerated
  - Side effects include nausea, diarrhea, anorexia, and weight loss
- Choose medications based on symptoms—depression, anxiety, psychosis
- Haloperidol
  - May modestly reduce aggression, but not agitation
  - Is associated with significant adverse effects
- Atypical antipsychotic agents, such as risperidone, olanzapine, and quetiapine, may be better tolerated than older agents but are more expensive
- Starting and target neuroleptic dosages are low (eg, haloperidol 0.5–2.0 mg; risperidone 0.25–2 mg)
- Risperidone and olanzapine may be associated with increased strokes
- Both haloperidol and atypical antipsychotic agents may increase mortality in older demented patients

THERAPEUTIC PROCEDURES

- Discontinue all nonessential drugs and correct, if possible, sensory deficits
- Exclude unrecognized delirium, pain, urinary obstruction, or fecal impaction
- Caregivers should speak simply to the patient, break down activities into simple component tasks, and use a "distract, not confront" approach

 OUTCOME

FOLLOW-UP

- Federal regulations require drug reduction efforts at least every 6 months if antipsychotic agents are used in a nursing home patient

COMPLICATIONS

- Clinicians should be alert for signs of elder abuse when working with stressed caregivers

PROGNOSIS

- The prevalence of fully reversible dementias is under 5%
- Life expectancy with Alzheimer's disease is typically 3–15 years
- Caregiver support, counseling, and respite care can prevent or delay nursing home placement

WHEN TO REFER

- Referral for neuropsychological testing may be helpful to distinguish dementia from depression, to diagnose dementia in persons of poor education or very high premorbid intellect, and to aid diagnosis when impairment is mild
- Referral to a geriatrician or neurologist is useful if the dementia does not have the classic features of Alzheimer's disease

WHEN TO ADMIT

- Dementia complicates other medical problems, and the threshold for admission should be lower

EVIDENCE

PRACTICE GUIDELINES

- American Academy of Family Physicians. Pharmacologic Treatment of Alzheimer's
- American Geriatrics Society: Dementia
- National Guideline Clearinghouse: Alzheimer's Management California Working Group for Alzheimer's Disease Management, 2002
- National Guideline Clearinghouse: American Academy of Neurology. Dementia

WEB SITES

- Alzheimer's Association
- American Geriatrics Society
- National Institute on Aging—Alzheimer's Disease Education and Referral Center

INFORMATION FOR PATIENTS

- Alzheimer's Association
- Alzheimer's Disease Education and Referral Center
- Alzheimer's Family Relief Program
- American Academy of Neurology

- JAMA patient page. Alzheimer disease. JAMA. 2001;286:2194. [PMID: 1175749]

REFERENCES

- Callahan CM et al. Effectiveness of collaborative care for older adults with Alzheimer disease in primary care: A randomized controlled trial. JAMA. 2006 May 10;295:2148–57. [PMID: 16684985]
- Courtney C et al. Long-term donepezil treatment in 565 patients with Alzheimer's disease (AD2000): randomized double-blind trial. Lancet. 2004 Jun 26; 363(9427):2105–15. [PMID: 15220031]
- Kaduszkiewicz H et al. Cholinesterase inhibitors for patients with Alzheimer's disease: systematic review of randomized clinical trials. BMJ. 2005 Aug 6; 331(7512):321–7. [PMID: 16081444]
- Schneider LS et al. Risk of death with atypical antipsychotic drug treatment for dementia; meta-analysis of randomized placebo controlled trials. JAMA. 2005 Oct 19;294(15):1934–43. [PMID: 16234500]
- Schneider LS et al; CATIE-AD Study Group. Effectiveness of atypical antipsychotic drugs in patients with Alzheimer's disease. N Engl J Med. 2006 Oct 12;355(15):1525–38. [PMID: 17035647]
- Vickrey BG et al. The effectiveness of a disease management intervention on quality and outcomes in dementia care. A randomized controlled trial. Ann Intern Med. 2006 Nov 21; 145(10):713–26. [PMID: 17116916]

Dengue

KEY FEATURES

- Extremely common togavirus infection transmitted by the bite of the *Aedes* mosquito
- Incubation period is typically 7–10 days (can be longer)
- Found throughout the tropics
- In United States, occurs in southern Texas and Puerto Rico and among travelers returning from the tropics

CLINICAL FINDINGS

- Usually nonspecific; self-limited febrile illness that typically lasts 3–7 days followed by a remission
- Severe dengue associated with fevers, terrible body aches ("breakbone"), pharyngitis, hemorrhage, and shock
- Rash is very common in the remission period or early in a second febrile phase
- Rash has maculopapular, petechial, or other morphology, appears first on the hands and feet and spreads to the arms, legs, trunk, and neck, usually sparing the face
- Death seen in cases of dengue hemorrhagic fever and dengue shock syndrome

DIAGNOSIS

- Consider diagnosis in travelers recently returned from endemic areas
- Leukopenia is characteristic
- Thrombocytopenia is common in the hemorrhagic form of the disease
- Rapid serologic testing is available

TREATMENT

- No specific antiviral therapy
- Supportive measures, including analgesics (avoiding agents with platelet dysfunction) and hydration
- Prevention: a vaccine has been developed but is not yet available commercially
- Mosquito control measures

Depression

KEY FEATURES

ESSENTIALS OF DIAGNOSIS

- In most depressions
  - Lowered mood, from mild sadness to intense guilt, worthlessness, and hopelessness
  - Difficulty in thinking and concentration, with rumination and indecision
  - Loss of interest, with diminished involvement in activities
  - Somatic complaints
  - Disrupted, reduced, or excessive sleep
  - Loss of energy, appetite, and sex drive
  - Anxiety
- In some severe depressions
  - Psychomotor disturbance: retardation or agitation
  - Delusions of a hypochondriacal or persecutory nature
  - Withdrawal from activities
  - Suicidal ideation

GENERAL CONSIDERATIONS

- Sadness and grief are normal responses to loss; depression is not
- Unlike grief, depression is marked by a disturbance of self-esteem, with a sense of guilt and worthlessness
- Dysthymia is a chronic depressive disturbance with symptoms generally milder than in a major depressive episode

DEMOGRAPHICS

- Up to 30% of primary care patients have depressive symptoms

CLINICAL FINDINGS

SYMPTOMS AND SIGNS

- Anhedonia
- Withdrawal from activities
- Feelings of guilt
- Poor concentration and cognitive dysfunction
- Anxiety
- Chronic fatigue and somatic complaints
- Diurnal variation with improvement as the day progresses
- Vegetative signs
  - Insomnia
  - Anorexia
  - Constipation
- Occasionally, severe agitation and psychotic ideation
- Atypical features
  - Hypersomnia
  - Overeating
  - Lethargy
  - Rejection sensitivity
- Unlike normal sadness and grief, depression often produces frustration and irritation in the clinician

DIFFERENTIAL DIAGNOSIS

- Bipolar disorder or cyclothymia
- Adjustment disorder with depressed mood
- Dysthymia
- Premenstrual dysphoric disorder

- Major depression with postpartum onset: usually 2 weeks to 6 months postpartum
- Seasonal affective disorder
  - Carbohydrate craving
  - Lethargy
  - Hyperphagia
  - Hypersomnia

 ## DIAGNOSIS

LABORATORY TESTS

- Complete blood cell count
- Thyroid-stimulating hormone
- Folate
- Toxicology screen may be indicated

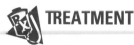 ## TREATMENT

MEDICATIONS

- See Table 148 and Figure 11
- Selective serotonin reuptake inhibitors (SSRIs) and atypical antidepressants
  - Generally lack anticholinergic or cardiovascular side effects
  - Most are activating and should be given in the morning
  - Some patients may experience sedation with paroxetine, fluvoxamine, and mirtazapine
  - Clinical response varies from 2 to 6 weeks
  - Common side effects are headache, nausea, tinnitus, insomnia, nervousness
  - Sexual side effects are very common and may respond to sildenafil
  - "Serotonin syndrome" may occur when taken in conjunction with monoamine oxidase inhibitors or selegiline
  - With the exception of paroxetine, this class should be tapered over weeks to months to avoid a withdrawal syndrome
  - Fluoxetine, fluvoxamine, sertraline, and venlafaxine appear to be safe in pregnancy; paroxetine carries a black box warning for possible teratogenecity
    □ Their use should be weighed against the risks of an untreated depression in the mother
- Tricyclic antidepressants (TCAs)
  - Mainstay of treatment before SSRIs
  - Clinical response lags several weeks
  - Start at low dose and increase by 25 mg weekly to avoid sedation and anticholinergic side effects
  - Overdose can be serious

- Monoamine oxidase inhibitors (MAOIs)
  - Commonly cause orthostatic hypotension and sympathomimetic effects
  - Third-line agents due to dietary restrictions and drug–drug interactions
  - However, with the availability of selegilene, which is a skin patch, the dietary restrictions are not necessary in the lowest dosage strength (6 mg/24h)
- Potential for withdrawal syndromes requires gradual tapering
- Drug selection influenced by any history of prior responses
- If response is inadequate, can either switch to a second agent or try augmenting the first agent according to the STAR*D study
- Lithium should be added when a second drug fails to produce a response
- Thyroid drug (liothyronine 25 mcg/day) may be added as augmentative therapy if a second agent fails
- Stimulants such as dextroamphetamine (5–30 mg/day) and methylphenidate (10–45 mg/day) can be used for short-term treatment of medically ill and geriatric patients or in refractory cases

THERAPEUTIC PROCEDURES

- Electroconvulsive therapy (ECT) is the most effective (70–85%) treatment for severe depression
  - Indications are contraindications to medications or depression refractory to medications
  - Most common side effects are headache and memory disturbances, which are usually short-lived
- Vagal nerve stimulation is approved for treatment of chronic refractory depression, though there is limited clinical experience
- Psychological
  - Medication and psychotherapy are more effective than either modality alone
  - Psychotherapy is seldom possible in the acute phase of severe depression
- Social
  - In depressions involving alcohol abuse, early involvement in recovery programs is important to future success
  - Family, employers, and friends can help mobilize a recently depressed patient

 ## OUTCOME

FOLLOW-UP

- Medication trials should be monitored every 1–2 weeks until 6 weeks, when the

effectiveness of the medication can be assessed
- If successful, medications should be continued for 6–12 months before tapering is considered
- Medications should be continued indefinitely in patients with their first episode before age 20, more than two episodes after age 40, or a single episode after age 50
- Tapering of medications should occur gradually over several months

COMPLICATIONS

- A lifetime risk of 10–15% of suicide among patients with depression
- Four major groups who attempt suicide
  - Those who are overwhelmed by problems in living
  - Those who are clearly attempting to control others
  - Those with severe depressions
  - Those with psychotic illness

PROGNOSIS

- Patients frequently respond well to a full trial of drug treatment

WHEN TO REFER

- When depression is refractory to antidepressant therapy
- When depression is moderate to severe
- When suicidality or significant loss of function is present
- With active psychosis or history of mania

WHEN TO ADMIT

- Patients at risk for suicide
- Complex treatment modalities are required

PREVENTION

- Patients at risk for suicide should receive medications in small amounts
- Guns and drugs should be removed from the patient's house
- High-risk patients should be asked not to drive

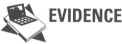 ## EVIDENCE

PRACTICE GUIDELINES

- Brigham and Young's Women's Hospital, 2001

WEB SITE

- American Psychiatric Association

INFORMATION FOR PATIENTS

- American Academy of Family Physicians: Depression in Women
- American Psychiatric Association
- JAMA patient page. Depression. JAMA. 2003;289:3198. [PMID: 12813126]
- JAMA patient page. Postpartum depression. JAMA 2002;287:802. [PMID: 11862958]
- JAMA patient page. Treating depression with electroconvulsive therapy. JAMA. 2001;285:1390. [PMID: 11280331]

REFERENCES

- Cohen LS et al. Relapse of major depression during pregnancy in women who maintain or discontinue antidepressant treatment. JAMA. 2006 Feb 1; 295(5):499–507. [PMID: 16449615]
- Fava M et al. Efficacy and safety of sildenafil in men with serotonergic antidepressant-associated erectile dysfunction: results from a randomized, double-blind, placebo-controlled trial. J Clin Psychiatry. 2006 Feb;67(2):240–6. [PMID: 16566619]
- Rush AJ et al. Acute and longer-term outcomes in depressed outpatients requiring one or several treatment steps: a STAR*D report. Am J Psychiatry. 2006 Nov;163(11):1905–17. [PMID: 17074942]
- Weissman et al. Remissions in maternal depression and child psychopathology: STAR*D-child report. JAMA. 2006 Mar 22;295(12):1389–98. [PMID: 16551710]
- Williams M et al. Paroxetine (Paxil) and congenital malformations. CMAJ. 2005 Nov 22;173(11):1320–1. [PMID: 16272192]

Depression in Elderly

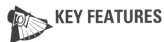 **KEY FEATURES**

ESSENTIALS OF DIAGNOSIS

- Older patients often present without complaining of depressed mood
- Somatization is a frequent presentation
- Older people not meeting diagnostic criteria for major depression may still have clinically significant depressive symptoms

GENERAL CONSIDERATIONS

- Compared with younger patients, geriatric patients with depression are
  - More likely to have somatic complaints
  - Less likely to report depressed mood or feelings of guilt
  - More likely to experience delusions
- Depression may be an early symptom of neurodegenerative condition, such as dementia

DEMOGRAPHICS

- Depressive symptoms, often related to loss, disease, and life changes, may be present in more than one-quarter of elders
- Depression is particularly common in hospitalized and institutionalized elders
- Older single men have highest suicide rate of any demographic group

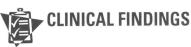 **CLINICAL FINDINGS**

SYMPTOMS AND SIGNS

- *DSM-IV* diagnosis requires at least five of the following symptoms for a diagnosis of major depression
  - Low mood (must be one of the symptoms)
  - Diminished interest or pleasure in most activities (must be one of the symptoms)
  - Significant weight loss or weight gain
  - Insomnia or hypersomnia
  - Fatigue
  - Feelings of worthlessness or guilt
  - Diminished ability to think or concentrate
  - Recurrent thoughts of death

DIFFERENTIAL DIAGNOSIS

- Substance-induced mood disorder (alcoholism)
- Bipolar disorder
- Grief reaction

 DIAGNOSIS

LABORATORY TESTS

- Complete blood cell count; liver, thyroid, and renal function; and calcium; urinalysis; and ECG may be helpful to rule out medical problems presenting as or contributing to depression

DIAGNOSTIC PROCEDURES

- A simple two-question screen is at least 96% sensitive for detecting major depression
  - "Over the last month, have you often been bothered by feeling sad, depressed or hopeless?"
  - "During the last month, have you often been bothered by little interest or pleasure in doing things?"
- Positive responses can be followed up with more comprehensive interviews such as the Yesavage's Geriatric Depression Scale (Table 43)
- Ask patients and their family members about medication use, including
  - Corticosteroids
  - Benzodiazepines
  - Cimetidine
  - β-Blockers
  - Clonidine

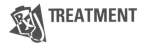 **TREATMENT**

MEDICATIONS

- Longer trials of antidepressants (at least 9 weeks) may be needed in elderly patients than in younger ones
- The major classes of antidepressants (tricyclics, selective serotonin reuptake inhibitors, monoamine oxidase inhibitors) have comparable efficacy in older adults
- Choice of an antidepressant should be based on side effect profile, pharmacokinetics, previous response, and cost
- Cognitive behavioral therapy can improve outcomes alone or in combination with pharmacologic therapy
- Electroconvulsive therapy should be considered in case of severe or refractory depression
- See Depression for more detailed description of individual classes of antidepressants

 OUTCOME

FOLLOW-UP

- Since recurrence of major depression is common among elders, monitor any elder with a history of depression closely and consider longer-term maintenance therapy
- Close follow-up of a patient with a recent diagnosis of depression, with frequent assessment of mental status and neurologic examination, may disclose an additional or alternative diagnosis

COMPLICATIONS

- Risk of suicide is highest in the geriatric age group

PROGNOSIS

- Chances for recovery are good, but it often takes several weeks to respond to an antidepressant
- Patients not responding to one antidepressant will often respond to another agent

WHEN TO REFER

- Suicidal ideation
- Possibility of bipolar disorder
- Unresponsive to treatment
- Coexisting substance use disorder

WHEN TO ADMIT

- Suicidal ideation, especially if active plan and/or patient will not contract to seek assistance if thoughts worsen
- Patient unable to care for self
- Psychotic symptoms

PREVENTION

- Some evidence suggests increasing social activity may be helpful
- Rates of recurrence are high; a high index of suspicion is required in a patient with a previous episode

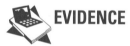

EVIDENCE

PRACTICE GUIDELINES

- American Psychiatric Association
- National Guideline Clearinghouse: The John A. Hartford Foundation, 2003

WEB SITES

- American Psychiatric Association
- ECT On-Line
- Psychopharmacology Tips
- The American Geriatrics Society

INFORMATION FOR PATIENTS

- American Academy of Family Physicians
- JAMA patient page. Depression. JAMA. 2000;284:1606. [PMID: 11032513]
- JAMA patient page. Psychiatric illness in older adults. JAMA. 2000;283:2886. [PMID: 10896524]

REFERENCES

- Hunkeler EM et al. Long term outcomes from the IMPACT randomized trial for depressed elderly patients in pri-mary care. BMJ. 2006 Feb 4; 332(7536):259–63. [PMID: 16428253]
- Reynolds CF 3rd et al. Maintenance treatment of major depression in old age. N Engl J Med. 2006 Mar 16; 354(11):1130-8. [PMID: 16540613]

Dermatitis, Atopic

KEY FEATURES

ESSENTIALS OF DIAGNOSIS

- Pruritic, exudative, or lichenified eruption on face, neck, upper trunk, wrists, hands, antecubital and popliteal folds
- Personal or family history of allergies or asthma
- Peripheral eosinophilia, increased IgE—not needed for the diagnosis

GENERAL CONSIDERATIONS

- Also known as eczema
- A chronic or intermittent pruritic, exudative, or lichenified eruption with typical distribution
- Poor prognostic factors for persistence: onset early in childhood, early generalized disease, asthma
- Personal or family history of allergic manifestations (eg, asthma, allergic rhinitis, atopic dermatitis)

CLINICAL FINDINGS

SYMPTOMS AND SIGNS

- Distribution of lesions is characteristic: face, neck, and upper trunk ("monk's cowl"), bends of elbows and knee
- Looks different at different ages and in different races, but most patients have scaly dry skin at some point
- Acute flares may present with red patches that are weepy, shiny, or lichenified and plaques and papules
- Fissures, crusts, erosions, or pustules indicate staphylococcal infection so dicloxacillin or first-generation cephalosporins may help in flares
- Pigmented persons tend to present with a papular eruption, and hypopigmented patches (pityriasis alba) are commonly seen on the cheeks and extremities

---

DIFFERENTIAL DIAGNOSIS

- Seborrheic dermatitis
- Contact dermatitis
- Impetigo
- Psoriasis
- Lichen simplex chronicus (circumscribed neurodermatitis)

DIAGNOSIS

LABORATORY TESTS

- Clinical diagnostic criteria
  - Pruritus
  - Typical morphology and distribution (flexural lichenification)
  - Tendency toward chronicity
- Also helpful
  - Personal or family history of atopic disease
  - Xerosis-ichthyosis
  - Facial pallor with infraorbital darkening
  - Fissures under the ear lobes
  - Tendency toward hand dermatitis
  - Tendency toward repeated skin infections
  - Nipple eczema
  - Elevated serum IgE

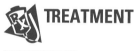

TREATMENT

MEDICATIONS

Local treatments
- Corticosteroids
  - Apply sparingly two to four times daily
  - Begin with hydrocortisone, Aclovate, or Desonide and use triamcinolone 0.1% for short periods
  - Taper when the dermatitis clears to avoid both tachyphylaxis, corticosteroid side effects, and to prevent rebounds
- Doxepin cream 5%
  - May use up to four times daily
  - Best applied simultaneously with the topical corticosteroid
  - Stinging and drowsiness occur in 25%
- Tacrolimus ointment (Protopic)
  - Effective as a first-line steroid-sparing agent
  - Available in 0.03% and 0.1% and applied twice daily
  - Burning on application occurs in about half but may resolve with continued treatment
  - Does not appear to cause corticosteroid side effects
  - Safe on the face and eyelids

- Pimecrolimus (Elidel) cream 1% is similar but burns less
- Use tacrolimus and pimecrolimus sparingly and for as brief a time as possible

Systemic and adjuvant therapies

- Immunosuppressives, oral antipruritic agents, and phototherapy

Treatment by stage of dermatitis

- Acute weeping lesions
  – Use saline or aluminum subacetate solution (Domeboro tablets) or colloidal oatmeal (Aveeno; dispense one box) as soothing or astringent soaks or wet dressings for 10–30 min two to four times a day
    □ Lesions on extremities may be bandaged for protection at night
- Tacrolimus may not be tolerated; systemic corticosteroids are last resort
- Subacute or scaly lesions (lesions are dry but still red and pruritic)
  – Mid- to high-potency corticosteroids
    □ In ointment form if tolerated—creams if not
    □ Should be continued until scaling and elevated skin lesions are cleared and itching is decreased
    □ Then, begin a 2- to 4-week taper with topical corticosteroids

OUTCOME

COMPLICATIONS

- Treatment complications
  – Monitor for skin atrophy
  – Eczema herpeticum, a generalized herpes simplex infection manifested by monomorphic vesicles, crusts, or erosions superimposed on atopic dermatitis or other extensive eczematous processes
- Smallpox vaccination is absolutely contraindicated in patients with atopic dermatitis or a history thereof because of the risk of eczema vaccinatum
- Atopic dermatitis patients may develop generalized vaccinia by contact with recent vaccine recipients who still have pustular or crusted vaccination sites

PROGNOSIS

- Runs a chronic or intermittent course
- Affected adults may have only hand dermatitis
- Poor prognostic factors for persistence into adulthood: onset early in childhood, early generalized disease, and asthma; only 40–60% of these patients have lasting remissions

WHEN TO REFER

- If there is a question about the diagnosis, if recommended therapy is ineffective, or if specialized treatment is necessary

PREVENTION

- Avoid things that dry or irritate the skin: low humidity and dry air
- Other triggers: sweating, overbathing, animal danders, scratchy fabrics
- Do not bathe more than once daily and use soap only on armpits, groin, and feet
- After rinsing, pat the skin dry (not rub) and then, before it dries completely, cover with a thin film of emollient such as Aquaphor, Eucerin, Vaseline
  – Triceram cream is a less greasy moisturizer and anti-inflammatory but is much more expensive

EVIDENCE

PRACTICE GUIDELINES

- Leung DY et al. Disease management of atopic dermatitis: an updated practice parameter. Joint Task Force on Practice Parameters. Ann Allergy Asthma Immunol. 2004;93(3 Suppl 2):S1. [PMID: 15478395]
- Hanifin JM et al. Guidelines of care for atopic dermatitis, developed in accordance with the American Academy of Dermatology (AAD)/American Academy of Dermatology Association "Administrative Regulations for Evidence-Based Clinical Practice Guidelines." J Am Acad Dermatol. 2004; 50:391. [PMID: 14988682]

WEB SITE

- American Academy of Dermatology

INFORMATION FOR PATIENTS

- American Academy of Dermatology: What is Eczema?
- National Eczema Association for Science and Education: All About Atopic Dermatitis
- National Institute of Arthritis and Musculoskeletal and Skin Diseases: Atopic Dermatitis

REFERENCES

- Akdis CA et al; European Academy of Allergology and Clinical Immunology/ American Academy of Allergy, Asthma and Immunology. Diagnosis and treatment of atopic dermatitis in children and adults: European Academy of Allergology and Clinical Immunology/ American Academy of Allergy, Asthma and Immunology/PRACTALL Consensus Report. J Allergy Clin Immunol. 2006 Jul;118(1):152–69. [PMID: 16815151]
- Boguniewicz M et al. Atopic dermatitis. J Allergy Clin Immunol. 2006 Jul; 118(1)40–3. [PMID: 16815136]
- Brown S et al. Atopic and non-atopic eczema. BMJ. 2006 Mar 11; 332(7541):584–8. [PMID: 16528081]
- Williams HC. Clinical practice. Atopic dermatitis. N Engl J Med. 2005 Jun 2; 352(22):2314–24. [PMID: 15930422]

Dermatitis, Contact

KEY FEATURES

ESSENTIALS OF DIAGNOSIS

- Erythema and edema, with pruritus, often followed by vesicles and bullae in an area of contact with a suspected agent
- Later, weeping, crusting, or secondary infection
- A history of previous reaction to suspected contactant
- Patch test with agent positive

GENERAL CONSIDERATIONS

- An acute or chronic dermatitis that results from direct skin contact with chemicals or allergens
- **Irritant contact dermatitis**
  – Eighty percent of cases are due to excessive exposure to or additive effects of primary or universal irritants such as soaps, detergents, or organic solvents
  – Only small number of cases are due to contact allergy, such as poison ivy or poison oak
- **Allergic contact dermatitis**
  – Occupational exposure is an important cause
  – The most common topicals causing allergic rashes include antimicrobials (especially neomycin), antihistamines, anesthetics (benzocaine), hair dyes, preservatives (eg, parabens), latex, and adhesive tape
- Weeping and crusting are typically due to allergic and not irritant dermatitis, which often appears red and scaly

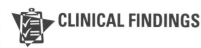

CLINICAL FINDINGS

SYMPTOMS AND SIGNS

- The acute phase is characterized by tiny vesicles and weepy and crusted lesions
- Resolving or chronic contact dermatitis presents with scaling, erythema, and possibly thickened skin; itching, burning, and stinging may be severe
- The lesions, distributed on exposed parts or in bizarre asymmetric patterns, consist of erythematous macules, papules, and vesicles
- The affected area is often hot and swollen, with exudation and crusting, simulating and at times complicated by infection
- The pattern of the eruption may be diagnostic (eg, typical linear streaked vesicles on the extremities in poison oak or ivy dermatitis)
- The location will often suggest the cause
  - Scalp involvement suggests hair dyes, sprays, or tonics
  - Face involvement, creams, cosmetics, soaps, shaving materials, nail polish; neck involvement, jewelry, hair dyes, etc

DIFFERENTIAL DIAGNOSIS

- Impetigo
- Scabies
- Dermatophytid reaction (allergy or sensitivity to fungi)
- Atopic dermatitis
- Pompholyx
- Asymmetric distribution, blotchy erythema around the face, linear lesions, and a history of exposure help distinguish contact dermatitis from other skin lesions
- The most commonly confused diagnosis is impetigo, in which case Gram stain and culture will rule out impetigo or secondary infection (impetiginization)

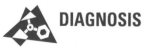

DIAGNOSIS

LABORATORY TESTS

- During the acute episode, patch testing cannot be performed
- After the episode has cleared, the patch test may be useful but not all potential allergens are available for testing
- In the event of a positive reaction, the clinical relevance of the chemical agent to the dermatitis must be determined

DIAGNOSTIC PROCEDURES

- If itching is generalized, then consider scabies

TREATMENT

- See Table 150
- Vesicular and weepy lesions often require systemic corticosteroid therapy
- Localized involvement (except on the face) can often be managed with topical agents
- Irritant contact dermatitis is treated by protection from the irritant and use of topical corticosteroids as for atopic dermatitis

Local measures
- Acute weeping dermatitis
  - Compresses are most often used
  - Calamine or starch shake lotions can be used between wet dressings, especially for intertriginous areas or when oozing is not marked
  - Lesions on the extremities may be bandaged with wet dressings for 30–60 min several times a day
  - High potency topical corticosteroids in gel or cream form (fluocinonide, clobetasol, or halobetasol) may help suppress acute contact dermatitis and relieve itching
  - Then, taper the number of applications per day or use a mid-potency corticosteroid such as triamcinolone 0.1% cream to prevent rebound of the dermatitis
  - A soothing formulation is 0.1% triamcinolone acetonide in Sarna lotion (0.5% camphor, 0.5% menthol, 0.5% phenol)
- Subacute dermatitis (subsiding)
  - Mid-potency (triamcinolone 0.1%) to high-potency corticosteroids (amcinonide, fluocinonide, desoximetasone) are the mainstays of therapy
- Chronic dermatitis (dry and lichenified)
  - High- to super-potency corticosteroids are used in ointment form

Systemic therapy
- For acute severe cases, give oral prednisone for 12–21 days
- Prednisone, 60 mg for 4–7 days, 40 mg for 4–7 days, and 20 mg for 4–7 days without a further taper is one useful regimen or dispense 78 5-mg pills to be taken 12 the first day, 11 the second day, and so on
- The key is to use enough corticosteroid (and as early as possible) to achieve a clinical effect and to taper slowly enough to avoid rebound
- A Medrol Dosepak (methylprednisolone) with 5 days of medication is inappropriate on both counts

OUTCOME

PROGNOSIS

- Self-limited if reexposure is prevented but often takes 2–3 weeks for full resolution

WHEN TO REFER

- Occupational allergic contact dermatitis should be referred to a dermatologist

PREVENTION

- Prompt and thorough removal of allergens by washing with water or solvents or other chemical agents may be effective if done very shortly after exposure to poison oak or ivy
- Several barrier creams (eg, Stokogard, Ivy Shield) offer some protection to patients at high risk for poison oak and ivy dermatitis if applied before exposure
- Iodoquinol cream (Vioform) may benefit nickel allergic patients
- Ingestion of rhus antigen is of limited clinical value for the induction of tolerance
- The mainstay of prevention is identification of agents causing the dermatitis and avoidance of exposure or use of protective clothing and gloves

EVIDENCE

PRACTICE GUIDELINES

- Bourke J et al. Guidelines for care of contact dermatitis. Br J Dermatol. 2001;145:877. [PMID: 11899139]

WEB SITE

- American Academy of Dermatology

INFORMATION FOR PATIENTS

- Mayo Clinic: Dermatitis
- MedlinePlus: Contact Dermatitis

REFERENCES

- Craig K et al. What is the best duration of steroid therapy for contact dermatitis (rhus)? J Fam Pract. 2006 Feb; 55(2):166–7. [PMID: 16451787]
- Mark BJ et al. Allergic contact dermatitis. Med Clin North Am. 2006 Jan; 90(1):169–85. [PMID: 16310529]

Dermatitis, Seborrheic

KEY FEATURES

- An acute or chronic papulosquamous dermatitis that often coexists with psoriasis
- The tendency is to lifelong recurrences, with outbreaks lasting weeks, months, or years

CLINICAL FINDINGS

- Greasy scales and underlying erythema
- Scalp, central face, presternal, interscapular areas, umbilicus, and body folds
- They occur on sun-exposed parts of the body in persons of fair complexion
- Differential diagnosis
  - Psoriasis
  - Atopic dermatitis (eczema)
  - Tinea capitis
  - Contact dermatitis
  - Tinea versicolor
  - Pityriasis rosea

DIAGNOSIS

- Clinical

TREATMENT

Scalp
- Shampoos that contain zinc pyrithione or selenium daily
- These may be alternated with ketoconazole shampoo (1% or 2%) used twice weekly
- Tar shampoos
- Topical corticosteroid solutions or lotions twice daily

Facial
- A mild corticosteroid (hydrocortisone 1%, alclometasone, desonide) used intermittently and not near the eyes
- Add ketoconazole (Nizoral) 2% cream BID if control is not obtained with intermittent topical corticosteroid use
- Topical tacrolimus (Protopic) and pimecrolimus (Elidel) are steroid-sparing alternatives
  - Only use when other agents are ineffective

- Use in a limited area for a brief time
- Avoid these agents for patients with known immunosuppression, HIV infection, bone marrow and organ transplantation, lymphoma, at high risk for lymphoma, and those with a prior history of lymphoma

Nonhairy/intertriginous areas
- 1% or 2.5% hydrocortisone, desonide, or alclometasone dipropionate cream twice weekly for maintenance
- Ketoconazole cream may be added
- Tacrolimus or pimecrolimus

Diabetes Insipidus

KEY FEATURES

ESSENTIALS OF DIAGNOSIS

- Polyuria (2–20 L/day); polydipsia
- Urine specific gravity usually < 1.006 during ad libitum fluid intake
- Urine is otherwise normal
- Vasopressin reduces urinary output except in nephrogenic diabetes insipidus (DI)

GENERAL CONSIDERATIONS

- Uncommon disease caused by a deficiency of or resistance to vasopressin

Deficiency of vasopressin
- Primary DI
  - No lesion on MRI of pituitary and hypothalamus
  - May be familial or idiopathic
- Secondary DI from damage to hypothalamus or pituitary stalk by
  - Tumor
  - Anoxic encephalopathy
  - Surgical or accidental trauma
  - Infection (eg, encephalitis, tuberculosis, syphilis)
  - Sarcoidosis
  - Multifocal Langerhans cell granulomatosis ("histiocytosis X")
- Metastases to pituitary cause DI more than pituitary adenomas (33% vs. 1%)
- Vasopressinase-induced DI may occur in last trimester of pregnancy and postpartum, often associated with oligohydramnios, preeclampsia, or hepatic dysfunction

"Nephrogenic" DI
- Due to defect in kidney tubules that interferes with water reabsorption

- Polyuria is unresponsive to vasopressin and patients have normal vasopressin secretion
- Congenital nephrogenic DI is
  - X-linked
  - Present from birth
  - Due to defective expression of renal vasopressin V2 receptors or vasopressin-sensitive water channels
- Acquired form is less severe and is seen in
  - Pyelonephritis
  - Amyloidosis
  - Multiple myeloma
  - Hypokalemia
  - Sjögren's syndrome
  - Sickle cell anemia
  - Hypercalcemia
  - Recovery from acute tubular necrosis
- May be caused by drugs
  - Corticosteroids
  - Diuretics
  - Demeclocycline
  - Tetracycline
  - Lithium
  - Foscarnet
  - Methicillin

DEMOGRAPHICS

- In familial autosomal dominant central DI, symptoms begin at about age 2 years

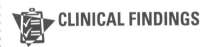
CLINICAL FINDINGS

SYMPTOMS AND SIGNS

- Intense thirst, especially for ice water
- Polyuria
- 2 L to 20 L of fluid ingested daily, with corresponding urine volumes
- Although most patients maintain fluid balance, dehydration and hypernatremia occur if patients are unable to drink or if hypothalamic thirst center is damaged by shock, anoxia, or tumor
- Partial DI presents with less intense symptoms and should be suspected in unremitting enuresis
- Wolfram syndrome
  - DI can occur in this rare, autosomal-recessive disorder
  - Also known by the acronym DIDMOAD (diabetes insipidus, type 1 diabetes mellitus, optic atrophy, and deafness)
  - Manifestations usually present in childhood but may not occur until adulthood, along with depression and cognitive problems

DIFFERENTIAL DIAGNOSIS

- Central versus nephrogenic DI
- Osmotic diuresis, eg, diabetes mellitus
- Polyuria from Cushing's syndrome, corticosteroids, or lithium
- Excessive fluid intake
  - Iatrogenic (IV fluids)
  - Psychogenic polydipsia

 DIAGNOSIS

LABORATORY TESTS

- 24-h urine collection for volume (< 2 L/day rules out DI), creatinine (to ensure accurate collection and assess creatinine clearance)
- Serum for osmolality, glucose, potassium (hypokalemia causes polyuria), sodium, uric acid
- Urinalysis: low specific gravity but is otherwise normal, no glucosuria
- Serum osmolality greater than urine osmolality
- Hypernatremia if access to water restricted or if hypothalamic thirst center damaged
- In nephrogenic DI, serum vasopressin is high during modest fluid restriction
- Hyperuricemia implicates central DI
- "Vasopressin challenge test" if suspect central DI
  - Desmopressin acetate, 0.05–0.1 mL (5–10 mcg) intranasally or 1 mcg SQ or IV, measuring urine volume for 12 h prior to and 12 h after administration
  - Obtain serum sodium immediately if symptoms of hyponatremia
  - Patients with central DI notice reduction in thirst and polyuria
  - Serum sodium remains normal except in some salt-losing conditions
  - If marginal response, desmopressin dosage is doubled

IMAGING STUDIES

- In nonfamilial central DI, MRI of pituitary and hypothalamus to exclude mass lesions

DIAGNOSTIC PROCEDURES

- Diagnosis of DI as cause of polyuria or hypernatremia mostly requires clinical judgment

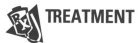 **TREATMENT**

MEDICATIONS

- Mild cases require only adequate fluid intake
- Reduction of aggravating factors (eg, corticosteroids) improves polyuria
- Desmopressin is treatment of choice for central DI or DI of pregnancy or postpartum
  - Intranasal
    □ Start at 0.05–0.1 mL (100 mcg/mL solution) q12–24h
    □ Then, individualize according to thirst and polyuria
    □ May cause sinusitis
  - Parenteral: dose is 1–4 mcg IV, IM, or SQ q12–24h PRN thirst or hypernatremia
  - Oral
    □ Available as 0.1- and 0.2-mg tablets given in a starting dose of 0.05 mg twice daily and increased to a maximum of 0.4 mg q8h, if required
    □ Particularly useful for patients with sinusitis from the nasal preparation
    □ Mild increases in hepatic enzymes, gastrointestinal symptoms, and asthenia may occur
- Hyponatremia is uncommon if minimum effective doses are used and occasional thirst is allowed
- Central and nephrogenic DI: hydrochlorothiazide 50–100 mg/day (with potassium supplement or amiloride) produces partial response
- Nephrogenic DI: indomethacin, 50 mg PO q8h, or combined indomethacin-hydrochlorothiazide, indomethacin-desmopressin, or indomethacin-amiloride
- Psychotherapy for patients with compulsive water drinking; if drug therapy is needed, thioridazine and lithium are best avoided since they cause polyuria

 OUTCOME

COMPLICATIONS

- Without water, excessive urinary output leads to severe dehydration
- Patients with impaired thirst mechanism are prone to hypernatremia, particularly when impaired mentation causes them to forget to take desmopressin
- With desmopressin acetate therapy, there is risk of water intoxication
- Desmopressin may cause nasal irritation, sinusitis, agitation, erythromelalgia

PROGNOSIS

- Chronic central DI is more an inconvenience than a dire medical condition
- Desmopressin treatment allows normal sleep and activity
- Central DI appearing after pituitary surgery usually remits after days to weeks but may be permanent if upper pituitary stalk is cut
- Central DI is made transiently worse by corticosteroids in high doses frequently given perioperatively
- Hypernatremia can occur, especially when thirst center is damaged
- Central DI itself does not reduce life expectancy if hypothalamic thirst center is intact. Prognosis is that of underlying disorder

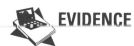 **EVIDENCE**

PRACTICE GUIDELINES

- Singer PA et al. Postoperative endocrine management of pituitary tumors. Neurosurg Clin North Am. 2003;14:123. [PMID: 12690984]

WEB SITES

- Diabetes Insipidus Foundation
- MedlinePlus—Diabetes insipidus
- Nephrogenic Diabetes Insipidus Foundation

INFORMATION FOR PATIENTS

- Mayo Clinic—Diabetes insipidus
- MedlinePlus—Diabetes insipidus
- NIDDK/NIH—Diabetes insipidus

REFERENCES

- Smith CJA et al. Phenotype-genotype correlations in a series of Wolfram syndrome families. Diabetes Care. 2004 Aug;27(8):2003–9. [PMID: 15277431]
- Verbalis JG. Disorders of body water homeostasis. Best Pract Res Clin Endocrinol Metab. 2003 Dec;17(4):471–503. [PMID: 14687585]

Diabetes Mellitus, Gestational

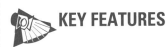

KEY FEATURES

ESSENTIALS OF DIAGNOSIS

- Euglycemia should be established before pregnancy
- Fasting and preprandial glucose values are lower during pregnancy in both diabetic and nondiabetic women
- During pregnancy, euglycemia is 60–80 mg/dL while fasting and 30–45 min before meals and < 120 mg/dL 2 h after meals
- At least two abnormal values on a 3-h glucose tolerance test (GTT)

GENERAL CONSIDERATIONS

- Pregnancy is a natural state of insulin resistance from placental lactogen and elevated circulating estrogens and progesterone
- Depending on the population screened, a significant proportion may evidence glucose intolerance, which can have implications for adverse fetal outcome
- Type 1 diabetics express particular HLA haplotypes with anti-islet cell antibodies
- Type 2 diabetics have minimal risk of ketoacidosis

DEMOGRAPHICS

- Women at higher risk include those of Hispanic, African-American, Native American, Asian, Pacific Island, or Indigenous Australian ancestry
- Prior history of gestational diabetes
- Prior history of adverse pregnancy outcome
- First-degree relative with diabetes mellitus
- Body mass index ≥ 30

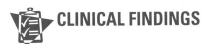 **CLINICAL FINDINGS**

SYMPTOMS AND SIGNS

- Polyuria and thirst
- Weakness or fatigue
- Recurrent blurred vision
- Macrosomia
- Polyhydramnios
- Often asymptomatic

DIFFERENTIAL DIAGNOSIS

- Drugs: corticosteriods, thiazides, tacrolimus
- Diabetes insipidus
- Psychogenic polydipsia
- Nondiabetic glycosuria (benign)

 DIAGNOSIS

LABORATORY TESTS

- See Table 140
- The target for glycemic control during pregnancy is euglycemia of 60–80 mg/dL while fasting and 30–45 min before meals and < 120 mg/dL 2 h after meals
- Glycated hemoglobin levels help determine the quality of glucose control both before and during pregnancy
- Glucose challenge test at 24–28 weeks with 50 g oral glucose load and venous sample 1 h later
- Cut-off value of 130 mg/dL or higher requires follow-up with 3-h GTT
- Normal values for glucose challenge test are fasting blood sugar ≤ 95 mg/dL; 1 h ≤ 180 mg/dL; 2 h ≤ 155 mg/dL; 3 h ≤ 140 mg/dL
- Two or more abnormal values required for diagnosis of gestational diabetes

 TREATMENT

MEDICATIONS

Before pregnancy
- Subcutaneous insulin in a split-dose regimen with frequent dosage adjustments
- Patients taking some oral agents prior to pregnancy should be switched to insulin but glyburide may be safe and effective in pregnancy

During pregnancy
- 15% of patients with gestational diabetes require insulin during pregnancy
- Dietary therapy with 1800–2200 kcal/day
- Insulin therapy for persistent fasting blood sugar at ≥ 90 mg/dL or 2 h postprandial values of ≥ 120 mg/dL
- Glyburide may be safe and effective in pregnancy
- Continuous insulin pump therapy is very useful in type 1 diabetes mellitus

SURGERY

- Cesarean sections are performed for obstetric indications

THERAPEUTIC PROCEDURES

- The risk of fetal demise in the third trimester (stillbirth) and neonatal death increases with the level of hyperglycemia. Consequently, pregnant women with diabetes must receive regular antepartum fetal testing (nonstress testing, contraction stress testing, biophysical profile) during the third trimester
- **Timing of delivery**
  - Dictated by the quality of diabetic control, the presence or absence of medical complications, and fetal status
  - The goal is to reach 39 weeks (38 completed weeks) and then proceed with delivery
  - Confirmation of lung maturity is necessary only for delivery prior to 39 weeks

 OUTCOME

FOLLOW-UP

- Patients should be evaluated 6–8 weeks postpartum by a 2-h oral GTT (75 g glucose load)
- Following delivery, insulin dosage needs to be adjusted down to prepregnancy levels

COMPLICATIONS

- Infants of diabetic mothers are at risk for macrosomia
- Congenital anomalies result from hyperglycemia during the first 4–8 weeks of pregnancy. They occur in 4–10% of diabetic pregnancies (two to three times the rate in nondiabetic pregnancies)
- Euglycemia in the early weeks of pregnancy, when organogenesis is occurring, reduces the rate of anomalies to near-normal levels. Even so, because euglycemia is not consistently achieved, congenital anomalies are the principal cause of perinatal fetal deaths in diabetic pregnancies
- Hydramnios, preeclampsia-eclampsia, infections, and prematurity are increased even in carefully managed diabetic pregnancies

PROGNOSIS

- Pregnancy does not appear to alter the long-term consequences of diabetes, but retinopathy and nephropathy may first appear or become worse during pregnancy

WHEN TO REFER

- All women with diabetes should receive prepregnancy management by providers experienced in diabetic pregnancies

WHEN TO ADMIT

- Failed intensive outpatient management of hypoglycemia or hyperglycemia
- Diagnosis of ketoacidosis
- Major complication of pregnancy

PREVENTION

- Prepregnancy HbA$_{1c}$ levels of < 7% should be achieved to reduce the incidence of congenital anomalies

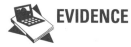

EVIDENCE

PRACTICE GUIDELINES

- American Academy of Family Physicians
- National Guideline Clearinghouse
  - American Diabetes Association, 2004
  - US Preventive Services Task Force, 2003

WEB SITES

- American Academy of Family Physicians
- American Diabetes Association

INFORMATION FOR PATIENTS

- American Academy of Family Physicians
- American Diabetes Association
- National Institute of Child Health and Human Development
- Patient Information for Obstetrics and Gynecology

REFERENCES

- ACOG Practice Bulletin. Clinical Management Guidelines for Obstetrician-Gynecologists. Number 60, March 2005. Pregestational diabetes mellitus. Obstet Gynecol. 2005 Mar; 105(3):675–85. [PMID: 15738045]
- Crowther CA et al; Australian Carbohydrate Intolerance Study in Pregnant Women (ACHOIS) Trial Group. Effect of treatment of gestational diabetes mellitus on pregnancy outcomes. N Engl J Med. 2005 Jun 16;352(24):2477–86. [PMID: 15951574]
- Langer O et al. A comparison of glyburide and insulin in women with gestational diabetes mellitus. N Engl J Med. 2000 Oct 19;343(16):1134–8. [PMID: 11036118]

Diabetes Mellitus, Type 1

KEY FEATURES

ESSENTIALS OF DIAGNOSIS

- Polyuria, polydipsia, and weight loss associated with random plasma glucose ≥ 200 mg/dL
- Plasma glucose ≥ 126 mg/dL after an overnight fast, documented on more than one occasion
- Ketonemia, ketonuria, or both

GENERAL CONSIDERATIONS

- Caused by pancreatic islet B-cell destruction
- Destruction immune-mediated in > 90% of cases and idiopathic in the remainder
- About 95% of type 1 patients possess either HLA-DR3 or HLA-DR4 compared with 45–50% of white controls. HLA-DQB1*0302 is an even more specific marker for susceptibility
- As many as 85% are positive for islet cell antibodies, antiglutamic acid decarboxylase (GAD), anti-insulin, and anti-ICA 512 (tyrosine phosphatase) antibodies at diagnosis
- The rate of pancreatic B-cell destruction ranges from rapid to slow
- Prone to ketoacidosis
- Serum C-peptide negative 1–5 years after diagnosis; plasma glucagon is elevated

DEMOGRAPHICS

- Occurs mainly in 10- to 14-year-olds but may occur in adults, especially when hyperglycemia first appears in the nonobese or elderly
- Incidence
  - Highest in Scandinavia
  - In Finland, yearly incidence per 100,000 10- to 14-year-olds is 37
  - Lowest incidence is < 1 per 100,000 per year in China and parts of South America
  - In the United States, average is 15 per 100,000
  - Incidences are higher in states densely populated with persons of Scandinavian descent such as Minnesota
  - The global incidence is increasing, with an annual increase of ~3%

- An estimated 18.2 million Americans have diabetes mellitus, of whom ~1 million have type 1 diabetes

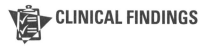

CLINICAL FINDINGS

SYMPTOMS AND SIGNS

- Increased thirst (polydipsia)
- Increased urination (polyuria)
- Increased appetite (polyphagia) with weight loss
- Ketoacidosis
- Paresthesias
- Recurrent blurred vision
- Vulvovaginitis or pruritus
- Nocturnal enuresis
- Postural hypotension from lowered plasma volume

DIFFERENTIAL DIAGNOSIS

- Type 2 diabetes
- Hyperglycemia resulting from other causes (corticosteroids, Cushing's syndrome, glucagonoma, acromegaly, pheochromocytoma, pentamidine)
- Metabolic acidosis of other causes (alcoholic ketoacidosis)
- Nondiabetic glycosuria (renal glycosuria)

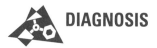

DIAGNOSIS

LABORATORY TESTS

- Fasting plasma glucose > 126 mg/dL or > 200 mg/dL 2 h after glucose load (Table 25)
- Ketonemia, ketonuria, or both
- Glucosuria (Clinistix, Diastix)
- Ketonuria (Acetest, Ketostix)
- Glycosylated hemoglobin (hemoglobin A$_{1c}$) reflects glycemic control over preceding 8–12 weeks
- Serum fructosamine
  - Reflects glycemic control over preceding 2 weeks
  - Helpful in presence of abnormal hemoglobins or in ascertaining glycemic control at time of conception among diabetic women
- Lipoprotein abnormalities; unlike in type 2 diabetes, moderately deficient control of hyperglycemia in type 1 diabetes is associated with only slight elevation of low-density lipoprotein (LDL) cholesterol and serum triglycerides and minimal change in high-density lipoprotein (HDL) cholesterol

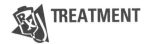

TREATMENT

MEDICATIONS

- Tables 27 and 28
- Regular insulin (a U500 concentration is available for use in patients who are very resistant)
- Rapidly-acting insulin analogs: insulin lispro, insulin aspart, insulin glulisine
- Intermediate-acting insulin purified: Neutral protamine Hagedorn (NPH)
- Premixed insulins
  - 70% NPH/30% regular (70/30 insulin)
  - 50% NPH/50% regular (50/50 insulin)
  - 70% insulin lispro protamine/30% insulin lispro (Humalog Mix 75/25)
  - 50% insulin lispro protamine/50% insulin lispro (Humalog Mix 50/50)
  - 70% insulin aspart protamine/30% insulin aspart (Novolog Mix 70/30)
- Long-acting insulins purified: insulin glargine, insulin detemir
- Inhaled insulin (1-mg or 3-mg blister packs—1 mg inhaled is equivalent to 3 units subcutaneously)
- Pramlintide (islet amyloid polypeptide analog)

SURGERY

- Infuse intraoperatively and in immediate postoperative period: D5 0.9% saline with 20 mEq KCl IV at 100–200 mL/h. Infuse regular human insulin (25 U/250 mL 0.9% saline) into IV tubing at 1–3 U/h
- Monitor blood glucose hourly and adjust infusion for target glucose levels 100–190 mg/dL
- Patients receiving simultaneous pancreas and kidney transplants have 85% chance of pancreatic graft survival and 92% chance of renal graft survival after 1 year. Solitary pancreas transplant only for recurrent life-threatening metabolic instability
- Islet transplantation is minimally invasive (data on long-term efficacy are lacking); application is limited by need for multiple donors; potent long-term immunotherapy; decline in insulin secretion with time

THERAPEUTIC PROCEDURES

- Eucaloric healthy diet. Limit cholesterol to 300 mg QD and protein to 10% of total calories
- Treat microalbuminuria with angiotensin-converting enzyme (ACE)-I inhibitor to retard diabetic nephropathy
- Treat hypertension and hyperlipidemia (reduce LDL to < 100 mg/dL)
- Attempts have been made to prolong the partial clinical remission ("honeymoon") using drugs that may induce immune tolerance

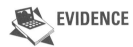

OUTCOME

FOLLOW-UP

- Glycemic control of HbA_{1c} to no higher than 2% above upper limits of normal has 60% reduction in risk of diabetic retinopathy, nephropathy, and neuropathy

COMPLICATIONS

- Diabetic ketoacidosis
- Hypoglycemia and altered awareness of hypoglycemia
- Diabetic retinopathy, cataracts
- Nephropathy
- Neuropathy
- Diabetic atherothrombosis (coronary artery disease, peripheral vascular disease)
- Lipodystrophy at injection sites

PROGNOSIS

- The Diabetes Control and Complications Trial (DCCT) showed that the poor prognosis for 40% of patients with type 1 diabetes is markedly improved by optimal care
- Patients can have a full life
- Tight control (mean HbA_{1c} 7.2%, normal: < 6%) in the DCCT was associated with a threefold greater risk of serious hypoglycemia as well as greater weight gain. However, no deaths occurred because of hypoglycemia, and no evidence of posthypoglycemic cognitive damage was detected
- Subsequent renal failure predicted by microalbuminuria > 30 µg/min in timed overnight urine collection. Risk decreased by treatment with ACE-I

WHEN TO REFER

- Team educational approach is critical. Enlist nutritionist
- Poorly controlled diabetes

WHEN TO ADMIT

- Altered mental status
- Diabetic ketoacidosis
- Marked volume disorders
- Marked electrolyte disorders
- Unstable comorbid conditions

PREVENTION

- Acetylsalicylic acid (aspirin) 81–325 mg (enteric coated) PO daily to reduce risk of diabetic atherothrombosis without increasing risk of vitreous bleeding
- Instruction in personal hygiene, in particular, care of feet, skin, and teeth
- Yearly diabetic eye examination
- Patient self-management training
- Self-monitoring of blood glucose
- Exercise

EVIDENCE

PRACTICE GUIDELINES

- American Association of Clinical Endocrinologists
- American Diabetes Association. Clinical practice recommendations. Diabetes Care. 2002;25(Suppl 1):S1.

WEB SITES

- American Diabetes Association
- CDC Diabetes Public Health Resource
- Joslin Diabetes Center

INFORMATION FOR PATIENTS

- American Academy of Family Physicians: Diabetes: Type 1
- American Diabetes Association: Type 1 Diabetes
- NIH—National Diabetes Education Program
- Torpy JM et al. JAMA patient page: Type 1 diabetes. JAMA. 2003; 290:2216. [PMID: 14570956]

REFERENCES

- American Diabetes Association: Standards of Medical Care in Diabetes. Diabetes Care. 2006;29:476. [PMID: 16482699]
- Daneman D. Type 1 diabetes. Lancet. 2006;367:847. [PMID: 16530579]
- Harris R et al. Screening adults for type 2 diabetes: a review of the evidence for the U.S. Preventive Services Task Force. Ann Intern Med. 2003;138:215. [PMID: 12558362]

Diabetes Mellitus, Type 2

KEY FEATURES

ESSENTIALS OF DIAGNOSIS

- Typically > 40 years of age
- Obesity
- Polyuria and polydipsia
- Candidal vaginitis sometimes an initial manifestation
- Often few or no symptoms
- After an overnight fast, plasma glucose ≥ 126 mg/dL more than once
- After 75 g oral glucose, diagnostic values are ≥ 200 mg/dL 2 h after the oral glucose
- Often associated with hypertension, dyslipidemia, and atherosclerosis

GENERAL CONSIDERATIONS

- Circulating endogenous insulin is sufficient to prevent ketoacidosis but inadequate to prevent hyperglycemia from tissue insensitivity
- Strong genetic influences
- Prevalence of obesity in type 2 diabetes mellitus
  - 30% in Chinese and Japanese
  - 60–70% in North Americans, Europeans, and Africans
  - Nearly 100% in Pima Indians and Pacific Islanders from Nauru or Samoa
- Enhancers of insulin resistance are aging, sedentary lifestyle, and abdominal-visceral obesity
- Abdominal fat, with an abnormally high waist–hip ratio, is generally associated with obesity in type 2 diabetes. This visceral obesity correlates with insulin resistance, whereas subcutaneous fat seems to have less of an association
- Both the tissue resistance to insulin and the impaired B-cell response to glucose are further aggravated by increased hyperglycemia, and both defects improve with decreased hyperglycemia

DEMOGRAPHICS

- 17.2 million Americans have type 2 diabetes
- Traditionally occurred in middle-aged adults but now more frequently encountered in children and adolescents
- No gender predominance

CLINICAL FINDINGS

SYMPTOMS AND SIGNS

- Polyuria
- Increased thirst (polydipsia)
- Weakness or fatigue
- Recurrent blurred vision
- Vulvovaginitis or pruritus
- Peripheral neuropathy
- Often asymptomatic

DIFFERENTIAL DIAGNOSIS

Hyperglycemia
- Endocrinopathies
  - Type 1 diabetes mellitus
  - Cushing's syndrome
  - Acromegaly
  - Pheochromocytoma
  - Glucagonoma
  - Somatostatinoma
- Drugs
  - Corticosteroids
  - Thiazides
  - Phenytoin
  - Niacin
  - Oral contraceptives
  - Pentamidine
- Pancreatic insufficiency
  - Subtotal pancreatectomy
  - Chronic pancreatitis
  - Hemochromatosis ("bronze diabetes")
  - Cystic fibrosis
  - Hemosiderosis
- Other
  - Gestational diabetes
  - Cirrhosis
  - Schmidt's syndrome (polyglandular failure: Addison's disease, autoimmune thyroiditis, diabetes)

Polyuria
- Diabetes insipidus

Hypercalcemia
- Psychogenic polydipsia

Nondiabetic glycosuria (benign)
- Genetic
- Fanconi's syndrome
- Chronic renal failure
- Pregnancy

DIAGNOSIS

LABORATORY TESTS

- Fasting plasma glucose ≥ 126 mg/dL or ≥ 200 mg/dL 2 h after glucose load (Table 25)
- Glucosuria (Clinistix, Diastix)

- Ketonuria on occasion without ketonemia (Acetest, Ketostix)
- Glycosylated hemoglobin (HbA$_{1c}$) reflects glycemic control over preceding 8–12 weeks
- Serum fructosamine
  - Reflects glycemic control over preceding 2 weeks
  - Helpful in the presence of abnormal hemoglobins and in ascertaining glycemic control at time of conception among diabetic women
- Lipoprotein abnormalities in obese persons with type 2 diabetes include
  - High serum triglyceride (300–400 mg/dL)
  - Low high-density lipoprotein (HDL) cholesterol (< 30 mg/dL)
  - A qualitative change in low-density lipoprotein (LDL) particles
- These abnormalities differ from type 1 diabetes, which is associated with only slight elevation of LDL cholesterol and serum triglycerides and minimal change in HDL cholesterol

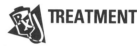

TREATMENT

MEDICATIONS

- Tables 26 and 27
- Drugs that stimulate insulin secretion
  - Sulfonylureas
  - Meglitinide analogs
  - D-phenylalanine derivative
- Drugs that alter insulin action
  - Metformin
  - Thiazolidinediones
- Drugs that principally affect glucose absorption: α-glucosidase inhibitors
- Drugs that mimic incretin effect: exenatide, sitagliptin
- Others: pramlintide (islet amyloid polypeptide analog)
- Insulin: indicated for persons with type 2 diabetes with insulinopenia and hyperglycemia unresponsive to diet and oral hypoglycemic agents
- Preprandial rapid-acting insulin plus basal insulin replacement with an intermediate- or long-acting insulin used to attain acceptable control of blood glucose (Table 27)
- Combination oral agents: several drug combinations of thiazolidinediones with metformin or sulfonylureas; sulfonylureas with metformin are available but these limit optimal dose adjustment of individual drugs

NONPHARMACOLOGIC APPROACH

Diet

- Limitations
  - Cholesterol to 300 mg once daily
  - Protein intake to 10% of total calories

SURGERY

Major surgery

- During major surgery, insulin is necessary for most persons with type 2 diabetes, even if not previously taking insulin
- Infuse IV intraoperatively and in the immediate postoperative period: 1 L D_5W with 20 mEq KCl and 10 U regular insulin at rate of ~100 mL/h
- Monitor blood glucose hourly and adjust infusion for target glucose levels 100–250 mg/dL. If blood glucose remains > 250 mg/dL after 1–2 h, increase insulin infusion to 15 U/L

Minor surgery

- Regular human insulin or rapidly-acting insulin analog SQ PRN to maintain glucose < 250 mg/dL

 OUTCOME

FOLLOW-UP

- Self-monitoring
- HbA_{1c} quarterly
- Screen for microalbuminuria annually
- Serum lipids
- Feet examination annually
- Diabetic eye examination annually
- Treatment goals
  - Self-monitored blood glucose, 80–120 mg/dL before meals; 100–140 mg/dL at bedtime; < 180 mg/dL 1.5–2.0 h postprandially
  - HbA_{1c} < 7.0%

COMPLICATIONS

- Hypoglycemia
- Ocular (diabetic cataracts and retinopathy)
- Diabetic nephropathy (microalbuminuria, progressive diabetic nephropathy)
- Gangrene of the feet
- Diabetic neuropathy
  - Peripheral neuropathy
  - Distal symmetric polyneuropathy
  - Isolated peripheral neuropathy
  - Painful diabetic neuropathy
  - Autonomic neuropathy
- Skin and mucous membranes
  - Pyogenic infections

- Eruptive xanthomas from hypertriglyceridemia associated with poor glucose control
- Necrobiosis lipoidica diabeticorum
- Shin spots
- Intertriginous candida
- Vulvovaginitis

WHEN TO REFER

- Team-oriented educational approach, including a nutritionist, is critical
- Poorly controlled diabetes

WHEN TO ADMIT

- Altered mental status
- Diabetic ketoacidosis
- Marked volume disorders
- Marked electrolyte disorders
- Unstable comorbid conditions

PROGNOSIS

- Antihypertensive control to a mean of 144/82 mm Hg had beneficial effects on all microvascular and all diabetes-related end points in the United Kingdom Prospective Diabetes Study

PREVENTION

- Goal of therapy is to prevent acute illness and reduce risk of long-term complications
- Lifestyle modifications can prevent or slow the development of diabetes
- Daily vigorous exercise prevents accumulation of visceral fat, which can prevent the development of diabetes
- Screen with fasting glucose at 3-year intervals beginning at age 45; screen earlier and more frequently if risk factors present

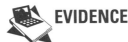 **EVIDENCE**

PRACTICE GUIDELINES

- American Association of Clinical Endocrinologists: Medical Guidelines for the Management of Diabetes Mellitus
- National Guideline Clearinghouse: Adult Diabetes Clinical Practice Guidelines
- National Guideline Clearinghouse: Standards of Medical Care in Diabetes

WEB SITES

- American Diabetes Association
- Centers for Disease Control and Prevention: Diabetes Public Health Resource
- Joslin Diabetes Center

INFORMATION FOR PATIENTS

- American Diabetes Association: Type 2 Diabetes
- JAMA patient page. Managing type 2 diabetes. JAMA. 2000;283:288.
- Joslin Diabetes Center: Joslin's Online Diabetes Library
- NIH: National Diabetes Education Program
- Stevens LM. JAMA patient page: The ABCs of diabetes. JAMA. 2002; 287:2608. [PMID: 12025825]

REFERENCES

- American Diabetes Association. Clinical practice recommendations. Diabetes Care. 2006;29(Suppl 1):S1.
- DeFronzo RA et al. Effects of exenatide (exendin-4) on glycemic control and weight over 30 weeks in metformin-treated patients with type 2 diabetes. Diabetes Care. 2005 May;28(5):1092–100. [PMID: 15855572]
- Mooradian AD et al. Narrative review: a rational approach to starting insulin therapy. Ann Intern Med. 2006 Jul 18; 145(2):125–34. [PMID: 16847295]
- UK Prospective Diabetes Study Group. Effect of intensive blood-glucose control with metformin on complications in overweight patients with type 2 diabetes. Lancet. 1998;352:854. [PMID: 9742977]

Diabetic Ketoacidosis

 KEY FEATURES

ESSENTIALS OF DIAGNOSIS

- Hyperglycemia > 250 mg/dL
- Acidosis with blood pH < 7.3
- Serum bicarbonate < 15 mEq/L
- Serum positive for ketones

GENERAL CONSIDERATIONS

- May be the initial manifestation of type 1 diabetes
- Commonly occurs with poor compliance in type 1 diabetics, particularly when episodes are recurrent
- Develops in type 1 diabetics with increased insulin requirements during

infection, trauma, myocardial infarction, or surgery

- May develop in type 2 diabetics under severe stress such as sepsis or trauma
- Common serious complication of insulin pump therapy

DEMOGRAPHICS

- Incidence is 5 to 8 episodes per 1000 diabetic persons annually
- Incidence in insulin pump therapy is 1 per 80 patient-months of treatment

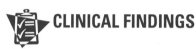

CLINICAL FINDINGS

SYMPTOMS AND SIGNS

- May begin with a day or more of polyuria, polydipsia, marked fatigue, nausea and vomiting and, finally, mental stupor that can progress to coma
- Dehydration, possible stupor
- Rapid deep breathing and a "fruity" breath odor of acetone
- Hypotension with tachycardia indicates profound fluid and electrolyte depletion
- Mild hypothermia usually present; elevated or even a normal temperature may suggest infection
- Abdominal pain and tenderness in the absence of abdominal disease; conversely, cholecystitis or pancreatitis may occur with minimal symptoms and signs

DIFFERENTIAL DIAGNOSIS

- Lactic acidosis in type 1 diabetics, including the use of metformin
- Alcoholic ketoacidosis
- Hypoglycemia
- Hyperglycemic hyperosmolar state
- Uremia
- Starvation ketoacidosis
- Salicylate poisoning

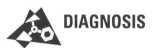

DIAGNOSIS

LABORATORY TESTS

- 4+ glycosuria, hyperglycemia
- Strong ketonuria and ketonemia (acetoacetic acid is measured by nitroprusside reagents [Acetest and Ketostix]; the more prevalent β-hydroxybutyric acid has no ketone group and is therefore not detected by conventional nitroprusside tests)
- Anion-gap ketoacidosis
- Serum potassium often elevated despite total body potassium depletion

- Elevated serum amylase from salivary as well as pancreatic amylase. An elevated serum amylase is not specific for acute pancreatitis
- Serum lipase may be useful if the diagnosis of pancreatitis is being seriously considered
- Leukocytosis up to 25,000/μL with a left shift may occur with or without associated infection
- Hyperchloremic metabolic acidosis can develop during initial therapy, as keto acids are lost in the urine and a portion of the bicarbonate deficit is replaced with chloride ions from the saline therapy. This relatively benign condition reverses over a day once IV saline is stopped

 TREATMENT

MEDICATIONS

Regular insulin

- Initially in severe ketoacidosis, use only regular insulin
- Begin with loading dose of 0.1 unit/kg as IV bolus, followed by 0.1 unit/kg/h, continuously infused or given hourly as an IM injection
- "Piggy-back" insulin into the fluid line so the rate of fluid replacement can be changed without altering the insulin delivery rate
- If plasma glucose level fails to fall at least 10% in the first hour, give repeat loading dose

Fluids

- Fluid deficit is usually 4–5 L. In the first hour, give at least 1 L of 0.9% saline to reexpand contracted vascular volume
- Then, can switch to 0.45% saline at a rate of 300–500 mL/h, depending on the severity of the dehydration and the cardiac and renal status. When blood glucose falls to < 250 mg/dL, use 5% **glucose** solutions to maintain blood glucose 200–300 mg/dL while continuing insulin to clear ketonemia
- Failure to give enough volume replacement (at least 3–4 L in 8 h) to restore normal perfusion affects satisfactory recovery
- Excessive fluid replacement (more than 5 L in 8 h) may contribute to acute respiratory distress syndrome or cerebral edema

Electrolytes

- Use **NaHCO₃** only for pH < 7.1. For arterial pH 6.9–7.0, add 1 ampule of 7.5% NaHCO₃ (44 mEq/L) to 200 mL

of sterile water and administer intravenously at a rate of 200 mL/h

- If the pH is below 6.9, use 2 ampules of NaHCO₃ (88 mEq) in 400 mL of sterile water and administer at the same rate of 200 mL/h
- For each ampule of NaHCO₃, add 15 mEq/L of KCl as long as the serum potassium does not exceed 5.5 mEq/L
- Stop bicarbonate when pH reaches 7.1

- Total body **potassium** loss from polyuria and vomiting may be several hundred milliequivalents

- However, initial serum potassium is usually normal or high because of extracellular shifts from acidosis
- Potassium infusion 20–30 mEq/h should begin 2–3 h after beginning therapy, or sooner if initial serum potassium is low
- Defer potassium replacement if serum potassium remains above 5 mEq/L, as in renal insufficiency

- **Phosphate** replacement is seldom required. However, if severe hypophosphatemia of < 0.35 mmol/L (< 1 mg/dL) develops during insulin therapy, a small amount of phosphate can be replaced as the potassium salt

- To minimize the risk of tetany from an overload of phosphate replacement, an average deficit of 40–50 mmol phosphate should be replaced by intravenous infusion at a rate not to exceed 3 mmol/h
- A stock solution (Abbott Laboratories) provides a mixture of 1.12 g KH₂PO₄ and 1.18 g K₂HPO₄ in a 5-mL single-dose vial representing 22 mEq potassium and 15 mmol phosphate (27 mEq); 5 mL of this stock solution in 2 L of 0.45% saline or 5% dextrose in water, infused at 400 mL/h, will replace the phosphate at the optimal rate of 3 mmol/h and provide 4.4 mEq potassium per hour
- If serum phosphate remains below 0.35 mmol/L (1 mg/dL), repeat a 5-h infusion of potassium phosphate at a rate of 3 mmol/h

THERAPEUTIC PROCEDURES

- Use a flow sheet listing vital signs, time sequence of laboratory values (arterial pH, plasma glucose, acetone, bicarbonate, serum urea nitrogen, electrolytes, serum osmolality) in relation to therapy
- Carefully monitor serum potassium during fluid replacement

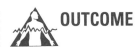

OUTCOME

COMPLICATIONS

- Acute myocardial infarction and infarction of the bowel following prolonged hypotension
- Renal failure, especially with prior kidney dysfunction
- Cerebral edema occurs rarely
  - Best prevented by avoiding sudden reversal of marked hyperglycemia
  - Maintaining glycemic levels of 200–300 mg/dL for the initial 24 h after correction of severe hyperglycemia reduces this risk

PROGNOSIS

- Life-threatening medical emergency with a mortality rate just under 5% in individuals younger than 40 years, but with a more serious prognosis in the elderly, who have mortality rates over 20%

WHEN TO REFER

- Recurrent diabetic ketoacidosis
- Poor compliance

WHEN TO ADMIT

- Severe ketosis, hyperosmolality
- An intensive care unit or step-down unit is preferable for more severe cases

PREVENTION

- The patient should contact a provider for persistent ketonuria
- Compliance is particularly important for juvenile-onset diabetics, particularly in the teen years. Intensive family counseling may be needed
- Urine ketones should be measured with signs of infection or in insulin pump-treated patients when capillary blood glucose is persistently high

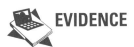

EVIDENCE

PRACTICE GUIDELINES

- National Guideline Clearinghouse: American Diabetes Association, 2004

WEB SITES

- American Diabetes Association
- Centers for Disease Control and Prevention: Diabetes
- Joslin Diabetes Center

INFORMATION FOR PATIENTS

- American Diabetes Association
- JAMA patient page. The ABCs of diabetes. JAMA. 2002;287:2608. [PMID: 12025825]
- National Institutes of Health
- NIH: National Diabetes Education Program (multiple languages available)

REFERENCE

- Kitabchi AE et al. Management of hyperglycemic crises in patients with diabetes. Diabetes Care. 2001 Jan; 24(1):131–53. [PMID: 11194218]

Diarrhea, Acute

KEY FEATURES

ESSENTIALS OF DIAGNOSIS

- Diarrhea is acute in onset with a duration of < 2–3 weeks
- Severity ranges from mild, self-limited to severe, life-threatening

GENERAL CONSIDERATIONS

- Most commonly caused by infectious agents, bacterial toxins, or drugs (Table 66)
- Recent illnesses in family members suggests infectious diarrhea
- Community outbreaks (schools, nursing homes, cruise ships) suggest viral etiology or common food source
- Ingestion of improperly stored or prepared food implicates toxin-secreting or invasive bacteria
- Exposure to unpurified water suggests *Giardia, Cryptosporidium,* or *Cyclospora*
- Recent travel abroad suggests "traveler's diarrhea"
- Antibiotic administration suggests *Clostridium difficile* colitis
- HIV infection or sexually transmitted diseases suggest AIDS-associated diarrhea
- Proctitis and rectal discharge suggest gonorrhea, syphilis, lymphogranuloma venereum, and herpes simplex

Noninflammatory diarrhea

- Fecal leukocytes and blood are absent
- Diarrhea may be voluminous with periumbilical cramps, nausea, or vomiting

- Usually arises from small bowel due to a toxin-producing bacterium or other agents (viruses, *Giardia*)
- Prominent vomiting suggests viral enteritis or *Staphylococcus aureus* food poisoning
- May cause dehydration, hypokalemia, and metabolic acidosis

Inflammatory diarrhea

- Fecal leukocytes are present; blood mixed with stool may also be present (dysentery)
- Diarrhea usually arises from colon, is small volume (< 1 L/day), with left lower quadrant cramps, urgency, and tenesmus
- Usually caused by invasive organisms (shigellosis, salmonellosis, *Campylobacter,* or *Yersinia* infection, amebiasis, cytomegalovirus) or a toxin (*C difficile, Escherichia coli* O157:H7)

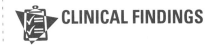

CLINICAL FINDINGS

SYMPTOMS AND SIGNS

- Increased stool frequency or liquidity
- Rectal discharge suggests proctitis
- Periumbilical cramps, bloating, nausea, or vomiting suggest noninflammatory diarrhea
- Fever, left lower quadrant cramps, urgency, and tenesmus suggest inflammatory diarrhea
- Physical examination may reveal abdominal tenderness, peritonitis

DIFFERENTIAL DIAGNOSIS

- Infectious: noninflammatory (non-bloody)
  - Viruses: Norwalk virus, rotavirus, adenoviruses, astrovirus, coronavirus
  - Preformed toxin (food poisoning): *S aureus, Bacillus cereus, Clostridium perfringens*
  - Toxin production: enterotoxigenic *E coli, Vibrio cholerae, Vibrio parahaemolyticus*
  - Protozoa: *Giardia lamblia, Cryptosporidium, Cyclospora, Isospora*
- Infectious: invasive or inflammatory
  - *Shigella, Salmonella, Campylobacter,* enteroinvasive *E coli, E coli* O157:H7, *Yersinia enterocolitica, C difficile* (eg, pseudomembranous colitis), *Entamoeba histolytica, Neisseria gonorrhoeae, Listeria monocytogenes*
- Associated with unprotected anal intercourse
  - *N gonorrhoeae*
  - Syphilis

- Lymphogranuloma venereum
- Herpes simplex
- Noninfectious
  - Drug reaction, especially antibiotics
  - Ulcerative colitis, Crohn's disease (inflammatory)
  - Ischemic colitis (inflammatory)
  - Fecal impaction (stool may leak around impaction)
  - Laxative abuse
  - Radiation colitis (inflammatory)
  - Emotional stress

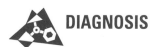 **DIAGNOSIS**

LABORATORY TESTS

- Noninflammatory diarrhea
  - 90% mild, self-limited, resolving within 7 days
  - Stool cultures positive in < 3%; therefore, initial symptomatic treatment given for mild symptoms
  - If diarrhea worsens or persists for > 7–10 days, send stools for leukocytes or lactoferrin, cultures, ova and parasites (3 samples), *Giardia* antigen
- Diarrhea that requires prompt evaluation
  - Inflammatory diarrhea: fever (> 38.5°C), blood or pus in diarrhea, or abdominal pain
  - Passage of six or more unformed stools in 24 hours
  - Profuse watery diarrhea and dehydration
  - Frail older patients
  - Immunocompromised patients (AIDS, posttransplantation)
  - Stool culture with serotyping if *E coli* O157:H7 is suspected
- Stool wet mount or antigen detection test for amebiasis in sexually active homosexuals, those with recent travel, and those whose bacterial cultures are negative
- Stool *C difficile* toxin assay if recent history of antibiotic exposure or hospitalization
- Rectal swab cultures for *Chlamydia*, *N gonorrhoeae*, and herpes simplex virus in sexually active patients with suspected proctitis

DIAGNOSTIC PROCEDURES

- In > 90% of cases, acute diarrhea is mild and self-limited, and diagnostic investigation is unnecessary
- Prompt sigmoidoscopy for severe proctitis (tenesmus, discharge, rectal pain) or for suspected *C difficile* colitis, ulcerative colitis, or ischemic colitis

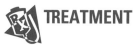 **TREATMENT**

MEDICATIONS

- Antidiarrheal agents may be used safely in mild to moderate noninflammatory diarrhea but should not be used in bloody diarrhea, high fever, or systemic toxicity
  - Loperamide, 4 mg PO initially, followed by 2 mg after each loose stool (maximum: 16 mg/24 hours)
  - Bismuth subsalicylate (Pepto-Bismol), 2 tablets or 30 mL PO QID
  - Diphenoxylate with atropine (anticholinergic) contraindicated in acute diarrhea because of the rare precipitation of toxic megacolon
- Empiric antibiotic treatment recommended with moderate to severe fever, tenesmus, or bloody stools or the presence of fecal leukocytes while the stool bacterial culture is incubating
  - Fluoroquinolones (eg, ciprofloxacin 500 mg, ofloxacin 400 mg, or norfloxacin 400 mg, PO BID) for 5–7 days
  - Trimethoprim-sulfamethoxazole, 160/800 mg PO BID, or doxycycline, 100 mg PO BID
- Specific antimicrobial treatment is recommended in
  - Shigellosis
  - Cholera
  - Extraintestinal salmonellosis
  - Traveler's diarrhea
  - *C difficile* infection
  - Giardiasis
  - Amebiasis
  - Gonorrhea, syphilis, chlamydiosis, and herpes simplex infection
- Antibiotics not recommended in nontyphoid *Salmonella*, *Campylobacter*, *Aeromonas*, *Yersinia*, or *E coli* O157:H7 infection except in severe disease

THERAPEUTIC PROCEDURES

- Diet
  - Adequate oral fluids containing carbohydrates and electrolytes
  - Avoidance of high-fiber foods, fats, milk products, caffeine, and alcohol
- Rehydration
  - Oral electrolyte solutions (eg, Pedialyte, Gatorade)
  - Intravenous fluids (lactated Ringer's injection) for severe dehydration

 OUTCOME

WHEN TO ADMIT

- Patients with fever > 38.5°C, severe dehydration, toxicity, or marked abdominal pain, rebound tenderness
- Frail and elderly patients
- Immunocompromised patients

PREVENTION

- When traveling, eat only "peeled, packaged, and piping hot" foods

 EVIDENCE

PRACTICE GUIDELINES

- Manatsathit S et al. Guideline for the management of acute diarrhea in adults. J Gastroenterol Hepatol. 2002;17 Suppl:S54. [PMID: 12000594]
- National Guideline Clearinghouse
- Practice guidelines for the management of infectious diarrhea. Infectious Diseases Society of America, 2001

INFORMATION FOR PATIENTS

- Centers for Disease Control and Prevention
- Mayo Clinic

REFERENCE

- Thielman NM et al. Clinical practice. Acute infectious diarrhea. N Engl J Med. 2004 Jan 1;350(1):38–47. [PMID: 14702426]

Diarrhea, Chronic

 KEY FEATURES

ESSENTIALS OF DIAGNOSIS

- Defined as increased stool frequency (> 3 bowel movements/day) or liquidity persisting for > 3 weeks
- Classification
  - Osmotic diarrhea
  - Secretory diarrhea
  - Inflammatory conditions
  - Malabsorption syndromes
  - Motility disorders
  - Chronic infections
  - Miscellaneous

GENERAL CONSIDERATIONS

- Osmotic diarrheas resolve during fasting
- Secretory diarrhea is caused by increased intestinal secretion or decreased absorption with little change in stool output during fasting
- Motility disorders are secondary to systemic disorders or surgery that lead to rapid transit or to stasis of intestinal contents with bacterial overgrowth, malabsorption
- Immunocompromised patients are susceptible to *Microsporidia, Cryptosporidium*, cytomegalovirus, *Isospora belli, Cyclospora*, and *Mycobacterium avium-intracellulare* infections
- Factitious diarrhea is caused by surreptitious laxative abuse or dilution of stool

DEMOGRAPHICS

- Lactase deficiency
  - Occurs in 75% of nonwhite adults and 25% of whites
  - May be acquired with viral gastroenteritis, medical illness, or gastrointestinal surgery

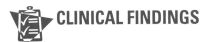 **CLINICAL FINDINGS**

SYMPTOMS AND SIGNS

- Osmotic diarrheas
  - Abdominal distention
  - Bloating
  - Flatulence due to increased colonic gas production
- Secretory diarrhea
  - High-volume (> 1 L/day) watery diarrhea
  - Dehydration
  - Electrolyte imbalance
- Inflammatory conditions
  - Abdominal pain
  - Fever
  - Weight loss
  - Hematochezia
- Malabsorption syndromes
  - Weight loss
  - Osmotic diarrhea
  - Nutritional deficiencies

DIFFERENTIAL DIAGNOSIS

- Common
  - Irritable bowel syndrome
  - Parasites
  - Caffeine
  - Laxative abuse
- Osmotic
  - Lactase deficiency

  - Medications: antacids, lactulose, sorbitol, olestra
  - Factitious: magnesium-containing antacids or laxatives
- Secretory
  - Hormonal: Zollinger-Ellison syndrome (gastrinoma), carcinoid, VI-Poma, medullary thyroid carcinoma, adrenal insufficiency
  - Laxative abuse: cascara, senna
  - Medications
- Inflammatory conditions
  - Inflammatory bowel disease
  - Microscopic colitis (lymphocytic or collagenous)
  - Cancer with obstruction and pseudodiarrhea
  - Radiation colitis
- Malabsorption
  - Small bowel: celiac sprue, Whipple's disease, tropical sprue, eosinophilic gastroenteritis, small bowel resection, Crohn's disease
  - Lymphatic obstruction: lymphoma, carcinoid, tuberculosis, *M avium-intracellulare* infection, Kaposi's sarcoma, sarcoidosis, retroperitoneal fibrosis
  - Pancreatic insufficiency: chronic pancreatitis, cystic fibrosis, pancreatic cancer
  - Bacterial overgrowth, eg, diabetes
  - Reduced bile salts: ileal resection, Crohn's disease, postcholecystectomy
- Motility disorders
  - Irritable bowel syndrome
  - Postsurgical: vagotomy, partial gastrectomy, blind loop with bacterial overgrowth
  - Systemic disease: diabetes mellitus, hyperthyroidism, scleroderma
  - Caffeine or alcohol use
- Chronic infections
  - Parasites: giardiasis, amebiasis, strongyloidiasis

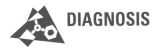 **DIAGNOSIS**

LABORATORY TESTS

- Obtain complete blood cell count, serum electrolytes, liver enzymes, calcium, phosphorus, albumin, thyroid-stimulating hormone
- Stool studies
  - Leukocytes or lactoferrin: implies inflammatory diarrhea
  - Ova and parasites (three specimens)
  - Fecal antigen studies for *Giardia* and *Entamoeba* more sensitive and specific
  - Modified acid-fast staining indicated for *Cryptosporidium* and *Cyclospora*

  - Stool osmotic gap: increased in osmotic diarrheas and malabsorption, normal in secretory, inflammatory diarrhea
  - 24-hour stool collection for weight and quantitative fecal fat
    - Stool weight > 300 g/24 hours confirms diarrhea
    - Stool weight > 1000–1500 g/24 hours suggests secretory diarrhea
    - Fecal fat > 10 g/24 hours indicates a malabsorption syndrome
  - Stool pH < 5.6 indicates carbohydrate malabsorption
  - Osmolality less than serum osmolality indicates factitious diarrhea
  - Laxative screen positive in laxative abuse
- If malabsorption suspected
  - Obtain serum folate, B_{12}, iron, vitamin A and D, prothrombin time
  - Serologic tests for celiac sprue: serum antiendomysial antibody or tissue transglutaminase antibody
- If secretory cause suspected
  - Obtain serum VIP (VIPoma), chromogranin A (carcinoid), calcitonin (medullary thyroid carcinoma), gastrin (Zollinger-Ellison syndrome), and glucagon
  - Urine 5-hydroxyindoleacetic acid (carcinoid), vanillmandelic acid, metanephrines (pheochromocytoma), and histamine determinations

IMAGING STUDIES

- Abdominal CT for suspected chronic pancreatitis, pancreatic cancer, neuroendocrine tumors
- Small intestinal barium radiography in suspected Crohn's disease, small bowel lymphoma, carcinoid, and jejunal diverticula
- Somatostatin receptor scintigraphy in suspected neuroendocrine tumors

DIAGNOSTIC PROCEDURES

- Sigmoidoscopy or colonoscopy with mucosal biopsy to diagnose inflammatory bowel disease, microscopic colitis, and melanosis coli
- Upper endoscopy with small bowel biopsy to diagnose suspected celiac sprue, Whipple's disease, and AIDS-related *Cryptosporidium, Microsporidia*, and *M avium-intracellulare* infection
- Breath hydrogen or ^{14}C-xylose breath tests to diagnose bacterial overgrowth

TREATMENT

MEDICATIONS

- Loperamide: 4 mg PO initially, then 2 mg after each loose stool (maximum: 16 mg/day)
- Diphenoxylate with atropine: 1 tablet PO TID–QID PRN
- Codeine 15–60 mg PO q4h; deodorized tincture of opium, 10–25 drops PO q6h PRN, safe in most patients with chronic, intractable diarrhea
- Clonidine, 0.1–0.6 mg PO BID, or a clonidine patch, 0.1–0.2 mg/day, helpful in secretory diarrheas, diabetic diarrhea, and cryptosporidiosis
- Octreotide, 50 mcg to 250 mcg SQ TID, for secretory diarrheas due to neuroendocrine tumors (VIPomas, carcinoid) and in some cases of AIDS-related diarrhea
- Cholestyramine resin, 4 g PO once to three times daily, in patients with bile salt–induced diarrhea secondary to intestinal resection or ileal disease

OUTCOME

COMPLICATIONS

- Dehydration
- Electrolyte abnormalities
- Malabsorption: weight loss, vitamin deficiencies

PROGNOSIS

- Cause is identifiable and treatable in almost all patients

WHEN TO ADMIT

- Secretory diarrhea with dehydration

EVIDENCE

PRACTICE GUIDELINES

- Thomas PD et al. Guidelines for the investigation of chronic diarrhoea, 2nd ed. Gut. 2003;52(Suppl 5):v1. [PMID: 12801941]

INFORMATION FOR PATIENTS

- Cleveland Clinic—Diarrhea
- JAMA patient page. Preventing dehydration from diarrhea. JAMA. 2001; 285:362. [PMID: 11236756]
- Mayo Clinic

REFERENCES

- Camilleri M. Chronic diarrhea: a review on pathophysiology and management for the clinical gastroenterologist. Clin Gastroenterol Hepatol. 2004 Mar; 2(3):198–206. [PMID: 15017602]
- Headstrom PD et al. Chronic diarrhea. Clin Gastroenterol Hepatol. 2005 Aug; 3(8):734–7. [PMID: 16234000]
- Schiller L. Chronic diarrhea. Gastroenterology. 2004 Jul;127(1):287–93. [PMID: 15236193]

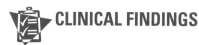

Digitalis Toxicity

KEY FEATURES

ESSENTIALS OF DIAGNOSIS

- Intoxication may result from
  - Acute single exposure
  - Chronic accumulation from accidental overmedication or renal insufficiency
- Hyperkalemia common after acute overdose
- Many different arrhythmias can occur

GENERAL CONSIDERATIONS

- Cardiac glycosides paralyze the Na^+-K^+-ATPase pump and have potent vagotonic effects
- Intracellular effects
  - Enhancement of calcium-dependent contractility
  - Shortening of the action potential duration
- Digoxin and ouabain are highly tissue bound, but digitoxin has a volume of distribution of just 0.6 L/kg, making it potentially accessible to enhanced removal procedures such as hemoperfusion or repeated doses of activated charcoal

DEMOGRAPHICS

- Older age and renal impairment are associated with greater risk of chronic digoxin toxicity

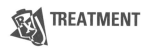

CLINICAL FINDINGS

SYMPTOMS AND SIGNS

Acute overdose

- Nausea and vomiting
- Bradycardia

- Atrioventricular (AV) block
- Junctional rhythm common in patients with underlying atrial fibrillation
- Hyperkalemia

Chronic overingestion

- Hypokalemia and hypomagnesia are more likely owing to concurrent diuretic treatment
- Ventricular arrhythmias; for example
  - Ectopy
  - Bidirectional ventricular tachycardia
  - Ventricular fibrillation

DIFFERENTIAL DIAGNOSIS

- β-Blocker overdose
- Calcium channel blocker overdose
- Cardiotoxic plant or animal ingestion
  - Oleander
  - Foxglove
  - Lily of the valley
  - Rhododendron
  - Toad venom

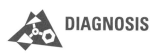

DIAGNOSIS

LABORATORY TESTS

- Serum digoxin level (**Note:** Levels drawn within 6 h of ingestion may be falsely elevated before complete tissue distribution)
- Serum potassium (frequent measures useful because they correlate with tissue effects)

DIAGNOSTIC PROCEDURES

- Continuous ECG monitoring
- Pacemaker may be needed

TREATMENT

MEDICATIONS

Emergency measures

- **Ventricular arrhythmias:** initially lidocaine, 2–3 mg/kg IV, or phenytoin, 10–15 mg/kg IV slowly over 30 min if digoxin-specific antibodies are not immediately available (see below)
- **Bradycardia:** initially atropine, 0.5–2.0 mg IV, or transcutaneous external cardiac pacemaker

Gut decontamination

- After acute overdose, administer activated charcoal, 60–100 g PO or via gastric tube, mixed in aqueous slurry
- Emesis not recommended because it may enhance vagotonic effects (eg, bradycardia, AV block)

Activated charcoal

- Repeated doses of activated charcoal, 20–30 g q3–4h, may speed elimination of digitoxin (but not digoxin) by adsorbing drug excreted into gut lumen (gut dialysis)
- Sorbitol or other cathartics should *not* be used with each dose; resulting large stool volumes may lead to dehydration or hypernatremia

Specific treatment

- Severe intoxication: administer digoxin-specific antibodies [digoxin immune Fab (ovine); Digibind]
- Digibind dose is estimated based on body burden of digoxin calculated from ingested dose or steady-state serum digoxin concentration
  - Ingested dose
    - Number of vials = ~1.5–2 × ingested dose (mg)
  - Serum concentration
    - Number of vials = serum digoxin (ng/mL) × body weight (kg) × 10^{-2}
    - **Note:** This is based on equilibrium digoxin level; after acute overdose, serum levels are falsely high before tissue distribution is complete, and overestimation of Digibind dose is likely
- Empiric dosing of Digibind
  - May be used if patient's condition is relatively stable and an underlying condition (eg, atrial fibrillation) suggests residual level of digitalis activity
  - Start with one or two vials and reassess clinical condition after 20–30 min
- **Note:** After administration of Digibind, serum digoxin levels may be falsely elevated depending on assay technique

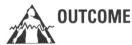 **OUTCOME**

FOLLOW-UP

- Monitor potassium levels and cardiac rhythm closely

COMPLICATIONS

- Cardiac arrest

WHEN TO ADMIT

- Symptomatic patients
- Asymptomatic patients after acute overdose, for monitoring at least several hours

PREVENTION

- Monitor renal function in elderly patients and obtain serum digoxin levels if symptoms of digoxin toxicity

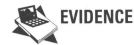 **EVIDENCE**

WEB SITE

- eMedicine: Toxicology Articles

INFORMATION FOR PATIENTS

- National Institutes of Health: Digitalis Toxicity
- MedlinePlus: Digitalis Medicines (Systemic)

REFERENCES

- Bateman DN. Digoxin-specific antibody fragments: how much and when? Toxicol Rev. 2004;23(3):135–43. [PMID: 15862081]
- Bauman JL et al. Mechanisms, manifestations, and management of digoxin toxicity in the modern era. Am J Cardiovasc Drugs. 2006;6(2):77–86. [PMID: 16555861]
- Roberts DM et al. Antidotes for acute cardenolide (cardiac glycoside) poisoning. Cochrane Database Syst Rev. 2006 Oct 18;(4):CD005490. [PMID: 17054261]

Discoid Lupus Erythematosus

 KEY FEATURES

ESSENTIALS OF DIAGNOSIS

- Localized red plaques, usually on the face
- Scaling, follicular plugging, atrophy, dyspigmentation, and telangiectasia of involved areas
- Histology distinctive
- Photosensitive

GENERAL CONSIDERATIONS

- Ten percent of patients with systemic lupus erythematosus (SLE) have discoid skin lesions, and 5% of patients with discoid lesions have SLE
- The disease is persistent but not life endangering unless systemic lupus intervenes, which is uncommon
- Treatment with antimalarials is effective in perhaps 60% of cases

 CLINICAL FINDINGS

SYMPTOMS AND SIGNS

- The lesions consist of dusky red, well-localized, single or multiple plaques, 5–20 mm in diameter, usually on the face; the scalp, external ears, and oral mucous membranes may be involved
- There is atrophy, telangiectasia, depigmentation, and follicular plugging
- The lesion may be covered by dry, horny, adherent scales
- On the scalp, permanent hair loss may occur

DIFFERENTIAL DIAGNOSIS

- Psoriasis
- Seborrheic dermatitis
- Acne rosacea
- Lupus vulgaris (cutaneous tuberculosis)
- Sarcoidosis
- Bowen's disease (squamous cell carcinoma in situ)
- Polymorphous light eruption
- Lichen planopilaris

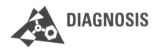 **DIAGNOSIS**

LABORATORY TESTS

- Diagnosis is based on the clinical appearance confirmed by skin biopsy in all cases

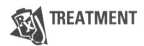 **TREATMENT**

MEDICATIONS

- See Table 150

General measures

- Protect from sunlight; use high-SPF (> 30) sunblock with UVB and UVA coverage daily
- Avoid using drugs that are potentially photosensitizing (eg, thiazides, piroxicam) when possible
- **Caution:** Do not use any form of radiation therapy

Local treatment

- High-potency corticosteroid creams applied each night and covered with air-tight plastic film (eg, Saran Wrap) or Cordran tape; or ultra-high-potency corticosteroid cream or ointment applied BID without occlusion

- Local infiltration
  - Triamcinolone acetonide suspension, 2.5–10 mg/mL, may be injected into the lesions once a month
  - This should be tried before systemic therapy

Systemic treatment

- Antimalarials
  - **Caution:** these drugs should be used only when the diagnosis is secure, because they have been associated with flares of psoriasis, which is in the differential diagnosis
  - They may also cause ocular changes, and ophthalmologic evaluation is required every 6 months
- Hydroxychloroquine sulfate, 0.2–0.4 g PO daily for several months
  - May be effective
  - Often used prior to chloroquine
  - A minimum 3-month trial is recommended
- Chloroquine sulfate, 250 mg daily, may be effective in some cases where hydroxychloroquine is not
- Quinacrine (Atabrine), 100 mg daily
  - May be the safest of the antimalarials, since eye damage has not been reported
  - It colors the skin yellow and is therefore not acceptable to some patients
  - May be added to the above antimalarials for incomplete responses
- Isotretinoin, 1 mg/kg/day
  - Effective in chronic or subacute cutaneous lupus erythematosus
  - Recurrences are prompt and predictable on discontinuation of therapy
- Thalidomide is effective in refractory cases in doses of 50–100 mg daily

THERAPEUTIC PROCEDURES

- Monitor for neuropathy if using thalidomide
- Because of the teratogenicity of isotretinoin and thalidomide, the drugs are used with caution in women of childbearing age using effective contraception with negative pregnancy tests before and during therapy

 OUTCOME

COMPLICATIONS

- Although the only morbidity may be cosmetic, this can be of overwhelming significance in more darkly pigmented patients with widespread disease
- Scarring alopecia can be prevented or lessened with close attention and aggressive therapy

PROGNOSIS

- The disease is persistent but not life endangering unless systemic lupus intervenes, which is uncommon
- Treatment with antimalarials is effective in perhaps 60% of cases

WHEN TO REFER

- If there is a question about the diagnosis, if recommended therapy is ineffective, or specialized treatment is necessary

 EVIDENCE

WEB SITES

- American Academy of Dermatology
- National Institute of Arthritis and Musculoskeletal and Skin Diseases
- University of Pennsylvania Dermatology Online Journal: Current Treatment of Cutaneous Lupus Erythematosus

INFORMATION FOR PATIENTS

- Lupus Foundation of America: Skin Disease In Lupus
- MedlinePlus: Lupus Interactive Tutorial
- National Institute of Arthritis and Musculoskeletal and Skin Diseases: Skin Care and Lupus

REFERENCE

- Callen JP. Cutaneous lupus erythematosus: a personal approach to management. Australas J Dermatol. 2006 Feb; 47(1)13–27. [PMID: 16405478]

Disseminated Intravascular Coagulation (DIC)

 KEY FEATURES

ESSENTIALS OF DIAGNOSIS

- Underlying serious illness
- Microangiopathic hemolytic anemia may be present
- Low fibrinogen, thrombocytopenia, fibrin degradation products, and prolonged prothrombin time (PT)

GENERAL CONSIDERATIONS

- If stimulus to coagulation is too great, control mechanisms are overwhelmed, leading to DIC
- Results from the presence of circulating thrombin (normally confined to localized area)
  - Thrombin cleaves fibrinogen to fibrin, stimulates platelet aggregation, activates factors V and VIII, and releases plasminogen activator, which generates plasmin
  - Plasmin cleaves fibrin, generating fibrin degradation products, and further inactivates factors V and VIII
- Thus, excess thrombin activity produces hypofibrinogenemia, thrombocytopenia, depletion of coagulation factors, and fibrinolysis
- Caused by a number of serious illnesses
  - Sepsis (especially with gram-negative bacteria)
  - Severe tissue injury (especially burns and head injury)
  - Obstetric complications (amniotic fluid embolism, septic abortion, retained fetus)
  - Cancer (acute promyelocytic leukemia, mucinous adenocarcinomas)
  - Major hemolytic transfusion reactions

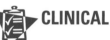 **CLINICAL FINDINGS**

SYMPTOMS AND SIGNS

- DIC leads to both bleeding and thrombosis; bleeding is far more common, but thrombosis may dominate
- Bleeding may occur at any site; spontaneous bleeding and oozing at venipuncture sites or wounds are important clues to diagnosis
- Thrombosis most commonly manifested by digital ischemia and gangrene, but catastrophic events such as renal cortical necrosis and hemorrhagic adrenal infarction may occur
- DIC may secondarily produce microangiopathic hemolytic anemia
- Subacute DIC occurs primarily in cancer; manifested primarily as recurrent superficial and deep venous thromboses (Trousseau's syndrome)

DIFFERENTIAL DIAGNOSIS

- Severe liver disease
- Thrombotic thrombocytopenic purpura
- Sepsis-induced thrombocytopenia or anemia
- Heparin-induced thrombocytopenia

- Other microangiopathic hemolytic anemia (eg, prosthetic valve hemolysis)

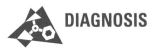

DIAGNOSIS

LABORATORY TESTS

- Serum fibrinogen low (may also occur in congenital hypofibrinogenemia, severe liver disease)
- Fibrin degradation products (eg, D-dimers) elevated (may also occur in hepatic dysfunction)
- Thrombocytopenia
- PT prolonged
- When baseline fibrinogen level is markedly elevated, initial level may be normal; because half-life is ~4 days, declining fibrinogen level suggests DIC
- Partial thromboplastin time (PTT) may or may not be prolonged
- Microangiopathic hemolytic anemia present in ~25% of cases, and peripheral blood smear shows fragmented red blood cells
- Antithrombin III levels may be markedly depleted
- When fibrinolysis is activated, levels of plasminogen and α_2-antiplasmin may be low
- Thrombocytopenia and D-dimer elevation are usually the only abnormalities in subacute DIC
- Fibrinogen level is normal, and PTT may be normal

TREATMENT

MEDICATIONS

- Replacement therapy alone if underlying cause is rapidly reversible
- Platelet transfusion to maintain platelet count > 30,000/mcL
- Cryoprecipitate to replace fibrinogen, aiming for plasma fibrinogen level of 150 mg/dL
- Fresh-frozen plasma may be required for coagulation factor deficiency
- Heparin
  - Dose is 500–750 U/h
  - Contraindicated when any increase in bleeding is unacceptable (neurosurgical procedures)
  - When DIC is producing serious clinical consequences and underlying cause not rapidly reversible, heparin may be necessary

- Successful therapy is indicated by rising fibrinogen level; it is not necessary to prolong PTT
- Must be used in combination with replacement therapy to prevent an unacceptable increase in bleeding
- Cannot be effective if antithrombin III is markedly depleted; measure antithrombin III level and if low, give fresh-frozen plasma to raise levels to > 50%
- Improvement in platelet count may lag by 1 week behind control of coagulopathy
- If heparin and replacement therapy does not control bleeding, ε-aminocaproic acid, 1 g IV every hour, is added to decrease rate of fibrinolysis, raise fibrinogen level, and control bleeding
- Aminocaproic acid should not be used without heparin in DIC because of risk of thrombosis

THERAPEUTIC PROCEDURES

- Treatment of underlying disorder
- Mild DIC requires no specific therapy

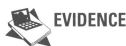

OUTCOME

PROGNOSIS

- Prognosis is that of the underlying disease

EVIDENCE

PRACTICE GUIDELINES

- Taylor FB et al. Towards definition, clinical and laboratory criteria, and a scoring system for disseminated intravascular coagulation. Thromb Haemost. 2001; 86:1327. [PMID: 11816725]

WEB SITE

- Postgraduate Medicine Online: Disseminated Intravascular Coagulation

INFORMATION FOR PATIENTS

- MedlinePlus: Disseminated Intravascular Coagulation

REFERENCES

- Franchini M et al. Update on the treatment of disseminated intravascular coagulation. Hematology. 2004 Apr; 9(2):81–5. [PMID: 15203862]
- Hoffmann JN et al. Effect of long-term and high-dose antithrombin supplementation on coagulation and fibrinoly-

sis in patients with severe sepsis. Crit Care Med. 2004 Sep;32(9):1851–9. [PMID: 15343012]

Diverticulitis

KEY FEATURES

ESSENTIALS OF DIAGNOSIS

- Intra-abdominal infection varies from microperforation (most common) with localized paracolic inflammation to macroperforation with either abscess or generalized peritonitis
- Acute abdominal pain and fever
- Left lower abdominal tenderness and mass
- Leukocytosis

GENERAL CONSIDERATIONS

- Diverticulosis
  - Present in 25% of adults over age 40
  - Increases with age
  - Most cases are asymptomatic
- Diverticulitis occurs in 10–20% of patients with diverticulosis

DEMOGRAPHICS

- Higher prevalence in societies with low fiber intake

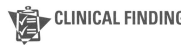

CLINICAL FINDINGS

SYMPTOMS AND SIGNS

- Abdominal pain, mild to moderate, aching, usually in the left lower quadrant
- Constipation or loose stools
- Nausea and vomiting
- Low-grade fever
- Left lower quadrant tenderness
- Palpable left lower quadrant mass
- Generalized abdominal pain and peritoneal signs in patients with free perforation

DIFFERENTIAL DIAGNOSIS

- Perforated colorectal cancer
- Infectious colitis, eg, *Campylobacter, Clostridium difficile*
- Inflammatory bowel disease
- Ischemic colitis
- Appendicitis

- Gynecologic
  - Pelvic inflammatory disease
  - Tuboovarian abscess
  - Ovarian torsion
  - Ruptured ectopic pregnancy or ovarian cyst
  - Mittelschmerz
  - Endometriosis
- Urinary calculus
- Gastroenteritis

 DIAGNOSIS

LABORATORY TESTS

- Leukocytosis, mild to moderate
- Stool occult blood test positive

IMAGING STUDIES

- Abdominal radiographs
- Barium enema
  - Contraindicated during acute attack
  - Perform only after resolution of clinical symptoms to document extent of diverticulosis or presence of fistula
- CT scan of the abdomen indicated
  - To confirm diagnosis
  - In patients who do not improve rapidly after 2–4 days of empiric therapy
  - In severe disease to diagnose abscess

DIAGNOSTIC PROCEDURES

- Colonoscopy
  - Contraindicated during acute attack
  - Perform only after resolution of clinical symptoms to document extent of diverticulitis and to exclude other clinical disorders
- Sigmoidoscopy with minimal air insufflation is sometimes required in acute disease to exclude other diagnoses

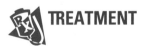 **TREATMENT**

MEDICATIONS

- Most patients can be managed with conservative measures
- Mild diverticulitis (mild symptoms and no peritoneal signs)
  - Clear liquid diet
  - Oral antibiotics targeting both anaerobic and aerobic (gram-negative) bacteria, such as amoxicillin and clavulanate potassium, 875 mg/125 mg PO BID; or metronidazole, 500 mg PO TID; plus either ciprofloxacin, 500 mg PO BID, or trimethoprim-sulfamethoxazole, 160/800 mg PO BID, for 7–10 days

- Severe diverticulitis (high fevers, leukocytosis, or peritoneal signs)
  - Nothing by mouth
  - Intravenous fluids
  - Nasogastric tube suction if ileus is present
  - Intravenous antibiotics targeting both anaerobic and aerobic (gram-negative) bacteria, such as either single-agent therapy with a second-generation cephalosporin (eg, cefoxitin), or piperacillin-tazobactam, or ticarcillin clavulanate; or combination therapy (eg, metronidazole or clindamycin plus an aminoglycoside) or third-generation cephalosporin (eg, ceftazidime, cefotaxime) for 7–10 days

SURGERY

- Surgical management is required in ~20–30% of cases
- Indications for surgery
  - Free peritonitis and large abscesses
  - Fistulas
  - Colonic obstruction
- Surgery in two stages for abscesses for which catheter drainage is not possible or helpful
  - Diseased colon is resected, temporary colostomy of proximal colon is created, and distal colonic stump is either closed (forming a Hartmann pouch) or exteriorized as a mucous fistula
  - Weeks later, colon is reconnected electively

THERAPEUTIC PROCEDURES

- Percutaneous catheter drainage of localized abdominal abscess, with subsequent single-stage elective surgical resection of diseased segment of colon

 OUTCOME

FOLLOW-UP

- Colonoscopy or barium enema 4–6 weeks after recovery from diverticulitis to diagnose extent of diverticulosis and to exclude colonic malignancy

COMPLICATIONS

- Fistula formation may involve the bladder, ureter, vagina, uterus, bowel, and abdominal wall
- Stricturing of the colon with partial or complete obstruction

PROGNOSIS

- Diverticulitis recurs in one-third

- Recurrent attacks warrant elective surgical resection

WHEN TO ADMIT

- Increasing pain, fever, or inability to tolerate oral fluids
- Severe diverticulitis and patients who are elderly or immunosuppressed or who have serious comorbid disease

PREVENTION

- High-fiber diet

 EVIDENCE

WEB SITE

- WebPath GI Pathology Index

INFORMATION FOR PATIENTS

- Cleveland Clinic—Diverticular disease
- Mayo Clinic—Diverticulitis
- National Digestive Diseases Information Clearinghouse—Colonoscopy

REFERENCES

- Mizuki A et al. The outpatient management of patients with acute mild-to-moderate colonic diverticulitis. Aliment Pharmacol Ther. 2005 Apr 1; 21(7):889–97. [PMID: 15801924]
- Petruzziello L et al. Review article: uncomplicated diverticular disease of the colon. Aliment Pharmacol Ther. 2006 May 15;23(10):1379–91. [PMID: 16669953]

Diverticulosis

 KEY FEATURES

- Incidence increases with age in Western societies
  - 5% at age < 40
  - 30% at age 60
  - 50% at age > 80
- Uncommon in developing countries
- Most are asymptomatic, discovered incidentally at sigmoidoscopy or colonoscopy or on barium enema
- Causes
  - Diet deficient in fiber
  - Abnormal motility
  - Hereditary factors

– Ehlers-Danlos syndrome
– Marfan's syndrome
– Scleroderma

 CLINICAL FINDINGS

- Nonspecific complaints
  - Chronic constipation
  - Abdominal pain
  - Fluctuating bowel habits
- Physical examination usually normal
  - May reveal mild left lower quadrant tenderness
- Complications occur in 33%, including lower GI bleeding and diverticulitis

 DIAGNOSIS

- Routine laboratory studies normal
- Barium enema best demonstrates diverticula
- Colonoscopy

 TREATMENT

- High-fiber diet or fiber supplements (bran powder, psyllium or methylcellulose 1–2 tbsp PO BID)

Down Syndrome

 KEY FEATURES

- Risk of an affected fetus being conceived increases exponentially with age of mother at conception and begins a marked rise after age 35
- At maternal age 45, risk is 1 in 40

 CLINICAL FINDINGS

- Usually diagnosed at birth
- Typical facial features: flat occiput, epicanthal folds, large tongue
- Hypotonia
- Single palmar crease
- Serious problems at birth or early in childhood, such as
  - Duodenal atresia

– Congenital heart disease (especially atrioventricular canal defects)
– Leukemia
- Mental retardation, although intelligence varies across a wide spectrum
- Alzheimer-like dementia in the fourth or fifth decade
- Affected patients who survive childhood have a reduced life expectancy

 DIAGNOSIS

- Cytogenetic analysis
- Most affected individuals have simple trisomy for chromosome 21
- Others have unbalanced translocations, usually resulting from a parent with a balanced translocation, incurring a substantial risk of Down syndrome in future offspring
- Can be detected in the early second trimester by
  - Screening maternal serum for α-fetoprotein and certain hormones (maternal serum multiple marker screening, MSMMS)
  - Observation of increased nuchal skin thickness on fetal ultrasonogram

 TREATMENT

- No treatment is effective for the mental impairment
- Duodenal atresia should be treated surgically
- Congenital heart disease should be treated as in any other patient

Dupuytren's Contracture

 KEY FEATURES

- Hyperplasia of the palmar fascia and related structures, with nodule formation and contracture
- Cause is unknown
- Occurs primarily in white men older than 50 yr. The incidence is higher among alcoholics and patients with chronic systemic disorders (especially cirrhosis)

- Also associated with systemic fibrosing syndrome, which includes Peyronie's disease, mediastinal and retroperitoneal fibrosis, and Riedel's struma

 CLINICAL FINDINGS

- Slowly progressive chronic disease
- Nodular or cord-like thickening of one or both hands, with the fourth and fifth fingers most commonly affected
- Tightness of the involved digits, with inability to satisfactorily extend the fingers
- The contracture is well tolerated because it exaggerates the normal position of function of the hand, although resulting cosmetic problems may be unappealing

 DIAGNOSIS

- Clinical findings outlined above

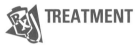 **TREATMENT**

- If the palmar nodule is growing rapidly, injections of triamcinolone into the nodule may be of benefit
- Surgical intervention is indicated in patients with significant flexion contractures, depending on the location, but recurrence is not uncommon

Dysmenorrhea

 KEY FEATURES

ESSENTIALS OF DIAGNOSIS

- **Primary dysmenorrhea** is menstrual pain associated with ovular cycles in the absence of pathologic findings
- **Secondary dysmenorrhea** is menstrual pain for which an organic cause exists, such as endometriosis

GENERAL CONSIDERATIONS

Primary dysmenorrhea
- The pain usually begins within 1–2 years after the menarche and may become more severe with time
- The pain is produced by uterine vasoconstriction, anoxia, and sustained contractions mediated by prostaglandins

DEMOGRAPHICS

Primary dysmenorrhea

- The frequency of cases increases up to age 20 and then decreases with age and markedly with parity
- Fifty to 75% of women are affected at some time, and 5–6% have incapacitating pain

Secondary dysmenorrhea

- It usually begins well after menarche, sometimes even as late as the third or fourth decade of life

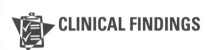 **CLINICAL FINDINGS**

SYMPTOMS AND SIGNS

Primary dysmenorrhea

- Pain is low, midline, wave-like, cramping pelvic pain often radiating to the back or inner thighs
- Cramps may last for 1 or more days and may be associated with nausea, diarrhea, headache, and flushing
- No pathologic findings on pelvic examination

Secondary dysmenorrhea

- The history and physical examination commonly suggest endometriosis or pelvic inflammatory disease

DIFFERENTIAL DIAGNOSIS

- Endometriosis
- Adenomyosis (uterine endometriosis)
- Pelvic inflammatory disease
- Uterine leiomyomas (fibroids)
- Intrauterine device (IUD)
- Pelvic pain syndrome
- Endometrial polyp
- Cervicitis
- Cervical stenosis
- Cystitis
- Interstitial cystitis

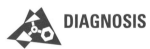 **DIAGNOSIS**

IMAGING STUDIES

- MRI is the most reliable method to detect submucous myomas

DIAGNOSTIC PROCEDURES

Secondary dysmenorrhea

- Laparoscopy is often needed to differentiate endometriosis from pelvic inflammatory disease

- Submucous myomas can be detected by saline infusion hysterography, by hysteroscopy, or by passing a sound or curette over the uterine cavity during D&C

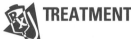 **TREATMENT**

MEDICATIONS

Primary dysmenorrhea

- Nonsteroidal anti-inflammatory drugs (ibuprofen, ketoprofen, mefenamic acid, naproxen) are generally helpful
- Drugs should be started at the onset of bleeding to avoid inadvertent drug use during early pregnancy
- Medication should be continued on a regular basis for 2–3 days
- Ovulation can be suppressed and dysmenorrhea usually prevented by
  - Oral contraceptives
  - Depot-medroxyprogesterone acetate
  - Levonorgestrel-containing IUD

Secondary dysmenorrhea

- Periodic use of analgesics, including the nonsteroidal anti-inflammatory drugs given for primary dysmenorrhea, may be beneficial
- Oral contraceptives may give relief, particularly in endometriosis
- Danazol and gonadotropin-releasing hormone agonists are effective in the treatment of endometriosis

SURGERY

- If disability is marked or prolonged, laparoscopy or exploratory laparotomy is usually warranted
- Definitive surgery depends on the degree of disability and the findings at operation

THERAPEUTIC PROCEDURES

- Cervical stenosis may result from induced abortion, creating crampy pain at the time of expected menses with no blood flow; this is easily cured by passing a sound into the uterine cavity after administering a paracervical block

 OUTCOME

WHEN TO REFER

- Standard therapy fails to relieve pain
- Suspicion of pelvic pathology, such as endometriosis

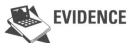 **EVIDENCE**

PRACTICE GUIDELINES

- University of Texas at Austin: Recommendations for the treatment of dysmenorrhea

INFORMATION FOR PATIENTS

- American College of Obstetricians and Gynecologists: Dysmenorrhea
- Mayo Clinic: Dysmenorrhea
- National Women's Health Information Center: Menstruation and the Menstrual Cycle
- University of Utah: Dysmenorrhea

REFERENCES

- French L. Dysmenorrhea. Am Fam Physician. 2005 Jan;71(2):285–91. [PMID: 15686299]
- Proctor M et al. Diagnosis and management of dysmenorrhoea. BMJ. 2006 May 13;332(7550):1134–8. [PMID: 16690671]

Dyspareunia (Painful Intercourse)

 KEY FEATURES

GENERAL CONSIDERATIONS

Etiology

- Vulvovaginitis: inflammation or infection of the vagina
- Vaginismus
  - Voluntary or involuntary contraction of muscles around the introitus
  - Results from fear, pain, sexual trauma, or having learned negative attitudes toward sex during childhood
- Insufficient lubrication of the vagina is a frequent cause of dyspareunia in postmenopausal women
- Infection, endometriosis, tumors, or other pathologic conditions: pain occurring with deep thrusting during coitus is usually due to acute or chronic infection of the cervix, uterus, or adnexa; endometriosis; adnexal tumors; or adhesions resulting from prior pelvic disease or operation
- Vulvodynia is the most frequent cause of dyspareunia in premenopausal women

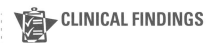

CLINICAL FINDINGS

SYMPTOMS AND SIGNS

- Questions related to sexual functioning should be asked as part of the reproductive history. Two helpful questions are, "Are you sexually active?" and "Are you having any sexual difficulties at this time?"
- During the pelvic examination, the patient should be placed in a half-sitting position and given a hand-held mirror and then asked to point out the site of pain and describe the type of pain
- Vulvovaginitis: areas of marked tenderness in the vulvar vestibule without visible inflammation
- Vulvodynia
  - A sensation of burning along with other symptoms including pain, itching, stinging, irritation, and rawness
  - Discomfort may be constant or intermittent, focal or diffuse, and experienced as either deep or superficial
  - Generally no physical findings except minimal erythema that may be associated with a subset of vulvodynia, vulvar vestibulitis

DIFFERENTIAL DIAGNOSIS

- Vulvodynia or vulvar vestibulitis
- Vaginismus
- Insufficient vaginal lubrication
- Atrophic vaginitis
- Vulvovaginitis, cervicitis, or pelvic inflammatory disease
- Endometriosis
- Lichen sclerosus
- Ovarian tumor
- Pelvic adhesions

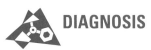

DIAGNOSIS

DIAGNOSTIC PROCEDURES

- Colposcopy to evaluate vulvovaginitis: areas of marked tenderness in the vulvar vestibule without visible inflammation occasionally show lesions resembling small condylomas

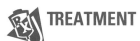

TREATMENT

THERAPEUTIC PROCEDURES

Vulvovaginitis
- Warty lesions on colposcopy or biopsy should be treated appropriately (see Vaginitis)

Vaginismus
- Sexual counseling and education may be useful
- Self-dilation, using a lubricated finger or test tubes of graduated sizes, may help. Before coitus (with adequate lubrication) is attempted, the patient and her partner should be able to painlessly introduce two fingers into the vagina

Insufficient lubrication of the vagina
- See Menopausal Syndrome
- For inadequate sexual arousal, sexual counseling is helpful
- Lubricants during sexual foreplay may be of use
- If lubrication remains inadequate, use estradiol vaginal ring worn continuously and replaced every 3 months. Concomitant progestin therapy is not needed with the ring
- Estrogen vaginal cream

Infection, endometriosis, tumors, or other pathologic conditions
- Temporarily abstain from coitus during treatment
- Consider hormonal or surgical treatment of endometriosis
- Dyspareunia from chronic pelvic inflammatory disease or extensive adhesions is difficult to treat without extirpative surgery. Couples can be advised to try coital positions that limit deep thrusting and to use manual and oral sexual techniques

Vulvodynia
- Difficult management since etiology unclear
- Surgical vestibulectomy has had success
- Antiviral, antifungal, corticosteroid, or anesthetic agents have varied success
- Pain control through behavioral therapy, biofeedback, or acupuncture has varied success
- Continuous genital burning or pain may be relieved with amitriptyline in gradually increasing doses from 10 mg PO QD to 75–100 mg PO QD

OUTCOME

WHEN TO REFER

- When symptoms persist despite first-line therapy
- For expertise in procedures

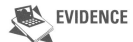

EVIDENCE

INFORMATION FOR PATIENTS

- American Academy of Family Physicians: Dyspareunia
- American Academy of Family Physicians: Vulvodynia
- American College of Obstetricians and Gynecologists: Pain During Intercourse
- Mayo Clinic: Vaginal Dryness
- MedlinePlus: Vaginismus
- MedlinePlus: Vulvovaginitis

REFERENCES

- Haefner HK et al. The vulvodynia guideline. J Low Genit Tract Dis. 2005 Jan;9(1):40–51. [PMID: 15870521]
- MacNeill C. Dyspareunia. Obstet Gynecol Clin N Am. 2006 Dec; 33(4):565–77. [PMID: 17116501]

Dyspepsia

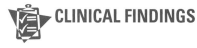

KEY FEATURES

ESSENTIALS OF DIAGNOSIS

- Pain or discomfort centered in the upper abdomen
- Upper abdominal fullness, early satiety, burning, bloating, belching, nausea, retching, or vomiting
- Heartburn (retrosternal burning) may also be present

GENERAL CONSIDERATIONS

- Functional dyspepsia is the most common cause

DEMOGRAPHICS

- Occurs in 25% of the adult population
- Accounts for 3% of office visits

CLINICAL FINDINGS

SYMPTOMS AND SIGNS

- History entails chronicity, location, and quality of the discomfort but has limited diagnostic utility
- "Alarm" features warrant endoscopy or abdominal imaging and include
  - Dysphagia

– Persistent vomiting
– Weight loss
– Organomegaly
– Abdominal mass
– Fecal occult blood

DIFFERENTIAL DIAGNOSIS

- "Indigestion" from overeating, high-fat foods, coffee
- Drugs
  – Aspirin
  – Nonsteroidal anti-inflammatory drugs (NSAIDs)
  – Antibiotics (eg, macrolides, metronidazole)
  – Diabetes drugs
  – Cholinesterase inhibitors
  – Corticosteroids
  – Digoxin
  – Iron
  – Theophylline
  – Opioids
- Gastroesophageal reflux (in 20%)
- Peptic ulcer disease (in 5–15% of cases)
- Gastroparesis
- Gastric cancer (in 1%)
- *Helicobacter pylori*
- Chronic pancreatitis or pancreatic cancer
- Lactase deficiency
- Malabsorption
- Parasitic infection, eg, *Giardia, Strongyloides, Ascaris*
- Cholelithiasis, choledocholithiasis, or cholangitis
- Abdominal or paraesophageal hernia
- Intra-abdominal malignancy
- Chronic mesenteric ischemia
- Pregnancy
- Metabolic conditions
  – Diabetes
  – Thyroid disease
  – Renal insufficiency
- Myocardial ischemia or pericarditis
- Physical or sexual abuse

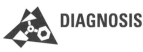 **DIAGNOSIS**

- Under age 55 without "alarm" signs of serious organic disease, perform noninvasive testing for *H pylori* (urea breath test, fecal antigen test, or serology); treat if positive
- If *H pylori* negative, or if symptoms persist after *H pylori* treatment, give trial of proton pump inhibitors for 4 weeks
- If symptoms persist or recur after empiric treatment, perform esophagogastroduodenoscopy (EGD)

- Over age 55 or any age with "alarm" signs of serious organic disease, perform upper endoscopy

LABORATORY TESTS

- Obtain complete blood cell count, serum electrolytes, liver enzymes, calcium, and thyroid-stimulating hormone

IMAGING STUDIES

- Abdominal ultrasonography indicated if pancreatic or biliary tract disease is suspected
- Abdominal CT scan indicated if pancreatic disease or intra-abdominal malignancy is suspected

DIAGNOSTIC PROCEDURES

- Upper endoscopy
  – Indicated in all patients with new-onset dyspepsia age > 55 years or of any age with symptoms of weight loss, dysphagia, recurrent vomiting, hematemesis, melena, or anemia
  – Helpful in reassuring patients concerned about serious underlying disease
- Noninvasive test for *H pylori*
  – IgG serology
  – Fecal antigen test
  – Urea breath test
- Gastric emptying studies indicated for recurrent vomiting
- Ambulatory esophageal pH testing if atypical gastroesophageal reflux is suspected

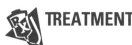 **TREATMENT**

MEDICATIONS

- Proton pump inhibitors benefit 10–15%
  – Omeprazole or rabeprazole, 20 mg
  – Esomeprazole or pantoprazole, 40 mg PO once daily, or lansoprazole, 30 mg PO once daily
  – Antidepressants (eg, desipramine or nortriptyline, 10–50 mg PO each night at bedtime)
- Prokinetic agent, metoclopramide 10 mg PO TID, improves symptoms
- *H pylori* eradication therapy benefits 5–10% (see *Helicobacter pylori* Gastritis)

THERAPEUTIC PROCEDURES

- Discontinue potentially offending medications if possible
- Reduce or discontinue alcohol and caffeine intake
- Psychotherapy and hypnotherapy beneficial in selected patients

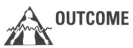 **OUTCOME**

FOLLOW-UP

- Reevaluate symptoms after 4 weeks of empiric management; if they persist or recur, further testing with EGD, possible imaging studies

PROGNOSIS

- Half to two-thirds of people affected have functional dyspepsia, ie, no demonstrable organic cause; symptoms may be chronic

WHEN TO REFER

- Dyspepsia with signs of serious organic disease
- Chronic dyspepsia unresponsive to routine therapies

WHEN TO ADMIT

- Signs of GI bleeding
- Protracted vomiting with dehydration

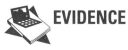 **EVIDENCE**

PRACTICE GUIDELINES

- American Gastroenterological Association Medical Position Statement. Evaluation of dyspepsia. Gastroenterology 2005;128:1838. [PMID: 15940619]
- Dyspepsia. Institute for Clinical Systems Improvement—Private Nonprofit Organization, 2003
- Eisen GM et al. The role of endoscopy in dyspepsia. Gastrointest Endosc. 2001;54:815. [PMID: 11726874]
- National Guideline Clearinghouse
- Talley NJ et al; Practice Parameters Committee of the American College of Gastroenterology. Guidelines for the management of dyspepsia. Am J Gastroenterol. 2005 Oct;100(10):2324–37. [PMID: 16181387]

INFORMATION FOR PATIENTS

- Cleveland Clinic—What is indigestion?
- Mayo Clinic—Nonulcer Dyspepsia

REFERENCES

- Gupta S et al. Management of nonsteroidal, anti-inflammatory, drug-associated dyspepsia. Gastroenterology. 2005 Nov;129(5):1711–9. [PMID: 16285968]

- Jarbol DE et al. Proton pump inhibitor or testing for *Helicobacter pylori* as the first step for patients presenting with dyspepsia? A cluster-randomized trial. Am J Gastroenterol. 2006 Jun; 101(6):1200–8. [PMID: 16771937]

- Moayyedi P et al. Can the clinical history distinguish between organic and functional dyspepsia? JAMA. 2006 Apr 5;295(13):1566–76. [PMID: 16595759]

- Veldhuyzen van Zanten S et al. Esomeprazole 40 mg once a day in patients with functional dyspepsia: the randomized, placebo-controlled "ENTER" trial. Am J Gastroenterol. 2006 Sep; 101(9):2096–106. [PMID: 16817845]

Echinococcosis

KEY FEATURES

ESSENTIALS OF DIAGNOSIS

- History of exposure to dogs or wild canines in an endemic area
- Large cystic lesions, most commonly of the liver or lung
- Positive serologic tests

GENERAL CONSIDERATIONS

- The principal species that infect humans
  - *Echinococcus granulosus,* which causes cystic hydatid disease
  - *Echinococcus multilocularis,* which causes alveolar hydatid disease
- Infection occurs when humans are intermediate hosts for canine tapeworms
- Transmitted by ingesting food contaminated with canine feces containing parasite eggs
- Eggs hatch in intestines to form oncospheres, which
  - Penetrate the mucosa
  - Enter the circulation
  - Encyst in specific organs as hydatid cysts
- *E granulosus* forms cysts most commonly in the liver (65%) and in the lungs (25%)
- However, cysts may develop in any organ, including
  - Brain
  - Bones
  - Skeletal muscles
  - Kidneys
  - Spleen
- Cysts are most commonly single and can persist and grow slowly for many years

DEMOGRAPHICS

- *E granulosus*
  - Transmitted by domestic dogs in areas with livestock (sheep, goats, camels, and horses) as intermediate hosts
  - Endemic in Africa, the Middle East, southern Europe, South America, central Asia, Australia, New Zealand, and the southwestern United States
- *E multilocularis*
  - Causes human disease much less commonly
  - Transmitted by wild canines
  - Endemic in northern forest areas of the northern hemisphere, including central Europe, Siberia, northern Ja-

pan, northwestern Canada, and western Alaska
- An increase in the fox population in Europe has been associated with an increase in human cases
- Other species that cause limited disease in humans are endemic in South America and China

CLINICAL FINDINGS

SYMPTOMS AND SIGNS

- Infections are commonly asymptomatic
- Infections may be noted incidentally on imaging studies or present with symptoms caused by an enlarging or superinfected mass
- Findings may include
  - Abdominal or chest pain
  - Biliary obstruction
  - Cholangitis
  - Portal hypertension
  - Cirrhosis
  - Bronchial obstruction leading to segmental lung collapse
  - Abscesses
- Cyst leakage or rupture may be accompanied by a severe allergic reaction, including fever and hypotension
- Seeding of cysts after rupture may extend the infection to new areas
- *E multilocularis* generally causes a more aggressive disease than *E granulosus,* with initial infection of the liver, but then local and distant spread commonly suggests a malignancy
- Obstructive findings in the liver and elsewhere develop with chronic infection

DIFFERENTIAL DIAGNOSIS

- Amebic or pyogenic liver abscess
- Malignant or benign tumor of liver or other involved organ
- Fascioliasis (sheep liver fluke)
- Clonorchiasis (Chinese liver fluke)
- Choledocholithiasis
- Congenital liver cyst or liver cyst associated with polycystic kidney disease
- Cavitary pulmonary tuberculosis
- Cysticercosis

DIAGNOSIS

LABORATORY TESTS

- Serologic tests
  - Include ELISA and immunoblot

- Offer sensitivity and specificity over 80% for *E granulosus* liver infections, but lower sensitivity for involvement of other organs
- May also distinguish the two major echinococcal infections

IMAGING STUDIES

- Diagnosis usually based on imaging studies
  - Ultrasonography
  - CT
  - MRI
- In *E granulosus* infection, a large cyst containing daughter cysts is highly suggestive of diagnosis
- In *E multilocularis* infection, imaging shows an irregular mass often with areas of calcification

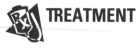

TREATMENT

MEDICATIONS

- Albendazole
  - Often used in conjunction with surgery
  - When used alone, 10–15 mg/kg/day orally has shown efficacy, with courses of 3 months or longer, in some cases with alternating cycles of treatment and rest
- Mebendazole (40–50 mg/kg/day orally) is an alternative
- Praziquantel may also be effective
- In some cases, medical therapy is begun, with surgery performed if disease persists after some months of therapy

SURGERY

- Treatment of cystic hydatid disease
  - Involves cautious surgical resection of cysts, with care not to rupture cysts during removal
  - Injection of a cysticidal agent is used to limit spread in the case of rupture
- Treatment of alveolar cyst disease
  - Generally relies on wide surgical resection of lesions
  - Therapy with albendazole before or during surgery may be beneficial and may also provide improvement or even cure in inoperable cases

THERAPEUTIC PROCEDURES

- Percutaneous aspiration, injection, and reaspiration (PAIR)
  - Can be used when cysts are inoperable
  - Patients receive antihelminthic therapy
  - Cyst is partially aspirated

– Scolicidal agent (eg, 95% ethanol or 0.5% cetrimide) injected after diagnostic confirmation
- Do not use PAIR if cysts communicate with biliary tract

 ## OUTCOME

FOLLOW-UP

- Liver function tests and complete blood cell counts should be monitored weekly when using albendazole

PROGNOSIS

- About 15% of untreated patients eventually die because of the disease or its complications
- 90% of patients with nonresectable masses die within 10 years
- 25% recurrence rates after surgery

WHEN TO REFER

- All patients

WHEN TO ADMIT

- Patients with symptomatic cysts
- Patients who will have percutaneous aspiration of cysts or surgery

PREVENTION

- In endemic areas, prevention is by prophylactic treatment of pet dogs with 5 mg/kg of praziquantel at monthly intervals to remove adult tapeworms and by health education to prevent feeding of offal to dogs

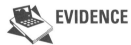 ## EVIDENCE

PRACTICE GUIDELINES

- Heath DD et al. Progress in control of hydatidosis using vaccination—a review of formulation and delivery of the vaccine and recommendations for practical use in control programmes. Acta Trop. 2003;85:133. [PMID: 12606090]

WEB SITE

- CDC—Division of Parasitic Diseases

INFORMATION FOR PATIENTS

- Centers for Disease Control and Prevention
- National Institutes of Health

REFERENCES

- Craig PS et al. Control of cystic echinococcosis/hydatidosis: 1863–2002. Adv Parasitol. 2006;61:443–508. [PMID: 16735171]
- Filippou D. Advances in liver echinococcosis: diagnosis and treatment. Clin Gastroenterol Hepatol. 2007 Feb; 5(2):152–9. [PMID: 17157079]
- Koulas SG et al. A 15-year experience (1988–2003) in the management of liver hydatidosis in northwestern Greece. Int Surg. 2006 Mar–Apr; 91(2):112–6. [PMID: 16774183]
- Schantz PM. Progress in diagnosis, treatment and elimination of echinococcosis and cysticercosis. Parasitol Int. 2006;55 Suppl:S7–S13. [PMID: 16386944]
- Smego RA Jr et al. Treatment options for hepatic cystic echinococcosis. Int J Infect Dis. 2005 Mar;9(2):69–76. [PMID: 15708321]
- Ulku R et al. Surgical treatment of pulmonary hydatid cysts: report of 139 cases. Int Surg. 2006 Mar–Apr; 91(2):77–81. [PMID: 16774176]

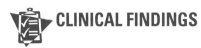 # Ectopic Pregnancy

 ## KEY FEATURES

ESSENTIALS OF DIAGNOSIS

- Amenorrhea or irregular bleeding and spotting
  – Pelvic pain, usually adnexal
  – Adnexal mass by clinical examination or ultrasound
  – Failure of serum level of human chorionic gonadotropin (hCG) to double every 48 h
- No intrauterine pregnancy on transvaginal ultrasound with serum hCG of ≥ 2000 mU/mL

GENERAL CONSIDERATIONS

- Occurs in about 1 of 150 live births, with 98% of cases being tubal pregnancies
- Implantation may also occur in the peritoneum or abdominal viscera, the ovary, and the cervix
- Undiagnosed or undetected ectopic pregnancy is the most common cause of first-trimester maternal death in the United States

DEMOGRAPHICS

- Conditions that prevent or retard migration of the fertilized ovum can predispose to ectopic implantation
- Specific risk factors
  – History of infertility
  – Pelvic inflammatory disease
  – Ruptured appendix
  – Prior tubal surgery

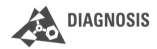 ## CLINICAL FINDINGS

SYMPTOMS AND SIGNS

- 40% of cases are acute
  – Sudden onset of severe, nonradiating, intermittent lancinating lower quadrant pain
  – Backache present during attacks
  – Shock in about 10%, often after pelvic examination
  – At least two-thirds of patients give a history of abnormal menstruation
- 60% of cases are chronic
  – Blood leaks from the tubal ampulla over days
  – Persistent vaginal spotting is reported
  – A pelvic mass is palpable
  – Abdominal distention and mild paralytic ileus are often present

DIFFERENTIAL DIAGNOSIS

- Acute appendicitis
- Intrauterine pregnancy (threatened abortion)
- Pelvic inflammatory disease
- Ruptured corpus luteum cyst or ovarian follicle
- Urinary calculi
- Tuboovarian abscess
- Gestational trophoblastic neoplasia, eg, hydatidiform mole
- Shock or sepsis due to other causes

 ## DIAGNOSIS

LABORATORY TESTS

- Complete blood cell count may show anemia and slight leukocytosis
- Serum hCG levels are lower than expected for a normal pregnancy of the same gestational age
- Serum hCG levels may rise slowly or plateau rather than double every 48 h as in viable early pregnancy or fall as in spontaneous abortion

IMAGING STUDIES

- Endovaginal ultrasound may identify the ectopic pregnancy
- An empty uterine cavity demonstrated by abdominal ultrasound with an hCG of 6500 mU/mL is virtually diagnostic

DIAGNOSTIC PROCEDURES

- Culdocentesis is rarely used in evaluation

 TREATMENT

MEDICATIONS

- Methotrexate (50 mg/m^2) IM is acceptable for early ectopic pregnancies < 3.5 cm and unruptured, without active bleeding
- Iron supplementation may be necessary for anemia during convalescence
- All Rh-negative patients should receive Rho(D) Ig (300 mcg)

SURGERY

- Laparoscopy is the surgical procedure of choice to both confirm and permit removal of an ectopic pregnancy without need for an exploratory laparotomy
- Salpingostomy with removal of the ectopic or partial salpingectomy can usually be performed laparoscopically
- Injection of indigo carmine into the uterine cavity with flow through the contralateral tube can demonstrate its patency

 OUTCOME

COMPLICATIONS

- Tubal infertility

PROGNOSIS

- Repeat tubal pregnancy occurs in 12%
- Early ultrasound confirmation of intrauterine gestation with next pregnancy

WHEN TO REFER

- For suggestive symptoms, laboratory tests, and especially ultrasound findings that support the diagnosis

WHEN TO ADMIT

- All suspected cases of ruptured ectopic pregnancy

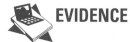 **EVIDENCE**

PRACTICE GUIDELINES

- ACOG Practice Bulletin. Medical management of tubal pregnancy Number 3, December 1998. Clinical management guidelines for obstetrician-gynecologists. American College of Obstetricians and Gynecologists. Int J Gynaecol Obstet. 1999;65:97. [PMID: 10390113]

WEB SITES

- Ectopic Pregnancy Demonstration Case

INFORMATION FOR PATIENTS

- March of Dimes: Ectopic and Molar Pregnancy
- MedlinePlus: Ectopic Pregnancy
- Nemours Foundation

REFERENCE

- Alleyassin A et al. Comparison of success rates in the medical management of ectopic pregnancy with single-dose and multiple-dose administration of methotrexate: a prospective, randomized clinical trial. Fertil Steril. 2006 Jun; 85(6):1661–6. [PMID: 16650421]

Edema, Lower Extremity

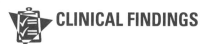 **KEY FEATURES**

ESSENTIALS OF DIAGNOSIS

- History of venous thromboembolism
- Lower extremity asymmetry
- Lower extremity pain
- Lower extremity dependence
- Skin findings
- Time course: acute or chronic edema

GENERAL CONSIDERATIONS

- Lower extremities can swell in response to
  - Increased venous or lymphatic pressures
  - Decreased intravascular oncotic pressure
  - Increased capillary leak
  - Local injury or infection
- Acute lower extremity edema: deep venous thrombosis (DVT)

- Other causes of acute edema
  - Ruptured popliteal cyst
  - Calf strain or trauma
  - Cellulitis
  - Drug therapy with calcium channel blockers (particularly felodipine and amlodipine), thioglitazones, and minoxidil
- Chronic venous insufficiency is the most common cause of chronic lower extremity edema, affecting up to 2% of the population
- Other causes of chronic edema
  - Postphlebitic syndrome with valvular incompetence
  - Congestive heart failure (CHF)
  - Cirrhosis
  - Drug therapy (as above)

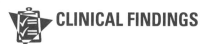 **CLINICAL FINDINGS**

SYMPTOMS AND SIGNS

- Most common symptom of chronic venous insufficiency is "heavy legs," followed by itching
- Assess heart, lungs, and abdomen for evidence of pulmonary hypertension (primary or secondary to chronic lung disease), CHF, or cirrhosis
- Size of both calves should be measured 10 cm below the tibial tuberosity
- Swelling of the entire leg or swelling of one leg > 3 cm more than the other suggests deep venous obstruction
- Elicit pitting and tenderness
- Chronic venous insufficiency skin findings range from hyperpigmentation and stasis dermatitis to lipodermatosclerosis and atrophie blanche to skin ulceration
- Stasis dermatitis: brawny, fibrotic skin changes
- Skin ulceration can occur, particularly in the medial malleolar area, when due to chronic venous insufficiency
- Other causes of medial malleolar skin ulceration
  - Arterial insufficiency
  - Vasculitis
  - Infections (including cutaneous diphtheria)
  - Cancer

DIFFERENTIAL DIAGNOSIS

- Cardiovascular
  - CHF (right-sided)
  - Pericardial effusion
  - Pericarditis
  - Tricuspid regurgitation
  - Tricuspid stenosis
  - Pulmonic stenosis

- Cor pulmonale
- Venous insufficiency (most common)
- Venous obstruction
- Noncardiovascular
  - Cirrhosis
  - Low albumin (nephrotic syndrome, malnutrition, protein-losing enteropathy)
  - Cellulitis
  - Premenstrual fluid retention
  - Drugs (vasodilators, eg, calcium channel blockers; salt-retaining medications, eg, nonsteroidal anti-inflammatory drugs, thiazolidinediones)
  - Musculoskeletal (Baker's cyst, gastrocnemius tear, compartment syndrome)
  - Lymphatic obstruction
  - Eclampsia
  - Hypothyroidism with myxedema
  - Filariasis
- Unilateral
  - DVT
  - Venous insufficiency
  - Baker's cyst
  - Cellulitis
  - Trauma
  - Lymphatic obstruction, eg, obstruction by pelvic tumor
  - Reflex sympathetic dystrophy

 DIAGNOSIS

LABORATORY TESTS

- Serum creatinine, blood urea nitrogen
- D-dimers
- Urinalysis
- Liver tests: alkaline phosphatase, aspartate aminotransferase, gamma glutamyl-transpeptidase, total bilirubin, albumin
- Thyroid-stimulating hormone

IMAGING STUDIES

- Color duplex ultrasonography of lower extremity
- Ankle-brachial pressure index (ABPI)

DIAGNOSTIC PROCEDURES

- Consider echocardiogram

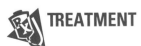 **TREATMENT**

THERAPEUTIC PROCEDURES

- Treatment should be guided by underlying etiology
- Avoid diuretic therapy in patients with chronic venous insufficiency unless

comorbid CHF or other fluid-retaining comorbid condition
- Edema resulting from calcium channel blocker therapy responds to concomitant therapy with angiotensin-converting enzyme inhibitors or angiotensin receptor blockers
- Mechanical measures effective in chronic venous insufficiency
  - Leg elevation, above the level of the heart, for 30 min three to four times daily and during sleep
  - Compression therapy with stockings and devices
- Refrain from using compression therapy if there are risk factors for or signs of peripheral arterial occlusive disease
- Horse chestnut seed extract is equivalent to compression therapy for mild to moderate chronic venous insufficiency

 OUTCOME

WHEN TO REFER

- Refer to vascular surgeon
  - Patients with chronic venous insufficiency in combination with peripheral arterial occlusive disease
  - Patients with nonhealing ulcers from chronic venous insufficiency or other causes

WHEN TO ADMIT

- Cellulitis requiring IV antibiotics
- Skin ulcers requiring grafting

 EVIDENCE

WEB SITES

- Vacek JL. Chronic Edema Curbside Consult. Postgraduate Medicine Online 2000;108.

INFORMATION FOR PATIENTS

- Harvard Medical School, InteliHealth: Edema
- Mayo Clinic: Foot Swelling During Air Travel
- National Lymphedema Network: Lymphedema Overview

REFERENCES

- Barwell JR et al. Comparison of surgery and compression with compression alone in chronic venous ulceration (ESCHAR study): randomised controlled trial. Lancet. 2004 Jun 5;363(9424):1854–9. [PMID: 15183623]
- Belcaro G et al. Prevention of edema, flight microangiopathy and venous thrombosis in long flights with elastic stockings. A randomized trial: the LONFLIT 4 Concorde Edema-SSL Study. Angiology. 2002 Nov–Dec; 53(6):635–45. [PMID: 12463616]
- Bergan JJ et al. Chronic Venous Disease. N Engl J Med. 2006 Aug 3; 355(5):488–98. [PMID: 16885552]
- Criqui MH et al. Chronic venous disease in an ethnically diverse population: the San Diego Population Study. Am J Epidemiol. 2003 Sep 1;158(5):448–56. [PMID: 12936900]
- Felty CL et al. Compression therapy for chronic venous insufficiency. Semin Vasc Surg. 2005 Mar;18(1):36–40. [PMID: 15791552]
- O'Brien JG et al. Treatment of edema. Am Fam Physician. 2005 Jun 1; 71(11):2111–7. [PMID: 15952439]

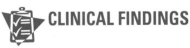

Effusions, Malignant, Pleural, Pericardial, & Peritoneal

KEY FEATURES

- Half of undiagnosed effusions in patients not known to have cancer are malignant
- Malignant effusions occur in pleural, pericardial, and peritoneal spaces
- Caused by direct neoplastic involvement of serous surface or obstruction of lymphatic drainage

CLINICAL FINDINGS

- Pleural, pericardial
  - Chest pain
  - Shortness of breath
  - Cough
- Pericardial
  - Hypotension
  - Muffled heart sounds
- Peritoneal: Abdominal distention

DIAGNOSIS

- Thoracentesis, pericardiocentesis, or paracentesis; send fluid for
  – Cytology
  – Cell count and differential
  – Protein content
  – Lactate dehydrogenase level
- Malignant effusions are generally bloody
- Chylous effusions occur with thoracic duct obstruction or enlarged mediastinal lymph nodes in lymphoma
- If pleural cytology is negative on two occasions but suspicion of tumor high, thoracoscopic pleural biopsy may be helpful
- Differential diagnosis
  – Congestive heart failure
  – Pulmonary embolism
  – Trauma
  – Infections
- Effusions are a complication of some chemotherapeutic agents

 TREATMENT

- Treatment of underlying malignancy is often ineffective in relieving effusions
- **Pleural:** Diuretics are used to minimize reexpansion pulmonary edema after thoracentesis
- Thoracentesis alone
  – Controls < 10% of pleural effusions
  – May be useful in conjunction with systemic chemotherapy
- Closed water-seal drainage with a chest tube for 3–4 days, followed by chemosclerosis with talc, bleomycin, or mitoxantrone, if necessary
- Indwelling pleural drainage catheter with a valve allows intermittent home drainage but only for patients with a limited life expectancy, because the risk of infection and blockage reduces long-term effectiveness
- Pleuroperitoneal shunting
  – Occasionally helpful
  – However, patient must pump shunt 100 times five times a day
- Pleurectomy
  – Effective
  – High complication rate, however, so rarely done
- **Pericardial**
  – Pericardial window or stripping achieves good control
  – Also useful for constrictive pericarditis after radiation therapy
- **Peritoneal**
  – Diuretics are used in initial treatment of small to moderate effusions and as

adjunctive treatment after large-volume paracentesis
  – Chemosclerosis less useful in malignant ascites though success has been reported using bleomycin, mitoxantrone, doxorubicin, thiotepa, and other agents

Endocarditis, Infective

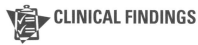 **KEY FEATURES**

ESSENTIALS OF DIAGNOSIS

- Preexisting organic heart lesion
- Fever
- New or changing heart murmur
- Evidence of systemic emboli
- Positive blood culture
- Evidence of vegetation on echocardiography

GENERAL CONSIDERATIONS

- Important factors that determine the clinical presentation
  – Nature of the infecting organism
  – Which valve is infected
  – Route of infection
- More virulent organisms, particularly *Staphylococcus aureus,* cause
  – Rapidly progressive and destructive infection
  – Acute febrile illnesses
  – Early embolization
  – Acute valvular regurgitation and myocardial abscess
- Subacute presentation
  – Viridans strains of streptococci, enterococci, and other gram-positive and gram-negative bacilli, yeasts, and fungi
  – Systemic and peripheral manifestations may predominate
- Patients may have underlying cardiac disease, but prevalence as a risk factor is decreasing
- The initiating event is colonization of the valve by bacteria during a transient or persistent bacteremia

Native valve endocarditis
- Most commonly due to
  – *S aureus* (~40%)
  – Viridans streptococci (~30%)
  – Enterococci (5–10%)

- Gram-negative organisms and fungi account for a small percentage
- Injection drug users
  – *S aureus* in at least 60% of cases and 80–90% of tricuspid valve infections
  – Enterococci and streptococci comprise the balance in about equal proportions

Prosthetic valve endocarditis
- **Early** infections (within 2 months of valve implantation) are commonly caused by
  – Staphylococci—both coagulase-positive and coagulase-negative
  – Gram-negative organisms and fungi
- **Late** prosthetic valve endocarditis
  – Resembles native valve endocarditis
  – Most cases caused by streptococci, though coagulase-negative staphylococci cause a significant proportion of cases

DEMOGRAPHICS

- Injection drug use
- Underlying valvular disease

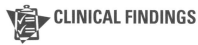 **CLINICAL FINDINGS**

SYMPTOMS AND SIGNS

- Most present with a febrile illness that has lasted several days to 2 weeks
- Heart murmurs
  – In most cases, heart murmurs are stable
  – Changing murmur is significant diagnostically, but it is the exception rather than the rule
- Characteristic peripheral lesions occur in up to 20–25% of patients
  – Petechiae (on the palate or conjunctiva or beneath the fingernails)
  – Subungual ("splinter") hemorrhages
  – Osler nodes (painful, violaceous raised lesions of the fingers, toes, or feet)
  – Janeway lesions (painless erythematous lesions of the palms or soles)
  – Roth spots (exudative lesions in the retina)

DIFFERENTIAL DIAGNOSIS

- Valvular abnormality without endocarditis
  – Rheumatic heart disease
  – Mitral valve prolapse
  – Bicuspid or calcific aortic valve
- Flow murmur (anemia, pregnancy, hyperthyroidism, sepsis)
- Atrial myxoma
- Noninfective endocarditis, eg, systemic lupus erythematosus (Libman-Saks

endocarditis), marantic endocarditis (nonbacterial thrombotic endocarditis)
- Hematuria due to other causes, such as
  - Glomerulonephritis
  - Renal cell carcinoma
- Acute rheumatic fever
- Vasculitis

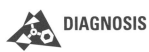 **DIAGNOSIS**

LABORATORY TESTS

- Blood culture
  - Most important diagnostic tool
  - To maximize the yield, obtain three sets of blood cultures at least 1 h apart before starting antibiotics
- In acute endocarditis, leukocytosis is common
- In subacute cases, anemia of chronic disease and a normal white blood cell count are the rule
- Hematuria and proteinuria as well as renal dysfunction may result from emboli or immunologically mediated glomerulonephritis
- **Duke criteria** for the diagnosis
  - Major criteria
    - Two positive blood cultures for a typical microorganism of infective endocarditis
    - Positive echocardiography (vegetation, myocardial abscess, or new partial dehiscence of a prosthetic valve)
    - New regurgitant murmur
  - Minor criteria
    - Presence of a predisposing condition
    - Fever > 38°C
    - Embolic disease
    - Immunologic phenomena (Osler nodes, Roth spots, glomerulonephritis, rheumatoid factor)
    - Positive blood cultures not meeting the major criteria or serologic evidence of active infection with an organism that causes endocarditis
  - A definite diagnosis is made with 80% accuracy if two major criteria, or one major criterion and three minor criteria, or five minor criteria are fulfilled
  - Possible endocarditis is defined as the presence of 1 major and 1 minor criterion, or three minor criteria
  - If these criteria thresholds are not met and either an alternative explanation for illness is identified or the patient has defervesced within 4 days, endocarditis is highly unlikely

IMAGING STUDIES

- Chest radiograph may show findings indicating an underlying cardiac abnormality and, in right-sided endocarditis, pulmonary infiltrates
- Echocardiography
  - Transthoracic echocardiography is 55–65% sensitive; therefore, it cannot rule out endocarditis but may confirm a clinical suspicion
  - Transesophageal echocardiography is 90% sensitive in detecting vegetations and is particularly useful for identifying valve ring abscesses, and pulmonary and prosthetic valve endocarditis

DIAGNOSTIC PROCEDURES

- The ECG is nondiagnostic. Changing conduction abnormalities suggest myocardial abscess formation

 TREATMENT

MEDICATIONS

- See Table 75

SURGERY

- Valvular regurgitation resulting in acute heart failure that does not resolve promptly after institution of medical therapy is an indication for valve replacement even if active infection is present, especially if the aortic valve is involved
- Infections that do not respond to appropriate antimicrobial therapy after 7–10 days (ie, persistent fevers, positive blood cultures despite therapy) are more likely to be eradicated if the valve is replaced
- Nearly always required for fungal endocarditis and is more often necessary with gram-negative bacilli
- Infection involving the sinus of Valsalva or produces septal abscesses
- Recurrent infection with the same organism often indicates that surgery is necessary, especially with infected prosthetic valves
- Continuing embolization when the infection is otherwise responding may be an indication for surgery

 OUTCOME

FOLLOW-UP

- Defervescence occurs in 3–4 days on average if infection is caused by
  - Viridans streptococci

- Enterococci
- Coagulase-negative staphylococci
- Patients may remain febrile for a week or more if infection is caused by
  - *S aureus*
  - *Pseudomonas aeruginosa*

COMPLICATIONS

- Destruction of infected heart valves
- Myocardial abscesses leading to conduction disturbances
- Systemic embolization
- Metastatic infections
- Mycotic aneurysms
- Right-sided endocarditis, which usually involves the tricuspid valve, often leads to septic pulmonary emboli, causing infarction and lung abscesses

PROGNOSIS

- Higher morbidity and mortality associated with nonstreptococcal etiology, aortic or prosthetic valvular infection

WHEN TO REFER

- Infectious diseases consultation recommended
- Patients with signs of heart failure should be referred for surgical evaluation

WHEN TO ADMIT

- Patients with evidence of heart failure
- Patients with a nonstreptococcal etiology
- For initiation of antimicrobial therapy in suspected, definite, or possible cases

PREVENTION

- Prophylactic antibiotics are given to patients with predisposing congenital or valvular anomalies who are to have any of a number of procedures (Tables 73 and 74)
- Current recommendations are given in Table 72

 EVIDENCE

PRACTICE GUIDELINES

- Baddour LM et al. Infective endocarditis: diagnosis, antimicrobial therapy, and management of complications: a statement for healthcare professionals from the Committee on Rheumatic Fever, Endocarditis, and Kawasaki Disease, Council on Cardiovascular Disease in the Young, and the Councils on Clinical Cardiology, Stroke, and Cardiovascular Surgery and Anesthesia, American Heart

Association: endorsed by the Infectious Diseases Society of America. Circulation. 2005 Jun 14;111(23):e394–434. Erratum in: Circulation. 2005;112:2373. [PMID: 15956145]

- Olaison L et al. Current best practices and guidelines indications for surgical intervention in infective endocarditis. Infect Dis Clin North Am. 2002; 16:453. [PMID: 12092482]
- Wilson W et al; American Heart Association. Prevention of infective endocarditis: guidelines from the American Heart Association: a guideline from the American Heart Association Rheumatic Fever, Endocarditis, and Kawasaki Disease Committee, Council on Cardiovascular Disease in the Young, and the Council on Clinical Cardiology, Council on Cardiovascular Surgery and Anesthesia, and the Quality of Care and Outcomes Research Interdisciplinary Working Group. Circulation. 2007 Oct 9; 116(15):1736–54. [PMID: 17446442]

WEB SITE

- CDC—Emerging Infectious Diseases

INFORMATION FOR PATIENTS

- American Heart Association
- Stevens LM. JAMA patient page: Endocarditis. JAMA. 2002;288:128. [PMID: 12109459]

REFERENCES

- Baddour LM et al. Infective endocarditis: diagnosis, antimicrobial therapy, and management of complications: a statement for healthcare professionals from the Committee on Rheumatic Fever, Endocarditis, and Kawasaki Disease, Council on Cardiovascular Disease in the Young, and the Councils on Clinical Cardiology, Stroke, and Cardiovascular Surgery and Anesthesia, American Heart Association: endorsed by the Infectious Diseases Society of America. Circulation. 2005 Jun 14;111(23):e394–434. Erratum in: Circulation. 2005;112:2373. [PMID: 15956145]
- Fowler VG Jr et al; ICE Investigators. *Staphylococcus aureus* endocarditis: a consequence of medical progress. JAMA. 2005 Jun 22;293(24):3012–21. [PMID: 15972563]
- Wilson W et al; American Heart Association. Prevention of infective endocarditis: guidelines from the American Heart Association: a guideline from the American Heart Association Rheumatic Fever, Endocarditis, and Kawasaki Disease Committee, Council on Cardiovascular

Disease in the Young, and the Council on Clinical Cardiology, Council on Cardiovascular Surgery and Anesthesia, and the Quality of Care and Outcomes Research Interdisciplinary Working Group. Circulation. 2007 Oct 9; 116(15):1736-54. [PMID: 17446442]

Endometrial Cancer

KEY FEATURES

ESSENTIALS OF DIAGNOSIS

- Abnormal bleeding is the presenting sign in 80% of cases
- Papanicolaou smear frequently negative
- After a negative pregnancy test, endometrial tissue is required to confirm the diagnosis

GENERAL CONSIDERATIONS

- Adenocarcinoma of the endometrium is the second most common cancer of the female genital tract

DEMOGRAPHICS

- Occurs most often in women 50–70 years of age
- History of unopposed estrogen in the past; this increased risk persists for 10 or more years after stopping the drug
- Obesity, nulliparity, diabetes, and polycystic ovaries with prolonged anovulation and the extended use of tamoxifen for the treatment of breast cancer are also risk factors

CLINICAL FINDINGS

SYMPTOMS AND SIGNS

- Vaginal bleeding
- Obstruction of the cervix with collection of pus (pyometra) or blood (hematometra) causing lower abdominal pain may occur
- However, pain generally occurs late in the disease, with metastases or infection

DIFFERENTIAL DIAGNOSIS

- Endometrial hyperplasia or proliferation
- Uterine leiomyomas (fibroids)

- Endometrial polyp
- Cervical cancer
- Atrophic endometrium
- Adenomyosis (uterine endometriosis)
- Atrophic vaginitis
- Ovarian tumor
- Leiomyosarcoma

DIAGNOSIS

LABORATORY TESTS

- Papanicolaou smears of the cervix occasionally show atypical endometrial cells but are an insensitive diagnostic tool

IMAGING STUDIES

- Vaginal ultrasonography may show thickness of the endometrium indicating hypertrophy and possible neoplastic change

DIAGNOSTIC PROCEDURES

- Endocervical and endometrial sampling is the only reliable means of diagnosis. Adequate specimens of each can usually be obtained during an office procedure with local anesthesia (paracervical block)
- Simultaneous hysteroscopy can localize polyps or other lesions within the uterine cavity
- Assess extent of disease with
  – Examination under anesthesia
  – Endometrial and endocervical sampling
  – Chest radiography
  – Intravenous urography
  – Cystoscopy
  – Sigmoidoscopy
  – Transvaginal sonography
  – MRI
- The staging is based on the surgical and pathologic evaluation

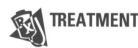

TREATMENT

MEDICATIONS

- Advanced or metastatic endometrial adenocarcinoma may be palliated with large doses of progestins, eg, medroxyprogesterone, 400 mg IM weekly, or megestrol acetate, 80–160 mg daily PO
- The role of chemotherapy alone or with irradiation is under investigation

SURGERY

- Treatment consists of total hysterectomy and bilateral salpingo-oophorectomy.

Peritoneal material for cytologic examination is routinely taken

THERAPEUTIC PROCEDURES

- Preliminary external irradiation or intracavitary radium therapy is indicated if the cancer is poorly differentiated or if the uterus is definitely enlarged in the absence of myomas

OUTCOME

FOLLOW-UP

- Examination every 3–4 months for 2 years, then every 6 months

COMPLICATIONS

- Related to therapy, radiation vs surgery

PROGNOSIS

- With early diagnosis and treatment, the 5-year survival is 80–85%

WHEN TO REFER

- All patients with carcinoma of the endometrium should be referred to a gynecologist
- If invasion deep into the myometrium has occurred or if sampled preaortic lymph nodes are positive for tumor, postoperative irradiation is indicated

PREVENTION

- Prompt endometrial sampling for patients who report abnormal menstrual bleeding or postmenopausal uterine bleeding will reveal many incipient as well as clinical cases of endometrial cancer
- Younger women with chronic anovulation are at risk for endometrial hyperplasia and subsequent endometrial cancer. They can reduce the risk of hyperplasia almost completely with the use of oral contraceptives or cyclic progestin therapy

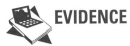

EVIDENCE

PRACTICE GUIDELINES

- American Cancer Society guidelines on testing for early endometrial cancer detection—update 2001
- American College of Obstetricians and Gynecologists. ACOG Practice Bulletin, Clinical Management Guidelines for Obstetrician-Gynecologists, No. 65, August 2005: Management of endome-

trial cancer. Obstet Gynecol. 2005 Aug; 106(2):413–25. [PMID: 16055605]
- Teng N et al; NCCN Endometrial Cancer and Uterine Sarcoma Practice Guidelines Panel. National Comprehensive Cancer Network: Uterine Cancers v.1.2004

WEB SITE

- National Cancer Institute: Endometrial Cancer Information for Patients and Health Professionals

INFORMATION FOR PATIENTS

- American Academy of Family Physicians: Endometrial Cancer
- American Cancer Society: Endometrial Cancer
- JAMA patient page. Endometrial cancer. JAMA. 2002;288:1678. [PMID: 12362917]
- MedlinePlus: Endometrial Cancer

REFERENCE

- Amant F et al. Endometrial cancer. Lancet 2005 Aug 6–12;366(9484):491–505. [PMID: 16084259]

Endometriosis

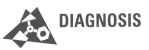

KEY FEATURES

ESSENTIALS OF DIAGNOSIS

- Pelvic pain related to menstrual cycle
- Dysmenorrhea
- Dyspareunia
- Increased frequency among infertile women

GENERAL CONSIDERATIONS

- An aberrant growth of endometrium outside the uterus, particularly in the dependent parts of the pelvis and in the ovaries
- Common cause of abnormal bleeding and secondary dysmenorrhea
- Its causes, pathogenesis, and natural course are poorly understood

DEMOGRAPHICS

- The prevalence in the United States is 6–10% among fertile women and four- to five-fold greater than that in infertile women

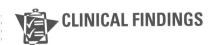

CLINICAL FINDINGS

SYMPTOMS AND SIGNS

- Aching pain tends to be constant, beginning 2–7 days before the onset of menses, and becomes increasingly severe until flow slackens
- Depending on the location and extent of the endometrial implants, infertility, dyspareunia, or rectal pain with bleeding may result
- Pelvic examination may disclose tender indurated nodules in the cul-de-sac

DIFFERENTIAL DIAGNOSIS

- Adenomyosis (uterine endometriosis)
- Pelvic inflammatory disease
- Uterine leiomyomas (fibroids)
- Primary dysmenorrhea
- Ovarian tumor
- Endometrial cancer
- Pelvic adhesions
- Irritable bowel syndrome
- Interstitial cystitis

DIAGNOSIS

IMAGING STUDIES

- Ultrasound examination will often reveal complex fluid-filled masses that cannot be distinguished from neoplasms
- MRI is more sensitive and specific than ultrasound, particularly in the diagnosis of retroperitoneal lesions

DIAGNOSTIC PROCEDURES

- The clinical diagnosis of endometriosis is presumptive and is usually confirmed by laparoscopy or laparotomy

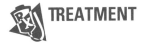

TREATMENT

MEDICATIONS

- Medications are designed to inhibit ovulation over 4–9 months to prevent cyclic stimulation of endometrial implants and induce atrophy
- The optimum duration of therapy is not known
- Gonadotropin-releasing hormone analogs
  - Nafarelin nasal spray, 0.2–0.4 mg BID, or long-acting injectable leuprolide acetate, 3.75 mg IM monthly, used for 6 months, suppress ovulation

– Side effects consisting of vasomotor symptoms and bone demineralization may be relieved by "add-back" therapy with norethindrone, 5–10 mg PO daily

- Danazol
  – Used for 4–6 months in the lowest dose necessary to suppress menstruation, usually 200–400 mg PO BID
  – Has a high incidence of androgenic side effects, including decreased breast size, weight gain, acne, and hirsutism
- Any of the combination oral contraceptives, the contraceptive patch, or the vaginal ring
  – May be used continuously for 6–12 months
  – Breakthrough bleeding can be treated with conjugated estrogens, 1.25 mg PO daily for 1 week, or estradiol, 2 mg PO daily for 1 week
- Medroxyprogesterone acetate
  – 100 mg IM every 2 weeks for four doses; then 100 mg IM every 4 weeks
  – Add oral estrogen or estradiol valerate, 30 mg IM, for breakthrough bleeding
  – Use for 6–9 months
- Low-dose oral contraceptives can also be given cyclically; prolonged suppression of ovulation will often inhibit further stimulation of residual endometriosis, especially if taken after one of the therapies mentioned above
- Analgesics, with or without codeine, may be needed during menses
- Nonsteroidal anti-inflammatory drugs may be helpful

SURGERY

- Surgical treatment of endometriosis—particularly extensive disease—is effective both in reducing pain and in promoting fertility
  – Laparoscopic ablation of endometrial implants along with uterine nerve ablation significantly reduces pain
  – Ablation of implants and, if necessary, removal of ovarian endometriomas enhance fertility, although subsequent pregnancy rates are related to the severity of disease
  – Women with disabling pain who no longer desire childbearing can be treated definitively with total abdominal hysterectomy and bilateral salpingo-oophorectomy (TAH-BSO)

THERAPEUTIC PROCEDURES

- The goal of medical treatment is to preserve the fertility of women wanting future pregnancies, ameliorate symp-

toms, and simplify future surgery or make it unnecessary

 OUTCOME

PROGNOSIS

- The prognosis for reproductive function in early or moderately advanced endometriosis is good with conservative therapy
- Bilateral ovariectomy is curative for patients with severe and extensive endometriosis with pain
- Following hysterectomy and oophorectomy, estrogen replacement therapy is indicated

WHEN TO REFER

- Refer to gynecologist for laparoscopic diagnosis and treatment

WHEN TO ADMIT

- Rarely necessary except in case of acute abdomen associated with a ruptured or bleeding endometrioma

 EVIDENCE

PRACTICE GUIDELINES

- ACOG Committee on Practice Bulletins. Medical management of endometriosis. Int J Gynaecol Obstet. 2000 Nov;71(2):183–96. [PMID: 11186465]

INFORMATION FOR PATIENTS

- American Association of Family Physicians: Endometriosis
- MedlinePlus: Endometriosis Interactive Tutorial
- MedlinePlus: Laparoscopy Interactive Tutorial
- National Institute of Child Health & Human Development: Endometriosis

REFERENCES

- Crosignani P et al. Advances in the management of endometriosis: an update for clinicians. Hum Reprod Update. 2006; 12:179–89. [PMID: 16280355]
- Kinkel K et al. Diagnosis of endometriosis with imaging: a review. Eur Radiol. 2006 Feb;16(2):285–98. [PMID: 16155722]

Epididymitis, Acute

 KEY FEATURES

- Painful enlargement of the epididymis, relieved by scrotal elevation
- Fever and irritative voiding symptoms are common
- In advanced cases, infection can spread to the testis and entire scrotal contents tender to palpation
- **Sexually transmitted** form
  – Typically in men under age 40
  – Associated with urethritis
  – Caused by *Chlamydia trachomatis* or *Neisseria gonorrhoeae*
- **Nonsexually transmitted** form
  – In older men, associated with urinary tract infections and prostatitis
  – Caused by gram-negative rods

 CLINICAL FINDINGS

- Symptoms can follow acute physical strain, trauma, or sexual activity
- Associated symptoms of urethritis and urethral discharge or cystitis (irritative voiding symptoms)
- Pain in the scrotum may radiate along the spermatic cord
- Fever and scrotal swelling
- Differential diagnosis
  – Tumors of the testis
  – Testicular torsion

 DIAGNOSIS

- Complete blood count: leukocytosis and left shift
- **Sexually transmitted** form
  – Perform Gram stain of urethral discharge
  – Results may show white cells and gram-negative intracellular diplococci (*N gonorrhoeae*) or white cells without visible organisms (nongonococcal urethritis, *C trachomatis*)
- **Nonsexually transmitted** form
  – Perform urinalysis
  – Results may show pyuria, bacteriuria, hematuria
  – Urine cultures may reveal pathogen

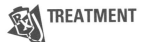

TREATMENT

- **Sexually transmitted** variety: antibiotics for 21 days, treat sexual partner also
- **Nonsexually transmitted** variety: antibiotics for 21–28 days
- Evaluate urinary tract to identify underlying disease
- Bed rest with scrotal elevation
- Prompt treatment usually results in a favorable outcome
- Delayed or inadequate treatment may result in epididymoorchitis, decreased fertility, abscess formation

Epilepsy

KEY FEATURES

ESSENTIALS OF DIAGNOSIS

- Recurrent seizures
- Epilepsy should not be diagnosed on the basis of a solitary seizure
- Characteristic electroencephalographic (EEG) changes may occur
- Postictal confusion or focal neurologic deficits may follow and last hours

GENERAL CONSIDERATIONS

- The most likely cause relates to the age of onset
- Idiopathic epilepsy onset is usually between the ages of 5 and 20 years
- Metabolic disorders may cause seizures
- Trauma is an important cause of seizures
  - Seizures in the first week after head injury do not imply that they will persist
  - Prophylactic anticonvulsant drugs have not been proven to reduce the incidence of posttraumatic epilepsy
- Tumors and other space-occupying lesions result in seizures that are often partial (focal), and most likely with frontal, parietal, or temporal lesions
- Vascular disease is the leading cause in patients aged 60 or older
- Alzheimer's disease and other degenerative disorders can cause seizures in later life
- CNS infections (meningitis, encephalitis, or brain abscess) must be considered in all age groups as potentially reversible causes of seizures

- Causes of secondary seizures
  - CNS vasculitis, eg, systemic lupus erythematosus
  - Febrile seizures in children younger than 5 years
  - Metabolic disorders, including withdrawal from alcohol or other CNS depressant drugs, hypoglycemia, hyperglycemia, uremia, and hyponatremia
  - Trauma
  - CNS infection
  - Degenerative disease, eg, Alzheimer's disease

DEMOGRAPHICS

- Epilepsy affects approximately 0.5% of the US population

CLINICAL FINDINGS

SYMPTOMS AND SIGNS

- See Table 132
- Nonspecific prodrome in some (headache, lethargy)
- The type of aura depends on the cerebral site of origin of the seizure, eg, gustatory or olfactory hallucinations or visual hallucinations with temporal or occipital lesions
- In most patients, seizures occur unpredictably
- Fever, sleep loss, alcohol, stress, or flashing lights may precipitate seizures
- Clinical examination may be normal interictally unless there is a structural cause for the seizures
- Immediately postictally there may be a focal deficit (Todd's paresis) or bilateral Babinski signs
- Focal signs postictally suggest focal CNS abnormality

DIFFERENTIAL DIAGNOSIS

- Syncope
- Cardiac arrhythmia
- Stroke or transient ischemic attack
- Pseudoseizure
- Panic attack
- Migraine
- Narcolepsy

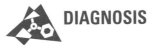

DIAGNOSIS

LABORATORY TESTS

- Complete blood count
- Serum glucose

- Liver and renal function tests
- Serologic tests for syphilis

IMAGING STUDIES

- All patients with progressive disorder and those with new onset of seizures should undergo CNS imaging
- Obtain an MRI if there are focal neurologic symptoms or signs, focal seizures, or a focal EEG disturbance

DIAGNOSTIC PROCEDURES

- History is key, including eyewitness accounts
- EEG
  - Abnormal in only about 60%
  - May support clinical diagnosis of epilepsy (paroxysmal spikes or sharp waves)
  - May guide prognosis
  - May help classify the seizure disorder
  - Important in evaluating candidates for surgical treatment
- Repeated Holter monitoring may be necessary to establish the diagnosis of cardiac arrhythmia

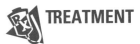

TREATMENT

MEDICATIONS

- Anticonvulsant drug treatment is generally not required for
  - A single seizure unless further attacks occur or investigations reveal some underlying untreatable pathology
  - Alcohol withdrawal seizures, which are self-limited
- Patients with alcohol withdrawal seizures should be observed in hospital for at least 24 hours
- See Table 133
- Anticonvulsant drug dose is gradually increased until seizures are controlled or side effects occur
- If seizures continue despite treatment at the maximal tolerated dose, a second drug is added and the first drug is then gradually withdrawn
- In most patients, control can be achieved with a single anticonvulsant drug
- Discontinue the medication only when the patient is seizure-free for at least 3 years
  - Dose reduction should be gradual over a period of weeks or months
  - If seizures recur, treatment is reinstituted with same drugs used previously
- A seizure recurrence after the medication is discontinued is more likely if
  - The patient did not respond to therapy initially

– Focal or multiple types of seizures
– EEG abnormalities persist

SURGERY

- Operative treatment or vagal nerve stimulation is best undertaken in specialized centers

THERAPEUTIC PROCEDURES

- Advise patients to avoid situations that may be dangerous or life-threatening if they have a seizure
- State laws may require clinicians to report to the public health department or department of motor vehicles any patients with seizures or other episodic lapses of consciousness

 OUTCOME

FOLLOW-UP

- Dosing should not be based simply on serum levels because some patients require levels that exceed the therapeutic range ("toxic levels") but tolerate these without ill effect
- In general, the dose of an antiepileptic agent is increased depending on clinical response, not serum drug level
- The trough drug level is then measured to provide a reference point for the maximum tolerated dose
- Measure serum drug levels when another drug is added to the therapeutic regimen and to assess compliance in poorly controlled patients
- Certain antiepileptic drugs may be teratogenic; epileptic women of childbearing potential require special care

COMPLICATIONS

- See Status Epilepticus
- Residual encephalopathy after prolonged seizures or poor control of seizures

PROGNOSIS

- The risk of seizure recurrence in different series varies between about 30% and 70%

WHEN TO ADMIT

- If status epilepticus
- If pseudoseizures are suspected, to a video monitoring unit
- If surgery is contemplated

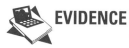 **EVIDENCE**

PRACTICE GUIDELINES

- American College of Emergency Physicians. Clinical policy: Critical issues in the evaluation and management of adult patients presenting to the emergency department with seizures. Ann Emerg Med. 2004;43:605. [PMID: 15111920]
- Hirtz D et al; American Academy of Neurology. Practice parameter: treatment of the child with a first unprovoked seizure: Report of the Quality Standards Subcommittee of the American Academy of Neurology and the Practice Committee of the Child Neurology Society. Neurology. 2003; 60:166. [PMID: 12552027]

INFORMATION FOR PATIENTS

- Epilepsy Foundation
- Epilepsy.com

REFERENCES

- Brathen G et al. EFNS guidelines on the diagnosis and management of alcohol-related seizures: report of a EFNS task force. Eur J Neurol. 2005 Aug;12(8):575–81. [PMID: 16053464]
- Chen JW et al. Status epilepticus: pathophysiology and management in adults. Lancet Neurol. 2006 Mar; 5(3):246–56. [PMID: 16488380]
- Duncan JS et al. Adult epilepsy. Lancet. 2006 Apr 1;367(9516):1087–100. [PMID: 16581409]
- Hitiris N et al. Modern antiepileptic drugs: guidelines and beyond. Curr Opin Neurol. 2006 Apr;19(2):175–80. [PMID: 16538093]
- Kelso AR et al. Advances in epilepsy. Br Med Bull. 2005 Apr 21;72:135–48. [PMID: 15845748]
- Vazquez B. Monotherapy in epilepsy: role of the newer antiepileptic drugs. Arch Neurol. 2004 Sep;61(9):1361–5. [PMID: 15364680]

Epistaxis

 KEY FEATURES

ESSENTIALS OF DIAGNOSIS

- Anterior nasal cavity bleeding is by far the most common type of epistaxis
- Most cases can be successfully treated by direct pressure on the bleeding site
- When this is inadequate, various nasal tamponade methods are usually effective

GENERAL CONSIDERATIONS

- **Anterior nasal cavity** bleeding originates from Kiesselbach's plexus, a vascular plexus on the anterior nasal septum
- **Posterior nasal cavity** bleeding
  – Originates from the posterior half of the inferior turbinate or the top of the nasal cavity
  – More commonly associated with atherosclerotic disease and hypertension
- Predisposing factors
  – Nasal trauma (eg, nose picking, forceful nose blowing, foreign body)
  – Drying of the nasal mucosa from low humidity or supplemental nasal oxygen
  – Allergic or viral rhinitis
  – Deviation of the nasal septum
  – Chronic sinusitis
  – Inhaled corticosteroids
  – Inhaled cocaine use
  – Alcohol use
  – Anticoagulation or antiplatelet medications (eg, aspirin, clopidogrel)
  – Hypertension
  – Atherosclerotic disease

DEMOGRAPHICS

- Only 5% of nasal bleeding originates in the posterior nasal cavity
- Less than 10% of nasal bleeding is caused by coagulopathy or tumor

 CLINICAL FINDINGS

SYMPTOMS AND SIGNS

- Bleeding from nostril or nasopharynx
- Posterior bleeding may present with hemoptysis or hematemesis

DIFFERENTIAL DIAGNOSIS

- Thrombocytopenia
- Idiopathic thrombocytopenic purpura
- Thrombotic thrombocytopenic purpura
- Hemophilia

- Hereditary hemorrhagic telangiectasia (Osler-Weber-Rendu syndrome)
- Polycythemia vera
- Leukemia
- Wegener's granulomatosis
- Nasal tumor

 ## DIAGNOSIS

LABORATORY TESTS

- Laboratory assessment of bleeding parameters (platelet count, coagulation studies) may be indicated, especially in recurrent cases

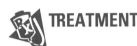 ## TREATMENT

- Most cases of anterior epistaxis may be successfully treated by direct pressure on the bleeding site

MEDICATIONS

- Short-acting topical nasal decongestants (eg, phenylephrine, 0.125–1% solution, one or two sprays), which act as vasoconstrictors, may be helpful
- When the bleeding does not readily subside, the nose should be examined to locate the bleeding site: topical 4% cocaine (or a topical decongestant [eg, oxymetazoline] and a topical anesthetic [eg, tetracaine]) applied either as a spray or on a cotton strip serves as an anesthetic and as a vasoconstricting agent

SURGERY

Posterior nasal bleeding

- Ligation of the nasal arterial supply (internal maxillary artery and ethmoid arteries) is a possible alternative to posterior nasal packing
- Ligation of the external carotid artery may be necessary

THERAPEUTIC PROCEDURES

Anterior nasal bleeding

- Compress the nasal alae firmly for 5–15 min
- Venous pressure is reduced in the sitting position, and leaning forward lessens the swallowing of blood
- Cauterize the bleeding site with silver nitrate, diathermy, or electrocautery
- Usually anterior packing will suffice if the bleeding has not stopped
  - Use several feet of lubricated iodoform packing systematically placed in

the floor of the nose and then the vault of the nose
  - Alternatively, there are various manufactured products designed for nasal tamponade

Posterior nasal bleeding

- Placement of a pack to occlude the choana before placement of a pack anteriorly
- Opioid analgesics reduce the discomfort and elevated blood pressure caused by a posterior pack
- Endovascular embolization of the internal maxillary artery is an alternative to surgical ligation in life-threatening hemorrhage
- Apply nasal saline to keep packing moist
- Administer antistaphylococcal antibiotics to limit possibility of toxic shock syndrome during the > 5 days pack must stay in place

 ## OUTCOME

FOLLOW-UP

- After control of the epistaxis, avoid vigorous exercise for several days
- Avoid hot or spicy foods and tobacco because they may cause vasodilation
- Once the acute episode has passed, carefully examine the nose and paranasal sinuses to rule out neoplasia
- Follow-up investigation of possible hypertension

COMPLICATIONS

- Sinusitis
- Aspiration or asphyxiation by blood

PROGNOSIS

- Generally self-limited with a good prognosis

WHEN TO REFER

- Refer to an otolaryngologist for persistent or recurrent bleeding
- If expertise in cauterization or localization of the bleeding site is needed
- For posterior nasal packing

WHEN TO ADMIT

- Because placing a nasal pack for posterior nasal bleeding is uncomfortable and requires oxygen supplementation to prevent hypoxia, hospitalization for several days is indicated

PREVENTION

- Avoiding nasal trauma, including nose picking
- Lubrication with petroleum jelly or bacitracin ointment
- Increased home humidity

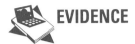 ## EVIDENCE

WEB SITES

- American Academy of Otolaryngology—Head and Neck Surgery: Management of Posterior Epistaxis Interactive Module
- Baylor College of Medicine Otolaryngology Resources

INFORMATION FOR PATIENTS

- American Academy of Family Physicians: Nosebleeds: What to Do When Your Nose Bleeds
- American Academy of Otolaryngology—Head and Neck Surgery: Nosebleeds
- MedlinePlus: Nosebleeds
  - MedlinePlus: Nosebleed Treatment

REFERENCES

- Klotz DA et al. Surgical management of posterior epistaxis: a changing paradigm. Laryngoscope. 2002 Sep; 112(9):1577–82. [PMID: 12352666]
- Randall DA. Epistaxis packing. Practical pointers for nosebleed control. Postgrad Med. 2006 Jun-Jul;119(1):77–82. [PMID: 16913650]
- Viehweg TL et al. Epistaxis: diagnosis and treatment. J Oral Maxillofac Surg. 2006 Mar;64(3):511–8. [PMID: 16487816]

Erectile Dysfunction

 ## KEY FEATURES

ESSENTIALS OF DIAGNOSIS

- Etiology is usually multifactorial
- Increasing incidence with older age
- Variety of treatment available, with multiple oral agents

GENERAL CONSIDERATIONS

- Consistent inability to maintain an erect penis with sufficient rigidity to allow sexual intercourse
- Loss of erections occurs from arterial, venous, neurogenic, or psychogenic causes
- Associated with concurrent medical problems (eg, diabetes mellitus), or radical pelvic or retroperitoneal surgery
- Antihypertensive medications
  - Centrally acting sympatholytics (methyldopa, clonidine, reserpine) can cause loss of erection
  - Vasodilators, α-blockers, and diuretics rarely do so
- Androgen deficiency causes both loss of libido and erections and lack of emission by decreasing prostatic and seminal vesicle secretions
- Loss of orgasm: if libido and erections are intact, usually of psychological origin
- Premature ejaculation
  - Anxiety related
  - Due to a new partner
  - Unreasonable expectations about performance
  - Emotional disorders
- Lack of emission (lack of antegrade seminal fluid during ejaculation) due to
  - Retrograde ejaculation or mechanical disruption of the bladder neck (eg, after transurethral resection of the prostate)
  - Androgen deficiency

DEMOGRAPHICS

- Affects 10 million American men; ~25% of men are > 65 years of age
- Most have an organic rather than psychogenic cause

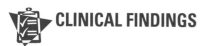 **CLINICAL FINDINGS**

SYMPTOMS AND SIGNS

- History: erectile dysfunction should be distinguished from problems with ejaculation, libido, and orgasm
- Degree of the dysfunction—chronic, occasional, or situational
- Timing of dysfunction
- Determine whether the patient ever has any normal erections, such as in early morning or during sleep
- Inquire about hyperlipidemia, hypertension, neurologic disease, diabetes mellitus, renal failure, adrenal and thyroid disorders, and depression
- Trauma to the pelvis, pelvic surgery, or peripheral vascular surgery
- Use of drugs, alcohol, tobacco, and recreational drugs
- Physical examination: secondary sexual characteristics
- Neurologic motor and sensory examination
- Peripheral vascular examination: palpation and quantification of lower extremity pulses
- Examination of genitalia, testicles, and prostate
- Evaluate for penile scarring, plaque formation (Peyronie's disease)

 DIAGNOSIS

LABORATORY TESTS

- Complete blood count
- Urinalysis
- Lipid profile
- Serum glucose, testosterone, luteinizing hormone/follicle-stimulating hormone (LH/FSH), and prolactin
- Serum testosterone and gonadotropin (LH/FSH) levels may help localize the site of disease

IMAGING STUDIES

- Diagnostic tests such as duplex ultrasound, penile cavernosography and pudendal arteriography can separate arterial from venous erectile dysfunction and help predict which patients may benefit from vascular surgery
- Cavernous arteries duplex ultrasound
  - If poor arterial inflow, perform pelvic arteriography before arterial reconstruction
  - If normal arterial inflow, probably venous leak
- Cavernosometry (measurement of flow required to maintain erection)
- Cavernosography (contrast study of the penis to determine site and extent of venous leak)

DIAGNOSTIC PROCEDURES

- Direct injection of vasoactive substances into the penis (prostaglandin E, papaverine, or a combination of drugs). Patients who respond with a rigid erection typically require no further vascular evaluation
- Nocturnal penile tumescence testing for frequency and rigidity in patients who fail to achieve an erection with injection of vasoactive substances

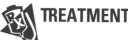 **TREATMENT**

MEDICATIONS

- Hormone replacement for documented androgen deficiency on endocrinologic evaluation, using testosterone injections (200 mg IM q3wks) or topical patches (2.5–10.0 mg/day), after prostate-specific antigen and digital rectal examination screening
- Alprostadil urethral suppository pellets (125, 250, 500, and 1000 mcg)
- PDE-5 inhibitors
  - Sildenafil, 50 mg; vardenafil, 5 mg; or tadalafil, 10 mg 1 h prior to anticipated sexual activity
  - Contraindicated in patients receiving nitrates
  - Some patients who do not respond to one PDE-5 inhibitor will respond to another

SURGERY

- Penile prosthesis: rigid, malleable, hinged, or inflatable
- Surgery for disorders of the arterial system
  - Vascular reconstruction
  - Endarterectomy and balloon dilation for proximal arterial occlusion
  - Arterial bypass procedures utilizing arterial (epigastric) or venous (deep dorsal vein) segments for distal occlusion
- Surgery for disorders of venous occlusion: ligation of certain veins (deep dorsal or emissary veins) or the crura of the corpora cavernosa

THERAPEUTIC PROCEDURES

- Vacuum constriction device: for patients with venous disorders of the penis and those who fail to achieve adequate erection with injection of vasoactive substances, use a vacuum device and rubber constriction band around proximal penis; complications are rare
- Behaviorally oriented sex therapy for men with no organic dysfunction

 OUTCOME

PROGNOSIS

- The majority of men suffering from erectile dysfunction can be managed successfully

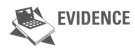

EVIDENCE

PRACTICE GUIDELINES

- Canadian Urological Association Guidelines Committee. Erectile dysfunction practice guidelines. Can J Urol. 2002;9:1583. [PMID: 12243654]
- Wespes E et al; European Association of Urology. Guidelines on erectile dysfunction. Eur Urol. 2002;41:1. [PMID: 11999460]

INFORMATION FOR PATIENTS

- Cleveland Clinic—Erectile dysfunction basics
- Mayo Clinic—Erectile dysfunction
- National Kidney and Urologic Diseases Information Clearinghouse

REFERENCES

- Basson R et al. Sexual sequelae of general medical disorders. Lancet. 2007 Feb 3;369(9559):409–24. [PMID: 17276781]
- Carson CC et al; Patient Response with Vardenafil in Sildenafil Non-Responders (PROVEN) Study Group. Erectile response with vardenafil in sildenafil nonresponders: a multicentre, double-blind, 12-week, flexible-dose, placebo-controlled erectile dysfunction clinical trial. BJU Int. 2004 Dec;94(9):1301–9. [PMID: 15610110]
- Lue TF. Erectile dysfunction. N Engl J Med. 2000 Jun 15;342(24):1802–13. [PMID: 10853004]
- Lue TF et al. Summary of recommendations on sexual dysfunctions in men. J Sex Med. 2004 Jul;1(1):6–23. [PMID: 16422979]
- Nehra A et al. Vardenafil improved patient satisfaction with erectile hardness, orgasmic function and sexual experience in men with erectile dysfunction following nerve sparing radical prostatectomy. J Urol. 2005 Jun; 173(6):2067–71. [PMID: 15879836]
- Seftel AD. Erectile dysfunction in the elderly: epidemiology, etiology and approaches to treatment. J Urol. 2003 Jun;169(6):1999–2007. [PMID: 12771705]

Erythema Multiforme

KEY FEATURES

ESSENTIALS OF DIAGNOSIS

- Sudden onset of symmetric erythematous skin lesions with history of recurrence
- May be macular, papular, urticarial, bullous, or purpuric
- "Target" lesions with clear centers and concentric erythematous rings or "iris" lesions may be noted in erythema multiforme (EM) minor; these are rare in drug-associated EM major (Stevens-Johnson syndrome)

GENERAL CONSIDERATIONS

- An acute inflammatory skin disease due to multiple causes
- EM is divided clinically into minor and major types based on the clinical findings
- ~90% of cases of EM minor follow outbreaks of herpes simplex
- **EM major** (Stevens-Johnson syndrome)
  – Toxicity and involvement of two or more mucosal surfaces (often oral and conjunctival)
  – Most often caused by drugs (sulfonamides, nonsteroidal anti-inflammatory drugs, and anticonvulsants)
  – Visceral involvement may occur, may be serious or even fatal
  – Main differential diagnosis is toxic epidermal necrolysis, and some regard this as a variant of the same disease
- EM may also present as recurring oral ulceration, with skin lesions present in only half of the cases, and is diagnosed by oral biopsy

CLINICAL FINDINGS

SYMPTOMS AND SIGNS

- EM major favors the trunk; EM minor on extensor surfaces, palms, soles, or mucous membranes
- Classic target lesion, most commonly seen in herpes-associated EM, consists of three concentric zones of color change, most often found acrally on the hands and feet

- Drug-associated EM is manifested by raised target-like lesions, with only two zones of color change and a central blister, or nondescript reddish or purpuric macules
- In EM major, mucous membrane ulcerations are present at two or more sites, causing pain on eating, swallowing, and urination
- Blisters are always worrisome and dictate the need for consultation

DIFFERENTIAL DIAGNOSIS

- EM minor: urticaria, drug eruption
  – Individual lesions of true urticaria itch, should come and go within 24 h, are usually responsive to antihistamines
- EM major in evolution
- Sweet's syndrome (acute febrile neutrophilic dermatosis)
- EM major
  – Paraneoplastic pemphigus
  – Pemphigus
  – Bullous pemphigoid
  – Bullous impetigo
  – Contact dermatitis
  – Dermatitis herpetiformis
  – Cicatricial pemphigoid
  – Linear IgA dermatosis
  – Pemphigus foliaceus
  – Porphyria cutanea tarda
  – Epidermolysis bullosa
  – Staphylococcus scalded skin syndrome
  – Herpes gestationis
  – Graft-versus-host disease

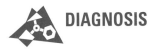

DIAGNOSIS

LABORATORY TESTS

- Blood tests are unhelpful

PROCEDURES

- Skin biopsy is diagnostic (direct immunofluorescence studies are negative)

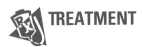

TREATMENT

MEDICATIONS

- See Table 150

EM major (Stevens-Johnson)

- No good data to support the use of corticosteroids, but they are still often prescribed
- If corticosteroids are to be tried in more severe cases, they should be used early, before blistering occurs, and in moderate to high doses (prednisone, 100–250 mg) and stopped within days if there is

no dramatic response; IGIV (0.75 g/kg/day for 4 days) has become standard treatment and can yield dramatic benefit if instituted early

- Oral and topical corticosteroids are useful in the oral variant of EM
- Antistaphylococcal antibiotics are used for secondary infection, which is uncommon
- Topical therapy is not very effective in this disease
- For oral lesions, 1% diphenhydramine elixir mixed with Kaopectate or with 1% dyclonine may be used as a mouth rinse several times daily

 OUTCOME

FOLLOW-UP

- Patients who begin to blister with EM major should be seen daily

COMPLICATIONS

- EM major
  - Extensive denudation, similar to an extensive burn
  - Corneal damage can result in permanent vision compromise and is the most frequent permanent sequela

PROGNOSIS

- EM major—visceral involvement may occur, may be serious or even fatal
- EM minor usually lasts 2–6 weeks and may recur
- Immediate discontinuation of the inciting medication (before blistering) improves prognosis and reduces risk of death

WHEN TO REFER

- Diagnosis or suspicion of EM major
- Consult ophthalmology early if the patient has any ocular symptoms or signs

WHEN TO ADMIT

- Patients need not be admitted unless mucosal involvement interferes with hydration and nutrition; extensive denudation of skin (> 30% BSA) is best treated in a burn unit

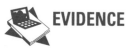 **EVIDENCE**

WEB SITES

- American Academy of Dermatology
- Dermatlas, Johns Hopkins University School of Medicine: Erythema Multiforme Images

INFORMATION FOR PATIENTS

- Mayo Clinic: Stevens-Johnson Syndrome
- MedlinePlus: Erythema Multiforme
- University of Maryland Medical Center: Erythema Multiforme

REFERENCES

- Faye O et al. Treatment of epidermal necrolysis with high-dose intravenous immunoglobulins (IV Ig): clinical experience to date. Drugs. 2005;65(15):2085–90. [PMID: 16225365]
- Fein JD et al. Images in clinical medicine. Stevens-Johnson syndrome. N Engl J Med. 2005 Apr 21;352(16):1696. [PMID: 15843672]
- Hynes AY et al. Controversy in the use of high-dose systemic steroids in the acute care of patients with Stevens-Johnson syndrome. Int Ophthalmol Clin. 2005 Fall;45(4):25–48. [PMID: 16199965]

Erythema Nodosum

 KEY FEATURES

ESSENTIALS OF DIAGNOSIS

- Painful red nodules without ulceration on anterior aspects of legs
- Slow regression over several weeks to resemble contusions
- Women are predominantly affected by a ratio of 4–8:1 over men
- Some cases associated with infection or drug sensitivity

GENERAL CONSIDERATIONS

- The disease may be associated with various infectious and noninfectious conditions
  - Infection: streptococcal, coccidioidomycosis, other fungal (eg, histoplasmosis, blastomycosis), tuberculosis, syphilis, *Yersinia enterocolitica*
  - Other: sarcoidosis, medications (eg, oral contraceptives), inflammatory bowel disease, pregnancy, lymphoma, or leukemia

 CLINICAL FINDINGS

SYMPTOMS AND SIGNS

- The swellings are exquisitely tender and may be preceded by fever, malaise, and arthralgia
- They are most often located on the anterior surfaces of the legs below the knees but may occur (rarely) on the arms, trunk, and face
- The lesions, 1–10 cm in diameter, are at first pink to red; with regression, all the various hues seen in a contusion can be observed

DIFFERENTIAL DIAGNOSIS

- Erythema induratum (associated with tuberculosis)
- Nodular vasculitis
- Erythema multiforme
- Lupus panniculitis
- Poststeroid panniculitis
- Contusions or bruises
- Sweet's syndrome (acute febrile neutrophilic dermatosis)
- Subcutaneous fat necrosis (associated with pancreatitis)

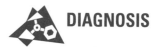 **DIAGNOSIS**

LABORATORY TESTS

- Evaluation of patients should include
  - Careful history and physical examination for prior upper respiratory infection or diarrheal illness
  - Symptoms of any deep fungal infection endemic to the area
  - Chest radiograph
  - Partial protein derivative (PPD)
  - Two consecutive ASO titers at 2- to 4-week intervals

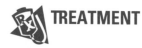 **TREATMENT**

MEDICATIONS

- See Table 150
- First identify and treat the underlying cause
- Primary therapy is with nonsteroidal anti-inflammatory drugs
- Saturated solution of potassium iodide, 5–15 drops TID, may result in prompt involution in many cases
- Systemic therapy directed against the lesions themselves may include use of corticosteroids unless contraindicated by associated infection

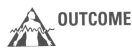

OUTCOME

PROGNOSIS

- It usually lasts about 6 weeks and may recur
- If no underlying cause is found, a significant underlying illness (usually sarcoidosis) will develop in only a small percentage of patients over the next year

WHEN TO REFER

- If there is a question about the diagnosis, if recommended therapy is ineffective, or specialized treatment is necessary

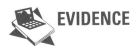

EVIDENCE

WEB SITES

- American Academy of Dermatology
- Dermatlas, Johns Hopkins University School of Medicine: Erythema Nodosum Images
- Requena L et al. Erythema Nodosum. Dermatology Online Journal

INFORMATION FOR PATIENTS

- American Osteopathic College of Dermatology: Erythema Nodosum
- MedlinePlus: Erythema Nodosum
- University of Maryland Medical Center: Erythema Nodosum

REFERENCES

- Campen RB et al. Case records of the Massachusetts General Hospital. Case 25-2006. A 41-year-old woman with painful subcutaneous nodules. N Engl J Med. 2006 Aug 17;355(7):714–22. [PMID: 16914708]
- Chew GY et al. Erythema induratum: a case of mistaken identity. Med J Aust. 2005 Nov 21;183(10):534. [PMID: 16296968]

Esophageal Cancer

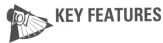

KEY FEATURES

ESSENTIALS OF DIAGNOSIS

- Progressive solid food dysphagia
- Weight loss

- Endoscopy with biopsy establishes diagnosis

GENERAL CONSIDERATIONS

- Two histologic types
  - Squamous cell carcinoma: occurs throughout esophagus; half occur in distal third
  - Adenocarcinoma: almost all occur in distal third of esophagus
- Squamous cell cancer risk factors
  - Chronic alcohol and tobacco use
  - Tylosis
  - Achalasia
  - Caustic-induced esophageal stricture
  - Other head and neck cancers
  - High incidence in certain regions of China, Southeast Asia
- Adenocarcinoma risk factors
  - Barrett's metaplasia due to chronic gastroesophageal reflux
  - Obesity

DEMOGRAPHICS

- Occurs usually in persons between 50 and 70 years of age
- Ratio of men to women is 3:1

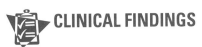

CLINICAL FINDINGS

SYMPTOMS AND SIGNS

- Solid food dysphagia (> 90%)
- Odynophagia
- Significant weight loss
- Coughing on swallowing or recurrent pneumonia suggests tracheoesophageal fistula from local tumor extension
- Chest or back pain mediastinal extension
- Hoarseness suggests recurrent laryngeal nerve involvement
- Physical examination often unrevealing
- Supraclavicular or cervical lymphadenopathy hepatomegaly suggests metastatic disease

DIFFERENTIAL DIAGNOSIS

- Peptic stricture
- Achalasia
- Adenocarcinoma of gastric cardia with esophageal involvement
- Esophageal web, ring (eg, Schatzki's), or diverticulum

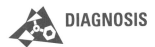

DIAGNOSIS

LABORATORY TESTS

- Anemia related to chronic disease or occult blood loss
- Elevated aminotransferase or alkaline phosphatase if hepatic metastases
- Hypoalbuminemia

IMAGING STUDIES

- Chest radiographs may show adenopathy
- Barium esophagogram
- CT of the chest and liver for evaluation of metastases, lymphadenopathy

DIAGNOSTIC PROCEDURES

- Upper endoscopy with biopsy
- Endoscopic ultrasonography with guided fine-needle aspiration (FNA) of lymph nodes is superior to CT for evaluating local extension and lymph node involvement
- TNM classification

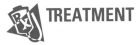

TREATMENT

MEDICATIONS

- Chemotherapy (cisplatin and fluorouracil) plus radiation therapy for patients with "curable" disease who are poor surgical candidates

SURGERY

- Surgery alone for stage I and stage IIA cancer; two options:
  - Transhiatal esophagectomy with anastomosis of the stomach to the cervical esophagus
  - Transthoracic excision of the esophagus with nodal resection; has higher perioperative morbidity and mortality but possible improved 5-year survival
- Surgery with neoadjuvant chemotherapy (cisplatin and fluorouracil) and radiation therapy for patients with stage IIB and stage IIIA cancer is used in some centers, though benefits of neoadjuvant therapy unproven

THERAPEUTIC PROCEDURES

- Palliative therapy for patients with extensive local tumor spread (T4) or distant metastases (M1), ie, most patients with stage IIIB and stage IV tumors
  - Radiation therapy
  - Peroral placement of expandable permanent wire stents

– Application of endoscopic laser therapy
– Photodynamic therapy
• Complications of stents, perforation, migration, and tumor ingrowth occur in 20–40%
• Photodynamic therapy
  – Uses a photosensitizing agent (porfimer sodium) in combination with low-power 630-nm laser irradiation delivered endoscopically
  – Side effects include skin photosensitivity for 4–6 weeks and esophageal stricture

OUTCOME

COMPLICATIONS

• Invasion of mediastinal structures
• Tracheoesophageal fistula

PROGNOSIS

• Overall 5-year survival rate is < 15%
• Most patients have advanced disease on presentation

WHEN TO REFER

• Dehydration due to dysphagia
• Palliative care

PREVENTION

• Adenocarcinoma: endoscopic surveillance every 3–5 years in patients with Barrett's esophagus to detect dysplasia, carcinoma
• Squamous cell carcinoma
  – Eliminate cigarettes
  – In endemic regions, endoscopic screening may be warranted

EVIDENCE

PRACTICE GUIDELINES

• Allum WH et al. Guidelines for the management of oesophageal and gastric cancer. Gut. 2002;50(9 Suppl 5):v1. [PMID: 12049068]
• American Gastroenterological Association Medical Position Statement: role of the gastroenterologist in the management of esophageal carcinoma. Gastroenterology. 2005;128:1468. [PMID: 15887128]
• Wong RK et al. Combined modality radiotherapy and chemotherapy in nonsurgical management of localized carcinoma of the esophagus: a practice guideline. Int J Radiat Oncol Biol Phys. 2003;55:930. [PMID: 12605971]

INFORMATION FOR PATIENTS

• Cleveland Clinic—Esophageal cancer
• National Cancer Institute

REFERENCES

• Cunningham D et al; MAGIC Trial Participants. Perioperative chemotherapy versus surgery for resectable gastroesophageal cancer. N Engl J Med. 2006 Jul 6;355(1):11–20. [PMID: 16822992]
• Malthaner RA et al. Preoperative chemotherapy for resectable thoracic esophageal cancer. Cochrane Database Rev. 2006 Jul 19;3:CD001556. [PMID: 16855972]
• Wang KK et al; American Gastroenterological Association. American Gastroenterological Association medical position statement: Role of the gastroenterologist in the management of esophageal carcinoma. Gastroenterology. 2005 May; 128(5):1468–70. [PMID: 15887128]
• Wang KK et al. American Gastroenterological Association Technical Review on the role of the gastroenterologist in the management of esophageal carcinoma. Gastroenterology. 2005 May; 128(5):1471–505. [PMID: 15887129]

Esophageal Varices

KEY FEATURES

ESSENTIALS OF DIAGNOSIS

• Dilated submucosal veins in patients with portal hypertension
• Develop in 50% of patients with cirrhosis
• Upper gastrointestinal bleeding develops in one-third

GENERAL CONSIDERATIONS

• Bleeding most commonly occurs in the distal 5 cm of the esophagus
• Approximately 50% of patients with cirrhosis have esophageal varices
• Serious bleeding develops in one-third of patients with varices

DEMOGRAPHICS

• Portal hypertension of any cause; most commonly due to cirrhosis

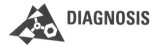

CLINICAL FINDINGS

SYMPTOMS AND SIGNS

• Acute gastrointestinal hemorrhage, usually severe, resulting in hypovolemia, postural vital signs, or shock

DIFFERENTIAL DIAGNOSIS

• Alcoholic gastritis
• Mallory-Weiss syndrome
• Portal hypertensive gastropathy
• Peptic ulcer disease
• Gastric or duodenal varices (rare)
• Vascular ectasias (angiodysplasias), eg, idiopathic arteriovenous malformation, CREST syndrome, hereditary hemorrhagic telangiectasia

DIAGNOSIS

LABORATORY TESTS

• Complete blood cell count, platelet count, prothrombin time, INR, type and cross-match
• Serum liver enzymes
• Creatinine, blood urea nitrogen

DIAGNOSTIC PROCEDURES

• Emergent upper endoscopy after the patient's hemodynamic status has been stabilized is diagnostic

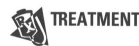

TREATMENT

MEDICATIONS

• Vasoactive agents
  – Octreotide infusion (50 mcg IV bolus followed by 50 mcg/h IV) reduces splanchnic and hepatic blood flow and portal pressures
  – Terlipressin (not available in the United States) causes significant reduction in portal and variceal pressures and, where available, may be preferred over octreotide
• Combined vasoactive agents and endoscopic therapy (band ligation or sclerotherapy)
  – Superior to either modality alone in controlling acute bleeding and early rebleeding
  – May improve survival

- Vitamin K subcutaneously
- Quinolone antibiotics (ciprofloxacin, 400 mg BID; levofloxacin, 500 mg once daily; or gatifloxacin, 400 mg once daily; either IV or PO) for 7–10 days reduce risk of serious infections from 50% to 10–20%
- Lactulose 30–45 mL/h PO until evacuation occurs, then reduced to 15–45 mL/h q8–12h as needed to promote 2–3 bowel movements daily for hepatic encephalopathy
- After bleeding stops, administer β-blockers to reduce portal pressure
  - Propranolol, 20–60 mg PO BID; long-acting propranolol, 60–80 mg PO once daily; or nadolol, 40 mg PO once daily
  - Gradually increase dosage until heart rate falls by 25% or reaches 55 beats/min

SURGERY

- Transvenous intrahepatic portosystemic shunt (TIPS) is indicated in the 5–10% of patients with acute variceal bleeding that cannot be controlled with pharmacologic and endoscopic therapy
- TIPS can control acute hemorrhage in > 90%; however, mortality approaches 40%, especially in an actively bleeding patient with renal insufficiency, bilirubin > 3.0 mg/dL, or requirement for ventilatory or blood pressure support
- TIPS reserved for patients who
  - Have recurrent (≥ 2) episodes of variceal bleeding who have failed endoscopic or pharmacologic therapies, and who have gastric varices or portal hypertensive gastropathy
  - Are noncompliant with other therapies
  - Live in remote locations (without access to emergency care)
- Emergency portosystemic shunt, eg, selective distal splenorenal shunt, surgery can decompress portal hypertension, but is associated with a 40–60% mortality rate, so seldom performed
- Liver transplantation

THERAPEUTIC PROCEDURES

- Initial management involves rapid assessment and acute resuscitation with fluids or blood products
- Transfusion of fresh frozen plasma or platelets to patients with INRs > 1.8–2.0 or platelet counts < 50,000/mcL in the presence of active bleeding
- Mechanical tamponade with nasogastric tubes containing large gastric and esophageal balloons (Minnesota or Sengstaken-Blakemore tubes)
  - Provides initial control of active variceal hemorrhage in 60–90% of patients
  - However, rebleeding occurs in 50%
- Acute endoscopic treatment with either banding or sclerotherapy
  - Either modality arrests active bleeding in 90% of patients
  - Although banding more widely used, sclerotherapy preferred by some endoscopists for actively bleeding patients (in whom visualization for banding may be difficult)
  - Reduces the chance of early recurrent bleeding by half (from 70% to 35%)
- Repeat banding at intervals of 1–2 weeks until the varices are obliterated or reduced to a small size
- Long-term treatment with banding achieves lower rates of rebleeding, complications, and death than sclerotherapy

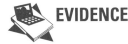

OUTCOME

FOLLOW-UP

- Stenosis and thrombosis of the TIPS occur in the majority over time with a consequent risk of rebleeding; monitor shunt periodically with Doppler ultrasonography or hepatic venography
- After obliteration of varices by endoscopic banding or sclerotherapy, repeat endoscopy every 6–12 months

COMPLICATIONS

- Encephalopathy occurs in 35% after TIPS
- Hepatic failure may occur after TIPS
- Sclerotherapy complications occur in 20–30% and include
  - Chest pain
  - Fever
  - Bacteremia
  - Esophageal ulceration, stricture, and perforation
- Complications of mechanical tamponade include
  - Esophageal and oral ulcerations
  - Perforation
  - Aspiration
  - Airway obstruction

PROGNOSIS

- Mortality rate within 2 weeks after an acute bleeding episode is 20%
- Mortality rate at 2 years is 60% due to recurrent bleeding or progression of chronic liver disease

WHEN TO ADMIT

- All patients with variceal hemorrhage

PREVENTION

- Risk of rebleeding is 50–70% without further therapy
- Long-term treatment with nonselective β-adrenergic blockers and/or band ligation reduces rebleeding to 20–50%
- Some but not all studies suggest a lower risk of rebleeding with band ligation than with nonselective β-adrenergic blockers (propranolol, nadolol)
- Compliant patients with well compensative liver disease may be optimal candidates for nonselective β-adrenergic blockers alone

EVIDENCE

PRACTICE GUIDELINES

- Quershi W et al. ASGE Guideline: the role of endoscopy in the management of variceal hemorrhage; updated July 2005. Gastrointest Endosc. 2005; 62:651. [PMID: 16244673]

WEB SITE

- WebPath Gastrointestinal Pathology Index

INFORMATION FOR PATIENTS

- American Academy of Family Physicians
- Cleveland Clinic—Variceal bleeding management procedures

REFERENCES

- Boyer T et al; American Association for the Study of Liver Diseases. The role of transjugular intrahepatic portosystemic shunt in the management of portal hypertension. Hepatology. 2005 Feb; 41(2):386–400. [PMID: 15660434]
- D'Amico G et al. Hepatic vein pressure gradient reduction and prevention of variceal bleeding in cirrhosis: a systematic review. Gastroenterology. 2006 Nov; 131(5):1611–24. [PMID: 17101332]
- De la Pena J et al. Variceal ligation plus nadolol compared with ligation for prophylaxis of variceal rebleeding: a multicenter trial. Hepatology. 2005 Mar; 41(3):572–8. [PMID: 15726659]
- Gotzsche PC et al. Somatostatin analogues for acute bleeding oesophageal varices. Cochrane Database Syst Rev. 2005 Jan 25;(1):CD000193. [PMID: 15674868]
- Jutabha R et al. Randomized study comparing banding and propranolol to

prevent initial variceal hemorrhage in cirrhotics with high-risk esophageal varices. Gastroenterology. 2005 Apr; 128(4):870–81. [PMID: 15825071]

- Khuroo MS et al. Meta-analysis: endoscopic variceal ligation for primary prophylaxis of oesophageal variceal bleeding. Aliment Pharmacol Ther. 2005 Feb 15; 21(4):347–61. [PMID: 15709985]
- Qureshi W et al; Standards of Practice Committee. ASGE Guideline: the role of endoscopy in the management of variceal hemorrhage, updated July 2005. Gastrointest Endosc. 2005 Nov; 62(5):651–5. [PMID: 16246673]
- Sarin SK et al. Endoscopic variceal ligation plus propranolol versus endoscopic variceal ligation alone in primary prophylaxis of variceal bleeding. Am J Gastroenterol. 2005 Apr;100(4):797–804. [PMID: 15784021]

Esophagitis, Pill-Induced

KEY FEATURES

- Various medications may injure the esophagus through direct, prolonged mucosal contact
- Most commonly implicated: alendronate, clindamycin, doxycycline, iron, NSAIDs, potassium chloride tablets, quinidine, risedronate, tetracycline, trimethoprim-sulfamethoxazole, vitamin C, zalcitabine, and zidovudine
- Injury is most likely to occur if pills are swallowed without water or while supine
- Hospitalized or bed-bound patients are at greater risk

CLINICAL FINDINGS

- Severe retrosternal chest pain
- Odynophagia
- Dysphagia

DIAGNOSIS

- Endoscopy reveals one or several discrete, shallow or deep ulcers
- Severe esophagitis with stricture, hemorrhage, or perforation

TREATMENT

- Prevention by instructing patients to take pills with 4 oz water and to remain upright for 30 minutes after ingestion
- Known offending agents should not be given to patients with esophageal dysmotility, dysphagia, or strictures

Eustachian Tube Dysfunction

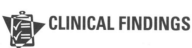

KEY FEATURES

ESSENTIALS OF DIAGNOSIS

- Aural fullness
- Fluctuating hearing
- Discomfort with barometric pressure change
- At risk for serous otitis media

GENERAL CONSIDERATIONS

- The tube that connects the middle ear to the nasopharynx—the eustachian tube—provides ventilation and drainage for the middle ear cleft
- The eustachian tube is normally closed, opening only during the act of swallowing or yawning

Hypofunctioning (narrowed) eustachian tube

- When eustachian tube function is compromised, air trapped within the middle ear becomes absorbed and negative pressure results
- The most common causes are diseases associated with edema of the tubal lining, such as viral upper respiratory tract infections and allergy

Overly patent (patulous) eustachian tube

- A relatively uncommon problem that may be quite distressing
- May develop during rapid weight loss or may be idiopathic

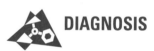

CLINICAL FINDINGS

SYMPTOMS AND SIGNS

Hypofunctioning eustachian tube

- Usually there is a sense of fullness in the ear and mild to moderate impairment of hearing

- When the tube is only partially blocked, swallowing or yawning may elicit a popping or crackling sound
- Examination reveals retraction of the tympanic membrane and decreased mobility on pneumatic otoscopy

Overly patent (patulous) eustachian tube

- Sensation of fullness in the ear
- Autophony, an exaggerated ability to hear oneself breathe and speak
- In contrast to a hypofunctioning eustachian tube, the aural pressure is often made worse by exertion and may diminish during an upper respiratory tract infection
- Although physical examination is usually normal, respiratory excursions of the tympanic membrane may occasionally be detected during vigorous breathing

DIFFERENTIAL DIAGNOSIS

- Cerumen impaction (ear wax)
- Acute or chronic otitis media
- Temporomandibular joint dysfunction
- Paget's disease
- Head trauma

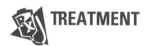

DIAGNOSIS

DIAGNOSTIC PROCEDURES

- Clinical diagnosis

TREATMENT

MEDICATIONS

Hypofunctioning eustachian tube

- Systemic and intranasal decongestants (eg, pseudoephedrine, 60 mg PO q4h; oxymetazoline, 0.05% spray q8–12h) combined with autoinflation by forced exhalation against closed nostrils may hasten relief
- Allergic patients may also benefit from desensitization or intranasal corticosteroids (eg, beclomethasone dipropionate, two sprays in each nostril BID for 2–6 weeks)

Overly patent (patulous) eustachian tube

- Avoidance of decongestant products

SURGERY

Hypofunctioning eustachian tube

- In medically refractory tube hypofunction, insertion of a tympanostomy tube is often helpful

Overly patent (patulous) eustachian tube

- Rarely, surgical narrowing of the eustachian tube is indicated, and the same is true of insertion of a ventilating tube to reduce the outward stretch of the ear drum during phonation

THERAPEUTIC PROCEDURES

- Autoinflation should not be recommended to patients with active intranasal infection, because this maneuver may precipitate middle ear infection

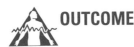

OUTCOME

PROGNOSIS

- Following a viral illness, this disorder is usually transient, lasting days to weeks

WHEN TO REFER

- Refer to an otolaryngologist if symptoms persist despite medical therapy or if there is persistent hearing loss

PREVENTION

- Avoid long-term decongestant use
- Avoid exacerbants of air travel, rapid altitudinal change, and underwater diving
- Control associated sinonasal disease

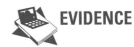

EVIDENCE

WEB SITE

- Baylor College of Medicine: Otolaryngology Resources

INFORMATION FOR PATIENTS

- MedlinePlus: Eustachian Tube Patency
- McKinley Health Center, University of Illinois: Eustachian Tube Dysfunction
- Vestibular Disorders Association: Inner Ear Anatomy

REFERENCES

- Grimmer JF et al. Update on Eustachian tube dysfunction and the patulous eustachian tube. Curr Opin Otolaryngol Head Neck Surg. 2005 Oct;13(5):277–82. [PMID: 16160520]
- Seibert JW et al. Eustachian tube function and the middle ear. Otolaryngol Clin North Am. 2006 Dec;39(6):1221–35. [PMID: 17097443]

Falls in Elderly

 KEY FEATURES

ESSENTIALS OF DIAGNOSIS

- Falls in older people are rarely due to a single cause
- Medications are a common and potentially reversible cause of falls in elders

GENERAL CONSIDERATIONS

Causes of falls

- Visual impairment
- Gait impairment due to
  - Podiatric disorder (ingrown nail, ulcer)
  - Arthritis
  - Muscular weakness (myopathy, deconditioning)
  - Sensory ataxia (diabetic neuropathy, vitamin B$_{12}$ deficiency)
  - Other neurologic disorders (parkinsonism, Alzheimer's disease, spinal stenosis, multiple sclerosis, cerebellar ataxia)
- Environmental hazards (poor lighting, stairs, rugs, uneven floors)
- Medications and polypharmacy (benzodiazepines, opioids, phenothiazines, antidepressants, diuretics)
- Alcohol
- Orthostatic or postprandial hypotension
- Vertigo, presyncope, syncope, or dysequilibrium
- Acute medical illness (pneumonia, myocardial infarction, anemia, hyponatremia)
- Other contributing factors
  - Urinary urgency
  - Peripheral edema
  - Insomnia
  - Footwear

DEMOGRAPHICS

- 30% of community-dwelling elderly fall each year, including 50% of people over age 80; of those who fall 25% have serious injuries
- About 5% of falls result in fracture
- 50% of those who fall are unable to get up without assistance
- Falls are the sixth leading cause of death for older people

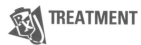 **CLINICAL FINDINGS**

SYMPTOMS AND SIGNS

Gait and balance tests

- "Up and Go Test"
  - Patient is asked to stand from a sitting position without using the hands, walk 10 feet, turn around, walk back, and sit down
  - Test performance is qualitative: normal vs abnormal
  - Patient should be timed during the test: 10–15 seconds is considered normal
  - Times longer than 20 seconds are often associated with other functional impairments
- Tinetti Gait and Balance Assessment
  - Includes aspects of both the "Up and Go Test" and Romberg test
  - Is most often used for formal testing
  - Evaluates step length, height, width, symmetry, and continuity
  - Evaluates steadiness with eyes closed and with gentle sternal nudge
  - Evaluates posture, sway, and use of mobility aids
- Romberg test
  - Is there steadiness when patient stands with eyes closed?
- When turning are steps continuous or discontinuous?
- Is balance maintained when the patient is pushed lightly on the sternum?

Vision

- A formal vision and eye examination should be considered a standard part of an assessment of elders who fall

 DIAGNOSIS

LABORATORY TESTS

- Laboratory and other diagnostic tests should be directed by the history and physical examination
- Most patients who fall should be assessed for osteoporosis risk

DIAGNOSTIC PROCEDURES

- Every older person should be asked about falls; many will not volunteer such information
- Review circumstances of falls, including associated symptoms, location, and exacerbating factors
- Review medications, including over-the-counter sleeping aids
- Review substance use history
- Ask about urinary symptoms
- Examine for postural hypotension
- Examine for peripheral edema
- Ask about vision

 TREATMENT

MEDICATIONS

- Eliminate all nonessential medications that can interfere with gait, cause somnolence or urinary urgency

THERAPEUTIC PROCEDURES

- Home safety check: generally reimbursed by third-party payers, including Medicare
- For patients with repeated falls, make available phones at floor level, a portable phone, or a lightweight radio call system
- Exercise programs
  - Resistance training and balance retraining reduced risk of falling
  - Tai Chi programs have also shown modest benefits
  - Physicial therapy can instruct in balance, strength, use of assistive devices, and getting up from the floor after a fall
- Use of an anatomically designed external hip protector reduces hip fracture risk in frail elders but is often poorly tolerated
- Evaluate for osteoporosis, and treat when present

OUTCOME

COMPLICATIONS

- Fractures, commonly of the wrist, hip, and vertebrae
- Loss of confidence and independence and self-restricted activity because of fear of repeated falls
- Nursing home placement
- Chronic subdural hematoma
  - Consider in an elderly patient who presents with new neurologic symptoms or signs, particularly obtundation
  - Headache is uncommon
- Dehydration, electrolyte imbalance, pressure sores, hypothermia, and rhabdomyolysis in patients who are unable to get up from a fall

PROGNOSIS

- Patients who fall are at high risk for subsequent falls
- Falls are associated with a higher risk of nursing home placement

There is a high mortality rate (approximately 20% in 1 year) in elderly women with hip fractures

WHEN TO REFER

- Refer for a home safety check any elderly individual with a history of falls or balance or gait abnormalities
- Consider referral to a physical therapist for gait assessment and training (how to get up from a fall and training with special devices)
- An interdisciplinary geriatrics assessment can be useful

PREVENTION

- It is likely that maintenance of physical activity and muscle strength will help prevent falls
- Remedy home hazards
- Evaluate gait and make interventions when abnormal
- Regular vision evaluation
- Evaluate for osteoporosis and treat when present
- Some evidence suggests that vitamin D (700–800 IU daily) and possibly calcium (1000 mg) will help prevent fractures

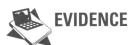 **EVIDENCE**

PRACTICE GUIDELINES

- American Geriatrics Society
- National Guideline Clearinghouse
  - University of Iowa Gerontologic Nursing Research Center, 2004

WEB SITES

- AARP Guide to Internet Resources on Aging
- Administration on Aging
- ACOVE

INFORMATION FOR PATIENTS

- American Academy of Family Physicians
- JAMA patient page. Fall-induced injuries. JAMA. 1999;281:1962. [PMID: 10349902]
- JAMA patient page. Hip fractures. JAMA. 2001;285:2814. [PMID: 11419423]

REFERENCES

- Bischoff-Ferrari HA et al. Effect of Vitamin D on falls: a meta-analysis. JAMA. 2004 Apr 28;291(16):1999–2006. [PMID: 15113819]

- Tinetti ME. Clinical practice. Preventing falls in elderly persons. N Engl J Med. 2003 Jan 2;348(1):42–9. [PMID: 12510042]

Familial Adenomatous Polyposis

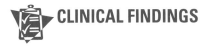 **KEY FEATURES**

ESSENTIALS OF DIAGNOSIS

- Hundreds to thousands of colorectal polyps evident on sigmoidoscopy or colonoscopy
- Mutation of adenomatous polyposis coli (*APC*) gene on 5q21 in 90% of affected patients; mutation in *MYH* present in some remaining patients

GENERAL CONSIDERATIONS

- Classic form of familial adenomatous polyposis (FAP) characterized by development of hundreds to thousands of colorectal polyps
- Other gastrointestinal tumors include
  - Benign gastric fundic gland polyps
  - Duodenal (especially periampullary) adenomas
  - Adenocarcinomas
- Extraintestinal manifestations include
  - Skin soft tissue tumors
  - Desmoid tumors
  - Osteomas
  - Congenital hypertrophy of retinal pigment
- Most commonly caused by autosomal dominant inheritance of mutation in *APC* gene; location of mutation affects number of polyps formed and extracolonic features
- An attenuated variant of FAP has been recognized in which an average of only 25 polyps (range of 0–500) develop
- FAP due to *MYH* mutation is inherited in an autosomal recessive fashion
- Mutations in the *MYH* gene have been identified in patients with classic and attenuated forms of FAP who do not have mutations of the *APC* gene

DEMOGRAPHICS

- Affects 1:10,000 people
- Accounts for 0.5% of colorectal cancers

- Colorectal polyps develop at mean age of 15 and cancers, by age 40
- Persons with FAP due to *MYH* mutation may have no family history of colorectal cancer
- Colorectal cancer inevitable by age 50 unless prophylactic colectomy performed

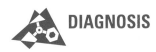 **CLINICAL FINDINGS**

SYMPTOMS AND SIGNS

- Iron deficiency anemia
- Hematochezia
- Obstipation due to obstructing colonic carcinoma
- Jaundice due to ampullary neoplasm or metastases to liver
- Weight loss if metastatic disease

DIFFERENTIAL DIAGNOSIS

- Sporadic colorectal cancer
- Inflammatory bowel disease with multiple inflammatory polyps
- Other nonadenomatous polyposis syndromes: Peutz-Jeghers syndrome, juvenile polyposis
- Hereditary nonpolyposis colorectal cancer also is an inherited autosomal dominant condition associated with early-onset colorectal cancer but few adenomatous polyps

DIAGNOSIS

IMAGING STUDIES

- No imaging necessary in most cases
- Abdominal CT for evaluation of colorectal cancer or periampullary neoplasms
- Endoscopic ultrasonography and endoscopic retrograde cholangiopancreatography (ERCP) for evaluation of periampullary neoplasms

DIAGNOSTIC PROCEDURES

- Genetic counseling followed by testing (*APC* and possibly *MYH*) of first-degree relatives of patients with FAP, preferably at age 10–12; a negative result is considered true negative only if one affected member has a positive result
- Genetic counseling followed by testing in patients with > 20–100 polyps (without family history) to detect de novo classic or attenuated FAP
- Endoscopic screening beginning at age 12 for family members with *APC* muta-

tion or for all family members, when known mutation not identified

- Classic FAP: sigmoidoscopy every year
- Attenuated FAP: colonoscopy every 2 years
- Upper endoscopy to look for periampullary tumors every 1–3 years, beginning at age 25

TREATMENT
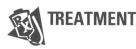

MEDICATIONS

- Nonsteroidal anti-inflammatory drugs (NSAIDs), including sulindac 150 mg PO BID and celecoxib 400 mg PO BID, prevent or induce regression of polyps in duodenum and rectum (after subtotal colectomy)

SURGERY

- Complete proctocolectomy with ileoanal pouch anastamosis or subtotal colectomy with ileorectal anastamosis is recommended after the development of polyposis, usually before age 20
- Ileorectal anastamosis affords superior bowel function but has 10% risk of rectal cancer
- Duodenal resection for patients with multiple or large periampullary adenomas, especially with dysplasia

THERAPEUTIC PROCEDURES

- For patients with retained rectum, sigmoidoscopy for surveillance and fulguration of polyps recommended every 6 months
- Endoscopic biopsy, removal, or fulguration of duodenal polyps and selected ampullary adenomas

OUTCOME
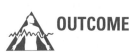

FOLLOW-UP

- For patients with subtotal colectomy, surveillance sigmoidoscopy every 6 months

COMPLICATIONS

- Desmoid tumors (mesenteric fibrosis) develop in some kindreds (especially after surgery) causing obstruction and constriction of the intestines, mesenteric circulation, and ureters; these tumors cause death in > 10%

PROGNOSIS

- For patients with ileorectal anastamosis, completion proctectomy is required in 10–20% due to development of rectal cancer
- Duodenal cancer occurs in 5–10%

WHEN TO REFER

- Genetic counseling and testing should be performed by trained counselor or geneticist
- Ileoanal pouch should be performed by colorectal surgeon
- Surveillance of rectal pouch and duodenum should be performed by therapeutic gastroenterologist
- Patients with desmoid tumors

EVIDENCE

PRACTICE GUIDELINES

- American Gastroenterological Association Technical Review. Hereditary colorectal cancer and genetic testing. Gastroenterology. 2001;121:198. [PMID: 11438509]

WEB SITES

- Cleveland Clinic Inherited Colorectal Cancer Registries
- Johns Hopkins Medical Institution Gastroenterology & Hepatology Resource Center

INFORMATION FOR PATIENTS

- Johns Hopkins Guide for Patients and Families: Familial Adenomatous Polyposis
- National Library of Medicine Genetics Home Reference: Familial adenomatous polyposis

REFERENCES

- Burt R et al. Genetic testing for inherited colon cancer. Gastroenterology. 2005 May;128(6):1696–716. [PMID: 15887160]
- Galiatsatos P et al. Familial adenomatous polyposis. Am J Gastroenterol. 2006 Feb;101(2):385–98. [PMID: 16454848]
- Maple JT et al. Genetics of colonic polyposis. Clin Gastroenterol Hepatol. 2006 Jul;4(7):831–5. [PMID: 16797242]

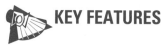

Fatty Liver Disease, Nonalcoholic

KEY FEATURES

ESSENTIALS OF DIAGNOSIS

- Often asymptomatic
- Elevated aminotransferase levels and/or hepatomegaly
- Macrovesicular or microvesicular steatosis, or both on liver biopsy

GENERAL CONSIDERATIONS

Nonalcoholic fatty liver disease (NAFLD)

- Besides ethanol, hepatic macrovascular steatosis can be caused by obesity, diabetes mellitus, and hypertriglyceridemia
- These features are a hallmark of the insulin resistance (metabolic) syndrome

Nonalcoholic steatohepatitis (NASH)

- Results from progression of macrovascular steatosis to steatohepatitis and fibrosis
- Characterized histologically by macrovesicular steatosis of NAFLD with
  - Focal infiltration by polymorphonuclear neutrophils
  - Mallory's hyalin
  - Histologic features are indistinguishable from alcoholic hepatitis

Other causes of fatty liver disease

- Cushing's syndrome
- Starvation or rapid weight loss
- Hypobetalipoproteinemia
- Obstructive sleep apnea
- Total parenteral nutrition
- Corticosteroids, amiodarone, tamoxifen, irinotecan, oxaliplatin
- Wilson's disease
- Jejunoileal bypass
- Poisons: carbon tetrachloride, yellow phosphorus

Causes of microvesicular steatosis

- Reye's syndrome, valproic acid toxicity, tetracycline, acute fatty liver of pregnancy
- Women in whom fatty liver of pregnancy develops often have a defect in fatty acid oxidation due to reduced long-chain 3-hydroxyacyl-CoA dehydrogenase activity

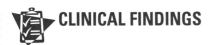

CLINICAL FINDINGS

SYMPTOMS AND SIGNS

- Hepatomegaly is present in 75% of patients with NASH, but the stigmata of chronic liver disease are uncommon

DIFFERENTIAL DIAGNOSIS

- Alcoholic fatty liver disease
- Hepatitis, eg, viral, alcoholic, toxic
- Cirrhosis
- Congestive heart failure
- Hepatocellular carcinoma or metastatic cancer

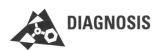

DIAGNOSIS

LABORATORY TESTS

- There may be mildly elevated aminotransferase and alkaline phosphatase levels
- In contrast to alcoholic liver disease,
  - Ratio of alanine aminotransferase (ALT) to aspartate aminotransferase (AST) is almost always > 1 in NASH
  - However, it decreases to < 1 as advanced fibrosis and cirrhosis develop

IMAGING STUDIES

- Fat in liver may be demonstrated on ultrasound, CT, or MRI
- These imaging methods are insensitive for detecting inflammation and fibrosis

DIAGNOSTIC PROCEDURES

- Percutaneous liver biopsy
  - Diagnostic
  - Only way to assess the degree of inflammation and fibrosis
  - Risks of the procedure must be balanced against the impact of the added information on management decisions and assessment of prognosis

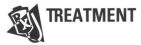

TREATMENT

MEDICATIONS

- Metformin, thiazolidinediones, vitamin E, orlistat, betaine, and recombinant human leptin may reverse fatty liver and are under study
- Supplemental choline may reverse fatty liver associated with total parenteral nutrition
- Ursodeoxycholic acid, 12–15 mg/kg/day, has not consistently resulted in biochemical and histologic improvement

SURGERY

- Gastric bypass may be considered in patients with a body mass index > 35 kg/m^2

THERAPEUTIC PROCEDURES

- Fatty liver is readily reversible with discontinuation of alcohol or treatment of other underlying conditions
- Weight loss, dietary fat restriction, and exercise can often improve liver tests and steatosis in obese patients with fatty liver

OUTCOME

COMPLICATIONS

- Risk factors for advanced hepatic fibrosis and cirrhosis
  - Older age
  - Obesity
  - Diabetes

PROGNOSIS

- NASH may be associated with hepatic fibrosis in 40% of cases; cirrhosis develops in 9–25%; and decompensated cirrhosis occurs in 30–50% of patients over 10 years
- Hepatocellular carcinoma in cirrhosis caused by NASH can occur
- NASH may account for many cases of cryptogenic cirrhosis and can recur following liver transplantation
- Mortality in patients with fatty liver is more likely to result from malignancy or ischemic heart disease than from liver disease

WHEN TO REFER

- For progressive liver diasease
- For liver biopsy

PREVENTION

- Avoid alcohol
- Maintain ideal weight
- Exercise
- Avoid hypertriglyceridemia

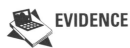

EVIDENCE

PRACTICE GUIDELINES

- National Guideline Clearinghouse

WEB SITES

- Diseases of the Liver
- Pathology Index

INFORMATION FOR PATIENTS

- American Liver Foundation
- Mayo Clinic
- Patient Information

REFERENCES

- Belfort R et al. A placebo-controlled trial of pioglitazone in subjects with nonalcoholic steatohepatitis. N Engl J Med. 2006 Nov 30;355(22):2297–307. [PMID: 17135584]
- Comar KM et al. Review article: drug therapy for non-alcoholic fatty liver disease. Aliment Pharmacol Ther. 2006 Jan 15;23(2):207–15. [PMID: 16393299]
- Dufour JF et al. Randomized placebo-controlled trial of ursodeoxycholic acid with vitamin E in nonalcoholic steatohepatitis. Clin Gastroenterol Hepatol. 2006 Dec;4(12):1537–43. [PMID: 17162245]

Fever

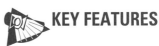

KEY FEATURES

ESSENTIALS OF DIAGNOSIS

- Localizing symptoms
- Weight loss
- Joint pain
- Injection substance use
- Immunosuppression or neutropenia
- History of cancer
- Travel

GENERAL CONSIDERATIONS

- Fever is a regulated rise to a new "set point" of body temperature mediated by pyrogenic cytokines
- The fever pattern is of marginal value, except for the relapsing fever of malaria, borreliosis, and lymphoma, especially Hodgkin's disease
- Most febrile illnesses are
  - Due to common infections
  - Short lived
  - Relatively easy to diagnose
- The term FUO ("fever of undetermined origin") refers to cases of unexplained fever exceeding 38.3°C on several occasions for at least 3 weeks in patients without neutropenia or immunosuppression

- In HIV-infected individuals, prolonged unexplained fever is usually due to infections
  - Disseminated *Mycobacterium avium*
  - *Pneumocystis jiroveci*
  - Cytomegalovirus
  - Disseminated histoplasmosis
- Lymphoma is another common cause of prolonged FUO in HIV-infected persons
- In the returned traveler, consider
  - Malaria
  - Dysentery
  - Hepatitis
  - Dengue fever

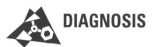 **CLINICAL FINDINGS**

SYMPTOMS AND SIGNS

- Fever is defined as an elevated body temperature exceeding 38.3°C
- The average normal oral body temperature taken in mid morning is 36.7°C (range 36.0–37.4°C)
- The normal rectal or vaginal temperature is 0.5°C higher; the axillary temperature is 0.5°C lower
- Rectal is more reliable than oral temperature, particularly in mouth breathers or in tachypneic states
- The normal diurnal temperature variation is 0.5–1.0°C—lowest in the early morning and highest in the evening
- There is a slight sustained temperature rise following ovulation, during the menstrual cycle, and in the first trimester of pregnancy

DIFFERENTIAL DIAGNOSIS

Common causes
- Infections
  - Bacterial
  - Viral
  - Rickettsial
  - Fungal
  - Parasitic
- Autoimmune diseases
- Central nervous system diseases
  - Head trauma
  - Mass lesions
- Malignant disease
  - Renal cell carcinoma
  - Primary or metastatic liver cancer
  - Leukemia
  - Lymphoma
- Cardiovascular diseases
  - Myocardial infarction
  - Thrombophlebitis
  - Pulmonary embolism

- Gastrointestinal diseases
  - Inflammatory bowel disease
  - Alcoholic hepatitis
  - Granulomatous hepatitis
- Miscellaneous diseases
  - Drug fever
  - Sarcoidosis
  - Familial Mediterranean fever
  - Tissue injury
  - Hematoma
  - Factitious fever

Hyperthermia
- Peripheral thermoregulatory disorders
  - Heat stroke
  - Malignant hyperthermia of anesthesia
  - Malignant neuroleptic syndrome

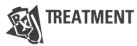 **DIAGNOSIS**

LABORATORY TESTS

- Complete blood cell count with differential
- Urinalysis
- Erythrocyte sedimentation rate (ESR) or C-reactive protein level
- Liver tests (alkaline phosphatase, aspartate aminotransferase, gamma-glutamyl transpeptidase, total bilirubin)
- Blood and urine cultures

IMAGING STUDIES

- Chest radiograph
- Abdominal ultrasound and CT scan
- Radionuclide-labeled leukocyte, gallium-67, and radiolabeled human immunoglobulin tests

DIAGNOSTIC PROCEDURES

- Temporal artery biopsy in patients aged ≥ 60 with elevated ESR

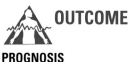 **TREATMENT**

MEDICATIONS

- Antipyretic therapy with aspirin or acetaminophen, 325–650 mg PO q4h
- After obtaining blood and urine cultures, empiric broad-spectrum antibiotic therapy is indicated in patients
  - Who are likely to have a clinically significant infection
  - Who are clinically unstable
  - Who have hemodynamic instability
  - Who have neutropenia (neutrophils < 500/mcL)
  - Who are asplenic (from surgery or sickle cell disease)

  - Who are immunosuppressed (including persons taking systemic corticosteroids, azathioprine, cyclosporine, or other immunosuppressive medications, and those who are HIV infected)
- If a fungal infection is suspected, add fluconazole or amphotericin B

THERAPEUTIC PROCEDURES

- Most fever is well tolerated
- When temperature is < 40°C, symptomatic treatment
- When temperature is > 41°C, emergent management of hyperthermia is indicated
  - Alcohol sponges
  - Cold sponges
  - Ice bags
  - Ice-water enemas
  - Ice baths

OUTCOME

PROGNOSIS

- After extensive evaluation
  - 25% of patients with FUO have chronic or indolent infection
  - 25% have autoimmune disease
  - 10% have malignancy
  - The remainder have miscellaneous other disorders or no definitive diagnosis
- Long-term follow-up of patients with initially undiagnosed FUO demonstrates that
  - 50% become symptom-free during evaluation
  - 20% reach a definitive diagnosis (usually within 2 months)
  - 30% have persistent or recurring fever for months or years

WHEN TO REFER

- When patients have prolonged unexplained fever, including FUO, refer to infectious disease expert

WHEN TO ADMIT

- Admit for empiric broad-spectrum antibiotic therapy patients who
  - Are likely to have a clinically significant infection
  - Are clinically unstable
  - Have hemodynamic instability
  - Have neutropenia
  - Are asplenic
  - Are immunosuppressed

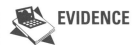

EVIDENCE

PRACTICE GUIDELINES

- Wade JC et al. NCCN Fever and Neutropenia Practice Guidelines Panel. NCCN: Fever and neutropenia. Cancer Control. 2001;8(6 Suppl 2):16. [PMID: 11760554]

WEB SITES

- Centers for Disease Control and Prevention
- National Institute of Allergy and Infectious Diseases/National Institutes of Health
- World Health Organization

INFORMATION FOR PATIENTS

- Mayo Clinic: Fever
- MedlinePlus: Fever

REFERENCES

- Roth AR et al. Approach to the adult patient with fever of unknown origin. Am Fam Physician. 2003 Dec 1; 68(11):2223–8. [PMID: 14677667]
- Rusyniak DE et al. Toxin-induced hyperthermic syndromes. Med Clin North Am. 2005 Nov;89(6):1277–96. [PMID: 16227063]
- Vanderschueren S et al. From prolonged febrile illness to fever of unknown origin: the challenge continues. Arch Intern Med. 2003 May 12;163(9):1033–41. [PMID: 12742800]
- Watson JT et al. Clinical characteristics and functional outcomes of West Nile fever. Ann Intern Med. 2004 Sep 7; 141(5):360–5. [PMID: 15353427]
- Woolery WA et al. Fever of unknown origin: keys to determining the etiology in older patients. Geriatrics. 2004 Oct; 59(10):41–5. [PMID: 15508555]

Fever of Unknown Origin (FUO)

 KEY FEATURES

ESSENTIALS OF DIAGNOSIS

- At least 3 weeks of illness with fever > 38.3°C on several occasions, and no diagnosis after 3 outpatient visits or 3 days of hospitalization
- **Hospital-associated FUO**
  - Occurs in a hospitalized patient with fever of ≥ 38.3°C on several occasions, due to a process not present or incubating at admission, in whom initial cultures are negative
  - Diagnosis remains unknown after 3 days of investigation
- **Neutropenic FUO**
  - Fever of ≥ 38.3°C in a patient on several occasions with < 500 neutrophils per microliter in whom initial cultures are negative
  - Diagnosis remains uncertain after 3 days
- **HIV-associated FUO**
  - Occurs in HIV-positive patients with fever of ≥ 38.3°C who have been febrile for 4 weeks or more as an outpatient or 3 days as an inpatient
  - Diagnosis remains uncertain after 3 days of investigation with at least 2 days for cultures to incubate
- Although not usually considered separately, **FUO in solid organ transplant** recipients is a common scenario with a unique differential diagnosis (see below)

GENERAL CONSIDERATIONS

Common causes

- Most cases represent unusual manifestations of common diseases and not rare or exotic diseases—eg, tuberculosis and HIV (primary infection or opportunistic infection) are more common causes than Whipple's disease
- A thorough history—including family, occupational, social (sexual practices, use of injection drugs), dietary (unpasteurized products, raw meat), exposures (animals, chemicals), and travel—may give clues to the diagnosis

Age of patient

- Infections (25–40% of cases) and cancer (25–40% of cases) account for the majority of FUOs
- In the elderly (> 65 years of age), 25–30% of all FUOs are due to multisystem immune-mediated diseases such as temporal arteritis, polymyalgia rheumatica, sarcoidosis, rheumatoid arthritis, Wegener's granulomatosis

Duration of fever

- Granulomatous diseases (granulomatous hepatitis, Crohn's disease, ulcerative colitis) and factitious fever are more likely if fever has been present for ≥ 6 months
- One-fourth of patients who report being febrile for ≥ 6 months have no true fever. Instead, the usual normal circadian variation in temperature (temperature 0.5–1.0°C higher in the afternoon than in the morning) is interpreted as abnormal
- Episodic or recurrent fever patients who meet the criteria for FUO but have fever-free periods of 2 weeks or longer are similar to those with prolonged fever
  - Infection, malignancy, and autoimmune disorders account for 20–25% of such fevers, whereas other diseases (Crohn's disease, familial Mediterranean fever, allergic alveolitis) account for another 25%
  - ~50% remain undiagnosed but have a benign course with eventual resolution of symptoms

Immunologic status

- In neutropenia, fungal infections and occult bacterial infection are important causes of FUO
- In organ transplant patients or others taking immunosuppressive medications, common causes of fever include
  - Cytomegalovirus (CMV) infections
  - Fungal infections
  - Nocardiosis
  - *Pneumocystis jiroveci* pneumonia
  - Mycobacterial infections
- Noninfectious causes, such as posttransplant lymphoproliferative disease, can also cause prolonged fever

Posttransplant

- Infections immediately after transplant often involve the transplanted organ
- After lung transplantation
  - Pneumonia
  - Mediastinitis
- After liver transplantation
  - Intra-abdominal abscess
  - Cholangitis
  - Peritonitis
- After renal transplantation
  - Urinary tract infections
  - Perinephric abscesses
  - Infected lymphoceles
- In contrast to solid organ transplants, in bone marrow transplant patients the source of fever cannot be found in 60–70% of patients
- Most infections that occur in the first 2–4 weeks are related either to
  - The operative procedure and to hospitalization itself (wound infection, IV catheter infection, urinary tract infection from a Foley catheter) or
  - The transplanted organ
- Infections that occur between the first and sixth months are often related to immunosuppression
  - Reactivated herpes simplex, varicella-zoster, and CMV infections are quite common

- Opportunistic infections with fungi (*Candida, Aspergillus, Cryptococcus, Pneumocystis,* and others), *Listeria monocytogenes, Nocardia,* and *Toxoplasma* are also common
- After 6 months, when immunosuppression has been reduced to maintenance levels, infections that are found in any population occur

Classification of causes of FUO

- Most patients with FUO will fit into one of five categories
  - Infection
  - Neoplasms
  - Autoimmune disorders
  - Miscellaneous causes
  - Undiagnosed FUO
- Despite extensive evaluation, the diagnosis remains elusive in 10–15% of patients
  - In about 75%, the fever abates spontaneously and the clinician never knows the cause
  - In the remainder, more classic manifestations of the underlying disease appear

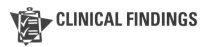 CLINICAL FINDINGS

SYMPTOMS AND SIGNS

- Document the fever in order to exclude factitious (self-induced) fever
- Tachycardia, chills, and piloerection generally accompany fever
- Repeated physical examination may reveal subtle, evanescent clinical findings, such as a rash

DIFFERENTIAL DIAGNOSIS

- **Infection**
  - Tuberculosis
  - Endocarditis
  - Osteomyelitis
  - Urinary tract infection
  - Sinusitis
  - Occult abscess (eg, intra-abdominal, dental, brain)
  - Cholangitis
  - Primary HIV
  - Epstein-Barr virus
  - CMV
  - Systemic mycosis
  - Toxoplasmosis
  - Brucellosis
  - Q fever
  - Cat scratch disease
  - Salmonellosis
  - Malaria
- **Neoplasm**
  - Hodgkin's and non-Hodgkin's lymphoma
  - Leukemia
  - Primary or metastatic liver cancer
  - Renal cell carcinoma
  - Atrial myxoma
  - Posttransplant lymphoproliferative disease
- **Autoimmune**
  - Adult Still's disease
  - Systemic lupus erythematosus
  - Cryoglobulinemia
  - Polyarteritis nodosa
  - Temporal (giant cell) arteritis
  - Polymyalgia rheumatica
  - Wegener's granulomatosis
- **Miscellaneous causes**
  - Drug fever
  - Sarcoidosis
  - Alcoholic or granulomatous hepatitis
  - Crohn's disease
  - Ulcerative colitis
  - Factitious fever
  - Thyroiditis
  - Hematoma
  - Recurrent pulmonary emboli
  - Hypersensitivity pneumonitis
  - Familial Mediterranean fever
  - Whipple's disease
  - Transplant rejection
  - Organ ischemia and necrosis
  - Thrombophlebitis

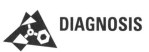 DIAGNOSIS

LABORATORY TESTS

- Perform culture on the following fluids preferably when antibiotics have not been taken for several days, and hold in the laboratory for 2 weeks to detect slow-growing organisms
  - Blood
  - Urine
  - Sputum
  - Stool
  - Cerebrospinal fluid
  - Morning gastric aspirates (if one suspects tuberculosis)
- Cultures on special media are requested for
  - *Legionella*
  - *Bartonella*
  - Nutritionally deficient streptococci
- "Screening tests" with immunologic or microbiologic serologies ("febrile agglutinins") are not useful
- A single elevated titer rarely is diagnostic of an infection; a fourfold rise or fall in titer confirms a specific cause
- Direct examination of blood smears may establish a diagnosis of malaria or relapsing fever (*Borrelia*)

IMAGING STUDIES

- Chest radiograph in all patients
- Use targeted studies (eg, sinus films, gallbladder studies) when symptoms, signs, or a history suggest disease in these body regions
- CT scan of the abdomen and pelvis is particularly useful for looking at the liver, spleen, and retroperitoneum
  - An abnormal CT scan often leads to a specific diagnosis
  - A normal CT scan is not quite as useful
- MRI is generally better than CT for lesions of the nervous system and is useful in diagnosing some vasculitides
- Ultrasound is sensitive for lesions of the kidney, pancreas, and biliary tree
- Radionuclide scans are not very helpful when used as screening tests
- A gallium or PET scan may be more helpful than an indium-labeled white blood cell scan because gallium and (18)fluorodeoxyglucose detect infection, inflammation, and neoplasm whereas indium is only useful for infection

DIAGNOSTIC PROCEDURES

- Echocardiography if endocarditis or atrial myxoma is being considered
- Transesophageal echocardiography is more sensitive than surface echocardiography for detecting valvular lesions
- Invasive procedures are often required for diagnosis
- Any abnormal finding should be aggressively evaluated
  - Headache calls for lumbar puncture
  - Skin from a rash should be biopsied
  - Enlarged lymph nodes should be aspirated or biopsied for cytology and culture
- Bone marrow aspiration with biopsy is a relatively low-yield procedure (except in HIV-positive patients, in whom mycobacterial infection is a common cause of FUO), but is low-risk and should be done if other less invasive tests have not yielded a diagnosis
- Liver biopsy will yield a specific diagnosis in 10–15% of FUO patients
- Consider laparotomy or laparoscopy in the deteriorating patient if the diagnosis is elusive despite extensive evaluation

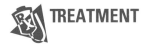

TREATMENT

MEDICATIONS

- Therapeutic trials are indicated if a diagnosis is strongly suspected—eg, antituberculous drugs
- However, if there is no clinical response in several weeks, it is imperative to stop therapy and reevaluate the patient
- In the seriously ill or rapidly deteriorating patient, empiric therapy is often given
- Antituberculosis medications (particularly in the elderly or foreign-born) and broad-spectrum antibiotics are reasonable in this setting (Table 63)
- Empiric administration of corticosteroids should be discouraged; they can suppress fever and exacerbate many infections that cause FUO

OUTCOME

WHEN TO REFER

- If patients remain symptomatic without a diagnosis after initial cultural and radiographic evaluation

WHEN TO ADMIT

- Patients who are clinically deteriorating with symptoms that are interfering with daily activity
- Progressive debilitating weight loss

EVIDENCE

PRACTICE GUIDELINES

- American Academy of Family Physicians
- Infectious Diseases Society of America
- Wade JC et al: NCCN Fever and Neutropenia Practice Guidelines Panel. NCCN: Fever and neutropenia. Cancer Control 2001;8(6 suppl 2):16. [PMID: 11760554]

INFORMATION FOR PATIENTS

- National Cancer Institute
- The National Institutes of Health

REFERENCES

- Bleeker-Rovers et al. A prospective multicenter study on fever of unknown origin: the yield of a structured diagnostic protocol. Medicine. 2007 Jan;86(1):26–38. [PMID: 17220753]
- Crispin JC et al. Adult-onset Still disease as the cause of fever of unknown origin. Medicine (Baltimore). 2005 Nov;84(6):331–7. [PMID: 16267408]
- Knockaert DC et al. Fever of unknown origin in adults: 40 years on. J Intern Med. 2003 Mar;253(3):263–75. [PMID: 12603493]
- Mourad O et al. A comprehensive evidence-based approach to fever of unknown origin. Arch Intern Med. 2003 Mar 10;163(5):545–51. [PMID: 12622601]
- Ozaras R et al. Is laparotomy necessary in the diagnosis of fever of unknown origin? Acta Chir Belg. 2005 Feb; 105(1):89–92. [PMID: 15790210]
- Woolery WA et al. Fever of unknown origin: keys to determining the etiology in older patients. Geriatrics. 2004 Oct; 59(10):41–5. [PMID: 15508555]
- Zernone T. Fever of unknown origin in adults: evaluation of 144 cases in a non-university hospital. Scand J Infect Dis. 2006;38(8):632–8. [PMID: 16857607]

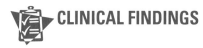

Fibrocystic Condition, Breast

KEY FEATURES

ESSENTIALS OF DIAGNOSIS

- Painful, often multiple bilateral masses of the breasts
- Pain and size often increase premenstrually

GENERAL CONSIDERATIONS

- Most frequent lesion of the breast
- Estrogen hormone is considered a causative factor
- Encompasses a wide variety of benign histologic changes
- Always associated with benign changes in the breast epithelium
- Microscopic findings include
  - Cysts (gross and microscopic)
  - Papillomatosis
  - Adenosis
  - Fibrosis
  - Ductal epithelial hyperplasia
- Risk factor for breast cancer only if ductal epithelial hyperplasia is present, especially when atypia is present

DEMOGRAPHICS

- Occurs most commonly in women age 30–50
- Rare in postmenopausal women not receiving hormonal replacement therapy

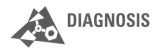

CLINICAL FINDINGS

SYMPTOMS AND SIGNS

- Generally painful mass or masses but may be asymptomatic
- Serous nipple discharge may be present
- Rapid fluctuation in size of masses is common

DIFFERENTIAL DIAGNOSIS

- Breast cancer
- Fibroadenoma
- Lipoma
- Breast abscess
- Intraductal papilloma

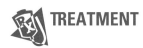

DIAGNOSIS

IMAGING STUDIES

- Mammography may be helpful but is often limited due to radiodensity of breast tissue in young women
- Breast ultrasonography is useful in differentiating cystic from solid mass

DIAGNOSTIC PROCEDURES

- Suspicious lesions should be biopsied
- Fine-needle aspiration cytology may be used, but if mass does not resolve over several months, it must be excised

TREATMENT

MEDICATIONS

- Gamolenic acid, 3 g PO BID
- Vitamin E, 400 IU PO once daily (anecdotal data)
- Danazol, 100–200 mg PO BID, for severe pain, but is rarely used due to side effects (acne, hirsutism, edema)
- Postmenopausal women receiving hormone replacement therapy may stop hormones to reduce pain

SURGERY

- Total or subcutaneous mastectomy or extensive removal of breast tissue is rarely, if ever, indicated for fibrocystic breast disease

THERAPEUTIC PROCEDURES

- Aspiration of a discrete mass suggestive of a cyst is indicated in order to alleviate pain and, more importantly, to confirm the cystic nature of the mass
- Diet
  - Low-fat diet or decreasing dietary fat intake may reduce painful symptoms
  - The role of caffeine consumption remains controversial
  - Many patients report relief of symptoms after giving up coffee, tea, and chocolate

 OUTCOME

FOLLOW-UP

- Reexamine at intervals
- Women with proliferative or atypical epithelium on biopsy should be monitored carefully by physical examination and mammography for development of breast cancer; consider tamoxifen chemoprevention
- The patient should be advised to examine her own breasts each month just after menstruation and to inform her physician if a mass appears
- Excisional biopsy should be performed
  - If no fluid is obtained or if fluid is bloody on aspiration
  - If a mass persists after aspiration
  - If at any time during follow-up a persistent lump is noted

COMPLICATIONS

- Risk of breast cancer in women with proliferative or atypical changes in the epithelium is higher than in women in general

PROGNOSIS

- Exacerbations of pain, tenderness, and cyst formation may occur at any time until menopause
- After menopause, symptoms usually subside, except in patients receiving hormone replacement therapy

PREVENTION

- Avoid trauma
- Avoid caffeine (anecdotal data)
- Wear supportive bra night and day

 EVIDENCE

PRACTICE GUIDELINES

- Heisey R et al. Management of palpable breast lumps. Consensus guideline for family physicians. Can Fam Physician. 1999;45:1926. [PMID: 10463093]

WEB SITE

- American Academy of Family Physicians: Breast Problems in Women Flowchart

INFORMATION FOR PATIENTS

- American College of Obstetricians and Gynecologists: Fibrocystic Breast Changes
- MedlinePlus: Fibrocystic Breast Disease
- National Cancer Institute: Understanding Breast Changes

REFERENCES

- Lucas JH et al. Breast cyst aspiration. Am Fam Physician. 2003 Nov 15; 68(10):1983–6. [PMID: 14655807]
- Morrow M. The evaluation of common breast problems. Am Fam Physician. 2000 Apr 15;61(8):2371–8. [PMID: 10794579]
- Olawaiye A et al. Mastalgia: a review of management. J Reprod Med. 2005 Dec; 50(12):933–9. [PMID: 16444894]
- Qureshi S et al. Topical nonsteroidal anti-inflammatory drugs versus oil of evening primrose in the treatment of mastalgia. Surgeon. 2005 Feb;3(1):7–10. [PMID: 15789786]
- Terry MB et al. Lifetime alcohol intake and breast cancer risk. Ann Epidemiol. 2006 Mar;16(3):230–40. [PMID: 16230024]

Fibromyalgia

 KEY FEATURES

- One of the most common rheumatic syndromes in ambulatory medicine
- Although many of the clinical features of the two conditions overlap, musculoskeletal pain predominates in fibromyalgia and lassitude dominates chronic fatigue syndrome
- Cause is unknown

 CLINICAL FINDINGS

- Chronic aching pain and stiffness, often involving the entire body but with prominence of pain around neck, shoulders, low back, and hips
- Fatigue, sleep disorders, subjective numbness, chronic headaches, and irritable bowel symptoms are common
- Physical examination is normal except for "trigger points" of pain produced by palpation of various areas such as
  - The trapezius
  - The medial fat pad of the knee
  - The lateral epicondyle of the elbow

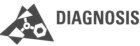 DIAGNOSIS

- Diagnosis of exclusion
- Thyroid function tests are useful because hypothyroidism can produce a secondary fibromyalgia syndrome
- Polymyositis produces weakness rather than pain
- Polymyalgia rheumatica
  - Produces shoulder and girdle pain
  - Is associated with an elevated sedimentation rate and anemia
  - Occurs after age 50

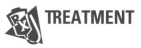 TREATMENT

- Patients can be comforted that they have a syndrome treatable by specific, though imperfect, therapies and that the course is not progressive
- Amitriptyline, fluoxetine, chlorpromazine, or cyclobenzaprine reduce symptoms in some patients
- Amitriptyline is initiated at a dosage of 10 mg PO at bedtime and gradually increased to 40–50 mg depending on efficacy and toxicity
- Exercise programs are also beneficial
- Opioids, NSAIDs, and corticosteroids are ineffective

Focal Segmental Glomerular Sclerosis

KEY FEATURES

- Idiopathic or secondary to heroin use, morbid obesity, HIV infection

CLINICAL FINDINGS

- Nephrotic syndrome
- Microscopic hematuria in 80%
- Hypertension
- Decreased renal function at diagnosis in 25–50%

DIAGNOSIS

- Renal biopsy
  - Light microscopy shows focal segmental glomerular sclerosis
  - Immunofluorescence shows IgM and C3
  - Electron microscopy shows fusion of epithelial foot processes

TREATMENT

- Nephrology consultation
- Prednisone, 1.0–1.5 mg/kg/day PO for up to 4 mo followed by a slow taper
- Remission in > 50% of patients, most within 5–9 mo
- Cytotoxic drug therapy produces remission in < 20% of those refractory to corticosteroids

Folic Acid Deficiency

KEY FEATURES

- Folic acid present in most fruits and vegetables (especially citrus fruits and green leafy vegetables)

- Daily requirements of 50–100 mcg/day usually met in the diet
- Total body stores of folate enough to supply requirements for 2–3 mo
- Most common cause of folate deficiency is inadequate dietary intake, which occurs in
  - Alcoholics
  - Anorectic patients
  - Persons who do not eat fresh fruits and vegetables
  - Those who overcook food
- Other causes
  - Decreased absorption (tropical sprue; drugs, eg, phenytoin, sulfasalazine, trimethoprim-sulfamethoxazole)
  - Increased requirement (chronic hemolytic anemia, pregnancy, exfoliative skin disease)
  - Loss (dialysis)
  - Inhibition of reduction to active form (methotrexate)

CLINICAL FINDINGS

- Megaloblastic anemia, which may be severe
- Glossitis and vague GI disturbances (eg, anorexia, diarrhea)
- No neurologic abnormalities, unlike vitamin B_{12} deficiency

DIAGNOSIS

- Megaloblastic anemia identical to that in vitamin B_{12} deficiency (eg, macro-ovalocytes, hypersegmented neutrophils (see Vitamin B_{12} Deficiency)
- Red blood cell folate level < 150 ng/mL
- Serum vitamin B_{12} level normal
- Distinguish from anemia of liver disease (macrocytic anemia with target cells but no megaloblastic changes)

TREATMENT

- Folic acid, 1 mg PO once daily, for patients with folate deficiency or increased folate requirements
- Rapid improvement in sense of well-being, reticulocytosis in 5–7 days, and total correction of hematologic abnormalities within 2 months

Folliculitis

KEY FEATURES

ESSENTIALS OF DIAGNOSIS

- Itching and burning in hairy areas
- Pustules in the hair follicles

GENERAL CONSIDERATIONS

- May be more common in diabetic persons
- Multiple types
  - Bacterial (usually staphylococcal)
  - Sycosis (chronic on head and neck)
  - Gram-negative (eg, if on antibiotics for acne)
  - Hot tub folliculitis
  - Herpes folliculitis
  - Due to oils, occlusion, perspiration, or rubbing
  - *Malassezia furfur* (on back) "steroid acne"
  - Eosinophilic folliculitis (in AIDS)
- **Gram-negative folliculitis**
  - *Klebsiella*
  - *Enterobacter*
  - *Escherichia coli*
  - *Proteus*
- **"Hot tub folliculitis"**
  - Caused by *Pseudomonas aeruginosa*
- **Nonbacterial folliculitis**
  - May be caused by oils that are irritating to the follicle
  - May be encountered in the workplace (machinists) or at home (various cosmetics and cocoa butter or coconut oils)
- Folliculitis may also be caused by occlusion, perspiration, and rubbing, such as that resulting from tight jeans and other heavy fabrics on the upper legs
- **Eosinophilic folliculitis**
  - A form of sterile folliculitis
- **Pseudofolliculitis**
  - Caused by ingrowing hairs in the beard area
  - It may be treated by growing a beard, by using chemical depilatories, or by shaving with a foil-guard razor
  - Laser hair removal is dramatically beneficial in patients with pseudofolliculitis, requires limited maintenance, and can be done on patients of any skin color
  - Pseudofolliculitis is a true medical indication for such a procedure and should not be considered cosmetic

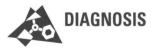 **CLINICAL FINDINGS**

SYMPTOMS AND SIGNS

- The symptoms range from slight burning and tenderness to intense itching
- The lesions consist of pustules of hair follicles
- **Sycosis**
  - Deep-seated, chronic, recalcitrant lesion on the head and neck
- **Gram-negative folliculitis**
  - May develop during antibiotic treatment of acne
  - May present as a flare of acne pustules or nodules
- **"Hot tub folliculitis"**
  - Characterized by pruritic or tender follicular or pustular lesions occurring within 1–4 days after bathing in a hot tub, whirlpool, or public swimming pool
  - Rarely, systemic infections may result
- Folliculitis on the back that looks like acne but does not respond to acne therapy may be caused by the yeast *M furfur*; this infection may require biopsy for diagnosis
- Folliculitis—so-called steroid acne— may be seen during topical or systemic corticosteroid therapy
- **Eosinophilic folliculitis**
  - Consisting of urticarial papules with prominent eosinophilic infiltration
  - Common in patients with AIDS
- **Pseudofolliculitis**
  - Caused by ingrowing hairs in the beard area
  - In this entity, the papules and pustules are located at the side of and not in follicles

DIFFERENTIAL DIAGNOSIS

- Acne vulgaris
- Miliaria (heat rash)
- Impetigo
- Tinea
- Pseudofolliculitis barbae (ingrown beard hairs)
- Hidradenitis suppurativa

 DIAGNOSIS

LABORATORY TESTS

- Clinical diagnosis

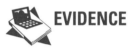 **TREATMENT**

MEDICATIONS

- See Table 150

Local measures

- Anhydrous ethyl alcohol containing 6.25% aluminum chloride (Xerac AC), applied to lesions and environs, may be helpful, especially for chronic folliculitis of the buttocks

Specific measures

- Systemic antibiotics may be tried if the skin infection is resistant to local treatment, if it is extensive or severe and accompanied by a febrile reaction, if it is complicated, or if it involves the nose or upper lip
- Extended periods of treatment (4–8 weeks or more) with antistaphylococcal antibiotics are required in some cases
- Hot tub *Pseudomonas* folliculitis virtually always resolves without treatment but may be treated with ciprofloxacin, 500 mg PO BID for 5 days
- Gram-negative folliculitis in acne patients may be treated with isotretinoin in compliance with all precautions for that medication
- Folliculitis due to *M furfur* is treated with topical 2.5% selenium sulfide, 15 min daily for 3 weeks, or with ketoconazole, 200 mg PO once daily for 7–14 days
- Eosinophilic folliculitis
  - May be treated initially by the combination of potent topical corticosteroids and oral antihistamines
  - In more severe cases, treatment is with one of the following
    - Topical permethrin (application for 12 h every other night for 6 weeks)
    - Itraconazole, 200–400 mg daily
    - UVB or PUVA phototherapy
    - Isotretinoin, 0.5 mg/kg/day for up to 5 months
  - A remission may be induced by some of these therapies, but long-term treatment may be required

OUTCOME

COMPLICATIONS

- Abscess formation is the major complication of bacterial folliculitis

PROGNOSIS

- Bacterial folliculitis is occasionally stubborn and persistent, requiring prolonged or intermittent courses of antibiotics
- Steroid folliculitis is treatable by acne therapy and resolves as corticosteroids are discontinued

WHEN TO REFER

- If there is a question about the diagnosis, if recommended therapy is ineffective, or if specialized treatment is necessary

PREVENTION

- Correct any predisposing local causes (eg, irritations of a mechanical or chemical nature)
- Control of blood glucose in diabetes may reduce the number of these infections; be sure that the water in hot tubs and spas is treated properly
- If staphylococcal folliculitis is persistent, treatment of nasal or perineal carriage with rifampin, 600 mg daily for 5 days, or with topical mupirocin ointment 2% twice daily for 5 days, may help
- Chronic oral clindamycin, 150–300 mg/day, is also effective in preventing recurrent staphylococcal folliculitis and furunculosis

EVIDENCE

WEB SITES

- American Academy of Dermatology
- Dermatlas, Johns Hopkins University School of Medicine: Folliculitis Images

INFORMATION FOR PATIENTS

- American Academy of Family Physicians: *Staphylococcus aureus* Infections
- Mayo Clinic: Folliculitis
- MedlinePlus: Folliculitis
- MedlinePlus: Hot Tub Folliculitis

REFERENCE

- Rajendran PM et al. Eosinophilic folliculitis: before and after the introduction of antiretroviral therapy. Arch Dermatol. 2005 Oct;141(10):1227–31. [PMID: 16230559]

Fragile X Mental Retardation

 KEY FEATURES

- Accounts for more cases of retardation in males than any condition except Down syndrome
- Inherited as an X-linked condition
- About 1 in 4000–6000 males is affected
- Heterozygous women have variable phenoytpes that range from mental retardation to premature ovarian failure to essentially normal, in large part dependent on the number of repeated trinucleotides present

 CLINICAL FINDINGS

- Affected males have
  - Macro-orchidism (enlarged testes) after puberty
  - Large ears and a prominent jaw, high-pitched voice, and mental retardation
  - Evidence of a mild connective tissue defect, with joint hypermobility and mitral valve prolapse
- Affected (heterozygous) women show no physical signs other than premature ovarian failure (early menopause), but they may have learning difficulties or frank retardation
- Premutation carriers (men and women with 55–200 CGG repeats) may develop ataxia and tremor as older adults

 DIAGNOSIS

- Cytogenetic studies demonstrate a small gap, or fragile site, near the tip of the long arm of the X chromosome
- Fragile site is due to expansion of a trinucleotide repeat (CGG) near a gene called *FMR1*
- One *FMR1* allele with ≥ 200 repeats results in mental retardation in virtually all men and learning difficulties in 60% of women
- Clinical DNA diagnosis for the number of CGG repeats can be performed for any male or female who has unexplained mental retardation
- Prenatal DNA diagnosis can be performed

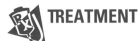 **TREATMENT**

- None

Furunculosis

 KEY FEATURES

ESSENTIALS OF DIAGNOSIS

- Extremely painful inflammatory swelling based on a hair follicle that forms an abscess
- Predisposing condition (diabetes mellitus, HIV disease, injection drug use) sometimes present
- Coagulase-positive *Staphylococcus aureus* is the causative organism

GENERAL CONSIDERATIONS

- A furuncle (boil) is a deep-seated infection (abscess) involving the entire hair follicle and adjacent subcutaneous tissue
- The most common sites of occurrence are the hairy parts exposed to irritation and friction, pressure, or moisture
- Because the lesions are autoinoculable, they are often multiple
- A carbuncle consists of several furuncles developing in adjoining hair follicles and coalescing to form a conglomerate, deeply situated mass with multiple drainage points

DEMOGRAPHICS

- Predisposing cause usually not found
- However, diabetes mellitus (especially if using insulin injections), injection drug use, allergy injections, and HIV disease all increase the risk of staphylococcal infections by increasing the rate of nasal carriage

 CLINICAL FINDINGS

SYMPTOMS AND SIGNS

Furuncle
- Rounded or conical abscesses on the hairy parts exposed to irritation and friction, pressure, or moisture
- Lesions are often multiple and pain and tenderness may be prominent
- Gradually enlarges, becomes fluctuant, and then softens and opens spontane-

ously after a few days to 1–2 weeks to discharge a core of necrotic tissue and pus
- Infection of the soft tissue around the nails (paronychia) may be due to staphylococci when it is acute; other organisms may be involved, including *Candida* and herpes simplex (herpetic whitlow)

Carbuncle
- Consists of several furuncles in adjoining hair follicles and coalescing to form a deeply situated mass with multiple drainage points

DIFFERENTIAL DIAGNOSIS

- Inflamed sebaceous (epidermal inclusion) cyst
  - Suddenly becomes red, tender, and expands greatly in size over 1 to a few days
  - History of prior cyst in the same location, the presence of a clearly visible cyst orifice, and the extrusion of malodorous cheesy rather than purulent material helps in the diagnosis
- Acne vulgaris
- Tinea profunda (deep tinea of hair follicle)
- Sporotrichosis
- Blastomycosis
- Hidradenitis suppurativa
  - Recurrent tender sterile abscesses in the axillae, groin, on the buttocks, or below the breasts
  - Presence of old scars or sinus tracts plus negative cultures suggests this diagnosis
- Anthrax
- Tularemia

 DIAGNOSIS

LABORATORY TESTS

- Leukocytosis may occur, but a white blood cell count is rarely required
- Although *S aureus* is almost always the cause, pus should be cultured, especially in immunocompromised patients, to rule out methicillin-resistant *S aureus* or other bacteria

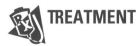 **TREATMENT**

MEDICATIONS

- Systemic antibiotics
  - Sodium dicloxacillin or cephalexin, 1 g PO daily in divided doses for 10 days, is usually effective
  - Erythromycin in similar doses may be used in penicillin-allergic individuals in communities with low prevalence

of erythromycin-resistant staphylococci or if the particular isolate is sensitive
– Ciprofloxacin, 500 mg PO BID, is effective against strains of staphylococci resistant to other antibiotics
- Recurrent furunculosis may be effectively treated with a combination of dicloxacillin, 250–500 mg PO QID for 2–4 weeks, and rifampin, 300 mg PO BID for 5 days, during this period
- Long-term clindamycin, 150–300 mg PO once daily for 1–2 months, may also cure recurrent furunculosis
- Applications of topical 2% mupirocin to the nares, axillae, and anogenital areas twice daily for 5 days eliminates the staphylococcal carrier state

SURGERY

- Incision and drainage, recommended for all loculated collections, is a mainstay of therapy
- Use surgical incision and débridement **after** the lesions are "mature"
- Incision and drainage of an acute staphylococcal paronychia

THERAPEUTIC PROCEDURES

- Immobilize the part and avoid overmanipulation of inflamed areas
- Use moist heat to help larger lesions "localize"
- For a paronychia, inserting a flat metal spatula or sharpened hardwood stick into the nail fold where it adjoins the nail will release pus from a mature lesion

 OUTCOME

FOLLOW-UP

Recurrent furunculosis

- Culture of the anterior nares may identify chronic staphylococcal carriage in recurrent infections
- Family members and intimate contacts may need evaluation for staphylococcal carrier state and perhaps concomitant treatment

PROGNOSIS

- Recurrent crops may occur for months or years

WHEN TO REFER

- If there is a question about the diagnosis, if recommended therapy is ineffective, or if specialized treatment is necessary

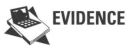 **EVIDENCE**

WEB SITE

- American Academy of Dermatology

INFORMATION FOR PATIENTS

- American Osteopathic College of Dermatology: Boils
- Mayo Clinic: Boils and Carbuncles
- MedlinePlus: Carbunculosis
- MedlinePlus: Furuncle

REFERENCES

- Embil JM et al. A man with recurrent furunculosis. CMAJ. 2006 Jul 18; 175(2):143. [PMID: 16804121]
- Zetola N et al. Community-acquired methicillin-resistant *Staphylococcus aureus*: an emerging threat. Lancet Infect Dis. 2005 May;5(5):275–86. [PMID: 15854883]

Galactorrhea

KEY FEATURES

- Lactation that occurs without breast-feeding
- Usual cause: hyperprolactinemia
- Nipple stimulation and nipple rings can increase prolactin
- Idiopathic (benign) galactorrhea
  - Many parous women can express a small amount of breast milk
  - Prolactin level is normal
- Normal breast milk may vary in color, but bloody discharge raises suspicion of cancer

CLINICAL FINDINGS

- Unilateral or bilateral milky nipple discharge
- Oligomenorrhea, amenorrhea, or infertility
- Pituitary prolactinomas may co-secrete growth hormone, causing acromegaly
- Large pituitary tumors may cause
  - Headaches
  - Visual field defects
  - Pituitary insufficiency (hypogonadism, hypothyroidism, adrenal insufficiency, growth hormone deficiency)

DIAGNOSIS

- Evaluation is required when
  - Amount is significant
  - Present in a nulliparous woman
  - Associated with amenorrhea, headache, visual field abnormalities, or other symptoms of endocrinopathy
- Serum prolactin level is elevated
- Urine or serum hCG is elevated if pregnancy causes galactorrhea
- TSH high if hypothyroidism causes hyperprolactinemia
- MRI of the pituitary and hypothalamus indicated for nonpregnant patients when
  - Prolactin is persistently elevated with no discernible cause
  - Patient has headaches or visual field defects

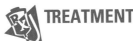

TREATMENT

- Reassure if prolactin is normal or if parous woman
- Correct underlying cause of elevated prolactin
- Discontinue potentially offending medications, and recheck in a few weeks
- Cabergoline or bromocriptine can reduce galactorrhea regardless of cause; not to be used postpartum
- See Hyperprolactinemia

Gastric Cancer

KEY FEATURES

ESSENTIALS OF DIAGNOSIS

- Dyspeptic symptoms with weight loss in patients age > 40
- Iron deficiency anemia; occult blood in stools
- Abnormality on upper gastrointestinal series or endoscopy

GENERAL CONSIDERATIONS

- Gastric adenocarcinoma is the most common cancer worldwide
- Most gastric cancers arise in the antrum
- Chronic *Helicobacter pylori* gastritis is the major risk factor
- However, among individuals chronically infected with *H pylori*, gastric carcinoma will develop in < 1%
- Other risk factors
  - Gastric adenomas
  - Chronic atrophic gastritis with intestinal metaplasia
  - Pernicious anemia
  - Partial gastric resection > 15 years previously

DEMOGRAPHICS

- Incidence in the United States has declined by two-thirds over the last 30 years
- Currently, 20,000 cases annually in the United States
- Uncommon under age 40; mean age at diagnosis is 63 years
- Men affected twice as often as women
- Incidence is higher in Hispanics, African Americans, and Asian Americans

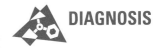

CLINICAL FINDINGS

SYMPTOMS AND SIGNS

- Generally asymptomatic or nonspecific symptoms until advanced disease
- Dyspepsia, vague epigastric pain, anorexia, early satiety, and weight loss
- Acute upper gastrointestinal bleeding with hematemesis or melena
- Postprandial vomiting suggests gastric outlet obstruction
- Progressive dysphagia suggests lower esophageal obstruction
- Physical examination rarely helpful
- Gastric mass is palpated in < 20%
- Lymphadenopathy: left supraclavicular lymph node (Virchow's node), umbilical nodule (Sister Mary Joseph nodule)
- Rigid rectal shelf (Blumer's shelf)
- Ovarian metastases (Krukenberg tumor)

DIFFERENTIAL DIAGNOSIS

- Benign gastric ulcers
- Lymphoma
- Menetrier's disease

DIAGNOSIS

LABORATORY TESTS

- Guaiac-positive stools
- Iron deficiency anemia or anemia of chronic disease
- Liver function test abnormalities if metastatic spread
- Serologic markers (eg, carcinoembryonic antigen) not helpful

IMAGING STUDIES

- Barium upper gastrointestinal series when endoscopy is not readily available
- Upper gastrointestinal series may not detect small or superficial lesions and cannot reliably distinguish benign from malignant ulcerations
- Preoperative evaluation with abdominal CT and endoscopic ultrasonography

DIAGNOSTIC PROCEDURES

- Upper endoscopy with biopsy and cytologic brushings
- Staging by TNM system
  - Stage I: T1N0, T1N1, T2N0, all M0
  - Stage II: T1N2, T2N1, T3N0, all M0
  - Stage III: T2N2, T3N1, T4N0, all M0
  - Stage IV: T4N2M0, any M1

- After preoperative staging, about two-thirds found to have localized disease (ie, stages I–III)

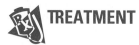 **TREATMENT**

MEDICATIONS

- Single-agent or combination chemotherapy with fluorouracil, doxorubicin, and cisplatin or mitomycin may provide palliation in up to 30%
- Patients with stage III tumors undergoing curative resection may be considered for postoperative adjuvant chemoradiotherapy

SURGERY

- For patients with clinically localized disease (stages I–III), surgical exploration
  - Patients with confirmed localized disease should undergo radical surgical resection with curative intent
  - Approximately 25% will be found to have locally unresectable tumors or peritoneal, hepatic, or distant lymph node metastases, and "curative" surgical resection is not warranted
- Palliative resection of the tumor
  - Can reduce the risk of bleeding and obstruction
  - Lead to improved quality of life
  - Improve survival
- For patients with unresectable disease, gastrojejunostomy can prevent obstruction

THERAPEUTIC PROCEDURES

- After careful staging (including endoscopic ultrasonography), small (< 3 cm), early intramucosal gastric cancers may be amenable to endoscopic mucosal resection
- Endoscopic laser or stent therapy, radiation therapy, or angiographic embolization can palliate bleeding or obstruction from unresected tumors

 OUTCOME

FOLLOW-UP

- After surgical therapy, further follow-up is determined by clinical course
- Routine follow-up not recommended

COMPLICATIONS

- Acute or chronic gastrointestinal blood loss
- Gastric outlet obstruction
- Carcinomatosis with ascites, small bowel obstruction

PROGNOSIS

- Survival related to tumor stage, location, and histologic features
- Overall long-term survival is < 15%
- Stage I and stage II tumors resected for cure have a > 50% long-term survival
- Patients with stage III tumors have a < 20% long-term survival
- Tumors of the diffuse and signet ring type have a worse prognosis than those of the intestinal type
- Tumors of the proximal stomach (fundus and cardia) have 5-year survival of < 15%, a far worse prognosis than distal lesions

WHEN TO REFER

- Patients with a confirmed diagnosis of gastric adenocarcinoma should be evaluated by a general surgeon or oncologist

WHEN TO ADMIT

- Acute upper gastrointestinal bleeding
- Vomiting and dehydration

PREVENTION

- In Japan, population-based endoscopic screening is performed
- At present, population-based testing and treating of *H pylori* as a chemopreventive measure to reduce the incidence of gastric adenocarcinoma is not recommended

 EVIDENCE

PRACTICE GUIDELINES

- Dicken BJ et al. Gastric adenocarcinoma: review and consideration for future directions. Ann Surg. 2005; 241:27. [PMID: 15478858]
- Earle CC et al. Neoadjuvant or adjuvant therapy for resectable gastric cancer? A practice guideline. Can J Surg. 2002; 45:438. [PMID: 12500920]

WEB SITE

- WebPath GI Pathology Index

INFORMATION FOR PATIENTS

- Cleveland Clinic—Stomach cancer
- Mayo Clinic—Stomach cancer
- MedlinePlus—Gastric cancer

REFERENCES

- Dicken BJ et al. Gastric adenocarcinoma: review and considerations for future directions. Ann Surg. 2005 Jan; 241(1):27–39. [PMID: 15621988]
- Hazard L et al. Role of radiation therapy in gastric adenocarcinoma. World J Gastroenterol. 2006 Mar 14; 12(10):1511–20. [PMID: 16570342]
- McCulloch P et al. Extended versus limited lymph node dissection technique for adenocarcinoma of the stomach. Cochrane Database Syst Rev. 2004 Oct 18;(4):CD001964. [PMID: 15495024]
- Melfertheiner P et al. *Helicobacter pylori* eradication has the potential to prevent gastric cancer: a state-of-the-art critique. Am J Gastroenterol. 2005 Sep; 100(9):2100–15. [PMID: 16128957]

Gastritis, Erosive & Hemorrhagic

KEY FEATURES

ESSENTIALS OF DIAGNOSIS

- Hematemesis, "coffee grounds" emesis, or melena; usually not significant bleeding
- Often asymptomatic; may cause epigastric pain, anorexia, nausea, and vomiting
- Occurs most commonly in alcoholics, critically ill patients, or patients taking nonsteroidal anti-inflammatory drugs (NSAIDs)

GENERAL CONSIDERATIONS

- Most common causes
  - Drugs (especially NSAIDs)
  - Alcohol
  - Stress due to severe medical or surgical illness
  - Portal hypertension ("portal gastropathy")
- Uncommon causes
  - Caustic ingestion
  - Radiation

DEMOGRAPHICS

- Patients using NSAIDs, especially aspirin, short- or long-term
- Heavy alcohol ingestion
- Critically ill ICU patients with major risk factors
  - Coagulopathy
  - Mechanical ventilation
  - Sepsis
  - Trauma

– Burns
– CNS injury
– Hepatic or renal failure

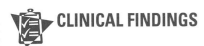 **CLINICAL FINDINGS**

SYMPTOMS AND SIGNS

- Often asymptomatic
- Symptoms, when they occur, include dyspepsia, anorexia, epigastric pain, nausea, and vomiting
- Upper gastrointestinal (GI) bleeding, hematemesis, "coffee grounds" emesis, or melena
- Bleeding is not usually hemodynamically significant

DIFFERENTIAL DIAGNOSIS

- Epigastric pain suggests
  – Peptic ulcer
  – Gastroesophageal reflux
  – Gastric cancer
  – Biliary tract disease
  – Food poisoning
  – Viral gastroenteritis
  – Functional dyspepsia
- Severe pain suggests
  – Perforated or penetrating ulcer
  – Pancreatic disease
  – Esophageal rupture
  – Ruptured aortic aneurysm
  – Gastric volvulus
  – Myocardial ischemia
- Upper GI bleeding suggests
  – Peptic ulcer disease
  – Esophageal varices
  – Mallory-Weiss tear
  – Arteriovenous malformations

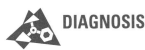 **DIAGNOSIS**

LABORATORY TESTS

- Hematocrit is low if significant bleeding
- Iron deficiency

IMAGING STUDIES

- Upper endoscopy for dyspepsia or upper GI bleeding is diagnostic
  – Erythema
  – Subepithelial petechiae
  – Erosion
- Barium upper GI series is insensitive because abnormalities are confined to the mucosa

DIAGNOSTIC PROCEDURES

- Nasogastric tube placement reveals bloody aspirate

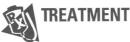 **TREATMENT**

MEDICATIONS

- Treatment of clinically significant upper GI bleeding due to stress-related gastritis, alcoholic gastritis, or NSAID gastritis
  – Proton pump inhibitors may be used; however, efficacy and optimal dosing strategy are unknown
  – Esomeprazole, lansoprazole, or pantoprazole 30–60 mg IV BID may be given initially, increased as necessary to maintain intragastric pH > 4.0
- Empiric treatment of dyspepsia (without alarm symptoms) caused by NSAIDs
  – Proton pump inhibitor (omeprazole, 20 mg PO once daily; rabeprazole, 20 mg PO once daily; esomeprazole, 40 mg PO once daily; lansoprazole 30 mg PO once daily; or pantoprazole, 40 mg PO once daily) for 2–4 weeks
  – H$_2$-receptor antagonists or sucralfate may also be effective
- Treatment of dyspepsia or minor upper GI hemorrhage caused by alcoholic gastritis: oral H$_2$-receptor antagonists or proton pump inhibitor for 2–4 weeks
- Portal hypertensive gastropathy
  – Nonselective β-blocker (propranolol or nadolol)
  – Dose adjusted to reduce resting heart rate to < 60 beats/minute

THERAPEUTIC PROCEDURES

- Portal hypertensive gastropathy: portal decompressive procedures, eg, transvenous intrahepatic portosystemic shunts, are sometimes required for acute hemorrhage

 OUTCOME

COMPLICATIONS

- Acute upper GI hemorrhage
- Chronic GI blood loss with anemia

WHEN TO REFER

- NSAID gastritis with persistent dyspepsia despite discontinuation of NSAIDs or empiric therapy
- All patients with alarm symptoms (severe pain, weight loss, vomiting, anemia, melena) should be referred for upper endoscopy
- Clinically significant acute upper GI hemorrhage

WHEN TO ADMIT

- NSAID gastritis
  – Acute upper GI hemorrhage
  – Severe dyspepsia with concern for complicated peptic ulcer disease or alternative diagnosis
- Alcoholic gastritis with protracted vomiting and/or acute upper GI hemorrhage or signs of alcohol withdrawal
- Portal hypertensive gastropathy with acute upper GI hemorrhage

PREVENTION

- Stress gastritis
  – Prophylactic therapy warranted only in high-risk ICU patients
  – Optimal approach uncertain
  – H$_2$-receptor antagonist infusions at a dose sufficient to maintain intragastric pH > 4.0
  – Cimetidine (900–1200 mg), ranitidine (150 mg), or famotidine (20 mg) by continuous IV infusion over 24 hours
  – Immediate-release omeprazole suspension (40 mg initially and 8 hours later on day 1, then daily) given orally or per nasogastric tube may be preferred due to ease of administration, comparable efficacy, and lower cost
  – IV proton pump inhibitors (pantoprazole) are more expensive than H$_2$-receptor agonists and omeprazole suspension; efficacy and optimal dosage not yet established
  – Sucralfate suspension 1 g QID
- NSAID gastritis
  – Patients at high risk for NSAID-induced complications should receive cotherapy with an oral proton pump inhibitor (eg, omeprazole or rabeprazole 20 mg, lansoprazole 30 mg, or esomeprazole or pantoprazole 40 mg once daily) or misoprostol, 200 mcg PO QID
  – Alternatively, a cyclooxygenase (COX)-2 selective agent should be used (celecoxib)
  – Use of low-dose aspirin negates safety of COX-2 selective agent
  – High-risk patients should be tested for *Helicobacter pylori* and treated if positive

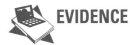 **EVIDENCE**

PRACTICE GUIDELINES

- Gupta S et al. Management of nonsteroidal, anti-inflammatory, drug-associated dyspepsia. Gastroenterology. 2005 Nov; 129(5):1711–9. [PMID: 16285968]
- National Guideline Clearinghouse

INFORMATION FOR PATIENTS

- Mayo Clinic
- MedlinePlus—Acute gastritis
- MedlinePlus—Chronic gastritis

REFERENCES

- Conrad SA et al. Randomized, double-blind comparison of immediate-release omeprazole suspension versus intravenous cimetidine for the prevention of upper gastrointestinal bleeding in critically ill patients. Crit Care Med. 2005 Apr;33(4):760–5. [PMID: 15818102]
- Harty RF et al. Stress ulcer bleeding. Curr Treat Options Gastroenterol. 2006 Apr;9(2):157–66. [PMID: 16539876]
- Hawkey C et al; NASA1 SPACE1 Study Group. Improvement with esomeprazole in patients with upper gastrointestinal symptoms taking non-steroidal antiinflammatory drugs, including selective COX-2 inhibitors. Am J Gastroenterol. 2005 May;100(5):1028–36. [PMID: 15842575]
- Stollman N et al. Pathophysiology and prophylaxis of stress ulcer in intensive care unit patients. J Crit Care. 2005 Mar;20(1):35–45. [PMID: 16015515]

Gastroesophageal Reflux Disease (GERD)

 KEY FEATURES

ESSENTIALS OF DIAGNOSIS

- Heartburn exacerbated by meals, bending, or recumbency
- Endoscopy demonstrates esophageal abnormalities in < 50% of patients

GENERAL CONSIDERATIONS

- Affects 20% of adults, who report at least weekly episodes of heartburn
- Up to 10% complain of daily symptoms
- Most patients have mild disease
- Esophageal mucosal damage (reflux esophagitis) develops in up to 50%
- Few develop serious complications
- Patients with uncomplicated disease treated empirically without diagnostic studies
- Investigation is required for patients with complicated disease and in those unresponsive to empiric therapy
- Pathogenesis includes
  - Relaxation or incompetence of lower esophageal sphincter
  - Hiatal hernia
  - Abnormal acid clearance (esophageal peristalsis), eg, scleroderma
  - Impaired salivation (exacerbates GERD), eg, Sjögren's syndrome, anticholinergics, radiation
  - Delayed gastric emptying (exacerbates GERD), eg, gastroparesis

DEMOGRAPHICS

- Increased in whites
- High prevalence in North America and Europe
- Increased in pregnancy

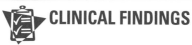 **CLINICAL FINDINGS**

SYMPTOMS AND SIGNS

- Heartburn, most often 30–60 minutes after meals and upon reclining, with relief from antacids
- Regurgitation—spontaneous reflux of sour or bitter gastric contents into the mouth
- Dysphagia common due to inflammation, impaired motility, or stricture
- Atypical manifestations
  - Asthma
  - Chronic cough
  - Chronic laryngitis
  - Sore throat
  - Noncardiac chest pain
- Gradual development of solid food dysphagia progressive over months to years suggests stricture formation
- Physical examination normal

DIFFERENTIAL DIAGNOSIS

- Angina pectoris
- Peptic ulcer disease, gastritis, nonulcer dyspepsia
- Infectious esophagitis: *Candida*, herpes simplex virus, cytomegalovirus
- Pill-induced esophagitis
- Esophageal motility disorders, eg, achalasia, esophageal spasm, scleroderma
- Zollinger-Ellison syndrome (gastrinoma) may cause severe esophagitis due to acid hypersecretion

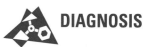 **DIAGNOSIS**

LABORATORY TESTS

- Laboratory test results are normal

IMAGING STUDIES

- Upper endoscopy reveals visible mucosal abnormalities (erythema, friability, and erosions) in 50%
- Endoscopy is indicated
  - In patients who have not responded to empiric medical management
  - In patients with symptoms suggesting complicated disease (dysphagia, odynophagia, occult or overt bleeding, or iron deficiency anemia)
  - In patients who have long-standing (> 5 years) symptoms to look for Barrett's esophagus
  - To differentiate peptic stricture from other benign or malignant causes of dysphagia
- Barium esophagography
  - Insensitive for diagnosis of GERD or detection of mucosal abnormalities
  - Useful for detection of esophageal stricture in patients with dysphagia

DIAGNOSTIC PROCEDURES

- Clinical diagnosis has sensitivity of 80%; specificity, 70%
- In patients with typical GERD symptoms without complications, empiric medical management recommended without diagnostic procedures
- Ambulatory esophageal pH monitoring
  - Best study to document acid reflux, but unnecessary in most patients
  - Indications
    - Document abnormal esophageal acid exposure in a patient being considered for antireflux surgery who has a normal endoscopy
    - Evaluate patients with a normal endoscopy who have reflux symptoms unresponsive to proton pump inhibitor
    - Detect association between reflux and atypical symptoms

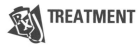 **TREATMENT**

MEDICATIONS

- Mild, occasional symptoms
  - Antacids provide rapid but short-term relief
  - Nonprescription H_2-receptor antagonists
    - Cimetidine, 200 mg

□ Ranitidine and nizatidine, 75 mg
□ Famotidine, 10 mg
□ Taken before meals may prevent symptoms
□ If taken after symptoms develop, symptom relief within 60 minutes

• For symptoms occurring > 1–2 times per week, either
  – H₂-receptor antagonists (for 8–12 weeks)
    □ Nizatidine, 150 mg PO BID
    □ Famotidine, 20 mg PO BID
    □ Cimetidine, 400–800 mg PO BID
  – Proton pump inhibitors (for 8–12 weeks)
    □ Omeprazole or rabeprazole, 20 mg PO once daily
    □ Esomeprazole, 40 mg PO once daily
    □ Lansoprazole, 30 mg PO once daily
    □ Pantoprazole, 40 mg PO once daily
  – After initial course of therapy, occasional symptom relapses may be treated with intermittent therapy for 2–4 weeks or until symptoms resolve ("on demand" therapy)

• For patients with documented erosive esophagitis, proton pump inhibitors provide effective symptom relief and healing (> 80–95%)

• Continuous "maintenance" proton pump inhibitor therapy
  – Omeprazole or rabeprazole, 20 mg PO once daily
  – Esomeprazole, 20–40 mg PO once daily
  – Lansoprazole, 15–30 mg PO once daily
  – Pantoprazole, 40 mg once daily
  – Should be given to patients with erosive esophagitis, Barrett's esophagus, or peptic stricture, or to those with frequent symptom relapse off therapy

• Unresponsive disease
  – 10–20% of patients with symptoms do not respond to once-daily doses of proton pump inhibitors
  – 5% of patients do not respond to taking twice-daily doses or to a change to a different proton pump inhibitor
  – Promotility drugs (metoclopramide, bethanechol) reduce reflux, but side effects preclude long-term use

SURGERY

• Surgical fundoplication produces relief in > 85% of properly selected patients, 10-year success rates 60–90%

• Laparoscopic fundoplication has low complication rates

• Among of patients undergoing fundoplication
  – > 50% require continued acid-suppression medication

– New dysphagia, bloating, increased flatulence, or dyspepsia develops in > 30%

• Surgery is recommended
  – For otherwise healthy patients with extraesophageal manifestations of reflux
  – For those with severe reflux who are unwilling to accept lifelong medical therapy
  – For patients with erosive disease who are intolerant of or resistant to proton pump inhibitors

THERAPEUTIC PROCEDURES

• Lifestyle modifications
• Reduce meal size
• Avoid bending over after meals
• Avoid lying down within 3 hours after meals
• Avoid acidic foods (tomato, citrus, spicy foods, coffee) and agents that relax the lower esophageal sphincter or delay gastric emptying (fatty foods, peppermint, chocolate, alcohol, and smoking)
• Weight reduction
• Elevate the head of the bed
• Dilation of peptic stricture effective in up to 90% of symptomatic patients

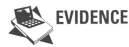

OUTCOME

FOLLOW-UP

• After discontinuation of therapy, relapse of symptoms occurs in 80% of patients within 1 year—most within the first 3 months
• Barrett's esophagus (intestinal metaplasia) is present in up to 10% of patients with chronic reflux
• Patients with Barrett's should undergo endoscopic surveillance with mucosal biopsies every 3–5 years
• Patients with low-grade dysplasia are treated with aggressive medical management and endoscopic surveillance every 6–12 months
• For patients with high-grade dysplasia, options include
  – Surgical esophagectomy
  – Endoscopic surveillance every 3 months
  – Endoscopic mucosal resection of focal lesions
  – Photodynamic ablation

COMPLICATIONS

• GERD
  – Stricture formation in ~10% (effectively treated with dilation)

– Acid-peptic ulceration
– Erosive, or hemorrhagic esophagitis
• Barrett's esophagus
  – Increased annual incidence of esophageal adenocarcinoma to 0.5%
  – A 40-fold risk compared with patients without Barrett's
  – High grade dysplasia: 15–40% risk of progression to adenocarcinoma

PROGNOSIS

• Heartburn symptoms can be controlled in almost all patients with intermittent or long-term therapy
• Symptoms of regurgitation, bloating, dyspepsia may persist despite acid-reduction therapy

WHEN TO REFER

• Complicated disease: dysphagia, weight loss, fecal-occult positive stool, anemia
• Symptoms that persist despite proton pump inhibitor therapy
• Candidates for fundoplication

WHEN TO ADMIT

• Seldom required

EVIDENCE

PRACTICE GUIDELINES

• National Guideline Clearinghouse
• Sampliner RE. Practice Parameters Committee of the American College of Gastroenterology. Updated guidelines for the diagnosis, surveillance, and therapy of Barrett's esophagus. Am J Gastroenterol. 2002;97:1888. [PMID: 12190150]

INFORMATION FOR PATIENTS

• Mayo Clinic
• NIH Patient Education Institute—Gastroesophageal reflux disease
• Society of Thoracic Surgeons

REFERENCES

• Belafsky PC. PRO: Empiric treatment with PPIs is not appropriate without testing. Am J Gastroenterol. 2006 Jan; 101(1):6–8. [PMID: 16405525]
• DeVault K. A BALANCING VIEW: Empiric PPI therapy remains the champ, but not by a knock out! Am J Gastroenterol. 2006 Jan;101(1):10–1. [PMID: 16405527]
• Gralnek I et al. Esomeprazole versus other proton pump inhibitors in erosive esophagitis: a meta-analysis of random-

ized clinical trials. Clin Gastroenterol Hepatol. 2006 Dec;4(12):1452–8. [PMID: 17162239]

- Irwin RS. Chronic cough due to gastro-esophageal reflux disease: ACCP evidence-based guidelines. Chest. 2006 Jan;129(1 Suppl):80S–94S. [PMID: 16428697]

- Peters FP et al. Endoscopic treatment of high-grade dysplasia and early stage cancer in Barrett's esophagus. Gastrointest Endosc. 2005 Apr;61(4):506–14. [PMID: 15812401]

- Rice TW. Pro: esophagectomy is indicated in high-grade dysplasia in Barrett's esophagus. Am J Gastroenterol. 2006 Oct; 101(10):2177–9. [PMID: 17032178]

- Sharma P et al. Dysplasia and cancer in a large multicenter cohort of patients with Barrett's esophagus. Clin Gastroenterol Hepatol. 2006 May;4(5):566–72. [PMID: 16630761]

- Sontag S. Con: surgery for Barrett's with flat HGD—no! Am J Gastroenterol. 2006 Oct;101(10):2180–3. [PMID: 17032179]

- Spechler S. Thermal ablation of Barrett's esophagus: a heated debate. Am J Gastroenterol. 2006 Aug;101(8):1770–2. [PMID: 16928252]

Gastrointestinal Bleeding, Acute Lower

KEY FEATURES

ESSENTIALS OF DIAGNOSIS

- Hematochezia usually present
- Stable patients can be evaluated by colonoscopy
- Massive active bleeding calls for evaluation with upper endoscopy, or nuclear technetium-labeled red blood cell scan, and/or angiography

GENERAL CONSIDERATIONS

- Lower GI bleeding defined as that arising below the ligament of Treitz, ie, small intestine or colon; > 95% of cases from the colon
- Lower tract bleeding
  - 25% less common than upper tract bleeding

- Tends to have a more benign course
- Is less likely to present with shock or orthostasis (< 20%) or to require transfusions (< 40%)
- Spontaneous cessation in > 85%; hospital mortality in < 3%
- Most common causes in patients < 50 years
  - Infectious colitis
  - Anorectal disease
  - Inflammatory bowel disease
- Most common causes in patients > 50 years
  - Diverticulosis (50% of cases)
  - Vascular ectasias (5–10%)
  - Neoplasms (polyps or carcinoma) (10%)
  - Ischemia
  - Radiation-induced proctitis
  - Solitary rectal ulcer
  - Nonsteroidal anti-inflammatory drug (NSAID)-induced ulcers
  - Small bowel diverticula
  - Colonic varices
- In 20% of cases, no source of bleeding can be identified
- Diverticulosis
  - Acute, painless, large-volume maroon or bright red hematochezia occurs in 3–5%, often associated with the use of NSAIDs
  - Bleeding more commonly originates on the right side
  - > 95% require fewer than 4 units of blood transfusion
  - Bleeding subsides spontaneously in 80% but may recur in up to 25% of patients
- Vascular ectasias (angiodysplasias)
  - Painless bleeding ranging from melena or hematochezia to occult blood loss
  - Bleeding most commonly originates in the cecum and ascending colon
  - Causes: congenital; hereditary hemorrhagic telangiectasia; autoimmune disorders, typically scleroderma
- Neoplasms: benign polyps and carcinoma cause chronic occult blood loss or intermittent anorectal hematochezia
- Anorectal disease
  - Small amounts of bright red blood noted on the toilet paper, streaking of the stool, or dripping into the toilet bowl
  - Painless bleeding with internal hemorrhoids
  - Pain with bleeding suggests anal fissure
- Ischemic colitis
  - Hematochezia or bloody diarrhea associated with mild cramps
  - In most cases, bleeding is mild and self-limited

DEMOGRAPHICS

- Lower tract bleeding is more common in older men
- Diverticular bleeding is more common in patients > 50 years
- Angiodysplasia bleeding is more common in patients > 70 years and with chronic renal failure
- Ischemic colitis is most commonly seen
  - In older patients due to atherosclerotic disease—postoperatively after ileo-aortic or abdominal aortic aneurysm surgery
  - In younger patients due to vasculitis, coagulation disorders, estrogen therapy, and long-distance running

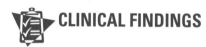 CLINICAL FINDINGS

SYMPTOMS AND SIGNS

- Brown stools mixed or streaked with blood suggest rectosigmoid or anal source
- Painless large-volume bleeding suggests a colonic source (diverticular bleeding or vascular ectasias)
- Maroon stools suggest a right colon or small intestine source
- Black stools (melena) suggest a source proximal to the ligament of Treitz, but dark maroon stools arising from small intestine or right colon may be misinterpreted as "melena"
- Bright red blood per rectum occurs uncommonly with upper tract bleeding and almost always in the setting of massive hemorrhage with shock
- Bloody diarrhea associated with cramping abdominal pain, urgency, or tenesmus suggests inflammatory bowel disease (especially ulcerative colitis), infectious colitis, or ischemic colitis

DIFFERENTIAL DIAGNOSIS

- Diverticulosis
- Vascular ectasias (angiodysplasias), eg, idiopathic arteriovenous malformation, CREST syndrome, hereditary hemorrhagic telangiectasias
- Colonic polyps
- Colorectal cancer
- Inflammatory bowel disease
- Hemorrhoids
- Anal fissure
- Ischemic colitis
- Infectious colitis
- Radiation colitis or proctitis
- NSAID-induced ulcers of small bowel or right colon

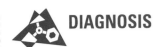

DIAGNOSIS

LABORATORY TESTS

- Complete blood cell count, platelet count, prothrombin time, INR
- Serum creatinine, blood urea nitrogen
- Type and cross-match

IMAGING STUDIES

- Nuclear technetium-labeled red blood cell scan in patients with massive bleeding
- Selective mesenteric angiography in patients with massive bleeding or positive technetium scans

DIAGNOSTIC PROCEDURES

- Nasogastric tube aspiration to exclude upper tract source
- Anoscopy
- Colonoscopy in patients in whom bleeding has ceased or in patients with moderate active bleeding immediately after rapid purge with 4–12 L polyethylene glycol solution to clear colon (rapid purge colonoscopy)
- Small intestine push enteroscopy or video capsule imaging in patients with unexplained recurrent hemorrhage of obscure origin, suspected from the small intestine
- Upper endoscopy in massive hemotochezia to exclude upper GI source

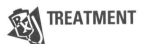

TREATMENT

SURGERY

- Surgery indicated in patients with ongoing bleeding that requires > 4–6 units of blood transfusion within 24 hours or > 10 total units
- Limited resection of the bleeding segment of small intestine or colon, if possible
- Total abdominal colectomy with ileorectal anastomosis, if bleeding site cannot be precisely identified

THERAPEUTIC PROCEDURES

- Therapeutic colonoscopy: high-risk lesions (eg, diverticulum with active bleeding or a visible vessel, or a vascular ectasia) can be treated endoscopically with saline or epinephrine injection, cautery (bipolar or heater probe), or application of metallic clips
- Angiography: selective mesenteric arterial infusion of vasoconstrictors (eg, vasopressin) and/or embolization of

actively bleeding arteriole controls hemorrhage in up to 90%

OUTCOME

COMPLICATIONS

- Complications of angiography occur in 3% and include
  - Atherosclerotic emboli
  - Thrombosis
  - Localized bowel infarction
- Operative mortality for continuous or recurrent hemorrhage is 3–15% owing to comorbid illness

PROGNOSIS

- 25% with diverticular hemorrhage have recurrent bleeding

WHEN TO ADMIT

- Patients with mild, intermittent bleeding suggesting anorectal source (blood on toilet paper, dripping in bowl) may be evaluated as outpatients
- All patients with significant hematochezia require admission

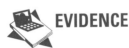

EVIDENCE

PRACTICE GUIDELINES

- Davila RE et al; Standards of Practice Committee. ASGE Guideline: the role of endoscopy in the patient with lower-GI bleeding. Gastrointest Endosc. 2005 Nov;62(5):656–60. [PMID: 16246674]
- Eisen GM et al. Standards of Practice Committee. An annotated algorithmic approach to acute lower gastrointestinal bleeding. Gastrointest Endosc. 2001; 53:859. [PMID: 11375618]

INFORMATION FOR PATIENTS

- MedlinePlus—Gastrointestinal bleeding
- National Digestive Diseases Information Clearinghouse

REFERENCES

- Green BT et al. Lower gastrointestinal bleeding management. Gastroenterol Clin North Am. 2005 Dec;34(4):665–78. [PMID: 16303576]
- Jensen D. Management of patients with severe hematochezia—with all current evidence available. Am J Gastroenterol. 2005 Nov;100(11):2403–6. [PMID: 16279892]

- Khanna A et al. Embolization as first-line therapy for diverticulosis-related massive lower gastrointestinal bleeding: evidence from a meta-analysis. J Gastrointest Surg. 2005 Mar;9(3):343–52. [PMID: 15749594]
- Strate LL et al. Validation of a clinical prediction rule for severe acute lower intestinal bleeding. Am J Gastroenterol. 2005 Aug;100(8):1821–7. [PMID: 16086720]
- Villavicencio R et al. Efficacy and complications of argon plasma coagulation for hematochezia related to radiation therapy. Gastrointest Endosc. 2002 Jan; 55(1):70–4. [PMID: 11756918]

Gastrointestinal Bleeding, Acute Upper

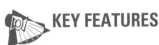

KEY FEATURES

ESSENTIALS OF DIAGNOSIS

- Hematemesis (bright red blood or "coffee grounds")
- Melena in most cases; hematochezia in massive upper GI bleeding
- Use volume (hemodynamic) status to determine severity of blood loss; hematocrit is a poor early indicator of blood loss
- Endoscopy is diagnostic and may be therapeutic

GENERAL CONSIDERATIONS

- Most common presentation is hematemesis or melena; hematochezia in 10% of cases
- Hematemesis is either bright red blood or brown "coffee grounds" material
- Melena develops after as little as 50–100 mL of blood loss
- Hematochezia requires > 1000 mL of blood loss
- Upper GI bleeding is self-limited in 80% of cases; urgent medical therapy and endoscopic evaluation are required in the remainder
- Bleeding > 48 hours prior to presentation carries a low risk of recurrent bleeding
- Peptic ulcers account for ~50% of cases

- Portal hypertension bleeding (10–20% of cases) occurs from varices (most commonly esophageal)
- Mallory-Weiss tears are lacerations of the gastroesophageal junction (5–10% of cases)
- Vascular anomalies, vascular ectasias (angiodysplasias) (7% of cases) occur in hereditary hemorrhagic telangiectasia, CREST syndrome, or sporadically, with increased incidence in chronic renal failure
- Gastric neoplasms (1% of cases)
- Erosive gastritis (< 5% of cases) due to nonsteroidal anti-inflammatory drugs (NSAIDs), alcohol, or severe medical or surgical illness (stress gastritis)

DEMOGRAPHICS

- 250,000 hospitalizations a year in the United States

 CLINICAL FINDINGS

SYMPTOMS AND SIGNS

- Signs of chronic liver disease implicate bleeding due to portal hypertension, but a different lesion is identified in 25–50% of patients with cirrhosis
- Dyspepsia, NSAID use, or history of previous peptic ulcer suggests peptic ulcer disease
- Heavy alcohol ingestion or retching suggests a Mallory-Weiss tear

DIFFERENTIAL DIAGNOSIS

- Hemoptysis
- Peptic ulcer disease
- Esophageal or gastric varices
- Erosive gastritis, eg, NSAIDs, alcohol, stress
- Mallory-Weiss syndrome
- Portal hypertensive gastropathy
- Vascular ectasias (angiodysplasias), eg, idiopathic arteriovenous malformation, CREST syndrome, hereditary hemorrhagic telangiectasias
- Gastric cancer
- Rare causes
  - Erosive esophagitis
  - Duodenal varices
  - Aortoenteric fistula
  - Dieulafoy's lesion (aberrant gastric submucosal artery)
  - Hemobilia (blood in biliary tree), eg, iatrogenic, malignancy
  - Pancreatic cancer
  - Hemosuccus pancreaticus (pancreatic pseudoaneurysm)

 DIAGNOSIS

LABORATORY TESTS

- Complete blood cell count
- Platelet count
- Prothrombin time
- INR
- Serum creatinine
- Liver enzymes and serologies
- Type and cross-matching for 2–4 units or more of packed red blood cells
- Hematocrit is not a reliable indicator of the severity of acute bleeding

DIAGNOSTIC PROCEDURES

- Assess volume (hemodynamic) status
  - Systolic blood pressure
  - Heart rate
  - Postural hypotension
- Upper endoscopy after the patient is hemodynamically stable
  - To identify the source of bleeding
  - To determine the risk of rebleeding
  - To render endoscopic therapy such as cautery or injection of a sclerosant or epinephrine or application of a rubber band or metallic clips

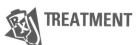 **TREATMENT**

MEDICATIONS

- IV proton pump inhibitor (eg, esomeprazole or pantoprazole 80-mg IV bolus, followed by 8 mg/hour continuous infusion for 72 hours) in patients admitted for active bleeding
- High doses of oral proton pump inhibitors (eg, omeprazole or esomeprazole, 40 mg PO BID, or lansoprazole, 60 mg PO BID for 5 days)
  - May also be effective
  - Commonly given to patients with suspected peptic ulcer bleeding in emergency department before endoscopy
- Octreotide, 100-mcg bolus, followed by 50–100 mcg/hour, for bleeding related to portal hypertension

SURGERY

- Surgery is required in < 5% of patients with peptic ulcer disease hemorrhage that cannot be controlled with endoscopic therapy

THERAPEUTIC PROCEDURES

- Insert two 18-gauge or larger intravenous lines

- In patients without hemodynamic compromise or overt active bleeding, aggressive fluid repletion can be delayed until extent of bleeding clarified
- Patients with hemodynamic compromise should be given 0.9% saline or lactated Ringer's injection and cross-matched blood
- Nasogastric tube placed for aspiration
- Blood replacement to maintain a hematocrit of 25–28%
- In the absence of continued bleeding, the hematocrit should rise 3% for each unit of transfused packed red cells
- Transfuse blood in patients with brisk active bleeding regardless of the hematocrit
- Transfuse platelets if platelet count < 50,000/mcL or if impaired platelet function due to aspirin or clopidogrel use
- Uremic patients with active bleeding should be given 1–2 doses of desmopressin (DDAVP), 0.3 mcg/kg IV at 12- to 24-hour intervals
- Fresh frozen plasma should be given for actively bleeding patients with a coagulopathy and an INR > 1.5
- In massive bleeding, 1 unit of fresh frozen plasma should be given for each 5 units of packed red blood cells transfused
- Intra-arterial embolization or vasopressin indicated (rarely) in patients who are poor operative risks and with persistent bleeding from ulcers, angiomas, or Mallory-Weiss tears in whom endoscopic therapy has failed
- Transvenous intrahepatic portosystemic shunts (TIPS) to decompress the portal venous system and control acute variceal bleeding are indicated in patients in whom endoscopic modalities have failed

 OUTCOME

PROGNOSIS

- Mortality rate is 10%, even higher in patients age > 60
- Hemorrhage from peptic ulcers has an overall mortality rate of 4%
- Portal hypertension has a hospital mortality rate of 15–40%; if untreated, 50% will rebleed during hospitalization; mortality rate of 60–80% at 1–4 years

WHEN TO REFER

- Refer to gastroenterologist for endoscopy
- Refer to surgeon for uncontrollable, life-threatening hemorrhage

WHEN TO ADMIT

- Very low-risk patients who meet following criteria do not require hospital admission and can be evaluated as outpatients
  - No serious comorbid medical illnesses or advanced liver disease and normal hemodynamic status
  - No evidence of overt bleeding (hematemesis or melena) within 48 hours
  - Negative nasogastric lavage
  - Normal laboratory tests
- Low- to moderate-risk patients are admitted to hospital
  - Upper endoscopy after appropriate stabilization and further treatment
  - Based on findings, may then be discharged and monitored as outpatients
- High-risk patients with any of the following require ICU admission
  - Active bleeding manifested by hematemesis or bright red blood on nasogastric aspirate
  - Shock
  - Persistent hemodynamic derangement despite fluid resuscitation
  - Serious comorbid medical illness
  - Evidence of advanced liver disease

EVIDENCE

PRACTICE GUIDELINES

- Barkun A et al. A Canadian clinical practice algorithm for the management of patients with nonvariceal upper gastrointestinal bleeding. Can J Gastroenterol. 2004;18:605. [PMID: 15497000]
- Eisen GM et al; American Society for Gastrointestinal Endoscopy. Standards of Practice Committee: An annotated algorithmic approach to upper gastrointestinal bleeding. Gastrointest Endosc. 2001;53:853. [PMID: 11375617]

INFORMATION FOR PATIENTS

- American College of Gastroenterology
- MedlinePlus—Gastrointestinal bleeding
- National Digestive Diseases Information Clearinghouse

REFERENCES

- Bardou M et al. Meta-analysis: proton-pump inhibition in high-risk patients with acute peptic ulcer bleeding. Aliment Pharmacol Ther. 2005 Mar 15; 21(6):677–86. [PMID: 15771753]
- Carbonell N et al. Erythromycin infusion prior to endoscopy for acute upper gastrointestinal bleeding: a randomized, controlled, double-blind trial. Am J Gastroenterol. 2006 Jun;101(6):1211–5. [PMID: 16771939]
- Das A et al. Prediction of outcome of acute GI hemorrhage: a review of risk scores and predictive models. Gastrointest Endosc. 2004 Jul;60(1):85–93. [PMID: 15229431]
- Esrailian E et al. Nonvariceal upper gastrointestinal bleeding: epidemiology and diagnosis. Gastroenterol Clin North Am. 2005 Dec;34(4):589–605. [PMID: 16303572]
- Targownik LA et al. Trends in management and outcomes of acute nonvariceal upper gastrointestinal bleeding: 1993–2003. Clin Gastroenterol Hepatol. 2006 Dec;4(12):1459-1466. [PMID: 17101296]

Gastroparesis

KEY FEATURES

- Chronic condition characterized by intermittent, waxing and waning symptoms of nausea, bloating, early satiety, and vomiting in the absence of any mechanical lesions
- Caused by
  - Endocrine disorders (diabetes mellitus, hypothyroidism, cortisol deficiency)
  - Postsurgical (vagotomy, partial gastric resection, fundoplication, gastric bypass, Whipple procedure)
  - Neurologic conditions (Parkinson's disease, muscular and myotonic dystrophy, autonomic dysfunction, multiple sclerosis, postpolio syndrome, porphyria)
  - Rheumatologic conditions (progressive systemic sclerosis)
  - Infections (postviral, Chagas' disease)
  - Amyloidosis
  - Paraneoplastic syndromes
  - Medications
  - Anorexia nervosa
- Cause may not always be identified

CLINICAL FINDINGS

- Manifestations of gastroparesis may be chronic or intermittent
- Early satiety, bloating, nausea, and postprandial vomiting (1–3 hours after meals)

DIAGNOSIS

- Abdominal radiography shows dilatation of the stomach
- Endoscopy or barium radiography (upper GI series) excludes mechanical obstruction
- Gastric scintigraphy with a low-fat solid meal assesses gastric emptying
- Gastric retention of 60% after 2 hours or more than 10% after 4 hours is abnormal

TREATMENT

- No specific therapy
- Acute exacerbations: Nasogastric suction and IV fluids, correction of electrolyte disturbance
- Long-term treatment: Small, frequent meals low in fiber, milk, gas-forming foods, and fat
- Jejunal feeding via external feeding tube or jejunostomy if oral feeding cannot meet nutritional needs
- Parenteral nutrition seldom required unless there is a diffuse gastric and intestinal motility disorder
- Avoid opioids, anticholinergics
- In persons with diabetes, maintain glucose levels < 200 mg/dL
- Metoclopramide, 5–20 mg PO QID or 5–10 mg IV or SQ before meals, and erythromycin, 125–250 mg PO BID or 3 mg/kg IV q8h
- Gastric decompression: Patients with severe gastroparesis may require placement of a percutaneous endoscopic gastrostomy (PEG) to decompress the stomach
- Gastric pacing with internally implanted neurostimulators

Gaucher Disease

KEY FEATURES

- Caused by a deficiency of β-glucocerebrosidase, leading to an accumulation of sphingolipid within phagocytic cells throughout the body
- Inherited as an autosomal recessive
- Over 200 mutations have been found
- Most common in people of Ashkenazi Jewish ancestry

- Two uncommon forms of Gaucher's disease, types II and III, involve neurologic accumulation of sphingolipid and neurologic problems
- Type II is of infantile onset and has a poor prognosis

 CLINICAL FINDINGS

- Anemia and thrombocytopenia are common and primarily due to hypersplenism, but marrow infiltration with Gaucher cells may be a contributing factor
- Cortical erosions of bones, especially vertebrae and femur, are due to local infarctions
- Bone pain, termed "crises" reminiscent of pain seen in sickle cell disease

 DIAGNOSIS

- Bone marrow aspirates reveal typical Gaucher cells, which have an eccentric nucleus and periodic acid-Schiff–positive inclusions, along with wrinkled cytoplasm and inclusion bodies of a fibrillar type
- Serum acid phosphatase elevated
- Deficient glucocerebrosidase activity in leukocytes confirms diagnosis

 TREATMENT

- Supportive treatment of bone pain; avoid fracture risk
- Splenectomy for thrombocytopenia
- Enzyme replacement therapy
- Imiglucerase
  - Recombinant form of the enzyme glucocerebrosidase
  - Dosage: 30 units/kg/mo IV
  - Reduces total body stores of glycolipid
  - Improves orthopedic and hematologic, but not neurologic, manifestations

Giardiasis

 KEY FEATURES

ESSENTIALS OF DIAGNOSIS

- Acute diarrhea, which may be profuse and watery

- Chronic diarrhea with greasy, malodorous stools
- Abdominal cramps, distention, flatulence, and malaise
- Cysts or trophozoites in stools

GENERAL CONSIDERATIONS

- This upper small intestine infection is caused by the flagellate *Giardia lamblia* (also called *G intestinalis* and *G duodenalis*)
- The organism occurs in feces as a flagellated trophozoite and as a cyst
  - Only the cyst form is infectious by the oral route
  - Trophozoites are destroyed by gastric acidity
- Reservoirs for infection
  - Humans
  - Dogs, cats, beavers, and other mammals are implicated but not confirmed
- Under moist, cool conditions, cysts can survive in the environment for weeks to months
- Transmission occurs as a result of
  - Fecal contamination of water or food
  - Person-to-person contact
  - Anal-oral sexual content
- Infectious dose is low, requiring as few as 10 cysts
- Hypogammaglobulinemia, low secretory IgA levels in the gut, achlorhydria, and malnutrition favor development of infection

DEMOGRAPHICS

- The parasite occurs worldwide, especially in areas with poor sanitation
- In the United States and Europe, the infection is the most common intestinal protozoal pathogen
- US estimate is 100,000 to 2.5 million new infections leading to 5000 hospital admissions yearly
- Groups at special risk include
  - Travelers to endemic areas
  - Persons who swallow contaminated water during recreation or wilderness travel
  - Men who have sex with men
  - Persons with impaired immunity
- Multiple cases are common in households, children's day care centers, and residential facilities
- Outbreaks occur from contamination of water supplies

 CLINICAL FINDINGS

SYMPTOMS AND SIGNS

- About 50% of infected persons have no discernable infection and about 10% become asymptomatic cyst passers
- Acute diarrheal syndrome develops in 25–50% of persons
- Incubation period is usually 1–3 weeks but may be longer

Acute infection

- May resolve spontaneously but is commonly followed by chronic diarrhea
- May begin gradually or suddenly
- May last days or weeks and is usually self-limited but cyst excretion may be prolonged
- Cysts may not be detected in the stool at the onset of the illness
- The initial illness may include profuse watery diarrhea
- Hospitalization may be required due to dehydration, particularly in young children

Chronic infection

- Abdominal cramps, bloating, flatulence, nausea, malaise, and anorexia are typical
- Malabsorption may also be present
- Fever and vomiting are uncommon
- Diarrhea
  - Usually not severe
  - May be daily or recurrent
  - Intervening periods may include constipation
- Stools are greasy or frothy and foul smelling, without blood, pus, or mucus
- Weight loss is frequent

DIFFERENTIAL DIAGNOSIS

- Viral or bacterial gastroenteritis
- Amebiasis
- Lactase deficiency
- Irritable bowel syndrome
- Malabsorption due to other causes, eg, celiac sprue
- Laxative abuse
- Crohn's disease
- Cryptosporidiosis

 DIAGNOSIS

LABORATORY TESTS

- Stool is generally without blood or leukocytes
- Diagnosis is made by the identification of trophozoites or cysts in stool

- A wet mount of liquid stool may identify motile trophozoites
- Stained fixed specimens may show cysts or trophozoites
- Sensitivity of stool analysis is not ideal, estimated at 50–80% for a single specimen and over 90% for three specimens
- Antigen assays may be simpler and cheaper than repeated stool examinations, but these tests will not identify other stool pathogens
- Multiple tests, which identify antigens of trophozoites or cysts, are generally quite sensitive (85–98%) and specific (90–100%)

DIAGNOSTIC PROCEDURES

- Sampling of duodenal contents with a string test or biopsy is no longer generally recommended, but biopsies may be helpful in very ill or immunocompromised patients

 TREATMENT

MEDICATIONS

- Metronidazole (250 mg orally TID for 5–7 days) or tinidazole (2 g orally once)
  - Treatments of choice
  - Tinidazole appears to be equally efficacious and has the advantage of single-dose therapy
  - Cure rates for single courses are typically about 80–95%
  - Side effects include transient nausea, vomiting, epigastric discomfort, headache, metallic taste
- Nitazoxanide
  - Recently approved in the United States for the treatment of children but is also used in adults (500 mg orally BID for 3 days)
  - Generally well tolerated but may cause mild gastrointestinal side effects
- Other drugs
  - Furazolidone (100 mg orally QID for 7 days) is about as effective as the other drugs but causes gastrointestinal side effects
  - Albendazole (400 mg orally daily for 5 days) appears to have similar efficacy but has been less studied
  - Paromomycin (500 mg orally TID for 7 days) appears to have somewhat lower efficacy but may be the safest drug in pregnant women

THERAPEUTIC PROCEDURES

- All household contacts and children exposed in day care should be tested

- Treatment of asymptomatic patients should be considered since they can transmit the infection
- In the presence of a presumptive diagnosis but negative diagnostic studies, an empiric course of treatment is sometimes appropriate

 OUTCOME

PREVENTION

- Since community water chlorination (0.4 mg/L) is relatively ineffective for inactivating cysts, filtration is required
- For wilderness or international travelers, adequate measures include
  - Bringing water to a boil for 1 min
  - Filtering water with a pore size < 1 mcm
- In day care centers, appropriate disposal of diapers and frequent hand washing are essential

 EVIDENCE

PRACTICE GUIDELINES

- National Guideline Clearinghouse

WEB SITE

- CDC—Division of Parasitic Diseases

INFORMATION FOR PATIENTS

- American Academy of Family Physicians
- Centers for Disease Control and Prevention
- CDC—Division of Parasitic Diseases

REFERENCES

- Ali SA et al. *Giardia intestinalis*. Curr Opin Infect Dis. 2003 Oct;16(5):453–60. [PMID: 14501998]
- Bailey JM et al. Nitazoxanide treatment for giardiasis and cryptosporidiosis in children. Ann Pharmacother. 2004 Apr;38(4):634–40. [PMID: 14990779]
- Huang DB et al. An updated review on *Cryptosporidium* and *Giardia*. Gastroenterol Clin North Am. 2006 Jun;35(2):291–314. [PMID: 16880067]
- Karabay O et al. Albendazole versus metronidazole treatment of adult giardiasis: An open randomized clinical study. World J Gastroenterol. 2004 Apr 15;10(8):1215–7. [PMID: 15069729]

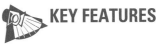 # Glomerulonephritis

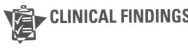 KEY FEATURES

ESSENTIALS OF DIAGNOSIS

- Acute kidney insufficiency
- Edema
- Hypertension
- Hematuria (with or without dysmorphic red cells, red blood cell casts)
- Mild to moderate proteinuria

GENERAL CONSIDERATIONS

- A relatively uncommon cause of acute renal failure, ~5% of cases of hospitalized intrinsic renal failure
- Acute glomerulonephritis usually signifies an inflammatory process causing renal dysfunction over days to weeks that may or may not resolve (Table 87)
- Inflammatory glomerular lesions include mesangioproliferative, focal and diffuse proliferative, and crescentic lesions
- Rapidly progressive acute glomerulonephritis can cause permanent damage to glomeruli if not identified and treated rapidly

Causes of glomerulonephritis

- Immune complex
  - IgA nephropathy
  - Endocarditis
  - Systemic lupus erythematosus
  - Cryoglobulinemia (often associated with hepatitis C)
  - Postinfectious glomerulonephritis
  - Membranoproliferative glomerulonephritis
- Pauci-immune (ANCA⁺)
  - Wegener's granulomatosis
  - Churg-Strauss syndrome
  - Microscopic polyarteritis
- Antiglomerular basement membrane (GBM)
  - Goodpasture's disease
  - Anti-GBM glomerulonephritis

CLINICAL FINDINGS

SYMPTOMS AND SIGNS

- Hypertension
- Edema, first in body parts with low tissue tension such as periorbital and scrotal regions
- Dark urine

DIFFERENTIAL DIAGNOSIS

- Acute interstitial nephritis (AIN)
- Acute tubular necrosis (ATN)

DIAGNOSIS

LABORATORY TESTS

- Urinalysis dipstick
  - Hematuria, moderate proteinuria (usually < 3 g/day)
  - Microscopic: abnormal urinary sediment with cellular elements such as red cells, red cell casts, and white cells
- 24-h urine for protein excretion and creatinine clearance
- Urine creatinine clearance is an unreliable marker of glomerular filtration rate in cases of rapidly changing serum creatinine values
- Fractional excretion of sodium is usually low (< 1%), unless renal tubular dysfunction is marked
- Complement levels (C3, C4, CH_{50}), ASO titer, anti-GBM antibody levels, ANA titers, cryoglobulins, hepatitis B surface antigen and hepatitis C virus antibody, C3 nephritic factor, ANCA

IMAGING STUDIES

- Renal ultrasound

DIAGNOSTIC PROCEDURES

- Renal biopsy: Type of glomerulonephritis can be categorized according to the light microscopy immunofluorescence pattern and electron microscopy appearance

TREATMENT

MEDICATIONS

- Corticosteroids in high dose and cytotoxic agents such as cyclophosphamide, depending on the nature and severity of disease
- Antihypertensive agents
- Diuretics and restriction of salt and water for fluid overload
- Angiotensin-converting enzyme inhibitors and angiotensin II receptor blockers

THERAPEUTIC PROCEDURES

- Specific therapies aimed at the underlying cause
- Dialysis as needed

OUTCOME

FOLLOW-UP

- With nephrologist as dictated by specific disease

COMPLICATIONS

- Chronic kidney disease

WHEN TO REFER

- Any evidence of possible glomerulonephritis

WHEN TO ADMIT

- Any acute or rapidly progressive symptoms (days to weeks) may be cause for admission depending on the disease

EVIDENCE

PRACTICE GUIDELINES

- Singapore Ministry of Health: Glomerulonephritis, 2001
- Tomino Y et al. Clinical guidelines for immunoglobulin A (IgA) nephropathy in Japan, second version. Clin Exp Nephrol. 2003;7:93. [PMID: 14586726]

WEB SITE

- National Kidney and Urologic Diseases Information Clearinghouse

INFORMATION FOR PATIENTS

- Mayo Clinic: Glomerulonephritis
- MedlinePlus: Glomerulonephritis
- National Kidney Foundation: Glomerulonephritis
- National Kidney and Urologic Diseases Information Clearinghouse: Glomerular Diseases

REFERENCES

- Cantarovich F et al. High-dose furosemide for established ARF: a prospective, randomized, double-blind, placebo-controlled, multicenter trial. Am J Kidney Dis. 2004 Sep;44(3):402–9. [PMID: 15332212]
- Esson ML et al. Diagnosis and treatment of acute tubular necrosis. Ann Intern Med. 2002 Nov 5;137(9):744–52. [PMID: 12416948]
- Kodner CM et al. Diagnosis and management of acute interstitial nephritis. Am Fam Physician. 2003 Jun 15; 67(12):2527–34. [PMID: 12825841]
- Mehta R et al. Diuretics, mortality, and nonrecovery of renal function in acute renal failure. JAMA. 2002 Nov 27; 288(20):2547–53. [PMID: 12444861]
- Merten GJ et al. Prevention of contrast-induced nephropathy with sodium bicarbonate: a randomized controlled trial. JAMA. 2004 May 19; 291(19):2328–34. [PMID: 15150204]
- Parmet S et al. JAMA patient page. Acute renal failure. JAMA. 2002 Nov 27;288(20):2634. [PMID: 12444873]
- Perazella MA. Drug-induced renal failure: update on new medications and unique mechanisms of nephrotoxicity. Am J Med Sci. 2003 Jun;325(6):349–62. [PMID: 12811231]
- Vinen CS et al. Acute glomerulonephritis. Postgrad Med J. 2003 Apr; 79(930):206–13. [PMID: 12743337]
- Warnock DG. Towards a definition and classification of acute kidney injury. J Am Soc Nephrol. 2005 Nov; 16(11):3149–50. [PMID: 16207828]
- Weisbord S et al. Radiocontrast-induced acute renal failure. J Intensive Care Med. 2005 Mar–Apr;20(2):63–75. [PMID: 15855219]

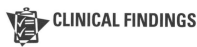

Glomerulonephritis, Membranoproliferative

KEY FEATURES

- Idiopathic or secondary to immune complex or paraprotein deposition and thrombotic microangiopathic glomerulonephritides
- Presents with nephritic or nephrotic features
- Most patients are older than 30 years
- Two major subgroups: type I and type II; type II less common than type I

CLINICAL FINDINGS

Type I
- History of recent upper respiratory tract infection in ~33%
- Nephrotic syndrome

Type II
- Glomerulonephritis findings

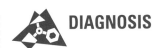

DIAGNOSIS

Type I

- Serum complement levels are low
- Renal biopsy
  - Light microscopy shows glomerular basement membrane is thickened by immune complex deposition, abnormal mesangial cell proliferation, "splitting" appearance to the capillary wall
  - Immunofluorescence shows IgG, IgM, and granular deposits of C3, C1q, and C4

Type II

- Renal biopsy
  - Light microscopy findings similar to type I
  - However, electron microscopy shows dense deposit of homogeneous material replacing part of the glomerular basement membrane
- C3 nephritic factor, a circulating IgG antibody, found in serum

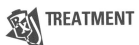

TREATMENT

- Treatment is controversial
- Corticosteroid therapy
- Antiplatelet drugs: aspirin, 500–975 mg/day, plus dipyridamole, 225 mg/day
- In the past, 50% of patients progressed to end-stage renal disease in 10 years; fewer do so now with introduction of more aggressive therapy
- Prognosis less favorable with type II disease, early renal insufficiency, hypertension, and persistent nephrotic syndrome
- Renal transplantation, but both types may recur thereafter

Glomerulonephritis, Postinfectious

KEY FEATURES

- Causes include
  - Infection from nephritogenic group A β-hemolytic streptococci, especially type 12
  - Bacteremia (eg, *Staphylococcus aureus* sepsis)
  - Infective endocarditis
  - Shunt infections
  - Hepatitis B
  - Cytomegalovirus infection
  - Infectious mononucleosis
  - Coccidioidomycosis
  - Malaria
  - Toxoplasmosis

CLINICAL FINDINGS

- Oliguria
- Edema
- Hypertension, variable
- Proteinuria

DIAGNOSIS

- Serum complement levels are low
- Antistreptolysin O (ASO) titers sometimes high
- Urinalysis: cola-colored urine, with red blood cells, red cell casts, and proteinuria
- 24-h urine protein < 3.5 g/day
- Renal biopsy
  - Light microscopy shows diffuse proliferative glomerulonephritis
  - Immunofluorescence shows IgG and C3 in a granular pattern in the mesangium and along the capillary basement membrane
  - Electron microscopy shows large, dense subepithelial deposits or "humps"

TREATMENT

- Supportive measures
- Antibiotics, as indicated for infection
- Antihypertensive medications
- Salt and water restriction
- Diuretics

Glossitis & Glossodynia

KEY FEATURES

- **Glossitis**
  - Inflammation of the tongue with loss of filiform papillae leads to glossitis
  - May be secondary to nutritional deficiencies (eg, niacin, riboflavin, iron, or vitamin E), drug reactions, dehydration, irritants, food and liquids, and possibly autoimmune reactions or psoriasis
- **Glossodynia**
  - Burning and pain of the tongue; it may occur with or without glossitis
  - It has been associated with diabetes mellitus, drugs (eg, diuretics), tobacco, xerostomia, and candidiasis as well as the causes of glossitis
  - Periodontal disease is not a factor

CLINICAL FINDINGS

- Rarely painful
- Glossitis: red, smooth-surfaced tongue

DIAGNOSIS

- Clinical

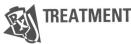

TREATMENT

- **Glossitis**
  - If the primary cause cannot be treated, consider empiric nutritional replacement therapy
- **Glossodynia**
  - Reassurance that there is no infection or tumor
  - Anxiolytic medications and evaluation of possible psychological status may be useful
  - Treating possible underlying causes, changing long-term medications to alternative ones, and smoking cessation may resolve symptoms
  - Consider an empiric trial of gabapentin for symptom control

Glucose-6-Phosphate Dehydrogenase Deficiency

KEY FEATURES

- Hereditary enzyme defect causes episodic hemolytic anemia from RBC's decreased ability to deal with oxidative stresses

- Hemoglobin may become oxidized, forming precipitants (Heinz bodies) which cause membrane damage, leading to removal of RBCs by spleen
- X-linked recessive disorder affects 10–15% of black American males, who have a variant G6PD (A–) with 15% of normal enzyme activity; in addition, enzyme activity declines rapidly as RBC ages past 40 days
- Mediterranean variants have extremely low enzyme activity
- Female carriers are affected when unusually high percentage of cells producing normal enzyme are inactivated (rare)

 CLINICAL FINDINGS

- Usually healthy, without chronic hemolytic anemia or splenomegaly
- Hemolysis occurs at time of infection or exposure to certain drugs
- Common drugs initiating hemolysis
  - Dapsone
  - Primaquine
  - Quinidine
  - Quinine
  - Sulfonamides
  - Nitrofurantoin
- Hemolytic episode self-limited, even with continued use of offending drug, because older RBCs (with low G6PD activity) removed and replaced with young RBCs (with adequate G6PD activity)
- Chronic hemolytic anemia in severe G6PD deficiency (eg, Mediterranean variants)

 DIAGNOSIS

- Coombs test is negative
- Blood is normal between hemolytic episodes
- Reticulocytosis and increased indirect bilirubin during hemolytic episodes
- G6PD enzyme assays low, especially in severe cases of G6PD deficiency
- G6PD enzyme assays may be misleadingly normal if performed shortly after hemolytic episode when enzyme-deficient RBCs have been removed
- RBC smear, although not diagnostic, may reveal "bite" cell
- Heinz bodies may be seen on peripheral blood smear with crystal violet stain

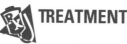 **TREATMENT**

- Avoid known oxidant drugs
- Otherwise, no treatment necessary

Goiter, Endemic

 KEY FEATURES

ESSENTIALS OF DIAGNOSIS

- Common in regions of the world with low-iodine diets
- Goiters may become multinodular and grow to great size
- Most adults with endemic goiter are euthyroid; however, some are hypothyroid or hyperthyroid
- Impaired cognition and hearing may be subtle or severe in congenital hypothyroidism

GENERAL CONSIDERATIONS

- Up to 0.5% of iodine-deficient populations have full-blown cretinism; less severe manifestations of congenital hypothyroidism more common
- Causes
  - Iodine deficiency (most common)
  - Certain foods (eg, sorghum, millet, maize, cassava)
  - Mineral deficiencies (selenium, iron)
  - Water pollutants
  - Congenital partial defects in thyroid enzyme activity
- Increase in size of thyroid nodules and emergence of new nodules in pregnancy

DEMOGRAPHICS

- ~5% of world's population have goiters
- Of these, 75% occur in areas of iodine deficiency
  - Such areas found in 115 countries, mostly developing nations
  - However, also found in Europe, eg, in Pescopagano, Italy, 60% of adults have goiters, with hyperthyroidism in 2.9%; overt hypothyroidism in 0.2% and subclinical hypothyroidism in 3.8%; thyroid cancer in < 0.1%

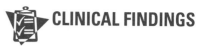 **CLINICAL FINDINGS**

SYMPTOMS AND SIGNS

- Thyroid may become multinodular and very large
- Growth often occurs during pregnancy and may cause compressive symptoms
- Substernal goiters usually asymptomatic but can cause
  - Tracheal compression
  - Respiratory distress
  - Dysphagia
  - Superior vena cava syndrome
  - Phrenic or recurrent laryngeal nerve palsy, or Horner's syndrome
  - Gastrointestinal bleeding from esophageal varices
  - Pleural or pericardial effusions (rare)
- Cerebral ischemia and stroke can result from arterial compression or thyrocervical steal syndrome
- Malignancy in < 1%
- Some patients with goiter become hypothyroid
- Other patients become thyrotoxic as goiter grows and becomes more autonomous, especially if iodine added to diet
- Congenital hypothyroidism
  - Isolated deafness
  - Short stature
  - Impaired mentation

DIFFERENTIAL DIAGNOSIS

- Benign multinodular goiter
- Pregnancy (in areas of iodine deficiency)
- Graves' disease
- Hashimoto's thyroiditis
- Subacute (de Quervain's) thyroiditis
- Drugs causing hypothyroidism
  - Lithium
  - Amiodarone
  - Propylthiouracil
  - Methimazole
  - Phenylbutazone
  - Sulfonamides
  - Interferon-α
  - Iodide
- Infiltrating disease, eg, malignancy, sarcoidosis
- Suppurative thyroiditis
- Riedel's thyroiditis

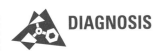

DIAGNOSIS

LABORATORY TESTS

- Serum thyroxine and thyroid-stimulating hormone (TSH) usually normal
  - TSH low if multinodular goiter becomes autonomous in presence of sufficient iodine for thyroid hormone synthesis, causing hyperthyroidism
  - TSH high in hypothyroidism
- Serum levels of antithyroid antibodies usually undetectable or low
- Serum thyroglobulin often elevated

IMAGING STUDIES

- Thyroid radioactive iodine uptake usually elevated, but may be normal if iodine intake has improved

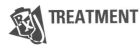

TREATMENT

MEDICATIONS

- Dietary iodine supplementation (eg, addition of potassium iodide to table salt)
  - Greatly reduces prevalence of endemic goiter and cretinism but is less effective in shrinking established goiter
  - Increases risk of autoimmune thyroid dysfunction, which may result in hypothyroidism or hyperthyroidism
  - Excessive iodine intake may increase risk of goiter
- Concurrent deficiencies in both vitamin A and iodine increase the risk of endemic goiter and concurrent repletion of both iodine and vitamin A reduces the risk of goiter in endemic regions
- Thyroxine supplementation
  - Can shrink goiters and reduce risk of further goiter growth
  - However, may induce hyperthyroidism in individuals with autonomous multinodular goiters
  - Thyroxine suppression should not be started in patients with suppressed TSH levels

SURGERY

- Thyroidectomy indicated for cosmesis, compressive symptoms, or thyrotoxicosis in adults with very large multinodular goiters

PROCEDURES

- Patients may be treated with ^{131}I for large compressive goiters

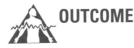

OUTCOME

FOLLOW-UP

- Partial thyroidectomy is followed by a high goiter recurrence rate in iodine-deficient geographic areas, so total thyroidectomy is preferred when surgery is indicated

COMPLICATIONS

- Initiating iodine supplementation in a geographic area causes increased frequency of hyperthyroidism in first year, followed by greatly reduced rates of toxic nodular goiter and Graves' disease thereafter
- Rarely, Graves' disease may develop in patients treated with ^{131}I 3–10 months after treatment
- Goiters may become multinodular and grow to great size

WHEN TO REFER

- Refer to endocrinologist for hyperthyroidism, enlarging goiter, suspicious nodules
- Refer to thyroid surgeon for thyroidectomy for cosmesis, compressive symptoms, or thyrotoxicosis in adults with very large multinodular goiters

WHEN TO ADMIT

- Thyroidectomy
- ^{131}I treatment

PREVENTION

- Dietary iodine supplementation started in Switzerland in 1922 with addition of potassium iodide to table salt
- Current level of supplementation in the United States is 20 mg potassium iodide per kg salt
- Iodized salt has greatly reduced incidence of endemic goiter. Unfortunately, many iodine-deficient countries have inadequate programs for iodine supplementation
- Minimum dietary requirement for iodine is about 50 mcg daily
  - Optimal iodine intake is 150–300 mcg daily
  - Iodine sufficiency is demonstrated by urinary iodide excretion > 10 mcg/dL

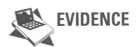

EVIDENCE

PRACTICE GUIDELINES

- American Association of Clinical Endocrinologists medical guidelines for clinical practice for the evaluation and treatment of hyperthyroidism and hypothyroidism. American Association of Clinical Endocrinologists, American College of Endocrinology—Medical Specialty Society, 2002

WEB SITES

- American Association of Clinical Endocrinologists
- Thyroid Disease Manager site

INFORMATION FOR PATIENTS

- Merck Manual
- Program Against Micronutrient Malnutrition—Emory University

REFERENCES

- Bellantone R et al. Predictive factors for recurrence after thyroid lobectomy for unilateral non-toxic goiter in an endemic area: results of a multivariate analysis. Surgery. 2004 Dec; 136(6):1247–51. [PMID: 15657583]
- Valentino R et al. Screening a coastal population in Southern Italy: iodine deficiency and prevalence of goitre, nutritional aspects and cardiovascular risk factors. Nutr Metab Cardiovasc Dis. 2004 Feb;14(1):15–9. [PMID: 15053159]

Gonococcal Infections

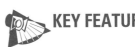

KEY FEATURES

ESSENTIALS OF DIAGNOSIS

- Purulent and profuse urethral discharge, especially in men, with dysuria, yielding positive smear
- In men
  - Epididymitis
  - Prostatitis
  - Periurethral inflammation
  - Proctitis
  - Pharyngeal infection

- In women
  - Asymptomatic or cervicitis with purulent discharge
  - Vaginitis, salpingitis, proctitis also occur
- Disseminated disease
  - Fever
  - Rash
  - Tenosynovitis
  - Septic arthritis
- Gram-negative intracellular diplococci seen in a smear or cultured from any site, particularly the urethra, cervix, pharynx, and rectum

GENERAL CONSIDERATIONS

- Gonorrhea is caused by *Neisseria gonorrhoeae*, a gram-negative diplococcus

DEMOGRAPHICS

- Gonorrhea is transmitted as a result of sexual activity and has its greatest incidence in the 15- to 29-year-old age group

 ## CLINICAL FINDINGS

SYMPTOMS AND SIGNS

- Asymptomatic infection is common and occurs in both sexes
- Atypical sites of primary infection (eg, the pharynx or rectum) must always be considered

Urethritis

- In men
  - Initially, burning on urination and a serous or milky discharge
  - One to 3 days later, more pronounced urethral pain and the discharge becomes yellow, creamy, and profuse, sometimes blood tinged
  - May regress and become chronic or progress to involve the prostate, epididymis, and periurethral glands with acute, painful inflammation
  - Rectal infection is common in homosexual men
- In women
  - Dysuria
  - Urinary frequency and urgency

Cervicitis

- Infection may be asymptomatic, with only slightly increased vaginal discharge and moderate cervicitis on examination
- Infection often becomes symptomatic during menses
- Vaginitis and cervicitis with purulent discharge and inflammation of Bartholin's glands are common

- Infection may remain as a chronic cervicitis
- It may progress to involve the uterus and tubes with acute and chronic salpingitis and with ultimate scarring of tubes and sterility
- In pelvic inflammatory disease, anaerobes and chlamydiae often accompany gonococci

Conjunctivitis

- Direct inoculation of gonococci into the conjunctival sac occurs by autoinoculation from a genital infection
- The purulent conjunctivitis may rapidly progress to panophthalmitis and loss of the eye unless treated promptly

DIFFERENTIAL DIAGNOSIS

- Nongonococcal urethritis, eg, *Chlamydia, Ureaplasma urealyticum*
- Septic arthritis of other bacterial cause
- Reactive arthritis (Reiter's syndrome)
- Vaginal discharge due to candidiasis, bacterial vaginosis, or trichomoniasis
- Chronic meningococcemia

 ## DIAGNOSIS

LABORATORY TESTS

- In men, Gram stain of urethral discharge, especially during the first week after onset, typically shows gram-negative diplococci in polymorphonuclear leukocytes
- Gram stain is less often positive in women
- Culture is the diagnostic gold standard, particularly when the Gram stain is negative
- Nucleic acid amplification tests
  - Detects *N gonorrhoeae* in cervical and urethral swab specimens and in urine, allowing for rapid diagnosis of gonococcal infection
  - Sensitivity and specificity are comparable or superior to culture of swab specimens

 ## TREATMENT

MEDICATIONS

- For urethritis or cervicitis
  - Treatment of choice is either ceftriaxone, 125 mg IM, or cefpodoxime, 400 mg PO as a single dose
  - Resistance to fluoroquinolone is increasing and fluoroquinolones are no longer recommended

  - Since coexistent chlamydial infection is common, also treat with doxycycline, 100 mg PO BID for 7 days, or a single 1-g oral dose of azithromycin
- Salpingitis, prostatitis, bacteremia, arthritis, and other complications due to susceptible strains
  - Initial therapy
    - Ceftriaxone, 1 g IV once daily
    - A fluoroquinolone (eg, ciprofloxacin, 400 mg IV q12h), provided the isolate is susceptible
    - Spectinomycin, 2 g IM q12h
  - At least a week total duration of therapy, which may be completed with an oral regimen such as
    - Cefpodoxime, 200–400 mg PO q12h
    - Levofloxacin, 500 mg once daily

THERAPEUTIC PROCEDURES

- Therapy typically is administered before antimicrobial susceptibilities are known
- All sexual partners should be treated

 ## OUTCOME

COMPLICATIONS

Disseminated disease

- Systemic complications follow the dissemination of gonococci from the primary site via the bloodstream
- Gonococcal bacteremia is associated with
  - Intermittent fever
  - Arthralgia
  - Skin lesions ranging from maculopapular to pustular, which tend to be few in number and peripherally located

WHEN TO REFER

- Report all cases to the public health department for tracing of contacts

WHEN TO ADMIT

- Most cases of pelvic inflammatory disease (perhaps not the mild cases)
- All cases of suspected or proven disseminated disease

PREVENTION

- The condom, if properly used, can reduce the risk of infection
- Effective drugs taken in therapeutic doses within 24 h of exposure can abort an infection

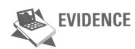

EVIDENCE

PRACTICE GUIDELINES

- Centers for Disease Control and Prevention. Sexually transmitted disease treatment guidelines 2002.

REFERENCE

- Workowski KA et al; Centers for Disease Control and Prevention. Sexually transmitted diseases treatment guidelines, 2006. MMWR Recomm Rep. 2006 Aug 4;55(RR-11):1–94. [PMID: 16888612]

Goodpasture's Syndrome, Pulmonary

KEY FEATURES

ESSENTIALS OF DIAGNOSIS

- Triad of pulmonary hemorrhage, circulating anti-glomerular basement membrane (GBM) antibody, and glomerulonephritis due to anti-GBM
- Up to one-third of patients with anti-GBM glomerulonephritis have no evidence of lung injury

GENERAL CONSIDERATIONS

- Clinical constellation of recurrent pulmonary alveolar hemorrhage with rapidly progressive glomerulonephritis
- Injury mediated by anti-GBM antibody
- ~10% of patients with rapidly progressive acute glomerulonephritis have anti-GBM
- Associated with influenza A infection, hydrocarbon solvent exposure, and HLA-DR2 and -B7 antigens

DEMOGRAPHICS

- Incidence in males ~6 times that in females
- Occurs most commonly in the second and third decades

CLINICAL FINDINGS

SYMPTOMS AND SIGNS

- Usually presents with hemoptysis, though pulmonary hemorrhage may be occult
- Dyspnea, cough, hypoxemia, and bilateral alveolar opacities are typical
- Iron deficiency anemia
- Microscopic hematuria
- Upper respiratory tract infection precedes onset in 20–60% of cases
- Possible respiratory failure
- Hypertension
- Edema

DIFFERENTIAL DIAGNOSIS

- Severe congestive heart failure (pulmonary edema and prerenal azotemia)
- Renal failure (with hypervolemia and pulmonary edema)
- Microscopic polyangiitis (polyarteritis nodosa)
- Systemic lupus erythematosus
- Henoch-Schönlein purpura
- Wegener's granulomatosis
- Legionnaire's disease
- Renal vein thrombosis with pulmonary embolism

DIAGNOSIS

LABORATORY TESTS

- Circulating anti-GBM antibody in serum in > 90%
- Iron deficiency anemia
- Complement levels are normal
- Sputum contains hemosiderin-laden macrophages
- Diffusion capacity of carbon monoxide may be markedly increased

IMAGING STUDIES

- Chest radiographs show shifting alveolar opacities

DIAGNOSTIC PROCEDURES

- Biopsy demonstrates characteristic linear IgG deposits in glomeruli or alveoli by immunofluorescence

TREATMENT

MEDICATIONS

- Treatment is a combination of plasma exchange therapy to remove circulating antibodies and administration of immunosuppressive drugs (corticosteroids and cyclophosphamide) to prevent formation of new antibodies
- Give methylprednisolone, 30 mg/kg IV once daily for 3 days followed by oral prednisone at 1 mg/kg/day **and** oral cyclophosphamide, 2 mg/kg/day

THERAPEUTIC PROCEDURES

- Plasmapheresis, performed daily for up to 2 weeks, in combination with the corticosteroids and cyclophosphamide

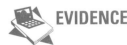

OUTCOME

FOLLOW-UP

- Anti-GBM antibody levels should decrease as the clinical course improves

COMPLICATIONS

- Renal failure
- Respiratory failure

PROGNOSIS

- Prognosis poor in patients with oliguria and serum creatinine > 6–7 mg/dL

WHEN TO REFER

- Patients should be referred to a pulmonologist, rheumatologist, or nephrologist

WHEN TO ADMIT

- Respiratory insufficiency
- Progressive or severe renal disease

EVIDENCE

INFORMATION FOR PATIENTS

- National Institutes of Health
- National Kidney and Urologic Diseases Information Clearinghouse

REFERENCE

- Collard HR et al. Diffuse alveolar hemorrhage. Clin Chest Med. 2004 Sep; 25(3):583–92. [PMID: 15331194]

Gouty Arthritis

KEY FEATURES

ESSENTIALS OF DIAGNOSIS

- Acute onset, typically nocturnal
- Usually monarticular, often involving the first metatarsophalangeal (MTP) joint
- Polyarticular involvement more common with long-standing disease
- Hyperuricemia in most; identification of urate crystals in joint fluid or tophi is diagnostic
- Dramatic therapeutic response to non-steroidal anti-inflammatory drugs

GENERAL CONSIDERATIONS

- A metabolic disease of heterogeneous nature, often familial, associated with abnormal amounts of urates in the body and characterized early by a recurring acute arthritis, usually monarticular, and later by chronic deforming arthritis
- **Secondary gout** is from acquired causes of hyperuricemia
  - Medication use (diuretics, low-dose aspirin, cyclosporine, and niacin)
  - Myeloproliferative disorders, multiple myeloma, hemoglobinopathies
  - Chronic renal disease
  - Hypothyroidism, psoriasis, sarcoidosis, and lead poisoning
- Alcohol ingestion promotes hyperuricemia by increasing urate production and decreasing the renal excretion of uric acid
- Hospitalized patients frequently suffer attacks of gout because of changes in diet (eg, inability to take oral feedings following abdominal surgery) or medications that lead either to rapid reductions or increases in the serum urate level

DEMOGRAPHICS

- Especially common in Pacific Islanders, eg, Filipinos and Samoans
- Rarely caused by a specifically determined genetic aberration (eg, Lesch-Nyhan syndrome)
- 90% of patients with primary gout are men, usually over 30 years of age
- In women, the onset is typically post-menopausal

CLINICAL FINDINGS
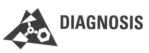

SYMPTOMS AND SIGNS

- **Sudden onset of arthritis**
  - Frequently nocturnal
  - Either without apparent precipitating cause or following rapid fluctuations in serum urate levels
  - The MTP joint of the great toe is the most susceptible joint ("podagra")
  - Other joints, especially those of the feet, ankles, and knees, are also commonly affected
  - May develop in periarticular soft tissues such as the arch of the foot
- **As the attack progresses**
  - The pain becomes intense
  - The involved joints are swollen and exquisitely tender
  - The overlying skin is tense, warm, and dusky red
  - Fever is common
- Tophi
  - May be found in cartilage, external ears, hands, feet, olecranon, prepatellar bursae, tendons, and bone
  - They are usually seen only after several attacks of acute arthritis
- Asymptomatic periods of months or years commonly follow the initial attack
- After years of recurrent severe monarthritis attacks, gout can evolve into a chronic, deforming polyarthritis of upper and lower extremities that mimics rheumatoid arthritis

DIFFERENTIAL DIAGNOSIS

Arthritis
- Cellulitis
- Septic arthritis
- Pseudogout
- Rheumatoid arthritis
- Reactive arthritis
- Osteoarthritis
- Chronic lead poisoning (saturnine gout)
- Palindromic rheumatism

Podagra
- Trauma
- Cellulitis
- Sarcoidosis
- Pseudogout
- Psoriatic arthritis
- Bursitis of first MTP joint (inflamed bunion)

Tophi
- Rheumatoid nodules
- Erythema nodosum
- Gout

- Coccidioidomycosis
- Endocarditis (Osler nodes)
- Sarcoidosis
- Polyarteritis nodosa

DIAGNOSIS
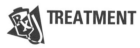

LABORATORY TESTS

- The serum uric acid is elevated (> 7.5 mg/dL) in 95% of patients who have serial measurements during the course of an attack
- However, a single uric acid determination is normal in up to 25% of cases, so it does not exclude gout

IMAGING STUDIES

- Early in the disease, radiographs show no changes
- Later, punched-out erosions with an overhanging rim of cortical bone ("rat bite") develop. When these are adjacent to a soft tissue tophus, they are diagnostic of gout

DIAGNOSTIC PROCEDURES

- Identification of sodium urate crystals in joint fluid or material aspirated from a tophus establishes the diagnosis
- The crystals, which may be extracellular or found within neutrophils, are needle-like and negatively birefringent when examined by polarized light microscopy

TREATMENT

MEDICATIONS

Asymptomatic hyperuricemia
- Should not be treated
- Uric acid–lowering drugs are not necessary until arthritis, renal calculi, or tophi become apparent

Acute attack
- **Nonsteroidal anti-inflammatory drugs** are the treatment of choice
- The pain of an acute attack may require **opioids**. Aspirin should be avoided since it aggravates hyperuricemia
- For monarticular gout, **intra-articular corticosteroid administration** (eg, triamcinolone, 10–40 mg depending on the size of the joint) is most effective
- For polyarticular gout, **corticosteroids** may be given intravenously (eg, methylprednisolone, 40 mg/day tapered off over 7 days) or orally (eg, prednisone, 40–60 mg/day tapered off over 7 days)

SURGERY

- Surgical excision of large tophi rarely offers mechanical improvement in selected deformities

THERAPEUTIC PROCEDURES

- Corticosteroid injections for acute monarticular disease
- Bed rest is important and should be continued for about 24 h after the acute attack has subsided. Early ambulation may precipitate a recurrence
- Treat the acute arthritis first and hyperuricemia later, if at all. Sudden reduction of serum uric acid often precipitates further gouty arthritis

 OUTCOME

FOLLOW-UP

- Maintain uric acid level within the normal range in nontophaceous gout
- Maintain serum uric acid below 5.0 mg/dL in tophaceous gout

COMPLICATIONS

- Chronic tophaceous arthritis can occur after repeated attacks of inadequately treated acute gout
- Uric acid kidney stones (5–10% of patients)
  - Hyperuricemia correlates highly with the likelihood of developing stones
  - The risk of stone formation reaching 50% with a serum urate level above 13 mg/dL
- Chronic urate nephropathy. Although progressive renal failure occurs in a substantial percentage of patients with chronic gout, the etiologic role of hyperuricemia is controversial, because there are numerous confounding risk factors for renal failure

PROGNOSIS

- Untreated, the acute attack may last from a few days to several weeks, but proper treatment quickly terminates the attack
- The intervals between acute attacks vary up to years, but the asymptomatic periods often become shorter if the disease progresses

WHEN TO REFER

- Refer to a rheumatologist if the patient has recurrent attacks despite treatment

WHEN TO ADMIT

- For suspected or proven superimposed septic arthritis

PREVENTION

- Potentially reversible causes of hyperuricemia
  - High-purine diet
  - Obesity
  - Frequent alcohol consumption
  - Use of certain medications (diuretics, niacin, low-dose aspirin)
- Colchicine, 0.6 mg PO once or twice daily
  - Can be used to prevent future attacks
  - Frequently prescribed to prevent attacks when probenecid or allopurinol is being initiated
- Two classes of drugs can lower uric acid levels in patients with frequent arthritis, tophaceous deposits, or renal damage
  - Probenecid, 1–2 g PO daily, is the principal uricosuric drug, which cannot be used if the creatinine is > 2 mg/dL
  - Allopurinol, 100–300 mg/day PO based on renal function
    - Promptly lowers plasma urate and urinary uric acid concentrations and facilitates tophus mobilization
    - Most common sign of hypersensitivity to allopurinol (occurring in 2% of cases) is a pruritic rash that may progress to toxic epidermal necrolysis
    - Vasculitis and hepatitis are other rare complications

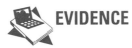 **EVIDENCE**

PRACTICE GUIDELINES

- Zhang W et al; EULAR Standing Committee for International Clinical Studies Including Therapeutics. EULAR evidence based recommendations for gout. Part I: Diagnosis. Report of a task force of the Standing Committee for International Clinical Studies Including Therapeutics (ESCISIT). Ann Rheum Dis. 2006 Oct;65(10):1301–11. [PMID: 16707533]
- Zhang w et al; EULAR Standing Committee for International Clinical Studies Including Therapeutics. EULAR evidence based recommendations for gout. Part II: Management. Report of a task force of the EULAR Standing Committee for International Clinical Studies Including Therapeutics (ESCISIT). Ann Rheum Dis. 2006 Oct; 65(10):1312–24. [PMID: 16707532]

WEB SITE

- American College of Rheumatology

INFORMATION FOR PATIENTS

- National Institute of Arthritis and Musculoskeletal and Skin Disease

Guillain-Barré Syndrome

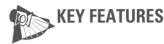 **KEY FEATURES**

ESSENTIALS OF DIAGNOSIS

- Acute or subacute progressive polyradiculoneuropathy
- Usually ascending, symmetric weakness
- Paresthesias are more variable

GENERAL CONSIDERATIONS

- A symmetric sensory, motor, or mixed deficit, often most marked distally
- Probably has an immunologic basis, but the mechanism is unclear

DEMOGRAPHICS

- Sometimes follows infections, innoculations, or surgical procedures
- There is an association with preceding *Campylobacter jejuni* enteritis

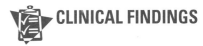 **CLINICAL FINDINGS**

SYMPTOMS AND SIGNS

Motor symptoms

- The main complaint is of weakness
  - Varies widely in severity in different patients
  - Often has a proximal emphasis and symmetric distribution
  - Usually begins in the legs, spreading to a variable extent but frequently involving the arms and often one or both sides of the face
  - The muscles of respiration or deglutition may also be affected

Sensory symptoms

- Sensory symptoms are usually less conspicuous than motor ones, but distal paresthesias and dysesthesias are common, and neuropathic or radicular pain is present in many patients

Autonomic symptoms

- Autonomic disturbances are common, may be severe, and are sometimes life-threatening; they include the following
  - Tachycardia

– Cardiac rhythm irregularities
– Hypotension or hypertension
– Facial flushing
– Abnormalities of sweating
– Pulmonary dysfunction
– Impaired sphincter control

DIFFERENTIAL DIAGNOSIS

- Chronic inflammatory demyelinating polyneuropathy (CIDP)
- Porphyria
- Diphtheritic neuropathy
- Toxic neuropathy, eg, lead, mercury, organophosphates, hexacarbon solvents
- Poliomyelitis
- Botulism
- Tick paralysis
- Spinal cord lesion
- Transverse myelitis
- West Nile virus infection
- Periodic paralysis syndrome

DIAGNOSIS

LABORATORY TESTS

- The cerebrospinal fluid characteristically contains a high protein concentration with a normal cell content, but this change may take 2 or 3 weeks to develop

DIAGNOSTIC PROCEDURES

- Electrophysiologic (nerve conduction) studies may reveal marked abnormalities, which do not necessarily parallel the clinical disorder in their temporal course
- Pathologic examination shows primary demyelination or, less commonly, axonal degeneration

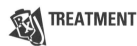

TREATMENT

MEDICATIONS

- Marked hypotension may respond to volume replacement or pressor agents
- IV immunoglobulin (400 mg/kg/day for 5 days) is helpful and imposes less stress on the cardiovascular system than plasmapheresis
- Low-dose heparin to prevent pulmonary embolism should be considered
- Prednisone is ineffective and may prolong recovery time

THERAPEUTIC PROCEDURES

- Respiratory toilet and chest physical therapy help prevent atelectasis

- Plasmapheresis is of value
  - Best performed within the first few days of illness
  - Best reserved for clinically severe or rapidly progressive cases or those with ventilatory impairment

OUTCOME

FOLLOW-UP

- Monitor spirometry
  - Patients should be admitted to intensive care units if their forced vital capacity is declining
  - Intubation is considered if the forced vital capacity reaches 15 mL/kg, dyspnea becomes evident, or oxygen saturation declines

PROGNOSIS

- Most patients eventually make a good recovery
  - However, recovery may take many months
  - About 20% of patients have residual disability
- Approximately 3% of patients have one or more clinically similar relapses, sometimes several years after the initial illness

WHEN TO ADMIT

- Decline in forced vital capacity; patients may need intensive care unit admission

EVIDENCE

PRACTICE GUIDELINES

- National Guideline Clearinghouse

WEB SITE

- Neuromuscular Disease Center

INFORMATION FOR PATIENTS

- National Institute of Neurological Disorders and Stroke
- The Mayo Clinic

REFERENCES

- Hughes RA et al. Corticosteroids for Guillain-Barré syndrome. Cochrane Database Syst Rev. 2006 Apr 19; (2):CD001446. [PMID: 16625544]
- Hughes RA et al. Guillain-Barré syndrome. Lancet. 2005 Nov 5;366(9497): 1653–66. [PMID: 16271648]

Gynecomastia

KEY FEATURES

ESSENTIALS OF DIAGNOSIS

- Glandular enlargement of the male breast
- **Fatty** gynecomastia typically diffuse and nontender
- **Glandular** gynecomastia "lumpy" and may be tender
- Must be distinguished from tumors or mastitis

GENERAL CONSIDERATIONS

Causes
- Endocrine
  - Hyperprolactinemia of any cause
  - Hyperthyroidism
  - Klinefelter's syndrome
  - Hypogonadism
- Systemic disease: chronic liver or renal disease
- Neoplasm
  - Testicular
  - Adrenal
  - Lung
  - Liver
- Drugs (selected)
  - Alcohol, marijuana
  - Amiodarone
  - Cimetidine, omeprazole
  - Diazepam
  - Digoxin
  - Estrogens, progestins, testosterone
  - Finasteride
  - Flutamide
  - Isoniazid
  - Ketoconazole
  - Opioids
  - Protease inhibitors and antiretrovirals
  - Spironolactone
  - Tricyclic antidepressants
  - Eating necks of poultry that have been fed estrogen
- HIV infection treated with highly active antiretroviral therapy (HAART), especially efavirenz or didanosine; breast enlargement resolves spontaneously in 73% within 9 months

DEMOGRAPHICS

- Common in puberty, especially in boys taller and heavier than average
- Common among elderly men
- Common in obesity
- Develops in ~50% of athletes who abuse androgens and anabolic steroids
- Family history of malignancy

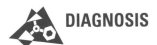

CLINICAL FINDINGS

SYMPTOMS AND SIGNS

- Female-appearing male breast
- Graded according to severity: I (mild), II (moderate), III (severe)
- Breast enlargement may be
  - Fatty
    - Usually diffuse
    - Nontender
  - Glandular
    - Asymmetric or unilateral, "lumpy"
    - Glandular enlargement beneath the areola may be tender
- Nipple discharge may be present
- Pubertal gynecomastia: tender discoid enlargement of breast tissue beneath areola, 2–3 cm in diameter
- Testicular examination may reveal tumor

DIFFERENTIAL DIAGNOSIS

- Breast cancer
- Fatty breast enlargement of obesity
- Breast abscess (mastitis)
- Metastatic cancer, eg, prostate
- Treatment of prostate cancer with gonadotropin-releasing hormone agonists/antagonists or antiandrogens

DIAGNOSIS

LABORATORY TESTS

- Serum prolactin elevated if gynecomastia caused by hyperprolactinemia
- Detectable serum β-human chorionic gonadotropin (hCG) implicates testicular tumor (germ cell or Sertoli cell) or other malignancy (usually lung or liver)
- However, low detectable levels (β-hCG < 5 mU/mL) may occur in primary hypogonadism if assay cross-reacts with luteinizing hormone (LH)
- Low serum testosterone, high serum LH in primary hypogonadism
- High testosterone, high LH in partial androgen resistance
- Serum estradiol usually normal but may be increased by
  - Testicular tumors
  - Increased β-hCG
  - Liver disease
  - Obesity
  - Adrenal tumors (rare)
- Serum thyroid-stimulating hormone low in hyperthyroidism

- Karyotype (for Klinefelter's syndrome) indicated in men with persistent gynecomastia without obvious cause

IMAGING STUDIES

- Chest radiograph or lung CT if lung cancer or metastases suspected
- Testicular ultrasound if detectable β-hCG or mass on examination
- CT or MRI of abdomen and pelvis if detectable β-hCG and no mass on testicular examination or ultrasound
- Mammography for large tumor to exclude breast cancer

DIAGNOSTIC PROCEDURES

- Fine-needle aspiration of suspicious masses, especially when unilateral or asymmetric, to distinguish gynecomastia from cancer or mastitis

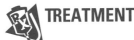

TREATMENT

MEDICATIONS

- Treatment of underlying condition
- Discontinue potentially offending medications if possible (eg, discontinue spironolactone and substitute eplerenone)
- Medications used to treat gynecomastia can produce adverse reactions; treat gynecomastia only if it is a troubling and persistent problem
- For painful or persistent glandular, rather than diffuse fatty, gynecomastia (> 12 months)
  - Raloxifene, 60 mg PO once daily, may be more effective than tamoxifen
  - Aromatase inhibitors (eg, letrozole, anastrozole, exemestane)
    - Marginally effective
    - Should not ordinarily be used for adolescent boys since long-term therapy may prevent epiphyseal fusion

SURGERY

- Surgery is reserved for persistent or severe gynecomastia, since results are often disappointing
- Endoscopically assisted transaxillary liposuction and subcutaneous mastectomy may produce acceptable results

OUTCOME

PROGNOSIS

- Pubertal and idiopathic gynecomastia usually subside spontaneously within 1–2 years

- Drug-induced gynecomastia resolves after offending drug is discontinued

PREVENTION

- Avoidance of androgen and anabolic steroid abuse

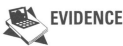

EVIDENCE

PRACTICE GUIDELINES

- Daniels IR et al. Gynaecomastia. Eur J Surg. 2001;167:885. [PMID: 11841077]
- Dicker AP. The safety and tolerability of low-dose irradiation for the management of gynaecomastia caused by anti-androgen monotherapy. Lancet Oncol. 2003;4:30. [PMID: 12517537]
- Fruhstorfer BH et al. A systematic approach to the surgical treatment of gynaecomastia. Br J Plast Surg. 2003; 56:237. [PMID: 12859919]

INFORMATION FOR PATIENTS

- American Academy of Family Physicians—Gynecomastia: when breasts form in males
- Mayo Clinic
- MedlinePlus—Gynecomastia
- University of Iowa Plastic Surgery

REFERENCES

- Lawrence SE et al. Beneficial effects of raloxifene and tamoxifen in the treatment of pubertal gynecomastia. J Pediatr. 2004 Jul;145(1):71–6. [PMID: 15238910]
- Mira JA et al; Grupo Andaluz para el Estudio de las Enfermedades Infecciosas. Gynaecomastia in HIV-infected men on highly active antiretroviral therapy: association with efavirenz and didanosine treatment. Antivir Ther. 2004 Aug;9(4):511–7. [PMID: 15456082]
- Ramon Y et al. Multimodality gynecomastia repair by cross-chest power-assisted superficial liposuction combined with endoscopic-assisted pull-through excision. Ann Plast Surg. 2005 Dec;55(6):591–4. [PMID: 16327457]
- Rhoden EL et al. Treatment of testosterone-induced gynecomastia with the aromatase inhibitor, anastrozole. Int J Impot Res. 2004 Feb;16(1):95–7. [PMID: 14963480]

Head & Neck Cancer

KEY FEATURES

ESSENTIALS OF DIAGNOSIS

- New and persistent (> 2 weeks duration) hoarseness in a smoker
- Persistent throat or ear pain, especially with swallowing
- Neck mass
- Hemoptysis
- Stridor or other symptoms of a compromised airway

GENERAL CONSIDERATIONS

- Head and neck examination in patients with concerning symptoms or signs or unexplained weight loss, especially in those over 45 who smoke tobacco or drink immoderately
- Examination components include the following
  - A systematic intraoral, pharyngeal, and laryngeal examination (including the lateral tongue, floor of the mouth, gingiva, buccal area, palate, tonsillar fossae, and indirect or fiberoptic examination of the pharynx and larynx)
  - Palpation of the neck for enlarged lymph nodes

DEMOGRAPHICS

- Occurs predominantly in heavy smokers and/or those with significant alcohol use
- Most common in men between ages 50 and 70
- About 13,000 new cases seen each year in the United States
- Nasopharyngeal cancer most common in southern Chinese ancestry

CLINICAL FINDINGS

SYMPTOMS AND SIGNS

- Persistent (> 2 weeks) throat or ear pain (referred otalgia)
- Weight loss
- Blood in the throat or mouth
- Change in speech/voice quality (including hoarseness or dysarthria)
- Dysphagia
- Airway compromise

- Visible mass (as seen on oral examination or indirect or fiberoptic pharyngoscopy)
- Palpable mass in base of tongue or tonsil
- Neck adenopathy (usually hard)

DIFFERENTIAL DIAGNOSIS

Oropharynx mass
- Occasionally a tumor can be misdiagnosed as a peritonsillar abscess

Laryngeal mass
- Vocal cord nodules
- Papillomas or granulomas
- Leukoplakia, as in the oral cavity, requires clarification clinically or by biopsy as judged by an experienced clinician

Oral mass
- Aphthous ulcer (canker sore, ulcerative stomatitis)
- See Leukoplakia & Erythroplakia and Lichen Planus for additional differential diagnosis

Nasopharynx mass
- Occasional benign cysts can mimic a tumor

DIAGNOSIS

LABORATORY TESTS

- Complete blood cell count, liver function tests

IMAGING STUDIES

- MRI is preferred to CT for staging, except laryngeal lesions
- Chest radiograph
- Chest CT may be indicated if there is concern for a second primary mass in the lung or for lung metastases
- PET or PET-CT may be helpful

DIAGNOSTIC PROCEDURES

- Laryngoscopy
- Fine-needle aspiration biopsy may confirm the presence of the carcinoma and the histologic type, but caution and clinical judgment should be exercised in interpreting an apparently negative result

TREATMENT

MEDICATIONS

- Cisplatin as a radiosensitizer during radiation therapy

- Other chemotherapy agents, including 5-fluorouracil, taxanes, carboplatinol, as well as methotrexate
- Management of associated **pain** is critically important and often includes opioids with short (3 h) and long (8–72 h) duration of effect, nonsteroidal anti-inflammatory agents, COX-2 inhibitor, and gabapentin
- See Tables 7 and 8

SURGERY

- **Small tumors** are often best treated with a sole modality of either function-sparing surgery or radiation, depending on the site of the primary tumor
- **Large nonoropharyngeal tumors** often are best treated with surgery and postoperative irradiation

THERAPEUTIC PROCEDURES

- Treatment depends on tumor site, TNM stage, prior treatment, and patient comorbidities (such as cardiovascular and lung disease)
- There must be careful weighing of the side effects of treatment options
- **Oropharyngeal tumors** (eg, base of the tongue and tonsil fossa) are usually best treated with radiation and often concomitant chemotherapy regardless of extent of primary and nodal disease
- **T1–2 laryngeal tumors** are best treated with radiation, endoscopic resection, or open partial resection
- **More advanced laryngeal tumors** are treated with chemoradiation or extended partial laryngeal surgery, both intended to avoid a permanent laryngeal stoma
- For **unresectable recurrent disease** and distant metastases, weigh the benefits of chemotherapy and possibly palliative radiation therapy

OUTCOME

FOLLOW-UP

- Monitor for recurrent squamous cell carcinoma or new primary tumor is key; incidence of second tumors: ~3–4%/ year
- Examine clinically q4–6 weeks in year 1, q8–10 weeks in year 2, q3–4 months thereafter for several years
- PET scans at 3 months postradiation therapy and baseline posttreatment MRIs for subsequent surveillance
- Strategies for DNA or protein molecular markers under investigation

COMPLICATIONS

- Airway compromise, requiring tracheotomy
- Bleeding associated with surface ulceration
- Erosion into major artery can lead to life-threatening oral or neck hemorrhage
- Dysphagia and odynophagia may lead to weight loss, requiring gastrostomy tube
- Failure to recognize early tumors results in more extensive intervention, with greater operative risks

PROGNOSIS

- Correlated with TNM staging, including specific site of disease, extent of primary tumor, nodal stage, presence of distant metastases
- Overall, 65% of head and neck cancers are cured; prognosis ranges from > 90% for early tongue and early larynx lesions to very poor for unresectable neck disease or distant metastases

WHEN TO REFER

- Specialty referral should be sought early for diagnosis and treatment
- Indirect or fiberoptic examination of the nasopharynx, oropharynx, hypopharynx, and larynx by otolaryngologist–head and neck surgeon should be considered with oral erythroplakia, unexplained throat or ear pain, unexplained oral or nasal bleeding, firm neck mass, or visible oral cavity or oropharyngeal mass

WHEN TO ADMIT

- Airway compromise, hemorrhage, dehydration
- Institute effective pain management regimen for severe pain

PREVENTION

- Smoking cessation and alcohol abatement programs helpful

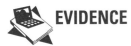

EVIDENCE

PRACTICE GUIDELINES

- Forastiere AA et al; NCCN Head and Neck Cancers Practice Guidelines Panel. National Comprehensive Cancer Network: Head and Neck Cancers v.1.2004.
- Pfister DG et al. American Society of Clinical Oncology clinical practice guideline for the use of larynx-preservation strategies in the treatment of laryngeal cancer. J Clin Oncol. 2006 Aug 1; 24(22):3693–704. [PMID: 16832122]

WEB SITE

- National Cancer Institute: Head and Neck Cancers

INFORMATION FOR PATIENTS

- American Academy of Otolaryngology: Head and Neck Surgery: Head and Neck Cancer
- American Cancer Society
- National Cancer Institute: Head and Neck Cancer: Q & A

REFERENCES

- Bernier J et al. Postoperative irradiation with or without concomitant chemotherapy for locally advanced head and neck cancer. N Engl J Med. 2004 May 6;350(19):1945–52. [PMID: 15128894]
- Forastiere AA et al. Concurrent chemotherapy and radiotherapy for organ preservation in advanced laryngeal cancer. N Engl J Med. 2003 Nov 27; 349(22):2091–8. [PMID: 14645636]
- Ganly I et al. Results of surgical salvage after failure of definitive radiation therapy for early-stage squamous cell carcinoma of the glottic larynx. Arch Otolaryngol Head Neck Surg. 2006 Jan; 132(1):59–66. [PMID: 16415431]
- Hoffman HT et al. Laryngeal cancer in the United States: changes in demographics, patterns of care, and survival. Laryngoscope. 2006 Sep;116(9 Pt 2 Suppl 111):1–13. [PMID: 16946667]
- Loughran S et al. Quality of life and voice following endoscopic resection or radiotherapy for early glottic cancer. Clin Otolaryngol. 2005 Feb;30(1):42–7. [PMID: 15748189]
- Sessions DG et al. Supraglottic laryngeal cancer: analysis of treatment results. Laryngoscope. 2005 Aug;115(8):1402–10. [PMID: 16094113]
- Yamazaki H et al. Radiotherapy for early glottic carcinoma (T1N0M0): results of prospective randomized study of radiation fraction size and overall treatment time. Int J Radiat Oncol Biol Phys. 2006 Jan 1;64(1):77–82. [PMID 16169681]

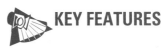

Head Injury

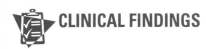

KEY FEATURES

ESSENTIALS OF DIAGNOSIS

- Absence of skull fracture does not exclude the possibility of severe head injury
- In many elderly patients, there may not be a known history of head trauma
- Occasionally, head injury, often trivial, precedes symptoms by several weeks

GENERAL CONSIDERATIONS

- Some guide to prognosis is provided by the mental status
  - Loss of consciousness for more than 1 or 2 min implies a worse prognosis than otherwise
- The degree of retrograde and posttraumatic amnesia provides an indication of the severity of injury and thus of the prognosis

DEMOGRAPHICS

- Trauma is the most common cause of death in young people, and head injury accounts for almost half of these trauma-related deaths

CLINICAL FINDINGS

SYMPTOMS AND SIGNS

- See Table 136
- Special attention should be given to the level of consciousness and extent of any brainstem dysfunction
- Clinical signs of basilar skull fracture
  - Bruising about the orbit (raccoon sign)
  - Blood in the external auditory meatus (Battle's sign)
  - Leakage of cerebrospinal fluid (which can be identified by its glucose content) from the ear or nose
- **Chronic subdural hemorrhage**
  - Head injury, often subtle, may precede the onset of symptoms by several weeks
  - Mental changes, such as slowness, drowsiness, headache, confusion, memory disturbances, personality change, or even dementia, may occur
  - Focal neurologic deficits such as hemiparesis or hemisensory disturbance are less common

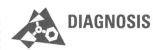

DIAGNOSIS

IMAGING STUDIES

- See Table 136
- Cervical spine radiographs (especially in the lateral projection) should always be obtained in
  - Comatose patients
  - Patients with severe neck pain or a deficit possibly related to cord compression
- CT scanning
  - Can demonstrate intracranial hemorrhage
  - May also provide evidence of cerebral edema and displacement of midline structures
- Skull radiographs or CT scans may provide evidence of fractures

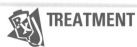

TREATMENT

MEDICATIONS

- Measures to reduce intracranial pressure include
  - Induced hyperventilation
  - IV mannitol infusion
  - IV furosemide
  - Corticosteroids provide no benefit in this context
- Conservative treatment is often helpful if there is any leakage of cerebrospinal fluid
  - Elevate the head
  - Restrict fluids
  - Administer acetazolamide (250 mg QID)
- Antibiotics should be prescribed if infection occurs
- No clear evidence that prophylactic anticonvulsant therapy reduces the incidence of posttraumatic seizures

SURGERY

- Scalp lacerations and depressed or compound depressed skull fractures should be treated surgically as appropriate
- Surgical evacuation of intracranial hematomas may be needed to prevent cerebral compression and herniation
- If leakage of cerebrospinal fluid continues for more than a few days, lumbar subarachnoid drainage may be necessary

THERAPEUTIC PROCEDURES

- Simple skull fractures require no specific treatment

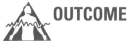

OUTCOME

FOLLOW-UP

- If admission to the hospital is declined, family members should be given clear instructions about the need for, and manner of, checking on them at regular (hourly) intervals and for obtaining additional medical help if necessary

COMPLICATIONS

- Increased intracranial pressure from
  - Seizures
  - Dilutional hyponatremia
  - Cerebral edema
  - Intracranial hematoma requiring surgical evacuation
- Chronic subdural hemorrhage
- Normal-pressure hydrocephalus
- Posttraumatic seizure disorder
- Posttraumatic headache

PROGNOSIS

- Depends on the site and severity of brain damage

WHEN TO ADMIT

- Patients who have lost consciousness for 2 min or more following head injury should be admitted to the hospital for observation
- Patients with focal neurologic deficits, lethargy, or skull fractures

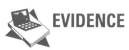

EVIDENCE

PRACTICE GUIDELINES

- Kamerling SN et al. Mild traumatic brain injury in children: practice guidelines for emergency department and hospitalized patients. The Trauma Program, The Children's Hospital of Philadelphia, University of Pennsylvania School of Medicine. Pediatr Emerg Care. 2003;19:431. [PMID: 14676497]
- National Guideline Clearinghouse

INFORMATION FOR PATIENTS

- National Institute of Neurological Disorders and Stroke
- Parmet S et al. JAMA patient page. Concussion in sports. JAMA. 2003; 290:2628. [PMID: 14625340]
- Torpy JM et al. Traumatic brain injury. JAMA. 2003;289:3038. [PMID: 12799412]

REFERENCES

- Vincent JL et al. Primer on medical management of severe brain injury. Crit Care Med. 2005 Jun;33(6):1392–9. [PMID: 15942361]
- Winter CD et al. A review of the current management of severe traumatic brain injury. Surgeon. 2005 Oct;3(5):329–37. [PMID: 16245652]

Headache

KEY FEATURES

ESSENTIALS OF DIAGNOSIS

- Severe headache in a previously well patient is more likely than chronic headache to relate to an intracranial disorder such as hemorrhage, meningitis, or mass lesion
- Headaches worse on awakening may indicate sinusitis or intracranial mass

GENERAL CONSIDERATIONS

- Chronic headaches are commonly due to migraine, tension, or depression, but may be related to intracranial pathology
- Possibility of underlying structural lesions is important because about one-third of patients with brain tumors have a primary complaint of headache

CLINICAL FINDINGS

SYMPTOMS AND SIGNS

Tension headache
- Often pulsating or throbbing
- Bandlike pain is common
- Sense of tightness or pressure is common
- Worsens with stress and at end of day

Migraine
- Often pulsating or throbbing
- May be ocular or periorbital ice pick–like pain
- Lateralized pain is common

Cluster headache
- Ocular or ice pick–like pain
- Lateralized pain is common
- Tends to occur at the same time each day or night

Cranial neuralgias
- Sharp lancinating pain may be suggestive
- Pain localized to one of the divisions of the trigeminal nerve or to the external auditory meatus or pharynx, respectively, in trigeminal or glossopharyngeal neuralgia

Sinusitis-related headache
- May cause tenderness of overlying skin and bone

Intracranial mass lesion–related headache
- Typically dull or steady pain
- Pain may be worse in the morning
- Pain may be localized or general

DIFFERENTIAL DIAGNOSIS

Intracranial
- Migraine
- Cluster headache
- Brain tumor
- Subarachnoid hemorrhage
- Meningitis
- Brain abscess
- Temporal (giant cell) arteritis
- Hypertension
- Caffeine, alcohol, or drug withdrawal
- Pseudotumor cerebri
- Subdural hemorrhage
- Cerebral ischemia
- Arterial dissection (carotid or vertebral)
- Arteriovenous malformation
- Head injury
- Lumbar puncture
- Venous sinus thrombosis (intracranial venous thrombosis)
- Postlumbar puncture
- Carbon monoxide poisoning

Extracranial
- Systemic infections
- Tension headache
- Cervical arthritis
- Glaucoma
- Dental abscess
- Sinusitis
- Otitis media
- Temporomandibular joint (TMJ) syndrome
- Depression
- Somatoform disorder (somatization)
- Trigeminal neuralgia
- Glossopharyngeal neuralgia

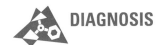 **DIAGNOSIS**

LABORATORY TESTS
- Cerebrospinal fluid examination if a meningeal infection or subarachnoid hemorrhage is considered

IMAGING STUDIES
- Cranial MRI or CT scan to exclude an intracranial mass lesion in patients with
  - A progressive headache disorder
  - New onset of headache in middle or later life
  - Headaches that disturb sleep or are related to exertion
  - Headaches that are associated with neurologic symptoms or a focal neurologic deficit

DIAGNOSTIC PROCEDURES
- Inquire about precipitating and exacerbating factors
- Precipitating factors include recent sinusitis or hay fever, dental surgery, head injury, and symptoms suggestive of a systemic viral infection
- Alcohol is a precipitating factor for cluster headache
- Chewing as a precipitating factor is associated with TMJ dysfunction, trigeminal or glossopharyngeal neuralgia, and giant cell arteritis
- Cough-induced headache occurs with structural lesions of the posterior fossa, but a specific cause is frequently unidentifiable
- Exacerbating factors for migraine include emotional stress, fatigue, foods containing nitrite or tyramine, and menses

 TREATMENT

- See specific headache disorder: Headache, Tension; Headache, Migraine; Polymyalgia Rheumatica & Giant Cell Arteritis; Cough

 OUTCOME

WHEN TO REFER
- If expertise in evaluation or treatment is needed

WHEN TO ADMIT
- Depends on the underlying cause (eg, mass lesion, intracerebral bleed)

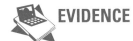 **EVIDENCE**

PRACTICE GUIDELINES
- American Academy of Neurology
- Lewis DW et al. Practice parameter: evaluation of children and adolescents with recurrent headaches: report of the Quality Standards Subcommittee of the American Academy of Neurology and the Practice Committee of the Child Neurology Society. Neurology. 2002; 59:490. [PMID: 12196640]
- National Guideline Clearinghouse

INFORMATION FOR PATIENTS
- JAMA patient page. Tension headache. JAMA. 2001;285:2282. [PMID: 11368044]
- National Institute of Neurological Disorders and Stroke
- Parmet S et al. JAMA patient page. Headaches. JAMA. 2003 Mar 19; 289(11):1462. [PMID: 12636471]

REFERENCES
- Capobianco DJ et al. Diagnosis and treatment of cluster headache. Semin Neurol. 2006 Apr;26(2):242–59. [PMID: 16628535]
- Friedman BW et al. A trial of metoclopramide vs. sumatriptan for the emergency department treatment of migraines. Neurology. 2005 Feb 8; 64(3):463–8. [PMID: 15699376]
- Goadsby PJ. Recent advances in understanding migraine mechanisms, molecules and therapeutics. Trends Mol Med. 2007 Jan;13(1):39–44. [PMID: 17141570]
- Linde K et al. Acupuncture for patients with migraine: a randomized controlled trial. JAMA. 2005 May 4; 293(17):2118–25. [PMID: 15870415]
- May A. Cluster headache: pathogenesis, diagnosis, and management. Lancet. 2005 Sep 3-9;366(9488):843–55. [PMID: 16139660]
- Schoenen J et al. Headache with focal neurological signs or symptoms: a complicated differential diagnosis. Lancet Neurol. 2004 Apr;3(4):237–45. [PMID: 15039036]

Headache, Acute

 KEY FEATURES

ESSENTIALS OF DIAGNOSIS

- Age > 50 years
- Rapid onset with severe intensity
- History of hypertension or HIV
- Fever, hypertension
- Trauma
- Vision changes
- Neurologic findings (mental status changes, motor or sensory deficits)

GENERAL CONSIDERATIONS

- In the emergency department, 1% of patients with acute headache have a life threatening condition
- In the physician's office, the prevalence of life-threatening conditions is much lower

 CLINICAL FINDINGS

SYMPTOMS AND SIGNS

- Sudden-onset headache that reaches maximal and severe intensity within seconds or a few minutes ("thunderclap headache") suggests subarachnoid hemorrhage
- Headache with uncontrolled hypertension should prompt search for other manifestations of "hypertensive urgency or emergency" (See Hypertensive Urgencies & Emergencies)
- Headache and hypertension in pregnancy may be due to preeclampsia
- Episodic headache with hypertension, palpitations, and sweats may be due to pheochromocytoma
- Physical examination should include
    - Vital signs
    - Neurologic examination
    - Vision/fundoscopic examination
    - Kernig and Brudzinski signs
- Patients ≥ 60 years old should be examined for scalp or temporal artery tenderness
- Diminished visual acuity suggests
    - Glaucoma
    - Temporal arteritis
    - Optic neuritis
- Ophthalmoplegia or visual field defects suggest
    - Venous sinus thrombosis
    - Tumor
    - Aneurysm
- Afferent pupillary defects occur with intracranial masses or optic neuritis
- Ipsilateral ptosis and miosis (Horner's syndrome) occur with carotid artery dissection
- Papilledema or absent retinal venous pulsation or both occur with elevated intracranial pressure

DIFFERENTIAL DIAGNOSIS

- Causes of headache that require immediate treatment
    - Imminent or completed vascular events (intracranial hemorrhage, thrombosis, vasculitis, malignant hypertension, arterial dissection, or aneurysm)
    - Infections (abscess, encephalitis, meningitis)
    - Intracranial masses causing intracranial hypertension
    - Preeclampsia
    - Carbon monoxide poisoning

 DIAGNOSIS

LABORATORY TESTS

- Cerebrospinal fluid (CSF) Gram stain
- White blood cell count with differential
- Red blood cell count
- Glucose
- Total protein
- Bacterial culture
- VDRL
- Erythrocyte sedimentation rate
- Urinalysis
- In suspected cases, obtain CSF polymerase chain reaction test for herpes simplex 2
- In HIV-infected patients, obtain CSF cryptococcal antigen, acid-fast bacillus stain and culture, and complement fixation and culture for coccidioidomycosis

IMAGING STUDIES

- Sinus CT scan or radiograph
- Noncontrast head CT immediately, followed by contrast head CT later
- In HIV-infected patients, new-onset headache warrants CT with and without contrast or MRI
- For clinical features associated with acute headache that warrant urgent or emergent neuroimaging (Table 129)
- Perform neuroimaging prior to lumbar puncture in acute headache with abnormal neurologic examination, abnormal mental status, abnormal fundoscopic examination (papilledema; loss of venous pulsations)
- Perform neuroimaging emergently in acute headache with abnormal neurologic examination, abnormal mental status, "thunderclap headache"
- Perform neuroimaging urgently in acute headache with HIV infection, age > 50 years (despite normal neurologic examination)

DIAGNOSTIC PROCEDURES

- Lumbar puncture
- If high suspicion for subarachnoid hemorrhage or aneurysm, lumbar puncture followed by cerebral angiography

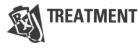 **TREATMENT**

- Treatment should be guided by the underlying etiology

MEDICATIONS

- Nonsteroidal anti-inflammatory drugs (Table 1)
- Migraine therapy (Table 130)
- Opioid agonist analgesics (Table 2)
- Clinical response to analgesics does not exclude life-threatening causes of acute headache

 OUTCOME

WHEN TO REFER

- Refer patients to the emergency department
    - Age > 50 years
    - Rapid onset with severe intensity
    - History of hypertension or HIV
    - Fever, hypertension
    - Trauma
    - Vision changes
    - Neurologic findings (mental status changes, motor or sensory deficits)

PREVENTION

- Prophylactic treatment of migraine (Table 130)

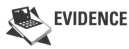 **EVIDENCE**

PRACTICE GUIDELINES

- American College of Emergency Physicians (ACEP). Clinical policy: critical issues in the evaluation and management of patients presenting to the emergency department with acute headache, 2002.

- National Guideline Clearinghouse

WEB SITES

- American Academy of Neurology
- Cleveland Clinic

INFORMATION FOR PATIENTS

- Parmet S et al. JAMA patient page. Headaches. JAMA. 2003;289:1462. [PMID: 12636471]

REFERENCES

- Beck E et al: Management of cluster headache. Am Fam Physician. 2005 Feb 15;71(4):717–24. [PMID: 15742909]
- Detsky ME et al. Does this patient have migraine? JAMA. 2006 Sep 13; 296(10):1274–83. [PMID: 16968852]
- Dodik DW. Chronic daily headache. N Engl J Med. 2006 Jan 12;354(2):158–65. [PMID: 16407511]
- Gladstein J. Headache. Med Clin North Am. 2006 Mar;90(2):275–90. [PMID: 16448875]
- van de Beek D et al. Clinical features and prognostic factors in adults with bacterial meningitis. N Engl J Med. 2004 Oct 28;351(18):1849–59. [PMID: 15509818]
- van Gijn J et al. Subarachnoid hemorrhage. Lancet. 2007 Jan 27; 369(9558):306–18. [PMID: 17258671]

Headache, Cluster

KEY FEATURES

- Affects mainly middle-aged men
- May relate to a vascular headache or a disturbance of a serotonergic mechanism
- There is often no family history of headache or migraine

CLINICAL FINDINGS

- Severe unilateral periorbital pain occurring daily for several weeks
  - Often accompanied by ipsilateral nasal congestion, rhinorrhea, redness of the eye, lacrimation, or Horner's syndrome
- Episodes often occur at night and last for less than 2 h
- Precipitants of an attack
  - Alcohol
  - Stress
  - Glare
  - Specific foods
- Spontaneous remission occurs, and the patient remains well for weeks or months before another bout occurs
- Typical attacks may occur without remission; this variant is chronic cluster headache

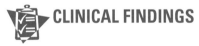

TREATMENT

- Sumatriptan, 6 mg SQ or 20-mg/spray intranasally, or inhalation of 100% oxygen (7 L/min for 15 min) may be effective
- Dihydroergotamine (1–2 mg IM or IV) is sometimes used
- Butorphanol tartrate nasal spray, 1 mg (1 spray in 1 nostril), repeated after 60–90 min if necessary, may help
- For prophylaxis, give ergotamine tartrate as rectal suppositories (0.5–1.0 mg HS or BID), PO (2 mg once daily), or by SQ injection (0.25 mg TID for 5 days per week)
- Other potentially helpful prophylactic agents include
  - Valproate (750–1500 mg PO daily)
  - Cyproheptadine
  - Lithium carbonate (monitored by plasma lithium determination)
  - Prednisone (20–40 mg PO daily or on alternate days for 2 weeks, followed by gradual withdrawal)
  - Verapamil (240–480 mg PO daily)
  - Topiramate (25–200 mg PO daily)

Headache, Migraine

KEY FEATURES

ESSENTIALS OF DIAGNOSIS

- Headache, usually pulsatile
- May be accompanied by
  - Nausea
  - Vomiting
  - Photophobia
  - Phonophobia
- Transient neurologic symptoms (typically visual) may precede the headache of classic migraine
- No preceding aura is common

GENERAL CONSIDERATIONS

- The pathophysiology probably relates to serotonin and to dilation and excessive pulsation of the branches of the external carotid artery
- Focal disturbances of neurologic function
  - May precede or accompany the headaches (classic migraines)
  - Have been attributed to constriction of branches of the internal carotid artery
- Attacks may be triggered by
  - Emotional or physical stress
  - Lack or excess of sleep
  - Missed meals
  - Specific foods (eg, chocolate)
  - Alcoholic beverages
  - Menstruation
  - Use of oral contraceptives

DEMOGRAPHICS

- Patients often give a family history of migraine

CLINICAL FINDINGS

SYMPTOMS AND SIGNS

Classic migraine

- Lateralized throbbing headache that occurs episodically following its onset in adolescence or early adult life
- Visual disturbances occur quite commonly and may consist of
  - Field defects
  - Luminous visual hallucinations, such as stars, sparks, unformed light flashes (photopsia), geometric patterns, or zigzags of light
  - Some combination of field defects and luminous hallucinations (scintillating scotomas)
- Other focal disturbances
  - Aphasia or numbness
  - Tingling
  - Clumsiness
  - Weakness in a circumscribed distribution

Common migraine

- Commonly bilateral and periorbital
- Visual disturbances and other focal neurologic deficits do not occur

Basilar artery migraine

- Blindness or disturbances throughout both visual fields are accompanied or followed by
  - Dysarthria
  - Dysequilibrium
  - Tinnitus
  - Perioral and distal paresthesias
- Blindness or visual disturbances sometimes followed by
  - Transient loss or impairment of consciousness or a confusional state
  - This, in turn, is followed by a throbbing (usually occipital) headache, often with nausea and vomiting

Ophthalmoplegic migraine

- Lateralized pain, often about the eye, is accompanied by
  - Nausea
  - Vomiting
  - Diplopia due to transient external ophthalmoplegia
- Ophthalmic division of the fifth nerve has also been affected in some patients

Migraine equivalent

- In rare instances, the neurologic or somatic disturbance accompanying typical migrainous headaches becomes the sole manifestation of an attack without headaches occurring ("migraine equivalent")

DIFFERENTIAL DIAGNOSIS

- Other causes of headache
- Cluster headache
- Brain tumor
- Temporal (giant cell) arteritis
- Sinusitis
- Subarachnoid hemorrhage
- Pseudotumor cerebri
- Transient ischemic attack

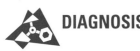 **DIAGNOSIS**

IMAGING STUDIES

- Changes in brainstem regions involved in sensory modulation may be seen, suggesting that migraine relates to failure of normal sensory processing

DIAGNOSTIC PROCEDURES

- Inquire about precipitating and exacerbating factors
- Inquire about family history

 TREATMENT

MEDICATIONS

- A simple analgesic (eg, aspirin) taken right away often provides relief
- However, treatment with extracranial vasoconstrictors or other drugs is sometimes necessary
- Cafergot, a combination of ergotamine tartrate (1 mg) and caffeine (100 mg), is often particularly helpful
  - One or two tablets are taken at the onset of headache or warning symptoms, followed by one tablet every 30 min
  - If necessary, up to six tablets per attack and ten tablets per week can be taken
  - Cafergot can be given rectally as suppositories containing 2 mg of ergotamine (one-half to one suppository per dose)
- Sumatriptan is a rapidly effective agent for aborting attacks when given subcutaneously by an autoinjection device (4–6 mg SQ once, may repeat q2h × 1 if needed; maximum dose 12 mg/24h)
- Zolmitriptan is effective for acute treatment
  - Optimal initial oral dose is 5 mg
  - Relief usually occurs within 1 h
  - May repeat q2h × 1 if needed
  - Maximum dose is 10 mg/24h
  - Can also be taken by nasal spray
    - 5 mg in one nostril × 1; may repeat q2h × 1
    - Maximum dose is 10 mg/24h
- Other triptans are available
  - Rizatriptan (5–10 mg PO once, may repeat dose q2h × 2 if needed; maximum dose 30 mg/24h, 15 mg/24h if taking propranolol)
  - Naratriptan (1–2.5 mg PO once, may repeat × 1 after 4h if needed; maximum dose 5 mg/24h)
  - Almotriptan (6.25–12.5 mg PO once, may repeat q2h × 1 if needed; maximum dose 25 mg/24h)
  - Eletriptan (20–40 mg PO once, any repeat q2h × 1 if needed; maximum dose 80 mg/24 h) is useful for immediate therapy
  - Frovatriptan has longer half-life than eletriptan; helps patients with prolonged attacks (2.5 mg PO once, may repeat q2h × 1; maximum dose 7.5 mg/24 h)
- Triptans
  - Should be avoided in pregnancy and in patients with risk factors for stroke
  - Are contraindicated in patients with coronary or peripheral vascular disease
  - May cause nausea or vomiting
- Narcotic analgesics, such as meperidine 100 mg IM or butorphanol tartrate by nasal spray (1 mg/ spray in one nostril, repeated after 3 or 4 h if necessary), are needed in rare instances

THERAPEUTIC PROCEDURES

- Management of migraine consists of avoidance of any precipitating factors, together with prophylactic or symptomatic pharmacologic treatment if necessary
- During acute attacks, many patients find it helpful to rest in a quiet, darkened room until symptoms subside

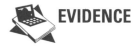 **OUTCOME**

COMPLICATIONS

- Serotonin syndrome (potentially fatal agitation, confusion, fever, incoordination, vomiting, tachycardia, alterations in blood pressure) may develop when triptans are used with selective serotonin or serotonin/norepinephrine reuptake inhibitors
- Very rarely, the patient may be left with a permanent neurologic deficit following a migrainous attack

PREVENTION

- Prophylactic treatment may be necessary if migrainous headaches occur more frequently than two or three times a month (see Table 130)
- Several drugs may have to be tried in turn before the headaches are brought under control
- Once a drug has been found to help, it should be continued for several months
- If the patient remains headache free, the dose can then be tapered and the drug eventually withdrawn

EVIDENCE

PRACTICE GUIDELINES

- American Academy of Neurology
- National Guideline Clearinghouse

INFORMATION FOR PATIENTS

- The Mayo Clinic
- Parmet S et al. JAMA patient page. Headaches. JAMA. 2003 Mar 19; 289(11):1462. [PMID: 12636471]

REFERENCES

- Friedman BW et al. A trial of metoclopramide vs. sumatriptan for the emergency department treatment of migraines. Neurology. 2005 Feb 8; 64(3):463–8. [PMID: 15699376]
- Goadsby PJ. Recent advances in understanding migraine mechanisms, molecules and therapeutics. Trends Mol Med. 2007 Jan;13(1):39–44. [PMID: 17141570]

Headache, Tension

 KEY FEATURES

- Constant daily headaches that are often vise-like or tight in quality
- May be exacerbated by emotional stress, fatigue, noise, or glare
- Patients also frequently complain of poor concentration and other vague nonspecific symptoms

 CLINICAL FINDINGS

- Usually generalized
- May be most intense about the neck or back of the head
- Not associated with focal neurologic symptoms

 DIAGNOSIS

- Diagnosis is made after exclusion of other causes of headache (see individual diagnoses, eg, Sinusitis, Acute)

 TREATMENT

- When treatment with simple analgesics is not effective, a trial of antimigrainous agents (see Headache, Migraine) is worthwhile
- Techniques to induce relaxation are also useful and include massage, hot baths, and biofeedback
- Exploration of underlying causes of chronic anxiety is often rewarding
- Anecdotal reports of beneficial responses to local injection of botulinum toxin type A have been published

Hearing Loss

 KEY FEATURES

ESSENTIALS OF DIAGNOSIS

- Three main types of hearing loss
  - Conductive
  - Sensory
  - Neural
- Most commonly caused by cerumen impaction or transient auditory tube dysfunction associated with upper respiratory tract infection

GENERAL CONSIDERATIONS

Conductive loss
- Four mechanisms, each resulting in impairment of the passage of sound vibrations to the inner ear
  - Obstruction (eg, cerumen impaction)
  - Mass loading (eg, middle ear effusion)
  - Stiffness effect (eg, otosclerosis)
  - Discontinuity (eg, ossicular disruption)
- Generally more correctable than sensory and neural losses

Sensory loss
- Common causes include
  - Excessive noise exposure
  - Head trauma
  - Systemic diseases, such as diabetes mellitus

Neural hearing loss
- Occurs with lesions involving the eighth nerve, auditory nuclei, ascending tracts, or auditory cortex
- It is the least common clinically recognized cause of hearing loss
- Causes include
  - Acoustic neuroma
  - Multiple sclerosis
  - Cerebrovascular disease

DEMOGRAPHICS

- Nearly 30 million Americans have impaired hearing
- For the elderly—the largest group affected—excessive noise, drugs, toxins, and heredity are the most frequent contributing factors

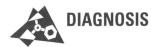 **CLINICAL FINDINGS**

SYMPTOMS AND SIGNS

- Reduction in hearing level

- **Weber test**
  - A 512-Hz tuning fork is placed on the forehead or front teeth
  - In conductive losses, the sound appears louder in the poorer hearing ear, whereas in sensorineural losses it radiates to the better side
- **Rinne test**
  - A 512-Hz tuning fork is placed alternately on the mastoid bone and in front of the ear canal
  - In conductive losses, bone conduction exceeds air conduction, whereas in sensorineural losses the opposite is true

DIFFERENTIAL DIAGNOSIS

Conductive (external or middle ear)
- Cerumen impaction (ear wax)
- Transient auditory tube dysfunction
- Acute or chronic otitis media
- Mastoiditis
- Otosclerosis
- Disruption of ossicles
- Trauma or barotrauma
- Glomus tympanicum (middle ear tumor)
- Paget's disease

Sensory
- Presbycusis (age related)
- Excessive noise exposure
- Ménière's disease (endolymphatic hydrops)
- Labyrinthitis
- Head trauma
- Ototoxicity
- Occlusion of ipsilateral auditory artery
- Hereditary hearing loss
- Autoimmune
  - Systemic lupus erythematosus
  - Wegener's granulomatosis
  - Cogan's syndrome
- Other systemic causes
  - Diabetes
  - Hypothyroidism
  - Hyperlipidemia
  - Renal failure
  - Infections

Neural
- Acoustic neuroma
- Multiple sclerosis
- Cerebrovascular disease

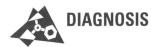 **DIAGNOSIS**

DIAGNOSTIC PROCEDURES

- Formal audiometric studies are performed in a soundproofed room

- Pure-tone thresholds in decibels (dB) are obtained over the range of 250–8000 Hz (the main speech frequencies are between 500 and 3000 Hz) for both air and bone conduction
- **Conductive losses** create a gap between the air and bone thresholds
- In **sensorineural losses** both air and bone thresholds are equally diminished
- The threshold of normal hearing is from 0 to 20 dB, which corresponds to the loudness of a soft whisper
- Hearing loss threshold
  - Mild hearing loss is indicated by a threshold of 20–40 dB (soft spoken voice)
  - Moderate loss has a threshold of 40–60 dB (normal spoken voice)
  - Severe loss has a threshold of 60–80 dB (loud spoken voice)
  - Profound loss has a threshold of 80 dB (shout)
- The clarity of hearing is often impaired in sensorineural hearing loss; this is evaluated by speech discrimination testing, which is reported as percentage correct (90–100% is normal)
- The site of the lesion responsible for sensorineural loss—whether it lies in the cochlea or in the central auditory system—may be determined with auditory brainstem-evoked responses

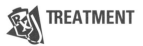 **TREATMENT**

SURGERY

- The cochlear implant—an electronic device that is surgically implanted to stimulate the auditory nerve—offers socially beneficial auditory rehabilitation to most adults with acquired deafness
- Many types of conductive hearing loss (eg, otosclerosis, tympanic membrane perforation, ossicular discontinuity) are surgically remediable
- Hearing aids
  - There is much interest in the development of semi-implantable and fully implantable hearing aids
  - A variety of devices are under development that deliver vibrations—usually via either a rare earth magnet or a piezoceramic crystal—directly to the ossicular chain
  - An alternative strategy, the bone-anchored hearing aid, uses an oscillating post drilled into the mastoid; this technology shows promise in surgically uncorrectable conductive hearing loss and as well as in unilateral sensorineural deafness

THERAPEUTIC PROCEDURES

- Hearing aids
- Assistive devices such as telephone amplifiers and infrared devices for use with television, theaters, and auditoriums (eg, Senheiser)

 OUTCOME

WHEN TO REFER

- Every patient who complains of a hearing loss should be referred for audiologic evaluation unless the cause is easily remediable (eg, cerumen impaction, otitis media)

 EVIDENCE

PRACTICE GUIDELINES

- ACOEM Noise and Hearing Conservation Committee. ACOEM evidence-based statement: noise-induced hearing loss. J Occup Environ Med. 2003; 45:579. [PMID: 12802210]

WEB SITES

- American Academy of Otolaryngology—Head and Neck Surgery: Sensorineural Hearing Loss Interactive Module
- Baylor College of Medicine Otolaryngology Resources

INFORMATION FOR PATIENTS

- American Speech-Language-Hearing Association: Types of Hearing Loss
- MedlinePlus: Hearing Loss Interactive Tutorial
- NIH Senior Health: Hearing Loss
- Occupation Safety & Health Administration: Noise and Hearing Conservation
- Parmet S et al. JAMA patient page. Adult hearing loss. JAMA. 2003; 289:2020. [PMID: 12697805]

REFERENCES

- Angeli SI et al. Etiologic diagnosis of sensorineural hearing loss in adults. Otolaryngol Head Neck Surg. 2005 Jun;132(5):890–5. [PMID: 15944560]
- Bagai A et al. Does this patient have hearing impairment? JAMA. 2006 Jan 25;295(4):416–28. [PMID: 16434632]
- Jackler RK. A 73-year-old man with hearing loss. JAMA. 2003 Mar 26; 289(12):1557–65. [PMID: 12672773]

Heat Exposure Syndromes

 KEY FEATURES

ESSENTIALS OF DIAGNOSIS

- Four medical disorders can result
  - Heat syncope
  - Heat cramps
  - Heat exhaustion
  - Heat stroke

GENERAL CONSIDERATIONS

Heat syncope
- Sudden unconsciousness from cutaneous vasodilation and volume depletion
- Typically occurs immediately following vigorous physical activity

Heat cramps
- Slow, painful muscle contractions of the skeletal muscles most heavily used
- Typically occurs immediately following vigorous physical activity
- Fluid and electrolyte depletion is cause

Heat exhaustion
- Results from prolonged strenuous activity with inadequate salt intake in a hot environment
- Characterized by dehydration, sodium depletion, or isotonic fluid loss with accompanying cardiovascular changes
- May progress to heat stroke if sweating ceases

Heat stroke
- A life-threatening medical emergency resulting from failure of the thermoregulatory mechanism
- Classic heat stroke occurs in patients with compromised homeostatic mechanisms
- Exertional heat stroke occurs in healthy persons undergoing strenuous exertion in a thermally stressful environment

DEMOGRAPHICS

- Persons at greatest risk for heat stroke
  - Very young
  - Elderly (age > 65)
  - Chronically ill
  - Patients taking medications (eg, anticholinergics, antihistamines, phenothiazines) that interfere with heat-dissipating mechanisms
- Heat stroke occurs in unconditioned amateurs participating in strenuous athletic activities

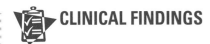 CLINICAL FINDINGS

SYMPTOMS AND SIGNS

Heat syncope

- Systolic blood pressure usually < 100 mm Hg; weak pulse
- Skin typically cool, moist

Heat cramps

- Muscle spasms last 1–3 min
- Muscles tender; may be twitching
- Skin moist, cool
- Victim alert, with stable vital signs, but may be agitated and complain of pain
- Body temperature may be normal or slightly increased

Heat exhaustion

- Prolonged symptoms and rectal temperature > 37.8°C, increased pulse (> 150% of patient's normal) and moist skin
- Symptoms associated with heat syncope and heat cramps may be present
- Patient may be thirsty and weak, with CNS symptoms (eg, headache, fatigue)
- Anxiety, paresthesias, impaired judgement, hysteria, psychosis (in cases chiefly caused by water depletion)
- Hyperventilation secondary to heat exhaustion can lead to respiratory alkalosis

Heat stroke

- Core temperature usually > 41°C
- Cerebral dysfunction with impaired consciousness, fever, absence of sweating
- Skin hot; initially covered with perspiration, later dries
- Pulse initially strong
- Blood pressure may be slightly elevated at first, but hypotension develops later
- Hyperventilation may lead to respiratory alkalosis
- Exertional heat stroke may present with sudden collapse and loss of consciousness followed by irrational behavior
- 25% of victims have prodromal symptoms (dizziness, weakness, nausea, confusion, disorientation, drowsiness, irrational behavior)

DIFFERENTIAL DIAGNOSIS

Heat stroke

- Neuroleptic malignant syndrome
- Malignant hyperthermia (anesthetic associated)
- Serotonin syndrome (eg, selective serotonin reuptake inhibitors used with monoamine oxidase inhibitor [MAOI])
- Other drugs
  – Anticholinergics
  – Antihistamines
  – Tricyclic antidepressants
  – MAOIs
  – Salicylates
  – Amphetamines
  – Cocaine
- Thyrotoxicosis
- Prolonged seizures

 DIAGNOSIS

LABORATORY TESTS

- **Muscle cramps**
  – Low serum sodium
  – Hemoconcentration
  – Elevated urea and creatinine
- **Heat stroke**
  – Hemoconcentration
  – Leukocytosis
  – Elevated blood urea nitrogen (BUN)
  – Hyperuricemia
  – Acid-base abnormalities (eg, lactic acidosis)
  – Decreased serum potassium, sodium, calcium, and phosphorus
  – Urine is concentrated, with elevated protein, tubular casts, and myoglobinuria
  – Thrombocytopenia, increased bleeding and clotting times, fibrinolysis, and consumption coagulopathy may also be present
  – Rhabdomyolysis and myocardial, hepatic, or renal damage may be identified by elevated serum creatine kinase and aminotransferase levels and BUN and by the presence of anuria, proteinuria, and hematuria

DIAGNOSTIC PROCEDURES

- In **heat stroke**, ECG findings may include ST–T changes consistent with myocardial ischemia

 TREATMENT

MEDICATIONS

Heat stroke

- Antipyretics (aspirin, acetaminophen) have no effect on environmentally induced hyperthermia and are contraindicated
- 5% dextrose in 0.45% or 0.9% saline should be administered for fluid replacement
- Fluid administration to ensure a high urinary output (> 50 mL/h), mannitol administration (0.25 mg/kg), and alkalinizing the urine (IV bicarbonate administration, 250 mL of 4%) are recommended to reduce risk of renal failure from rhabdomyolysis

THERAPEUTIC PROCEDURES

Heat syncope

- Place patient at recumbency in a cool place, with fluids PO (or IV if necessary)

Heat cramps

- Place patient in a cool environment and give saline solution, 4 tsp of salt per gallon of water PO, to replace both salt and water
- *Because of their slower absorption, salt tablets are not recommended*
- The victim may have to rest for 1–3 days with continued dietary salt supplementation before returning to work or resuming strenuous activity in the heat

Heat exhaustion

- Place patient in a cool environment, provide adequate hydration (1–2 L over 2–4 h), salt replenishment—orally, if possible—and active cooling (eg, fans, ice packs) if necessary
- Physiological saline or isotonic glucose solution should be administered IV when oral administration is not appropriate
- IV 3% (hypertonic) saline may be necessary if sodium depletion is severe
- At least 24 h of rest is suggested

Heat stroke

- See Hyperthermia
- Aim to reduce the core temperature rapidly (within 1 h) and control the secondary effects
- Continue treatment until rectal temperature drops to 39°C
- Fluid output should be monitored by an indwelling urinary catheter

 OUTCOME

FOLLOW-UP

- Because sensitivity to high environmental temperature may persist for prolonged periods following an episode of heat stroke, immediate reexposure should be avoided

COMPLICATIONS

- Hypovolemic and cardiogenic shock
- Renal failure from rhabdomyolysis, hypokalemia, cardiac arrhythmias, coagulopathy, and hepatic failure
- Hypokalemia may not appear until rehydration

PROGNOSIS

- Heat stroke is associated with high mortality

WHEN TO ADMIT

- All patients with heat syncope, exhaustion, or stroke
- Patients with heat cramps if sustained fluid and electrolyte replacement is needed

PREVENTION

- Athletic competition is not recommended when the wet bulb globe temperature (WBGT) index exceeds 26–28°C
- Workers and athletes need acclimatization for hot temperatures and should drink water or balanced electrolyte fluids frequently
- Protective cooled suits have been used successfully in industry for prolonged work in environments up to 60°C

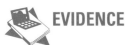

EVIDENCE

INFORMATION FOR PATIENTS

- American Red Cross: Heat-Related Illness
- Centers for Disease Control and Prevention
- MedlinePlus: Heat Emergencies
- National Institute for Occupational Safety and Health: Working in Hot Environments

REFERENCES

- Glazer JL. Management of heatstroke and heat exhaustion. Am Fam Physician. 2005 Jun 1;71(11):2133–40. [PMID: 15952443]
- Misset B et al. Mortality of patients with heatstroke admitted to intensive care units during the 2003 heat wave in France: a national multiple-center risk-factor study. Crit Care Med. 2006 Apr; 34(4):1087–92. [PMID: 16484920]
- Seto CK et al. Environmental illness in athletes. Clin Sports Med. 2005 Jul; 24(3):695–718, x. [PMID: 16004926]
- Smith JE. Cooling methods used in the treatment of exertional heat illness. Br J Sports Med. 2005 Aug;39(8):503–7. [PMID: 16046331]
- Sucholeiki R. Heatstroke. Semin Neurol. 2005 Sep;25(3):307–14. [PMID: 16170743]

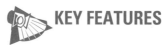

Helicobacter pylori Gastritis

KEY FEATURES

ESSENTIALS OF DIAGNOSIS

- *Helicobacter pylori* is a spiral gram-negative rod that causes gastric mucosal inflammation

GENERAL CONSIDERATIONS

- Acute infection causes a transient illness of nausea and abdominal pain for several days associated with acute histologic gastritis with polymorphonuclear neutrophils
- After these symptoms resolve, the majority progress to chronic infection with chronic, diffuse mucosal inflammation characterized by polymorphonuclear neutrophils and lymphocytes
- Eradication achieved with antibiotics in > 85% leads to resolution of the chronic gastritis
- Majority of those with chronic infection are asymptomatic and suffer no sequelae, but a peptic ulcer develops in ~15%
- Risk of gastric adenocarcinoma and low-grade B cell gastric lymphoma (mucosa-associated lymphoid tissue lymphoma, or MALToma) is increased 3.5- to 20-fold

DEMOGRAPHICS

- Infection usually acquired in childhood through person-to-person spread
- In the United States, the prevalence of infection is < 10% in nonimmigrants younger than 30 years to > 50% in those older than 60 years
- Prevalence is higher in nonwhites and immigrants from developing countries

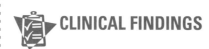

CLINICAL FINDINGS

SYMPTOMS AND SIGNS

- Acute infection: transient epigastric pain, nausea, vomiting
- Chronic infection
  - Usually asymptomatic
  - Symptoms arise in patients in whom peptic ulcer disease or gastric cancer develops
  - Controversial whether chronic infection may cause dyspepsia

DIFFERENTIAL DIAGNOSIS

- Peptic ulcer disease
- Functional dyspepsia
- Gastroesophageal reflux disease or hiatal hernia
- Biliary disease or pancreatitis
- Gastric or pancreatic cancer
- Viral gastroenteritis
- "Indigestion" from overeating, high-fat foods, coffee
- Angina pectoris

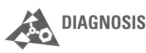

DIAGNOSIS

LABORATORY TESTS

Noninvasive testing for H pylori

- Fecal antigen, urea breath tests, or serologic tests are recommended as the most cost-effective initial tests
- Fecal antigen immunoassay and ^{13}C-urea breath tests
  - Have sensitivity and specificity of > 95%
  - Positive test indicates active infection
  - Although more expensive than serology, they may be more cost-effective because they reduce unnecessary treatment in patients without active infection
- Laboratory-based serologic ELISA test
  - Has overall accuracy of 80%
  - Positive test does not necessarily imply ongoing active infection
  - After eradication with antibiotics, antibody levels decline to undetectable levels in 50% of patients by 12–18 months
- Proton pump inhibitors significantly reduce the sensitivity of urea breath tests and fecal antigen assays (but not serologic tests) and should be discontinued 14 days prior to testing

Endoscopic testing for H pylori

- Gastric biopsy specimens can detect *H pylori* organisms on histology and can be tested for active infection by urease production (sensitivity and specificity of 90%)

DIAGNOSTIC PROCEDURES

- Upper endoscopy with biopsy for urease production and/or histology is diagnostic
- In patients under age 55 years with dyspepsia without signs of complications (dysphagia, weight loss, vomiting, anemia), empiric testing and treating for *H pylori* are recommended
- In patients over age 55 years with chronic dyspepsia or patients of any age

with signs of complications (dysphagia, weight loss, vomiting, anemia), endoscopy is recommended to exclude other organic disease

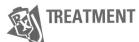

TREATMENT

MEDICATIONS

- Treat with anti–*H pylori* regimen for 10–14 days with one of the following
  - Triple-therapy: proton pump inhibitor: omeprazole, 20 mg PO BID; lansoprazole, 30 mg PO BID; rabeprazole, 20 mg PO BID; pantoprazole, 40 mg PO BID; or esomeprazole, 40 mg PO QD; **plus** clarithromycin, 500 mg PO BID and amoxicillin, 1 g PO BID **or** metronidazole, 500 mg PO BID (in penicillin-allergic patients)
  - Quadruple-therapy: proton pump inhibitor: omeprazole, 20 mg PO BID; lansoprazole, 30 mg PO BID; rabeprazole, 20 mg PO BID; or pantoprazole, 40 mg PO BID; **plus** bismuth subsalicylate two tablets PO QID, **plus** tetracycline, 500 mg PO QID **plus** metronidazole, 250 mg PO QID
  - Quadruple therapy is recommended for patients who did not respond to initial attempt at eradication with triple-therapy
- Proton pump inhibitors should be administered before meals
- Avoid metronidazole regimens in areas of known high resistance or in patients who did not respond to a course of treatment that included metronidazole

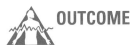

OUTCOME

FOLLOW-UP

- After antibiotic therapy, routine follow-up not recommended
- In patients with history of peptic ulcer disease with complications (bleeding) successful eradication should be confirmed with urea breath test or fecal antigen test

PROGNOSIS

- All recommended treatment regimens achieve > 85% eradication
- Risk of reinfection with *H pylori* is only 1%/year

WHEN TO REFER

- Patients with persistent infection after one or two attempts at treatment should be referred to a gastroenterologist or infectious disease specialist

WHEN TO ADMIT

- Complications of *H pylori*–associated peptic ulcer disease

EVIDENCE

PRACTICE GUIDELINES

- Caselli M et al; Cervia Working Group. "Cervia Working Group Report": guidelines on the diagnosis and treatment of *Helicobacter pylori* infection. Dig Liver Dis. 2001;33:75. [PMID: 11303980]
- Hunt R et al. Canadian Helicobacter Study Group Consensus Conference: update on the management of *Helicobacter pylori*—an evidence-based evaluation of six topics relevant to clinical outcomes in patients evaluated for *H pylori* infection. Can J Gastroenterol. 2004;18:547. [PMID: 15457293]
- Malfertheiner P et al. Current concepts in the management of *Helicobacter pylori* infection—the Maastricht 2-2000 Consensus Report. Aliment Pharmacol Ther. 2002;16:167. [PMID: 11860399]
- National Guideline Clearinghouse

WEB SITE

- CDC—*H pylori*: The key to cure for most ulcer patients

INFORMATION FOR PATIENTS

- Uptodate—*Helicobacter pylori* infection and treatment

REFERENCES

- Axon A. *Helicobacter pylori*. What do we still need to know? J Clin Gastroenterol. 2006 Jan;40(1):15–9. [PMID: 16340627]
- Byzer P et al. Treatment of *Helicobacter pylori*. Helicobacter. 2005;10(Suppl 1):40–6. [PMID: 16178970]
- Gillen D et al. Gastroduodenal disease, *Helicobacter pylori,* and genetic polymorphisms. Clin Gastroenterol Hepatol. 2005 Dec;3(12):1180–6. [PMID: 16361041]
- Moayyedi P et al. Eradication of *Helicobacter pylori* for non-ulcer dyspepsia. Cochrance Database Syst Rev. 2005 Jan 25;(1):CD002096. [PMID: 15674892]
- Vakil N. *Helicobacter pylori* treatment: a practical approach. Am J Gastroenerol.

2006 Mar;101(3):497–9. [PMID: 16542285]

Hemochromatosis

KEY FEATURES

ESSENTIALS OF DIAGNOSIS

- Usually diagnosed because of elevated iron saturation or serum ferritin or a family history
- Most patients are asymptomatic
- Hepatic abnormalities and cirrhosis, congestive heart failure, hypogonadism, and arthritis
- The disease is rarely recognized clinically before the fifth decade

GENERAL CONSIDERATIONS

- Increased accumulation of iron as hemosiderin in the liver, pancreas, heart, adrenals, testes, pituitary, and kidneys
- Cirrhosis is more likely to develop in affected persons who drink alcohol excessively or have obesity-related steatosis
- Autosomal recessive disease
- About 85% of persons with well-established hemochromatosis are homozygous for the *C282Y* mutation
- Population studies have shown an increased prevalence of liver disease but not of diabetes, arthritis, or heart disease in *C282Y* homozygotes
- Hemochromatosis develops in 1–2% of *C282Y/H63D* compound heterozygotes
- Heterozygotes do not develop cirrhosis in the absence of associated disorders such as viral hepatitis or nonalcoholic fatty liver disease

DEMOGRAPHICS

- The frequency of the gene mutation
  - Averages 7% in Northern European and North American white populations, resulting in a 0.5% frequency of homozygotes (of whom 40–70% will develop iron overload and even fewer will develop clinical symptoms)
  - Uncommon in African-American and Asian-American populations

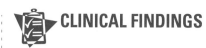

CLINICAL FINDINGS

SYMPTOMS AND SIGNS

- The onset is usually after age 50—earlier in men than in women
- Early symptoms are nonspecific (eg, fatigue, arthralgias)

Later clinical manifestations

- Arthropathy, hepatomegaly, and evidence of hepatic insufficiency
- Skin pigmentation (combination of slate gray due to iron and brown due to melanin, sometimes resulting in a bronze color)
- Cardiac enlargement with or without heart failure or conduction defects, diabetes mellitus with its complications, and impotence in men
- Bleeding from esophageal varices
- A variant presentation in young patients is characterized by cardiac dysfunction, hypogonadotropic hypogonadism, and a high mortality rate and is not associated with the *C282Y* mutation

DIFFERENTIAL DIAGNOSIS

- Hepatomegaly due to other causes, eg, fatty liver
- Diabetes mellitus due to other causes, eg, Cushing's syndrome
- Cardiac infiltrative disease due to other causes, eg, amyloidosis, sarcoidosis
- Arthritis due to other causes, eg, rheumatoid arthritis, pseudogout
- Hyperpigmentation due to other causes, eg, hyperbilirubinemia
- Cirrhosis due to other causes

DIAGNOSIS

LABORATORY TESTS

- Mildly abnormal liver tests (aspartate aminotransferase [AST], alkaline phosphatase)
- An elevated plasma iron with > 50% transferrin saturation in men and 45% in women (after an overnight fast)
- An elevated serum ferritin (although a normal iron saturation and a normal ferritin do not exclude the diagnosis)
- Testing for *HFE* mutations is indicated in any patient with evidence of iron overload and in siblings of patients with confirmed hemochromatosis

IMAGING STUDIES

- CT and MRI may show changes consistent with iron overload of the liver

- However, these techniques are not sensitive enough for screening

DIAGNOSTIC PROCEDURES

- The liver biopsy characteristically shows
  - Extensive iron deposition in hepatocytes and in bile ducts
  - Hepatic iron index—hepatic iron content per gram of liver converted to micromoles and divided by the patient's age—generally > 1.9
- In patients who are homozygous for *C282Y*, liver biopsy is often indicated to determine whether cirrhosis is present (found in 5% of patients with hemochromatosis identified by screening in a primary care setting)
- However, biopsy can be deferred when patients
  - Are younger than 40 years
  - Have serum ferritin level < 1000 mcg/L
  - Have normal serum AST level
  - Do not have hepatomegaly
- Likelihood of cirrhosis is low in these individuals
- Liver biopsy is also indicated when iron overload is suspected even though the patient is not homozygous for *C282Y*

TREATMENT

MEDICATIONS

- The chelating agent deferoxamine
  - Indicated for patients with hemochromatosis and anemia or for those with secondary iron overload due to thalassemia who cannot tolerate phlebotomies
  - Administer IV or SQ in a dose of 20–40 mg/kg/day infused over 24 h
  - Treatment is painful and time consuming
  - Can mobilize 30 mg of iron per day
- Deferasirox, 20 mg/kg once daily
  - An oral chelating agent
  - Used to treat iron overload due to blood transfusions

SURGERY

- Liver transplantation for advanced cirrhosis
  - Associated with severe iron overload, including hemochromatosis
  - Has been reported to lead to survival rates that are lower than those for other types of liver disease because of cardiac complications and an increased risk of infections

THERAPEUTIC PROCEDURES

- Early diagnosis and treatment in the precirrhotic phase are of great importance
- Avoid foods rich in iron (such as red meat), alcohol, vitamin C, raw shellfish, and supplemental iron
- Phlebotomies
  - Initially, weekly 1 or 2 units of blood (each containing about 250 mg of iron)
  - Continue for up to 2–3 years to achieve depletion of iron stores
  - Process is monitored by hematocrit and serum iron determinations
  - When iron store depletion is achieved (iron saturation < 50% and serum ferritin level < 50 mcg/L), maintenance phlebotomies (every 2–4 months) are continued
- Complications of hemochromatosis—arthropathy, diabetes, heart disease, portal hypertension, and hypopituitarism—also require treatment

OUTCOME

COMPLICATIONS

- Patients are at increased risk for infection with *Vibrio vulnificus*, *Listeria monocytogenes*, *Yersinia enterocolitica*, and other siderophilic organisms
- Arthropathy, diabetes, heart disease, portal hypertension, and hypopituitarism
- In patients in whom cirrhosis develops, there is a 15–20% incidence of hepatocellular carcinoma

PROGNOSIS

- The course of the disease is favorably altered by phlebotomy therapy
- In precirrhotic patients, cirrhosis may be prevented
- Cardiac conduction defects and insulin requirements improve with treatment
- In patients with cirrhosis, varices may reverse, and the risk of variceal bleeding declines
- However, cirrhotic patients must be monitored for the development of hepatocellular carcinoma

WHEN TO REFER

- All patients should be referred to a hepatologist or hematologist

PREVENTION

- Genetic testing is recommended for all first-degree family members of the proband

- Children of an affected person (*C282Y* homozygote) need to be screened only if the patient's spouse carries the *C282Y* or *H63D* mutation
- Screening all white men over age 30 or all adults over age 20 by measurement of the transferrin saturation or possibly the unbound iron-binding capacity has been recommended by some, but the value of screening is uncertain
- Screening is recommended for patients with arthritis, impotence, and late-onset type 1 diabetes mellitus

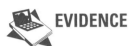

EVIDENCE

PRACTICE GUIDELINES

- National Guideline Clearinghouse
- Qaseem A et al. Screening for hereditary hemochromatosis: a clinical practice guideline from the American College of Physicians. Ann Intern Med. 2005; 143:517. [PMID: 16204164]

WEB SITES

- Diseases of the Liver
- Hepatic Ultrasound Images
- Liver Tutorials Visualization and Volume Measurement
- Pathology Index

INFORMATION FOR PATIENTS

- Mayo Clinic
- National Digestive Diseases Information Clearinghouse

REFERENCES

- Adams PC. Review article: the modern diagnosis and management of haemochromatosis. Aliment Pharmacol Ther. 2006 Jun 15;23(12):1681–91. [PMID: 16817911]
- Falize L et al. Reversibility of hepatic fibrosis in treated genetic hemochromatosis: a study of 36 cases. Hepatology. 2006 Aug;44(2):472–7. [PMID: 16871557]
- Walsh A et al. The clinical relevance of compound heterozygosity for the *C282Y* and *H63D* substitutions in hemochromatosis. Clin Gastroenterol Hepatol. 2006 Nov;4(11):1403–10. [PMID: 16979952]
- Whitlock EP et al. Screening for hereditary hemochromatosis: a systematic review for the U.S. Preventive Services Task Force. Ann Intern Med. 2006 Aug 1;145(3):209–23. [PMID: 16880463]

Hemoglobinuria, Paroxysmal Nocturnal

KEY FEATURES

- Acquired clonal stem cell disorder causing abnormal sensitivity of RBC membrane to lysis by complement
- Defect involves increased binding of C3b and increased vulnerability to lysis by complement
- Suspect diagnosis in confusing cases of hemolytic anemia or pancytopenia

CLINICAL FINDINGS

- Hemoglobinuria (reddish-brown urine), particularly in first morning urine
- Anemia
- Increased susceptibility to thrombosis, especially of mesenteric and hepatic veins
- May progress to aplastic anemia, myelodysplasia, or acute myelogenous leukemia

DIAGNOSIS

- Flow cytometric assays may confirm diagnosis by demonstrating absence of CD59
- Anemia of variable severity
- Reticulocytosis may or may not be present
- Urine hemosiderin test may indicate episodic intravascular hemolysis
- Serum lactate dehydrogenase characteristically elevated
- Iron deficiency common because of chronic iron loss from hemoglobinuria
- WBC and platelet count may be low
- Bone marrow morphology variable; may show generalized hypoplasia or erythroid hyperplasia

TREATMENT

- Iron replacement often indicated for iron deficiency; may improve anemia but also may cause transient increase in hemolysis

- Prednisone, including alternate-day regimens, may be effective in decreasing hemolysis
- Allogeneic bone marrow transplantation for severe cases and cases of transformation to myelodysplasia
- Anticoagulation may be needed if thrombosis present
- Eculizumab
  - Investigational anti-complement C5 antibody
  - Has been shown to be effective in reducing hemolysis and transfusion requirements

Hemolytic-Uremic Syndrome

KEY FEATURES

ESSENTIALS OF DIAGNOSIS

- Microangiopathic hemolytic anemia
- Thrombocytopenia
- Renal failure
- Elevated serum lactate dehydrogenase (LDH)
- Normal coagulation tests
- Absence of neurologic abnormalities

GENERAL CONSIDERATIONS

- Disorder consisting of microangiopathic hemolytic anemia, thrombocytopenia, and renal failure due to microangiopathy
- Cause is unknown, but some cases are related to deficiency in ADAMTS13, a protein that cleaves von Willebrand factor
- Similar to thrombotic thrombocytopenic purpura (TTP) except different vascular beds involved
  - Pathogenesis probably similar
  - Platelet-agglutinating factor found in plasma may be involved
- In children, hemolytic-uremic syndrome (HUS) frequently occurs after diarrheal illness due to *Shigella, Salmonella, Escherichia coli* strain O157:H7, or viruses
- In adults, often precipitated by estrogen use or postpartum state
- May occur as delayed complication of autologous bone marrow or stem cell transplantation, or of cyclosporine or tacrolimus as immunosuppression in allogeneic transplantation

- Familial (hereditary) HUS: family members have recurrent episodes over several years

CLINICAL FINDINGS

SYMPTOMS AND SIGNS

- Symptoms of anemia, bleeding, or renal failure
- Renal failure may or may not be oliguric
- No neurologic manifestations other than those due to uremia

DIFFERENTIAL DIAGNOSIS

- Disseminated intravascular coagulation
- TTP
- Preeclampsia-eclampsia
- Vasculitis
- Acute glomerulonephritis

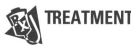

DIAGNOSIS

LABORATORY TESTS

- Microangiopathic hemolytic anemia
- Thrombocytopenia, but often less severe than in TTP
- Peripheral blood smear should show striking red blood cell fragmentation
- LDH usually elevated out of proportion to degree of hemolysis
- Coombs test negative
- Coagulation tests normal except elevated fibrin degradation products

DIAGNOSTIC PROCEDURES

- Kidney biopsy shows endothelial hyaline thrombi in afferent arterioles and glomeruli
- Ischemic necrosis in renal cortex may occur with obstruction from intravascular coagulation

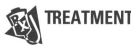

TREATMENT

THERAPEUTIC PROCEDURES

- Treatment of choice (as in TTP): large-volume plasmapheresis with fresh-frozen replacement (exchange of up to 80 mL/kg), repeated daily until remission is achieved
- In children, HUS is almost always self-limited and requires only conservative management of acute renal failure
- In adults, high rate of permanent renal insufficiency and death without treatment

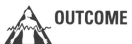

OUTCOME

COMPLICATIONS

- Chronic renal insufficiency

PROGNOSIS

- Mortality rate of childhood form is low (< 5%)
- Prognosis in adults remains unclear; without effective therapy, up to 40% have died, and 80% have had chronic renal insufficiency
- Early institution of aggressive therapy with plasmapheresis promises to be beneficial
- Survival and correction of hematologic abnormalities are the rule, but restoration of renal function requires early treatment

EVIDENCE

PRACTICE GUIDELINES

- Allford SL et al; Haemostasis and Thrombosis Task Force, British Committee for Standards in Haematology. Guidelines on the diagnosis and management of the thrombotic microangiopathic haemolytic anaemias. Br J Haematol. 2003;120:556. [PMID: 12588343]

WEB SITE

- National Organization of Rare Disorders: Hemolytic Uremic Syndrome

INFORMATION FOR PATIENTS

- MedlinePlus: Hemolytic Uremic Syndrome
- National Kidney and Urologic Diseases Information Clearinghouse: Hemolytic Uremic Syndrome
- National Kidney Foundation: Hemolytic Uremic Syndrome

REFERENCES

- Garg AX et al. Long-term renal prognosis of diarrhea-associated hemolytic uremic syndrome: a systematic review, meta-analysis, and meta-regression. JAMA. 2003 Sep 10;290(10):1360–70. [PMID: 12966129]
- Vesely SK et al. ADAMTS13 activity in thrombotic thrombocytopenic purpura-hemolytic uremic syndrome: relation to presenting features and clinical outcomes in a prospective cohort of 142 patients. Blood. 2003 Jul 1;102(1):60–8. [PMID: 12637323]

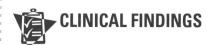

Hemophilia A

KEY FEATURES

ESSENTIALS OF DIAGNOSIS

- X-linked recessive pattern of inheritance with only males affected
- Factor VIII coagulant (VIII:C) activity low
- Factor VIII antigen normal
- Spontaneous hemarthroses

GENERAL CONSIDERATIONS

- Hemophilia A (classic hemophilia, factor VIII deficiency hemophilia) is a hereditary bleeding disorder caused by deficiency of coagulation factor VIII (VIII:C)
- Factor VIII coagulant protein usually quantitatively reduced, but defective coagulant protein is present on immunoassay in small number of cases
- Hemophilia classified as
  - Severe, if factor VIII:C levels < 1%
  - Moderate, if 1–5%
  - Mild, if levels > 5%
- X-linked recessive disease
- Families tend to breed true in severity of hemophilia
- Many hemophiliacs acquired HIV infection via factor VIII concentrate; many have developed AIDS
- HIV-associated immune thrombocytopenia may aggravate bleeding tendency

DEMOGRAPHICS

- Most common severe bleeding disorder and second most common congenital bleeding disorder, after von Willebrand's disease
- ~1 in 10,000 males affected
- Rarely, female carriers clinically affected if their normal X chromosomes are disproportionately inactivated
- Females may also be affected if they are offspring of hemophiliac father and carrier mother

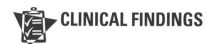

CLINICAL FINDINGS

SYMPTOMS AND SIGNS

- Bleeding tendency, with severity in proportion to factor VIII:C levels
- Mild hemophilia: bleeding only after major trauma or surgery

- Moderately severe hemophilia: bleeding with mild trauma or surgery
- Severe hemophilia: spontaneous bleeding
- Bleeding may occur anywhere, but most commonly into joints (knees, ankles, elbows), muscles, and gastrointestinal tract
- Spontaneous hemarthroses virtually diagnostic of hemophilia

DIFFERENTIAL DIAGNOSIS

- Hcmophilia B
- von Willebrand's disease
- Disseminated intravascular coagulation
- Heparin administration
- Acquired factor deficiency or inhibitors (eg, paraproteins with anti-VIII or anti-IX activity)

 DIAGNOSIS

LABORATORY TESTS

- Partial thromboplastin time (PTT) prolonged
- Other coagulation tests, including prothrombin time, bleeding time, and serum fibrinogen level, are normal
- Factor VIII:C levels reduced, but measurements of von Willebrand factor are normal
- If plasma from a hemophiliac patient is mixed with normal plasma, PTT becomes normal; failure of PTT to normalize in such a mixing test is diagnostic of factor VIII inhibitor
- Platelet count below normal in a hemophiliac should raise suspicion of HIV-associated immune thrombocytopenia

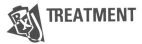 **TREATMENT**

MEDICATIONS

- Infusion of factor VIII concentrates is standard treatment
- Recombinant factor VIII appears safe and effective, though expensive, and imposes no risk of transmitting HIV or other viruses
- New heat-treated factor VIII concentrates also appear very safe
- Desired plasma level of factor VIII depends on bleeding severity
  - For minor bleeding, raise factor VI-II:C levels to 25% with one infusion
  - For moderate bleeding (eg, deep muscle hematoma), raise level initially to 50% and maintain level > 25% with repeated infusion for 2–3 days

- For major bleeding, raise level to 100% and maintain level > 50% continuously for 10–14 days
- Factor VIII concentrate dose is 60 U/kg (~4000 U for 70-kg individual); to raise level to 25% requires 1000 U; half-life of factor VIII:C is ~12 h
- To raise level to 100%, initial dose is 60 U/kg, followed by 30 U/kg q12h
  - During surgery, verify initial rise in factor VIII lcvels
  - If levels fail to rise, suspect presence of factor VIII inhibitor
- Desmopressin, 0.3 mcg/kg IV q24h, may be useful in preparing patients with mild hemophilia for minor surgical procedures; causes release of factor VIII:C and raises factor VIII:C levels twofold to threefold for several hours
- For persistent bleeding after use of either desmopressin or factor VIII concentrate, use ε-aminocaproic acid (EACA; Amicar), 4 g PO q4h for several days
- Avoid aspirin

THERAPEUTIC PROCEDURES

- Treat patients with head injuries (with or without neurologic signs) emergently as for major bleeding

 OUTCOME

COMPLICATIONS

- Arthritis from recurrent joint bleeding
- Hepatitis B and C and HIV infection from recurrent transfusion (incidence decreasing)

PROGNOSIS

- Prognosis markedly improved by availability of factor VIII replacement
- Major limiting factor is disability from recurrent joint bleeding
- Hemophiliacs with hepatitis B or C or HIV have worse prognosis associated with those disorders
- ~15% develop inhibitors to factor VIII and thus cannot be adequately supported with factor VIII

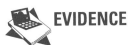 **EVIDENCE**

PRACTICE GUIDELINES

- Hay CR. The 2000 United Kingdom Haemophilia Centre Doctors' Organisation (UKHCDO) inhibitor guidelines. Pathophysiol Haemost Thromb. 2002; 32(Suppl 1):19. [PMID: 12214141]

- Kasper CK. Protocols for the treatment of haemophilia and von Willebrand disease. Haemophilia. 2000;6(Suppl 1):84. [PMID: 10982273]
- United Kingdom Haemophilia Centre Doctors' Organisation. Guidelines on the selection and use of therapeutic products to treat haemophilia and other hereditary bleeding disorders. Haemophilia. 2003;9:1. [PMID: 12558775]

WEB SITES

- National Library of Medicine Genetics Home Reference: Hemophilia
- National Hemophilia Foundation
- World Federation of Hemophilia

INFORMATION FOR PATIENTS

- National Heart, Lung, and Blood Institute: Hemophilia
- National Hemophilia Foundation: Hemophilia A
- World Federation of Hemophilia: What Is Hemophilia?

REFERENCES

- Goudemand J et al; FVIII-LFB and Recombinant FVIII study groups. Influence of the type of factor VIII concentrate on the incidence of factor VIII inhibitors in previously untreated patients with severe hemophilia A. Blood. 2006 Jan 1;107(1):46–51. [PMID: 16166584]
- Lillicrap D. The role of immunomodulation in the management of factor VIII inhibitors. Hematology Am Soc Hematol Educ Program. 2006:421–5. [PMID: 17124093]

Hemophilia B

 KEY FEATURES

ESSENTIALS OF DIAGNOSIS

- X-linked recessive inheritance, with only males affected
- Factor IX coagulant activity levels low
- Spontaneous hemarthroses

GENERAL CONSIDERATIONS

- Hemophilia B (Christmas disease, factor IX hemophilia) is a hereditary bleeding disorder caused by deficiency of coagulation factor IX

- Factor IX is usually quantitatively reduced, but an abnormally functioning molecule is detectable immunologically in one-third of cases
- One-seventh as common as hemophilia A (factor VIII deficiency) but otherwise clinically and genetically identical

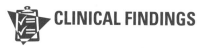 **CLINICAL FINDINGS**

SYMPTOMS AND SIGNS

- Bleeding tendency, with severity in proportion to factor IX levels
- Mild hemophilia: bleeding only after major trauma or surgery
- Moderately severe hemophilia: bleeding with mild trauma or surgery
- Severe hemophilia: spontaneous bleeding
- Bleeding may occur anywhere, but most commonly into joints (knees, ankles, elbows), muscles, and gastrointestinal tract
- Spontaneous hemarthroses virtually diagnostic of hemophilia

DIFFERENTIAL DIAGNOSIS

- Hemophilia A
- von Willebrand's disease
- Disseminated intravascular coagulation
- Heparin administration
- Acquired factor deficiency or inhibitor (eg, paraproteins with anti-VIII or anti-IX activity)

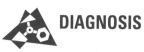 **DIAGNOSIS**

LABORATORY TESTS

- Partial thromboplastin time (PTT) prolonged
- Factor IX coagulant activity levels are low when measured by specific factor assays, but measurements of von Willebrand factor are normal
- Other coagulation tests, including prothrombin time, bleeding time, and serum fibrinogen level, are normal
- If plasma from hemophiliac patient is mixed with normal plasma, PTT becomes normal; failure of PTT to normalize in such a mixing test is diagnostic of factor IX inhibitor
- Platelet count below normal in a hemophiliac should raise suspicion of HIV-associated immune thrombocytopenia

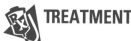 **TREATMENT**

MEDICATIONS

- Infusion of factor IX concentrates, heat-treated to reduce likelihood of HIV transmission, is standard treatment
- Factor VIII concentrates are ineffective
- Factor IX concentrate dose is 80 U/kg (~6000 units) to achieve 100% level; half-life is 18 h
- For major surgery, give 80 U/kg initially, followed by 40 U/kg q18h; measure factor IX levels to ensure that expected levels are achieved and that factor IX inhibitor is not present
- Unlike factor VIII concentrates, factor IX concentrates contain other proteins, including activated coagulating factors that appear to contribute to risk of thrombosis with recurrent usage; more care is thus needed in deciding to use these concentrates
- Desmopressin is not useful in hemophilia B
- Avoid aspirin

 OUTCOME

COMPLICATIONS

- Risk of thrombosis with recurrent factor IX concentrate usage

PROGNOSIS

- Prognosis markedly improved by availability of factor IX replacement
- Major limiting factor is disability from recurrent joint bleeding
- Hemophiliacs with hepatitis B or C or HIV have worse prognosis associated with those disorders
- ~2.5% develop inhibitors to factor IX and thus cannot be adequately supported with factor IX

 EVIDENCE

PRACTICE GUIDELINES

- Hay CR. The 2000 United Kingdom Haemophilia Centre Doctors' Organisation (UKHCDO) inhibitor guidelines. Pathophysiol Haemost Thromb. 2002; 32(Suppl 1):19. [PMID: 12214141]
- United Kingdom Haemophilia Centre Doctors' Organisation. Guidelines on the selection and use of therapeutic products to treat haemophilia and other hereditary bleeding disorders. Haemophilia. 2003;9:1. [PMID: 12558775]

WEB SITES

- National Library of Medicine Genetics Home Reference: Hemophilia
- National Hemophilia Foundation
- World Federation of Hemophilia

INFORMATION FOR PATIENTS

- National Heart, Lung, and Blood Institute: Hemophilia
- National Hemophilia Foundation: Hemophilia B
- World Federation of Hemophilia: What Is Hemophilia?

REFERENCE

- Shapiro AD et al. The safety and efficacy of recombinant human blood coagulation factor IX in previously untreated patients with severe or moderately severe hemophilia B. Blood. 2005 Jan 15;105(2):518-25. [PMID: 15383463]

Hemoptysis

 KEY FEATURES

- Expectoration of blood originating below the vocal cords
- Massive hemoptysis
  - > 200–600 mL of blood/24 hours
  - Hemodynamic or airway compromise
- Causes can be classified anatomically
  - Airway (bronchitis, bronchiectasis, malignancy)
  - Pulmonary vasculature (left ventricular failure, mitral stenosis, pulmonary embolism, arteriovenous malformation [AVM])
  - Parenchymal (pneumonia, inhalation of crack cocaine, or autoimmune diseases)

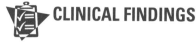 **CLINICAL FINDINGS**

- Blood-tinged sputum to frank blood
- Dyspnea may be mild or severe
- Hypoxemia may be present

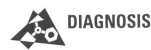

DIAGNOSIS

- Chest radiograph may demonstrate the cause
- High-resolution CT of the chest can diagnose bronchiectasis and AVM as well as many malignancies and other disorders
- Bronchoscopy is indicated when there is a suspicion of malignancy or a normal chest radiograph

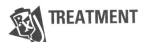

TREATMENT

- In massive hemoptysis, airway protection and circulatory support are first steps
- Patients should be placed in decubitus position with affected lung down
- Rigid bronchoscopy and surgical consultation are necessary in uncontrollable hemorrhage
- Bronchoscopy and angiography can localize lesions
- Angiographic embolization is initially effective in 85% of cases, although 20% rebleed in 1 year

Hemorrhoids

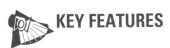

KEY FEATURES

ESSENTIALS OF DIAGNOSIS

- Bright red blood per rectum
- Protrusion of tissue from anus, with discomfort
- Characteristic findings on external anal inspection and anoscopy

GENERAL CONSIDERATIONS

- Internal hemorrhoids are a plexus of superior hemorrhoidal veins located above the dentate line that are covered by mucosa
- External hemorrhoids arise from the inferior hemorrhoidal veins located below the dentate line and are covered with squamous epithelium of the anal canal or perianal region
- Causes include
  - Straining at stool
  - Constipation
  - Prolonged sitting
  - Pregnancy
  - Obesity
  - Low-fiber diet

DEMOGRAPHICS

- Prevalence increases with
  - Advancing age
  - Chronic constipation with straining
  - Pregnancy
  - Weight-lifting

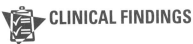

CLINICAL FINDINGS

SYMPTOMS AND SIGNS

- Bright red blood per rectum
  - Streaks of blood visible on toilet paper or stool, or bright red blood that drips
  - Rarely severe enough to cause anemia
- Mucoid discharge
- Internal hemorrhoids
  - May gradually enlarge and protrude
  - Prolapsed hemorrhoids appear as protuberant purple nodules covered by mucosa
  - Discomfort and pain are unusual, occurring only when there is extensive inflammation and thrombosis of irreducible tissue
- External hemorrhoids
  - Readily visible on perianal inspection or may protrude through the anus with gentle straining
  - Usually asymptomatic, though may interfere with perianal hygiene
  - Acute thrombosis causes severe pain; appears as an exquisitely painful, tense and bluish perianal nodule covered with skin that may be up to several centimeters in size

DIFFERENTIAL DIAGNOSIS

- Rectal prolapse
- Anal fissure
- Anal skin tag
- Perianal fistula or abscess, eg, Crohn's disease
- Infectious proctitis, eg, gonorrhea
- Anogenital warts (condyloma acuminata)
- Perianal pruritus
- Proctalgia fugax or levator ani syndrome
- Lower gastrointestinal bleeding due to other cause, eg, diverticulosis, polyps, colorectal cancer

DIAGNOSIS

DIAGNOSTIC PROCEDURES

- Anoscopy: visualization of internal hemorrhoids
- Grading
  - I: No prolapse
  - II: Prolapse with defecation; spontaneously reduces
  - III: Prolapse with defecation or other times; requires manual reduction
  - IV: Permanently prolapsed mucosal tissue; visible externally

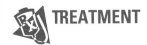

TREATMENT

SURGERY

- Surgical excision (hemorrhoidectomy) for patients with grade IV hemorrhoids with persistent bleeding or discomfort

THERAPEUTIC PROCEDURES

- Injection sclerotherapy for symptomatic grade I–II hemorrhoids
- Rubber band ligation, bipolar cautery or infrared photocoagulation for symptomatic grade I–III hemorrhoids; choice dictated by operator preference

Conservative measures
- High-fiber diet
- Increase fluid intake
- Application of a cotton ball tucked next to the anal opening after bowel movements for mucoid discharge
- Symptomatic relief of prolapsed hemorrhoids by suppositories (eg, Anusol with or without hydrocortisone)
- Warm sitz baths

Thrombosed external hemorrhoid
- Warm sitz baths
- Analgesics
- Ointments
- Incision to remove the clot may hasten symptomatic relief

OUTCOME

FOLLOW-UP

- Bleeding usually subsides after 1–3 sessions of sclerotherapy or rubber band ligation

COMPLICATIONS

- Sclerotherapy or rubber band ligation rarely complicated by bleeding or life-threatening pelvic cellulitis; early signs are worsening anal pain radiating to legs, or difficulty with urination

PROGNOSIS

- Recurrence is common after injection sclerosis or banding

WHEN TO REFER

- Refer to surgeon or gastroenterologist for injection sclerosis, banding, or hemorrhoidectomy

WHEN TO ADMIT

- Severe bleeding with anemia (rare)
- Incarcerated, thrombosed grade IV internal hemorrhoids
- Pelvic cellulitis after banding or sclerotherapy

PREVENTION

- High-fiber diet
- Stool softeners to prevent straining at stool

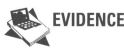

EVIDENCE

PRACTICE GUIDELINES

- Clinical Practice Committee, American Gastroenterological Association. American Gastroenterological Association medical position statement: Diagnosis and treatment of hemorrhoids. Gastroenterology. 2004;126:1461. [PMID: 15131806]
- Madoff RD et al. American Gastroenterological Association technical review on the diagnosis and treatment of hemorrhoids. Gastroenterology. 2004; 126:1463. [PMID: 15131807]
- Surgical management of hemorrhoids. Society for Surgery of the Alimentary Tract, Inc., 2000

INFORMATION FOR PATIENTS

- American Academy of Family Physicians
- Mayo Clinic—Hemorrhoids
- MedlinePlus—Hemorrhoids
- NIH Patient Education Institute—Hemorrhoid Surgery

REFERENCES

- Alonso-Coello P et al. Fiber for the treatment of hemorrhoid compications: a systematic review and meta-analysis. Am J Gastroenterol. 2006 Jan; 101(1):181–8. [PMID: 16405552]

- Longman RJ et al. A prospective study of outcome from rubber band ligation of piles. Colorectal Dis. 2006 Feb; 8(2):145–8. [PMID: 16412076]
- Madoff RD et al. American Gastroenterological Association technical review on the diagnosis and treatment of hemorrhoids. Gastroenterology. 2004 May; 126(5):1463–73. [PMID: 15131807]

Henoch-Schönlein Purpura

KEY FEATURES

- The most common systemic vasculitis in children
- Occurs in adults as well

CLINICAL FINDINGS

- Purpuric skin lesions typically located on the lower extremities; may also be seen on the hands, arms, trunk, and buttocks
- Joint symptoms are present in most patients; the knees and ankles are most commonly involved
- Abdominal pain secondary to vasculitis of the intestinal tract is often associated with gastrointestinal bleeding
- Hematuria signals the presence of a glomerular lesion that is usually reversible, although it occasionally may progress to renal insufficiency

DIAGNOSIS

- Skin biopsy can demonstrate leukocytoclastic vasculitis with IgA deposition
- Kidney biopsy reveals segmental glomerulonephritis with crescents and mesangial deposition of IgA
- Differential diagnosis
  - Immune thrombocytopenic purpura
  - Meningococcemia
  - Rocky Mountain spotted fever
  - Rheumatoid arthritis (including juvenile form)
  - Polyarteritis nodosa
  - Endocarditis
  - Cryoglobulinemia

TREATMENT

- Usually self-limited, lasting 1–6 weeks, and subsiding without sequelae if renal involvement is not severe
- Chronic courses with persistent or intermittent skin disease are more likely to occur in adults than children
- The efficacy of treatment is not well established

Hepatic Encephalopathy

KEY FEATURES

ESSENTIALS OF DIAGNOSIS

- Stage 1: day-night reversal, mild confusion, somnolence
- Stage 2: confusion, drowsiness
- Stage 3: stupor
- Stage 4: coma

GENERAL CONSIDERATIONS

- A state of disordered central nervous system function resulting from failure of the liver to detoxify noxious agents of gut origin because of hepatocellular dysfunction and portosystemic shunting
- Ammonia is the most readily identified toxin but is not solely responsible for the disturbed mental status
- Precipitants of hepatic encephalopathy
  - Gastrointestinal (GI) bleeding—increases the protein in the bowel and rapidly precipitates hepatic encephalopathy
  - Constipation
  - Alkalosis
  - Potassium deficiency induced by diuretics
  - Opioids, hypnotics, and sedatives
  - Medications containing ammonium or amino compounds
  - Paracentesis with attendant hypovolemia
  - Hepatic or systemic infection
  - Portosystemic shunts (including transjugular intrahepatic portosystemic shunts)

DEMOGRAPHICS

- Alcoholic liver disease and chronic hepatitis C are the most common etiologies of cirrhosis

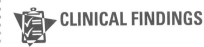 **CLINICAL FINDINGS**

SYMPTOMS AND SIGNS

- Metabolic encephalopathy characterized by
  - Day–night reversal
  - Asterixis, tremor, dysarthria
  - Delirium
  - Drowsiness, stupor, and ultimately coma
- In patients with cirrhosis, may be precipitated by an acute hepatocellular insult or an episode of GI bleeding
- Clinical diagnosis supported by asterixis, elevated serum ammonia with exclusion of other causes of delirium
- Minimal hepatic encephalopathy is characterized by mild cognitive and psychomotor deficits

DIFFERENTIAL DIAGNOSIS

- Metabolic encephalopathy, especially hyponatremia, hypoglycemia, or renal failure
- Central nervous system infection
- Altered mental status from medication effects, particularly if they are hepatically metabolized

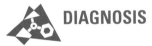 **DIAGNOSIS**

LABORATORY TESTS

- Liver biochemical tests often consistent with advanced chronic liver disease
- Serum (and cerebrospinal fluid) ammonia level is generally elevated
- Role of neuroimaging tests (eg, cerebral positron emission tomography, magnetic resonance spectroscopy) is evolving

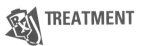 **TREATMENT**

MEDICATIONS

- Purge blood from the GI tract with 120 mL of magnesium citrate by mouth or nasogastric (NG) tube q3–4h until the stool is free of gross blood, or by administration of lactulose
- Lactulose
  - Initial dose is 30 mL PO TID or QID

- Titrate so that two or three soft stools per day are produced
- Administer rectally if patient cannot take orally: lactulose 300 mL in 700 mL of saline or sorbitol as a retention enema for 30–60 min; it may be repeated q4–6h
- Neomycin sulfate, 0.5–1 g PO q6 or 12h for 7 days
  - Controls the ammonia-producing intestinal flora
  - Side effects include diarrhea, malabsorption, superinfection, ototoxicity, and nephrotoxicity, usually only after prolonged use
- Alternative antibiotics
  - Rifaximin, 1200 mg PO once daily
  - Vancomycin, 1 g PO BID
  - Metronidazole, 250 mg PO TID
- Patients who do not respond to lactulose may improve with a 1-week course of an antibiotic in addition to lactulose
- Avoid opioids, tranquilizers, and sedatives metabolized or excreted by the liver
- If agitation is marked, oxazepam, 10–30 mg (not metabolized by the liver) may be given cautiously PO or by NG tube
- Correct zinc deficiency, if present, with oral zinc sulfate, 600 mg/day in divided doses
- Sodium benzoate, 10 g once daily, and ornithine aspartate, 9 g TID, may lower blood ammonia levels, but less is known about these drugs than lactulose
- Flumazenil is effective in about 30% of severe hepatic encephalopathy, but the drug is short-acting and intravenous administration is required

THERAPEUTIC PROCEDURES

- Withhold dietary protein during acute episodes
- When the patient resumes oral intake, protein intake should be restricted to 60–80 g/day as tolerated, and vegetable protein is better tolerated than meat protein
- Use of special dietary supplements enriched with branched-chain amino acids is usually unnecessary except in occasional patients who are intolerant of standard protein supplements

 OUTCOME

COMPLICATIONS

- Hypernatremia can develop from intensive lactulose use

WHEN TO ADMIT

- Inability to care for self or follow medical instructions

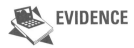 **EVIDENCE**

PRACTICE GUIDELINES

- Blei AT et al. Hepatic encephalopathy. Am J Gastroenterol. 2001;96:1968. [PMID: 11467622]

WEB SITES

- Acute Liver Failure: Case study
- Diseases of the Liver
- Hepatic Ultrasound Images
- Pathology Index

INFORMATION FOR PATIENTS

- National Institute of Neurological Disorders and Stroke
- National Institutes of Health

REFERENCE

- Córdoba J et al. Treatment of hepatic encephalopathy. Lancet. 2005; 365:1384. [PMID: 15836879]

Hepatic Failure, Acute

 KEY FEATURES

ESSENTIALS OF DIAGNOSIS

- May be fulminant or subfulminant and both carry an equally poor prognosis
- Acetaminophen and idiosyncratic drug reactions are the most common causes

GENERAL CONSIDERATIONS

- In fulminant hepatic failure, encephalopathy and coagulopathy develop within 8 weeks after the onset of acute liver disease
- Subfulminant hepatic failure occurs when encephalopathy and coagulopathy appear between 8 weeks and 6 months after the onset of acute liver disease
- Acetaminophen toxicity accounts for 40% of cases; idiosyncratic drug reactions are second

- Among cases caused by acetaminophen
  – 44% are due to suicide attempts
  – 48% are due to unintentional overdose (the threshold for liver failure is lowered by chronic alcohol use)

Etiology

- Acetaminophen toxicity
- Idiosyncratic drug reactions
- Poisonous mushrooms
- Viral hepatitis
- Shock
- Hyperthermia or hypothermia
- Budd-Chiari syndrome
- Malignancy (especially lymphomas)
- Wilson's disease
- Reye's syndrome
- Fatty liver of pregnancy and other disorders of fatty acid oxidation
- Autoimmune hepatitis
- Parvovirus B19 infection
- Grand mal seizures (rarely)

DEMOGRAPHICS

- Most cases in the United States are caused by
  – Acetaminophen toxicity
  – Idiosyncratic drug reactions
  – Acute viral hepatitis, especially hepatitis B
  – Some cases are due to hepatitis A or unknown (non-ABCDE) viruses
- In endemic areas, hepatitis D and hepatitis E cause acute hepatic failure
- Hepatitis C is a rare cause of acute hepatic failure; acute hepatitis A or B superimposed on chronic hepatitis C has a high risk of fulminant hepatitis

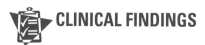 CLINICAL FINDINGS

SYMPTOMS AND SIGNS

- Jaundice may be absent or minimal early
- Hepatic encephalopathy
- Coagulopathy
- Ultimately symptoms and signs of increased intracranial pressure may develop
- High risk of infection, especially with gram-positive organisms

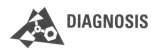 DIAGNOSIS

LABORATORY TESTS

- Severe hepatocellular damage (Table 90)
- Coagulopathy

- Elevated serum ammonia
- Low factor V levels (correlate with outcome)
- In acetaminophen toxicity, serum aminotransferase levels are often towering (> 5000 units/L), and diagnosis is aided by detection of acetaminophen-protein adducts in serum
- In acute hepatic failure due to microvesicular steatosis (eg, Reye's syndrome), serum aminotransferase elevations may be modest (< 300 units/L)

IMAGING STUDIES

- Head CT can help rule out or detect cerebral edema

 TREATMENT

MEDICATIONS

- Prophylactic antibiotic therapy
  – Decreases the risk of infection in 90% of patients
  – No effect on survival
  – Not routinely recommended
- For suspected sepsis, broad coverage is indicated
- The most frequent isolates
  – *Staphylococcus aureus*
  – *Streptococcus* species
  – Coliforms
  – *Candida* species (later in disease course)
- Acetylcysteine
  – Acetaminophen toxicity is an indication for early administration
  – Improves cerebral blood flow and oxygenation in fulminant hepatic failure due to any cause
  – Dosage is 140 mg/kg PO followed by 70 mg/kg PO q4h for an additional 17 doses or 150 mg/kg in 5% dextrose IV over 15 minutes followed by 50 mg/kg over 4 hours and then 100 mg/kg over 16 hours)
  – Can prolong the prothrombin time leading to the erroneous perception that liver failure is worsening
- Penicillin G (300,000 to 1 million units/kg/day IV) or silibinin (silymarin, not licensed in the United States) is given for mushroom poisoning
- Nucleoside analogs are recommended for fulminant hepatitis B (see Hepatitis B, Chronic)
- Lactulose is administered for encephalopathy (see Cirrhosis)
- Mannitol, 100–200 mL of a 20% solution by IV infusion over 10 min, may decrease cerebral edema but should be used with caution in renal failure

---

- IV hypertonic saline may also reduce intracranial pressure
- If these measures fail, hypothermia to 33.1°C or short-acting barbiturates may reduce intracranial pressure
- The value of hyperventilation and IV prostaglandin E_1 is uncertain

SURGERY

- Early transfer to a liver transplantation center is essential

THERAPEUTIC PROCEDURES

- The treatment is directed toward correcting metabolic abnormalities, which include
  – Coagulation defects
  – Electrolyte and acid-base disturbances
  – Renal failure
  – Hypoglycemia
  – Encephalopathy
- The Molecular Adsorbents Recirculating System (MARS), hepatic-assist devices using living hepatocytes, extracorporeal whole liver perfusion, hepatocyte transplantation, and liver xenografts have shown promise

 OUTCOME

FOLLOW-UP

- Extradural sensors are placed to monitor intracranial pressure for impending cerebral edema
- Monitor for disseminated intravascular coagulopathy
- Monitor renal function, acid-base status

PROGNOSIS

- The mortality rate of fulminant hepatitis with severe encephalopathy is as high as 80%
- The outlook is especially poor in patients younger than 10 and older than 40 years of age and in those with an idiosyncratic drug reaction
- Other adverse prognostic factors
  – Serum bilirubin level > 18 mg/dL
  – INR > 6.5
  – Onset of encephalopathy more than 7 days after the onset of jaundice
  – Low factor V level (< 20% of normal)
- Acetaminophen-induced fulminant hepatic failure
  – Transplant-free survival is 65%
  – Only 8% of affected patients require transplantation
  – Indicators of a poor outcome
    □ Acidosis (pH < 7.3)
    □ INR > 6.5

- □ Azotemia (serum creatinine ≥ 3.4 mg/dL)
- □ Hyperphosphatemia (> 1.2 mmol/L)
- □ Elevated blood ammonia level (> 124 mcmol/L)
- □ Elevated blood lactate level (> 3.5 mmol/L)
- – A rising serum alpha-fetoprotein level predicts a favorable outcome
- Emergency liver transplantation is considered for patients with stage 2 to stage 3 encephalopathy and is associated with an 80% survival rate at 1 year

WHEN TO REFER

- Refer to a liver transplantation center early

WHEN TO ADMIT

- Any patient with acute liver disease and encephalopathy

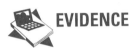 **EVIDENCE**

PRACTICE GUIDELINES

- Polson J et al. AASLD position paper: the management of acute liver failure. Hepatology. 2005;41:1179. [PMID: 15841455]

WEB SITES

- Acute Liver Failure: Case study
- Diseases of the Liver
- Hepatic Ultrasound Images
- Liver Tutorials Visualization and Volume Measurement
- Pathology Index

INFORMATION FOR PATIENTS

- National Institutes of Health

REFERENCES

- Davern TJ 2nd et al. Measurement of serum acetaminophen-protein adducts in patients with acute liver failure. Gastroenterology. 2006 Mar;130(3):687–94. [PMID: 16530510]
- Khan SA et al. Acute liver failure: a review. Clin Liver Dis. 2006 May; 10(2):239–58. [PMID: 16971260]
- O'Grady J. Personal view: current role of artificial liver support devices. Aliment Pharmacol Ther. 2006 Jun 1; 23(11):1549–57. [PMID: 16696802]
- Rutherford A et al; Acute Liver Failure Study Group. Influence of high body mass index on outcome in acute liver failure. Clin Gastroenterol Hepatol. 2006 Dec;4(12):1544–9. [PMID: 16996806]

Hepatic Vein Obstruction (Budd-Chiari Syndrome)

 KEY FEATURES

ESSENTIALS OF DIAGNOSIS

- Right upper quadrant pain and tenderness
- Ascites
- Imaging study showing occlusion/absence of flow in the hepatic vein(s) or inferior vena cava
- Similar picture in sinusoidal obstruction syndrome (venoocclusive disease) but major hepatic veins are patent

GENERAL CONSIDERATIONS

- Cases in India, China, and South Africa
  - Often the result of occlusion of the hepatic portion of the inferior vena cava, presumably due to prior thrombosis
  - Clinical presentation is mild but the course is frequently complicated by hepatocellular carcinoma
- Sinusoidal obstruction syndrome
  - Occlusion of terminal venules and sinusoids that mimics Budd-Chiari syndrome clinically
  - Is common in patients who have undergone bone marrow transplantation, particularly those with pretransplant aminotransferase elevations or fever during cytoreductive therapy with cyclophosphamide, azathioprine, carmustine, busulfan, or etoposide
  - Also common in those receiving high-dose cytoreductive therapy or high-dose total body irradiation
  - Can be caused by some cytotoxic agents and "bush teas" (pyrrolizidine alkaloids)

Etiologies

- Hypercoagulable state
- Caval webs
- Myeloproliferative disease, eg, polycythemia vera
- Right-sided congestive heart failure (CHF) or constrictive pericarditis
- Neoplasm compressing the hepatic vein
- Paroxysmal nocturnal hemoglobinuria
- Behçet's syndrome
- Oral contraceptives or pregnancy

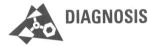 **CLINICAL FINDINGS**

SYMPTOMS AND SIGNS

- Presentation may be fulminant, acute, subacute, or chronic; an insidious (subacute) onset is most common
- Tender, painful hepatic enlargement
- Jaundice; splenomegaly; and ascites
- With advanced disease, bleeding varices and hepatic coma may be evident
- Hepatopulmonary syndrome may occur

DIFFERENTIAL DIAGNOSIS

- Cholecystitis
- Shock liver
- Cirrhosis
- Hepatic congestion from right-sided CHF
- Metastatic cancer involving the liver

 DIAGNOSIS

LABORATORY TESTS

- Liver function test abnormalities are nonspecific
- Jaundice may or may not be present
- Very high alanine aminotransferase/aspartate aminotransferase levels (ALT/AST) (> 1000 units/L) suggest occlusion of hepatic and portal veins
- Signs of decompensated liver disease (low albumin, coagulopathy) indicate poor prognosis

IMAGING STUDIES

- Hepatic imaging studies may show a prominent caudate lobe, since its venous drainage may not be occluded
- Contrast-enhanced, color or pulsed-Doppler ultrasonography
  - Screening test of choice
  - Has a sensitivity of 85% for detecting evidence of hepatic venous or inferior vena caval thrombosis
- MRI and caval venography can delineate caval webs and occluded hepatic veins

DIAGNOSTIC PROCEDURES

- Percutaneous liver biopsy
  - Frequently shows a characteristic centrilobular congestion
  - Often contraindicated in sinusoidal obstruction syndrome because of thrombocytopenia, and the diagnosis is based on clinical findings

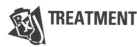

TREATMENT

MEDICATIONS

- Lifelong anticoagulation and treatment of the underlying myeloproliferative disease is often required
- Antiplatelet therapy with aspirin and hydroxyurea may be an alternative to warfarin in myeloproliferative disorders

SURGERY

- Surgical decompression (side-to-side portacaval, mesocaval, or mesoatrial shunt) of the congested liver
  - May be required to relieve persistent hepatic congestion
  - Transjugular intrahepatic portosystemic shunt (TIPS) is not feasible
- Consider liver transplantation for
  - Fulminant hepatic failure
  - Cirrhosis and hepatocellular dysfunction
  - Failed portosystemic shunt

THERAPEUTIC PROCEDURES

- Treat ascites with fluid and salt restriction and diuretics (see Ascites)
- Treatable causes of Budd-Chiari syndrome should be sought
- Prompt recognition and treatment of an underlying hematologic disorder may avoid the need for surgery
- Rarely, thrombolytic therapy may be attempted within 2 weeks of acute hepatic vein thrombosis
- In cases of unresolved hepatic congestion, placement of a TIPS may be feasible, although late TIPS dysfunction is common
- Balloon angioplasty, in some cases with placement of an intravascular metallic stent, is preferred in inferior vena caval web and is being performed increasingly when there is a short segment of thrombosis in the hepatic vein

OUTCOME

COMPLICATIONS

- Liver failure
- Cirrhosis
- Spontaneous bacterial peritonitis (less common than in cirrhosis alone)

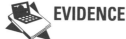

EVIDENCE

WEB SITES

- Diseases of the Liver
- Pathology Index

INFORMATION FOR PATIENTS

- American Liver Foundation
- National Institutes of Health

REFERENCES

- Helmy A. Review article: updates in the pathogenesis and therapy of hepatic sinusoidal obstruction syndrome. Aliment Pharmacol Ther. 2006 Jan 1; 23(1):11–25. [PMID: 16393276]
- Patel RK et al. Prevalence of the activating JAK2 tyrosine kinase mutation V617F in the Budd-Chiari syndrome. Gastroenterology. 2006 Jun; 130(7):2031–8. [PMID: 16762626]
- Plessier A et al. Aiming at minimal invasiveness as a therapeutic strategy for Budd-Chiari syndrome. Hepatology. 2006 Nov;44(5):1308–16. [PMID: 17058215]

Hepatitis A

KEY FEATURES

ESSENTIALS OF DIAGNOSIS

- Prodrome of anorexia, nausea, vomiting, malaise, aversion to smoking
- Fever, enlarged and tender liver, jaundice
- Normal to low white blood cell count
- Abnormal liver tests, especially markedly elevated aminotransferases
- Hepatitis can be caused by many drugs, toxic agents, and viruses, and the clinical manifestations may be similar

GENERAL CONSIDERATIONS

- Transmission of hepatitis A virus (HAV) is by the fecal-oral route
- The incubation period averages 30 days
- HAV is excreted in feces for up to 2 weeks before the clinical illness and rarely persists in feces after the first week of illness
- There is no carrier state

DEMOGRAPHICS

- HAV spread is favored by crowding and poor sanitation
- Common source outbreaks result from contaminated water or food
- Outbreaks among injection drug users have been reported
- Since introduction of HAV vaccine in 1995, the incidence rate of HAV infection has declined by 76% in United States

CLINICAL FINDINGS

SYMPTOMS AND SIGNS

- Onset may be abrupt or insidious
- General malaise, myalgia, arthralgia, easy fatigability, upper respiratory symptoms, and anorexia
- A distaste for smoking, paralleling anorexia, may occur early
- Nausea and vomiting are frequent, and diarrhea or constipation may occur
- Defervescence and a fall in pulse rate often coincide with the onset of jaundice
- Abdominal pain
  - Usually mild and constant in the right upper quadrant or epigastrium
  - Often aggravated by jarring or exertion
  - Rarely severe enough to simulate cholecystitis
- Jaundice
  - Never develops in most patients
  - Occurs after 5–10 days but may appear at the same time as the initial symptoms
  - With its onset, prodromal symptoms often worsen, followed by progressive clinical improvement
  - Stools may be acholic
- Hepatomegaly—rarely marked—is present in over 50% of cases. Liver tenderness is usually present
- Splenomegaly occurs in 15% of patients
- Soft, enlarged lymph nodes—especially in the cervical or epitrochlear areas—may occur
- The acute illness usually subsides over 2–3 weeks
- Complete clinical and laboratory recovery by 9 weeks
- Clinical, biochemical, and serologic recovery may be followed by one or two relapses, but recovery is the rule
- A protracted course has been reported to be associated with HLA *DRB1*1301*

DIFFERENTIAL DIAGNOSIS

- Hepatitis B, C, D, E, G (rarely, if ever, causes frank hepatitis) viruses
- Unidentified agents account for a small percentage of cases of apparent acute viral hepatitis
- The TT virus is in up to 7.5% of blood donors, but this virus is not known to cause liver disease
- A related virus known as SEN-V has been found in 2% of U.S. blood donors, is transmitted by transfusion, and may account for some cases of transfusion-associated non-ABCDE hepatitis
- In immunocompromised and rare immunocompetent persons, consider cytomegalovirus, Epstein-Barr virus, and herpes simplex virus
- Severe acute respiratory syndrome (SARS) may be associated with high serum aminotransferase elevations

 DIAGNOSIS

LABORATORY TESTS

- Antibody to hepatitis A (anti-HAV) appears early in the course of the illness (Figure 5)
- Both IgM and IgG anti-HAV are detectable in serum soon after the onset
- Peak titers of IgM anti-HAV occur during the first week of clinical disease and disappear within 3–6 months
- Detection of IgM anti-HAV is an excellent test for diagnosing acute hepatitis A (but is not indicated in evaluation of asymptomatic patients with persistent aminotransferase elevations)
- Titers of IgG anti-HAV peak after 1 month of the disease and may persist for years
- IgG anti-HAV indicates previous exposure to HAV, noninfectivity, and immunity. In the United States, about 30% of the population have serologic evidence of previous infection
- The white blood cell count is normal to low, especially in the preicteric phase. Large atypical lymphocytes may occasionally be seen
- Mild proteinuria is common, and bilirubinuria often precedes the appearance of jaundice
- Strikingly elevated aspartate or alanine aminotransferases occur early, followed by elevations of bilirubin and alkaline phosphatase; in a small number of patients, the latter persist after aminotransferase levels have normalized
- Cholestasis is occasionally marked

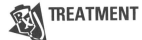 **TREATMENT**

MEDICATIONS

- If nausea and vomiting are pronounced or if oral intake is substantially decreased, IV 10% glucose is indicated
- Small doses of oxazepam are safe, as metabolism is not hepatic; morphine sulfate is avoided
- Corticosteroids produce no benefit

THERAPEUTIC PROCEDURES

- Bed rest is recommended only for marked symptoms
- Dietary management consists of palatable meals as tolerated, without overfeeding; breakfast is usually best tolerated
- Strenuous physical exertion, alcohol, and hepatotoxic agents are avoided

 OUTCOME

COMPLICATIONS

- Fulminant hepatitis A is uncommon; the frequency is increased when hepatitis A occurs in a patient with chronic hepatitis C

PROGNOSIS

- Generally, clinical recovery is complete in 3–6 weeks
- Does not cause chronic liver disease, though it may persist for up to 1 year, and clinical and biochemical relapses may occur before full recovery
- The mortality rate is less than 0.2%

WHEN TO ADMIT

- Intractable nausea and vomiting and need for parenteral fluids
- Severe coagulopathy (eg, prothrombin time > 20 s)
- Encephalopathy

PREVENTION

- Strict isolation is not necessary, but hand washing after bowel movements is required
- Thorough hand washing by anyone who may contact contaminated utensils, bedding, or clothing is essential

Immune globulin

- Give to all *close* (eg, household) personal contacts and consider giving it to persons who consume food prepared by an infected food handler
- The recommended dose, 0.02 mL/kg IM, is protective if administered during incubation

Vaccination

- Two effective inactivated hepatitis A vaccines are recommended for
  - Persons living in or traveling to endemic areas (including military personnel)
  - Patients with chronic liver disease on diagnosis
  - Persons with clotting-factor disorders who are treated with concentrates
  - Homosexual and bisexual men
  - Animal handlers
  - Illicit drug users
  - Sewage workers
  - Food handlers
  - Children and caregivers in day care centers and institutions
- Routine vaccination is advised for children in states with a high incidence of hepatitis A and has been recommended for all children ages 1 to 2 in the United States by the Advisory Committee on Immunization Practices of the Centers for Disease Control and Prevention (Tables 67 and 68)
- HAV vaccine is effective in the prevention of secondary spread to household contacts of primary cases
- The recommended dose for adults
  - 1 mL (1440 ELISA units) of Havrix (GlaxoSmithKline) or 0.5 mL (50 units) of Vaqta (Merck) IM
  - Follow with a booster dose at 6–18 months
- A combined hepatitis A and B vaccine (Twinrix, GlaxoSmithKline) is available

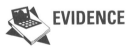 **EVIDENCE**

INFORMATION FOR PATIENTS

- Centers for Disease Control and Prevention
- Hepatitis Information Network
- National Digestive Diseases Information Clearinghouse

REFERENCE

- Advisory Committee on Immunization Practices (ACIP); Fiore AE et al. Prevention of hepatitis A through active or passive immunization: recommendations of the Advisory Committee on Immunization Practices (ACIP). MMWR Recomm Rep. 2006 May 19;55(RR-7):1–23. [PMID: 16708058]

Hepatitis B, Acute

KEY FEATURES

ESSENTIALS OF DIAGNOSIS

- Prodrome of anorexia, nausea, vomiting, malaise, aversion to smoking
- Fever, tender hapatomegaly, jaundice
- Markedly elevated aminotransferases early in the course
- Liver biopsy shows hepatocellular necrosis and mononuclear infiltrate but is rarely indicated

GENERAL CONSIDERATIONS

- Hepatitis B virus (HBV) contains an inner core protein (hepatitis B core antigen, HBcAg) and outer surface coat (hepatitis B surface antigen, HBsAg)
- The incubation period is 6 weeks to 6 months (average 3 months)
- The onset of HBV is more insidious and the aminotransferase levels higher on average than in hepatitis A virus (HAV) infection
- Eight genotypes of HBV (A–H) have been identified
- Hepatitis can be caused by many drugs, toxic agents, and viruses; the clinical manifestations of which may be similar

DEMOGRAPHICS

- HBV is usually transmitted by
  - Infected blood or blood products
  - Sexual contact
- It is present in saliva, semen, and vaginal secretions
- HBsAg-positive mothers may transmit HBV at delivery
- The risk of chronic infection in the infant approaches 90% if the mother is HBeAg positive (about 7% of HIV-infected persons are coinfected with HBV)
- HBV is prevalent in homosexuals and injection drug users, but most cases result from heterosexual transmission
- Incidence has decreased by over 75% since the 1980s
- Groups at risk include
  - Patients and staff at hemodialysis centers
  - Physicians, dentists, and nurses
  - Personnel working in clinical and pathology laboratories and blood banks
- The risk of HBV infection from a blood transfusion is < 1 in 60,000 units transfused in the United States

 CLINICAL FINDINGS

SYMPTOMS AND SIGNS

- Onset may be abrupt or insidious
- Malaise, myalgia, arthralgia, fatigability, upper respiratory symptoms, anorexia, and a distaste for smoking
- Nausea and vomiting, diarrhea or constipation
- Low-grade fever is generally present; serum sickness may be seen
- Abdominal pain is usually mild and constant in the right upper quadrant or epigastrium
- Defervescence and a fall in pulse rate coincide with the onset of jaundice
- Jaundice occurs after 5–10 days but may appear at the same time as the initial symptoms; it never develops in most patients
- Often worsening of the prodromal symptoms, followed by progressive clinical improvement
- The acute illness usually subsides over 2–3 weeks
- Complete clinical and laboratory recovery by 16 weeks
- In 5–10% of cases, the course may be more protracted, but < 1% will have a fulminant course
- Hepatitis B may become chronic

DIFFERENTIAL DIAGNOSIS

- Acute and chronic hepatitis ACDE
- The TT virus (TTV) is found in up to 7.5% of blood donors and is readily transmitted by blood transfusions, but an association with liver disease is not established
- The SEN-V virus is found in 2% of U.S. blood donors, is transmitted by transfusion, and may account for transfusion-associated non-ABCDE hepatitis
- Cytomegalovirus, Epstein-Barr virus, and herpes simplex virus, particularly in immunocompromised persons

 DIAGNOSIS

LABORATORY TESTS

- See Table 91 and Figure 7

HBsAg
- Appears before biochemical evidence of liver disease, and persists throughout the clinical illness
- After the acute illness, it may be associated with chronic hepatitis

Anti-HBs
- Appears after clearance of HBsAg and after successful vaccination against hepatitis B
- Signals recovery from HBV infection, noninfectivity, and immunity

Anti-HBc
- IgM anti-HBc appears shortly after HBsAg is detected. (HBcAg alone does not appear in serum)
  - Its presence in acute hepatitis indicates a diagnosis of acute hepatitis B
  - It fills the rare serologic gap when HBsAg has cleared but anti-HBs is not yet detectable
  - Can persist for 6 months or more and reappear during flares of chronic hepatitis B
- IgG anti-HBc also appears during acute hepatitis B but persists indefinitely
- In asymptomatic blood donors, an isolated anti-HBc with no other positive HBV serologic results may represent a falsely positive result or latent infection

HBeAg
- Found only in HBsAg-positive serum and indicates viral replication and infectivity
- Persistence beyond 3 months indicates an increased likelihood of chronic hepatitis B
- Its disappearance is often followed by the appearance of anti-HBe, generally signifying diminished viral replication and decreased infectivity

HBV DNA
- Generally parallels the presence of HBeAg, though HBV DNA is a more sensitive and precise marker of viral replication and infectivity
- Very low levels of HBV DNA are detectable only by PCR
  - May persist in serum after recovery from acute hepatitis B
  - However, HBV DNA is bound to IgG and is rarely infectious

Other laboratory tests
- Normal to low white blood cell count and large atypical lymphocytes
- Mild proteinuria is common
- Bilirubinuria often precedes the appearance of jaundice
- Elevated aspartate or alanine aminotransferase occurs early, followed by elevations of bilirubin and alkaline phosphatase
- Marked prolongation of prothrombin time in severe hepatitis correlates with increased mortality

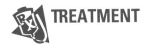 **TREATMENT**

MEDICATIONS

- If nausea and vomiting are pronounced or oral intake is substantially decreased, give 10% glucose IV
- Small doses of oxazepam are safe, as metabolism is not hepatic; morphine sulfate is avoided
- Corticosteroids have no benefit and may be harmful

THERAPEUTIC PROCEDURES

- Bed rest only for severe symptoms
- Dietary management consists of palatable meals as tolerated, without overfeeding
- Strenuous physical exertion, alcohol, and hepatotoxic agents are avoided

 OUTCOME

COMPLICATIONS

- See Hepatic Failure, Acute
- See Hepatitis B, Chronic

PROGNOSIS

- The risk of fulminant hepatitis is < 1%, with a 60% mortality rate
- Following acute hepatitis B
  - HBV infection persists in 1–2% of immunocompetent persons
  - Risk is higher in immunocompromised persons
- Chronic hepatitis B, particularly when HBV infection is acquired early in life and viral replication persists
  - Confers a substantial risk of cirrhosis and hepatocellular carcinoma (up to 25–40%)
  - Men are at greater risk than women
- HBV may be associated with
  - Serum sickness
  - Glomerulonephritis
  - Polyarteritis nodosa
- Universal vaccination of neonates in countries endemic for HBV reduces the incidence of hepatocellular carcinoma

WHEN TO ADMIT

- Intractable nausea and vomiting and need for parenteral fluids
- Encephalopathy or severe coagulopathy (prothrombin time > 20 s), which indicates impending acute hepatic failure

PREVENTION

- Strict isolation of patients is not necessary, but thorough hand washing by medical staff is essential
- Screening of donated blood for HBsAg and anti-HBc has reduced the risk of transfusion-associated hepatitis markedly
- Test pregnant women for HBsAg
- Counsel patients to practice safe sex
- Vaccinate against HAV (after prescreening for prior immunity) in those with chronic hepatitis B

Hepatitis B immune globulin (HBIG)

- May be protective, or attenuate the severity of illness, if given within 7 days after exposure (dose is 0.06 mL/kg body weight) followed by HBV vaccine
- Use this approach after exposure to HBsAg-contaminated material via mucous membranes or breaks in the skin, after sexual contact, and for infants born to HBsAg-positive mothers (in combination with the vaccine series)

Vaccination

- The current vaccines are recombinant-derived
- CDC recommends universal vaccination of infants and children (Table 67) and all at-risk adults
- Over 90% of recipients mount protective antibody to hepatitis B
- Give 10–20 mcg initially (depending on the formulation), repeated again at 1 and 6 months, but alternative schedules are approved, including accelerated schedules of 0, 1, 2, and 12 months
- Check postimmunization anti-HBs titers if need to document seroconversion
- Protection appears to be excellent—at least for 15 years—even if the titer of anti-HBs wanes
- Booster reimmunization is not routinely recommended but is advised for immunocompromised persons in whom anti-HBs titers fall below 10 mIU/mL (Table 68)
- For vaccine nonresponders, three additional vaccine doses may elicit seroprotective anti-HBs levels in 30–50%

 EVIDENCE

PRACTICE GUIDELINES

- National Guideline Clearinghouse

INFORMATION FOR PATIENTS

- Hepatitis Information Network
- Mayo Clinic

REFERENCE

- Mast EE et al; Advisory Committee on Immunization Practices (ACIP) Centers for Disease Control and Prevention (CDC). A comprehensive immunization strategy to eliminate transmission of hepatitis B virus infection in the United States: recommendations of the Advisory Committee on Immunization Practices (ACIP) Part II: immunization of adults. MMWR Recomm Rep. 2006 Dec 8;55(RR-16):1–33. [PMID: 17159833]

Hepatitis B, Chronic

KEY FEATURES

ESSENTIALS OF DIAGNOSIS

- Chronic inflammatory reaction of the liver of more than 3–6 months duration
- Persistently abnormal serum aminotransferase levels and detectable hepatitis B surface antigen (HBsAg)
- Liver biopsy shows features of chronic hepatitis, ground-glass hepatocytes

GENERAL CONSIDERATIONS

- Early in the course, hepatitis Be antigen (HBeAg) and hepatitis B virus (HBV) DNA are present in serum
  - Indicative of active viral replications and necroinflammatory activity in the liver
  - These persons are at risk for progression to cirrhosis and for hepatocellular carcinoma
  - Low-level IgM anti-HBc is also present in about 70%
- Clinical and biochemical improvement may coincide with
  - Disappearance of HBeAg and HBV DNA from serum
  - Appearance of anti-HBe
  - Integration of the HBV genome into the host genome in infected hepatocytes
- If cirrhosis has not yet developed, such persons are at a lower risk for cirrhosis and hepatocellular carcinoma
- Chronic hepatitis is characterized
  - On the basis of the etiology

- The grade of portal, periportal, and lobular inflammation (minimal, mild, moderate, or severe)
- The stage of fibrosis (none, mild, moderate, severe, cirrhosis)

DEMOGRAPHICS

- Chronic hepatitis B afflicts nearly 400 million people worldwide and 1.25 million (predominantly males) in the United States

 CLINICAL FINDINGS

SYMPTOMS AND SIGNS

- Clinically indistinguishable from chronic hepatitis due to other causes

DIFFERENTIAL DIAGNOSIS

- Hepatitis C and D (delta)
- Autoimmune hepatitis
- α_1-Antiprotease deficiency
- Drug-induced chronic hepatitis
- Wilson's disease

 DIAGNOSIS

LABORATORY TESTS

- Elevated serum aminotransferase levels; in approximately 40% of cases, serum aminotransferase levels remain normal
- Elevated serum bilirubin level, low albumin level, and prolonged prothrombin time reflect advanced disease (severe inflammation or cirrhosis, or both)
- Table 91 and Figure 7
- Replicative phase (HBeAg-positive chronic hepatitis B): HBeAg and HBV DNA level $\geq 10^5$ copies/mL in serum
- Nonreplicative phase: anti-HBe and HBV DNA level $< 10^5$ copies/mL in serum
- Precore mutant (HBeAg-negative chronic hepatitis B): anti-HBe and HBV DNA level $\geq 10^5$ copies/mL in serum

DIAGNOSTIC PROCEDURES

- Liver biopsy may be indicated for diagnosis, staging, and predicting response to therapy

 TREATMENT

MEDICATIONS

- Treat active viral replication (HBV DNA > 10^5 copies/mL in serum)
  - Use peginterferon alfa-2a, 180 mcg SQ weekly for 48 weeks
- In the past, recombinant human interferon alfa-2b has been used: 5 million units/day or 10 million units three times a week SQ for 4–6 months
- Lamivudine, 100 mg PO daily as a single dose
  - May be used instead of interferon and is much better tolerated
  - Can be used in decompensated cirrhosis
  - May be effective in rapidly progressive hepatitis B ("fibrosing cholestatic hepatitis") following organ transplantation
  - Relapse is frequent when lamivudine is stopped
  - Long-term treatment is associated with a high rate of viral resistance
- Combined use of interferon/peginterferon and a nucleoside analog such as lamivudine offers no advantage over the use of either drug alone
- Adefovir, 10 mg PO once a day, a nucleotide analog, has activity against wild-type and lamivudine-resistant HBV
  - Resistance to this drug is less common than with lamivudine
  - Nephrotoxicity rarely can develop, especially if there is underlying renal dysfunction
- Telbivudine, daily dose of 600 mg PO, is more potent than either lamivudine or adefovir, but resistance may develop and patients who are resistant to lamivudine may also be resistant to telbivudine
- Entecavir, 0.5 mg PO once a day (or 1 mg PO once a day in patients with cirrhosis or resistance to lamivudine), is also effective against wild-type and lamivudine-resistant HBV; preferred first-line treatment
- Tenofovir has activity against HBV
  - However, it is not approved in the United States for the treatment of HBV infection
  - It is useful as part of an antiretroviral regimen in patients coinfected with HIV
- Because of the high rate of resistance to lamivudine, adefovir and entecavir are preferred nucleoside (or nucleotide) analogs for HBV infection
- A nucleoside or nucleotide analog is recommended for inactive HBV carriers before starting immunosuppressive therapy or cancer chemotherapy to prevent reactivation
- Side effects are frequent with interferon/peginterferon
  - Flu-like symptoms
  - Malaise
  - Weight loss
- Depression
- Thyroid disease
- Cytopenias
- Side effects are infrequent with nucleoside/nucleotide analogs

THERAPEUTIC PROCEDURES

- Activity is modified according to symptoms; bed rest is not necessary
- The diet should be well balanced, without limitations other than sodium or protein restriction if dictated by fluid overload or encephalopathy

 OUTCOME

COMPLICATIONS

- Cirrhosis
- Hepatocellular carcinoma
- Extrahepatic: polyarteritis nodosa, membranous glomerulonephritis

PROGNOSIS

- Interferon and peginterferon
  - Up to 40% of patients with HBeAg-positive chronic hepatitis B will respond with sustained normalization of aminotransferase levels, disappearance of HBeAg and HBV DNA from serum, appearance of anti-HBe, and improved survival
  - Response is most likely with a low HBV DNA level and high aminotransferase levels
  - Over 60% of the responders may eventually clear HBsAg from serum and liver, develop anti-HBs in serum, and be cured. Relapses are uncommon in such complete responders
  - HBeAg-negative chronic hepatitis B (precore mutant) has a response rate of 60% after 48 weeks of therapy with peginterferon, but durability of response is unclear
  - The response is poor in patients with HIV coinfection and autoimmune diseases
- Lamivudine, adefovir, entecavir
  - Suppress HBV DNA in serum in 60–80% of patients; entecavir is most effective
  - Improve liver histology in at least 60% of patients, and lead to normal alanine aminotransferase levels in over 40% and HBeAg seroconversion in around 20% of patients after 1 year of therapy
  - With lamivudine, 15–30% of responders experience a generally mild relapse during treatment as a result of mutation in the polymerase gene of

HBV DNA that confers resistance to lamivudine
– The rate of resistance increases to 70% at 5 years
– Resistance to adefovir occurs in up to 29% of patients treated for 5 years
– Resistance to entecavir is thus far uncommon
– Hepatitis may recur when the drug is stopped
– Indefinite treatment may be required when HBeAg seroconversion does not ensue
– Rates of complete response—as well as resistance to lamivudine—increase with longer duration of therapy

WHEN TO ADMIT

- Decompensated liver disease (eg, severe coagulopathy, variceal bleeding, severe ascites)

PREVENTION

- Strict isolation of patients is not necessary, but hand washing after bowel movements is required
- Thorough hand washing by anyone who may contact contaminated utensils, bedding, or clothing is essential
- Screening of donated blood for HBsAg and anti-HBc has reduced the risk of transfusion-associated hepatitis markedly
- Pregnant women should be tested for HBsAg
- Persons with HBV should practice safe sex
- Vaccinate against HAV (after prescreening for prior immunity) in those with chronic hepatitis B

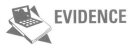 **EVIDENCE**

PRACTICE GUIDELINES

- National Guideline Clearinghouse

INFORMATION FOR PATIENTS

- Centers for Disease Control and Prevention
- Mayo Clinic
- Patient Information

REFERENCES

- Chang TT et al; BEHoLD AI463022 Study Group. A comparison of entecavir versus lamivudine for HBeAg-positive chronic hepatitis B. N Engl J Med. 2006 Mar 9;354(10):1001–10. [PMID: 16525137]
- Keeffe EB et al. A treatment algorithm for the management of chronic hepatitis

B virus infection in the United States: an update. Clin Gastroenterol Hepatol. 2006 Aug;4(8):936–62. [PMID: 16844425]
- Yeo W et al. Diagnosis, prevention and management of hepatitis B virus reactivation during anticancer therapy. Hepatology. 2006 Feb;43(2):209–20. [PMID: 16440366]

Hepatitis C, Acute

 KEY FEATURES

ESSENTIALS OF DIAGNOSIS

- Often asymptomatic
- Prodrome of anorexia, nausea, vomiting, malaise, aversion to smoking
- Fever, enlarged and tender liver, jaundice
- Markedly elevated aminotransferases early in the course
- Liver biopsy shows hepatocellular necrosis and mononuclear infiltrate
- Source of infection in many is unknown

GENERAL CONSIDERATIONS

- The hepatitis C virus (HCV) is a single-stranded RNA virus (hepacivirus) with properties similar to those of flavivirus
- At least six major genotypes of HCV have been identified
- Coinfection is found in at least 30% of persons infected with HIV
- HIV leads to more rapid progression of chronic hepatitis C to cirrhosis
- Anti-HCV is not protective; in patients with acute or chronic hepatitis, its presence in serum generally signifies that HCV is the cause

DEMOGRAPHICS

- There are more than 2.7 million HCV carriers in the United States and another 1.3 million previously exposed persons who have cleared the virus
- In the past, HCV caused over 90% of cases of posttransfusion hepatitis, yet only 4% of cases of hepatitis C were attributable to blood transfusions
- Over 50% of cases are transmitted by injection drug use
- Intranasal cocaine use, body piercing, tatoos, and hemodialysis may be risk factors

- The risk of sexual and maternal-neonatal transmission is low and may be greatest in those with high circulating levels of HCV RNA
  – Multiple sexual partners may increase the risk of HCV infection
  – Transmission via breast-feeding has not been documented
- Nosocomial transmission may occur via
  – Multidose vials of saline
  – Reuse of disposable syringes
  – Contamination of shared saline bags

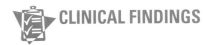 **CLINICAL FINDINGS**

SYMPTOMS AND SIGNS

- The incubation period averages 6–7 weeks
- Clinical illness
  – Often mild
  – Usually asymptomatic
  – Characterized by waxing and waning aminotransferase elevations and a high rate (> 80%) of chronic hepatitis
- Slight neurocognitive impairment may occur with chronic hepatitis C
- Hepatic steatosis is a particular feature of infection with HCV genotype 3

DIFFERENTIAL DIAGNOSIS

- Hepatitis A, B, D, E virus
- Hepatitis G virus (HGV) rarely, if ever, causes frank hepatitis
- TT virus (TTV)
  – Found in up to 7.5% of blood donors
  – Readily transmitted by blood transfusions
  – However, an association between this virus and liver disease has not been established
- A related virus known as SEN-V has been found in 2% of U.S. blood donors
  – It is transmitted by transfusion
  – May account for some cases of transfusion-associated non-ABCDE hepatitis
- Cytomegalovirus, Epstein-Barr virus, and herpes simplex virus, particularly in immunocompromised hosts

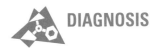 **DIAGNOSIS**

LABORATORY TESTS

- Antibodies to HCV (Figure 6)
  – The immunoassay has moderate sensitivity (false-negatives) for the diagnosis early in the course and in healthy blood donors and low speci-

ficity (false-positives) in persons with elevated γ-globulin levels

– In these situations, a diagnosis of hepatitis C may be confirmed by use of an assay for HCV RNA and, in some cases, a supplemental recombinant immunoblot assay (RIBA) for anti-HCV

- Most RIBA-positive persons are potentially infectious, as confirmed by use of polymerase chain reaction-based tests to detect HCV RNA
- Occasional persons are found to have anti-HCV in serum, confirmed by RIBA, without HCV RNA in serum, suggesting recovery from HCV infection in the past
- In pregnant patients, serum aminotransferase levels frequently normalize despite persistence of viremia, only to increase again after delivery
- The white blood cell count is normal to low, especially in the preicteric phase
- Large atypical lymphocytes may occasionally be seen
- Mild proteinuria is common, and bilirubinuria often precedes the appearance of jaundice
- Elevated aspartate or alanine aminotransferase levels occur early, followed by elevations of bilirubin and alkaline phosphatase; in a small number of patients, the latter persist after aminotransferase levels have normalized

 TREATMENT

MEDICATIONS

- If nausea and vomiting are pronounced or if oral intake is substantially decreased, 10% IV glucose is indicated
- Small doses of oxazepam are safe, as metabolism is not hepatic; morphine sulfate is avoided
- Corticosteroids have no benefit
- Treatment with interferon alfa or peginterferon can be considered when HCV RNA has not cleared from serum in 3–4 months (doses as for chronic hepatitis C)
- If HCV RNA has not cleared after 3 months of therapy, ribavirin can be added

THERAPEUTIC PROCEDURES

- Bed rest is recommended only if symptoms are marked
- Dietary management consists of palatable meals as tolerated, without overfeeding; breakfast is usually best tolerated
- Strenuous physical exertion, alcohol, and hepatotoxic agents are avoided

 OUTCOME

COMPLICATIONS

- Mixed cryoglobulinemia and membranoproliferative glomerulonephritis
- Possibly lichen planus, autoimmune thyroiditis, lymphocytic sialadenitis, idiopathic pulmonary fibrosis, sporadic porphyria cutanea tarda, monoclonal gammopathies, and probably lymphoma
- The risk of type 2 diabetes mellitus is increased with chronic hepatitis C

PROGNOSIS

- In most patients, clinical recovery is complete in 3–6 months
- Liver function returns to normal, though aminotransferase elevations persist in most patients in whom chronic hepatitis C ensues
- The mortality rate is < 1%, but the rate is higher in older people
- Fulminant hepatitis C is rare in the United States
- Chronic hepatitis develops in as many as 80% of all persons with acute hepatitis C, which in many cases progresses very slowly
- Cirrhosis develops in up to 30% of those with chronic hepatitis C; the risk is higher in patients coinfected with both HCV and HBV or with HCV and HIV
- Patients with cirrhosis are at risk for hepatocellular carcinoma at a rate of 3–5% per year

WHEN TO ADMIT

- Intractable nausea and vomiting and need for parenteral fluids
- Encephalopathy or severe coagulopathy indicate impending acute hepatic failure, and hospitalization is necessary

PREVENTION

- Strict isolation of patients is not necessary, but hand washing after bowel movements is required
- Thorough hand washing by anyone who may contact contaminated utensils, bedding, or clothing is essential
- Testing blood for HCV has helped reduce the risk of transfusion-associated hepatitis C

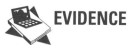 **EVIDENCE**

PRACTICE GUIDELINES

- National Guideline Clearinghouse

WEB SITE

- Hepatitis C: Case study

INFORMATION FOR PATIENTS

- Centers for Disease Control and Prevention
- Torpy JM et al. JAMA patient page. Hepatitis C. JAMA. 2003;289:2450. [PMID: 12746370]

REFERENCES

- Armstrong GL et al. The prevalence of hepatitis C virus infection in the United States, 1999 through 2002. Ann Intern Med. 2006 May 16;144(10):705–14. [PMID: 16702586]
- Kamal SM et al. Duration of peginterferon therapy in acute hepatitis C: a randomized trial. Hepatology. 2006 May; 43(5):923–31. [PMID: 16628640]
- Prati D. Transmission of hepatitis C by blood transfusions and other medical procedures: a global review. J Hepatol. 2006 Oct;45(4):607–16. [PMID: 16901579]

Hepatitis C, Chronic

KEY FEATURES

ESSENTIALS OF DIAGNOSIS

- Chronic inflammatory reaction of the liver of more than 3–6 months duration
- Persistently abnormal serum aminotransferase levels and antibody to hepatitis C virus (HCV) in serum
- Liver biopsy shows features of chronic hepatitis, often with portal lymphoid nodules and interface hepatitis

GENERAL CONSIDERATIONS

- Chronic hepatitis is characterized on
  – The basis of the etiology
  – The grade of portal, periportal, and lobular inflammation (minimal, mild, moderate, or severe)

– The stage of fibrosis (none, mild, moderate, severe, cirrhosis)
- HCV may be the most common etiology of chronic hepatitis
- HCV coinfection is found in 30% of persons infected with HIV
- Anti-HCV is not protective; in chronic hepatitis its presence in serum signifies that HCV is the cause
- At least six major genotypes of HCV have been identified

DEMOGRAPHICS

- Chronic hepatitis C develops in up to 85% of patients with acute hepatitis C
- There are more than 2.7 million HCV carriers in the United States and another 1.3 million previously exposed persons who have cleared the virus
- HCV was responsible for over 90% of cases of posttransfusion hepatitis; yet only 4% of cases of hepatitis C were attributable to blood transfusions
- Over 50% of cases are transmitted by injection drug use
- The risk of sexual and maternal-neonatal transmission is low and may be greatest in those with high circulating levels of HCV RNA
- Multiple sexual partners may increase the risk of HCV infection

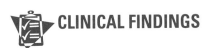

CLINICAL FINDINGS

SYMPTOMS AND SIGNS

- Clinically indistinguishable from chronic hepatitis due to other causes
- In approximately 40% of cases, serum aminotransferase levels are persistently normal
- Slight neurocognitive impairment has been reported

DIFFERENTIAL DIAGNOSIS

- Hepatitis B and D (delta agent)
- Autoimmune hepatitis
- α_1-Antiprotease deficiency
- Drug-induced hepatitis
- Hemochromatosis
- Wilson's disease

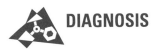

DIAGNOSIS

LABORATORY TESTS

- Serum anti-HCV by enzyme immunoassay (EIA) is present (Figure 6)

- HCV RNA level and HCV genotype help predict response to therapy
- Level of viremia does not correlate with degree of hepatic inflammation or fibrosis
- In rare cases of negative anti-HCV EIA, HCV RNA is detected by polymerase chain reaction (PCR)
- Hepatic steatosis (fatty liver) is a particular feature of infection with HCV genotype 3

DIAGNOSTIC PROCEDURES

- Liver biopsy is indicated in patients offered treatment for diagnosis, staging, and predicting response to therapy

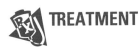 **TREATMENT**

MEDICATIONS

- Two peginterferon formulations are available
  – Peginterferon alfa-2b, with a 12-kDa polyethylene glycol (PEG), in a dose of 1.5 mcg/kg weekly
  – Peginterferon alfa-2a, with a 40-kDa PEG, in a dose of 180 mcg once per week for 48 weeks
- When ribavirin is used with **peginterferon alfa-2b**
  – Dose of ribavirin is based on the patient's weight
  – May range from 800 mg to 1400 mg daily in two divided doses
- When ribavirin is used with **peginterferon alfa-2a**
  – Daily ribavirin dose is 1000 mg or 1200 mg depending on the patient's weight (less than or greater than 75 kg)
- Treat cirrhosis or a high viral level in serum (> 400,000 IU/mL) for 48 weeks
- Treat genotype 1 for 48 weeks if the level of viremia is reduced by 2 logs at 12 weeks; otherwise discontinue
- Treat genotypes 2 or 3, without cirrhosis, and with low levels of viremia (< 2–3.5×10^6 copies/mL) for 24 weeks with a decreased dose of ribavirin of 800 mg in a split dose
- Peginterferon alfa with ribavirin may be effective treatment for **cryoglobulinemia** associated with chronic hepatitis C
- Asymptomatic "chronic carriers" with normal serum aminotransferase levels respond as well to treatment as do patients with elevated aminotransferase levels
- Coinfection of HCV and HIV may benefit from treatment of HCV
- Treatment with peginterferon alfa plus ribavirin
  – Costly

– Side effects (flu-like symptoms) are almost universal
– More serious toxicity includes psychiatric symptoms (irritability, depression), thyroid dysfunction, and bone marrow suppression
- Contraindications for interferon therapy
  – Pregnancy and breast-feeding
  – Decompensated cirrhosis
  – Profound cytopenias
  – Severe psychiatric disorders
  – Autoimmune diseases
- Ribavirin should be avoided in
  – Persons over age 65
  – Persons in whom hemolysis could pose a risk of angina or stroke
- Rash, itching, headache, cough, and shortness of breath also occur with ribavirin
- Lactic acidosis is a concern if also taking highly active antiretroviral therapy for HIV
- Occasionally, erythropoietin and granulocyte colony-stimulating factor are used to treat therapy-induced anemia and leukopenia, respectively
- "Consensus" interferon (a synthetic recombinant interferon, also known as alfacon), 15 mcg/day SQ for 48 weeks, plus ribavirin, may be effective in some nonresponders to peginterferon and ribavirin

THERAPEUTIC PROCEDURES

- Activity is modified according to symptoms; bed rest is not necessary
- The diet should be well balanced, without limitations other than sodium or protein restriction if dictated by fluid overload or encephalopathy
- Generally offer treatment if
  – Patient under age 70
  – More than minor fibrosis is present on liver biopsy findings
- Because of high response rates to treatment with HCV genotype 2 or 3 infection, treatment may be initiated without a liver biopsy

 OUTCOME

FOLLOW-UP

- Peginterferon alfa plus ribavirin therapy
  – Obtain a blood cell count at weeks 1, 2, and 4 after therapy is started and monthly thereafter
- Ribavirin therapy
  – Monitor for hemolysis
  – Because of teratogenic concerns, patients must practice strict contracep-

tion until 6 months after conclusion of therapy

COMPLICATIONS

- Cryoglobulinemia and membranoproliferative glomerulonephritis
- The following may be related to chronic hepatitis C
  - Lichen planus
  - Autoimmune thyroiditis
  - Lymphocytic sialadenitis
  - Idiopathic pulmonary fibrosis
  - Porphyria cutanea tarda
  - Lymphoma
  - Monoclonal gammopathy
- Type 2 diabetes mellitus

PROGNOSIS

- Up to 80% of acute hepatitis C becomes chronic hepatitis, which in many cases progresses very slowly
- Most patients with persistently normal serum aminotransferase levels have mild chronic hepatitis with slow or absent progression to cirrhosis
- However, cirrhosis is present in 10% of these patients
- Progression to cirrhosis occurs in 20% of affected patients after 20 years, with an increased risk in men, those who drink more than 50 g of alcohol daily, and possibly those who acquire HCV infection after age 40
- Immunosuppressed persons (hypogammaglobulinemia, HIV infection with a low CD4 count, or organ transplant recipients receiving immunosuppressants) progress more rapidly to cirrhosis than immunocompetent persons
- Hepatocellular carcinoma develops in cirrhosis at a rate of 3–5% per year
- Peginterferon plus ribavarin
  - Probably improves survival and quality of life
  - Is cost-effective
  - Retards and even reverses fibrosis
  - May reduce the risk of hepatocellular carcinoma in responders
- Factors predicting an increased chance of response include
  - Absence of advanced fibrosis on liver biopsy (though treatment is not contraindicated by compensated cirrhosis)
  - Low serum HCV RNA levels
  - Infection by genotypes of HCV other than 1a, 1b, or 4

WHEN TO ADMIT

- Rarely necessary
- Only in advanced cirrhosis with decompensation

PREVENTION

- Strict isolation of patients is not necessary, but hand washing after bowel movements is required
- Thorough hand washing by anyone who may contact contaminated utensils, bedding, or clothing is essential
- Testing of donated blood for HCV has helped reduce the risk of transfusion-associated hepatitis C from 10% a decade ago to about 1 in 2 million units today

EVIDENCE

PRACTICE GUIDELINES

- Dienstag JL et al. American Gastroenterological Association medical position statement on the management of hepatitis C. Gastroenterology. 2006 Jan; 130(1):231–64. [PMID: 16401486]
- National Guideline Clearinghouse

WEB SITES

- Hepatitis C: Case Study
- Viral Hepatitis

INFORMATION FOR PATIENTS

- Centers for Disease Control and Prevention
- Torpy JM et al. JAMA patient page. Hepatitis C. JAMA. 2003;289:2450. [PMID: 12746370]

REFERENCE

- Hoofnagle JH et al. Peginterferon and ribavirin for chronic hepatitis C. N Engl J Med. 2006 Dec 7;355(23):2444–51. [PMID: 17151366]

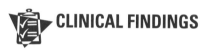

Hepatitis, Autoimmune

 KEY FEATURES

ESSENTIALS OF DIAGNOSIS

- Usually young to middle-aged women
- Chronic hepatitis with high serum globulins
- Antinuclear antibody (+ANA) and/or smooth muscle antibody
- Responds to corticosteroids

GENERAL CONSIDERATIONS

- The onset is usually insidious
- However, up to 40% present with an acute (occasionally fulminant) attack of hepatitis
- Some cases follow a viral illness such as
  - Hepatitis A
  - Epstein-Barr infection
  - Measles
  - Exposure to a toxin or drug, such as nitrofurantoin
- There are at least three types of autoimmune hepatitis, distinguished by autoantibodies

DEMOGRAPHICS

- Though usually a disease of young women, autoimmune hepatitis can occur in either sex at any age
- Affected younger persons are often positive for HLA-B8 and -DR3; older patients are often positive for HLA-DR4
- The principal susceptibility allele among white Americans and northern Europeans is HLA *DRB1*0301*; HLA *DRB1*0401* is a secondary but independent risk factor

CLINICAL FINDINGS

SYMPTOMS AND SIGNS

- Typically, a healthy-appearing young woman with multiple spider nevi, cutaneous striae, acne, hirsutism, and hepatomegaly
- Amenorrhea may be a presenting feature
- Extrahepatic features
  - Arthritis
  - Sjögren's syndrome
  - Thyroiditis
  - Nephritis
  - Ulcerative colitis
  - Coombs-positive hemolytic anemia

DIFFERENTIAL DIAGNOSIS

- Chronic viral hepatitis
- Primary biliary cirrhosis
- Primary sclerosing cholangitis
- Wilson's disease
- Hemochromatosis
- Drug-induced liver disease
- α_1-Antiprotease deficiency

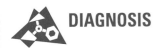 **DIAGNOSIS**

LABORATORY TESTS

- The serum bilirubin is usually increased, but 20% are anicteric
- Serum aminotransferase levels may be > 1000 units/L
- Type I (classic) autoimmune hepatitis
  - ANA or smooth muscle antibody (either or both) is detected in serum
  - Serum γ-globulin levels are typically elevated (up to 5–6 g/dL)
    - In this setting, the enzyme immunoassay for antibody to hepatitis C virus may be falsely positive
    - Other antibodies, including antineutrophil cytoplasmic antibodies (ANCA), may be found
- Type II
  - Seen more often in Europe
  - Characterized by circulating antibody to liver–kidney microsomes (anti-LKM1)—directed against cytochrome P450 2D6—or anti-liver cytosol type 1—directed against formiminotransferase—without antismooth muscle antibody or ANA
  - Can be seen in patients with autoimmune polyglandular syndrome type 1
- Type III
  - Characterized by antibodies to soluble liver antigen/liver pancreas (anti-SLA/LP)
  - May represent a variant of type I characterized by severe disease, high relapse rate after treatment, and absence of the usual antibodies (ANA and smooth muscle antibody)
  - Anti-SLA/LP antibodies appear to be directed against a transfer RNA complex responsible for incorporating selenocysteine into peptide chains

 TREATMENT

MEDICATIONS

- Prednisone
  - With or without azathioprine improves symptoms and reduces hepatic inflammation
  - Indicated for symptomatic patients with at least a tenfold elevation of aminotransferases (or fivefold if the serum globulins are elevated at least twofold)
  - Asymptomatic patients with modest enzyme elevations may also be treated, but most asymptomatic patients have mild disease histologically and do not require immunosuppressive therapy
  - Initally, give 30 mg PO daily with azathioprine (or mercaptopurine), 50 mg/day PO
  - Taper after 1 week to 20 mg/day and again after 2 or 3 weeks to 15 mg/day
  - Ultimately, a maintenance dose of 10 mg/day is achieved

SURGERY

- Liver transplantation may be required for treatment failures, and the disease has been recognized to recur in up to one-third of transplanted livers (and rarely to develop de novo) as immunosuppression is reduced

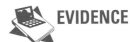 **OUTCOME**

FOLLOW-UP

- Monitor blood cell counts weekly for the first 2 months of azathioprine therapy and monthly thereafter because of the small risk of bone marrow suppression
- Once clinical, biochemical, and histologic remission is achieved (usually after at least 18 months of treatment), therapy may be withdrawn
  - Subsequent relapse rate is 50–90%
  - Relapses may again be treated in the same manner as the initial episode, with the same remission rate
- After successful treatment of a relapse
  - Treat indefinitely with azathioprine up to 2 mg/kg or the lowest dose of prednisone needed to maintain aminotransferase levels as close to normal as possible
  - Another attempt at withdrawing therapy may be considered in patients remaining in remission long term (eg, ≥ 4 years)
- Budesonide, a corticosteroid with less toxicity than prednisone, does not appear to be effective in maintaining remission
- Nonresponders to prednisone and azathioprine may be considered for a trial of cyclosporine, tacrolimus, or methotrexate
- Mycophenolate mofetil is effective when there is no response to azathioprine or it is not tolerated

COMPLICATIONS

- Concurrent primary biliary cirrhosis or primary sclerosing cholangitis
  - Occurs in up to 15% of patients
  - Liver biopsy is indicated for diagnosis and to determine the need for treatment
- Progression to cirrhosis and liver failure is an indication for liver transplantation

PROGNOSIS

- With immunosuppressive therapy, there is prompt symptomatic improvement but biochemical improvement is more gradual, with normalization of serum aminotransferase levels after several months in many cases
- Histologic resolution of inflammation may require 18–24 months, the time at which repeat liver biopsy is recommended
- Fibrosis may reverse after apparent biochemical and histologic remission
- The overall response rate is at least 80%
- Failure of aminotransferase levels to normalize invariably predicts lack of histologic resolution

PREVENTION

- Monitor bone density, particularly with corticosteroid use, for osteoporosis

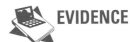 **EVIDENCE**

PRACTICE GUIDELINES

- Czaja AJ et al. American Association for the Study of Liver Disease. Diagnosis and treatment of autoimmune hepatitis. Hepatology. 2002;36:479. [PMID: 12143059]
- National Guideline Clearinghouse

WEB SITES

- Diseases of the Liver
- Hepatic Ultrasound Images
- Pathology Index

INFORMATION FOR PATIENTS

- National Institute of Diabetes and Digestive and Kidney Diseases
- National Institutes of Health

REFERENCES

- Czaja AJ et al. Distinctive clinical phenotype and treatment outcome of type I autoimmune hepatitis in the elderly. Hepatology. 2006 Mar;43(3):532–8. [PMID: 16496338]
- Heneghan MA et al. Utility of thiopurine methyltransferase genotyping and phenotyping, and measurement of azathioprine metabolites in the management of patients with autoimmune hepatitis. J Hepatol. 2006 Oct; 45(4):584–91. [PMID: 16876902]

• Krawitt EL. Autoimmune hepatitis. N Engl J Med. 2006 Jan 5;354(1):54–66. [PMID: 16394302]

Hepatitis, Drug- or Toxin-Induced

 KEY FEATURES

ESSENTIALS OF DIAGNOSIS

- Can mimic viral hepatitis, biliary tract obstruction, or other types of liver disease
- Clinicians must inquire about the use of many therapeutic agents, including over-the-counter "natural" and "herbal" products in any patient with liver disease

GENERAL CONSIDERATIONS

- Drug toxicity may be categorized on the basis of pathogenesis or histologic appearance

Direct hepatotoxic group

- Dose-related severity
- A latent period following exposure
- Susceptibility in all individuals
- Examples include
  - Acetaminophen (toxicity enhanced by fasting and chronic alcohol use)
  - Alcohol
  - Carbon tetrachloride
  - Chloroform
  - Heavy metals
  - Mercaptopurine
  - Niacin
  - Plant alkaloids
  - Phosphorus
  - Tetracyclines
  - Valproic acid
  - Vitamin A
- Statins may cause elevated serum aminotransferase levels (like all cholesterol-lowering agents) but rarely cause true hepatitis
- Coadministration of a second agent may increase the toxicity of the first (eg, isoniazid and rifampin, acetaminophen and alcohol)

Idiosyncratic reactions

- Reactions are sporadic, not dose-related, and occasionally are associated with fever and eosinophilia
- May have genetic predisposition

- Examples include
  - Amiodarone
  - Aspirin
  - Carbamazepine
  - Chloramphenicol
  - Diclofenac
  - Disulfuram
  - Duloxetine
  - Ezetimibe
  - Flutamide
  - Halothane
  - Isoniazid
  - Ketoconazole
  - Lamotrigine
  - Methyldopa
  - Oxacillin
  - Phenytoin
  - Pyrazinamide
  - Quinidine
  - Rofecoxib (withdrawn from the market in the United States)
  - Streptomycin
  - Troglitazone (withdrawn from the market in the United States)
  - Less commonly other thiazolidinediones, and perhaps tacrine

Cholestatic reactions

- **Noninflammatory**
  - Following drugs cause cholestasis: estrogens, anabolic steroids containing an alkyl or ethinyl group at carbon 17, indinavir, mercaptopurine, methyltestosterone, cyclosporine
- **Inflammatory**
  - Inflammation of portal areas with bile duct injury (cholangitis), often with allergic features such as eosinophilia: amoxicillin-clavulanic acid, azathioprine, azithromycin, captopril, cephalosporins, chlorothiazide, chlorpromazine, chlorpropamide, erythromycin, penicillamine, prochlorperazine, semisynthetic penicillins (eg, cloxacillin), and sulfadiazine

Acute or chronic hepatitis

- Can be clinically and histologically indistinguishable from autoimmune hepatitis
  - Aspirin
  - Isoniazid (increased risk in hepatitis B virus carriers)
  - Methyldopa
  - Minocycline
  - Nitrofurantoin
  - Nonsteroidal anti-inflammatory drugs
  - Propylthiouracil
- Can occur with
  - Cocaine
  - Ecstasy
  - Efavirenz
  - Nevirapine
  - Ritonavir
  - Sulfonamides

  - Telithromycin
  - Troglitazone (withdrawn from the market in the United States)
  - Zafirlukast
  - Various herbal and alternative remedies (eg, chaparral, germander, jin bu huan, skullcap)

Other reactions

- Fatty liver, macrovesicular
  - Alcohol
  - Amiodarone
  - Corticosteroids
  - Irinotecan
  - Oxaliplatin (possibly)
  - Methotrexate
- Fatty liver, microvesicular
  - Didanosine
  - Stavudine
  - Tetracyclines
  - Valproic acid
  - Zidovudine
- Granulomas
  - Allopurinol
  - Quinidine
  - Quinine
  - Phenylbutazone
  - Phenytoin
- Fibrosis and cirrhosis: methotrexate, vitamin A
- Sinusoidal obstruction syndrome (venoocclusive disease)
  - Antineoplastic agents (pre-bone marrow transplant)
  - Pyrrolizidine alkaloids (eg, Comfrey)
- Peliosis hepatis (blood-filled cavities)
  - Anabolic steroids
  - Azathioprine
  - Oral contraceptive steroids
- Neoplasms
  - Oral contraceptive steroids, estrogens (hepatic adenoma but not focal nodular hyperplasia)
  - Vinyl chloride (angiosarcoma)

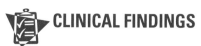 **CLINICAL FINDINGS**

SYMPTOMS AND SIGNS

- Can mimic all types of liver disease

DIFFERENTIAL DIAGNOSIS

Causes of acute hepatitis

- Viral
  - Hepatitis A, B, C, D (in presence of B), and E
  - Infectious mononucleosis
  - Cytomegalovirus
  - Herpes simplex virus
  - Parvovirus B19
- Other infections, eg, leptospirosis, secondary syphilis, brucellosis, Q fever

- Vascular
  - Right-sided congestive heart failure
  - Shock (ischemic) liver
  - Portal vein thrombosis
  - Budd-Chiari syndrome
- Metabolic
  - Wilson's disease
  - Acute fatty liver of pregnancy
  - Reye's syndrome
- Autoimmune hepatitis
- Lymphoma or metastatic cancer

Causes of cholestasis

- Extrahepatic
  - Choledocholithiasis
  - Pancreatic tumor
  - Biliary stricture
  - Primary sclerosing cholangitis (intrahepatic and extrahepatic)
- Intrahepatic
  - Primary biliary cirrhosis
  - Autoimmune cholangitis
  - Infiltrative disease (eg, tuberculosis, sarcoidosis, lymphoma, amyloidosis)
  - Drugs

DIAGNOSIS

DIAGNOSTIC PROCEDURES

- Inquire about the use of potentially hepatotoxic drugs or exposure to hepatotoxins

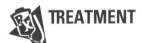

TREATMENT

MEDICATIONS

- Removing the offending agent is critical
- Corticosteroids are rarely, if ever, indicated

SURGERY

- Liver transplantation in rare instances of acute liver failure

THERAPEUTIC PROCEDURES

- Supportive treatment: see specific hepatitis etiology

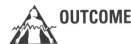

OUTCOME

FOLLOW-UP

- Monitor liver function tests until sustained improvement is seen

PROGNOSIS

- In patients with drug-induced hepatitis, development of jaundice is associated with a mortality rate of 10%

COMPLICATIONS

- Complications are those of liver disease of any etiology and include
  - Hypoprothrombinemia
  - Ascites
  - Edema
  - Portal hypertension
  - Variceal bleeding
  - Spontaneous bacterial peritonitis

WHEN TO ADMIT

- Intractable nausea and vomiting and need for parenteral fluids
- Encephalopathy or severe coagulopathy indicates impending acute hepatic failure, and hospitalization is mandatory

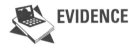

EVIDENCE

PRACTICE GUIDELINES

- Centers for Disease Control and Prevention (CDC); American Thoracic Society. Update: adverse event data and revised American Thoracic Society/CDC recommendations against the use of rifampin and pyrazinamide for treatment of latent tuberculosis infection–United States, 2003. MMWR Morb Mortal Wkly Rep. 2003;52:735. [PMID: 12904741]

WEB SITES

- Diseases of the Liver
- Pathology Index

INFORMATION FOR PATIENTS

- National Institutes of Health

REFERENCES

- Andrade RJ et al. Outcome of acute idiosyncratic drug-induced liver injury: long-term follow-up in a hepatotoxicity registry. Hepatology. 2006 Dec; 44(6):1581–8. [PMID: 17133470]
- Navarro VJ et al. Current concepts: drug-related hepatotoxicity. N Engl J Med. 2006 Feb 16;354(7):731–9. [PMID: 16481640]
- Watkins PB et al. Drug-induced liver injury: summary of a single-topic clinical research conference. Hepatology. 2006 Mar;43(3):618–31. [PMID: 16496329]

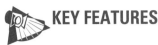

Hepatocellular Carcinoma

KEY FEATURES

ESSENTIALS OF DIAGNOSIS

- Hepatocellular carcinoma: malignant neoplasm of the liver that arises from parenchymal cells
- Cholangiocarcinoma: malignant neoplasm that originates in the ductular cells

GENERAL CONSIDERATIONS

- Risk factors
  - Cirrhosis in general, including nonalcoholic fatty liver disease, and hepatitis B or C in particular
  - In Africa and Asia, hepatitis B is of major etiologic significance
  - In the West and Japan, hepatitis C and alcoholic cirrhosis are most common
  - Hemochromatosis, aflatoxin exposure (associated with mutation of the *TP53* gene), α_1-antiprotease (α_1-antitrypsin) deficiency, and tyrosinemia
- In patients with cirrhosis, additional risk factors include
  - Male gender
  - Age > 55
  - Nonwhite ethnicity
  - Diabetes mellitus, hypothyroidism, being overweight
  - Prothrombin time < 75% of control
  - Platelets < 75,000/mcL
  - TIPS
- Fibrolamellar variant of hepatocellular carcinoma
  - Occurs in young women
  - Characterized by a distinctive histologic picture, absence of risk factors, and indolent course
- Histologically, hepatocellular carcinoma is made up of cords or sheets of cells that roughly resemble the hepatic parenchyma; blood vessels such as portal or hepatic veins are commonly involved by tumor
- Staging in the TNM classification
  - T0: there is no evidence of primary tumor
  - T1: solitary tumor without vascular invasion
  - T2: solitary tumor with vascular invasion or multiple tumors none > 5 cm
  - T3: multiple tumors > 5 cm or a tumor involving a major branch of the portal or hepatic vein(s)

– T4: tumor(s) with direct invasion of adjacent organs other than the gallbladder or with perforation of the visceral peritoneum

DEMOGRAPHICS

• Incidence is rising in the United States and western countries because of the high prevalence of chronic hepatitis C infection

CLINICAL FINDINGS

SYMPTOMS AND SIGNS

• May be unsuspected until there is deterioration in a cirrhotic patient who was formerly stable
• Cachexia, weakness, and weight loss are associated symptoms
• The sudden appearance of ascites, which may be bloody, suggests portal or hepatic vein thrombosis by tumor or bleeding from the necrotic tumor
• There may be a tender enlargement of the liver, occasionally with a palpable mass
• In Africa, young patients typically present with a rapidly expanding abdominal mass. Auscultation may reveal a bruit over the tumor or a friction rub when the process has extended to the surface of the liver

DIFFERENTIAL DIAGNOSIS

• Metastatic cancer
• Benign liver tumors
  – Hemangioma
  – Adenoma
  – Focal nodular hyperplasia
• Pyogenic or amebic liver abscess

DIAGNOSIS

LABORATORY TESTS

• There may be leukocytosis, as opposed to the leukopenia that is frequently encountered in cirrhotic patients
• Anemia is common
• However, hematocrit is normal or elevated one-third of patients from tumor elaboration of erythropoietin
• Sudden and sustained elevation of the serum alkaline phosphatase in a formerly stable patient is common
• Hepatitis B surface antigen in most cases in endemic areas
• In the United States, anti-hepatitis C virus (HCV) is in up to 40% of cases

• α-Fetoprotein levels
  – Elevated in up to 70% of patients in western countries (though the sensitivity is lower in African-Americans)
  – However, mild elevations are also often seen in patients with chronic hepatitis
• Serum levels of des-γ-carboxy prothrombin
  – Elevated in up to 90% of patients
  – Also may be elevated in patients with vitamin K deficiency, chronic hepatitis, and metastatic cancer
  – Test is not widely used in United States
• Cytologic study of ascitic fluid rarely reveals malignant cells

IMAGING STUDIES

• Multiphasic helical CT scanning with and without intravenous contrast or MRI is preferred for the location and vascularity of the tumor
• Ultrasound is less sensitive but is used to screen for hepatic nodules in high-risk patients
• Contrast-enhanced ultrasound has a sensitivity and specificity approaching those of multiphasic helical CT

DIAGNOSTIC PROCEDURES

• Liver biopsy
  – Diagnostic, though seeding of the needle tract by tumor is a potential risk (< 3%)
  – Can be deferred if imaging studies and α-fetoprotein levels are diagnostic or if surgical resection is planned

TREATMENT

MEDICATIONS

• Chemotherapy, hormonal therapy with tamoxifen, and long-acting octreotide have not been shown to prolong life
• Adaptive immunotherapy and treatment of underlying chronic viral hepatitis may lower postsurgical recurrence rates

SURGERY

• Liver transplantation
  – May achieve a better recurrence-free survival than resection with well-compensated cirrhosis and small tumors (Milan criteria: one tumor < 5 cm or three or fewer tumors each < 3 cm in diameter)
  – However, often impractical because of the donor organ shortage; living

donor liver transplantation may be considered in these cases
  – May be appropriate for small unresectable tumors in a patient with advanced cirrhosis, with reported 5-year survival rates of up to 75%
• Laparoscopic liver resection has been performed in selected cases

THERAPEUTIC PROCEDURES

• If the disease progresses despite treatment, meticulous efforts at palliative care are essential
• Severe pain may develop due to expansion of the liver capsule by the tumor and require concerted efforts at pain management, including opioid use
• Chemoembolization via the hepatic artery
  – May be palliative
  – May prolong survival in patients with large or multifocal tumor in the absence of vascular invasion or extrahepatic spread
• Injection of absolute ethanol into, radiofrequency ablation of, or cryotherapy of small tumors (< 3 cm) may prolong survival; these are reasonable alternatives to surgical resection in some patients and may provide a "bridge" to liver transplantation
• Radiofrequency ablation is superior to ethanol injection for tumors > 2 cm

OUTCOME

PROGNOSIS

• In the United States, overall 1- and 5-year survival rates for hepatocellular carcinoma are 23% and 5%, respectively
• Attempts at surgical resection are usually fruitless if concomitant cirrhosis is present and if the tumor is multifocal
• Surgical resection of solitary hepatocellular carcinomas may result in cure if liver function is preserved (Child class A or possibly B)
• 5-year survival rates rise to 56% for patients with localized resectable disease (T1, T2, T3, selected T4; N0; M0) but are almost nil for those with localized unresectable or advanced disease
• The fibrolamellar variant has a better prognosis than conventional hepatocellular carcinoma

PREVENTION

• Although the standard approach for patients with chronic hepatitis B or cirrhosis caused by HCV or alcohol is α-fetoprotein testing and ultrasonography every 6 months, the value of α-fetoprotein screening has been questioned

- The risk of hepatocellular carcinoma with cirrhosis is 3–5% a year

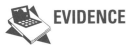

EVIDENCE

PRACTICE GUIDELINES

- British Society of Gastroenterology

WEB SITES

- Hepatic Ultrasound Images
- Liver Tutorials Visualization and Volume Measurement

INFORMATION FOR PATIENTS

- American Cancer Society
- National Cancer Institute

REFERENCES

- Cillo U et al. Prospective validation of the Barcelona Clinic Liver Cancer staging system. J Hepatol. 2006 Apr; 44(4):723–31. [PMID: 16488051]
- El-Serag HB et al. The association between diabetes and hepatocellular carcinoma: a systematic review of epidemiologic evidence. Clin Gastroenterol Hepatol. 2006 Mar;4(3):369–80. [PMID: 16527702]
- Llovet JM. Hepatocellular carcinoma: patients with increasing alpha-fetoprotein but no mass on ultrasound. Clin Gastroenterol Hepatol. 2006 Jan; 4(1):29–35. [PMID: 16431301]
- Lopez PM et al. Systematic review: evidence-based management of hepatocellular carcinoma—an updated analysis of randomized controlled trials. Aliment Pharmacol Ther. 2006 Jun 1; 23(11):1535–47. [PMID: 16696801]

Hepatopathy, Ischemic

KEY FEATURES

- Caused by an acute fall in cardiac output (eg, acute myocardial infarction or arrhythmia)
- Usually in a patient with passive congestion of the liver

CLINICAL FINDINGS

- Typically follows hypotension, but clinical hypotension may be absent
- Precipitating event can be arterial hypoxemia due to
  - Respiratory failure
  - Septic shock
  - Severe anemia
  - Heat stroke
  - Carbon monoxide poisoning
  - Cocaine use
  - Bacterial endocarditis
- In severe cases, encephalopathy may develop
- Mortality rate resulting from the underlying disease is high
- In patients who recover, aminotransferase levels return to normal quickly, usually within 1 week, in contrast to viral hepatitis
- In chronic passive congestion
  - Hepatojugular reflux is present
  - With tricuspid regurgitation, the liver may be pulsatile
- Ascites may be out of proportion to peripheral edema in patients with right-sided heart failure

DIAGNOSIS

- Hallmarks of ischemic hepatopathy
  - Rapid elevation of serum aminotransferase levels (often > 5000 units/L)
  - Early rapid rise in serum lactate dehydrogenase level
  - Elevations of serum alkaline phosphatase and bilirubin are usually mild
  - Prothrombin time may be prolonged
- In passive congestion of the liver caused by right-sided heart failure
  - Serum bilirubin level may be elevated, occasionally as high as 40 mg/dL, resulting partly from hypoxia of perivenular hepatocytes
  - Serum alkaline phosphatase levels are normal or slightly elevated
- Ascites caused by heart failure generally has
  - High serum ascites-albumin gradient (> 1.1)
  - Protein content of more than 2.5 g/dL

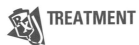

TREATMENT

- Supportive. Treat underlying cardiac disease

Hepatopulmonary Syndrome

KEY FEATURES

- Characteristic triad
  - Chronic liver disease
  - Increased alveolar-arterial gradient at room air
  - Intrapulmonary vascular dilations or arteriovenous communications that result in a right-to-left intrapulmonary shunt

CLINICAL FINDINGS

- Dyspnea (platypnea) and arterial deoxygenation (orthodeoxia) are greater in the upright position than in the recumbent position
- Suspect diagnosis in a cirrhotic patient with a pulse oximetry level ≤ 97%

DIAGNOSIS

- Contrast-enhanced echocardiography is a sensitive screening test for detecting pulmonary vascular dilations, whereas macroaggregated albumin lung perfusion scanning is more specific and is used to confirm the diagnosis
- High-resolution CT may be useful for detecting dilated pulmonary vessels that may be amenable to embolization

TREATMENT

- Medical therapy has been disappointing
- However, IV methylene blue and oral garlic powder may improve oxygenation by inhibiting nitric oxide–induced vasodilation
- The syndrome may reverse with liver transplantation
- Postoperative mortality is increased when the preoperative arterial oxygen tension is ≤ 50 mm Hg or with substantial intrapulmonary shunting
- Liver transplantation
  - Contraindicated in moderate to severe pulmonary hypertension (mean pulmonary pressure > 35 mm Hg)
  - Treatment with epoprostenol or bosentan may reduce pulmonary hy-

pertension, thereby facilitating transplantation
- TIPS may provide palliation in patients with hepatopulmonary syndrome awaiting transplantation

tem (MARS), a modified dialysis method that selectively removes albumin-bound substances
- Improvement may also follow TIPS placement
- Mortality is high without liver transplantation; death is due to complicating infection or hemorrhage

Hepatorenal Syndrome

 ## KEY FEATURES

- Diagnosed when other causes of renal disease have been excluded in the setting of end-stage liver disease

 ## CLINICAL FINDINGS

- Often precipitated by an acute decrease in cardiac output
- The pathogenesis involves intense renal vasoconstriction
- Histologically, the kidneys are normal
- **Type I:** serum creatinine doubles to a level > 2.5 mg/dL or the creatinine clearance halves to < 20 mL/min in fewer than 2 weeks
- **Type II:** chronic and slowly progressive

 ## DIAGNOSIS

- Azotemia, hyponatremia, oliguria, unremarkable urinary sediment, no proteinuria
- 24-h urinary sodium < 10 mEq
- Renal function fails to improve after IV infusion of 1.5 L of isotonic saline

 ## TREATMENT

- Improvement may follow IV infusion of
  - Albumin plus the long-acting vasoconstrictor ornipressin (but with a high rate of ischemic side effects)
  - Ornipressin and dopamine
  - Terlipressin (a long-acting vasopressin analog)
  - Norepinephrine
  - SQ octreotide and PO midodrine, an α-adrenergic drug
- Survival benefit has occurred with the molecular adsorbent recirculating sys-

Herpes Simplex Virus Infections

 ## KEY FEATURES

ESSENTIALS OF DIAGNOSIS

- Recurrent small grouped vesicles, especially in the orolabial and genital areas
- May follow minor infections, trauma, stress, or sun exposure
- Viral cultures and direct fluorescent antibody tests are positive

GENERAL CONSIDERATIONS

- The patient may have recurrent self-limited attacks, provoked by sun exposure, orofacial surgery, fever, or a viral infection
- Herpes simplex type 2 (HSV-2) causes lesions whose morphology and natural history are similar to those caused by herpes simplex type 1 (HSV-1) on the genitalia of both sexes; the infection is acquired by sexual contact
- Genital herpes may also be due to HSV-1

DEMOGRAPHICS

- Up to 85% of adults have serologic evidence of HSV-1 infections, most often acquired asymptomatically in childhood
- About 25% of the US population has serologic evidence of infection with HSV-2
- In monogamous heterosexual couples where one partner has HSV-2 infection, seroconversion of the noninfected partner occurs in 10% over a 1-year period
  - Up to 70% of such infections appeared to be transmitted during periods of asymptomatic shedding; uninfected female partners are at greater risk than males

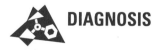 ## CLINICAL FINDINGS

SYMPTOMS AND SIGNS

- The principal symptoms are burning and stinging; neuralgia may precede or accompany attacks
- The lesions consist of small, grouped vesicles on an erythematous base that can occur anywhere but that most often occur on the vermillion border of the lips, the penile shaft, the labia, the perianal skin, and the buttocks
- Any erosion in genital region can be due to HSV-2 (or HSV-1)
- Regional lymph nodes may be swollen and tender
- The lesions usually crust and heal in 1 week
- Occasionally, primary infections may be manifested as severe gingivostomatitis
- Lesions, especially those on the genitalia are often clinically nonspecific fissures or erosions

DIFFERENTIAL DIAGNOSIS

- Impetigo
- Varicella (chickenpox)
- Herpes zoster (shingles)
- Scabies
- Trauma
- Genital lesions
  - Syphilis
  - Chancroid
  - Lymphogranuloma venereum
  - Behçet's syndrome
  - Fixed drug eruption
- Oral lesions
  - Aphthous ulcers
  - Herpangina (coxsackievirus)
  - Erythema multiforme
  - Pemphigus
  - Primary HIV infection
  - Candidiasis
  - Reactive arthritis
  - Systemic lupus erythematosus
  - Behçet's syndrome
  - Bullous pemphigoid

DIAGNOSIS

LABORATORY TESTS

- Viral cultures and direct fluorescent antibody tests are positive
- Herpes serology
  - Not used in the diagnosis of an acute genital ulcer
  - Can determine who is HSV infected and potentially infectious

– Such testing is very useful in couples in which only one partner reports a history of genital herpes
– Beware of laboratory variations in type of HSV serologies, and false-negatives with ELISA testing

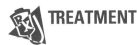 **TREATMENT**

MEDICATIONS

- **For first clinical episodes**
  – Acyclovir: 200 mg PO five times daily (or 800 mg TID)
  – Valacyclovir: 1000 mg BID
  – Famciclovir: 250 mg TID
  – Treatment is from 7–10 days depending on the severity of the outbreak
- **For recurrent herpes**
  – Generally milder symptoms than first episode and does not require therapy; when therapy is tried, it is of limited benefit, with studies finding a reduction in the average outbreak by only 12–24 h
  – Recurrent outbreaks may be treated with 5 days of acyclovir, 200 mg five times a day; 3 days of valacyclovir, 500 mg BID; or 5 days of famciclovir, 125 mg BID
  – For orolabial HSV, valacyclovir, 2 g BID for 1 day, is as effective as longer courses of therapy
  – For genital HSV, famciclovir 1.5 g as a single oral dose or 750 mg BID for 1 day is as effective as longer courses of treatment
  – The addition of a potent topical corticosteroid three times daily reduces the duration, size, and pain of orolabial herpes treated with an oral antiviral agent
- **For frequent or severe recurrences**
  – Suppressive treatment will reduce outbreaks by 85% and reduces viral shedding by more than 90%
  – The recommended suppressive doses, taken continuously, are acyclovir, 400 mg BID; valacyclovir, 500 mg once daily; or famciclovir, 125–250 mg BID
  – Long-term suppression appears very safe, and after 5–7 years a substantial proportion of patients can discontinue treatment
  – Suppression of outbreaks and asymptomatic shedding reduces rate of transmission by about 50%
- **Local measures:** topical antiviral therapy is not significantly effective

 OUTCOME

COMPLICATIONS

- Pyoderma
- Eczema herpeticum
- Herpetic whitlow
- Herpes gladiatorum (epidemic herpes in wrestlers transmitted by contact)
- Esophagitis
- Neonatal infection
- Keratitis
- Encephalitis
- Recurrent attacks lasting several days

PROGNOSIS

- Recurrent attacks last several days and patients generally recover without sequelae

WHEN TO REFER

- Refractory cases not responding to oral antiviral therapy

PREVENTION

- Sunscreens are very useful adjuncts in preventing sun-induced recurrences
- Prophylactic use of oral acyclovir
  – May prevent recurrence
  – Dosage is 200 mg five times daily beginning 24 h prior to ultraviolet light exposure, dental surgery, or orolabial cosmetic surgery; comparable doses are 500 mg BID for valacyclovir and 250 mg BID for famciclovir
- Suppressive therapy with valacyclovir 500 mg once daily significantly reduces the risk of transmission of genital herpes among heterosexual, HSV-2-discordant couples
- Barrier protection is not completely effective, since shedding occurs from widespread areas of the perineum not covered by condoms

 EVIDENCE

PRACTICE GUIDELINES

- Association for Genitourinary Medicine, Medical Society for the Study of Venereal Disease (London). 2002 national guideline for the management of genital herpes
- Centers for Disease Control and Prevention: Diseases characterized by genital ulcers. Sexually transmitted diseases treatment guidelines. 2006

WEB SITES

- American Social Health Association: National Herpes Resource Center
- Centers for Disease Control and Prevention

INFORMATION FOR PATIENTS

- American Association of Family Physicians: Herpes: What It Is and How to Deal With It
- American Social Health Association: Herpes: Get the Facts
- Mayo Clinic: Cold Sores
- National Institute of Allergy and Infectious Disease: Genital Herpes

REFERENCES

- Barton SE. Reducing the transmission of genital herpes. BMJ. 2005 Jan 22; 330(7484):157–8. [PMID: 15661761]
- Beauman JG. Genital herpes: a review. Am Fam Physician. 2005 Oct 15; 72(8):1527–34. [PMID: 16273819]
- Geretti AM. Genital herpes. Sex Transm Infect. 2006 Dec;82 Suppl 4:iv31–iv34. [PMID: 17151051]
- Spruance S et al. Short-course therapy for recurrent genital herpes and herpes labialis. J Fam Pract. 2007 Jan; 56(1):30–6. [PMID: 17217895]

Herpes Zoster

KEY FEATURES

ESSENTIALS OF DIAGNOSIS

- Pain along the course of a nerve followed by painful grouped vesicular lesions
- Involvement is unilateral; some lesions (fewer than 20) may occur outside the affected dermatome
- Lesions are usually on face or trunk
- Tzanck smear positive, especially in vesicular lesions

GENERAL CONSIDERATIONS

- An acute vesicular eruption due to the varicella-zoster virus
- It usually occurs in adults
- With rare exceptions, patients suffer only one attack

- Dermatomal herpes zoster does not imply the presence of a visceral malignancy
- Generalized disease, however, raises the suspicion of an associated immunosuppressive disorder such as Hodgkin's disease or HIV infection
- Early (within 72 h after onset) and aggressive antiviral treatment of herpes zoster reduces the severity and duration of postherpetic neuralgia

DEMOGRAPHICS

- HIV-infected patients are 20 times more likely to develop zoster, often before other clinical findings of HIV disease are present

 CLINICAL FINDINGS

SYMPTOMS AND SIGNS

- Pain usually precedes the eruption by 48 h or more and may persist and actually increase in intensity after the lesions have disappeared
- The lesions consist of grouped, tense, deep-seated vesicles distributed unilaterally along a dermatome
- The most common distributions are on the trunk or face
- Up to 20 lesions may be found outside the affected dermatomes
- Regional lymph glands may be tender and swollen

DIFFERENTIAL DIAGNOSIS

- Contact dermatitis (eg, poison oak or ivy)
- Herpes simplex
- Erysipelas
- Prodromal pain mimics angina, peptic ulcer, appendicitis, biliary or renal colic

 DIAGNOSIS

- Clinical, including obtaining a history of HIV risk factors

LABORATORY TESTING

- HIV testing should be considered when appropriate, especially in zoster patients under 55 years of age

 TREATMENT

MEDICATIONS

- See Table 150

Immunocompetent person

- Antiviral therapy should be given to patients over age 55; younger patients with acute moderate to severe pain or rash may benefit from antiviral therapy
  - Administer famciclovir, 500 mg PO TID; valacyclovir, 1 g PO TID; or acyclovir, 800 mg five times daily; all for 7 days
  - Adjust the dose of antiviral agent if renal dysfunction
- Systemic corticosteroids
  - Effectively reduce acute pain, improve quality of life, and return patients more quickly to normal activities
  - Do not increase the risk of dissemination in immunocompetent hosts
  - If not contraindicated, administer a tapering 3-week course of prednisone, starting at 60 mg/day, for adjunctive benefit

Immunocompromised person

- Most immunocompromised patients are candidates for antiviral therapy
- Use same dosages of antiviral agents as listed above, but continue treatment until the lesions have completely crusted and are healed or almost healed (up to 2 weeks)
- Corticosteroids should not be given adjunctively since they increase the risk of dissemination
- Progression of disease may necessitate IV therapy with acyclovir, 10 mg/kg TID
  - After 3–4 days, oral therapy may be substituted if there has been a good response to IV therapy
  - Adverse effects include renal insufficiency from crystallization, nausea and vomiting, and abdominal pain
- Foscarnet, administered in a dosage of 40 mg/kg IV BID or TID, is indicated for treatment of acyclovir-resistant varicella-zoster virus infections

Local measures

- Calamine or starch shake lotions

Postherpetic neuralgia

- Capsaicin cream, 0.025–0.075%, applied TID-QID or lidocaine (Lidoderm) 5% topical patches, applied for up to 12 h/d
- Chronic postherpetic neuralgia may be relieved by regional blocks (stellate ganglion, epidural, local infiltration, or peripheral nerve), with or without corticosteroids added to the injections
- Amitriptyline, 25–75 mg PO HS, is the first-line oral therapy beyond simple analgesics
- Gabapentin, up to 3600 mg PO daily (starting at 300 mg TID), may be added for additional pain relief

THERAPEUTIC PROCEDURES

- Nerve blocks may help in the management of initial severe pain
- Patients should maintain good hydration, and elderly patients with reduced renal function should be monitored

 OUTCOME

COMPLICATIONS

- Sacral zoster may be associated with bladder and bowel dysfunction
- Persistent neuralgia, anesthesia or scarring of the affected area, facial or other nerve paralysis, and encephalitis may occur
- Postherpetic neuralgia is most common after involvement of the trigeminal region, and in patients over age 55
- Zoster ophthalmicus (V_1) can result in visual impairment

PROGNOSIS

- The skin eruption persists 2–3 weeks and usually does not recur
- Motor involvement in 2–3% may lead to temporary palsy
- Oral corticosteroids do not reduce the prevalence, severity, or duration of postherpetic neuralgia beyond that achieved by effective antiviral therapy

WHEN TO REFER

- Ophthalmologic consultation is vital for involvement of the first branch of the trigeminal nerve (V1)

PREVENTION

- The zoster vaccine markedly reduced morbidity from herpes zoster and postherpetic neuralgia among older adults
- Early and aggressive antiviral therapy for postherpetic neuralgia

 EVIDENCE

PRACTICE GUIDELINES

- Gross G et al. Herpes zoster guideline of the German Dermatology Society. J Clin Virol. 2003;26:277. [PMID: 12637076]

WEB SITES

- American Academy of Dermatology
- National Institute of Allergy and Infectious Disease

INFORMATION FOR PATIENTS

- American Academy of Dermatology: Herpes Zoster
- American Academy of Family Physicians: Shingles
- MedlinePlus: Shingles Interactive Tutorial
- National Institute on Aging: Shingles

REFERENCES

- Dworkin RH et al. Recommendations for the management of herpes zoster. Clin Infect Dis. 2007 Jan 1;44(Suppl 1):S1–S26. [PMID: 17143845]
- Hornberger J et al. Cost-effectiveness of a vaccine to prevent herpes zoster and postherpetic neuralgia in older adults. Ann Intern Med. 2006 Sep 5; 145(5):317–25. [PMID: 16954357]
- Oxman MN et al; Shingles Prevention Study Group. A vaccine to prevent herpes zoster and postherpetic neuralgia in older adults. N Engl J Med. 2005 Jun 2; 352(22):2271–84. [PMID: 15930418]

Hiccups

 KEY FEATURES

- Usually benign and self-limited but may be persistent and a sign of serious underlying illness
- Causes of self-limited hiccups
  - Gastric distention
  - Sudden temperature changes
  - Alcohol ingestion
  - Emotion
- Causes of recurrent or persistent hiccups
  - Neoplasms, infections, cerebrovascular accident, trauma
  - Uremia, hypocapnia (hyperventilation)
  - Irritation of the vagus or phrenic nerve
    □ Foreign body in ear, goiter, neoplasms
    □ Pneumonia, empyema, neoplasms, myocardial infarction, pericarditis, aneurysm, esophageal obstruction, reflux esophagitis
    □ Subphrenic abscess, hepatomegaly, hepatitis, cholecystitis, gastric distention, gastric neoplasm, pancreatitis, pancreatic malignancy
  - General anesthesia, postoperative
  - Psychogenic and idiopathic

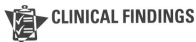 **CLINICAL FINDINGS**

- Detailed neurologic examination

 DIAGNOSIS

- Serum creatinine, liver enzymes
- Chest radiograph, chest fluoroscopy
- CT of the head, chest, abdomen
- Echocardiography
- Bronchoscopy
- Upper endoscopy

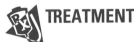 **TREATMENT**

Acute hiccups

- Irritating nasopharynx by catheter stimulation or tongue traction, lifting uvula with a spoon, or eating 1 tsp dry granulated sugar
- Interrupting respiratory cycle by
  - Breath holding
  - Valsalva's maneuver
  - Sneezing
  - Gasping
  - Rebreathing into bag
- Stimulating vagus nerve by carotid massage
- Irritating diaphragm by holding knees to chest or by continuous positive airway pressure during mechanical ventilation
- Relieving gastric distention by belching or insertion of a nasogastric tube

Chronic hiccups

- Chlorpromazine, 25–50 mg PO or IM TID–QID
- Anticonvulsants (phenytoin, carbamazepine)
- Benzodiazepines (lorazepam, diazepam)
- Metoclopramide
- Baclofen
- Occasionally general anesthesia

Hirsutism & Virilization

 KEY FEATURES

ESSENTIALS OF DIAGNOSIS

- Menstrual disorders, hirsutism, acne
- Virilization

- Occasionally, a palpable pelvic tumor
- Urinary 17-ketosteroids, serum dehydroepiandrosterone sulfate (DHEAS) and androstenedione elevated in adrenal disorders, variable in others
- Serum testosterone often elevated

GENERAL CONSIDERATIONS

- Major androgen is testosterone
- If serum testosterone is normal, an endocrine cause for hirsutism is extremely unlikely

Causes of hirsutism

- Idiopathic or familial—often hirsutism may be normal for genetic background
- Polycystic ovary syndrome—accounts for > 50% of cases
  - Affects 5% of premenopausal women in the United States
  - Associated with amenorrhea or oligomenorrhea, anovulation, and obesity
  - Insulin resistance and diabetes common
- Ovarian tumor (uncommon) and adrenal carcinoma (rare)
- Steroidogenic enzyme defects
  - ~2% of adult-onset hirsutism is due to partial defect in adrenal 21-hydroxylase
  - Rare patients with hyperandrogenism and hypertension have 11-hydroxylase deficiency
  - Patients with XY karyotype and deficiency of 17α-hydroxysteroid dehydrogenase-3 or 5α-reductase-2 may present as phenotypic girls in whom virilization develops at puberty
- Other rare causes
  - Acromegaly
  - ACTH-induced Cushing's syndrome
  - Adrenal carcinoma
  - Genetic cortisol resistance
  - Maternal virilization during pregnancy due to luteoma of pregnancy
  - Hyperreactio luteinalis
  - Diffuse stromal Leydig cell hyperplasia in postmenopausal women
  - Acquired hypertrichosis lanuginosa (diffuse fine hair growth on face and body in association with malignancy, especially colorectal cancer)
- Pharmacologic causes
  - Minoxidil
  - Cyclosporine
  - Phenytoin
  - Anabolic steroids
  - Diazoxide
  - Some progestins

DEMOGRAPHICS

- Most common in women with some Mediterranean ancestry

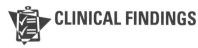 **CLINICAL FINDINGS**

SYMPTOMS AND SIGNS

- Increased sexual hair (chin, upper lip, abdomen, and chest)
- Acne due to increased sebaceous gland activity
- Menstrual irregularities, anovulation, and amenorrhea common
- Defeminization
  - Breast size decrease
  - Loss of feminine adipose tissue
- Virilization implicates presence of testosterone-producing neoplasm
  - Frontal balding
  - Muscularity
  - Clitoromegaly
  - Deepening of voice
- Hypertension seen in rare conditions with Cushing's syndrome, adrenal 11-hydroxylase deficiency, or cortisol resistance syndrome
- Ovarian enlargement may be cystic or neoplastic
- Polycystic ovary syndome associated with hypertension and hyperlipidemia

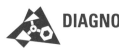 **DIAGNOSIS**

LABORATORY TESTS

- Serum androgens mainly useful to screen for rare occult adrenal or ovarian neoplasms
  - Serum testosterone > 200 ng/dL or free testosterone > 40 ng/dL indicates need for pelvic examination and ultrasound. If normal, perform adrenal CT scan
  - Serum androstenedione > 1000 ng/dL implicates ovarian or adrenal neoplasm
  - Milder elevations of testosterone or androstenedione are usually treated with oral contraceptives
  - Markedly elevated serum DHEAS (> 700 mcg/dL) implies adrenal source of androgen, usually adrenal hyperplasia and rarely adrenal carcinoma. Perform adrenal CT scan
- Unclear which patients (if any) with hyperandrogenism should be screened for "late-onset" 21-hydroxylase deficiency, where baseline 17-hydroxyprogesterone is usually > 300 ng/dL or stimulated level is > 1000 ng/dL (30–60 min after 0.25 mg IM cosyntropin)
- Signs of Cushing's syndrome should prompt screening

- Follicle-stimulating hormone (FSH) and luteinizing hormone (LH) elevated if amenorrhea is due to ovarian failure
- LH:FSH ratio > 2.0, hyperglycemia, and elevated fasting insulin level are common in polycystic ovary syndrome
- Selective venous sampling for testosterone may be required to diagnose small virilizing ovarian tumors not detected on ultrasound, MRI, or CT

IMAGING STUDIES

- Adrenal CT as described above
- Pelvic ultrasound or MRI to detect virilizing tumors of ovary
- Ultrasound shows polycystic ovaries in ~33% of normal young women, so test is not helpful in diagnosis of polycystic ovary syndrome

 TREATMENT

MEDICATIONS

- Spironolactone
  - 50–100 mg PO BID on days 5–25 of menstrual cycle or once daily if used concomitantly with oral contraceptive
  - Hyperkalemia or hyponatremia occur uncommonly
- Cyproterone acetate (not available in United States), 2 mg PO once daily; usually given with oral contraceptive
- Finasteride
  - 5 mg PO once daily modestly reduces hirsutism over 6 months—comparable results to spironolactone
  - Ineffective for androgenic alopecia in women
- Flutamide
  - 250 mg PO once daily
  - Used with oral contraceptive, likely more effective than spironolactone in improving hirsutism, acne, and male pattern baldness
  - Rarely hepatotoxic
- Oral contraceptives
  - Stimulate menses but less effective for hirsutism
  - Low-androgenic progestin (desogestrel, gestodene)-containing contraceptives are preferred
  - Addition of simvastatin may decrease serum free testosterone
- Metformin
  - 500–1000 mg PO BID for polycystic ovary syndrome with amenorrhea or oligomenorrhea may improve menstrual function, particularly in women with insulin resistance

  - Contraindicated in renal and liver disease
  - Does not cause hypoglycemia in nondiabetics
- Androgenic alopecia
  - Topical minoxidil 2% solution BID chronically to dry scalp
  - Hypertrichosis occurs in 3–5% (eg, on forehead, cheeks, upper lip, chin); usually resolves 1–6 months after drug stopped
- **Note: Give antiandrogen treatments only to nonpregnant women—use during pregnancy causes malformations and pseudohermaphroditism in male infants. Women taking antiandrogens should take oral contraceptives when indicated and avoid pregnancy**

SURGERY

- Resection of any testosterone-secreting ovarian or adrenal tumor
- Laparoscopic bilateral oophorectomy (if CT scan of adrenals and ovaries normal) indicated in postmenopausal women with severe hyperandrogenism, since small hilar cell tumors of ovary may not be visible on scans

THERAPEUTIC PROCEDURES

- Discontinue any potentially offending drugs
- Encourage shaving, depilatories, waxing, electrolysis, or bleaching, and laser therapy for hirsutism

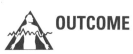 **OUTCOME**

FOLLOW-UP

- Check serum potassium and creatinine 1 month after starting spironolactone
- If testosterone elevated, follow serum testosterone during therapy or after surgery

PROGNOSIS

- Polycystic ovary syndrome: women frequently regain normal menstrual cycles with aging

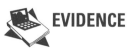 **EVIDENCE**

PRACTICE GUIDELINES

- Azziz R. The evaluation and management of hirsutism. Obstet Gynecol. 2003; 101(5 Pt 1):995. [PMID: 12738163]
- Claman P et al. SOGC clinical practice guidelines. Hirsutism: evaluation and treatment. J Obstet Gynaecol Can. 2002;24:62. [PMID: 12196888]

REFERENCES

- Azziz R et al. Androgen excess in women: experience with over 1000 consecutive patients. J Clin Endocrinol Metab. 2004 Feb;89(2):453–62. [PMID: 14764747]
- Ganie MA et al. Comparison of efficacy of spironolactone with metformin in the management of polycystic ovary syndrome: an open-label study. J Clin Endocrinol Metab. 2004 Jun; 89(6):2756–62. [PMID: 15181054]
- Murphy MK et al. Polycystic ovarian morphology in normal women does not predict the development of polycystic ovary syndrome. J Clin Endocrinol Metab. 2006 Oct;91(10):3878–84. [PMID: 16882750]
- Ortega-Gonzalez C et al. Responses of serum androgen and insulin resistance to metformin and pioglitazone in obese, insulin-resistant women with polycystic ovary syndrome. J Clin Endocrinol Metab. 2005 Mar;90(3):1360–5. [PMID: 15598674]
- Palomba S et al. Prospective parallel randomized, double-blind, double-dummy controlled clinical trial comparing clomiphene citrate and metformin as the first-line treatment for ovulation induction in nonobese anovulatory women with polycystic ovary syndrome. J Clin Endocrinol Metab. 2005 Jul; 90(7):4068–74. [PMID: 15840746]
- Rosenfield RL. Clinical practice. Hirsutism. N Engl J Med. 2005 Dec 15; 353(24):2578–88. [PMID: 16354894]

Histoplasmosis

KEY FEATURES

ESSENTIALS OF DIAGNOSIS

- Infection caused by *Histoplasma capsulatum*, a dimorphic fungus isolated from soil contaminated with bird or bat droppings in endemic areas
- Most patients asymptomatic; if symptomatic, respiratory illness most common
- Dissemination in profoundly immunocompromised patients

GENERAL CONSIDERATIONS

- Acute histoplasmosis frequently occurs in epidemics, often when soil containing infected bird or bat droppings is disturbed
- Infection presumably occurs by inhalation
- The organism proliferates and is carried hematogenously from lungs to other organs
- Dissemination common in AIDS patients, usually with CD4 counts < 100 cells/mcL, and in other immunocompromised patients, with poor prognosis

DEMOGRAPHICS

- Endemic areas
    - Central and eastern United States (especially Ohio River and Mississippi River valleys)
    - Eastern Canada
    - Mexico
    - Central America
    - South America
    - Africa
    - Southeast Asia
- Disseminated disease most often occurs as reactivation of prior infection but may reflect acute infection
- Chronic progressive pulmonary histoplasmosis occurs in older patients with chronic obstructive pulmonary disease

CLINICAL FINDINGS

SYMPTOMS AND SIGNS

- Most cases asymptomatic with no pulmonary symptoms or signs even in those who later have calcifications on chest radiograph
- Mild symptomatic illness: influenza-like illness, often lasting 1–4 days
- More severe illness: presents as atypical pneumonia, with fever, cough, and mild central chest pain for 5–15 days
- Physical examination usually normal
- Acute pulmonary histoplasmosis: marked prostration, fever, but few pulmonary complaints even when chest radiograph shows pneumonia
- Progressive pulmonary histoplasmosis occurs in patients with chronic pulmonary disease
    - Fever, weight loss, prostration
    - Dyspnea, cough
    - Upper lobe cavitation and fibrosis
- Mediastinal fibrosis thought to represent abnormal immune response to organisms in mediastinal lymph nodes
- Disseminated histoplasmosis occurs mainly in immunocompromised patients
    - Fever, weight loss, cough
    - Hepatomegaly, splenomegaly, lymphadenopathy
    - Gastrointestinal involvement with oral ulcers, intestinal lesions
    - Skin findings include papules, ulcers
    - Adrenal glands commonly involved
    - Meningitis and endocarditis rare
    - Shock occurs in severe cases

DIFFERENTIAL DIAGNOSIS

- Influenza
- Atypical pneumonia
- Tuberculosis
- Coccidioidomycosis
- Sarcoidosis
- Blastomycosis
- Pneumoconiosis
- *Pneumocystis jiroveci* pneumonia
- Lymphoma (including lymphocytic interstitial pneumonia)

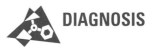

DIAGNOSIS

LABORATORY TESTS

- Elevations of alkaline phosphatase and lactate dehydrogenase (marked) and ferritin common
- Anemia of chronic disease in chronic progressive pulmonary histoplasmosis
- Sputum culture rarely positive except in chronic pulmonary histoplasmosis
- Pancytopenia from bone marrow involvement in disseminated disease
- Blood or bone marrow cultures positive in > 80% of disseminated disease in immunocompromised individuals
- Skin tests and serologic tests seldom diagnostic
- In acute pulmonary histoplasmosis: screening immunodiffusion test sensitivity 50%, complement fixation titers sensitivity ~80%, combination sensitivity up to 80% in immunocompromised
- Urine antigen test
    - Sensitivity > 90% for disseminated disease in AIDS
    - Useful to diagnose relapse
- Biopsy of affected organs with culture useful in disseminated disease

IMAGING STUDIES

- Lung and splenic calcifications on radiographs may reflect past infection
- Radiographic findings during acute illness are variable and nonspecific
- Disseminated disease in profoundly immunocompromised: chest radiograph may show a miliary pattern

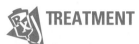 TREATMENT

MEDICATIONS

- Itraconazole is highly effective against *H capsulatum*
  - Oral itraconazole, 200–400 mg once daily for weeks to months, can be used for progressive pulmonary disease, mild to moderate non-meningeal disease
  - Response rates of ~80% can be expected
  - Due to variable absorption, some experts recommend measuring drug levels with peak value of 4–10 mcg/mL being sufficient
- Amphotericin B 0.7–1.0 mg/kg/day IV is used if patients
  - Cannot take itraconazole orally
  - Have not responded to itraconazole
  - Have meningitis
  - Have severe disseminated disease
- Oral itraconazole can replace amphotericin once patient is stable and afebrile, which usually occurs in 3–7 days
- Relapse rates are high, especially among HIV patients in the absence of immune reconstitution so itraconazole, 200 mg PO once daily, should be used in this situation indefinitely
  - After at least 12 months of itraconazole, secondary prophylaxis can be safely discontinued in HIV patients that have responded to antiretroviral therapy
- Treatment of endocarditis is difficult with removal of infected valve recommended along with maximal doses of amphotericin B and prolonged oral itraconazole
- Mediastinal fibrosis may not respond to antifungal therapy; itraconazole has shown the best efficacy in patients who have evidence of inflammation and not just fibrosis on biopsy of affected nodes
  - Surgery is not generally recommended in this condition because complications are common
  - Intravascular stents may be helpful in maintaining patency of central blood vessels

 OUTCOME

PROGNOSIS

- Acute histoplasmosis: lasts from 1 week to 6 months but is almost never fatal
- Progressive disseminated histoplasmosis: usually fatal within 6 weeks or less; more rapidly in immunocompromised

PREVENTION

- Recurrence of AIDS-related histoplasmosis is decreased with lifelong itraconazole, 200–400 mg PO once daily; it is possible to discontinue secondary prophylaxis following adequate treatment of histoplasmosis and a sustained CD4 cell response (> 150/mcL) to highly active antiretroviral therapy

 EVIDENCE

PRACTICE GUIDELINES

- Practice Guidelines from the Infectious Diseases Society of America
- AIDS Info. US Department of Health and Human Services, Public Health Service

WEB SITE

- Centers for Disease Control and Prevention—Division of Bacterial and Mycotic Diseases

INFORMATION FOR PATIENTS

- Centers for Disease Control and Prevention—Division of Bacterial and Mycotic Diseases
- Cleveland Clinic—OHS
- National Institute of Allergy and Infectious Diseases

REFERENCE

- Wheat LJ. Histoplasmosis: a review for physicians from non-endemic areas. Mycoses. 2006 Jul;49(4):274–82. [PMID: 16784440]

HIV Infection & AIDS

 KEY FEATURES

ESSENTIALS OF DIAGNOSIS

- Risk factors include
  - Sexual contact with an infected person
  - Parenteral exposure to infected blood by transfusion or needle sharing
  - Perinatal exposure
- Opportunistic infections
  - Due to diminished cellular immunity Often life-threatening
- Aggressive cancers, particularly Kaposi's sarcoma and extranodal lymphoma
- Neurologic manifestations
  - Dementia
  - Aseptic meningitis
  - Neuropathy

GENERAL CONSIDERATIONS

- Definition: Centers for Disease Control and Prevention AIDS case definition (Table 55)
- Etiology: HIV-1, a retrovirus

DEMOGRAPHICS

- In 2005, HIV infection in
  - ~40 million persons worldwide
  - ~950,000 Americans
- In 2005, AIDS in ~425,000 Americans
  - 52% are men who have sex with men
  - 15% are heterosexual male injection drug users
  - 9% are heterosexual male noninjection drug users
  - 23% are women, of whom 65% infected through heterosexual contact

 CLINICAL FINDINGS

SYMPTOMS AND SIGNS

- HIV-related infections and neoplasms affect virtually every organ
- Many HIV-infected persons remain asymptomatic for years even without antiretroviral therapy: mean of ~10 years between exposure to HIV and development of AIDS
- Symptoms protean and nonspecific
- Fever, night sweats, and weight loss
- Shortness of breath, cough, and fever from pneumonia

- Anorexia, nausea and vomiting, and increased metabolic rate contribute to weight loss
- Diarrhea from bacterial, viral, or parasitic infections
- Physical examination may be normal
- Conditions highly suggestive of HIV infection
  - Hairy leukoplakia of the tongue
  - Disseminated Kaposi's sarcoma
  - Cutaneous bacillary angiomatosis
  - Generalized lymphadenopathy early in infection
- **Ocular**
  - Cytomegalovirus (CMV)
  - Herpesvirus
  - Toxoplasmosis retinitis
- **Oral**
  - Candidiasis, pseudomembranous (removable white plaques) and erythematous (red friable plaques)
  - Hairy leukoplakia
  - Angular cheilitis
  - Gingivitis or periodontitis
  - Aphthous ulcers
  - Kaposi's sarcoma (usually on the hard palate)
  - Warts
- **Sinuses:** chronic sinusitis
- **Lungs**
  - Bacterial (eg, *Streptococcus pneumoniae, Haemophilus influenzae*)
  - Mycobacterial (eg, *Mycobacterium tuberculosis, Mycobacterium avium* complex [MAC])
  - Fungal (eg, *Pneumocystis jiroveci*)
  - Viral pneumonias
  - Noninfectious
    - Kaposi's sarcoma
    - Non-Hodgkin's lymphoma
    - Interstitial pneumonitis
- **Gastrointestinal**
  - Esophagitis (*Candida*, herpes simplex, CMV)
  - Gastropathy
  - Malabsorption
- **Enterocolitis**
  - Bacteria (*Campylobacter, Salmonella, Shigella*)
  - Viruses (CMV, adenovirus, HIV)
  - Protozoans (*Cryptosporidium, Entamoeba histolytica, Giardia, Isospora, Microsporidia*)
- **Hepatic**
  - Liver infections (mycobacterial, CMV, hepatitis B and C viruses) and neoplasms (lymphoma)
  - Medication-related hepatitis
- **Biliary**
  - Cholecystitis
  - Sclerosing cholangitis
  - Papillary stenosis (CMV, *Cryptosporidium*, and *Microsporidia*)

- **Central nervous system (CNS)**
  - Intracerebral space-occupying lesions
    - Toxoplasmosis
    - Bacterial and *Nocardia* abscesses
    - Cryptococcomas
    - Tuberculomas
  - HIV encephalopathy
  - Meningitis
  - CNS (non-Hodgkin's) lymphoma
  - Progressive multifocal leukoencephalopathy (PML)
- **Spinal cord:** HIV myelopathy
- **Peripheral nervous system**
  - Inflammatory polyneuropathies, sensory neuropathies, and mononeuropathies
  - CMV polyradiculopathy
  - Transverse myelitis (herpes zoster or CMV)
- **Endocrinologic**
  - Adrenal insufficiency from infection (eg, CMV and MAC), infiltration (Kaposi's sarcoma), hemorrhage, and presumed autoimmune injury
  - Isolated mineralocorticoid defect
  - Thyroid function test abnormalities (high T3, T4, and thyroxine-binding globulin, and low reverse-T3)
- **Gynecologic**
  - Vaginal candidiasis
  - Cervical dysplasia and carcinoma
  - Pelvic inflammatory disease
- **Malignancies**
  - Kaposi's sarcoma
  - Non-Hodgkin's and Hodgkin's lymphoma
  - Primary CNS lymphoma
  - Cervical dysplasia and invasive cervical carcinoma
  - Anal dysplasia and squamous cell carcinoma
- **Skin**
  - Viral
    - Herpes simplex
    - Herpes zoster
    - Molluscum contagiosum
  - Bacterial
    - *Staphylococcus* folliculitis, furuncles, bullous impetigo, dissemination with sepsis
    - Bacillary angiomatosis caused by *Bartonella henselae* and *Bartonella quintana*
  - Fungal
    - *Candida*
    - Dermatophytes
    - *Malassezia furfur/Pityrosporum ovale* seborrheic dermatitis
  - Neoplastic (Kaposi's sarcoma)
  - Nonspecific (psoriasis, severe pruritus, xerosis) dermatitides
- **Musculoskeletal**
  - Myopathy

- Arthritis of single or multiple joints, with or without effusions
- Reactive arthritis (Reiter's syndrome)
- Psoriatic arthritis
- Sicca syndrome
- Systemic lupus erythematosus

DIFFERENTIAL DIAGNOSIS

- Depends on mode of presentation
- **Constitutional symptoms**
  - Cancer
  - Tuberculosis
  - Endocarditis
  - Endocrinologic diseases (eg, hyperthyroidism)
- **Pulmonary processes**
  - Acute and chronic lung infections
  - Other causes of diffuse interstitial pulmonary infiltrates
- **Neurologic disease**
  - Causes of mental status changes
  - Causes of neuropathy
- **Diarrhea**
  - Infectious enterocolitis
  - Antibiotic-associated colitis
  - Inflammatory bowel disease
  - Malabsorptive symptoms

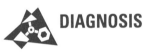 **DIAGNOSIS**

LABORATORY TESTS

- See Table 56
- HIV antibody by ELISA, confirmed by Western blot (sensitivity > 99.5%, specificity ~100%)
- ~95% of persons develop antibodies within 6 weeks after infection
- Absolute CD4 lymphocyte count: as counts decrease, risk of serious opportunistic infection increases

DIAGNOSTIC PROCEDURES

- For *P jiroveci* pneumonia
  - Arterial blood gases
  - Serum lactate dehydrogenase
  - Chest radiograph
  - Wright-Giemsa stain of induced sputum
  - Bronchoalveolar lavage
  - Diffusing capacity of carbon monoxide (DL_{CO})
  - High-resolution CT scan
- For CNS toxoplasmosis
  - Head CT scan
  - Stereotactic brain biopsy
- For cryptococcal meningitis
  - Cerebrospinal fluid (CSF) culture
  - CSF, serum cryptococcal antigen (CRAG)
- For HIV meningitis: CSF cell count

- For HIV myelopathy
  - Lumbar puncture
  - Head MRI or CT scan
- For AIDS dementia complex, depression: neuropsychiatric testing
- For myopathy
  - Serum creatine kinase
  - Muscle biopsy
- For hepatic dysfunction
  - Percutaneous liver biopsy
  - Blood culture
  - Biopsy of a more accessible site
- For enterocolitis
  - Stool culture and multiple ova and parasite examinations
  - Colonoscopy and biopsy

 TREATMENT

MEDICATIONS

- Fever: antipyretics
- Anorexia: megestrol acetate, 80 mg PO QID or dronabinol, 2.5–5.0 mg PO TID
- Weight loss
  - Food supplementation with high-calorie drinks
  - Growth hormone, 0.1 mg/kg/day SQ for 12 weeks, or anabolic steroids—oxandrolone, 15–20 mg PO in 2–4 divided doses
  - Testosterone enanthate or cypionate, 100–200 mg IM q2–4wk, or testosterone patches or gel
- Nausea
  - Prochlorperazine, 10 mg PO TID QAC
  - Metoclopramide, 10 mg PO TID QAC
  - Ondansetron, 8 mg PO TID QAC
  - Empiric oral antifungal agent
- Table 59 for antiretroviral treatment when CD4 count < 350 cells/mcL
- Table 58 for treatment of common opportunistic infections and malignancies

 OUTCOME

FOLLOW-UP

- CD4 cell counts every 3–6 months
- Viral load tests every 3–6 months, and 1 month after change in therapy
- Health care maintenance (Table 57)

PROGNOSIS

- The efficacy of antiretroviral treatments—especially protease inhibitors

and nonnucleoside reverse transcriptase inhibitors—has improved prognosis

WHEN TO REFER

- For advice regarding change of antiretroviral therapy, including interpretation of resistance tests
- For management of complicated opportunistic infections

WHEN TO ADMIT

- For new unexplained fever if bacterial infection requiring IV antibiotics is suspected
- For acute organ system dysfunction or acute change in mental status

PREVENTION

Primary prevention

- Precautions regarding sexual practices and injection drug use (safer sex, latex condoms, and clean needle use)
- Perinatal HIV prophylaxis
- Screening of blood products
- Infection control practices in the health care setting

Secondary prevention

- For *P jiroveci* pneumonia when CD4 counts < 200 cells/mcL, a CD4 lymphocyte percentage < 14%, or weight loss or oral candidiasis: trimethoprim-sulfamethoxazole, dapsone, or atovaquone (Table 60)
- For MAC infection when CD4 counts < 75–100 cells/mcL: azithromycin (1200 mg PO every week), or clarithromycin (500 mg PO BID)
- For *M tuberculosis* infection when positive PPD reactions > 5 mm of induration: isoniazid, 300 mg PO once daily plus pyridoxine, 50 mg PO once daily for 9–12 months
- For toxoplasmosis when positive IgG toxoplasma serology when CD4 counts < 100 cells/mcL: trimethoprim-sulfamethoxazole (1 double-strength tablet PO once daily), or pyrimethamine, 50 mg PO every week plus dapsone, 50 mg PO once daily plus leucovorin 25 mg PO every week

 EVIDENCE

PRACTICE GUIDELINES

- Department of Health and Human Services: Guidelines for the use of antiretroviral agents in HIV-infected adults and adolescents. October 2004.

WEB SITES

- Center for HIV Information, University of California—San Francisco
- National Institutes of Health—National Institute of Allergy and Infectious Diseases—Division of AIDS

INFORMATION FOR PATIENTS

- AIDS Info—US Department of Health and Human Services
- CDC—National AIDS Hotline: 1-800-342-AIDS
- JAMA Patient Page. HIV Infection: The Basics. JAMA 2004;292:296.
- MedlinePlus: Interactive AIDS tutorial

REFERENCE

- Gallant JE et al; Study 934 Group. Tenofovir DF, emtricitabine, and efavirenz vs. zidovudine, lamivudine, and efavirenz for HIV. N Engl J Med. 2006 Jan 19; 354(3):251–60. [PMID: 16421366]

Hoarseness, Dysphonia, & Stridor

KEY FEATURES

ESSENTIALS OF DIAGNOSIS

- The primary symptoms of laryngeal disease are hoarseness and stridor

GENERAL CONSIDERATIONS

- Hoarseness is caused by an abnormal vibration of the vocal cords

Acute hoarseness

- Acute laryngitis is thought to be viral in origin, although *Moraxella catarrhalis* and *Haemophilus influenzae* isolates from the nasopharynx occur at higher than expected frequencies

Persistent hoarseness

- Vocal cord nodules or polyps (from overuse of voice or improper use over extended periods of time) produce prolonged hoarseness
- Vocal cord polypoid changes (from vocal abuse, smoking, chemical industrial irritants, or hypothyroidism)
- Gastroesophageal reflux is a common cause of chronic hoarseness and should

be considered if other causes of abnormal laryngeal airflow (such as tumor) have been excluded by laryngoscopy; < 50% of patients have typical symptoms of heartburn and regurgitation

- In patients with a history of tobacco use, laryngeal cancer or lung cancer (leading to paralysis of a recurrent laryngeal nerve) must be strongly considered in persistent hoarseness

DEMOGRAPHICS

- Acute laryngitis is the most common cause of hoarseness

 CLINICAL FINDINGS

SYMPTOMS AND SIGNS

- The voice is "breathy" when too much air passes incompletely apposed vocal cords, as in unilateral vocal cord paralysis
- The voice is harsh when the vocal cords are stiff and vibrate irregularly, as is the case in laryngitis or malignancy
- Stridor, a high-pitched sound, is the result of turbulent airflow from a narrowed glottis
  - Airway narrowing at or above the vocal cords produces inspiratory stridor
  - Airway narrowing below the vocal cords produces either expiratory or biphasic stridor
- In gastroesophageal reflux-induced hoarseness, the voice is usually worse in the morning and improves during the day; associated symptoms include a feeling of a lump in the throat or an excessive desire for throat clearing

DIFFERENTIAL DIAGNOSIS

- Laryngitis
- Voice overuse
- Vocal cord nodules, polyps, or papillomas
- Intubation granulomas
- Laryngeal cancer
- Lung cancer
- Unilateral vocal cord paralysis
- Hypothyroidism
- Retrosternal goiter, thyroiditis, multinodular goiter, or thyroid carcinoma
- Gastroesophageal reflux
- Angioedema

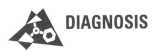 **DIAGNOSIS**

IMAGING STUDIES

- Consider chest radiograph for tumor

DIAGNOSTIC PROCEDURES

- Evaluation of an abnormal voice begins with obtaining a history of the circumstances preceding its onset and an examination of the airway
- Indirect or flexible laryngoscopy and at times videostrobolaryngoscopy
- In gastroesophageal reflux, nonresponders to medical management should undergo pH testing and manometry

 TREATMENT

MEDICATIONS

- Erythromycin may reduce the severity of hoarseness and cough in acute laryngitis

Vocal cord polypoid changes

- Attention to the underlying cause may resolve the problem
- Inhaled corticosteroid spray (eg, beclomethasone, 42 mcg/spray, or dexamethasone, 84 mcg/spray, BID or TID) may hasten resolution

Gastroesophageal reflux

- Empiric trial of a proton pump inhibitor at twice-daily dosing (eg, omeprazole, 20 mg PO BID) for 2–3 months is a practical alternative to an initial pH study
- If symptoms improve and cessation of therapy leads to recurrence of symptoms, resume a proton pump inhibitor at the lowest dose effective for remission, usually daily but at times on a demand basis
- H_2-receptor antagonists are generally less clinically effective

SURGERY

- Recalcitrant nodules or polyps may require excision

 OUTCOME

COMPLICATIONS

- In hoarseness from acute laryngitis, patients should avoid vigorous use of the voice (singing, shouting) while laryngitis is present to avoid formation of vocal nodules

PROGNOSIS

Acute laryngitis

- Self-limited
- May persist for 1–2 weeks after other symptoms of upper respiratory tract infection have cleared

Vocal nodules

- Benign condition

WHEN TO REFER

- All cases of stridor
- Rapid-onset stridor should be evaluated emergently

PREVENTION

- Prevent vocal abuse, particularly among singers
- Modification of voice habits to avoid formation of vocal cord nodules

 EVIDENCE

PRACTICE GUIDELINES

- Dejonckere PH et al. A basic protocol for functional assessment of voice pathology, especially for investigating the efficacy of (phonosurgical) treatments and evaluating new assessment techniques. Guideline elaborated by the Committee on Phoniatrics of the European Laryngological Society (ELS). Eur Arch Otorhinolaryngol. 2001;258:77. [PMID: 11307610]

WEB SITES

- American Academy of Otolaryngology—Head and Neck Surgery: Hoarseness Interactive Module
- Baylor College of Medicine Otolaryngology Resources: Laryngology

INFORMATION FOR PATIENTS

- American Academy of Otolaryngology—Head and Neck Surgery: Doctor, Why Am I Hoarse?
- American Academy of Otolaryngology—Head and Neck Surgery: Most Common Voice Disorders
- American Academy of Otolaryngology—Head and Neck Surgery: Understanding Vocal Cord Lesions: Nodules, Polyps, and Cysts

REFERENCES

- Grillone GA et al. Laryngeal dystonia. Otolaryngol Clin North Am. 2006 Feb; 39(1):87–100. [PMID: 16469657]
- Merati AL et al. Common movement disorders affecting the larynx: a report from the neurolaryngology committee of the AAO-HNS. Otolaryngol Head Neck Surg. 2005 Nov;133(5):654–65. [PMID: 16274788]
- Richardson BE et al. Clinical evaluation of vocal fold paralysis. Otolaryngol Clin

North Am. 2004 Feb;37(1):45–58.
[PMID: 15062686]

Hodgkin's Disease

KEY FEATURES

ESSENTIALS OF DIAGNOSIS

- Painless lymphadenopathy
- Constitutional symptoms may or may not be present
- Pathologic diagnosis by lymph node biopsy

GENERAL CONSIDERATIONS

- Group of cancers characterized by Reed-Sternberg cells in appropriate reactive cellular background
- Malignant cell is a B lymphocyte
- Divided into several pathologic subtypes
  - Lymphocyte predominance
  - Nodular sclerosis
  - Mixed cellularity
  - Lymphocyte depletion
- Tendency to arise within single lymph node areas and spread in orderly fashion to contiguous lymph nodes
- Widespread hematogenous dissemination only late in course

DEMOGRAPHICS

- Bimodal age distribution: one peak at age 20–30 and second peak at age > 50

 ## CLINICAL FINDINGS

SYMPTOMS AND SIGNS

- Painless lymphadenopathy (mass), commonly in neck
- Constitutional symptoms, eg, fever, weight loss, or night sweats, or generalized pruritus
- Pain in involved lymph node after alcohol ingestion is an unusual symptom

DIFFERENTIAL DIAGNOSIS

- Non-Hodgkin's lymphoma
- Tuberculous lymphadenitis (scrofula)
- Cat-scratch disease
- Sarcoidosis
- Metastatic cancer
- Drug-induced pseudolymphoma (eg, phenytoin)

 ## DIAGNOSIS

DIAGNOSTIC PROCEDURES

- Lymph node biopsy establishes pathologic diagnosis. Fine needle aspirate is not adequate
- Staging nomenclature (Ann Arbor)
  - Stage I, one lymph node region involved
  - Stage II, involvement of two lymph node areas on one side of diaphragm
  - Stage III, lymph node regions involved on both sides of diaphragm
  - Stage IV, disseminated disease with bone marrow or liver involvement
- In addition, designated as stage A if there is a lack of constitutional symptoms and stage B if there is a 10% weight loss over 6 months, fever, or night sweats ("B symptoms")

 ## TREATMENT

MEDICATIONS

- Combination chemotherapy for six to eight cycles, involving doxorubicin (Adriamycin), bleomycin, vincristine, and dacarbazine (ABVD) for most patients with advanced disease (see Table 7)
- New intensified chemotherapy programs are being tested
- Early stage disease, formerly treated primarily with radiation, is now commonly treated with short-course (ie, 4 cycles) of combination chemotherapy

THERAPEUTIC PROCEDURES

- All patients with both localized and disseminated disease should be treated with curative intent
- Radiation therapy is initial treatment only for patients with low-risk stage IA and IIA disease, and short-course chemotherapy may substitute
- High-dose chemotherapy with autologous stem cell transplantation is treatment of choice for relapse after initial chemotherapy

 ## OUTCOME

PROGNOSIS

- Excellent for stage IA or IIA disease treated by radiotherapy: 10-year survival rates > 80%
- Advanced disease: 5-year survival rates of 50–60%
- Prognosis is poorer in patients who
  - Are older
  - Have bulky disease
  - Have lymphocyte depletion or mixed cellularity Hodgkin's
- Prognosis for those with the lymphocyte-predominant form of the disease is better than in other subtypes
  - Cure seen in > 70% of those with disseminated disease
  - Limited treatment needed for those with early stage disease
- Recurrent disease after initial radiotherapy may still be curable with chemotherapy
- High-dose chemotherapy with autologous stem cell transplantation for relapse offers 35–50% chance of cure if disease is still chemotherapy sensitive

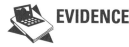 ## EVIDENCE

PRACTICE GUIDELINES

- Ferme C et al. Hodgkin's disease. Br J Cancer. 2001;84(Suppl 2):55. [PMID: 11355971]
- Hoppe RT et al. NCCN Hodgkin's Disease Practice Guidelines Panel. National Comprehensive Cancer Network: Hodgkin's Disease v.2.2005

WEB SITES

- National Cancer Institute: Adult Hodgkin's Lymphoma: Treatment

INFORMATION FOR PATIENTS

- American Cancer Society: What Is Hodgkin's Disease?
- Leukemia & Lymphoma Society: Hodgkin Lymphoma
- National Cancer Institute: Hodgkin's Disease

REFERENCES

- Bonadonna G et al. ABVD plus subtotal nodal versus involved-field radiotherapy in early-stage Hodgkin's disease: long-term results. J Clin Oncol. 2004 Jul 15;22(14):2835–41. [PMID: 15199092]
- Engert A et al. Hodgkin's lymphoma in elderly patients: a comprehensive retrospective analysis from the German Hodgkin's Study Group. J Clin Oncol. 2005 Aug 1;23(22):5052–60. [PMID: 15955904]
- Nogova L et al. Biology, clinical course and management of nodular lymphocyte-predominant hodgkin lymphoma. Hematology Am Soc Hematol Educ

Program. 2006:266–72. [PMID: 17124071]

• Re D et al. From Hodgkin disease to Hodgkin lymphoma: biologic insights and therapeutic potential. Blood. 2005 Jun 15;105(12):4553–60. [PMID: 15728122]

Hospital Acquired Infections

KEY FEATURES

ESSENTIALS OF DIAGNOSIS

• Hospital-associated infections are defined as those not present or incubating at the time of hospital admission and developing at least 48–72 hours after admission

• Hand washing is the easiest and most effective means of prevention and should be done routinely even when gloves are utilized

GENERAL CONSIDERATIONS

• Although most fevers are due to infections, about 25% of patients will have fever of noninfectious origin

• Many infections are a direct result of the use of invasive devices for monitoring or therapy such as
  – IV catheters
  – Foley catheters
  – Catheters placed by interventional radiology for drainage
  – Orotracheal tubes for ventilatory support

• Early removal of such devices reduces infection

• Patients in whom hospital-associated infections develop
  – Are often critically ill
  – Have been hospitalized for extended periods
  – Have received several courses of broad-spectrum antibiotic therapy

• As a result, the causative organisms are often multidrug resistant and different from those in community-acquired infections
  – *Staphylococcus aureus* and *Staphylococcus epidermidis* (a frequent cause of prosthetic device infection) may be resistant to nafcillin and cephalosporins and require vancomycin for therapy
  – *Enterococcus faecium* resistant to ampicillin and vancomycin
  – Gram-negative infections caused by *Pseudomonas, Citrobacter, Enterobacter, Acinetobacter*, and *Stenotrophomonas* may be resistant to most antibacterials

DEMOGRAPHICS

• In the United States, approximately 5% of patients who enter the hospital free of infection acquire a hospital-associated infection resulting in
  – Prolongation of the hospital stay
  – Increase in cost of care
  – Significant morbidity
  – 5% mortality rate

CLINICAL FINDINGS

SYMPTOMS AND SIGNS

• Those of the underlying disease

DIFFERENTIAL DIAGNOSIS

• Noninfectious
  – Drug fever
  – Nonspecific postoperative fevers (tissue damage or necrosis)
  – Hematoma
  – Pancreatitis
  – Pulmonary embolism
  – Myocardial infarction
  – Ischemic bowel
• Urinary tract infections
• Pneumonia
• Bacteremia, eg, indwelling catheter, wound, abscess, pneumonia, genitourinary or gastrointestinal tract
• Wound infection, eg, decubitus ulcer, *Clostridium difficile* colitis

DIAGNOSIS

LABORATORY TESTS

• Blood cultures are universally recommended

• A properly prepared sputum Gram stain and semi-quantitative sputum cultures may be useful in selected patients where there is a high pretest probability of pneumonia

• Unreliable or uninterpretable specimens are often obtained for culture that result in unnecessary use of antibiotics
  – The best example of this principle is the diagnosis of line-related or bloodstream infection in the febrile patient
  – Blood cultures from unidentified sites, a single blood culture from any site, or a blood culture through an existing line will often be positive for *S epidermidis* and will result in therapy with vancomycin
  – The likelihood that such a culture represents a true bacteremia is 10–20%

• Unless two separate venipuncture cultures are obtained—*not* through catheters—interpretation of results is impossible and unnecessary therapy is given

• A positive wound culture without signs of inflammation or infection, a positive sputum culture without pulmonary infiltrates on chest radiograph, or a positive urine culture in a catheterized patient without signs or symptoms of pyelonephritis are all likely to represent colonization, not infection

IMAGING STUDIES

• Chest radiographs frequently obtained

TREATMENT

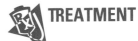

MEDICATIONS

• When choosing antibiotics to treat the seriously ill patient, consider the previous antimicrobial therapy the patient has received as well as the "local ecology"

• It is often necessary to institute therapy with vancomycin, a carbapenem, an aminoglycoside, or a fluoroquinolone until a specific agent is isolated and sensitivities are known

OUTCOME

FOLLOW-UP

• Monitoring of high-risk areas by hospital epidemiologists detects increases in infection rates early

WHEN TO REFER

• For persistent fevers or systemic toxicity despite treatment of underlying problem

PREVENTION

• Universal precautions against potential blood-borne transmissible disease

• Hepatitis A, hepatitis B, and varicella vaccines should be considered in the appropriate setting

• Peripheral IV lines should be replaced every 3 days and arterial lines every 4 days

- Lines in the central venous circulation (including those placed peripherally) can be left in indefinitely and are changed or removed when
  – They are clinically suspected of being infected
  – They are nonfunctional
  – They are no longer needed
- Silver alloy–impregnated Foley catheters reduce the incidence of catheter-associated bacteriuria, and antibiotic-impregnated (minocycline plus rifampin or chlorhexidine plus silver sulfadiazine) venous catheters reduce line infections and bacteremia
- Whether the increased cost of these devices justifies their routine use should be determined by individual institutions based on local infection rates
- Perioperative administration of chlorhexidine intranasal ointment and oropharyngeal rinse has been shown to reduce incidence of infection following surgery
- Attentive nursing care (positioning to prevent decubitus ulcers, wound care, elevating the head during tube feedings to prevent aspiration) is critical

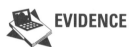

EVIDENCE

PRACTICE GUIDELINES

- American Thoracic Society; Infectious Diseases Society of America. Guidelines for the management of adults with hospital-acquired, ventilation-associated and healthcare-associated pneumonia. Am J Respir Crit Care Med. 2005; 171:388. [PMID: 15699079]
- National Guideline Clearinghouse
  – Guidelines for preventing health-care–associated pneumonia, 2003: CDC and the Healthcare Infection Control Practices Advisory Committee
  – Handwashing and antisepsis. APIC 1995
  – Hand hygiene. HICPAC/SHEA/APIC/IDSA, 2002

WEB SITE

- Centers for Disease Control and Prevention—National Nosocomial Infections Surveillance System

INFORMATION FOR PATIENTS

- National Institute of Allergy and Infectious Diseases
- National Institutes of Health

REFERENCES

- Canadian Critical Care Trials Group. A randomized trial of diagnostic tech-

niques for ventilator-associated pneumonia. N Engl J Med. 2006 Dec 21; 355(25):2619–30. [PMID: 17182987]
- Kollef MH. Prevention of hospital-associated pneumonia and ventilator-associated pneumonia. Crit Care Med. 2004 Jun; 32(6):1396–405. [PMID: 15187525]
- Pronovost P et al. An intervention to decrease catheter-related bloodstream infections in the ICU. N Engl J Med. 2006 Dec 28;355(26):2725–32. [PMID: 17192537]
- Raad I et al. Differential time to positivity: a useful method for diagnosing catheter-related bloodstream infections. Ann Intern Med. 2004 Jan 6; 140(1):18–25. [PMID: 14706968]
- Segers P et al. Prevention of nosocomial infection in cardiac surgery by decontamination of the nasopharynx and oropharynx with chlorhexidine gluconate: a randomized controlled trial. JAMA. 2006 Nov 22;296(20):2460–6. [PMID: 17119142]
- Vermeulen H et al. Diagnostic accuracy of routine postoperative body temperature measurements. Clin Infect Dis. 2005 May 15;40(10):1404–10. [PMID: 15844061]

Huntington Disease

KEY FEATURES

ESSENTIALS OF DIAGNOSIS

- Gradual onset and progression of chorea and dementia or behavioral change
- Family history of the disorder
- Responsible gene identified on chromosome 4

GENERAL CONSIDERATIONS

- Inherited in an autosomal dominant manner and occurs throughout the world, in all ethnic groups, with a prevalence rate of about 5 per 100,000
- The gene responsible for the disease has been located on the short arm of chromosome 4
  – There is an expanded and unstable CAG trinucleotide repeat at 4p16.3
  – Length of CAG trinucleotide repeat may have an effect on rate of progression

- Offspring should be offered genetic counseling
- Genetic testing permits presymptomatic detection and definitive diagnosis of the disease

CLINICAL FINDINGS

SYMPTOMS AND SIGNS

- Clinical onset is usually between 30 and 50 years of age
- **Initial symptoms**
  – May consist of either abnormal movements or intellectual changes
  – However, both ultimately occur
- Earliest **mental changes**
  – Often behavioral, with irritability, moodiness, antisocial behavior, or a psychiatric disturbance
  – However, a more obvious dementia subsequently develops
- **Dyskinesia**
  – May initially be no more than an apparent fidgetiness or restlessness
  – However, choreiform movements and some dystonic posturing eventually occur
- **Progressive rigidity** and **akinesia** (rather than chorea) sometimes occur in association with dementia, especially in cases with childhood onset

DIFFERENTIAL DIAGNOSIS

- Chorea developing with no family history of choreoathetosis should not be attributed to Huntington disease, at least not until other causes of chorea have been excluded clinically and by appropriate laboratory studies
- In younger patients, self-limiting Sydenham chorea develops after group A streptococcal infections on rare occasions
- Other nongenetic causes of chorea
  – Stroke
  – Systemic lupus erythematosus and related disorders
  – Paraneoplastic syndromes
  – Infection with HIV
  – Various medications
- If progressive intellectual failure is the sole presentation, it may not be possible to distinguish Huntington disease from other causes of dementia unless there is a characteristic family history or a dyskinesia develops
- Dentatorubral-pallidolysian atrophy
  – A clinically similar autosomal dominant disorder
  – Uncommon except in persons of Japanese ancestry

– Manifested by chorea, dementia, ataxia, and myoclonic epilepsy
– Due to a mutant gene mapping to 12p13.31

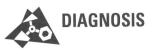

DIAGNOSIS

IMAGING STUDIES

- CT scanning usually demonstrates cerebral atrophy and atrophy of the caudate nucleus in established cases
- MRI and positron emission tomography (PET) have shown reduced glucose utilization in an anatomically normal caudate nucleus

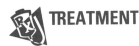

TREATMENT

MEDICATIONS

- Dopamine receptor blockers, such as phenothiazines or haloperidol, may control the dyskinesia and any behavioral disturbances
- Haloperidol
  – Initial dose is 1 mg PO once daily or BID
  – Dose is increased every 3 or 4 days, depending on the response
- Tetrabenazine
  – Depletes central monoamines
  – Widely used in Europe to treat dyskinesia but not available in the United States
- Reserpine
  – Similar in its actions to tetrabenazine and may be helpful
  – Daily dose is built up gradually to between 2 and 5 mg PO, depending on the response
- Behavioral disturbances may respond to clozapine
- Attempts to compensate for the relative gamma-aminobutyric acid (GABA) deficiency by enhancing central GABA activity or to compensate for the relative cholinergic underactivity by giving choline chloride have not been therapeutically helpful
- Cysteamine (a selective depleter of somatostatin in the brain) is currently under study

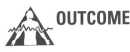

OUTCOME

PROGNOSIS

- There is no cure for Huntington disease
  – Progression cannot be halted
  – Treatment is purely symptomatic
- Usually fatal within 15–20 years

WHEN TO REFER

- All patients may benefit from practitioners with particular expertise in this area
- For genetic counseling of offspring

PREVENTION

- Genetic counseling is important to prevention

EVIDENCE

PRACTICE GUIDELINES

- International Huntington Association and the World Federation of Neurology Research Group on Huntington's Chorea. Guidelines for the molecular genetics predictive test in Huntington's disease. J Med Genet. 1994;31:555. [PMID: 7966192]

WEB SITE

- National Institute of Neurological Disorders and Stroke

INFORMATION FOR PATIENTS

- Huntington's Disease Society of America
- The Mayo Clinic

REFERENCES

- Cardoso F et al. Seminar on choreas. Lancet Neurol. 2006 Jul;5(7):589–602. [PMID: 16781989]
- Higgins DS. Huntington's disease. Curr Treat Options Neurol. 2006 May; 8(3):236–44. [PMID: 16569382]
- Rosenblatt A et al. The association of CAG repeat length with clinical progression in Huntington disease. Neurology. 2006 Apr 11;66(7):1016–20. [PMID: 16606912]

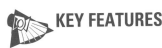

Hydatidiform Mole & Choriocarcinoma

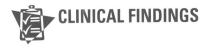

KEY FEATURES

ESSENTIALS OF DIAGNOSIS

- Uterine bleeding
- Pathologic demonstration of choriocarcinoma in samples of a pelvic or vaginal mass, or in a metastatic tumor
- Hydatidiform mole
  – Amenorrhea
  – Irregular uterine bleeding
  – Serum human chorionic gonadotropin (hCG)-β subunit > 40,000 mU/mL
  – Passage of grape-like clusters of enlarged edematous villi per vagina
  – Ultrasound of uterus with characteristic heterogeneous echogenic image and no fetus or placenta
  – Cytogenetic composition is 46,XX (85%) completely of paternal origin

GENERAL CONSIDERATIONS

- Hydatidiform mole, invasive mole, and choriocarcinoma comprise a spectrum of gestational trophoblastic neoplasia
- Partial moles generally show evidence of an embryo or gestational sac; are polypoid, slower-growing, and less symptomatic; and often present clinically as a missed abortion

DEMOGRAPHICS

- Highest rates of gestational trophoblastic neoplasia occur in some developing countries: 1/125 pregnancies in areas of Asia, 1/1500 pregnancies in the United States
- Risk factors include low socioeconomic status, a history of mole, and age below 18 or above 40

CLINICAL FINDINGS

SYMPTOMS AND SIGNS

- **Hydatidiform mole**
  – Excessive nausea and vomiting in over one-third of patients
  – Uterine bleeding beginning at 6–8 weeks is usual
  – In 20% of cases, the uterus appears larger than would be expected
  – Intact or collapsed grape-like clusters of enlarged villi (vesicles) may be passed
  – Bilaterally enlarged cystic ovaries may be palpable
  – Less commonly, preeclampsia-eclampsia may develop during the second trimester
- **Choriocarcinoma** may be manifested by continued or recurrent bleeding
  – After evacuation of a mole
  – Following delivery, abortion, or ectopic pregnancy
  – An ulcerative vaginal tumor, pelvic mass, or evidence of distant metastatic tumor may be observed

DIFFERENTIAL DIAGNOSIS

- Similarly elevated levels of serum hCG-β subunit are seen in multiple gestation
  - Spontaneous abortion
  - Ectopic pregnancy
  - Prolapsed uterine fibroid
  - Uterine leiomyomas (fibroids), endometrial polyp, or adenomyosis (uterine endometriosis)
  - Ovarian tumor
  - Cervical neoplasm or lesion

 DIAGNOSIS

LABORATORY TESTS

- Serum hCG-β subunit value > 40,000 mU/mL or a urinary hCG > 100,000 mU/mL over 24 h increases the likelihood of hydatidiform mole, though such values are occasionally seen with a normal pregnancy in multiple gestation

IMAGING STUDIES

- Ultrasound has replaced all other means of preoperative diagnosis of mole
- Ultrasound findings are multiple echoes indicating edematous villi within an enlarged uterus, and absent fetus and placenta
- Preoperative chest radiograph is required to evaluate for pulmonary metastases of trophoblast

DIAGNOSTIC PROCEDURES

- The diagnosis of choriocarcinoma is established by pathologic examination of curettings or biopsy

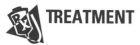 **TREATMENT**

MEDICATIONS

- Chemotherapy is indicated for mole if malignant tissue is discovered at surgery or during follow-up examination
- For low-risk patients with a good prognosis, give
  - Methotrexate, 0.4 mg/kg IM over a 5-day period, or
  - Dactinomycin, 10–12 mcg/kg/day IV over a 5-day period (Table 7)
  - The side effects usually are reversible in about 3 weeks and can be ameliorated by the administration of leucovorin (0.1 mg/kg); they include
    - Anorexia
    - Nausea and vomiting
    - Stomatitis
    - Rash

- Diarrhea
- Bone marrow depression
- Repeated courses of methotrexate 2 weeks apart generally are required to destroy the trophoblast and maintain a zero chorionic gonadotropin titer, as indicated by β-hCG determination
- β-Blockers should be used preoperatively to stabilize patients who have thyrotoxicosis as a result of their mole

SURGERY

- The uterus should be emptied as soon as a mole is diagnosed, preferably by suction
- Ovarian cysts should not be resected nor ovaries removed; spontaneous regression of theca lutein cysts will occur with elimination of the mole

 OUTCOME

FOLLOW-UP

- hCG levels should be negative for 6–12 months before conception is attempted
- In the pregnancy following a mole, hCG level should be checked 6 weeks postpartum
- Contraception should be prescribed to avoid the confusion of elevated hCG from a new pregnancy; oral contraceptive pills are preferred
- Weekly serum hCG levels are measured
- After two negative hCG levels are documented in succession, levels may be checked less frequently at intervals out to 1 year
- A plateau or rise in hCG levels mandates a repeat chest radiograph and D&C before chemotherapy

COMPLICATIONS

- Approximately 10% of women require further treatment after evacuation of the mole; choriocarcinoma develops in 5%
- hCG has minimal TSH–like activity; at very high levels, release of T_3 and T_4 may occur and cause hyperthyroidism, which resolves promptly after resection

PROGNOSIS

- Partial moles tend to follow a benign course
- Complete moles have a greater tendency to become choriocarcinomas
- 5-year survival after courses of chemotherapy, even when metastases have been demonstrated, can be expected in at least 85% of cases of choriocarcinoma

WHEN TO REFER

- Patients with a poor prognosis should be referred to a cancer center, where multiple-agent chemotherapy probably will be given

WHEN TO ADMIT

- Patients with excessive vaginal bleeding
- Patients passing vesicular tissue
- Patients with thyrotoxicosis
- Patients with symptomatic metastatic disease

EVIDENCE

PRACTICE GUIDELINES

- Benedet JL et al. FIGO staging classifications and clinical practice guidelines in the management of gynecologic cancers. FIGO Committee on Gynecologic Oncology. Int J Gynaecol Obstet. 2000; 70:209. [PMID: 11041682]
- Soper JT et al; American College of Obstetricians and Gynecologists. Diagnosis and treatment of gestational trophoblastic disease: ACOG Practice Bulletin No. 53. Gynecol Oncol. 2004; 93:575. [PMID: 15196847]

WEB SITE

- National Cancer Institute: Gestational Trophoblastic Disease Information for Patients and Health Professionals

INFORMATION FOR PATIENTS

- American Cancer Society: Gestational Trophoblastic Disease
- MedlinePlus: Gestational Trophoblastic Disease

REFERENCES

- Smith HO et al. Choriocarcinoma and gestational trophoblastic disease. Obstet Gynecol Clin North Am. 2005 Dec; 32(4):661–84. [PMID: 16310678]
- Soper JT. Gestational trophoblastic disease. Obstet Gynecol. 2006 Jul; 108(1):176–87. [PMID: 16816073]

Hyperaldosteronism, Primary

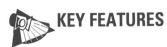

KEY FEATURES

ESSENTIALS OF DIAGNOSIS

- Hypertension
- Hypokalemia, alkalosis
- Polyuria, polydipsia
- Muscular weakness
- Plasma and urine aldosterone levels elevated and plasma renin level low

GENERAL CONSIDERATIONS

- Aldosterone stimulates renal tubule to reabsorb sodium and excrete potassium
- Causes
  - Unilateral adrenocortical adenoma (Conn's syndrome, 73%)
  - Bilateral cortical hyperplasia (27%)
    - May be corticosteroid suppressible due to an autosomal dominant genetic defect allowing ACTH stimulation of aldosterone production

DEMOGRAPHICS

- Classic hyperaldosteronism (with hypokalemia) accounts for ~0.7% of cases of hypertension
- Milder hyperaldosteronism, without hypokalemia, is more common, with a prevalence of 5–14% among hypertensive patients
- More common in women

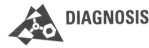

CLINICAL FINDINGS

SYMPTOMS AND SIGNS

- Hypertension ranging from mild to severe. Malignant hypertension rare
- Muscular weakness; episodic paralysis simulating periodic paralysis
- Fatigue and reduced stamina
- Paresthesias, sometimes with frank tetany
- Headache
- Polyuria and polydipsia
- Edema, common in secondary hyperaldosteronism, rare in primary hyperaldosteronism

DIFFERENTIAL DIAGNOSIS

- Essential hypertension
- Hypokalemic thyrotoxic periodic paralysis
- Renal vascular hypertension (hypertension and hypokalemia, but plasma renin activity is high)
- Hypokalemia due to other cause, eg, diuretics
- Secondary hyperaldosteronism (dehydration, heart failure)
- Congenital adrenal hyperplasia: 11β-hydroxylase deficiency, 17α-hydroxylase deficiency
- Cushing's syndrome
- Excessive real licorice ingestion
- Syndrome of cortisol resistance

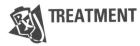

DIAGNOSIS

LABORATORY TESTS

- Discontinue all antihypertensives and remain off diuretics for 3 weeks
  - Persistent hypokalemia even after diuretics stopped
- Maintain high sodium intake (>120 mEq/day) during evaluation
- Obtain 24-h urine aldosterone, free cortisol, and creatinine
  - 24-h urine aldosterone > 20 mcg with low plasma renin activity (< 5 mcg/dL) indicates hyperaldosteronism
- Once hyperaldosteronism diagnosed, further testing to distinguish between resectable adrenal adenoma and nonsurgical adrenal hyperplasia
- Plasma 18-hydroxycorticosterone
  - > 85 ng/dL with adrenal neoplasms
  - Level < 85 ng/dL is nondiagnostic
- Plasma aldosterone is measured at 8 AM while patient is supine after overnight recumbency and again after 4 h upright
  - With adrenal adenoma, baseline aldosterone is usually > 25 ng/dL (695 pmol/L) and does not rise during upright posture
  - With hyperplasia, baseline aldosterone usually is < 20 ng/dL and rises during upright posture

IMAGING STUDIES

- Thin-section CT suggests discrete (> 1 cm diameter) adrenal adenoma in 60–80% of patients with laboratory findings suggesting adrenal adenoma

DIAGNOSTIC PROCEDURES

- Adrenal vein catheterization for aldosterone or during stimulation with cosyntropin. An adrenal vein to inferior vena cava gradient of > 5:1 confirms the adrenal location of the adenoma
- Dexamethasone-suppressed adrenal scan using ^{131}I-labeled 6-iodomethyl-19-norcholesterol may identify an aldosteronoma, but may yield misleading results

TREATMENT

MEDICATIONS

- Spironolactone
  - Treatment of choice for bilateral adrenal hyperplasia
  - Lifelong therapy is an option for patients with unilateral adrenal adenoma (Conn's syndrome) who are poor surgical candidates
- Potassium supplements are required
- Antihypertensive medications for hypertension in bilateral adrenal hyperplasia
  - Angiotensin receptor blockers or angiotensin-converting enzyme inhibitors preferred since they reduce renal potassium losses
  - Thiazides aggravate potassium loss
- Low-dose dexamethasone suppression is an alternative for bilateral adrenal hyperplasia

SURGERY

- Surgical resection (laparoscopic adrenalectomy) is treatment of choice for unilateral adrenal adenoma secreting aldosterone (Conn's syndrome)
- Bilateral adrenalectomy corrects hypokalemia but not hypertension and should *not* be performed for bilateral adrenal hyperplasia

OUTCOME

FOLLOW-UP

- Monitor electrolytes, blood pressure, renal function

COMPLICATIONS

- Complications of chronic hypertension
- Progressive renal damage is less reversible than in essential hypertension
- Hyperkalemia and hypotension from temporary postoperative hypoaldosteronism can occur from suppression of contralateral adrenal gland following unilateral adrenalectomy for Conn's syndrome
- Surgical morbidity is 7.1%; < 4.1% in major centers. Surgical mortality is rare

PROGNOSIS

- Hypertension remits after surgery in about two-thirds of cases but persists or returns despite surgery in one-third

- Prognosis much improved by early diagnosis and treatment
- Only 2% of aldosterone-secreting adrenal tumors are malignant

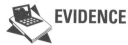 EVIDENCE

PRACTICE GUIDELINES

- Foo R et al. Hyperaldosteronism: recent concepts, diagnosis, and management. Postgrad Med J. 2001;77:639. [PMID: 11571370]
- Young WF Jr. Minireview: primary aldosteronism–changing concepts in diagnosis and treatment. Endocrinology. 2003; 144:2208. [PMID: 12746276]

WEB SITE

- Family Practice Notebook article on hyperaldosteronism

INFORMATION FOR PATIENTS

- MedlinePlus—Hyperaldosteronism—primary and secondary
- National Adrenal Disease Foundation

REFERENCES

- Tiu SC et al. The use of aldosterone-renin ratio as a diagnostic test for primary hyperaldosteronism and its test characteristics under different conditions of blood sampling. J Clin Endocrinol Metab. 2005 Jan;90(1):72–8. [PMID: 15483077]
- Vasan RS et al. Serum aldosterone and the incidence of hypertension in nonhypertensive persons. N Engl J Med. 2004 Jul 1;351(1):33–41. [PMID: 15229305]
- Young WF et al. Role for adrenal venous sampling in primary aldosteronism. Surgery. 2004 Dec;136(6):1227–35. [PMID: 15657580]

Hypercalcemia

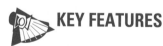 KEY FEATURES

ESSENTIALS OF DIAGNOSIS

- Primary hyperparathyroidism and malignancy account for 90% of all cases
- Asymptomatic, mild hypercalcemia (< 11 mg/dL) is usually due to primary hyperparathyroidism

- Hypercalcemia of malignancy is usually symptomatic and severe (≥ 15 mg/dL)
- Hypercalciuria usually precedes hypercalcemia

GENERAL CONSIDERATIONS

- Primary hyperparathyroidism is the most common cause of hypercalcemia in ambulatory patients
- Tumor production of parathyroid hormone–related protein (PTHrP)
  - Most common paraneoplastic endocrine syndrome, accounting for most cases of hypercalcemia among inpatients
  - The neoplasm is clinically apparent in nearly all cases when hypercalcemia is detected
- Chronic hypercalcemia (> 6 months) or some manifestations such as nephrolithiasis suggests a benign etiology
- Hypophosphatemia suggests elevated parathyroid hormone (PTH) or PTHrP
- Hypocalciuric hypercalcemia occurs in
  - Milk-alkali syndrome
  - Thiazide diuretic use
  - Familial hypocalciuric hypercalcemia
- Hypercalcemia can cause nephrogenic diabetes insipidus and volume depletion, which further worsen hypercalcemia

Etiology

- Increased intake or absorption
  - Milk-alkali syndrome
  - Vitamin D or A excess
- Endocrine disorders
  - Primary and secondary hyperparathyroidism
  - Chronic kidney disease stage 5D
  - Acromegaly
  - Adrenal insufficiency
  - Hyperthyroidism
- Neoplastic diseases
  - Tumor production of PTHrP (ovary, kidney, lung)
  - Multiple myeloma (osteoclast-activating factor)
- Other
  - Thiazide diuretics
  - Sarcoidosis and other granulomatous diseases
  - Paget's bone disease
  - Immobilization
  - Familial hypocalciuric hypercalcemia

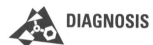 CLINICAL FINDINGS

SYMPTOMS AND SIGNS

- First, determine duration of hypercalcemia
- Look for neoplasm, particularly if hypercalcemia is acute (< 6 months)

- Symptoms usually occur if the serum calcium is > 12 mg/dL and tend to be more severe in acute hypercalcemia
- Constipation and polyuria occur regardless of cause of hypercalcemia
- Stupor, coma, and azotemia may develop in severe hypercalcemia
- Polyuria is absent in familial hypocalciuric hypercalcemia
- Ventricular extrasystoles and idioventricular rhythm occur and can be accentuated by digitalis

DIAGNOSIS

LABORATORY TESTS

- Serum calcium must be interpreted in relation to serum albumin level
- When albumin is low, serum Ca^{2+} concentration is depressed in a ratio of 0.8–1.0 mg/dL of Ca^{2+}: 1 g/dL of albumin
- The highest serum calcium levels (≥ 15 mg/dL) generally occur in malignancy
- A high serum chloride concentration and a low serum phosphate concentration (ratio > 33:1) suggest primary hyperparathyroidism because PTH decreases proximal tubular phosphate reabsorption
- A low serum chloride concentration with a high serum bicarbonate concentration, along with blood urea nitrogen and serum creatinine elevations, suggests milk-alkali syndrome
- Urinary calcium excretion
  - > 200 mg/day suggests hypercalciuria
  - < 100 mg/day suggests hypocalciuria
- Hypercalciuria from malignancy or from vitamin D therapy frequently results in hypercalcemia when volume depletion occurs
- Serum PTH and PTHrP levels help distinguish between malignancy-associated hypercalcemia (elevated PTHrP) and hyperparathyroidism (elevated PTH)
- Serum phosphate may or may not be low, depending on the cause
- A serum calcium × serum phosphorus product > 70 markedly increases the risk of nephrocalcinosis and soft tissue calcification

IMAGING STUDIES

- Chest radiograph: to exclude malignancy or granulomatous disease

DIAGNOSTIC PROCEDURE

- ECG: shortened QT interval

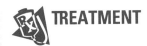 **TREATMENT**

MEDICATIONS

Emergency treatment

- Establish euvolemia to induce renal excretion of Na^+, which is accompanied by excretion of Ca^{2+}
- In dehydrated patients with normal cardiac and renal function, infuse 0.45% saline or 0.9% saline rapidly (250–500 mL/h)
- Administer IV furosemide (20–40 mg q2h) to prevent volume overload and enhance Ca^{2+} excretion
- Thiazides can actually worsen hypercalcemia (as can furosemide if inadequate saline is given)
- In the treatment of hypercalcemia of malignancy
  - Bisphosphonates are the mainstay
  - Zoledronic acid, 4-mg single 15-min IV infusion, with adequate hydration normalizes serum Ca^{2+} in 70% of patients in 3 days and can be repeated as necessary to control the hypercalcemia
- See Hyperparathyroidism

THERAPEUTIC PROCEDURES

- In emergency cases, dialysis with low or no calcium dialysate may be needed

 OUTCOME

FOLLOW-UP

- Monitor serum calcium at least every 6 months during medical therapy of hyperparathyroidism

COMPLICATIONS

- Pathologic fractures are more common in individuals with hyperthyroidism than the general population
- Renal stones
- Renal failure
- Peptic ulcer disease
- Pancreatitis
- Precipitation of calcium throughout the soft tissues
- Gestational hypercalcemia produces neonatal hypocalcemia

PROGNOSIS

- Depends on the underlying disease
- Poor prognosis in malignancy

WHEN TO REFER

- Early referral to an oncologist or nephrologist may aid in management

- Persistent hypercalcemia > 10.5 mg/dL even without symptoms

WHEN TO ADMIT

- Altered mental status
- Marked dehydration and hypotension
- Severe renal insufficiency

PREVENTION

- Prevent dehydration that can further aggravate hypercalcemia

 EVIDENCE

WEB SITE

- National Cancer Institute: Hypercalcemia

INFORMATION FOR PATIENTS

- American Association for Clinical Chemistry: Lab Tests Online: Calcium
- Mayo Clinic: Hypercalcemia
- National Cancer Institute: Hypercalcemia

REFERENCES

- Jacobs TP et al. Clinical review: Rare causes of hypercalcemia. J Clin Endocrinol Metab. 2005 Nov;90(11):6316–22. [PMID: 16131579]
- Lee CT et al. Hypercalcemia in the emergency department. Am J Med Sci. 2006 Mar;331(3):119–23. [PMID: 16538071]
- Stewart AF. Clinical practice. Hypercalcemia associated with cancer. N Engl J Med. 2005 Jan 27;352(4):373–9. [PMID: 15673803]

Hypercoagulable States

 KEY FEATURES

ESSENTIALS OF DIAGNOSIS

- Thrombosis

GENERAL CONSIDERATIONS

- There are both acquired and congenital causes of thrombosis (see Differential Diagnosis)
- The family history usually reveals hypercoagulable states if due to congenital

causes; events are often precipitated by trauma or pregnancy
- Cancer is associated with increased risk of both venous and arterial thrombosis
- Myeloproliferative disorders are associated with high incidence of thrombosis due to qualitative platelet abnormalities
- Venous thrombosis may occur in unusual locations, eg, mesenteric, hepatic, or splenic venous beds
- Arterial thrombosis may manifest as large-vessel occlusion (stroke, myocardial infarction) or microvascular events (burning in hands and feet)
- Heparin is associated with thrombocytopenia in ~10% of treatment courses; it is often modest and resolves spontaneously, but it may be severe and complicated by arterial thrombosis
- Warfarin-induced skin necrosis may occur in patients with undiagnosed protein C deficiency
  - Warfarin, by creating a vitamin K–dependent state, transiently depletes protein C (which has a short half-life) before it leads to anticoagulation
  - During this period of hypercoagulability, thrombosis of skin vessels may lead to infarction and necrosis

DEMOGRAPHICS

- Congenital hypercoagulable states often present during early adulthood rather than childhood

 CLINICAL FINDINGS

SYMPTOMS AND SIGNS

- Thrombosis
- Erythromelalgia (painful redness and burning of hands) in essential thrombocytosis

DIFFERENTIAL DIAGNOSIS

- Acquired causes of thrombosis
  - Immobility or postoperative state
  - Cancer
  - Inflammatory disorders, eg, ulcerative colitis
  - Myeloproliferative disorder, eg, polycythemia vera, essential thrombocytosis
  - Estrogens, pregnancy
  - Heparin-induced thrombocytopenia
  - Lupus anticoagulant
  - Anticardiolipin antibodies
  - Nephrotic syndrome
  - Paroxysmal nocturnal hemoglobinuria
  - Disseminated intravascular coagulation
  - Congestive heart failure

- Congenital causes of thrombosis
  - Activated protein C resistance, eg, factor V Leiden
  - Prothrombin 20210 mutation
  - Antithrombin III deficiency
  - Protein C deficiency
  - Protein S deficiency
  - Hyperhomocystinemia
  - Dysfibrinogenemia
  - Abnormal plasminogen

 DIAGNOSIS

LABORATORY TESTS

- Dysfibrinogenemia is diagnosed by a prolonged reptilase time
- Assays of antithrombin III, protein S, protein C, homocysteine, factor V Leiden

 TREATMENT

MEDICATIONS

- Preoperative low-dose heparin (5000 units SQ q8–12h) may reduce perioperative thrombosis risk
- Heparin, 10,000 units SQ q12h, may reduce thrombosis in hypercoagulable state associated with cancer
  - Low-molecular-weight heparin is more convenient, equally effective, and requires less laboratory monitoring
  - Warfarin is usually ineffective in cancer, most likely because of low-grade disseminated intravascular coagulation
- Aspirin, 325 mg PO QD
  - Helpful for thrombosis in myeloproliferative disease but may increase risk of bleeding
  - Effective for erythromelalgia
- Warfarin is effective and is often given indefinitely in congenital defects if complicated by thrombosis
- Warfarin-induced skin necrosis can be prevented by the use of heparin for 5–7 days until warfarin induces anticoagulation

 OUTCOME

FOLLOW-UP

- Screen family members for congenital defects (eg, deficiency of antithrombin III or vitamin K–dependent proteins C and S)

COMPLICATIONS

- Arterial thrombosis in heparin-induced thrombocytopenia

 EVIDENCE

PRACTICE GUIDELINES

- American College of Chest Physicians. The Seventh ACCP Conference on Antithrombotic and Thrombolytic Therapy: Evidence-Based Guidelines. Chest 2004;126(Suppl 3).
- College of American Pathologists Consensus Conference XXXVI. Diagnostic Issues in Thrombophilia. Arch Pathol Lab Med. 2002;126:1277. [PMID: 12421135]
- Haemostasis and Thrombosis Task Force, British Committee for Standards in Haematology. Investigation and management of heritable thrombophilia. Br J Haematol. 2001;114:512. [PMID: 11552975]

WEB SITE

- Deitcher SR et al. Hypercoagulable States. Cleveland Clinic 2003.

INFORMATION FOR PATIENTS

- American Academy of Family Physicians: Hypercoagulation
- MedlinePlus: Hypercoagulable States
- Parmet S et al. JAMA patient page. Pulmonary embolism. JAMA. 2003; 290:2898. [PMID: 14657080]

REFERENCES

- Bockenstedt PL. Management of hereditary hypercoagulable disorders. Hematology Am Soc Hematol Educ Program. 2006:444–9. [PMID: 17124097]
- Prandoni P. How I treat venous thromboembolism in patients with cancer. Blood. 2005 Dec 15;106(13):4027–33. [PMID: 16076870]
- Rieder MJ et al. Effect of VKORC1 haplotypes on transcriptional regulation and warfarin dose. N Engl J Med. 2005 Jun 2;352(22):2285–93. [PMID: 15930419]

 KEY FEATURES

ESSENTIALS OF DIAGNOSIS

- Hyperglycemia, serum glucose > 600 mg/dL
- Serum osmolality > 310 mOsm/kg
- No acidosis; blood pH > 7.3
- Serum bicarbonate > 15 mEq/L
- Normal anion gap (< 14 mEq/L)

GENERAL CONSIDERATIONS

- Frequently occurs with mild or occult diabetes mellitus
- Infection, myocardial infarction, stroke, or recent operation is often a precipitating event
- Drugs (phenytoin, diazoxide, corticosteroids, and diuretics) or procedures associated with glucose loading such as peritoneal dialysis can also precipitate the syndrome
- Renal insufficiency develops from hypovolemia, leading to increasingly higher blood glucose concentrations
- Underlying renal insufficiency or congestive heart failure is common, and the presence of either worsens the prognosis

DEMOGRAPHICS

- Rarer than diabetic ketoacidosis even in older age groups
- Affects middle-aged to elderly

 CLINICAL FINDINGS

SYMPTOMS AND SIGNS

- Onset may be insidious over days or weeks, with weakness, polyuria, and polydipsia
- The lack of features of ketoacidosis may retard recognition until dehydration becomes more profound than in ketoacidosis
- Fluid intake is usually reduced from inappropriate lack of thirst, nausea, or inaccessibility of fluids to bedridden patients
- Lethargy and confusion develop as serum osmolality exceeds 310 mOsm/kg;

coma can occur if osmolality exceeds 320–330 mOsm/kg
- Physical examination shows profound dehydration, lethargy, or coma without Kussmaul respirations

DIFFERENTIAL DIAGNOSIS

- Diabetic ketoacidosis
- Cerebrovascular accident or head trauma
- Hypoglycemia
- Sepsis
- Diabetes insipidus

 DIAGNOSIS

LABORATORY TESTS

- Severe hyperglycemia (serum glucose 600–2400 mg/dL)
- When dehydration is less severe, dilutional hyponatremia as well as urinary sodium losses may reduce serum sodium to 120–125 mEq/L
- As dehydration progresses, serum sodium can exceed 140 mEq/L, producing serum osmolality readings of 330–440 mOsm/kg
- Ketosis and acidosis are usually absent or mild
- Prerenal azotemia with blood urea nitrogen elevations > 100 mg/dL typical
- Rhabdomyolysis may be present

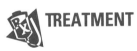 **TREATMENT**

MEDICATIONS

Saline

- Fluid replacement paramount to correct fluid deficits of 6–10 L
- In hypovolemic oliguric hypotension, initiate fluid resuscitation with isotonic 0.9% saline
- Otherwise, hypotonic (0.45%) saline preferred because of hyperosmolality
- As much as 4–6 L of fluid may be required in first 8–10 h
- Once blood glucose reaches 250 mg/dL, add 5% dextrose to either water, 0.45% saline solution, or 0.9% saline solution at a rate to maintain serum glucose levels of 250–300 mg/dL to reduce risk of cerebral edema
- Goal of fluid therapy is to restore urinary output to ≥ 50 mL/h

Insulin

- Less insulin is required than in diabetic ketoacidotic coma

- Fluid replacement alone can reduce hyperglycemia by increasing glomerular filtration and renal excretion of glucose
- Initial insulin dose of 0.15 U/kg is followed by insulin infusion of 1–2 U/h, titrated to lower blood glucose levels by 50–70 mg/dL/h

Potassium

- Add potassium chloride (10 mEq/L) to initial fluids if serum potassium is not elevated. Adjust subsequent potassium replacement based on serum potassium level

Phosphate

- If severe hypophosphatemia (serum phosphate < 1 mg/dL [0.35 mmol/L]) develops during therapy, phosphate replacement can be given as its potassium salt
- To minimize risk of tetany from phosphate replacement overload, average deficit of 40–50 mmol phosphate should be replaced by IV infusion not to exceed 3 mmol/h
  - A stock solution (Abbott) provides a mixture of 1.12 g KH_2PO_4 and 1.18 g K_2HPO_4 in a 5-mL single-dose vial representing 22 mEq potassium and 15 mmol phosphate (27 mEq)
  - 5 mL of this solution in 2 L of 0.45% saline or 5% dextrose in water, infused at 400 mL/h, will replace the phosphate at optimal rate of 3 mmol/h and provide 4.4 mEq potassium/h
- If serum phosphate remains < 0.35 mmol/L (1 mg/dL), repeat a 5-h infusion of potassium phosphate at 3 mmol/h

THERAPEUTIC PROCEDURES

- Using a flow sheet, document vital signs, time sequence of laboratory values (arterial pH, plasma glucose, acetone, bicarbonate, blood urea nitrogen, electrolytes, serum osmolality) in relation to therapy

 OUTCOME

PROGNOSIS

- The overall mortality rate is > 10 times that of diabetic ketoacidosis because of its higher incidence in older patients and greater dehydration
- When prompt therapy is instituted, the mortality rate can be reduced from nearly 50% to that related to the severity of coexistent disorders

WHEN TO ADMIT

- Altered mental status
- Severe volume depletion

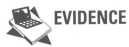 **EVIDENCE**

PRACTICE GUIDELINES

- American Diabetes Association: Hyperglycemic Crises in Patients with Diabetes Mellitus
- Joslin Diabetes Center: Hyperglycemic Emergencies for Adults, 2004
- National Guideline Clearinghouse: Hyperglycemic Crises in Diabetes, 2001

WEB SITES

- American Association of Diabetes Educators
- American Diabetes Association
- CDC Diabetes Public Health Resource

INFORMATION FOR PATIENTS

- American Diabetes Association: What Is Hyperosmolar Hyperglycemic Nonketotic Syndrome (HHNS)?
- National Institutes of Health: Diabetic Hyperglycemic Hyperosmolar Coma
- Stevens LM. JAMA patient page: The ABCs of diabetes. JAMA. 2002; 287:2608. [PMID: 12025825]

REFERENCE

- American Diabetes Association. Hyperglycemic crises in patients with diabetes mellitus. Diabetes Care. 2001 Jan; 24(1):154–61. [PMID: 11221603]

Hyperkalemia

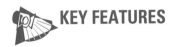 **KEY FEATURES**

ESSENTIALS OF DIAGNOSIS

- Serum potassium > 5.5 mEq/L
- ECG may be normal despite life-threatening hyperkalemia

GENERAL CONSIDERATIONS

- In acidosis, serum potassium concentration rises about 0.7 mEq/L for every decrease of 0.1 pH unit
- In the absence of acidosis
  - Serum potassium concentration rises about 1 mEq/L when there is a total body potassium excess of 1–4 mEq/kg
  - However, the higher the serum potassium concentration, the smaller the

excess necessary to raise the potassium levels further

- Hyperkalemia may develop with use of the following drugs, alone or in combination, even with normal renal function or only mild renal dysfunction
  - Angiotensin-converting enzyme (ACE) inhibitors
  - Angiotensin-receptor blockers
  - Potassium-sparing diuretics
- Life-threatening hyperkalemia can occur during combined therapy with ACE inhibitors and spironolactone or eplerenone, β-blockers
- Mild hyperkalemia that occurs in the absence of potassium-sparing drug therapy is usually due to type IV renal tubular acidosis
- Hyperkalemia occurs commonly in AIDS
  - Impaired renal excretion of potassium can be due to use of pentamidine or trimethoprim-sulfamethoxazole or to hyporeninemic hypoaldosteronism
  - An abnormality may occur in potassium redistribution between intracellular and extracellular compartments

Etiology

- **Spurious**
  - Leakage from erythrocytes, marked thrombocytosis or leukocytosis
  - Repeated fist clenching during phlebotomy
  - Specimen from arm with K⁺ infusion
- **Decreased excretion**
  - Renal failure
  - Renal secretory defects, eg, interstitial nephritis, sickle cell disease
  - Hyporeninemic hypoaldosteronism (type IV renal tubular acidosis), eg, diabetic nephropathy, heparin, AIDS; adrenal insufficiency
  - Drugs that inhibit K⁺ excretion (spironolactone, triamterene, ACE inhibitors, trimethoprim, nonsteroidal anti-inflammatory drugs)
- **Potassium shift out of cell**
  - Burns, rhabdomyolysis, hemolysis, severe infection, internal bleeding, vigorous exercise
  - Metabolic acidosis
  - Hypertonicity (solvent drag)
  - Insulin deficiency
  - Hyperkalemic periodic paralysis
  - Drugs: digitalis toxicity, β-adrenergic antagonists, succinylcholine, arginine
- **Excessive intake of K⁺**
  - Ingestion or iatrogenic

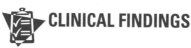

CLINICAL FINDINGS

SYMPTOMS AND SIGNS

- Frequently asymptomatic
- Muscle weakness and, rarely, flaccid paralysis
- Abdominal distention and diarrhea may occur

DIAGNOSIS

LABORATORY TESTS

- Measure plasma potassium rather than serum potassium to confirm that hyperkalemia is genuine
- Obtain serum electrolytes and creatinine
- Consider arterial blood gas

DIAGNOSTIC PROCEDURES

- ECG is not a sensitive method for detecting hyperkalemia, since nearly half of patients with a serum potassium level > 6.5 mEq/L will not manifest ECG changes

ECG Changes

- Peaked T waves
- Widening of the QRS complex
- Biphasic QRS–T complexes
- Inhibition of atrial depolarization despite normal conduction through usual pathways may occur
- Slow heart rate; ventricular fibrillation and cardiac arrest are terminal events

TREATMENT

MEDICATIONS

- Withhold potassium and give cation exchange resin (see Table 30)
- Glibenclamide can reverse severe hyperkalemia caused by such drugs as nicorandil, cyclosporine, isoflurane
- Emergent treatment is indicated if cardiac toxicity or muscular paralysis is present or if the hyperkalemia is severe (K⁺ > 6.5–7.0 mEq/L) even in the absence of ECG changes

THERAPEUTIC PROCEDURES

- Hemodialysis or peritoneal dialysis may be required to remove K⁺ in the presence of protracted kidney injury

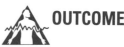

OUTCOME

FOLLOW-UP

- Monitor potassium frequently (q1–4h) during inpatient therapy for hyperkalemia

PROGNOSIS

- Depends on the underlying condition (renal failure)
- Drug-induced hyperkalemia is generally readily reversible with therapy

WHEN TO REFER

- Refer to a nephrologist if expertise is needed for treatment, particularly for emergent treatment or dialysis

WHEN TO ADMIT

- For serum potassium > 6.0 mEq/L
- For rapidly increasing serum potassium in the setting of acutely worsening comorbid condition (eg, acute renal failure, rhabdomyolysis)

PREVENTION

- Closely monitor serum potassium levels in patients with congestive heart failure and creatinine clearances < 30-60 mL/min who are treated with ACE inhibitors or potassium-sparing diuretics

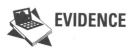

EVIDENCE

WEB SITE

- National Kidney Foundation

INFORMATION FOR PATIENTS

- Mayo Clinic: Hyperkalemia
- Mayo Clinic: Kidney Failure
- MedlinePlus: Hyperkalemia
- National Kidney and Urologic Diseases Information Clearinghouse: Renal Tubular Acidosis

REFERENCES

- de Denus S et al. Quantification of the risk and predictors of hyperkalemia in patients with left ventricular dysfunction: a retrospective analysis of the Studies of Left Ventricular Dysfunction (SOLVD) trials. Am Heart J. 2006 Oct; 152(4):705–12. [PMID: 16996842]
- Hebert LA. Optimizing ACE-inhibitor therapy for chronic kidney disease. N Engl J Med. 2006 Jan 12;354(2):189–91. [PMID: 16407515]

- Hollander-Rodriguez JC et al. Hyperkalemia. Am Fam Physician. 2006 Jan 15;73(2):283–90. [PMID: 16445274]
- Palmer BF. Managing hyperkalemia caused by inhibitors of the renin-angiotensin-aldosterone system. N Engl J Med. 2004 Aug 5;351(6):585–92. [PMID: 15295051]
- Singer M et al. Reversal of life-threatening, drug-related potassium-channel syndrome by glibenclamide. Lancet. 2005 May 28–Jun 3;365(9474):1873–5. [PMID: 15924984]

Hypernatremia

KEY FEATURES

ESSENTIALS OF DIAGNOSIS

- Serum sodium > 145 mEq/L
- Occurs most commonly when water intake is inadequate, eg, with altered mental status
- Urine osmolality helps determine whether the water loss is renal or nonrenal

GENERAL CONSIDERATIONS

- An intact thirst mechanism usually prevents hypernatremia
- Excess water loss can cause hypernatremia only when water intake is inadequate
- Rarely, excessive sodium intake may cause hypernatremia
- Hypernatremia in the presence of salt and water overload is uncommon but has been reported in very ill patients in the course of therapy

Etiology

- **Urine osmolality > 400 mosm/kg**
  - Nonrenal losses
    - Excessive sweating, burns
    - Insensible respiratory tract losses
    - Diarrhea, vomiting, nasogastric suctioning, osmotic cathartics (eg, lactulose)
  - Renal losses
    - Diuretics
    - Osmotic diuresis (eg, hyperglycemia, mannitol, urea)
    - Postobstructive diuresis
    - Diuretic phase of acute tubular necrosis
  - Hypertonic sodium gain
    - Salt intoxication (rare)
    - Hypertonic IV fluids, tube feeds, enema

- Primary hyperaldosteronism (hypernatremia usually mild and asymptomatic)
- **Urine osmolality < 250 mosm/kg**
  - Central diabetes insipidus: idiopathic, head trauma, CNS mass
  - Nephrogenic diabetes insipidus: lithium, demeclocycline, prolonged urinary tract infections, interstitial nephritis, hypercalcemia, hypokalemia, congenital

CLINICAL FINDINGS

SYMPTOMS AND SIGNS

- With dehydration, orthostatic hypotension and oliguria are typical findings
- Altered mental status
- With severe hyperosmolality, hyperthermia, delirium, and coma may be seen
- Symptoms in elderly may not be specific; recent change in consciousness is associated with poor prognosis

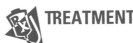

DIAGNOSIS

LABORATORY TESTS

- Urine osmolality > 400 mosm/kg when renal water-conserving ability is functioning
- Urine osmolality < 250 mosm/kg when renal water-conserving ability is impaired
- Serum osmolality invariably increased in the dehydrated state

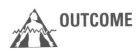

TREATMENT

MEDICATIONS

Type of fluid for replacement

- **Hypernatremia with hypovolemia**
  - Severe hypovolemia: give 0.9% saline (osmolality 308 mosm/kg) to restore volume deficit and treat hyperosmolality, followed by 0.45% saline to replace any remaining free water deficit
  - Milder hypovolemia: give 0.45% saline and 5% dextrose in water
- **Hypernatremia with euvolemia**
  - Encourage water drinking or give 5% dextrose and water to cause excretion of excess sodium in urine
  - If GFR is decreased, give diuretics to increase urinary sodium excretion; however, diuretics may impair renal concentrating ability, increasing

quantity of water that needs to be replaced
- **Hypernatremia with hypervolemia**
  - Give 5% dextrose in water to reduce hyperosmolality, though this will expand vascular volume
  - Administer loop diuretic (eg, furosemide, 0.5–1.0 mg/kg) IV to remove excess sodium
  - In severe renal injury, consider hemodialysis

Calculation of water deficit

- When calculating fluid replacement, add deficit and maintenance requirements to each 24-h replacement regimen
- **Acute hypernatremia**
  - In acute dehydration without much solute loss, free water loss is similar to weight loss
  - Initially, use 5% dextrose in water
  - As water deficit corrects, continue therapy with 0.45% saline with dextrose
- **Chronic hypernatremia**
  - Water deficit is calculated to restore normal osmolality for total body water (TBW)
  - Current TBW is 0.4–0.6 of current body weight
  - TBW correlates with muscle mass and therefore decreases with advancing age, cachexia, and dehydration and is lower in women than in men (Table 29)

THERAPEUTIC PROCEDURES

- Correct the cause of fluid loss, and replace water and, as needed, electrolytes
- Administer fluid therapy over 48-h period, aiming for decrease in serum sodium of 1 mEq/L/h (1 mmol/L/h)
- Add potassium and phosphate as indicated by serum levels; monitor other electrolytes often

OUTCOME

COMPLICATIONS

- If hypernatremia is too rapidly corrected, the osmotic imbalance may cause water to preferentially enter brain cells, causing cerebral edema and potentially severe neurologic impairment

WHEN TO REFER

- Severe hypernatremia, with serum Na$^+$ > 150 mEq/L

WHEN TO ADMIT

- Altered mental status

- Marked dehydation
- Hypernatremia with hypervolemia

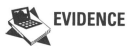

EVIDENCE

PRACTICE GUIDELINES

- American Medical Directors Association: Dehydration and Fluid Maintenance, 2001

WEB SITE

- Fall PJ. Hyponatremia and Hypernatremia: A Systematic Approach to Causes and Their Correction. Postgrad Med Online, 2000.

INFORMATION FOR PATIENTS

- MedlinePlus. Serum Sodium
- National Kidney and Urologic Diseases Information Clearinghouse: Diabetes Insipidus

REFERENCES

- Adrogue HJ et al. Hypernatremia. N Engl J Med. 2000 May 18;342(20):1493–9. [PMID: 10816188]
- Chassagne P et al. Clinical presentation of hypernatremia in elderly patients: a case control study. J Am Geriatr Soc. 2006 Aug;54(8):1225–30. [PMID: 16913989]
- Lin M et al. Disorders of water imbalance. Emerg Med Clin North Am. 2005 Aug;23(3):749–70. [PMID: 15982544]

Hyperpara-thyroidism

 KEY FEATURES

ESSENTIALS OF DIAGNOSIS

- Frequently incidentally detected by screening
- Renal stones, polyuria, hypertension, constipation, mental changes
- Bone pain
- Serum and urine calcium elevated; urine phosphate high with low or normal serum phosphate; alkaline phosphatase normal or elevated
- Elevated or high-normal serum parathyroid hormone (PTH) level

GENERAL CONSIDERATIONS

- Primary hyperparathyroidism
  - PTH hypersecretion usually due to parathyroid adenoma, less commonly hyperplasia or carcinoma (rare)
  - If age < 30 years, higher incidence of multiglandular disease (36%) and carcinoma (5%) responsible for hyperparathyroidism
- Secondary or tertiary hyperparathyroidism
  - Chronic renal failure: hyperphosphatemia and decreased renal vitamin D production decrease ionized calcium, thus stimulating the parathyroids
  - Renal osteodystrophy: bone disease of secondary hyperparathyroidism and renal failure
- Multiple endocrine neoplasia (MEN)
  - Parathyroid adenomas or hyperplasia can be familial (about 5%) and may be part of MEN types 1, 2A, and 2B
  - In MEN 1, multiglandular hyperparathyroidism is usually the initial manifestation and ultimately occurs in over 90% of affected individuals
  - Hyperparathyroidism in MEN 2A is less frequent that in MEN 1 and is usually milder
- Hyperparathyroidism-jaw tumor syndrome is autosomal dominant and associated with recurrent parathyroid ademonas (5% malignant), benign jaw tumors and renal cysts

DEMOGRAPHICS

- Incidence of primary hyperparathyroidism in adults is 0.1%
- More common in persons age > 50
- Ratio of M:F is 1:3

CLINICAL FINDINGS

SYMPTOMS AND SIGNS

- Frequently asymptomatic
- Symptoms include problems with "bones, stones, abdominal groans, psychic moans, fatigue"
- Bone pain and arthralgias are common
- Chronic cortical bone resorption due to excess PTH (osteitis fibrosa cystica) may cause pathologic fractures or cystic bone lesions (eg, "brown tumors" of jaw)
- Polyuria and polydipsia (from hypercalcemia-induced nephrogenic diabetes insipidus)
- Calcium-containing kidney stones
- Depression, intellectual weariness, and increased sleep requirement common

- Constipation, fatigue, anemia, weight loss, muscle weakness, pruritus, and paresthesias
- Anorexia, nausea, and vomiting in severe cases
- Hypertension
- Parathyroid adenomas rarely palpable; palpable mass usually a thyroid nodule
- Parathyroid carcinomas often palpable (50%)
- Pancreatitis occurs in 3%
- Psychosis or even coma in severe hypercalcemia
- Calcium phosphate deposition in corneas or soft tissues
- Jaw tumors in hyperparathyroidism-jaw tumor syndrome

DIFFERENTIAL DIAGNOSIS

- Hypercalcemia of malignancy
- Multiple myeloma
- Vitamin D intoxication
- Sarcoidosis, tuberculosis
- Hyperthyroidism
- Vitamin D deficiency (serum 25-OH Vit D < 20 ng/mL) can cause high serum PTH with normal serum calcium
- High-dose corticosteroid therapy in patients taking thiazide diuretics

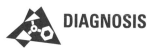 DIAGNOSIS

LABORATORY TESTS

- Serum calcium > 10.5 mg/dL
- Elevated or high-normal PTH confirms the diagnosis. Immunoradiometric assay (IRMA) is most specific and sensitive
- Serum phosphate often low (< 2.5 mg/dL)
- Serum phosphate high in secondary hyperparathyroidism (renal failure)
- Urine calcium excretion high or normal (average 250 mg/g creatinine), but low for degree of hypercalcemia
- Screen for familial benign hypocalciuric hypercalcemia with 24-h urine for calcium and creatinine. Discontinue thiazide diuretics prior to this test
- Urine phosphate high despite low to low normal serum phosphate
- Serum alkaline phosphatase elevated only if bone disease present
- Plasma chloride and uric acid may be elevated

IMAGING STUDIES

- Preoperative imaging may be unsuccessful due to small size of gland, but if successful, may allow limited surgery

- ^{99m}Tc-sestamibi/Tc-pertechnetate subtraction scintigraphy with SPECT recommended; has sensitivity of 87%, specificity 95%
- Neck ultrasound has sensitivity of 80%
- Combination of both tests has sensitivity of 94%, but sensitivity only 55% if multiglandular disease
- MRI and CT not as sensitive as ultrasound
- MRI or ultrasound for hyperparathyroidism reveals incidental small benign thyroid nodules in ~50%
- Bone radiographs
  - Usually normal and not required
  - However, may show demineralization, subperiosteal bone resorption, cysts throughout skeleton, mottling of skull, or pathologic fractures
- In renal osteodystrophy, bone radiographs may show
  - Ectopic calcifications around joints or soft tissue
  - Osteopenia
  - Osteitis fibrosa
  - Osteosclerosis
- Bone densitometry of wrist, hip, and spine

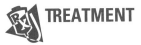 TREATMENT

MEDICATIONS

- Primary hyperparathyroidism
  - Intravenous bisphosphonates can temporarily treat hypercalcemia and relieve bone pain
  - Pamidronate, 30–90 mg IV over 2–4 h, or zoledronic acid, 2–4 mg IV over 15 min (expensive)
  - Oral bisphosphonates are ineffective
- Secondary or tertiary hyperparathyroidism of renal failure
  - Cinacalcet, 30–250 mg PO once daily, causes a drop of serum PTH levels to < 250 pg/mL in 41%
  - Paricalcitol, 0.04–0.1 mg/kg IV TIW, or doxercalciferol, 10 mg orally TIW after dialysis
    □ Increase to maximum of 20 mg TIW if PTH remains > 400 ng/L
    □ Hold for PTH < 100 ng/L
- Propranolol may prevent adverse cardiac effects of hypercalcemia
- Corticosteroid therapy is ineffective for hypercalcemia in hyperparathyroidism

SURGERY

- Parathyroidectomy for patients with symptomatic hyperparathyroidism, kidney stones, or bone disease

- Consider surgery for asymptomatic patients if
  - Serum calcium 1 mg/dL above normal if urine calcium excretion > 50 mg/24 h
  - Urine calcium > 400 mg/24 h
  - Cortical bone density > 2 SD below normal
  - Age < 50–60 years
  - Difficulty ensuring medical follow-up
  - Pregnancy (second trimester)
- Minimally invasive parathyroid surgery usually sufficient if adenoma identified preoperatively
- Subtotal parathyroidectomy ($3^1/_2$ glands removed) for patients with resistant parathyroid hyperplasia

THERAPEUTIC PROCEDURES

- Patients with mild, asymptomatic hyperparathyroidism are advised to
  - Keep active
  - Drink adequate fluids
  - Avoid immobilization
  - Avoid thiazides, large doses of vitamins D and A, calcium-containing antacids or supplements, and digitalis (hypercalcemia predisposes to toxicity)

 OUTCOME

FOLLOW-UP

- In mild, asymptomatic hyperparathyroidism, check
  - Serum calcium and albumin twice yearly
  - Renal function and urine calcium once yearly
  - Bone density (distal radius) every 2 years
- Postoperatively
  - Keep patients hospitalized overnight
  - Monitor serum calcium and PTH
  - Oral calcium and calcitriol 0.25 mg/day for 2 weeks helps prevent tetany
  - Treat symptomatic hypocalcemia with oral calcium carbonate and calcitriol 0.25–1.0 mcg PO once daily
  - Secondary hyperparathyroidism occurs in ~12% and is treated with calcium and vitamin D, usually for 3–6 months
  - Hyperthyroidism immediately following parathyroid surgery may require short-term propranolol

COMPLICATIONS

- Forearm and hip fractures
- Urinary tract infection due to obstruction by stones

- Confusion, renal failure, and soft tissue calcinosis from rapidly rising serum calcium
- Renal osteodystrophy from hyperphosphatemia
- Peptic ulcer and pancreatitis
- Pseudogout before or after surgery
- Disseminated calcification in skin, soft tissues, and arteries (calciphylaxis) can result in gangrene, arrhythmias, and respiratory failure

PROGNOSIS

- Asymptomatic mild hypercalcemia does not affect survival
- Resection of sporadic parathyroid adenoma generally results in cure
- Bones, despite severe cyst formation or fracture, heal if parathyroid tumor removed
- Significant renal damage may progress even after adenoma removal
- Parathyroid carcinoma tends to invade local structures and may metastasize; repeat surgical resections and radiation therapy can prolong life

WHEN TO REFER

- Refer to parathyroid surgeon for parathyroidectomy

WHEN TO ADMIT

- Patients with severe hypercalcemia for IV hydration

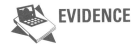 EVIDENCE

PRACTICE GUIDELINES

- Malone JP et al. Hyperparathyroidism and multiple endocrine neoplasia. Otolaryngol Clin North Am. 2004;37:715. [PMID: 15262511]

WEB SITES

- Allerheiligen D et al. Hyperthyroidism. American Family Physician, 1998.
- National Institute of Diabetes and Digestive and Kidney Diseases (NIDDK)

INFORMATION FOR PATIENTS

- American Academy of Family Physicians—Hyperparathyroidism

REFERENCES

- Block GA et al. Cinacalcet for secondary hyperparathyroidism in patients receiving hemodialysis. N Engl J Med. 2004

Apr 8;350(15):1516–25. [PMID: 15071126]

- Coburn JW et al. Doxercalciferol safely suppresses PTH levels in patients with secondary hyperparathyroidism associated with chronic kidney disease stages 3 and 4. Am J Kidney Dis. 2004 May; 43(5):877–90. [PMID: 15112179]
- Grey A et al. Vitamin D repletion in patients with primary hyperparathyroidism and coexistent vitamin D insufficiency. J Clin Endocrinol Metab. 2005 Apr;90(4):2122–6. [PMID: 15644400]
- Lambert LA et al. Surgical treatment of hyperparathyroidism in patients with multiple endocrine neoplasia type 1. Arch Surg. 2005 Apr;140(4):374–82. [PMID: 15841561]
- Peacock M et al. Cinacalcet hydrochloride maintains long-term normocalcemia in patients with primary hyperparathyroidism. J Clin Endocrinol Metab. 2005 Jan;90(1):135–41. [PMID: 15522938]
- Rao DS et al. Randomized controlled clinical trial of surgery versus no surgery in patients with mild asymptomatic primary hyperparathyroidism. J Clin Endocrinol Metab. 2004 Nov; 89(11):5415–22. [PMID: 15531491]

Hyperphosphatemia

 KEY FEATURES

- Serum phosphate > 4.5 mg/dL (> 1.45 mmol/L)
- Main cause is advanced chronic kidney disease (CKD) with insufficient urinary excretion of phosphorus
- Inadequately treated hyperphosphatemia in CKD leads to
  - Secondary hyperparathyroidism
  - Renal osteodystrophy
  - Extraosseous calcification of soft tissues

 CLINICAL FINDINGS

- Symptoms are those of the underlying disorders (eg, CKD, hypoparathyroidism)
- An elevated serum phosphate level in patients who have had prior MI

increases risk of cardiovascular events and death

 DIAGNOSIS

- Serum phosphate > 4.5 mg/dL (> 1.45 mmol/L)
- Other blood chemistry values are those of the underlying disease

 TREATMENT

- Treatment is that of the underlying disorder and of associated hypocalcemia if present
- In acute kidney injury and CKD, dialysis will reduce serum phosphate
- Phosphate binders (eg, calcium carbonate and sevelamer hydrochloride) reduce phosphate absorption
- Calcium carbonate
  - Administer 0.5–1.5 g PO TID with meals (500-mg tablets)
  - Preferred to aluminum hydroxide because of concerns about aluminum toxicity
- Sevelamer hydrochloride
  - Administer 800–1600 mg PO TID with meals (400- to 800-mg tablets and 403-mg capsules)
  - Does not contain calcium or aluminum and may be especially useful in hypercalcemia

Hyperprolactinemia

 KEY FEATURES

ESSENTIALS OF DIAGNOSIS

- Women
  - Menstrual cycle disturbances (oligomenorrhea, amenorrhea)
  - Galactorrhea
  - Infertility
  - Gynecomastia
- Men
  - Hypogonadism
  - Decreased libido and erectile dysfunction
  - Infertility

- CT scan or MRI often demonstrates pituitary adenoma

GENERAL CONSIDERATIONS

- Prolactin's main role is to induce lactation
- During pregnancy, prolactin increases from normal (< 20 ng/mL) to as high as 600 ng/mL
- Suckling stimulates continued production of prolactin
- Prolactin is mainly under inhibitory control by dopamine
- Elevated serum prolactin can be caused by numerous conditions
- Most prolactinomas are microadenomas (< 1 cm in diameter) that usually do not grow, even with pregnancy or oral contraceptives
- However, macroadenomas occur and can spread into cavernous sinuses, suprasellar areas, and rarely into sinsuses by eroding the sella floor

DEMOGRAPHICS

- Prolactin-secreting pituitary tumors more common in women
- Usually sporadic but rarely familial as part of multiple endocrine neoplasia type 1 (MEN-1)

 CLINICAL FINDINGS

SYMPTOMS AND SIGNS

- Hypogonadotropic hypogonadism
  - Men
    - Erectile dysfunction
    - Diminished libido
    - Sometimes gynecomastia, but never galactorrhea
  - Women
    - May have oligomenorrhea or amenorrhea, infertility, galactorrhea
    - 70% of women with secondary amenorrhea and galactorrhea have hyperprolactinemia
- Large pituitary tumors may cause headaches, visual field abnormalities
- Pituitary prolactinomas
  - May co-secrete growth hormone and cause acromegaly
  - Large tumors may cause
    - Pituitary insufficiency (hypogonadism)
    - Hypothyroidism
    - Adrenal insufficiency
    - Growth hormone deficiency

DIFFERENTIAL DIAGNOSIS

- Increased pituitary size is a normal variant in young women
- About 10% of hyperprolactinemic patients secrete macroprolactin, a relatively inactive "big prolactin"; pituitary MRI is normal in 78% of cases
- See Galactorrhea

DIAGNOSIS

LABORATORY TESTS

- Serum prolactin: If elevated, discontinue medications that increase prolactin, if possible, and recheck prolactin in a few weeks
- Urine or serum human chorionic gonadotropin to rule out pregnancy
- Serum thyroid-stimulating hormone high if hypothyroidism is cause
- Renal and liver chemistries abnormal in renal failure or cirrhosis
- Serum calcium elevated in hyperparathyroidism (MEN-1)
- Consider assay for macroprolactinemia if asymptomatic patient with no apparent cause for hyperprolactinemia
- Prolactin assay with serial dilutions in patients with macroprolactinomas (> 1 cm diameter)

IMAGING STUDIES

- MRI of pituitary and hypothalamus indicated for nonpregnant patients
  - With prolactin > 200 mg/dL
  - With headaches or visual field defects
  - With persistently elevated prolactin with no discernible cause
- Small prolactinomas may be demonstrated, but clear differentiation from normal variants not always possible

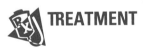

TREATMENT

MEDICATIONS

- Medical therapy is preferable, particularly for huge "macroprolactinomas"
- Dopamine agonists are initial treatment of choice and to restore normal sexual function and fertility
- Cabergoline
  - 0.25 mg PO once weekly for 1 week
  - Then, 0.25 mg twice weekly for 1 week
  - Then, 0.5 mg twice weekly

- Further increases may be required monthly, up to 1.5 mg twice weekly, based on serum prolactin
- Bromocriptine, 1.25–20.0 mg/day PO, is an alternative
- Quinagolide is a dopamine agonist for patients intolerant of or resistant to other agents
  - Not available in the United States
  - Dose: start at 0.075 mg/day PO, up to 0.6 mg/day
- Give dopamine agonists at bedtime to minimize side effects (fatigue, nausea, and orthostatic hypotension), which usually improve with dosage reduction and continued use
  - Psychiatric side effects occur, are not dose related, and may take weeks to resolve after dopamine agonist is discontinued
- Treat hypothyroidism with thyroxine
- Oral contraceptives or estrogen replacement
  - Safe for women with microprolactinomas who have amenorrhea or wish contraception
  - Minimal risk of stimulating adenoma enlargement
- Estrogens and testosterone
  - Can stimulate macroprolactinomas
  - Should not be used unless in full remission with medication or surgery

SURGERY

- Transsphenoidal resection may be urgently required for large tumors severely compromising visual fields or undergoing apoplexy
- Transsphenoidal selective resection of the pituitary adenoma is done electively for patients who fail dopamine agonists
- Craniotomy rarely indicated

THERAPEUTIC PROCEDURES

- Radiation therapy is reserved for macroadenomas that are growing despite medical therapy
- Focused radiation therapy with gamma knife or cyber knife is preferable
- Conventional radiation therapy carries high risk of eventual hypopituitarism and may also cause memory impairment, second tumors, and small-vessel ischemic strokes
- After radiation therapy, patients should take low-dose aspirin for life to reduce risk of stroke

OUTCOME

FOLLOW-UP

- Women with microadenomas may have dopamine agonists safely withdrawn during pregnancy
- Macroadenomas may enlarge during pregnancy; if therapy is withdrawn, they must be followed up clinically and with computer-assisted visual field perimetry
- After pituitary surgery or radiation, monitor serum prolactin every 3 months

COMPLICATIONS

- Macroadenomas can impair visual fields and cause hypopituitarism
- Untreated hypogonadism increases risk of osteoporosis

PROGNOSIS

- Fertility is usually promptly restored with dopamine agonists
- Discontinuing dopamine agonists after months or years usually results in reappearance of hyperprolactinemia, galactorrhea, and amenorrhea
- With dopamine agonist treatment for prolactinoma
  - Nearly half—even massive tumors— shrink by > 50%
  - Shrinkage of pituitary adenoma occurs early, but maximum effect may take up to a year
  - 90% have fall in serum prolactin to ≤ 10% pretreatment levels; 80% achieve normal serum prolactin level

EVIDENCE

PRACTICE GUIDELINES

- Leung AK et al. Diagnosis and management of galactorrhea. Am Fam Physician. 2004;70:543. [PMID: 15317441]
- Liu JK et al. Contemporary management of prolactinomas. Neurosurg Focus. 2004;16:E2. [PMID: 15191331]

WEB SITE

- E-Medicine Review Article

INFORMATION FOR PATIENTS

- NIDDK—Prolactinoma

REFERENCES

- Colao A et al. Outcome of cabergoline treatment in men with prolactinoma: effects of a 24-month treatment on prolactin levels, tumor mass, recovery of pituitary function, and semen analysis. J Clin Endocrinol Metab. 2004 Apr; 89(4):1704–11. [PMID: 15070934]

- Delgrange E. Cabergoline and mitral regurgitation. N Engl J Med. 2006 Jan 26;354(4):420. [PMID: 16436779]
- Gibney J et al. The impact on clinical practice of routine screening for macro-prolactin. J Clin Endocrinol Metab. 2005 Jul;90(7):3927–32. [PMID: 15811931]
- Haddad PM et al. Antipsychotic-induced hyperprolactinaemia: mechanisms, clinical features and management. Drugs. 2004;64(20):2291–314. [PMID: 15456328]
- Molitch ME. Medication-induced hyperprolactinemia. Mayo Clin Proc. 2005 Aug;80(8):1050–7. [PMID: 16092584]
- Sodi R et al. Testosterone replacement-induced hyperprolactinaemia: case report and review of the literature. Ann Clin Biochem. 2005 Mar;42(Pt 2):153–9. [PMID: 15829128]

Hypertension, Chronic

KEY FEATURES

ESSENTIALS OF DIAGNOSIS

- Usually asymptomatic
- Severe hypertension: occipital headache at awakening, blurry vision

GENERAL CONSIDERATIONS

- Mild to moderate hypertension nearly always asymptomatic
- Severe hypertension usually due to
  - Parenchymal renal disease
  - Endocrine abnormalities
  - Renal artery stenosis
  - Drug use
  - Abrupt cessation of antihypertensive medications
- Table 13 provides classification based on blood pressure (BP) measurements
- Resistant hypertension is defined as failure to reach BP control in patients adherent to full doses of a three-drug regimen (including a diuretic)
- Table 14 summarizes reasons for failure to reach BP control

DEMOGRAPHICS

- 66 million Americans affected
- 63% are aware of their condition
- 45% of those aware are receiving treatment
- 34% of all hypertensive patients have BP under control
- Incidence of hypertension increases with age
- More men than women in early life
- More women than men later in life
- More common in black Americans (up to 25%)

CLINICAL FINDINGS

SYMPTOMS AND SIGNS

- Usually asymptomatic
- Headaches are most frequent symptom but are nonspecific
- Elevated BP
- Loud A_2 on cardiac examination
- Retinal arteriolar narrowing with "silver-wiring," arteriovenous nicking
- Flame-shaped hemorrhages
- Laboratory findings usually normal

DIFFERENTIAL DIAGNOSIS

Primary (essential) hypertension
- "White-coat" hypertension
- BP cuff too small

Secondary hypertension
- Adrenal
  - Primary hyperaldosteronism
  - Cushing's syndrome
  - Pheochromocytoma
- Renal
  - Chronic renal disease
  - Renal artery stenosis (atherosclerotic or fibromuscular dysplasia)
- Other
  - Oral contraceptives
  - Alcohol
  - Nonsteroidal anti-inflammatory drugs
  - Pregnancy associated
  - Hypercalcemia
  - Hyperthyroidism
  - Obstructive sleep apnea
  - Obesity
  - Coarctation of the aorta
  - Acromegaly
  - Increased intracranial pressure
  - Cocaine or amphetamine use

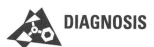 DIAGNOSIS

LABORATORY TESTS

- Urinalysis
- Serum creatinine, blood urea nitrogen
- Serum potassium
- Fasting blood glucose
- Cholesterol
- Hemoglobin
- Serum uric acid
- ECG
- When a secondary cause is suspected, consider
  - Chest radiograph
  - ECG
  - Plasma metanephrine levels
  - Plasma aldosterone concentration, plasma renin activity
  - Urine electrolytes

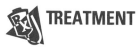 TREATMENT

MEDICATIONS

- Initiation of drug therapy based on level of BP, presence of target end-organ damage (Table 15), and overall cardiovascular risk profile: Figure 3
- Major risk factors include
  - Smoking
  - Dyslipidemia
  - Diabetes mellitus
  - Age > 60 years
  - Family history of cardiovascular disease
- Diuretics: Table 16
- β-Adrenergic blocking agents: Table 17
- Angiotensin-converting enzyme (ACE) inhibitors and angiotensin receptor blockers: Table 18
- Calcium channel-blocking agents: Table 19
- α-Adrenergic blockers, vasodilators, centrally acting agents: Table 20

THERAPEUTIC PROCEDURES

- Dietary changes (DASH diet): high in fruits and vegetables, low fat, low salt
- Weight reduction
- Alcohol restriction
- Salt reduction
- Adequate potassium intake
- Adequate calcium intake
- Increase physical activity
- Smoking cessation

- Aggressive risk factor management, including use of a statin, should be considered in all patients with hypertension
- Choice of antihypertensive medications determined by presence of compelling indications: Table 15
- Treatment strategies for persons with diabetics and hypertension and patients with chronic renal disease
  - Lower target BP of < 130/80 mm Hg, given high risk of cardiovascular events
  - Include ACE inhibitors or angiotensin receptor blockers as part of regimen
- In absence of compelling indications, choice of antihypertensive regimen guided by demographics and synergy (Figure 4)

 OUTCOME

FOLLOW-UP

- Frequent visits until BP is controlled
- Once controlled, visits can be infrequent, limited laboratory tests
- Lipid monitoring every year
- ECG every 2–4 years, depending on initial ECG

COMPLICATIONS

- Stroke
- Dementia
- Myocardial infarction
- Congestive heart failure
- Retinal vasculopathy
- Aortic dissection
- Renal disease, including proteinuria and nephrosclerosis

WHEN TO REFER

- If BP remains uncontrolled after three concurrent medications
- If patient has uncontrolled BP and symptoms and signs of end-organ damage

WHEN TO ADMIT

- Consider hospitalization if patient has very high BP and symptoms and signs of a hypertensive emergency (see Hypertensive Urgencies & Emergencies) including
  - Severe headache
  - Neurologic symptoms
  - Chest pain
  - Altered mental status
  - Acutely worsening renal failure

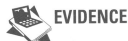 **EVIDENCE**

PRACTICE GUIDELINES

- Seventh report of the Joint National Committee on Prevention, Detection, Evaluation, and Treatment of High Blood Pressure. 2003.

WEB SITES

- American College of Cardiology
- American Society for Hypertension
- National Heart, Lung, and Blood Institute

INFORMATION FOR PATIENTS

- American Academy of Family Physicians: High Blood Pressure: Things You Can Do to Help Lower Yours
- American Heart Association: High Blood Pressure
- MedlinePlus: Hypertension Interactive Tutorial
- National Heart, Lung, and Blood Institute: High Blood Pressure
- National Heart, Lung, and Blood Institute: Your Guide to Lowering High Blood Pressure

REFERENCES

- Chobanian AV. Prehypertension revisited. Hypertension. 2006 Nov; 48(5):812–4. [PMID: 16982962]
- Chobanian AV et al. The Seventh Report of the Joint National Committee on prevention, detection, evaluation and treatment of high blood pressure: the JNC 7 report. JAMA. 2003; 289:2560. [PMID: 12748199]
- Cohen JD. Managing hypertension: state of the science. J Clin Hypertens (Greenwich). 2006 Oct;8(10 Suppl 3):5–11. [PMID: 17028478]
- Epstein M. Resistant hypertension: prevalence and evolving concepts. J Clin Hypertens (Greenwich). 2007 Jan;9(1 Suppl 1):2–6. [PMID: 17215648]
- Hemmelgarn BR et al. The 2006 Canadian Hypertension Education Program recommendations for the management of hypertension: Part I—Blood pressure measurement, diagnosis and assessment of risk. Can J Cardiol. 2006 May 15; 22(7):573–81. [PMID: 16755312]
- Khan NA et al. The 2006 Canadian Hypertension Education Program recommendations for the management of hypertension: Part II—Therapy. Can J Cardiol. 2006 May 15;22(7):583–93. [PMID: 16755313]
- Williams B et al; British Hypertension Society. Guidelines for management of hypertension: report of the fourth working party of the British Hypertension Society, 2004-BHS IV. J Hum Hypertens. 2004 Mar;18(3):139–85. [PMID: 14973512]

Hypertensive Urgencies & Emergencies

 KEY FEATURES

ESSENTIALS OF DIAGNOSIS

- Hypertensive crisis is typically defined as systolic blood pressure (BP) > 220 mm Hg or diastolic BP > 125 mm Hg
- However, the development of acute end organ damage depends on
  - Rate of rise in BP
  - Magnitude of increase in BP
  - Presence of underlying conditions

GENERAL CONSIDERATIONS

- Hypertensive urgency usually has systolic BP > 220 mm Hg or diastolic BP > 125 mm Hg without evidence of acute end-organ damage
- Hypertensive emergency defined as acute hypertensive injury to heart, brain, retina, kidneys, aorta and/or eclampsia
- Malignant hypertension typically occurs in the context of renal disease and is characterized by hemolysis and platelet consumption due to fibrinoid necrosis in arterioles

DEMOGRAPHICS

- Occurs in any age, gender, or racial/ethnic group
- Usually occurs in people with preexisting hypertension
- Often due to abrupt cessation of antihypertensive therapy
- Also occurs in setting of acute renal failure or use of high doses of sympathomimetics

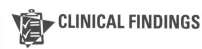

CLINICAL FINDINGS

SYMPTOMS AND SIGNS

- Symptoms depend on the end organ involved
- Headaches, irritability, confusion, and somnolence are signs of encephalopathy
- Chest pain or dyspnea occurs with cardiopulmonary involvement
- Back pain occurs with aortic dissection
- Blurry or diminished vision occurs with retinal involvement
- Cardiac examination may reveal low A_2, an S_4, or a murmur of aortic regurgitation
- Papilledema is indicative of elevated intracranial pressure
- Crackles on lung examination occur with congestive heart failure

DIFFERENTIAL DIAGNOSIS

- Any of the many causes of hypertension can lead to severe hypertension (see Hypertension, Chronic)
- The underlying causes most likely to present in this way include
  - Poorly controlled or undiagnosed hypertension
  - Withdrawal from antihypertensive medications
  - Chronic kidney disease
  - Renal artery stenosis (atherosclerotic or fibromuscular dysplasia)
  - Sympathomimetic drug use
  - Scleroderma crisis
  - Pheochromocytoma

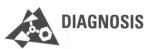

DIAGNOSIS

LABORATORY TESTS

- Complete blood cell count (microangiopathic smear with thrombocytopenia due to platelet consumption)
- Urinalysis
- Serum creatinine, blood urea nitrogen, troponin, creatine kinase
- ECG
- Chest radiograph
- Consider urine screen for cocaine

DIAGNOSTIC PROCEDURES

- If CNS symptoms, head CT to rule out bleed/infarct
- If chest pain, ECG (to rule out coronary syndrome), chest radiograph (thoracic aortic dissection)
- If renal dysfunction, renal ultrasound to rule out obstruction or chronic kidney disease

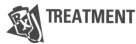

TREATMENT

MEDICATIONS

Hypertensive urgency

- Goal is to relieve symptoms and bring BP to reasonable level within 24–48 hours, aiming for gradual attainment of optimal control over several weeks
- Clonidine, captopril, metoprolol, and hydralazine are effective oral agents
- Avoid β-blockers if cocaine use
- Avoid angiotensin-converting enzyme (ACE) inhibitors if renal artery stenosis suspected
- Avoid short-acting dihydropyridine calcium channel blockers because BP reduction is often precipitous

Hypertensive emergency

- Treatment goal is to reduce mean arterial pressure by 25% in 1–2 h; then to reduce BP to 160/100 mm Hg over next 6–12 h
- If ischemic stroke, only treat if BP exceeds 220/120 mm Hg; aim to reduce by only 10–15%
- If thrombolytic agents are to be used to treat ischemic stroke, target BP is < 185/110 mm Hg
- Avoid excessive reduction in BP because this can lead to coronary, cerebral, or renal hypoperfusion
- Key to pharmacologic therapy is to use an agent with predictable, dose-dependent, transient effect
- Nitroprusside, labetalol, and nitroglycerin are most commonly used intravenously
- Fenoldopam, a peripheral dopamine agonist, is also effective
- ACE inhibitors are specifically indicated in scleroderma crisis

THERAPEUTIC PROCEDURES

- Treatment algorithm differs for hypertensive urgency and hypertensive emergency
- Goal is similar: reduce BP to "safe" range without causing end-organ damage
- Table 21 lists treatment options for hypertensive emergencies and urgencies
- In women who are pregnant or of childbearing age, preeclampsia or eclampsia should be excluded; if diagnosed, proper management plans should be instituted promptly

OUTCOME

FOLLOW-UP

- Patients with hypertensive urgency whose BP is brought under control should be seen within 48–72 h for a recheck of BP and tolerability of the antihypertensive regimen
- Patients with hypertensive emergency, once discharged from the hospital, should be followed-up in 48–72 h to ensure good compliance with BP medication and adequate BP control

COMPLICATIONS

- Stroke
- Myocardial infarction
- Congestive heart failure
- Retinal vasculopathy
- Aortic dissection
- Renal failure

WHEN TO REFER

- Refer patients with hypertensive urgency or emergency to expert in management of severe hypertension
- Hypertensive crises in pregnancy must be managed by expert in high-risk obstetrics

WHEN TO ADMIT

- Hospitalization for hypertensive urgency rarely needed
- Hospitalize all patients with hypertensive emergency, in particular patients with following
  - Encephalopathy
  - Neurologic deficits
  - Chest pain
  - Dyspnea
  - Papilledema
  - Hematuria
  - Renal dysfunction
  - ECG changes
  - Eclampsia
- Usually such patients need ICU admission for close monitoring of BP and clinical symptoms and signs

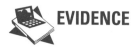

EVIDENCE

PRACTICE GUIDELINES

- American College of Obstetricians and Gynecologists. ACOG practice bulletin. Diagnosis and management of preeclampsia and eclampsia. Number 33, January 2002. Int J Gynaecol Obstet. 2002;77:67. [PMID: 12094777]

- Seventh report of the Joint National Committee on Prevention, Detection, Evaluation, and Treatment of High Blood Pressure. 2003.

WEB SITES

- American College of Cardiology
- Bales A. Hypertensive Crisis. Postgraduate Medicine Online 1999
- National Heart, Lung, and Blood Institute

INFORMATION FOR PATIENTS

- Mayo Clinic: Hypertensive Crisis
- MedlinePlus: Hypertension Interactive Tutorial

REFERENCES

- Flanigan JS et al. Hypertensive emergency and severe hypertension: what to treat, who to treat, and how to treat. Med Clin North Am. 2006 May; 90(3):439–51. [PMID: 16473099]
- Khanna A et al. Malignant hypertension presenting as hemolysis, thrombocytopenia, and renal failure. Rev Cardiovasc Med. 2003 Fall;4(4):255–9. [PMID: 14674379]
- Migneco A et al. Hypertensive crises: diagnosis and management in the emergency room. Eur Rev Med Pharmacol Sci. 2004 Jul–Aug;8(4):143–52. [PMID: 15636400]

Hyperthermia

KEY FEATURES

- A rapidly life-threatening complication
- May be due to poisoning by
  - Amphetamines (including ecstasy)
  - Atropine and other anticholinergic drugs
  - Cocaine
  - Salicylates
  - Strychnine
  - Tricyclic antidepressants
- Common causes
  - Multiple or prolonged seizures
  - Muscle hyperactivity
- Overdose of serotonin reuptake inhibitors (eg, fluoxetine, paroxetine) alone or combined with monoamine oxidase inhibitor may cause agitation, hyperactivity, hyperthermia (**serotonin syndrome**)
- Haloperidol and other antipsychotic agents can cause rigidity and hyperthermia (**neuroleptic malignant syndrome**)
- **Malignant hyperthermia** is associated with general anesthetic agents (rare)

 CLINICAL FINDINGS

- Severe hyperthermia (temperature > 40–41°C) may rapidly cause brain damage and multiorgan failure
- Rhabdomyolysis with elevated serum creatine kinase levels
- Metabolic acidosis
- Coagulopathy

 TREATMENT

- Remove clothing
- Spray with tepid water
- Fan patient
- Induce neuromuscular paralysis with nondepolarizing neuromuscular blocker (eg, vecuronium)
  - If rectal temperature not normal in 30–60 min
  - If there is significant muscle rigidity or hyperactivity
- Once paralyzed, patient must be intubated and mechanically ventilated
- With seizures, absence of visible muscular convulsive movements may give false impression that brain seizure activity has ceased; this must be confirmed by EEG
- Dantrolene
  - Give 2–5 mg/kg IV
  - May be effective for muscle rigidity unresponsive to neuromuscular blockade (ie, **malignant hyperthermia**)
- Bromocriptine, 2.5–7.5 mg PO daily, for **neuroleptic malignant syndrome**
- Cyproheptadine, 4 mg PO every hour for 3–4 doses, for **serotonin syndrome**

Hyperthyroidism

 KEY FEATURES

ESSENTIALS OF DIAGNOSIS

- Weight loss, heat intolerance, menstrual irregularity, tachycardia, tremor, stare
- In Graves' disease
  - Goiter (often with bruit)
  - Ophthalmopathy
- In primary hyperthyroidism
  - Increased free thyroxine (T_4) and triiodothyronine (T_3)
  - Low thyroid-stimulating hormone (TSH)

GENERAL CONSIDERATIONS

- Causes
  - Graves' disease (most common)
  - Autonomous toxic adenomas, single or multiple
  - Subacute de Quervain's thyroiditis: hyperthyroidism followed by hypothyroidism
  - Jodbasedow disease, or iodine-induced hyperthyroidism, may occur with multinodular goiters after significant iodine intake, radiographic contrast, or drugs, eg, amiodarone
  - Amiodarone-induced hyperthyroidism: can occur 4 months to 3 years after initiation of therapy and after discontinuation
  - Thyrotoxicosis factitia: excessive exogenous thyroid hormone
  - Hashimoto's thyroiditis may cause transient hyperthyroidism during initial phase and may occur postpartum
  - High serum human chorionic gonadotropin levels in first 4 months of pregnancy, molar pregnancy, choriocarcinoma, and testicular malignancies may cause thyrotoxicosis

CLINICAL FINDINGS

SYMPTOMS AND SIGNS

- Heat intolerance, sweating
- Frequent bowel movements
- Weight loss (or gain)
- Menstrual irregularities
- Nervousness, fine resting tremor
- Fatigue, weakness
- Muscle cramps, hyperreflexia
- Thyroid
  - Goiter (often with a bruit) in Graves' disease
  - Moderately enlarged, tender thyroid in subacute thyroiditis
- Eye
  - Upper eyelid retraction
  - Stare and lid lag
  - Ophthalmopathy (chemosis, conjunctivitis, and mild proptosis) in 20–40% of patients with Graves' disease
  - Diplopia may be due to coexistent myasthenia gravis

- Skin
  - Moist warm skin
  - Fine hair
  - Onycholysis
  - Dermopathy (myxedema) in 3% of patients with Graves' disease
- Heart
  - Palpitations or angina pectoris
  - Arrhythmias
    □ Sinus tachycardia
    □ Premature atrial contractions
    □ Atrial fibrillation or atrial tachycardia
  - Thyrotoxic cardiomyopathy due to thyrotoxicosis
  - (Rarely) heart failure
- Thyroid storm
- Hypokalemic paralysis (Asian or Native-American men)

DIFFERENTIAL DIAGNOSIS

- General anxiety, panic disorder, mania
- Other hypermetabolic state, eg, cancer, pheochromocytoma
- Exophthalmos due to other cause, eg, orbital tumor
- Atrial fibrillation due to other cause
- Acute psychiatric disorders (may falsely increase serum thyroxine)
- High estrogen states, eg, pregnancy
- Hypopituitarism
- Subclinical hyperthyroidism

 DIAGNOSIS

LABORATORY TESTS

- Sensitive TSH assay best test for thyrotoxicosis
- Serum T_3 and free T_4 usually increased
- T_4 sometimes normal but T_3 elevated
- Serum FT_3 (rather than T_3) in women, pregnant or taking oral estrogen
- Hypercalcemia
- Alkaline phosphatase increased
- Anemia, neutropenia
- Antibodies increased in most patients with Graves' disease include
  - TSH-R Ab[stim]
  - Antinuclear antibody (ANA)
  - Antithyroperoxidase or antithyroglobulin antibodies
  - ANA and anti-double-stranded DNA antibodies
- Erythrocyte sedimentation rate often elevated in subacute thyroiditis
- TSH elevated or normal despite thyrotoxicosis in TSH-secreting pituitary tumor

- Suppressed TSH and total T_4 > 20 mcg/dL or T_3 > 200 ng/dL to diagnose amiodarone-induced hyperthyroidism because high total T_4 and free T_4 common on amiodarone
- Type I amiodarone-induced thyrotoxicosis, diagnosable by elevated serum levels of thyroperoxidase Ab and TSH-R Ab

IMAGING STUDIES

- Thyroid radioactive iodine scan
  - Usually indicated for hyperthyroidism
  - High ^{123}I uptake in Graves' disease and toxic nodular goiter
  - Scan can detect toxic nodule or multinodular goiter
  - Low uptake characteristic of subacute thyroiditis and amiodarone-induced hyperthyroidism
- Color-flow Doppler: increased blood flow in type I and lower blood flow in type II amiodarone induced thyrotoxicosis
- Thyroid ultrasound can detect multinodular goiter

 TREATMENT

MEDICATIONS

Graves' disease
- Propranolol
  - 20 mg PO BID initially
  - Increase to 20–80 mg QID until improved tachycardia, tremor, diaphoresis, and anxiety
  - May then use propranolol LA 60–160 mg PO BID
  - Continue until hyperthyroidism resolved
- Thioureas (methimazole or propylthiouracil [PTU])
  - Generally used for
    □ Young adults
    □ Those with mild thyrotoxicosis, small goiters, or fear of radioiodine
    □ Preparing patients for surgery and elderly patients for ^{131}I treatment
  - Methimazole, 10–30 mg PO BID, reduce dose and give once daily as symptoms resolve and free T_4 normalizes
  - Methimazole preferred over PTU (rarely causes acute hepatic necrosis)
  - During pregnancy, use low doses of methimazole (5–15 mg/d) or PTU (50–150 mg/d) to avoid fetal hypothyroidism
  - During lactation, doses are methimazole, ≤ 20 mg/d, and PTU, ≤ 450 mg/d, taken just after breast-feeding

- Methimazole may be used long-term
- Agranulocytosis is an uncommon but serious complication
- Goiter occurs if prolonged hypothyroidism is allowed to develop in patient taking thioureas, but usually regresses rapidly with thyroid hormone replacement
- PTU, 300–600 mg PO divided QID, reduce dose and frequency as symptoms resolve and free T_4 normalizes
- Iodinated contrast agents (iopanoic acid [Telepaque] or ipodate sodium [Bilivist, Oragrafin])
  - 500 mg PO once or twice daily
  - Begin after thiourea is started

Subacute thyroiditis
- Propranolol for symptoms as above
- Ipodate sodium or iopanoic acid as above for 15–60 days

Amiodarone-induced thyrotoxicosis
- Methimazole, iopanoic acid, β-blockers, prednisone

Hypokalemic thyrotoxic paralysis
- Propranolol corrects hypokalemia, even in apathetic hyperthyroidism

Graves' ophthalmopathy
- For acute progressive exophthalmus, give prednisone 40–60 mg PO once daily
- For optic nerve compression, give prednisone 80–120 mg PO once daily
- Avoid smoking and thiazolidinediones

Atrial fibrillation
- Digoxin and β-blockers to control rate
- Warfarin
- Cardioversion unsuccessful until hyperthyroidism controlled

Thyrotoxic heart failure
- Aggressively control hyperthyroidism
- Use digoxin, angiotensin-converting enzyme inhibitors, angiotensin receptor blockers, diuretics

SURGERY

- Treat preoperatively with methimazole
- Six hours later, give ipodate sodium or iopanoic acid (500 mg PO BID) to accelerate euthyroidism and reduce thyroid vascularity
- Iodine (eg, Lugol's solution, 2–3 gtts PO daily for several days) also reduces vascularity
- Give propranolol preoperatively until serum T_3 or free T_3 is normal
- For thyrotoxic patients undergoing surgery, larger doses of propranolol are required perioperatively to reduce possibility of thyroid crisis

Graves' disease

- Thyroidectomy preferred over radioiodine for
  - Pregnant women whose thyrotoxicosis is not controlled with low-dose thioureas
  - Women desiring pregnancy in very near future
  - Patients with extremely large goiters
  - Those with suspected malignancy
  - Hartley-Dunhill operation
    - Procedure of choice
    - Total resection of one lobe and a subtotal resection of the other lobe, leaving about 4 g of thyroid tissue

Toxic solitary thyroid nodules

- Partial thyroidectomy for patients aged < 40
- [131]I for those aged > 40 years

THERAPEUTIC PROCEDURES

Graves' disease, toxic multinodular goiter

- Radioactive iodine (^{131}I) therapy
  - Patients usually only take propranolol
  - However, those with coronary disease, aged > 65 years, or severe hyperthyroidism are usually first rendered euthyroid with methimazole
  - Contraindicated in pregnancy
- Discontinue methimazole 4 days before ^{131}I treatment
- Methimazole given after ^{131}I for symptomatic hyperthyroidism until euthyroid

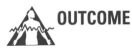 **OUTCOME**

FOLLOW-UP

- Check WBC periodically
  - In patients taking thioureas or in those with sore throat or febrile illness
- Free T_4 levels every 2–3 weeks during initial treatment
- Hypothyroidism common months to years after ^{131}I or subtotal thyroidectomy
- Lifelong clinical follow-up, with TSH and free T_4 measurements

COMPLICATIONS

- Osteoporosis, hypercalcemia
- Temporary decreased libido, decreased sperm count, gynecomastia
- Diplopia or loss of vision
- Total thyroidectomy: increased risk of hypoparathyroidism and damage to the recurrent laryngeal nerves
- Complications of thiourea therapy
  - Rash, nausea, agranulocytosis
  - Rarely, acute hepatic necrosis (PTU)

- Retrobulbar radiation, for Graves' exophthalmos, can cause radiation-induced retinopathy (usually subclinical) in about 5% of patients overall, mostly diabetics

PROGNOSIS

- Posttreatment hypothyroidism common, especially with ^{131}I or surgery
- Recurrence of hyperthyroidism occurs most commonly after thioureas (~50%)
- Subacute thyroiditis usually subsides spontaneously in weeks to months
- Graves' disease usually progresses, but may rarely subside spontaneously or even result in hypothyroidism
- Subtotal thyroidectomy of both lobes results in 9% recurrence of hyperthyroidism
- Despite treatment, increased risk of death from cardiovascular disease, stroke, and femur fracture in women
- Mortality of thyroid storm is high
- Subclinical hyperthyroidism: good prognosis; increased risk for bone loss

WHEN TO ADMIT

- Thyroid storm
- Hyperthyroidism-induced atrial fibrillation with severe tachycardia
- [131]I therapy or thyroidectomy

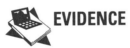 **EVIDENCE**

WEB SITE

- American Thyroid Association

REFERENCES

- Chi SY et al. A prospective, randomized comparison of bilateral subtotal thyroidectomy versus unilateral total and contralateral subtotal thyroidectomy for Graves' disease. World J Surg. 2005 Feb; 29(2):160–3. [PMID: 15650802]
- Cooper DS. Antithyroid drugs. N Engl J Med. 2005 Mar 3;352(9):905–17. [PMID: 15745981]
- Kahaly GJ et al. Randomized, single blind trial of intravenous versus oral steroid monotherapy in Graves' orbitopathy. J Clin Endocrinol Metab. 2005 Sep; 90(9):5234–40. [PMID: 15998777]
- Woeber KA. Observations concerning the natural history of subclinical hyperthyroidism. Thyroid. 2005 Jul; 15(7):687–91. [PMID: 16053385]

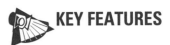

Hypocalcemia

KEY FEATURES

ESSENTIALS OF DIAGNOSIS

- Frequently mistaken for a neurologic disorder
- Mainly caused by insufficient action of parathyroid hormone (PTH) and/or vitamin D or by magnesium deficiency
- If the ionized calcium is normal despite a low total serum calcium, calcium metabolism is usually normal

GENERAL CONSIDERATIONS

- True hypocalcemia (decreased ionized calcium) implies insufficient action of PTH or active vitamin D
- The most common cause of low total serum calcium is hypoalbuminemia, correction of which is needed to accurately reflect the ionized calcium concentration
- The most common cause of true hypocalcemia is advanced stages of chronic kidney disease (CKD), in which there is decreased production of active vitamin D_3 and hyperphosphatemia
- Elderly hospitalized patients with low ionized serum calcium and hypophosphatemia, with or without an elevated serum PTH level, are likely deficient in vitamin D
- There is increased excitation of nerve and muscle cells, primarily affecting the neuromuscular and cardiovascular systems

Etiology

- **Decreased intake or absorption**
  - Malabsorption
  - Small bowel bypass
  - Vitamin D deficit, including 25-hydroxyvitamin D or 1,25-dihydroxyvitamin D
- **Increased loss**
  - Alcoholism
  - Chronic renal failure
  - Diuretic therapy
- **Endocrine disease**
  - Hypoparathyroidism
  - Sepsis
  - Pseudohypoparathyroidism
  - Calcitonin secretion from medullary carcinoma of the thyroid
  - Familial hypocalcemia
- **Physiologic causes**
  - Decreased serum albumin but normal ionized calcium
  - Decreased end-organ response to vitamin D

– Hyperphosphatemia
– Loop diuretics

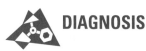

CLINICAL FINDINGS

SYMPTOMS AND SIGNS

- Extensive spasm of skeletal muscle causes cramps and tetany
- Laryngospasm with stridor can obstruct the airway
- Convulsions, paresthesias of lips and extremities, and abdominal pain
- **Chvostek's sign** (contraction of the facial muscle in response to tapping the facial nerve anterior to the ear)
- **Trousseau's sign** (carpal spasm occurring after occlusion of the brachial artery with a blood pressure cuff for 3 min) is usually readily elicited
- In chronic hypoparathyroidism, cataracts and calcification of basal ganglia of the brain may occur
- Ventricular arrhythmias if there is QT prolongation

DIAGNOSIS

LABORATORY TESTS

- When serum albumin concentration is < 4 g/dL, serum Ca^{2+} concentration is depressed in a ratio of 0.8–1.0 mg/dL of Ca^{2+} to 1 g/dL of albumin, but the physiologically active ionized calcium is normal
- In true hypocalcemia, the ionized serum calcium concentration is low (< 4.7 mg/dL or < 1.1 mmol/L)
- Serum phosphate is usually elevated in hypoparathyroidism or advanced stages of CKD, whereas it is suppressed in early-stages of CKD or vitamin D deficiency
- Serum Mg^{2+} is commonly low
- In respiratory alkalosis, total serum calcium is normal but ionized calcium is low

DIAGNOSTIC PROCEDURE

- ECG can show prolongation of the QT interval (as a result of lengthened ST segment)

TREATMENT

MEDICATIONS

Severe, symptomatic hypocalcemia

- In the presence of tetany, arrhythmias, or seizures, administer calcium gluco-
  nate 10% (10–20 mL) IV over 10–15 min
- Because of the short duration of action, calcium infusion is usually required; add 10–15 mg of calcium per kilogram body weight, or six to eight 10-mL vials of 10% calcium gluconate (558–744 mg of calcium), to 1 L of D_5W and infuse over 4–6 h
- Adjust the infusion rate to maintain the serum calcium level at 7.0–8.5 mg/dL

Asymptomatic hypocalcemia

- Oral calcium (1–2 g) and vitamin D preparations (Table 34)
- Calcium carbonate is well tolerated and less expensive than many other calcium tablets
- Check urinary calcium excretion after initiation of therapy because hypercalciuria (urine calcium excretion > 200 mg/day or urine calcium/urine creatinine ratio > 0.3) may impair kidney function in these patients
- The low serum Ca^{2+} associated with low serum albumin concentration does not require replacement therapy
- If serum Mg^{2+} is low, therapy must include replacement of magnesium, which by itself usually will correct hypocalcemia

OUTCOME

FOLLOW-UP

- Monitor the serum calcium level frequently (q4–6h) during calcium infusions for severe hypocalcemia

PROGNOSIS

- Depends on the underlying cause (eg, CKD)

WHEN TO REFER

- Refer early to a nephrologist if CKD is the underlying cause

WHEN TO ADMIT

- All symptomatic patients; intensive care unit admission may be needed
- If parenteral therapy is needed

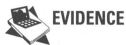

EVIDENCE

INFORMATION FOR PATIENTS

- American Association for Clinical Chemistry: Lab Tests Online: Calcium
- Mayo Clinic: Hypoparathyroidism
- Mayo Clinic: Kidney Failure
- MedlinePlus: Calcium Supplements (Systemic)
- MedlinePlus: Pseudohypoparathyroidism
- NIH Office of Dietary Supplements: Calcium Fact Sheet

REFERENCES

- Lyman D. Undiagnosed vitamin D deficiency in the hospitalized patient. Am Fam Physician. 2005 Jan 15;71(2):299–304. [PMID: 15686300]
- Murphy E et al. Disorders of calcium metabolism. Practitioner. 2006 Sep; 250(1686):4–6, 8. [PMID: 17036912]

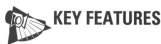

Hypoglycemic Disorders

KEY FEATURES

ESSENTIALS OF DIAGNOSIS

- Symptoms begin at plasma glucose levels of ~60 mg/dL, brain function impairment at ~50 mg/dL
- Two types of spontaneous hypoglycemia: fasting and postprandial
  - Fasting: Often subacute or chronic; usually presents with neuroglycopenia
  - Postprandial: Relatively acute, with symptoms of neurogenic autonomic discharge (sweating, palpitations, anxiety, tremulousness)

GENERAL CONSIDERATIONS

Fasting hypoglycemia

- Endocrine disorders (eg, hypopituitarism, Addison's disease, myxedema)
- Liver malfunction (eg, acute alcoholism, liver failure)
- End-stage chronic kidney disease on dialysis
- In absence of endocrine disorders, rule out hyperinsulinism from pancreatic B-cell tumors or surreptitious administration of insulin (or sulfonylureas) and hypoglycemia caused by non–insulin-producing extrapancreatic tumors
- Alcohol-related hypoglycemia
  - Due to hepatic glycogen depletion combined with alcohol-mediated inhibition of gluconeogenesis
  - Most common in malnourished alcohol abusers

– However, can occur in anyone unable to ingest food after an acute alcoholic episode followed by gastritis and vomiting
- Factitious hypoglycemia is due to surreptitious administration of insulin or sulfonylurea

Postprandial (reactive) hypoglycemia
- Postprandial hypoglycemia occurs either early (2–3 h after a meal) or late (3–5 h after eating)
- Early, or alimentary, hypoglycemia occurs when there is rapid discharge of ingested carbohydrate into the small bowel followed by rapid glucose absorption and hyperinsulinism
- Particularly associated with dumping syndrome after gastrectomy
- Rarely results from defective counterregulatory responses such as deficiencies of growth hormone, glucagon, cortisol, or autonomic responses
- Late postprandial hypoglycemia occurs in occult diabetes mellitus

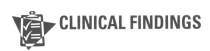 ## CLINICAL FINDINGS

SYMPTOMS AND SIGNS
- Whipple's triad is characteristic of hypoglycemia regardless of the cause
  – A history of hypoglycemic symptoms
  – An associated fasting blood glucose of ≤ 40 mg/dL
  – Immediate recovery on administration of glucose
- Weight gain can result from overeating to relieve symptoms
- Symptoms often develop in the early morning, after missing a meal, or occasionally after exercise
- Because of hypoglycemic unawareness, autonomic symptoms may be mild or late and the initial symptoms are due to neuroglycopenia
  – Blurred vision or diplopia
  – Headache
  – Feelings of detachment
  – Slurred speech
  – Weakness
- Personality changes may occur and range from anxiety to psychotic behavior
- Convulsions or coma may occur if symptoms are ignored and untreated

DIFFERENTIAL DIAGNOSIS
- Fasting hypoglycemia
  – Hyperinsulinism: pancreatic B-cell tumor and surreptitious insulin or sulfonylureas
  – Extrapancreatic tumors

- Postprandial early hypoglycemia: alimentary (eg, postgastrectomy)
- Postprandial late hypoglycemia: functional (increased vagal tone), occult diabetes mellitus
- Delayed insulin release resulting from B-cell dysfunction
  – Counterregulatory deficiency
  – Idiopathic
- Alcohol-related hypoglycemia
- Immunopathologic hypoglycemia: antibodies to insulin receptors, which act as agonists
- Pentamidine-induced hypoglycemia
- Islet hyperplasia (noninsulinoma pancreatogenous hypoglycemia syndrome)

 ## DIAGNOSIS

LABORATORY TESTS
- Serum insulin level ≥ 6 mcU/mL in RIA assay (≥ 3 mcU/mL in ICMA assay) in the presence of blood glucose values < 40 mg/dL is diagnostic of inappropriate hyperinsulinism. Besides insulinoma, other causes of hyperinsulinemic hypoglycemia must be considered, including factitious administration of insulin or sulfonylureas
- An elevated circulating proinsulin level (> 5 pmol/L) in the presence of fasting hypoglycemia is characteristic of most B-cell adenomas and does not occur in factitious hyperinsulinism
- In patients with epigastric distress, history of renal stones, or menstrual or erectile dysfunction, obtaining a serum calcium, gastrin, or prolactin level may be useful in screening for MEN-1 associated with insulinoma
- Prolonged fasting up to 72 h is done under hospital supervision until hypoglycemia is documented
  – In normal men, the blood glucose does not fall below 55–60 mg/dL during a 3-day fast
  – In normal premenopausal women who have fasted for only 24 h, however, the plasma glucose may fall normally to as low as 35 mg/dL. These women are not symptomatic, presumably owing to the development of sufficient ketonemia to supply energy needs to the brain
- Insulinoma patients become symptomatic when plasma glucose drops to subnormal levels, because inappropriate insulin secretion restricts ketone formation

 ## TREATMENT

MEDICATIONS

Inoperable pancreatic B-cell tumors
- Diazoxide, 300–600 mg PO once daily (along with a thiazide diuretic to control sodium retention)
- Octreotide, 50 mcg SQ BID

SURGERY
- Surgical treatment for endocrine tumors

THERAPEUTIC PROCEDURES

Inoperable pancreatic B-cell tumors
- Carbohydrate feeding every 2–3 h

Postprandial (reactive) hypoglycemia
- Frequent feedings with smaller portions of less rapidly assimilated carbohydrate combined with more slowly absorbed fat and protein

Functional alimentary hypoglycemia
- Support and mild sedation are mainstays of therapy
- Dietary manipulation is an adjunct: reduce proportion of carbohydrates in the diet, increase the frequency and reduce the size of the meals

 ## OUTCOME

COMPLICATIONS
- Indiscriminate use and overinterpretation of glucose tolerance tests have led to an overdiagnosis of functional hypoglycemia
- As many as one-third or more of normal individuals have blood glucose levels as low as 40–50 mg/dL with or without symptoms during a 4-h glucose tolerance test

 ## EVIDENCE

WEB SITES
- American Diabetes Association
- American Dietetic Association
- CDC Diabetes Public Health Resource
- Joslin Diabetes Center

INFORMATION FOR PATIENTS
- Joslin Diabetes Center: Is Low Blood Glucose (Hypoglycemia) Dangerous?
- Mayo Clinic: Hypoglycemia
- National Diabetes Information Clearinghouse

REFERENCES

- Frier BM. Managing hypoglycaemia. Practitioner. 2005;249:564. [PMID: 16108474]
- Grant CS. Insulinoma. Best Pract Res Clin Gastroenterol. 2005;19:783. [PMID: 16253900]
- Griffiths MJ et al. Adult spontaneous hypoglycaemia. Hosp Med. 2005; 66:277. [PMID: 15920857]
- Service FJ. Diagnostic approach to adults with hypoglycemic disorders. Endocrinol Metab Clin North Am. 1999;28:519. [PMID: 10500929]
- Tucker ON et al. The management of insulinoma. Br J Surg. 2006;93:264. [PMID: 16498592]

Hypogonadism, Male

 KEY FEATURES

ESSENTIALS OF DIAGNOSIS

- Diminished libido and erections
- Decreased growth of body hair
- Small or normal testes; serum or free testosterone decreased
- Luteinizing hormone (LH) and follicle-stimulating hormone (FSH)
  - Decrease in hypogonadotropic hypogonadism (insufficient gonadotropin secretion by pituitary)
  - Increase in hypergonadotropic hypogonadism (testicular failure)

GENERAL CONSIDERATIONS

- Caused by deficient testosterone secretion by the testes
- In hypogonadotropic form, FSH and LH deficiency may be isolated or accompanied by other pituitary hormone abnormalities

Hypogonadotropic hypogonadism

- Causes
  - Pituitary adenoma or hypopituitarism causing
    - Hyperprolactinemia
    - Cushing's syndrome
    - Adrenal insufficiency
    - Growth hormone excess or deficiency
    - Thyroid hormone excess or deficiency
  - Hemochromatosis
  - Estrogen-secreting tumor (testicular, adrenal)
  - Gonadotropin-releasing hormone agonist therapy, eg, leuprolide
  - Other drugs
    - Alcohol
    - Ketoconazole
    - Spironolactone
    - Marijuana
  - Anorexia nervosa, cirrhosis, other serious illness, or malnutrition
  - Kallmann's or Prader-Willi syndrome
  - Intrathecal opioid infusion
  - Congenital adrenal hypoplasia
  - Idiopathic

Hypergonadotropic hypogonadism

- Causes
  - Male climacteric (andropause)
  - Klinefelter's syndrome: at least one Y chromosome and at least two X chromosomes (47,XXY et al)
  - Orchitis, eg, mumps, gonorrhea, tuberculosis, leprosy
  - Testicular failure secondary to radiation therapy or chemotherapy
  - Autoimmune, uremia, testicular trauma or torsion, lymphoma, myotonic dystrophy, androgen insensitivity

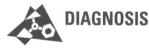 **CLINICAL FINDINGS**

SYMPTOMS AND SIGNS

- Delayed puberty if congenital or acquired during childhood
- Decreased libido with acquired hypogonadism in most
- Erectile dysfunction, hot sweats, fatigue, or depression
- Infertility, gynecomastia, headache (if pituitary tumor)
- Decreased body, axillary, beard, or pubic hair
- Loss of muscle mass and weight gain due to increased subcutaneous fat
- Testicular size, as assessed with orchidometer, may decrease but usually remains normal in length (> 6 cm) in postpubertal hypogonadotropic hypogonadism
- In Klinefelter's syndrome, manifestations are variable
  - Generally, testes normal in childhood, but usually become small, firm, fibrotic, and nontender in adolescence
  - Normal onset of puberty, variable degree of virilization, gynecomastia at puberty, tall stature with increased arm span
  - Patients with > 2 X or > 1 Y chromosomes are more prone to mental deficiency, clinodactyly, synostosis, poor social skills
- Testicular mass (Leydig cell tumor), trauma, infiltrative lesions (eg, lymphoma), or chronic infection (eg, leprosy, tuberculosis)
- Osteoporosis and fractures in chronic hypogonadism

DIFFERENTIAL DIAGNOSIS

- Erectile dysfunction due to other cause
  - Diabetes mellitus
  - Atherosclerosis
  - Stroke
  - Drugs
- Male infertility due to other cause
  - Cryptorchism
  - Retrograde ejaculation
- Gynecomastia due to other cause
  - Puberty
  - Chronic liver disease
  - Drugs
  - Malignancy
- Hypothyroidism (may also cause hypogonadism)
- Depression

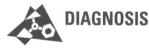 **DIAGNOSIS**

LABORATORY TESTS

- Total testosterone measured nonfasting in AM is low (may be 25–50% lower, below "normal range," if obtained fasting or in PM)
- Testosterone highest at age 20–30 years, slightly lower at 30–40 years; falls gradually but progressively after age 40
- Free testosterone useful in elderly men due to rising sex hormone-binding globulin (SHBG) with age
- Check serum LH and FSH levels if serum testosterone is low or borderline–low
- LH and FSH high in hypergonadotropic hypogonadism and low or inappropriately normal in hypogonadotropic hypogonadism

Hypogonadotropic hypogonadism

- Check serum prolactin: elevated in prolactinoma
- If gynecomastia, check serum androstenedione and estrone: both elevated in partial 17-ketosteroid reductase deficiency
- Check serum estradiol: elevated in cirrhosis and rare estrogen-secreting tumors (testicular Leydig cell tumor or adrenal carcinoma)
- If no clear cause for hypogonadotropic hypogonadism, check serum ferritin: elevated in hemochromatosis

Hypergonadotropic hypogonadism

- Check karyotyping or measurement of leukocyte X-inactive-specific transcriptase (XIST) by PCR for Klinefelter's syndrome

IMAGING STUDIES

- MRI of pituitary to evaluate for tumor or other lesion when no clear cause of hypogonadotropic hypogonadism
- Bone densitometry: reduced bone density in long-standing male hypogonadism

DIAGNOSTIC PROCEDURES

- Testicular biopsy is usually reserved for younger patients when reason for primary hypogonadism is unclear

 TREATMENT

MEDICATIONS

- Testosterone replacement is usual treatment
- Screen older men for prostate cancer before initiating testosterone therapy
- Topical testosterone 1% gel is available as Androgel (2.5-g and 5-g packets)
  - Starting dose is 5 g; dosage may be increased to maximum of 10.0 g/day if clinically indicated
  - Gel is applied once daily to clean, dry skin of shoulders, upper arms, or abdomen, not genitals
  - **Note:** Hands must be washed after gel application, site allowed to dry 5 minutes before dressing, and clothing worn during contact with women or children
- Transdermal testosterone is available in patch formulations applied once daily to different nongenital skin sites
  - Testoderm II, 5 mg/day leaves sticky residue but causes little skin irritation
  - Androderm, 2.5–10.0 mg/day adheres more tightly but may cause skin irritation
- Parenteral testosterone (enanthate or cypionate)
  - 300 mg IM q3wks or 200 mg IM q2wks, usually in gluteal area
  - Adjust dose per patient response
- Oral androgens (eg, methyltestosterone and fluoxymesterone) should not be used because
  - They predispose patients to peliosis hepatis, hepatic tumors, and hepatic dysfunction
  - Less effective than transdermal or parenteral testosterone

THERAPEUTIC PROCEDURES

- Men with mosaic Klinefelter's syndrome (eg, 46,XY/47,XXY) may be fertile
- Otherwise, infertility may be overcome by in vitro intracytoplasmic sperm injection (ICSI) into an ovum

 OUTCOME

FOLLOW-UP

- Reassess patient clinically and measure serum testosterone after initiation of testosterone replacement
- If clinical response is inadequate or serum testosterone is below normal, increase dose
- Monitor hematocrit due to risk of polycythemia

COMPLICATIONS

- Complication of hypogonadism: osteoporosis
- Complications of Klinefelter syndrome
  - Neoplasms including breast cancer
  - Chronic pulmonary disease
  - Varicosities of the legs
  - Diabetes mellitus (8%)
  - Impaired glucose tolerance without frank diabetes (19%)
- Side effects of testosterone replacement
  - Acne
  - Gynecomastia
  - Aggravation of sleep apnea
  - Reduced HDL cholesterol
- Side effects of oral androgens: cholestatic jaundice (1–2%), and liver tumors or peliosis hepatis rarely with long-term use
- Side effects of megestrol acetate
  - Increased appetite
  - Weight gain
  - Hyperglycemia
  - Hypertriglyceridemia

PROGNOSIS

- Prognosis of hypogonadism due to pituitary lesion is that of primary disease (eg, tumor, necrosis)
- Prognosis for restoration of virility is good if testosterone replacement is given

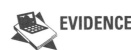 EVIDENCE

PRACTICE GUIDELINES

- AACE Medical Guidelines for Clinical Practice: Hypogonadism, 2002
- Morales A et al. International Society for the Study of the Aging Male. Investigation, treatment and monitoring of late-onset hypogonadism in males. Official recommendations of ISSAM. Aging Male. 2002;5:74. [PMID: 12198738]

WEB SITES

- The Pituitary Foundation
- Pituitary Network Association

INFORMATION FOR PATIENTS

- Mayo Clinic—Hypogonadism
- MedlinePlus: Hypogonadism

REFERENCES

- Bojesen A et al. Increased mortality in Klinefelter syndrome. J Clin Endocrinol Metab. 2004 Aug;89(8):3830–4. [PMID: 15292313]
- Greenstein A et al. Does sildenafil combined with testosterone gel improve erectile dysfunction in hypogonadal men in whom testosterone supplement therapy alone failed? J Urol. 2005 Feb; 173(2):530–2. [PMID: 15643239]
- Lanfranco F et al. Klinefelter's syndrome. Lancet. 2004 Jul 17–23;364(9430):273–83. [PMID: 15262106]
- Matsumoto AM et al. Serum testosterone assays—accuracy matters. J Clin Endocrinol Metab. 2004 Feb; 89(2):520–4. [PMID: 14764756]
- Rhoden EL et al. Risks of testosterone-replacement therapy and recommendations for monitoring. N Engl J Med. 2004 Jan 29;350(5):482–92. [PMID: 14749457]
- Wang C et al. Measurement of total serum testosterone in adult men: comparison of current laboratory methods versus liquid chromatography-tandem mass spectrometry. J Clin Endocrinol Metab. 2004 Feb;89(2):534–43. [PMID: 14764758]

Hypokalemia

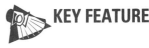 KEY FEATURES

ESSENTIALS OF DIAGNOSIS

- Serum K$^+$ < 3.5 mEq/L
- Severe hypokalemia may induce dangerous arrhythmias and rhabdomyolysis
- Transtubular potassium concentration gradient (TTKG) can distinguish renal from nonrenal loss of potassium

GENERAL CONSIDERATIONS

- Gastrointestinal loss due to infectious diarrhea is most common cause, especially in developing countries
- Potassium shift into the cell is transiently stimulated by insulin and glucose and facilitated by β-adrenergic stimulation
- α-Adrenergic stimulation blocks potassium shift into the cell
- Aldosterone, which facilitates urinary potassium excretion through enhanced potassium secretion at the distal renal tubules, is the most important regulator of body potassium content
- Magnesium is an important cofactor for potassium uptake and for maintenance of intracellular potassium levels
- Magnesium depletion should be suspected in persistent hypokalemia refractory to potassium repletion

Etiology

- **Potassium shift into cell**
  - Insulin excess, eg, postprandial
  - Alkalosis
  - β-Adrenergic agonists
  - Trauma (via epinephrine release)
  - Hypokalemic periodic paralysis
  - Barium or cesium intoxication
- **Renal potassium loss (urine K⁺ > 40 mEq/L)**
  - Increased aldosterone (mineralocorticoid) effects
    □ Primary hyperaldosteronism
    □ Secondary hyperaldosteronism (dehydration, heart failure)
    □ Renovascular or malignant hypertension
    □ Cushing's syndrome
    □ European licorice (inhibits cortisol)
    □ Renin-producing tumor
    □ Congenital abnormality of steroid metabolism (eg, adrenogenital syndrome, 17α-hydroxylase defect)
  - Increased flow of distal nephron
    □ Diuretics (furosemide, thiazides)
    □ Salt-losing nephropathy
  - Hypomagnesemia
    □ Unreabsorbable anion
    □ Carbenicillin, penicillin
  - Renal tubular acidosis (type I or II)
    □ Fanconi's syndrome
    □ Interstitial nephritis
    □ Metabolic alkalosis (bicarbonaturia)
  - Genetic disorder of the nephron
    □ Bartter's syndrome
    □ Liddle's syndrome
- **Extrarenal potassium loss (urine K⁺ < 20 mEq/L)**
  - Vomiting, diarrhea, laxative abuse
  - Villous adenoma, Zollinger-Ellison syndrome

 CLINICAL FINDINGS

SYMPTOMS AND SIGNS

- Muscular weakness, fatigue, and muscle cramps are common in mild to moderate hypokalemia
- Constipation or ileus may result from smooth muscle involvement
- Flaccid paralysis, hyporeflexia, hypercapnia, tetany, and rhabdomyolysis may be seen in severe hypokalemia (serum K⁺ < 2.5 mEq/L)
- Hypertension may result from aldosterone or mineralocorticoid excess

 DIAGNOSIS

LABORATORY TESTS

- Urinary potassium concentration is low (< 20 mEq/L) as a result of extrarenal loss and inappropriately high (> 40 mEq/L) with urinary losses
- Calculating TTKG is a rapid method to evaluate net potassium secretion

$$TTKG = \frac{Urine\ K^+/Plasma\ K^+}{Urine\ osm/Plasma\ osm}$$

- Hypokalemia with TTKG > 4 suggests renal potassium loss with increased distal K⁺ secretion
  - In such cases, plasma renin and aldosterone levels are helpful in differential diagnosis
  - The presence of nonabsorbed anions, including bicarbonate, also increases the TTKG

DIAGNOSTIC PROCEDURES

- ECG can show
  - Decreased amplitude and broadening of T waves
  - Prominent U waves
  - Premature ventricular contractions
  - Depressed ST segments

 TREATMENT

MEDICATIONS

- Oral potassium is the safest way to treat mild to moderate deficiency
- All potassium formulations are easily absorbed
- Dietary potassium is almost entirely coupled to phosphate—rather than chloride—and does not correct potassium loss associated with chloride depletion, such as from diuretics or vomiting

- In the setting of abnormal renal function and mild to moderate diuretic dosage
  - 20 mEq/day of oral potassium is generally sufficient to prevent hypokalemia
  - However, 40–100 mEq/day over a period of days to weeks is needed to treat hypokalemia and fully replete potassium stores
- Indications for IV potassium replacement
  - Severe hypokalemia
  - Inability to take oral supplementation
- For severe deficiency, potassium may be given through a peripheral IV line in a concentration that should not exceed 40 mEq/L at rates of up to 40 mEq/L/h
- Coexisting magnesium and potassium depletion can result in refractory hypokalemia despite potassium repletion if there is no magnesium repletion

 OUTCOME

FOLLOW-UP

- Monitor ECG continuously when infusing IV potassium for severe hypokalemia
- Check serum potassium level q3–6h

COMPLICATIONS

- Hypokalemia increases the likelihood of digitalis toxicity
- Hypokalemia induced by drug combinations, such as β₂-adrenergic agonists and diuretics, may impose a substantial risk

WHEN TO REFER

- Persistent hypokalemia (K⁺ < 3.0 mEq/L) or use of diuretics without any recent gastrointestinal losses

WHEN TO ADMIT

- For severe hypokalemia (K⁺ < 2.5 mEq/L)
- If IV potassium replacement is needed
- If cardiac monitoring is necessary during potassium replacement

PROGNOSIS

- Most hypokalemia will correct with replacement after 24–72 h

EVIDENCE

INFORMATION FOR PATIENTS

- MedlinePlus: Hyperaldosteronism
- MedlinePlus: Hypokalemia
- MedlinePlus: Potassium Drug Information

- National Kidney and Urologic Diseases Information Clearinghouse: Renal Tubular Acidosis

REFERENCES

- Coca SG et al. The cardiovascular implications of hypokalemia. Am J Kidney Dis. 2005 Feb;45(2):233–47. [PMID: 15685500]
- Groeneveld JH et al. An approach to the patient with severe hypokalemia: the potassium quiz. QJM. 2005 Apr; 98(4):305–16. [PMID: 15760922]
- Schaefer TJ et al. Disorders of potassium. Emerg Med Clin North Am. 2005 Aug; 23(3):723–47. [PMID: 15982543]
- Sherman FT. The 3 "hypo's" of hospitalization. Geriatrics. 2005 May;60(5):9–10. [PMID: 15877479]
- Welfare W et al. Challenges in managing profound hypokalemia. BMJ. 2002 Feb 2;324(7332):269–70. [PMID: 11823358]

Hypomagnesemia

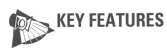 **KEY FEATURES**

ESSENTIALS OF DIAGNOSIS

- Causes neurologic symptoms and arrhythmias
- Serum concentration may be normal even in the presence of magnesium deficiency
- Check urinary magnesium excretion if depletion is suspected
- Impairs release of parathyroid hormone (PTH)

GENERAL CONSIDERATIONS

- Magnesium acts directly on the myoneural junction
- Hypomagnesemia-associated alteration of Ca^{2+}
  - Severe and prolonged magnesium depletion impairs secretion of PTH with consequent hypocalcemia
  - May also impair end-organ response to PTH

Etiology

- **Diminished absorption or intake**
  - Malabsorption
  - Chronic diarrhea
  - Laxative abuse
  - Prolonged gastrointestinal suction

  - Malnutrition
  - Alcoholism
  - Parenteral alimentation with inadequate Mg^{2+} content
- **Increased renal loss**
  - Diuretic therapy
  - Hyperaldosteronism
  - Barrter's syndrome
  - Hyperparathyroidism
  - Hyperthyroidism
  - Hypercalcemia
  - Volume expansion
  - Tubulointerstitial diseases
  - Drugs (aminoglycoside, cisplatin, amphotericin B, pentamidine)
- **Others**
  - Diabetes mellitus
  - Postparathyroidectomy (hungry bone syndrome)
  - Respiratory alkalosis
  - Pregnancy

DEMOGRAPHICS

- Nearly half of hospitalized patients for whom serum electrolytes are ordered have unrecognized hypomagnesemia
- Common causes
  - Large volumes of IV fluids
  - Diuretics
  - Cisplatin in cancer patients (with concomitant hypokalemia)
  - Administration of nephrotoxic agents, such as aminoglycosides and amphotericin B

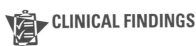 **CLINICAL FINDINGS**

SYMPTOMS AND SIGNS

- Weakness, muscle cramps, and tremor
- Marked neuromuscular and central nervous system hyperirritability
  - Tremors
  - Athetoid movements
  - Jerking
  - Nystagmus
  - Positive Babinski response
- Confusion and disorientation
- Hypertension, tachycardia, and ventricular arrhythmias

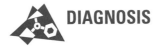 **DIAGNOSIS**

LABORATORY TESTS

- Urinary excretion of magnesium exceeding 10–30 mg/day or a fractional excretion more than 2% indicates renal magnesium wasting
- In calculating fractional excretion of magnesium, only 30% is protein

bound, thus 70% of circulating magnesium is filtered by the glomerulus
- Up to 40% of patients have hypokalemia and up to 50% have hypocalcemia
- PTH secretion is often suppressed

DIAGNOSTIC PROCEDURES

- ECG may show a prolonged QT interval because of lengthening of the ST segment

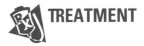 **TREATMENT**

MEDICATIONS

- **Symptomatic hypomagnesemia**
  - Infuse 1–2 g of magnesium sulfate immediately, followed by an infusion of 6 g of magnesium sulfate in at least 1 L of fluid over 24 h, repeated for up to 7 days
  - Magnesium sulfate may also be given IM in a dosage of 200–800 mg/day (8–33 mmol/day) in four divided doses
  - In magnesium replacement in a patient with renal insufficiency, reduce dose of magesium sulfate by 50–75%
- **Chronic hypomagnesemia**
  - Magnesium oxide, 250–500 mg PO once daily or BID, is useful for repleting stores
  - Hypokalemia and hypocalcemia of hypomagnesemia do not recover without magnesium supplementation
  - Thus, replacement of K^+ and Ca^{2+} are also required

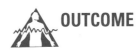 **OUTCOME**

FOLLOW-UP

- Monitor serum magnesium levels frequently (at least twice daily) and adjust dosage of magnesium supplementation to keep the level below 2.5 mmol/L
- Check tendon reflexes because hypermagnesemia causes hyporeflexia
- In patients with chronic kidney disease, replace magnesium cautiously to avoid hypermagnesemia

WHEN TO REFER

- Refer to an endocrinologist or nephrologist for consultation about repletion in the setting of marked neuromuscular symptoms or cardiac arrhythmia

WHEN TO ADMIT

- Confusion, disorientation

- Marked neuromuscular and central nervous system hyperirritability
- Need for intravenous replacement

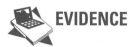

EVIDENCE

INFORMATION FOR PATIENTS

- American Association for Clinical Chemistry: Lab Tests Online: Magnesium
- MedlinePlus: Hypomagnesemia
- MedlinePlus: Magnesium Supplements (Systemic)
- NIH Office of Dietary Supplements: Magnesium

REFERENCES

- Mouw DR et al. Clinical inquiries. What are the causes of hypomagnesemia? J Fam Pract. 2005 Feb; 54(2):174–6. [PMID: 15689296]
- Tong GM et al. Magnesium deficiency in critical illness. J Intensive Care Med. 2005 Jan-Feb;20(1):3–17. [PMID: 15665255]

Hyponatremia

KEY FEATURES

ESSENTIALS OF DIAGNOSIS

- Serum Na⁺ < 130 mEq/L
- Most cases result from water imbalance, not sodium imbalance
- Assessment of extracellular fluid volume and measurement of serum osmolality are essential to determine etiology
- Treatment strategy should be based not only on etiology, but on the severity and speed of development

GENERAL CONSIDERATIONS

- Abnormal sodium balance is often associated with either volume depletion or edema formation
- Hospitalized patients treated with hypotonic fluid are at increased risk for hyponatremia

Etiology (Figure 8)

- **Isotonic hyponatremia or pseudohyponatremia**
  - Normal serum osmolality; artifact corrected in most US laboratories

- Hyperlipidemia
- Hyperproteinemia
- **Hypotonic hyponatremia (serum osmolality < 280 mosm/kg)**
  - Hypovolemic
    □ Extrarenal salt loss (U_{Na+} < 10 mEq/L): dehydration, diarrhea, vomiting, or third-spacing, as with ascites
    □ Renal salt loss (U_{Na+} > 20 mEq/L): diuretics, angiotensin-converting enzyme (ACE) inhibitors, angiotensin II receptor blockers (ARBs), salt-losing nephropathies, mineralocorticoid deficiency, cerebral sodium-wasting syndrome
  - Euvolemic
    □ Syndrome of inappropriate antidiuretic hormone (SIADH)
    □ Postoperative hyponatremia
    □ Hypothyroidism
    □ Psychogenic polydipsia
    □ Beer potomania
    □ Idiosyncratic drug reaction (thiazides, ACE inhibitors)
    □ Endurance exercise
  - Hypervolemic (edematous states)
    □ Congestive heart failure
    □ Liver disease
    □ Nephrotic syndrome (rare)
    □ Advanced renal failure
- **Hypertonic hyponatremia**
  - Serum osmolality > 295 mosm/kg
  - Hyperglycemia
  - Mannitol, sorbitol, glycerol, maltose
  - Radiocontrast agents

DEMOGRAPHICS

- Most common electrolyte abnormality observed in a general hospitalized population (~20% of patients)

CLINICAL FINDINGS

SYMPTOMS AND SIGNS

- Mild hyponatremia (plasma sodium 130–135 mEq/L) is usually asymptomatic
- Nausea and malaise can occur when the plasma sodium is < 125–130 mEq/L
- Headache, lethary, and disorientation are seen with plasma sodium levels of 115–120 mEq/L
- The most serious symptoms of severe and rapidly developing hyponatremia are
  - Seizure
  - Coma
  - Permanent brain damage
  - Respiratory arrest
  - Brainstem herniation
  - Death
- Natriuresis compensates for slight increase in volume from ADH secretion

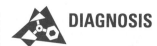

DIAGNOSIS

LABORATORY TESTS

- Measure serum and urine osmolality and assess patient's volume status (Figure 8)
- Urine Na⁺ helps distinguish renal from nonrenal causes of hyponatremia
- Urine Na⁺ > 20 mEq/L implies renal salt wasting
- Urine Na⁺ < 10 mEq/L or fractional excretion of Na⁺ < 1% (unless diuretics have been given) implies avid sodium retention by the kidney because of extrarenal fluid losses
- Fractional excretion of Na⁺ (%)

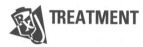

TREATMENT

MEDICATIONS

Hypovolemic hypotonic hyponatremia

- Replace lost volume with isotonic (0.9%) or half-normal (0.45%) saline or lactated Ringer's
- Adjust rate of correction to prevent cerebral damage (see below)
- Administer corticosteroids empirically if hypocortisolism is possible

Euvolemic hyponatremia

- See Syndrome of Inappropriate Antidiuretic Hormone
- **Symptomatic hyponatremia**
  - Initial goal: serum Na⁺ 125–130 mEq/L, guarding against overcorrection
  - Increase serum Na⁺ concentration by < 1–2 mEq/L/h and not > 25–30 mEq/L in the first 2 days to prevent central pontine myelinolysis; reduce rate to 0.5–1.0 mEq/L/h as neurologic symptoms improve
  - If CNS symptoms, treat hyponatremia rapidly at any level of serum Na⁺ concentration
  - Hypertonic (eg, 3%) saline plus furosemide (0.5–1.0 mg/kg IV)
    □ To determine how much 3% saline (513 mEq/L) to administer, obtain spot urinary Na⁺ after furosemide diuresis has begun
    □ Excreted Na⁺ is replaced with 3% saline, empirically begun at 1–2 mL/kg/h and then adjusted based on urinary output and urinary Na⁺
    □ For example, after furosemide, urine volume may be 400 mL/h and Na⁺ + K⁺ excretion 100 mEq/L; excreted Na⁺ + K⁺= 40 mEq/h, which is replaced with 78 mL/h of 3% saline (40 mEq/h divided by 513 mEq/L)

- **Asymptomatic hyponatremia**
  - Restrict water intake to 0.5–1.0 L/day; serum Na⁺ will gradually increase over days
  - Correction rate: < 0.5 mEq/L/h
  - No specific treatment needed for patients with reset osmostats
  - Isotonic 0.9% saline with furosemide in asymptomatic patients with serum Na⁺ < 120 mEq/L. Replace urinary Na⁺ and K⁺ losses as above
  - Demeclocycline, 300–600 mg PO BID
    - Inhibits effect of ADH on distal tubule
    - Useful for patients who cannot adhere to water restriction or need additional therapy
    - Onset of action may be 1 week, and concentrating ability may be permanently impaired
    - Therapy with demeclocycline in persons with cirrhosis increases risk of renal failure
  - Fludrocortisone for hyponatremia as part of cerebral salt-wasting syndrome
  - Selective renal vasopressin V2 antagonists
    - Conivaptan is used in hospitalized patients with euvolemic SIADH
    - Give as an IV loading dose of 20 mg delivered over 30 minutes, then as 20 mg continuously over 24 hours
    - Subsequent infusions may be administered every 1–3 days at 20–40 mg/day by continuous infusion

Hypervolemic hypotonic hyponatremia

- Treat underlying condition (eg, improve cardiac output) and restrict water (< 1–2 L daily)
- Diuretics
  - Can hasten water and salt excretion but may worsen hyponatremia
  - Caution patient not to increase free water intake
- Hypertonic 3% saline is potentially dangerous in volume-overloaded states, thus not generally recommended
  - If severe hyponatremia (serum Na⁺ < 110 mEq/L) and CNS symptoms, judicious administration of small amounts (100–200 mL) of 3% saline with diuretics may be necessary
- Consider emergency dialysis

 OUTCOME

FOLLOW-UP

- If symptomatic, measure serum Na⁺ ~q4h and observe patient closely

COMPLICATIONS

- Central pontine myelinolysis may occur from osmotically induced demyelination as a result of overly rapid correction of serum Na⁺ (an increase of > 1 mEq/L/h, or ≥ 25 mEq/L within first 24 h of therapy)
- Hypoxic-anoxic episodes during hyponatremia may contribute to demyelination

PROGNOSIS

- Premenopausal women in whom hyponatremic encephalopathy develops from rapidly acquired hyponatremia (eg, postoperative hyponatremia) are about 25 times more likely than postmenopausal women to suffer permanent brain damage or die

WHEN TO REFER

- Persistent hyponatremia despite therapy

WHEN TO ADMIT

- Symptomatic hyponatremia
- Serum Na⁺ < 120 mEq/L

 EVIDENCE

WEB SITE

- Fall PJ. Hyponatremia and Hypernatremia, A Systematic Approach to Causes and Their Correction. Postgraduate Medicine Online, 2000

INFORMATION FOR PATIENTS

- American Association for Clinical Chemistry: Lab Tests Online: Sodium
- Mayo Clinic: Low Blood Sodium in Older Adults
- MedlinePlus: Dilutional Hyponatremia (SIADH)
- MedlinePlus: Serum Sodium
- Penn State College of Medicine: Hyponatremia

REFERENCES

- Castello L et al. Hyponatremia in liver cirrhosis: pathophysiological principles of management. Dig Liver Dis. 2005 Feb;37(2):73–81. [PMID: 15733516]
- Goldsmith SR. Current treatments and novel pharmacologic treatments for hyponatremia in congestive heart failure. Am J Cardiol. 2005 May 2; 95(9A):14B–23B. [PMID: 15847853]
- Hoorn EJ et al. Diagnostic approach to a patient with hyponatremia: traditional versus physiology-based options. QJM. 2005 Jul;98(7):529–40. [PMID: 15955797]
- McDade G. Disorders of sodium balance: hyponatraemia and drug use (and abuse). BMJ. 2006 Apr 8; 332(7545):853. [PMID: 16601056]
- Reynolds RM et al. Disorders of sodium balance. BMJ. 2006 Mar 25;332(7543): 702–5. [PMID: 16565125]
- Riggs JE. Neurologic manifestations of electrolyte disturbances. Neurol Clin. 2002 Feb;20(1):227–39. [PMID: 11754308]

Hypoparathyroidism & Pseudohypoparathyroidism

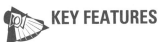 **KEY FEATURES**

ESSENTIALS OF DIAGNOSIS

- Carpopedal spasms, tingling of lips and hands, muscle cramps, psychological changes
- Positive Chvostek's sign and Trousseau's phenomenon
- Serum calcium low; serum phosphate high; alkaline phosphatase normal; urine calcium excretion reduced
- Serum magnesium may be low

GENERAL CONSIDERATIONS

- Causes
  - Post thyroidectomy (most common cause); usually transient but may be permanent
  - Parathyroid adenoma removal due to suppression of remaining parathyroids
  - DiGeorge's syndrome
  - Damage to gland by
    - Heavy metals, eg, copper (Wilson's disease), iron (hemochromatosis, transfusion hemosiderosis)
    - Granulomas
    - Sporadic autoimmunity
    - Riedel's thyroiditis
    - Tumors; infection; or neck irradiation (rare)
  - Magnesium deficiency, which prevents parathyroid hormone (PTH) secretion
  - Pseudohypoparathyroidism
    - Hypocalcemia and high PTH levels due to renal resistance to PTH from mutations in PTH receptor

□ Characterized by short stature, round face, obesity, short fourth metacarpals, ectopic bone formation, and mental retardation but without hypocalcemia

– Autosomal dominant hypocalcemia with hypocalciuria (ADHH)

□ Gain-of-function (constitutive activation) mutations of the calcium-sensing receptor (CaSR) gene essentially "fool" the parathyroid glands

□ Hypocalcemia without elevations in serum PTH levels

□ Characterized by hypocalcemic seizures in infancy

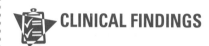# CLINICAL FINDINGS

SYMPTOMS AND SIGNS

- **Acute symptoms**

  – Tetany, with muscle cramps, irritability, carpopedal spasm, and convulsions

  – Tingling of circumoral area, hands, and feet

- **Chronic symptoms**

  – Lethargy
  – Personality changes
  – Anxiety
  – Blurred vision due to cataracts
  – Parkinsonism
  – Mental retardation

- Chvostek's sign (facial muscle contraction on tapping facial nerve in front of the ear)

- Trousseau's phenomenon (carpal spasm after application of blood pressure cuff)

- Cataracts

- Nails thin and brittle; skin dry and scaly, at times with candidiasis; hair loss (eyebrows)

- Deep tendon reflexes hyperactive

- Papilledema and elevated cerebrospinal fluid pressure occasionally

- Defective teeth if onset in childhood

DIFFERENTIAL DIAGNOSIS

- Pseudohypoparathyroidism (renal resistance to PTH)
- Vitamin D deficiency
- Acute pancreatitis
- Chronic renal failure
- Hypoalbuminemia
- Paresthesias or tetany due to respiratory alkalosis
- Familial hypocalcemia with hypercalciuria (normal serum PTH)
- Hypomagnesemia

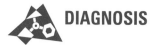# DIAGNOSIS

LABORATORY TESTS

- Low serum calcium

  – **Note:** serum calcium is largely bound to albumin. If hypoalbuminemia is present, obtain ionized calcium or correct calcium level for albumin level. Corrected Ca^{2+} = serum Ca^{2+} mg/dL + [$0.8 \times (4.0 - $albumin g/dL)]

- Serum phosphate high
- Alkaline phosphatase normal
- Urinary calcium low
- PTH level low
- Hypomagnesemia frequently accompanies hypocalcemia and may decrease parathyroid gland function

IMAGING STUDIES

- Skull radiographs or head CT may show basal ganglia calcifications
- Bone radiographs may show increased bone density
- Other radiographs may show cutaneous calcifications

DIAGNOSTIC PROCEDURES

- Slit-lamp examination may show early posterior lenticular cataract formation
- ECG shows prolonged QT interval and T-wave abnormalities

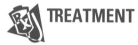# TREATMENT

MEDICATIONS

Emergency treatment for acute tetany

- Ensure adequate airway
- Calcium gluconate

  – 10–20 mL of 10% solution IV, given *slowly* until tetany ceases

  – Add 10–50 mL of calcium gluconate 10% to 1 L of D5W or saline by slow IV drip

  – Titrate to serum calcium of 8–9 mg/dL

- Oral calcium, 1–2 g daily as soon as possible

  – Liquid calcium carbonate (Titralac Plus), 500 mg/5 mL

  – Calcium citrate contains 21% calcium, but higher proportion is absorbed with less gastrointestinal intolerance

- Vitamin D derivatives to be given with oral calcium include

  – Calcitriol (1,25-dihydroxycholecalciferol), 0.25 to 4 mcg PO once daily

  – Ergocalciferol (vitamin D_2), 25,000–150,000 units PO once daily

  – Calcifediol (25-hydroxyvitamin D_3), 20 mcg PO once daily (Table 34)

- If hypomagnesemia is present,

  – Give $MgSO_4$ 1–2 g IV q6h *immediately*

  – Give magnesium oxide tablets, 600 mg 1–2 PO once daily, or combined magnesium and calcium preparation (dolomite, others) *long-term*

Maintenance treatment

- Calcium (1–2 g/day) and vitamin D supplementation (see above) to achieve slightly low but asymptomatic serum calcium (8.0–8.6 mg/dL) to minimize hypercalciuria and provide margin of safety against overdosage and hypercalcemia

- Calcitriol, 0.25 mcg PO every morning, titrated up to 0.5–2.0 mcg PO every morning, to achieve near normocalcemia in patients with chronic hypocalcemia

- Avoid phenothiazines in hypocalcemia; may precipitate extrapyramidal symptoms

- Avoid furosemide; may worsen hypocalcemia

SURGERY

- Transplantation of cryopreserved parathyroid tissue from prior surgery restores normocalcemia in ~23%

OUTCOME

FOLLOW-UP

- Monitor serum calcium at least every 3 months; keep serum calcium slightly low

- Monitor "spot" urine calcium to keep level < 30 mg/dL if possible

- Hypercalciuria may respond to oral hydrochlorothiazide, usually given with a potassium supplement

- Hypercalcemia developing in patients with previously stable, treated hypoparathyroidism may signal new onset of Addison's disease

COMPLICATIONS

- Stridor, especially with vocal cord palsy, may cause respiratory obstruction requiring tracheostomy

- Chronic hypoparathyroidism may be associated with autoimmune diseases, eg, sprue, pernicious anemia, or Addison's disease

- Cataract formation and calcification of the basal ganglia occur in long-standing cases; parkinsonism or choreoathetosis occasionally develops

- Nerve root compression due to ossification of paravertebral ligaments

- Seizures in untreated patients
- Nephrocalcinosis and impaired renal function if overtreatment with calcium and vitamin D

PROGNOSIS

- Prognosis good with prompt diagnosis and treatment
- Dental changes, cataracts, and brain calcifications permanent

WHEN TO REFER

- Refer all patients to endocrinologist for stable regimen

WHEN TO ADMIT

- Any symptomatic hypocalcemia

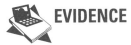 **EVIDENCE**

INFORMATION FOR PATIENTS

- Mayo Clinic—Hypoparathyroidism

REFERENCES

- Tartaglia F et al. Randomized study on oral administration of calcitriol to prevent symptomatic hypocalcemia after total thyroidectomy. Am J Surg. 2005 Sep;190(3):424–9. [PMID: 16105530]
- Tfelt-Hansen J et al. The calcium-sensing receptor in normal physiology and pathophysiology: a review. Crit Rev Clin Lab Sci. 2005;42(1):35–70. [PMID: 15697170]

Hypophosphatemia

 KEY FEATURES

ESSENTIALS OF DIAGNOSIS

- Serious depletion of body phosphate may exist with low, normal, or high serum phosphate levels
- May cause hypooxygenation and even rhabdomyolysis
- Reduced maximal tubular reabsorption rate of phosphate (TmP/GFR) indicates urinary phosphate loss

GENERAL CONSIDERATIONS

- Cellular uptake is stimulated by alkalemia, insulin, epinephrine, feeding, postparathy-roidectomy (hungry bone syndrome), and accelerated cell proliferation
- Alcoholism
  - In acute alcohol withdrawal, increased plasma insulin, epinephrine, and respiratory alkalosis promote intracellular shifts of phosphate
  - Vomiting, diarrhea, and poor dietary intake contribute to hypophosphatemia
  - In chronic alcohol use, there is a decreased renal threshold of phosphate excretion
- Parathyroid hormone (PTH) and fibroblast growth factor (FGF23) are the major factors that decreases TmP/GFR, leading to renal loss of phosphate
- In bronchospastic lung disease, hypophosphatemia can occur from
  - Theophylline (shifting phosphate intracellularly)
  - The phosphaturic effects of β-adrenergic agonists, loop diuretics, theophylline, and corticosteroids
- Therapy of hyperglycemia causes phosphate to accompany glucose intracellularly
- Moderate hypophosphatemia (1.0–2.5 mg/dL) occurs commonly in hospitalized patients and may not reflect decreased phosphate stores

Etiology

- Diminished supply or absorption
  - Starvation
  - Parenteral alimentation with inadequate phosphate content
  - Malabsorption
  - Vitamin D–resistant osteomalacia
- Increased loss
  - Phosphaturic drugs (diuretics, theophylline, bronchodilators, corticosteroids)
  - Hyperparathyroidism, hyperthyroidism
  - Renal tubular acidosis (eg, monoclonal gammopathy)
  - Alcoholism
  - Hypokalemic nephropathy
- Intracellular shift of phosphorus
  - Glucose administration
  - Drugs (anabolic steroids, estrogen, oral contraceptives)
  - Respiratory alkalosis
  - Salicylate poisoning
- Electrolyte abnormalities
  - Hypercalcemia
  - Hypomagnesemia
  - Metabolic alkalosis
- Abnormal losses followed by inadequate repletion
  - Diabetes mellitus with acidosis, especially during aggressive therapy
  - Recovery from starvation
  - Chronic alcoholism
  - Severe burns
- Inhibition of bone remodeling due to treatment with imatinib mesylate

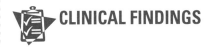 **CLINICAL FINDINGS**

SYMPTOMS AND SIGNS

- Moderate hypophosphatemia (1.0–2.5 mg/dL) is usually asymptomatic
- Severe hypophosphatemia (≤ 1 mg/dL) may cause muscle weakness
- Acute, severe hypophosphatemia (0.1–0.2 mg/dL)
  - Weakness from acute hemolytic anemia
  - Infection from impaired chemotaxis of leukocytes
  - Petechial hemorrhages from platelet dysfunction
  - Rhabdomyolysis
  - Encephalopathy (irritability, confusion, dysarthria, seizures, and coma)
  - Heart failure
- Chronic severe phosphate depletion causes anorexia, pain in muscles and bones, and fractures

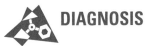 **DIAGNOSIS**

LABORATORY TESTS

- Serum phosphate < 2.5 mg/dL (< 0.8 mmol/L)
- Spot urine phosphate > 20 mg/dL suggests renal phosphate loss
- Normal TmP/GFR is 2.5–4.5 mg/dL
- TmP/GFR = [Serum Pi – (UPi × UV)]/ GFR
  - The main factors regulating TmP/GFR are PTH and phosphate intake
  - Increases of PTH or phosphate intake decreases TmP/GFR, so that more phosphate is excreted in the urine
- Lower values indicate urinary phosphate loss
- Hemolytic anemia may be present
- Elevated serum creatine kinase and myoglobinuria from rhabdomyolysis
- Renal glycosuria and hypouricemia together with hypophosphatemia indicate Fanconi's syndrome

IMAGING STUDIES

- In chronic depletion, radiographs and biopsies of bones show changes resembling those of osteomalacia

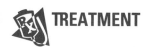

TREATMENT

MEDICATIONS

Oral replacement

- Acute hypocalcemia can occur with parenteral administration of phosphate; therefore, when possible, oral replacement of phosphate is preferable
- Use oral phosphate if the patient is asymptomatic and serum phosphorus is > 1 mg/dL
- Phosphate salts are available in skim milk (approximately 1 g/L [33 mmol/L])
- Sodium plus potassium phosphate tablets or capsules may be given to provide 0.5–1.0 g (18–32 mmol) per day
- Contraindications to phosphate salts
  - Hypoparathyroidism
  - Advanced stages of chronic kidney disease
  - Tissue damage and necrosis
  - Hypercalcemia

Intravenous replacement

- For asymptomatic patients with severe hypophosphatemia (serum phosphate 0.7–1.0 mg/dL) who cannot eat, infuse 279–310 mg (9–10 mmol)/12 h until the serum phosphate exceeds 1 mg/dL and then switch patient to oral therapy
- For symptomatic patients with severe hypophosphatemia (serum phosphate < 0.5–1.0 mg/dL) who cannot eat, give intravenous phosphorus up to 1 g in 1 L of fluid over 8–12 h
- Slow the infusion rate if hypotension occurs
- 3 g or more of phosphorus may be required over several days to replete body stores
- Parenteral phosphorus replacement carries potential of precipitating soft tissue calcification and nephrocalcinosis. Serum Ca^{2+} × serum PO_4 product > 70 markedly increases the risk
- A magnesium deficit often coexists and should be treated simultaneously

THERAPEUTIC PROCEDURES

- Mild hypophosphatemia usually resolves spontaneously with treatment of the underlying cause

OUTCOME

FOLLOW-UP

- Response to phosphate supplementation is not predictable

- During intravenous replacement of phosphate, monitor plasma phosphate, calcium and potassium q6h

WHEN TO REFER

- For consultation about etiology
- If expertise in phosphate repletion is needed, particularly with intravenous repletion

WHEN TO ADMIT

- Symptomatic hypophosphatemia
- Need for parenteral replacement

PREVENTION

- Include phosphate in repletion and maintenance fluids
- For parenteral alimentation
  - 620 mg (20 mmol) of phosphorus is required for every 1000 nonprotein kcal to maintain phosphate balance and to ensure anabolic function
  - A daily ration for prolonged parenteral fluid maintenance is 620–1240 mg (20–40 mmol) of phosphorus

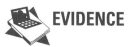

EVIDENCE

INFORMATION FOR PATIENTS

- American Association for Clinical Chemistry: Phosphorus Test
- MedlinePlus: Hypophosphatemia
- MedlinePlus: Phosphates Drug Information
- National Institute on Alcoholism and Alcohol Abuse: Alcoholism—Getting the Facts

REFERENCES

- Amanzadeh J et al. Hypophosphatemia: an evidence-based approach to its clinical consequences and management. Nature Clin Prac Nephrol. 2006 Mar; 2(3):136–48. [PMID: 16932412]
- Berman E et al. Altered bone and mineral metabolism in patients receiving imatinib mesylate. N Engl J Med. 2006 May 11;354(19):2006–13. [PMID: 16687713]
- Gaasbeek A et al. Hypophosphatemia: an update on its etiology and treatment. Am J Med. 2005 Oct;118(10):1094–101. [PMID: 16194637]
- Sheldon GF. Treatment of hypophosphatemia. J Am Coll Surg. 2004 Jul; 199(1):171. [PMID: 15217649]

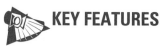

Hypopituitarism

KEY FEATURES

ESSENTIALS OF DIAGNOSIS

- Loss of one, all, or any combination of pituitary hormones
- ACTH deficiency reduces adrenal secretion of cortisol and testosterone; aldosterone secretion remains intact
- Luteinizing hormone (LH) and follicle-stimulating hormone (FSH) are secreted by the same pituitary cells, and their loss causes hypogonadism in men and women

GENERAL CONSIDERATIONS

- Caused by hypothalamic or pituitary dysfunction, including mass lesions (eg, pituitary adenomas, granulomas, Rathke's cleft cysts)
- May have single or multiple hormonal deficiencies of the anterior and posterior pituitary
- Pituitary tumor may be part of multiple endocrine neoplasia (type 1)
- Hypopituitarism without mass lesions may be due to
  - Idiopathic
  - Cranial radiation
  - Surgery
  - Encephalitis
  - Hemochromatosis
  - Autoimmune
  - Stroke
  - Post-CABG
  - Chronic epidural opioid infusion
  - X-linked congenital adrenal hypoplasia
  - Moderate to severe traumatic brain injury (Glasgow coma scale ≤ 13/15)
- About 55% of survivors of aneurysmal subarachnoid hemorrhage have at least one pituitary hormone deficiency
- Isolated hypogonadotrophic hypogonadism can occur in patients
  - With severe illness, malnutrition
  - Who take intrathecal opioids, methadone
  - Who perform extreme prolonged exercise (women)
  - Who are obese and have type 2 diabetes mellitus
  - With congenital adrenal hypoplasia
- Kallman's syndrome is the most common cause of congenital isolated gonadotropin deficiency
- Combined hypopituitarism can occur congenitally

CLINICAL FINDINGS

SYMPTOMS AND SIGNS

- Gonadotropin (LH and FSH) deficiency
  - Hypogonadism
  - Delayed adolescence, amenorrhea
  - Infertility, decreased libido
  - Loss of axillary, pubic, and body hair, especially with ACTH deficiency
  - Micropenis, cryptorchism
- TSH deficiency
  - Fatigue, weakness, weight gain
- ACTH deficiency of decreased cortisol with normal mineralocorticoid secretion
  - Weakness, weight loss, hypotension
  - Patients with partial ACTH deficiency have some cortisol secretion and may not have symptoms until stressed by illness or surgery
- Growth hormone (GH) deficiency
  - Obesity
  - Weakness
  - Reduced cardiac output
- ADH deficiency: Central diabetes insipidus with polyuria and polydipsia
- Oxytocin deficiency: No lactation
- Panhypopituitarism
  - Dry, pale, finely textured skin
  - Fine facial wrinkles and an apathetic countenance
- Congenital hypopituitarism
  - Growth failure due to GH and TSH deficiency
  - Lack of pubertal development occurs due to lack of FSH and LH
  - ACTH-cortisol deficiency occurs later, typically requiring corticosteroid therapy by age 18 years

DIFFERENTIAL DIAGNOSIS

- Anorexia nervosa or severe malnutrition (hypogonadotropic hypogonadism)
- Serious illness (hypogonadotropic hypogonadism, functional suppression of TSH and thyroxine [T_4])
- Severe malnutrition (hypogonadotropic hypogonadism)
- Primary hypothyroidism causes low T_4, high prolactin
- Addison's disease
- High-dose corticosteroids (secondary adrenal insufficiency)
- Low serum cortisol in critically ill patients due to low cortisol-binding globulin; free cortisol levels normal
- Triiodothyronine (T_3) administration can cause low TSH and low serum free T_4

DIAGNOSIS

LABORATORY TESTS

- Hyponatremia may occur, especially with combined ACTH and TSH deficiencies
- Fasting glucose may be low, potassium normal
- Low free T_4, TSH not elevated
- Low or low-normal testosterone, estradiol, LH, FSH
- Elevated prolactin in prolactinoma, acromegaly, hypothalamic disease
- ACTH stimulation test
  - Cosyntropin (synthetic ACTH analog), 0.25 mg IM or IV
  - Normally causes cortisol to rise to > 20 mcg/dL (550 nmol/L) in 30–60 min
  - ACTH deficiency causes adrenal atrophy and a deficient response
- Baseline ACTH low or normal in secondary hypoadrenalism; ACTH high in primary adrenal disease
- Basal cortisol ≥ 20 mcg/dL excludes adrenal insufficiency
- Metyrapone testing is unnecessary
- IGF-1 levels
  - Normal in 50% of adults with GH deficiency
  - Very low levels (< 84 mcg/L) indicate GH deficiency except in conditions that suppress IGF-1 (malnutrition, oral estrogen, hypothyroidism, uncontrolled diabetes mellitus, liver failure)
- Low serum levels of epinephrine and DHEA with ACTH-cortisol deficiency
- Screen for hemochromatosis with serum Fe, transferrin saturation, ferritin

IMAGING STUDIES

- MRI scan shows parasellar lesions

TREATMENT

MEDICATIONS

Secondary adrenal insufficiency

- Hydrocortisone, 15 mg PO every morning and 5–10 mg PO every night, or prednisone, 3 mg every morning and 2 mg every night PO once daily, or dexamethasone, 0.25 mg PO once daily
- Partial ACTH deficiency (basal morning serum cortisol > 8 mg/dL [220 mmol/L]) requires hydrocortisone maintenance doses of ~5 mg PO BID
- Some patients feel better with equivalent doses of prednisone 3.0–7.5 mg/day

- Monitor patients for manifestations of Cushing's syndrome or underreplacement. A serum WBC is useful, because a relative neutrophilia and lymphopenia can indicate overreplacement with corticosteroid, and vice versa
- Fludrocortisone is rarely needed
- Give additional hydrocortisone during stress
  - For mild illness, doses should be doubled or tripled
  - For trauma or surgery, 50 mg IM or IV q6h, then reduce to normal doses as stress subsides

Hypothyroidism

- Levothyroxine, 0.05–0.2 mg PO once daily after assessment for cortisol deficiency. Otherwise, may precipitate adrenal crisis
- Optimal replacement doses of thyroxine must be assessed by clinical evaluation
  - Serum free thyroxine levels may need to be in the high-normal or mildly elevated range for adequate replacement
  - Serum TSH assays are useless because levels are always low

Hypogonadism

- In women
  - Estrogen replacement (see Amenorrhea, Secondary & Menopause)
  - Clomiphene can induce ovulation
  - Oral dehydroepiandrosterone (USP-grade DHEA; 50 mg/d orally)
    - Increases sexual hair in 84%
    - Improves stamina in 70%
    - Improves sexual interest in 50%
- In men
  - Testosterone replacement (see Hypogonadism, Male)
  - To improve spermatogenesis, human chorionic gonadotropin (hCG), 2000–3000 units IM three times weekly, may be used with no testosterone
  - If sperm count remains low, FSH injections may be added

GH deficiency

- Somatotropin or somatrem (hGH) for symptomatic adults with severe GH deficiency, starting at 0.2 mg (0.6 IU) SC 3 × weekly or once daily
- Women who receive hGH should not take oral estrogen because this reduces hGH effect; topical estrogen is preferred
- Administer adequate hGH to maintain normal serum IGF-I levels
- Somatotropin discontinued if no improvement in energy, mentation, or visceral adiposity within 3–6 months at maximum tolerated dosage
- Do not administer hGH during major surgery or severe illness

Hyperprolactinemia
- Hypopituitarism from prolactin-secreting pituitary tumor may be reversible with bromocriptine, cabergoline, or quinagolide or with tumor resection (see Hyperprolactinemia)

Central diabetes insipidus
- Nasal desmopressin (DDAVP), 0.1 mL q12–24h
- Oral desmopressin, 0.1 or 0.2 mg q12–24h
- Parenteral desmopressin, 1–2 mcg IV SC q12–24h

SURGERY

- Transsphenoidal hypophysectomy for pituitary tumors sometimes reverses hypopituitarism

THERAPEUTIC PROCEDURES

- Radiation therapy for GH-secreting tumors, but increases risk of hypopituitarism

OUTCOME

FOLLOW-UP

- After pituitary surgery, postoperative hyponatremia is common. Check serum sodium frequently for 2 weeks
- Somatotropin therapy requires monitoring for side effects including hypertension, proliferative retinopathy

COMPLICATIONS

- Mass lesions may cause visual field deficits
- Radiation therapy increases risk of small vessel ischemic strokes and second tumors
- In craniopharyngioma, 16% have diabetes insipidus preoperatively and 60% postoperatively
- Hypothalamic damage may cause morbid obesity, cognitive and emotional problems
- GH deficiency increases cardiovascular morbidity
- Rarely, acute hemorrhage occurs in large pituitary tumors (pituitary apoplexy) causing rapid loss of vision and headache, requiring emergent decompression

PROGNOSIS

- Prognosis depends on primary cause
- Patients can recover from functional hypopituitarism, such as
  - Hypogonadism due to starvation or severe illness
  - ACTH suppression by corticosteroids

- TSH suppression by hyperthyroidism
- Intrathecal opioids

PREVENTION

- Patients with adrenal insufficiency should wear a medical ID bracelet

EVIDENCE

PRACTICE GUIDELINES

- Smith JC. Hormone replacement therapy in hypopituitarism. Expert Opin Pharmacother. 2004 May;5(5):1023–31. [PMID: 15155105]

WEB SITE

- Pituitary Network Association

INFORMATION FOR PATIENTS

- Mayo Clinic—Hypopituitarism

REFERENCES

- Agha A et al. Conventional glucocorticoid replacement overtreats adult hypopituitary patients with partial ACTH deficiency. Clin Endocrinol (Oxf). 2004 Jun;60(6):688–93. [PMID: 15163331]
- Agha A et al. The long-term predictive accuracy of the short synacthen (corticotropin) stimulation test for assessment of the hypothalamic-pituitary-adrenal axis. J Clin Endocrinol Metab. 2006 Jan;91(1):43–7. [PMID: 16249286]
- Brooke AM et al. Dehydroepiandrosterone improves psychological well-being in male and female hypopituitary patients on maintenance growth hormone replacement. J Clin Endocrinol Metab. 2006 Oct;91(10):3773–9. [PMID: 16849414]
- Leal-Cerro A et al. Prevalence of hypopituitarism and growth hormone deficiency in adults long-term after severe traumatic brain injury. Clin Endocrinol (Oxf). 2005 May;62(5):525–32. [PMID: 15853820]

Hypothermia

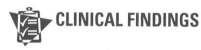

KEY FEATURES

ESSENTIALS OF DIAGNOSIS

- Systemic hypothermia is a reduction of core (rectal) body temperature below 35°C
- Oral temperatures are inaccurate; an esophageal or rectal probe that reads as low as 25°C is required

GENERAL CONSIDERATIONS

- In colder climates, elderly individuals living in inadequately heated housing are particularly susceptible
- Persons who are more vulnerable to accidental hypothermia
  - Those with comorbid conditions
  - Those who are using sedating or tranquilizing drugs
- Systemic hypothermia can be caused by
  - Prolonged postoperative hypothermia
  - Administration of large amounts of refrigerated stored blood (without rewarming)
- Therapeutic hypothermia can be used as adjunctive technique during neurosurgery to reduce postoperative neurologic sequelae

CLINICAL FINDINGS

SYMPTOMS AND SIGNS

Systemic hypothermia
- Early manifestations
  - Weakness
  - Drowsiness
  - Lethargy
  - Irritability
  - Confusion
  - Shivering
  - Impaired judgment and coordination
- The skin may appear blue or puffy
- At core temperatures below 35°C, the patient may become delirious, drowsy, or comatose and may stop breathing
- The pulse and blood pressure may be unobtainable, leading to the belief that the patient is dead

Hypothermia of the extremities
- Exposure of the extremities to cold produces immediate localized vasoconstriction followed by generalized vasoconstriction

- When the skin temperature falls to 25°C, the area becomes cyanotic
- At 15°C, there is a deceptively pink, well-oxygenated appearance to the skin. Tissue damage occurs at this temperature

DIFFERENTIAL DIAGNOSIS

- Infection
- Other cause of altered mental status (eg, hypoglycemia, drugs, stroke)
- Hypothyroidism
- Anorexia or malnutrition (poor fat stores)
- Adrenal insufficiency
- Burns
- Spinal cord injury

 DIAGNOSIS

LABORATORY TESTS

- Complete blood cell count
- Prothrombin time
- Partial thromboplastin time
- Serum electrolytes
- Blood urea nitrogen
- Serum creatinine
- Liver function tests
- Serum amylase
- Serum glucose
- pH level
- Arterial blood gases
- Urinalysis and urine volume

DIAGNOSTIC PROCEDURES

- ECG: cardiac arrhythmias and the pathognomonic J wave of Osborn, prominent in lateral precordial leads

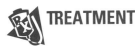 **TREATMENT**

THERAPEUTIC PROCEDURES

- **Mild hypothermia** (rectal temperature > 33°C) in healthy patients: warm bed or rapid passive rewarming with warm bath or warm packs and blankets
- **Moderate or severe hypothermia** (core temperatures < 33°C)
  - Establish cardiovascular support, acid-base balance, arterial oxygenation, and adequate intravascular volume before rewarming to minimize risk of organ infarction and "after-drop" (recurrent hypothermia)
  - Active external and internal rewarming
  - Once begun, CPR should continue until patient rewarmed to ≥ 32°C

Active external rewarming

- Heated blankets, warm baths, forced hot air
- Easier to monitor and perform diagnostic and therapeutic procedures using heated blankets
- Warm bath rewarming best done in tub of 40–42°C moving water (rewarming rate: ~1–2°C/h)
- When extracorporeal blood rewarming not an option, forced air rewarming (38–43°C) recommended
- Rewarming may cause marked peripheral dilation, predisposing to ventricular fibrillation and hypovolemic shock
- Antibiotics not routinely given

Active internal (core) rewarming

- Essential for severe hypothermia
- **Extracorporeal blood rewarming** (cardiopulmonary, venovenous, or arteriovenous femorofemoral bypass) treatment of choice, especially with cardiac arrest
- Without equipment for extracorporeal rewarming, left-sided thoracotomy followed by pericardial cavity irrigation with warmed saline and cardiac massage effective in systemic hypothermia < 28°C
- Thoracic lavage or hemodialysis also effective
- Repeated peritoneal dialysis with 2 L of warm (43°C) potassium-free dialysate solution exchanged every 10–12 min until core temperature raised to ~35°C
- Parenteral fluids (D_5 normal saline) warmed to 43°C
- Administer humidified air heated to 42°C through face mask or endotracheal tube
- Warm colonic and GI irrigations of less value
- Tracheal intubation for patients who are comatose or in respiratory failure

 OUTCOME

FOLLOW-UP

- Monitor cardiac rhythm
- Monitor core temperature (esophageal preferred over rectal) often during and after initial rewarming to avoid recurrent hypothermia

COMPLICATIONS

- Metabolic acidosis
- Hyperkalemia
- Pneumonia
- Pancreatitis
- Ventricular fibrillation
- Hypoglycemia or hyperglycemia
- Coagulopathy
- Renal failure
- Cardiac arrhythmias may occur, especially during rewarming
- Death usually caused by cardiac asystole, renal failure, or ventricular fibrillation

PROGNOSIS

- More than 75% of otherwise healthy patients may survive moderate or severe systemic hypothermia
- Prognosis is directly related to the severity of metabolic acidosis; if the pH is ≤ 6.6, the prognosis is poor
- The prognosis is grave if there are underlying predisposing causes or if treatment is delayed
- Neuropathic sequelae may persist for many years after the cold injury and include
  - Pain
  - Numbness
  - Tingling
  - Hyperhidrosis
  - Cold sensitivity of the extremities
  - Nerve conduction abnormalities

PREVENTION

- "Keep warm, keep moving, and keep dry"
- Tobacco and alcohol should be avoided
- Avoid cardiac, central vascular, or chest stimulation (eg, catheter, cannulas) unless essential because of the risk of inducing ventricular fibrillation

 EVIDENCE

PRACTICE GUIDELINES

- Brugger H et al; International Commission for Mountain Emergency Medicine. On-site treatment of avalanche victims ICAR-MEDCOM recommendation. High Alt Med Biol. 2002;3:421. [PMID: 12631429]
- Durrer B et al. The medical on-site treatment of hypothermia: ICAR-MEDCOM recommendation. High Alt Med Biol. 2003;4:99. [PMID: 12713717]
- European Resuscitation Council: Part 8: advanced challenges in resuscitation. Section 3: special challenges in ECC. 3A: hypothermia. Resuscitation. 2000; 46:267. [PMID: 10978806]

INFORMATION FOR PATIENTS

- Centers for Disease Control and Prevention: Extreme Cold: A Prevention Guide to Promote Your Personal Health and Safety
- Centers for Disease Control and Prevention: Winter Weather FAQs
- Mayo Clinic: Hypothermia

REFERENCES

- Kempainen RR et al. The evaluation and management of accidental hypothermia. Respir Care. 2004 Feb; 49(2):192–205. [PMID: 14744270]
- Ulrich AS et al. Hypothermia and localized cold injuries. Emerg Med Clin North Am. 2004 May;22(2):281–98. [PMID: 15163568]

Hypothyroidism (Myxedema)

KEY FEATURES

ESSENTIALS OF DIAGNOSIS

- Weakness, cold intolerance, constipation, depression, menorrhagia, hoarseness, dry skin, bradycardia
- Delayed return of deep tendon reflexes
- Serum free tetraiodothyronine (T_4) low
- Thyroid-stimulating hormone (TSH) elevated in primary hypothyroidism

GENERAL CONSIDERATIONS

- **Primary** hypothyroidism is due to thyroid gland disease
- **Secondary** hypothyroidism is due to lack of pituitary TSH
- **Maternal** hypothyroidism during pregnancy results in cognitive impairment in child
- Causes of **hypothyroidism with goiter**
  - Hashimoto's thyroiditis
  - Subacute (de Quervain's thyroiditis) (after initial hyperthyroidism)
  - Riedel's thyroiditis
  - Iodine deficiency
  - Genetic thyroid enzyme defects
  - Hepatitis C
  - Drugs:
    □ Lithium, amiodarone, propylthiouracil, methimazole, phenylbutazone, sulfonamides, interferon-α or β
  - Food goitrogens in iodide-deficient areas
  - Peripheral resistance to thyroid hormone
  - Infiltrating diseases
- Causes of **hypothyroidism without goiter**
  - Thyroid surgery, irradiation, or radioiodine treatment
  - Deficient pituitary TSH
  - Severe illness
- Radiation therapy to the head-neck-chest-shoulder region can cause hypothyroidism with or without goiter or thyroid cancer many years later
- "Subclinical" hypothyroidism, ie, clinically euthyroid individual with high TSH, normal T_4, occurs commonly in elderly women (~10% incidence)
- Amiodarone, due to high iodine content, causes clinical hypothyroidism in ~8%
- High iodine intake from other sources may also cause hypothyroidism, especially in those with underlying lymphocytic thyroiditis
- Myxedema is caused by interstitial accumulation of hydrophilic mucopolysaccharides, leading to fluid retention and lymphedema

CLINICAL FINDINGS

SYMPTOMS AND SIGNS

- **Early symptoms**
  - Fatigue, lethargy, weakness
  - Arthralgias, myalgias, muscle cramps
  - Cold intolerance
  - Constipation
  - Dry skin
  - Headache
  - Menorrhagia
- **Late symptoms**
  - Slow speech
  - Constipation
  - Peripheral edema
  - Pallor
  - Hoarseness
  - Decreased senses of taste, smell, and hearing
  - Muscle cramps, aches and pains
  - Dyspnea
  - Weight changes (usually gain, sometimes loss)
  - Amenorrhea or menorrhagia
  - Galactorrhea
  - Absent sweating
- **Early signs**
  - Thin, brittle nails, thinning of hair
  - Pallor
  - Poor turgor of mucosa
  - Delayed return of deep tendon reflexes

- **Late signs**
  - Goiter
  - Puffiness of face and eyelids
  - Carotenemia
  - Thinning of outer eyebrows
  - Tongue thickening
  - Hard pitting edema
  - Pleural, peritoneal, pericardial, and joint effusions
- **Myxedema coma**
  - Hypothermia, hypotension, hypoventilation, hypoxia, hypercapnia, hyponatremia
  - Convulsions and abnormal CNS signs
  - Often induced by
    □ Underlying infection
    □ Cardiac, respiratory, or CNS illness
    □ Cold exposure
    □ Drug use
- Cardiac enlargement due to pericardial effusion, bradycardia
- Hypothermia

DIFFERENTIAL DIAGNOSIS

- Conditions and drugs that cause a low serum T_4 or T_3 or high serum TSH in the absence of hypothyroidism
- The pituitary is often quite enlarged in primary hypothyroidism due to reversible hyperplasia of TSH-secreting cells; the concomitant hyperprolactinemia seen in hypothyroidism can lead to the mistaken diagnosis of a TSH-secreting or PRL-secreting pituitary adenoma

DIAGNOSIS

LABORATORY TESTS

- Serum TSH is increased in primary hypothyroidism but low or normal in secondary hypothyroidism (pituitary insufficiency)
- Free T_4 may be low or low normal
- Serum triiodothyronine (T_3) is not a good test for hypothyroidism
- Serum cholesterol, liver enzymes, creatine kinase, prolactin increased
- Hyponatremia occurs due to impaired renal tubular sodium reabsorption
- Hypoglycemia
- Anemia (with normal or increased mean corpuscular volume)
- Thyroperoxidase or thyroglobulin antibody titers usually high in hypothyroidism due to Hashimoto's thyroiditis
- During pregnancy in women with hypothyroidism taking replacement thyroxine, check serum TSH frequently (eg, every 1–2 months) to ensure adequate replacement

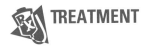 **TREATMENT**

MEDICATIONS

- Levothyroxine (T$_4$)
  - Treatment of choice after excluding adrenal insufficiency, which requires concurrent treatment
  - Starting dose
    - 50–100 mcg PO every morning if no coronary disease and age < 60 years
    - 100–150 mcg PO every morning if hypothyroid during pregnancy
    - 25–50 mcg PO every morning if coronary disease or age > 60
  - Dose titrated up by 25 mcg q1–3wks until patient is euthyroid, usually at 100–250 mcg every morning
  - Elevated TSH usually indicates underreplacement
  - Before increasing T$_4$ dosage, assess for angina, diarrhea, or malabsorption
  - Once a maintenance dose is determined, continue with the same brand owing to slight differences in absorption
  - T$_4$ requirements increase with oral estrogen therapy
  - Increase T$_4$ dose 30% as soon as pregnancy is confirmed
  - T$_4$ dosage requirements can rise, owing to increased hepatic metabolism of thyroxine induced by certain medications
    - Carbamazepine
    - Phenobarbitol
    - Phenytoin
    - Rifabutin
    - Rifampin
  - Suppressed TSH may indicate T$_4$ overreplacement
    - Assess for severe nonthyroidal illness
    - Assess medications (eg, nonsteroidal anti-inflammatory drugs, opioids, nifedipine, verapamil, corticosteroids)
  - T$_4$ requirements decrease postpartum, with menopause, or when switching from oral to transdermal estrogen therapy
  - Hypothyroid patients with ischemic heart disease should begin T$_4$ *after* coronary artery angioplasty or bypass
  - Avoid administration concurrently with binding substances, eg, iron, aluminum hydroxide antacids, calcium supplements, or soy milk; or with bile acid-binding resins (eg, cholestyramine)
- Hypothyroid patients taking T$_4$ typically have low serum T$_3$ levels (FT$_3$ levels during pregnancy or oral estrogen)
  - Addition of triiodothyronine (T$_3$, Cytomel) is controversial

- Amiodarone-induced hypothyroidism: treat with just enough T$_4$ to relieve symptoms
- **Myxedema coma**
  - Levothyroxine sodium, 400 mcg IV loading dose, then 100 mcg IV once daily
  - If hypothermic, warm only with blankets
  - If hypercapnic, mechanical ventilation
  - Treat infections aggressively
  - If adrenal insufficiency suspected, give hydrocortisone, 100 mg IV, then 25–50 mg q8h
- Myxedematous patients are unusually sensitive to opiates and may develop respiratory depression with typical doses

 OUTCOME

FOLLOW-UP

- Continue T$_4$ for life; reassess dosage requirements periodically clinically and with serum TSH
- Surveillance for atrial arrhythmias and for osteoporosis, especially in patients who require high doses of T$_4$
- Monitor patients with subclinical hypothyroidism for subtle signs (eg, fatigue, depression, hyperlipidemia)
- Clinical hypothyroidism later develops in ~18%

COMPLICATIONS

- Angina pectoris, congestive heart failure; may be precipitated by too rapid thyroid replacement
- Increased susceptibility to infection
- Megacolon in long-standing hypothyroidism
- Organic psychoses with paranoid delusions ("myxedema madness")
- Adrenal crisis precipitated by thyroid replacement
- Infertility (rare), miscarriage in untreated hypothyroidism
- Sellar enlargement and TSH-secreting tumors in untreated cases

PROGNOSIS

- Excellent prognosis with early treatment, but relapses may occur if treatment is interrupted
- Mortality rate for myxedema coma is high

WHEN TO REFER

- Difficulty titrating T$_4$ replacement to normal TSH or clinically euthyroid state

- Any patient with significant coronary disease needing T$_4$

WHEN TO ADMIT

- Suspected myxedema coma
- Hypercapnia

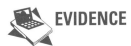 **EVIDENCE**

PRACTICE GUIDELINES

- Roberts CG et al. Hypothyroidism. Lancet. 2004;363:793. Comment in: Lancet 2004;363:1558. [PMID: 15016491]

WEB SITES

- American Thyroid Association
- Thyroid Disease Manager

INFORMATION FOR PATIENTS

- Mayo Clinic—Hypothyroidism
- Parmet S et al. JAMA patient page. Hypothyroidism. JAMA. 2003; 290:3024. [PMID: 14665665]

REFERENCES

- Alexander EK et al. Timing and magnitude of increases in levothyroxine requirements during pregnancy in women with hypothyroidism. N Engl J Med. 2004 Jul 15;351(3):241–9. [PMID: 15254282]
- Appelhof BC et al. Combined therapy with levothyroxine and liothyronine in two ratios, compared with levothyroxine monotherapy in primary hypothyroidism: a double-blind, randomized, controlled clinical trial. J Clin Endocrinol Metab. 2005 May;90(5):2666–74. [PMID: 15705921]
- Hennessey JV. Levothyroxine dosage and the limitations of current bioequivalence standards. Nat Clin Pract Endocrinol Metab. 2006 Sep;2(9):474–5. [PMID: 16957756]
- Roos A et al. The starting dose of levothyroxine in primary hypothyroidism treatment: a prospective, randomized, double-blind trial. Arch Intern Med. 2005 Aug 8–22;165(15):1714–20. [PMID: 16087818]
- Wekking EM et al. Cognitive functioning and well-being in euthyroid patients on thyroxine replacement therapy for primary hypothyroidism. Eur J Endocrinol. 2005 Dec;153(6):747–53. [PMID: 16322379]

Idiopathic (Autoimmune) Thrombocytopenic Purpura

 KEY FEATURES

ESSENTIALS OF DIAGNOSIS

- Isolated thrombocytopenia
- Other hematopoietic cell lines normal
- No systemic illness
- Spleen not palpable
- Normal bone marrow with normal or increased megakaryocytes

GENERAL CONSIDERATIONS

- Autoimmune disorder in which immunoglobulin G (IgG) autoantibody is formed that binds to platelets; it is unclear which antigen on platelet surface is involved
- Platelets are not destroyed by direct lysis; splenic macrophages bind to antibody-coated platelets
- Because the spleen is a major site of antibody production and platelet sequestration, splenectomy is highly effective therapy
- Hematologically identical to secondary thrombocytopenic purpura associated with systemic lupus erythematosus and chronic lymphocytic leukemia
- Childhood idiopathic thrombocytopenic purpura (ITP) is frequently precipitated by viral infection and usually self-limited
- Adult form is usually chronic and infrequently follows viral infection
- Higher incidence with HIV infection

DEMOGRAPHICS

- Disease of young persons: peak incidence between ages 20 and 50
- 2:1 female predominance

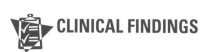 **CLINICAL FINDINGS**

SYMPTOMS AND SIGNS

- Patients are systemically well and usually are not febrile
- Mucosal or skin bleeding: epistaxis, oral bleeding or hemorrhagic bullae, menorrhagia, purpura, or petechiae
- No other abnormal physical findings
- Splenomegaly should lead to consideration of an alternative diagnosis

DIFFERENTIAL DIAGNOSIS

- Thrombotic thrombocytopenic purpura
- Acute leukemia
- Myelodysplastic syndrome
- Disseminated intravascular coagulation
- Early aplastic anemia
- Drug toxicity (eg, heparin, sulfonamides, thiazides, quinine)
- Alcohol abuse
- Hypersplenism
- Systemic lupus erythematosus

 DIAGNOSIS

LABORATORY TESTS

- Thrombocytopenia, which may be severe (< 10,000/mcL)
- Other counts are usually normal except for anemia resulting from bleeding or associated hemolysis
- Peripheral blood smear shows normal cell morphology except for slightly enlarged platelets (megathrombocytes)
- Coexistent autoimmune hemolytic anemia (Evans's syndrome) in ~10%
  - Associated with anemia, and peripheral smear showing reticulocytosis and spherocytes
  - Red blood cell fragmentation should not be seen
- Coagulation studies entirely normal

DIAGNOSTIC PROCEDURES

- Bone marrow aspiration and biopsy are normal, with normal or increased number of megakaryocytes

 TREATMENT

MEDICATIONS

- Initial treatment: prednisone, 1–2 mg/kg/day PO, gradually tapered after platelet count normalizes
- Normal platelet count is not necessary because risk of bleeding is small if platelet count is > 50,000/mcL
- High-dose IVIG, 1 g/kg for 1 or 2 days
  - Rapidly raises platelet count in 90%; platelet count rises within 1–5 days
  - Expensive and effect lasts only 1–2 weeks, so reserved for bleeding emergencies or preparing a severely thrombocytopenic patient for surgery
- Danazol, 600 mg/day, may be used if no response to prednisone and splenectomy
- Rituximab 325 mg/m² weekly for 4 weeks may be effective
- Non-cytotoxic immunosuppressive agents (eg, cyclosporine) may be used in refractory cases
- Cytotoxic immunosuppressive agents reserved for refractory cases

SURGERY

- Splenectomy
  - Definitive treatment; most adults ultimately undergo splenectomy
  - Indications
    □ No initial response to prednisone or unacceptably high doses required to maintain adequate platelet count
    □ Patient prefers surgery
  - Can be performed safely even with platelet counts < 10,000/mcL
  - Benefits 80% with either complete or partial remission
  - ITP may recur in 10–20% of cases

THERAPEUTIC PROCEDURES

- Few adults with ITP have spontaneous remissions; most require treatment
- High-dose immunosuppression and autologous stem cell transplantation for rare patients with severe and refractory ITP
- Platelet transfusions are reserved for life-threatening bleeding and are rarely used because exogenous platelets survive no better than the patient's own (only a few hours)

 OUTCOME

FOLLOW-UP

- With prednisone, bleeding often diminishes within 1 day; platelet count usually begins to rise within a week, and almost always within 3 weeks
- About 80% respond to prednisone, normalizing platelet count, but thrombocytopenia usually recurs if prednisone is completely withdrawn, so the aim is to find a dose that maintains adequate platelet count (> 50,000/mcL)
- About 50% of patients respond to danazol

COMPLICATIONS

- Major initial concern is cerebral hemorrhage, a risk when platelet count is < 5000/mcL
- Fatal bleeding is rare, even at very low platelet counts

PROGNOSIS

- Prognosis for remission is good
- Disease is usually initially controlled with prednisone; splenectomy offers definitive therapy

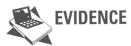 **EVIDENCE**

PRACTICE GUIDELINES

- British Committee for Standards in Haematology General Haematology Task Force. Guidelines for the investigation and management of idiopathic thrombocytopenic purpura in adults, children and in pregnancy. Br J Haematol. 2003;120:574. [PMID: 12588344]
- George JN et al. Idiopathic Thrombocytopenic Purpura. A Practice Guideline Developed by Explicit Methods for The American Society of Hematology 1996, reviewed 2001.

INFORMATION FOR PATIENTS

- National Heart, Lung, and Blood Institute: What Is Idiopathic Thrombocytopenic Purpura?
- Platelet Disorder Support Association: About ITP
- American Academy of Family Physicians: ITP
- National Institute of Diabetes & Digestive & Kidney Diseases

REFERENCES

- Beardsley DS. ITP in the 21st century. Hematology Am Soc Hematol Educ Program. 2006:402–7. [PMID: 17124090]
- Cines DB et al. How I treat idiopathic thrombocytopenic purpura (ITP). Blood. 2005 Oct 1;106(7):2244–51. [PMID: 15941913]
- Kojouri, K et al. Splenectomy for adult patients with idiopathic thrombocytopenia purpura: a systematic review to assess long-term platelet count responses, prediction of response, and surgical complications. Blood. 2004 Nov 1;104(9):2623–34. [PMID: 15217831]

Ileus, Acute Paralytic

 KEY FEATURES

ESSENTIALS OF DIAGNOSIS

- Precipitating factors
  - Surgery
  - Peritonitis
  - Electrolyte abnormalities
  - Severe medical illness
- Nausea, vomiting, obstipation, distention
- Minimal abdominal tenderness; decreased bowel sounds
- Plain abdominal radiography with gas and fluid distention in small and large bowel

GENERAL CONSIDERATIONS

- Neurogenic failure or loss of peristalsis in the intestine in the absence of any mechanical obstruction
- Common in hospitalized patients as a result of the following
  - Intra-abdominal processes, such as
    - Recent gastrointestinal or abdominal surgery
    - Peritoneal irritation (peritonitis, pancreatitis, ruptured viscus, hemorrhage)
  - Severe medical illness, such as
    - Pneumonia
    - Respiratory failure requiring intubation
    - Sepsis or severe infections
    - Uremia
    - Diabetic ketoacidosis
    - Electrolyte abnormalities (hypokalemia, hypercalcemia, hypomagnesemia, hypophosphatemia)
  - Medications, such as
    - Opioids
    - Anticholinergics
    - Phenothiazines

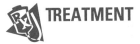 **CLINICAL FINDINGS**

SYMPTOMS AND SIGNS

- Mild diffuse, continuous abdominal discomfort
- Nausea and vomiting
- Generalized abdominal distention
- Minimal abdominal tenderness
- No signs of peritoneal irritation
- Bowel sounds are diminished to absent

DIFFERENTIAL DIAGNOSIS

- Mechanical obstruction of small intestine or proximal colon, eg, adhesions, volvulus, Crohn's disease
- Chronic intestinal pseudo-obstruction

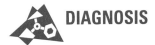 **DIAGNOSIS**

LABORATORY TESTS

- Obtain serum electrolytes, potassium, magnesium, phosphorus, and calcium

IMAGING STUDIES

- Plain abdominal radiography: air-fluid levels, distended gas-filled loops of small and large intestine
- Limited barium small bowel series or a CT scan can help exclude mechanical obstruction

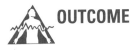 **TREATMENT**

THERAPEUTIC PROCEDURES

- Treat underlying primary medical or surgical illness
- Nasogastric suction for discomfort or vomiting
- Restrict oral intake, administer intravenous fluids
- Liberalize diet gradually as bowel function returns
- Minimize anticholinergic and opioid medications
- Peripheral nonopioid receptor antagonists reduce the duration of postoperative ileus; these agents are in clinical trials
- Severe or prolonged ileus requires nasogastric suction and infusion of parenteral fluids and electrolytes

OUTCOME

FOLLOW-UP

- Return of bowel function usually heralded by return of appetite and passage of flatus
- Serial plain film radiography and/or abdominal CT warranted for persistent or worsening symptoms to distinguish from mechanical obstruction

COMPLICATIONS

- Metabolic disturbances due to prolonged nasogastric suction (hypokalemia, metabolic alkalosis)

- Delayed nutritional intake complication of prolonged postoperative immobility

PROGNOSIS

- Ileus usually resolves within 48–72 h
- Following surgery, small intestinal motility normalizes first (within hours), followed by stomach (24–48 h) and colon (48–72 h)

WHEN TO REFER

- Persistent ileus lasting more than 3–5 days warrants further evaluation for underlying cause and to exclude mechanical obstruction

WHEN TO ADMIT

- All patients with ileus require admission for IV fluids

 EVIDENCE

PRACTICE GUIDELINES

- Bauer AJ et al. Ileus in critical illness: mechanisms and management. Curr Opin Crit Care. 2002;8:152. [PMID: 12386517]
- Holte K et al. Postoperative ileus: progress towards effective management. Drugs. 2002;62:2603. [PMID: 12466000]

INFORMATION FOR PATIENTS

- MedlinePlus—Intestinal obstruction

REFERENCE

- Tan EK et al. Meta-analysis: alvimpan vs. placebo in the treatment of post-operative ileus. Aliment Pharmacol Ther. 2007 Jan 1;25(1):47–57. [PMID: 17042776]

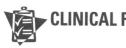 **Impetigo**

 KEY FEATURES

- A contagious and autoinoculable infection of the skin caused by staphylococci or rarely streptococci (or both)

 CLINICAL FINDINGS

- The lesions consist of macules, vesicles, bullae, pustules, and honey-colored gummy crusts that when removed leave denuded red areas
- The face and other exposed parts are most often affected
- Ecthyma is a deeper form of impetigo caused by staphylococci or streptococci, with ulceration and scarring; it occurs frequently on the legs and other covered areas

 DIAGNOSIS

- Culture confirms the diagnosis
- Differential diagnosis
  – Contact dermatitis (acute)
  – Herpes simplex

 TREATMENT

- Cephalexin, 250 mg PO QID
- Doxycycline, 100 mg PO BID, or trimethoprim/sulfamethoxazole, double-strength PO BID, can be used for penicillin allergy and methicillin-resistant *Staphylococcus aureus*
- Recurrent impetigo, which is due to nasal carriage of *S aureus*, is treated with rifampin, 600 mg PO once daily, or mupirocin intranasal ointment applied intranasally BID for 5 days
- Refer if questionable diagnosis or if therapy is ineffective

Infertility, Female

 KEY FEATURES

ESSENTIALS OF DIAGNOSIS

- Pregnancy does not result after 6–12 months of normal sexual activity without contraceptives

GENERAL CONSIDERATIONS

- About 25% of couples experience infertility at some point
- The incidence increases with age
- The male partner contributes to about 40% of cases of infertility, and a combination of male and female factors is common

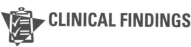 **CLINICAL FINDINGS**

SYMPTOMS AND SIGNS

- Obtain history of sexually transmitted disease or prior pregnancies
- Discuss ill effects of cigarettes, alcohol, and other recreational or prescription drugs on male fertility
- The gynecologic history should include
  – The menstrual pattern
  – Use and types of contraceptives, douches
  – Libido
  – Sexual technique
  – Frequency and success of coitus
  – Correlation of intercourse with time of ovulation
- Family history should inquire about family members with repeated abortions and maternal diethylstilbestrol use
- General physical and genital examinations for both partners

DIFFERENTIAL DIAGNOSIS

- Male factor infertility (hypogonadism, varicocele, alcohol or drug use, immotile cilia syndrome)
- Polycystic ovary syndrome
- Premature ovarian failure
- Hyperprolactinemia
- Hypothyroidism
- Inadequate luteal progesterone or short luteal phase
- Endometriosis
- Uterine leiomyomas (fibroids) or polyps
- Prior pelvic inflammatory disease
- Pelvic adhesions, eg, pelvic surgery, therapeutic abortion, ectopic pregnancy, septic abortion, intrauterine device use

DIAGNOSIS

DIAGNOSTIC PROCEDURES

Initial testing

- Complete blood cell count, urinalysis, cervical culture for *Chlamydia*, serologic test for syphilis, rubella antibody determination, and thyroid function tests
- A luteal phase serum progesterone above 3 ng/mL establishes ovulation
- Self-performed urine tests for the mid-cycle luteinizing hormone (LH) surge can enhance temperature observations relating to ovulation
- Coitus resulting in conception occurs during the 6-day period ending with the day of ovulation

- Before additional testing, an ejaculate from the male partner for semen analysis is obtained after sexual abstinence for at least 3 days
- Semen should be examined within 1–2 h after collection
  - Normal semen: volume, 3 mL; concentration, 20 million sperm per milliliter; motility, 50% after 2 h; and normal forms, 60%
  - If the sperm count is abnormal, search for exposure to environmental and workplace toxins, alcohol or drug abuse, and hypogonadism

Further testing
- Gross deficiencies of sperm (number, motility, or appearance) require a repeat semen analysis
- Zona-free hamster egg penetration tests evaluate the ability of the human sperm to fertilize an egg
- Obstruction of the uterine tubes requires either microsurgery or in vitro fertilization
- Absent or infrequent ovulation requires additional laboratory evaluation
  - Elevated follicle-stimulating hormone (FSH) and LH levels indicate ovarian failure causing premature menopause
  - Elevated LH levels in the presence of normal FSH levels confirm the presence of polycystic ovary syndrome
  - Elevation of blood prolactin (PRL) levels suggests pituitary microadenoma
- Major histocompatibility antigen typing of both partners can confirm HLA-B locus homozygosity, found in a greater percentage than expected among infertile couples
- Ultrasound monitoring of folliculogenesis may reveal unruptured luteinized follicles
- Endometrial biopsy in the luteal phase associated with simultaneous serum progesterone levels can be done to rule out luteal phase deficiency
- Hysterosalpingography
  - Can demonstrates uterine abnormalities (septa, polyps, submucous myomas) and tubal obstruction
  - A repeat x-ray film 24 hours later can confirm tubal patency if there is wide pelvic dispersion of the dye
  - Test has been associated with a subsequent increased pregnancy rate if an oil-based rather than water-soluble contrast medium is used
- Laparoscopy
  - Indicated if hysterosalpingography or history suggests tubal disease and IVF

is recommended as the primary treatment option
- In unexplained infertility, approximately 25% of women whose basic evaluation is normal have abnormal findings on laparoscopy explaining their infertility (eg, peritubal adhesions, endometriotic implants)

TREATMENT

MEDICATIONS

Induction of ovulation
- Clomiphene citrate
  - After a normal menstrual period or induction of withdrawal bleeding with progestin, give clomiphene 50 mg PO once daily for 5 days
  - If ovulation does not occur, increase dosage to 100 mg once daily for 5 days
  - If ovulation still does not occur, the course is repeated with 150 mg once daily for 5 days, and then 200 mg once daily for 5 days, with the addition of chorionic gonadotropin, 10,000 units IM, 7 days after clomiphene
- In the presence of increased androgen production (DHEA-S > 200 mcg/dL)
  - Addition of dexamethasone, 0.5 mg PO at bedtime, or prednisone, 5 mg PO at bedtime, improves the response to clomiphene
  - Dexamethasone should be discontinued after pregnancy is confirmed
- Bromocriptine
  - Used only if PRL levels are elevated and there is no withdrawal bleeding following progesterone administration (otherwise, clomiphene is used)
  - Initial dosage is 2.5 mg PO once daily, increased to two or three times daily in increments of 1.25 mg
  - Discontinue once pregnancy has occurred
- Human menopausal gonadotropins (hMG) or recombinant FSH is indicated in cases of hypogonadotropism and most other types of anovulation (exclusive of ovarian failure)
- Gonadotropin-releasing hormone (GnRH)—in hypothalamic amenorrhea unresponsive to clomiphene, subcutaneous pulsatile GnRH can be administered
- See Endometriosis for its treatment

SURGERY
- Fertility can be improved with excision of ovarian tumors or ovarian foci of

endometriosis, and microsurgical relief of tubal obstruction due to salpingitis
- Some cornual or fimbrial block can be relieved. Peritubal adhesions or endometriotic implants often can be treated via laparoscopy or via laparotomy
- Sperm characteristics are often improved following surgical treatment of varicocele in the male partner

THERAPEUTIC PROCEDURES
- Treat hypothyroidism or hyperthyroidism
- Give antibiotics for cervicitis if present
- In women with abnormal postcoital tests and demonstrated antisperm antibodies causing sperm agglutination or immobilization, condom use for up to 6 months may result in lower antibody levels and improved pregnancy rates
- Women who engage in vigorous athletic training often have low sex hormone levels; fertility improves with reduced exercise and some weight gain
- In cases of male partner azoospermia, artificial insemination by a donor usually results in pregnancy if female evaluation is normal

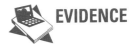

OUTCOME

PROGNOSIS
- The prognosis for normal pregnancy is good if minor disorders can be treated
- However, the prognosis for normal pregnancy is poor if the causes of infertility are severe, untreatable, or of prolonged duration (> 3 years)
- In the absence of identifiable causes of infertility, 60% of couples will achieve a pregnancy within 3 years
- Couples with unexplained infertility who do not achieve pregnancy within 3 years should be offered ovulation induction, assisted reproductive technology, or information about adoption

WHEN TO REFER
- Refer to reproductive endocrinologist for assisted reproductive techniques

EVIDENCE

PRACTICE GUIDELINES
- Brigham and Women's Hospital. Infertility. A guide to evaluation, treatment, and counseling. 2003

- Institute for Clinical Systems Improvement. Diagnosis and management of basic infertility. 2004

WEB SITE

- Centers for Disease Control and Prevention: Assisted Reproductive Technology Reports

INFORMATION FOR PATIENTS

- American Society for Reproductive Medicine: Patient Resources
- Mayo Clinic: Infertility
- MedlinePlus: Infertility
- National Infertility Association

REFERENCES

- Centers for Disease Control and Prevention, American Society for Reproductive Medicine: 2004 Assisted Reproductive Technology Success Rates. 2006, Atlanta, GA.
- Sutter P. Rational diagnosis and treatment in infertility. Best Pract Res Clin Obstet Gynecol. 2006 Oct;20(5):647–64. [PMID: 16769249]

Influenza

 KEY FEATURES

ESSENTIALS OF DIAGNOSIS

- Abrupt onset of fevers, chills, malaise, cough, arthralgias, and myalgias
- Although sporadic cases do occur, most cases of influenza occur as part of epidemics or pandemics, usually in the fall or winter seasons

GENERAL CONSIDERATIONS

- An orthomyxovirus transmitted by respiratory droplets
- Three antigenic subtypes have been described
  - Types A and B produce identical clinical symptoms
  - Type C produces milder disease
- Pandemics usually due to type A infections with significant antigenic shift (large genetic recombination of the virus)
- Influenza is difficult to diagnose in the absence of the epidemic because it resembles other viral illnesses

DEMOGRAPHICS

- 5000–250,000 cases annually in the United States
- Incidence highest in school-age children and young adults, students, prisoners, day care and health care workers; persons with asthma are at particular risk
- Complications occur most often in elderly, immunocompromised individuals

 CLINICAL FINDINGS

SYMPTOMS AND SIGNS

- Abrupt onset
- Fevers, chills, malaise with myalgias and headaches are common
- Nasal congestion, substernal tenderness, and nausea are not uncommon
- Fever typically lasts 3–5 days (range, 1–7 days)
- Sore throat, cervical lymphadenopathy, and nonproductive cough are usually present
- Leukopenia is common
- Leukocytosis may be a marker of secondary complications
- Proteinuria occasionally

DIFFERENTIAL DIAGNOSIS

- Common cold
- Primary bacterial pneumonia
- Infectious mononucleosis
- *Mycoplasma* infection
- Early Legionnaire's
- *Chlamydial pneumoniae* infection (TWAR)
- Acute HIV infection
- Meningitis
- In returning tropical traveler: malaria, dengue, typhoid

 DIAGNOSIS

LABORATORY TESTS

- Influenza virus can be isolated from throat or nasal washings sent for tissue culture
- Direct fluorescent antibody staining of washings can also make the diagnosis, though it cannot identify subtypes

DIAGNOSTIC PROCEDURES

- Usually diagnosed clinically when characteristic symptoms are found in the setting of an epidemic

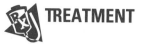 **TREATMENT**

MEDICATIONS

- Ribavirin (1.1 g/day, diluted to 20 mg/mL and delivered as particulate aerosol with oxygen over 12–18 hours a day for 3–7 days) helps severely ill patients with influenza A or B
- Amantadine and rimantadine no longer recommended because of high prevalence of resistant strains
- Zanamivir (inhaled) or oseltamivir (oral)
  - Effective at reducing the duration and severity of symptoms of influenza A and B
  - However, they are costly and must be started within 48 h of onset of symptoms to be effective
  - Zanamivir may cause bronchospasm in persons with asthma

THERAPEUTIC PROCEDURES

- Supportive measures with adequate hydration, analgesics, and rest

OUTCOME

COMPLICATIONS

- Influenza predisposes individuals to secondary bacterial infections of the respiratory tract, especially with pneumococcus and *Staphylococcus aureus*
- Pneumonia and purulent bronchitis are frequent complications
- Reye's syndrome, a severe form of hepatic failure, occurs rarely, particularly in young children given salicylates during influenza B or varicella infections

PROGNOSIS

- Most patients recover fully back to baseline health within 4–7 days
- Secondary complications can lengthen the course of illness and worsen the chances of a full recovery
- Poor outcomes usually occur in the elderly, often due to
  - Dehydration
  - Exacerbations of comorbid conditions
  - Secondary complications

WHEN TO REFER

- Refer when signs of secondary complications occur

WHEN TO ADMIT

- Consider hospitalization for signs of significant secondary complications, such as pneumonia or acute exacerbations of chronic bronchitis

PREVENTION

- Trivalent inactivated influenza vaccine is highly effective (85%) most years (Tables 67 and 68)
- Vaccination is recommended for persons who are older than 50 years or who have heart, lung, or other chronic diseases
- Vaccine should be avoided in patients with known hypersensitivity to eggs or its components
- Vaccine is not contraindicated in patients taking warfarin or corticosteroids, or in those with HIV infection
- The neuraminidase inhibitors (zanamivir or oseltamivir) can be used prophylactically for both influenza A and B
- Amantadine or rimantadine no longer used as prophylaxis because of high prevalence of resistant strains

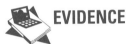 **EVIDENCE**

PRACTICE GUIDELINES

- National Guideline Clearinghouse
  - Prevention and control of influenza: recommendations of the Advisory Committee on Immunization Practices (ACIP)
  - Interim influenza vaccination recommendations—2004–05 influenza season
  - Influenza antiviral medications: 2004–05 interim chemoprophylaxis and treatment guidelines

WEB SITE

- Centers for Disease Control and Prevention

INFORMATION FOR PATIENTS

- Centers for Disease Control and Prevention Fact Sheet
- Torpy JM et al. JAMA patient page. Influenza. JAMA. 2004;292:2182. [PMID: 15523077]

REFERENCES

- Armstrong BG et al. Effect of influenza vaccination on excess deaths occurring during periods of high circulation of influenza: cohort study in elderly people. BMJ. 2004 Sep 18;329(7467):660. [PMID: 15313884]
- Advisory Committee on Immunization Practices. Prevention and Control of Influenza: recommendations of the Advisory Committee on Immunization Practices (ACIP). MMWR Recomm Rep. 2006 Jul 28;55(RR-10):1–42. [PMID: 16874296]
- Baz M et al. Characterization of multi-drug-resistant influenza A/H3N2 viruses shed during 1 year by an immunocompromised child. Clin Infect Dis. 2006 Dec 15;43(12):1555–61. [PMID: 17109288]
- Hayden FG et al. Antiviral management of seasonal and pandemic influenza. J Infect Dis. 2006 Nov 1;194(Suppl 2):S119–26. [PMID: 17163384]
- Kawai N et al. A comparison of the effectiveness of oseltamivir for the treatment of influenza A and influenza B: a Japanese multicenter study of the 2003–2004 and 2004–2005 influenza seasons. Clin Infect Dis. 2006 Aug 15; 43(4):439–44. [PMID: 16838232]
- Ohmit SE et al. Prevention of antigenically drifted influenza by inactivated and live attenuated vaccines. N Engl J Med. 2006 Dec 14;355(24):2513–22. [PMID: 17167134]
- Sugaya N et al. Lower clinical effectiveness of oseltamivir against influenza B contrasted with influenza A infection in children. Clin Infect Dis. 2007 Jan 15; 44(2):197–202. [PMID: 17173216]
- Thompson WW et al. Influenza-associated hospitalizations in the United States. JAMA. 2004 Sep 15; 292(11):1333–40. [PMID: 15367555]

Insomnia

 KEY FEATURES

ESSENTIALS OF DIAGNOSIS

- Transient episodes are usually of little significance
- Common factors
  - Stress
  - Caffeine
  - Physical discomfort
  - Daytime napping, early bedtime
- Psychiatric disorders are often associated with persistent insomnia

GENERAL CONSIDERATIONS

- **Sleep** consists of two distinct states
  - REM (rapid eye movement) sleep, also called dream sleep
- NREM (non-REM) sleep, is divided into stages 1, 2, 3, and 4
- Dreaming occurs mostly in REM and to a lesser extent in NREM sleep
- Sleep is a cyclic phenomenon, with four or five REM periods during the night accounting for about one-fourth of the total night's sleep ($1\frac{1}{2}$–2 hours)
- The first REM period occurs about 80–120 minutes after onset of sleep and lasts about 10 minutes
- Later REM periods are longer (15–40 minutes) and occur mostly in the last hours of sleep. Most stage 4 (deepest) sleep occurs in the first several hours
- **Age-related changes** in normal sleep include
  - An unchanging percentage of REM sleep
  - A marked decrease in stage 3 and stage 4 sleep
  - An increase in wakeful periods during the night
  - These normal changes, early bedtimes, and daytime naps contribute to the insomnia in older people
  - Variations in sleep patterns may be due to circumstances (eg, "jet lag") or to idiosyncratic patterns ("night owls") in persons with different "biological rhythms" who habitually go to bed late and sleep late in the AM
  - Creativity and rapidity of response to unfamiliar situations are impaired by loss of sleep
  - Desynchronization sleep disorder: rare; chronic difficulty in adapting to a 24-hour sleep-wake cycle; can be resynchronized by altering exposure to light
- **Depression** is usually associated with
  - Fragmented sleep
  - Decreased total sleep time
  - Earlier onset of REM sleep
  - A shift of REM activity to the first half of the night
  - Loss of slow-wave sleep
- **Manic disorders**
  - Sleeplessness is a cardinal feature and an important early sign of impending mania in bipolar cases
  - Total sleep time is decreased
  - Shortened REM latency and increased REM activity
- Sleep-related panic attacks occur in the transition from stage 2 to stage 3 sleep in some patients with a longer REM latency in the sleep pattern preceding the attacks
- **Abuse of alcohol**
  - May cause or be secondary to the sleep disturbance
  - There is a tendency to use alcohol as a means of getting to sleep without

realizing that it disrupts the normal sleep cycle

- *Acute alcohol intake*
  - Produces a decreased sleep latency with reduced REM sleep during the first half of the night
  - REM sleep is increased in the second half of the night, with an increase in total amount of slow-wave sleep (stages 3 and 4)
  - Vivid dreams and frequent awakenings are common
- *Chronic alcohol abuse*
  - Increases stage 1 and decreases REM sleep (most drugs delay or block REM sleep)
  - Symptoms persist for many months after the person has stopped drinking
- *Acute alcohol or other sedative withdrawal*
  - Delayed onset of sleep and REM rebound
  - Intermittent awakening during the night
- **Heavy smoking** (> 1 pack a day) causes difficulty falling asleep
- Excess intake of stimulants near bedtime of caffeine, cocaine, and other stimulants (eg, over-the-counter cold remedies) causes decreased total sleep time—mostly NREM sleep—with some increased sleep latency
- **Benzodiazepine sedative-hypnotics** tend to
  - Increase total sleep time
  - Decrease sleep latency
  - Decrease nocturnal awakening
  - Have variable effects on NREM sleep
  - Withdrawal causes just the opposite effects and results in continued use of the drug for the purpose of preventing withdrawal symptoms
- Antidepressants decrease REM sleep (with marked rebound on withdrawal in the form of nightmares) and have varying effects on NREM sleep
- REM sleep deprivation produces improvement in some depressions
- Persistent insomnias are also related to a wide variety of medical conditions, particularly delirium, pain, respiratory distress syndromes, uremia, asthma, and thyroid disorders
- Adequate analgesia and proper treatment of medical disorders reduce symptoms and decrease the need for sedatives

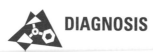 **CLINICAL FINDINGS**

SYMPTOMS AND SIGNS

- Difficulty getting to sleep or staying asleep
- Intermittent wakefulness during the night

- Early morning awakening
- Combinations of any of the latter

DIFFERENTIAL DIAGNOSIS

- Nocturia
  - Diuretics
  - Benign prostatic hyperplasia
  - Incontinence
  - Chronic heart failure
- Restless legs syndrome
- Medications
  - Corticosteroids
  - Selective serotonin reuptake inhibitors
  - Theophylline
  - Benzodiazepine withdrawal
- Circadian rhythm disorder

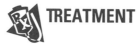 **DIAGNOSIS**

LABORATORY TESTS

- Consider thyroid-stimulating hormone

 TREATMENT

MEDICATIONS

- There are two broad classes of treatment, and the two may be combined
  - Psychological (cognitive-behavioral)
  - Pharmacologic
- Pharmacologic
  - In situations of acute distress, such as a grief reaction, pharmacologic measures may be most appropriate
  - These drugs are often effective for the elderly population and can be given in larger doses—twice what is prescribed for the elderly—in younger patients
    - Lorazepam 0.5 mg PO at bedtime
    - Eszopiclone 2–3 mg PO at bedtime
    - Temazepam 7.5–15.0 mg PO at bedtime
    - Zolpidem 5–10 mg PO at bedtime
    - Zaleplon 5–10 mg PO at bedtime
  - Longer-acting agents such as flurazepam (half-life of > 48 h) may accumulate in the elderly and lead to cognitive slowing, ataxia, falls, and somnolence
  - In general, it is appropriate to use medications for short courses of 1–2 weeks
  - Antihistamines such as diphenhydramine 25 mg PO at bedtime or hydroxyzine 25 mg PO at bedtime may be useful
    - Their anticholinergic effects may produce confusion or urinary symptoms in the elderly

- Trazodone 25–150 mg PO at bedtime is a non–habit-forming effective sleep medication in lower than antidepressant doses
  - Priapism is a rare side effect requiring emergent treatment
- Ramelteon helps with sleep onset and does not appear to have abuse potential
- Triazolam is popular because of its very short duration of action
  - It has been associated with dependency, transient psychotic reactions, anterograde amnesia, and rebound anxiety, therefore, it has been removed from the market in several European countries
  - If used, it must be prescribed only for short periods of time

THERAPEUTIC PROCEDURES

- With primary insomnia initial efforts should be psychologically based, particularly in the elderly
- Psychological
  - Educate the patient regarding good sleep hygiene
    - Go to bed only when sleepy
    - Use the bed and bedroom only for sleeping and sex
    - If still awake after 20 minutes, leave the bedroom and return only when sleepy
    - Get up at the same time every morning, regardless of the amount of sleep during the night
    - Discontinue caffeine and nicotine, at least in the evening if not completely
    - Establish a daily exercise regimen
    - Avoid alcohol because it may disrupt continuity of sleep
    - Limit fluids in the evening
    - Learn and practice relaxation techniques
  - Cognitive behavioral therapy for insomnia may be efficacious

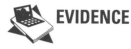 **OUTCOME**

PREVENTION

- Discontinue use of caffeine and nicotine
- Avoid alcohol
- Engage in regular exercise program

EVIDENCE

WEB SITES

- National Institutes of Health—National Heart, Lung, and Blood Institute
- National Sleep Foundation

INFORMATION FOR PATIENTS

- American Academy of Family Physicians
- JAMA patient page. Insomnia. JAMA. 2003;289:2602. [PMID: 12759329]
- National Institutes of Health—National Heart, Lung, and Blood Institute

REFERENCES

- Jindal RD et al. Maintenance treatment of insomnia: what can we learn from the depression literature? Am J Psychiatry. 2004 Jan;161(1):19–24. [PMID: 14702243]
- Johnson MW et al. Ramelteon: a novel hypnotic lacking abuse liability and sedative adverse affects. Arch Gen Psychiatry. 2006 Oct;63(10):1149-57. [PMID: 17015817]
- Siversten B et al. Cognitive behavioral therapy vs zopiclone for treatment of chronic primary insomnia in older adults: a randomized controlled trial. JAMA. 2006 Jun 28;295(24):2851-8. [PMID: 16804151]

Insulinoma

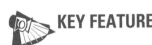 **KEY FEATURES**

ESSENTIALS OF DIAGNOSIS

- Fasting hypoglycemia rather than postprandial hypoglycemia
- Blood glucose < 40 mg/dL in an otherwise healthy-appearing person with central nervous dysfunction such as confusion or abnormal behavior
- Hypoglycemic unawareness is common

GENERAL CONSIDERATIONS

- Insulinoma is generally an adenoma of the islets of Langerhans
- Adenomas can be familial
- 90% of tumors are single and benign
- Multiple benign adenomas can occur, as can malignant tumors with functional metastases
- Multiple adenomas can occur with tumors of parathyroids and pituitary in multiple endocrine neoplasia type 1 (MEN-1)
- Rarely, B-cell hyperplasia can be a cause of fasting hypoglycemia
- Patients adapt to chronic (or recurrent) hypoglycemia by increasing their efficiency in transporting glucose across the blood–brain barrier, which masks awareness that their blood glucose is approaching critically low levels
  - Counterregulatory hormonal responses as well as neurogenic symptoms such as tremor, sweating, and palpitations are blunted during chronic (or recurrent) hypoglycemia

 CLINICAL FINDINGS

SYMPTOMS AND SIGNS

- Whipple's triad is characteristic of hypoglycemia regardless of the cause
  - A history of hypoglycemic symptoms
  - An associated fasting blood glucose of < 40 mg/dL
  - Immediate recovery on administration of glucose
- Symptoms often develop in the early morning, after missing a meal, or occasionally after exercise
- Initial CNS symptoms include
  - Blurred vision or diplopia
  - Headache
  - Feelings of detachment
  - Slurred speech
  - Weakness
- Convulsions or coma may occur
- Personality changes vary from anxiety to psychotic behavior
- Hypoglycemic unawareness is very common

DIFFERENTIAL DIAGNOSIS

- Hyperinsulinism from surreptitious insulin or sulfonylureas
- Extrapancreatic tumors
- Postprandial early hypoglycemia: alimentary disorders (dumping syndrome, postgastrectomy)
- Postprandial late hypoglycemia: functional (increased vagal tone), occult diabetes mellitus
- Delayed insulin release resulting from B-cell dysfunction
  - Counterregulatory deficiency
  - Idiopathic
- Alcohol-related hypoglycemia
- Immunopathologic hypoglycemia: antibodies to insulin receptors, which act as agonists
- Pentamidine-induced hypoglycemia

 DIAGNOSIS

LABORATORY TESTS

- Serum insulin level ≥ 6 mcU/mL in a radioimmunoassay (RIA) (≥ 3 mcU/mL in ICMA) in the presence of blood glucose values < 40 mg/dL is diagnostic of inappropriate hyperinsulinism suggestive of insulinoma
- An elevated circulating proinsulin level (> 5 pmol/L) in the presence of fasting hypoglycemia is characteristic of most B-cell adenomas and does not occur in factitious hyperinsulinism
- In patients with epigastric distress, history of renal stones, or menstrual or erectile dysfunction, serum calcium, gastrin, or prolactin level may be useful in screening for MEN-1 associated with insulinoma
- Prolonged fasting is done in hospital under supervision up to 72 h or until hypoglycemia is documented
  - In normal males, the blood glucose does not fall below 55–60 mg/dL during a 3-day fast
  - In normal premenopausal women who have fasted for only 24 h, the blood glucose may fall to as low as 35 mg/dL. These women are not symptomatic owing to the development of sufficient ketonemia to supply energy needs to the brain
- Insulinoma patients become symptomatic when blood glucose drops to subnormal levels, because inappropriate insulin secretion restricts ketone formation

IMAGING STUDIES

- Spiral CT angiography and endoscopic ultrasound may not identify insulinomas because of their small size
- If imaging studies are normal or inconclusive, tumor localization to the head, body or tail of the pancreas can be obtained by angiography combined with injections of calcium gluconate into the gastroduodenal, splenic and superior mesenteric arteries and insulin levels measured in the hepatic vein effluent
- The above studies, together with intraoperative ultrasonography and palpation, can identify up to 98% of insulinomas

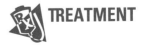 **TREATMENT**

MEDICATIONS

- Glucagon for hypoglycemic emergencies, but its benefit may be less than for diabetic hypoglycemia because of the concomitant insulin release from the tumor

- Diazoxide, 300–600 mg PO daily, along with a thiazide to control sodium retention
- Verapamil may inhibit insulin release from insulinoma cells; use if patient intolerant of diazoxide
- Octreotide, 50 mg SQ BID, is a synthetic analog of somatostatin; use when surgery fails to remove the source of hyperinsulinism
- Streptozocin can decrease insulin secretion in islet cell carcinomas; effective doses can be delivered via selective arterial catheter to decrease renal toxicity

SURGERY

- Laparoscopic surgery using ultrasonography and denucleation can be successful with a single insulinoma of the body or tail of the pancreas, but open surgery is necessary for insulinomas in the head of the pancreas

THERAPEUTIC PROCEDURES

- In islet cell carcinoma and in 5–10% of MEN-1 cases when surgical resection has not been curative, frequent feedings are necessary. Carbohydrate feedings every 2–3 h are usually effective in preventing hypoglycemia

 OUTCOME

COMPLICATIONS

- Irreversible brain damage from hypoglycemia
- Obesity may become a problem from frequent feeding
- Gastrointestinal upset, hirsutism, or edema from diazoxide

PROGNOSIS

- 90–95% cure at first surgical attempt for single benign adenoma when performed by a skilled surgeon
- Severe brain damage resulting from severe prolonged hypoglycemia is irreversible
- Significant increase in survival in streptozocin-treated patients with islet cell carcinoma, with reduction in tumor mass and decrease in hyperinsulinism

WHEN TO REFER

- Refer to endocrinologist to perform 72-h fast in hospital

- Refer to skilled surgeon for insulinoma resection

WHEN TO ADMIT

- For 72-h fast

 EVIDENCE

INFORMATION FOR PATIENTS

- Mayo Clinic: Hyperinsulinemia
- Medline Medical Encyclopedia: Insulinoma

REFERENCES

- Griffiths MJ et al. Adult spontaneous hypoglycaemia. Hosp Med. 2005 May; 66(5):277–83. [PMID: 15920857]
- Hirshberg B et al. Forty-eight-hour fast: the diagnostic test for insulinoma. J Clin Endocrinol Metab. 2000 Sep; 85(9):3222–6. [PMID: 10999812]
- Koch B. Selected topics of hypoglycemia care. Can Fam Physician. 2006 Apr; 52:466–71. [PMID: 16639972]
- Service FJ. Diagnostic approach to adults with hypoglycemic disorders. Endocrinol Metab Clin North Am. 1999 Sep;28(3):519–32. [PMID: 10500929]
- Tucker ON et al. The management of insulinoma. Br J Surg. 2006 Mar; 93(3):264–75. [PMID: 16498592]

Irritable Bowel Syndrome

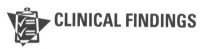 **KEY FEATURES**

ESSENTIALS OF DIAGNOSIS

- Common chronic functional disorder characterized by abdominal pain or discomfort with alterations in bowel habits
- Limited evaluation to exclude organic causes of symptoms

GENERAL CONSIDERATIONS

- No definitive diagnostic study
- Idiopathic clinical entity characterized by some combination of chronic (> 3 months) lower abdominal symptoms and bowel complaints that may be continuous or intermittent

- Abdominal discomfort or pain that has two of the following three features
  - Relieved with defecation
  - Onset associated with a change in frequency of stool
  - Onset associated with a change in appearance of stool
- Other symptoms include
  - Abnormal stool frequency (more than three bowel movements per day or fewer than three per week)
  - Abnormal stool form (lumpy or hard; loose or watery)
  - Abnormal stool passage (straining, urgency, or feeling of incomplete evacuation)
  - Passage of mucus
  - Bloating or abdominal distention
- Other somatic or psychological complaints are common

DEMOGRAPHICS

- Affects up to 20% of the adult population
- Symptoms usually begin in late teens to early 20s

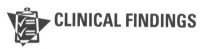 **CLINICAL FINDINGS**

SYMPTOMS AND SIGNS

- Symptoms for > 3 months
- Subjective abdominal distention; visible distention not clinically evident
- Abdominal pain, intermittent, crampy, in the lower abdomen, relieved by defecation, worsened by stress, worse for 1–2 h after meals
- More frequent or less frequent stools with the onset of abdominal pain
- Looser stools or harder stools with the onset of pain
- Constipation, diarrhea, or alternating constipation and diarrhea
- Mucus is common
- Physical examination usually is normal
- Abdominal tenderness in the lower abdomen is common, but not pronounced; physical examination is otherwise normal

DIFFERENTIAL DIAGNOSIS

- Inflammatory bowel disease
- Colonic neoplasia
- Celiac disease, bacterial overgrowth, lactase deficiency, and endometriosis
- Depression and anxiety
- Sexual and physical abuse
- Small bowel bacterial overgrowth reported by some investigators to occur

in up to 80% of patients with symptoms of irritable bowel syndrome; not confirmed by other investigators

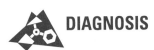

DIAGNOSIS

LABORATORY TESTS

- Diagnostic testing is not required initially in patients whose symptoms
  - Are compatible with irritable bowel syndrome
  - Do not suggest organic disease (nocturnal diarrhea, severe constipation or diarrhea, hematochezia, weight loss, fever, or family history of colon cancer or inflammatory bowel disease)
- However, further tests are warranted in patients whose symptoms do not improve after 2–4 weeks of empiric therapy
- Complete blood cell count, chemistry panel, serum albumin, stool occult blood test
- Thyroid function tests, erythrocyte sedimentation rate, C-reactive protein
- Celiac disease serologies (IgA tissue transglutaminase antibody or anti-endomysial antibody)
- Stool examination for ova and parasites if diarrhea
- D-[^{14}C]xylose, glucose or lactulose breath tests to screen for small bowel bacterial overgrowth

IMAGING STUDIES

- Colonoscopy or air-contrast barium enema for patients aged > 50 years to screen for colonic neoplasms
- Flexible sigmoidoscopy, colonoscopy, barium enema and/or barium small bowel series may be warranted in any patient whose symptoms do not respond to empiric therapy

DIAGNOSTIC PROCEDURES

- Diagnosis is established with compatible symptoms and the judicious use of tests to exclude organic disease

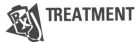

TREATMENT

MEDICATIONS

- Antispasmodic (anticholinergic) agents
  - Dicyclomine, 10–20 mg PO TID–QID
  - Hyoscyamine, 0.125 mg PO (or SL PRN) QID
  - Hyoscyamine, sustained-release 0.037 mg or 0.75 mg PO BID

- Commonly used despite a lack of good evidence demonstrating efficacy
- Antidiarrheal agents
  - Loperamide, 2 mg PO TID–QID
  - Diphenoxylate with atropine, 2.5 mg PO QID
- Fiber supplementation
  - Bran, psyllium, methylcellulose, or polycarbophil
  - May cause increased bloating
- Osmotic laxatives
  - Milk of magnesia
  - Polyethylene glycol
- Tricyclic and related antidepressants
  - Nortriptyline, desipramine, or imipramine
  - Begin at 10 mg PO every night at bedtime
  - Increase gradually to 25–50 mg PO every night at bedtime as tolerated
  - Trazodone, beginning at 50 mg PO every night at bedtime is an alternative
  - Not recommended for patients with predominant constipation
- Serotonin reuptake inhibitors
  - Sertraline, 50–150 mg PO once daily
  - Fluoxetine, 20–40 mg PO once daily
  - Not recommended for patients with predominant diarrhea
- Alosetran, 0.5–1 mg PO BID, for diarrhea as predominant symptom unresponsive to other conventional therapies
  - Restricted access in United States
  - May cause ischemic colitis in 4:1000 patients
- *Bifidobacterium infantis;* 10^8 bacteria/capsule PO daily
  - Probiotic reported to benefit a subset of patients in small controlled trials
  - Further study warranted
- Rifaximin, 400 mg TID for 10 days
  - Reported to benefit a subset of patients with small bowel bacterial overgrowth in small controlled trials
  - Further study warranted

THERAPEUTIC PROCEDURES

- Reassure patient
- Explain functional nature of the symptoms
- Behavioral modification with relaxation techniques, hypnotherapy

OUTCOME

FOLLOW-UP

- Regular visits helpful in reducing patient anxiety and overuse of the health care system

PROGNOSIS

- Symptoms usually chronic, but episodic; majority of affected patients learn to cope with their symptoms

WHEN TO REFER

- Persistent or worsening symptoms
- Signs of organic disease (blood per rectum, positive fecal occult blood, weight loss, severe pain)
- Signs of serious psychiatric disease or physical/sexual abuse

WHEN TO ADMIT

- Patients with irritable bowel syndrome have increased rate of hospitalizations and inappropriate abdominal surgeries for abdominal pain
- Avoid unnecessary hospitalizations and surgeries

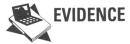

EVIDENCE

PRACTICE GUIDELINES

- American College of Gastroenterology Functional Gastrointestinal Disorders Task Force. Evidence-based position statement on the management of irritable bowel syndrome in North America. Am J Gastroenterol. 2002;97(11 Suppl):S1. [PMID: 12425585]
- American Gastroenterological Association medical position statement: irritable bowel syndrome. Gastroenteology. 2002;123:2105. [PMID: 12454865]

WEB SITES

- American Academy of Family Physicians—Irritable bowel syndrome: tips on controlling your symptoms
- Functional Brain-Gut Research Group
- International Foundation for Functional Gastrointestinal Disorders

INFORMATION FOR PATIENTS

- American Gastroenterological Association Patient Resource Services: Irritable bowel syndrome
- International Foundation for Functional Gastrointestinal Disorders (IFFGD): About Irritable Bowel Syndrome
- National Digestive Diseases Information Clearinghouse—What I Need to Know about Irritable Bowel Syndrome

REFERENCES

- Halpert A et al. Clinical response to tricyclic antidepressants in functional bowel disorders is not related to dosage. Am J Gastroenterol. 2005 Mar; 100(3):664–71. [PMID: 15743366]

• Halvorson HA et al. Postinfectious irritable bowel syndrome—a meta-analysis. Am J Gastroenterol. 2006 Aug; 101(8):1894–9. [PMID: 16928253]

• Pimentel M et al. The effect of a nonabsorbed oral antibiotic (rifaximin) on the symptoms of irritable bowel syndrome. Ann Intern Med. 2006 Oct 17; 145(8):557–63. [PMID: 17043337]

• Walters B et al. Detection of bacterial overgrowth in IBS using the lactulose H_2 breath test: comparison with ^{14}C-D-xylose and healthy controls. Am J Gastroenterol. 2005 Jul;100(7):1566–70. [PMID: 15984983]

• Whorwell PJ et al. Efficacy of encapsulated probiotic *Bifidobacterium infantis* 35624 in women with irritable bowel syndrome. Am J Gastroenterol. 2006 Jul;101(7):1581–90. [PMID: 16863564]

Jaundice

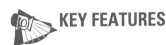

KEY FEATURES

ESSENTIALS OF DIAGNOSIS

- Results from accumulation of bilirubin in the body tissues; the cause may be hepatic or nonhepatic
- Hyperbilirubinemia may be due to abnormalities in the formation, transport, metabolism, and excretion of bilirubin

GENERAL CONSIDERATIONS

- Jaundice is caused by predominantly unconjugated or conjugated bilirubin in the serum
- In the absence of liver disease, hemolysis rarely elevates the serum bilirubin level to more than 7 mg/dL
- "Cholestasis" denotes retention of bile in the liver, and "cholestatic jaundice" implies conjugated hyperbilirubinemia from impaired bile flow

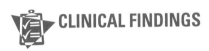

CLINICAL FINDINGS

Unconjugated hyperbilirubinemia
- Normal stool and urine color—no bilirubin in the urine
- Mild jaundice
- Splenomegaly occurs in hemolytic disorders except in sickle cell anemia

Conjugated hyperbilirubinemia
- Hereditary cholestatic syndromes or intrahepatic cholestasis
  - May be asymptomatic
  - Cholestasis is often accompanied by pruritus, light-colored stools, and jaundice
- Hepatocellular disease
  - Malaise, anorexia, low-grade fever, and right upper quadrant discomfort are frequent
  - Dark urine, jaundice and, in women, amenorrhea occur
  - An enlarged, tender liver; vascular spiders; palmar erythema; ascites; gynecomastia; sparse body hair; fetor hepaticus; and asterixis may be present, depending on the cause, severity, and chronicity of liver dysfunction

Biliary obstruction
- Right upper quadrant pain, weight loss (suggesting carcinoma), jaundice, dark urine, and light-colored stools

- Symptoms and signs may be intermittent if caused by stone, carcinoma of the ampulla, or cholangiocarcinoma
- Pain may be absent early in pancreatic cancer
- Stool occult blood suggests cancer of the ampulla
- Hepatomegaly and a palpable gallbladder (Courvoisier's sign) are characteristic, but are neither specific nor sensitive for pancreatic head tumor
- Fever and chills are more common in benign obstruction with associated cholangitis

DIFFERENTIAL DIAGNOSIS

- Obstructive hepatobiliary disease
- Hepatitis, eg, viral, alcoholic, toxic
- Hemochromatosis
- Cirrhosis

DIAGNOSIS

LABORATORY TESTS

- Table 90
- Elevated serum aspartate and alanine aminotransferase (AST, ALT) levels result from hepatocellular necrosis or inflammation, as in hepatitis
- ALT is more specific for the liver than AST, but an AST level at least twice that of the ALT is typical of alcoholic liver injury
- The ALT level is greater than the AST level in nonalcoholic fatty liver disease prior to the development of cirrhosis
- An isolated elevation of serum ALT may be seen in celiac disease
- Elevated alkaline phosphatase levels are seen in cholestasis or infiltrative liver disease (such as tumor or granuloma) [γ-glutamyl transpeptidase (GGT) also elevated]
- Alkaline phosphatase elevations of hepatic rather than bone, intestinal, or placental origin are confirmed by concomitant elevation of GGT or 5′-nucleotidase levels

IMAGING STUDIES

- Demonstration of dilated bile ducts by ultrasonography or CT scan indicates biliary obstruction (90–95% sensitivity)
- Ultrasonography, CT scan, and MRI may also demonstrate hepatomegaly, intrahepatic tumors, and portal hypertension
- The most sensitive techniques for detecting individual small hepatic

lesions in patients eligible for resection of metastases
  - Multiphasic helical or multislice CT
  - CT arterial portography, in which imaging follows IV contrast infusion via a catheter placed in the superior mesenteric artery
  - MRI with use of ferumoxides as contrast agents
  - Intraoperative ultrasonography
- Color Doppler ultrasound or contrast agents that produce microbubbles increase the sensitivity of transcutaneous ultrasound for detecting small neoplasms
- MRI is the most accurate technique for
  - Identifying isolated liver lesions, such as hemangiomas, focal nodular hyperplasia, or focal fatty infiltration
  - Detecting hepatic iron overload
- Because of its much lower cost, ultrasonography is preferable to CT or MRI as a screening test
- Ultrasonography can detect gallstones with a sensitivity of 95%
- Magnetic resonance cholangiopancreatography (MRCP) is a sensitive, noninvasive method for detecting bile duct stones, strictures, and dilation
- Endoscopic ultrasonography
  - Most sensitive test for detecting small lesions of the ampulla or pancreatic head and for detecting portal vein invasion by pancreatic cancer
  - It is also accurate in detecting or excluding bile duct stones

DIAGNOSTIC PROCEDURES

- Percutaneous liver biopsy
  - Definitive diagnostic method for determining the etiology and severity of the liver disease
  - Should be performed under ultrasound or CT guidance for suspected metastatic disease or a hepatic mass
  - A transjugular route can be used in patients with coagulopathy or ascites

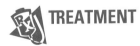

TREATMENT

THERAPEUTIC PROCEDURES

- Treatment of the causative etiology
- Uncomplicated obstructive jaundice responds to parenteral vitamin K
- Use endoscopic retrograde cholangiopancreatography (ERCP) or percutaneous transhepatic cholangiography (PTC)
  - To demonstrate pancreatic or ampullary causes of jaundice
  - To perform papillotomy and stone extraction

– To insert a stent through an obstructing lesion

 OUTCOME

COMPLICATIONS

- Complications of ERCP include pancreatitis in 5% of cases and, less commonly, cholangitis, bleeding, or duodenal perforation after papillotomy
- Severe complications of PTC occur in 3% of cases and include fever, bacteremia, bile peritonitis, and intraperitoneal hemorrhage

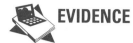 **EVIDENCE**

INFORMATION FOR PATIENTS

- National Institutes of Health

REFERENCES

- Brown RS Jr. Asymptomatic liver mass. Gastroenterology. 2006 Aug; 131(2):619–23. [PMID: 16890613]
- Chand N et al. Sepsis-induced cholestasis. Hepatology. 2007 Jan;45(1):230–41. [PMID: 17187426]
- Ioannou GN et al. Elevated serum alanine aminotransferase activity and calculated risk of coronary artery disease in the United States. Hepatology. 2006 May;43(5):1145–51. [PMID: 16628637]
- Mukherjee S et al. Noninvasive tests for liver fibrosis. Semin Liver Dis. 2006 Nov;26(4):337–47. [PMID: 17051448]
- Watkins PB et al. Aminotransferase elevations in healthy adults receiving 4 grams of acetaminophen daily: a randomized controlled trial. JAMA. 2006 Jul 5;296(1):8793. [PMID: 16820551]

Kaposi's Sarcoma

KEY FEATURES

ESSENTIALS OF DIAGNOSIS

- Human herpes virus 8 (HHV-8) or Kaposi's sarcoma–associated herpes virus (KSHV), is universally present in all forms of Kaposi's sarcoma
- It is a common infection in central Africa, is more common in Italy than in the United States, and is common in HIV-infected homosexual men and rare in HIV-infected hemophiliacs

GENERAL CONSIDERATIONS

- Before 1980 in the United States, this rare malignant skin lesion was seen mostly in elderly white men, had a chronic clinical course, and was rarely fatal
- Occurs endemically in an often aggressive form in young black men of equatorial Africa, but it is rare in American blacks
- The epidemiology of infection with HHV-8 or KSHV parallels the incidence of Kaposi's sarcoma in various risk groups and geographic regions

DEMOGRAPHICS

- The most common HIV-related malignancy

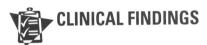 **CLINICAL FINDINGS**

SYMPTOMS AND SIGNS

- Red, purple, or dark plaques or nodules on cutaneous or mucosal surfaces
- Commonly involves the gastrointestinal tract, but in asymptomatic patients these lesions are not sought or treated

DIFFERENTIAL DIAGNOSIS

- Bacillary angiomatosis
- Hemangioma
- Vasculitis (palpable purpura)
- Dermatofibroma
- Pyogenic granuloma
- Prurigo nodularis
- Melanoma

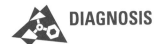 **DIAGNOSIS**

LABORATORY TESTS

- Based on appearance of skin lesions with confirmatory biopsy

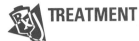 **TREATMENT**

MEDICATIONS

- Kaposi's sarcoma in the elderly
  - Palliative local therapy with intralesional chemotherapy or radiation is usually all that is required
- In the setting of iatrogenic immunosuppression
  - The treatment is primarily reduction of doses of immunosuppressive medications
- AIDS-associated Kaposi's
  - The patient should first be given effective anti-HIV antiretrovirals because in most cases this treatment alone is associated with improvement (see HIV Infection)
- Other therapeutic options include cryotherapy or intralesional vinblastine (0.1–0.5 mg/mL) for cosmetically objectionable lesions
- Systemic chemotherapy
  - Indicated for rapidly progressive skin disease (more than 10 new lesions per month), with edema or pain, and with symptomatic visceral disease or pulmonary disease
  - Liposomal doxorubicin is highly effective in controlling these cases and has considerably less toxicity—and greater efficacy—than anthracycline monotherapy or combination chemotherapeutic regimens

SURGERY

- Laser surgery for certain intraoral and pharyngeal lesions

THERAPEUTIC PROCEDURES

- Radiation therapy for accessible and space-occupying lesions

 OUTCOME

PROGNOSIS

- Pulmonary Kaposi's sarcoma may be life-threatening and is managed aggressively

WHEN TO REFER

- If there is a question about the diagnosis, if recommended therapy is ineffective, or if specialized treatment is necessary

WHEN TO ADMIT

- Respiratory insufficiency or other signs of systemic failure

 EVIDENCE

PRACTICE GUIDELINES

- Kaplan JE et al. Guidelines for preventing opportunistic infections among HIV-infected persons—2002. Recommendations of the U.S. Public Health Service and the Infectious Diseases Society of America. MMWR Recomm Rep. 2002;51:1.

WEB SITES

- American Academy of Dermatology
- National Cancer Institute: Kaposi's Sarcoma Treatment

INFORMATION FOR PATIENTS

- American Cancer Society: Kaposi's Sarcoma
- MedlinePlus: Kaposi's Sarcoma
- National Cancer Institute: Kaposi's Sarcoma

REFERENCES

- Bursics A et al. HHV-8 positive, HIV negative disseminated Kaposi's sarcoma complicating steroid dependent ulcerative colitis: a successfully treated case. Gut. 2005 Jul;54(7):1049–50. [PMID: 15951561]
- Fardet L et al. Treatment with taxanes of refractory or life-threatening Kaposi sarcoma not associated with human immunodeficiency virus infection. Cancer. 2006 Apr 15;106(8):1785–9. [PMID: 16534786]
- Gutman-Yassky E et al. Classic Kaposi sarcoma. Which KSHV-seropositive individuals are at risk? Cancer. 2006 Jan 15;106(2):413–9. [PMID: 16353205]
- Lim ST et al. Weekly docetaxel is safe and effective in the treatment of advanced-stage acquired immunodeficiency syndrome-related Kaposi sarcoma. Cancer. 2005 Jan 15; 103(2):417–21. [PMID: 15578686]

Kawasaki Disease

 KEY FEATURES

- Mucocutaneous lymph node syndrome
- Usually affects children age < 10, at times in an epidemic fashion
- No clear infectious cause identified

 CLINICAL FINDINGS

- Fever universal
- Bilateral nonexudative conjunctivitis
- Mucous membrane involvement
- Polymorphous rash
- Cervical lymphadenopathy

 DIAGNOSIS

- Clinical diagnosis, based on combination of findings
- Elevated erythrocyte sedimentation rate and C-reactive protein levels
- Coronary arteritis may develop, leading to myocardial infarction and arterial aneurysms

 TREATMENT

- High-dose aspirin (with tapering) is used indefinitely for coronary abnormalities; its utility in acute cases is questionable
- IV immunoglobulin
- Warfarin for coronary artery aneurysms
- Corticosteroids are used but controversial in refractory disease
- Limited case reports document successful use of infliximab in treating refractory disease
- Interventional catheter treatment, including stent implantation, for coronary arteritis

Klinefelter Syndrome

 KEY FEATURES

- Males with 1 extra X chromosome (XXY)
- Tall stature, gynecomastia, atrophic testes, infertility

 CLINICAL FINDINGS

- Boys are normal in appearance before puberty; after puberty, they have disproportionately long legs and arms, a female escutcheon, gynecomastia, and small testes
- Infertility resulting from azoospermia; the seminiferous tubules are hyalinized
- Mental retardation is somewhat more common than in the general population, and many have learning problems
- Higher risk of breast cancer
- Heightened risk of diabetes mellitus

 DIAGNOSIS

- Cytogenetic analysis

 TREATMENT

- Testosterone administration is advisable after puberty but will not restore fertility
- Intracytoplasmic sperm injection is possible using sperm obtained by testicular extraction

Knee, Overuse Syndromes

 KEY FEATURES

- Runners may develop a variety of painful overuse syndromes of the knee, particularly those who
  – Overtrain
  – Do not attain the proper level of conditioning before starting a running program
- Most of these conditions are forms of tendinitis or bursitis that can be diagnosed on examination
- The most common conditions include
  – Anserine bursitis
  – Iliotibial band syndrome
  – Popliteal and patellar tendinitis

 CLINICAL FINDINGS

- Symptoms worsen with continued running
- Anserine bursitis results in pain medial and inferior to the knee joint over the medial tibia
- The iliotibial band syndrome results in pain on the lateral side of the knee
- Patellar tendinitis, a cause of anterior knee discomfort, typically occurs at the tendon's insertion into the patella rather than at its more inferior insertion

 DIAGNOSIS

- Confirm the diagnoses by palpating the relevant sites around the knee
- Not associated with joint effusions or other signs of synovitis

 TREATMENT

- Rest and abstention from the associated physical activities for a period of days to weeks are essential
- Once the acute pain has subsided, a program of gentle stretching (particularly before resuming exercise) may prevent recurrence
- Corticosteroid with lidocaine injections may be useful when intense discomfort is present, but caution must be used when injecting corticosteroids into the region of a tendon since rupture may occur

Lead Poisoning

KEY FEATURES

- Toxicity is usually from subacute or chronic exposure to contaminated paint chips, dust, or fumes
- Acute ingestion of lead fishing weights or curtain weights can cause poisoning if they remain in the acidic gastric juice

CLINICAL FINDINGS

- Abdominal pain, constipation, headache, irritability
- Coma and convulsions in severe poisoning
- Chronic intoxication can cause learning disorders (in children) and motor neuropathy (eg, wristdrop)

DIAGNOSIS

- Blood lead level
- Microcytic anemia with basophilic stippling and elevated free erythrocyte protoporphyrin may be seen
- Can be misdiagnosed as porphyria

TREATMENT

- For recent ingestion, give activated charcoal, 60–100 g PO or via gastric tube, mixed in aqueous slurry (although efficacy is unknown)
- If a lead object is visible on abdominal x-ray, whole-bowel irrigation, endoscopy, or surgical removal may be necessary
- Consult a medical toxicologist or regional poison control center for advice about chelation
- For severe intoxication (encephalopathy or levels > 70–100 mcg/dL), give edetate calcium disodium (EDTA), 1500 mg/m²/kg/day (~50 mg/kg/day) in 4–6 divided doses or as a continuous IV infusion
- Dimercaprol, 4–5 mg/kg IM q4h for 5 days, is usually added if the patient is encephalopathic
- Less severe symptoms with blood lead levels between 55 and 69 mcg/dL may be treated with EDTA alone in dosages as above
- Succimer (dimercaptosuccinic acid), 10 mg/kg PO q8h for 5 days, then q12h for 2 weeks

Leiomyoma of the Uterus

KEY FEATURES

ESSENTIALS OF DIAGNOSIS

- Irregular enlargement of the uterus (may be asymptomatic)
- Heavy or irregular vaginal bleeding, dysmenorrhea
- Acute and recurrent pelvic pain if the tumor becomes twisted on its pedicle or infarcted
- Symptoms due to pressure on neighboring organs (large tumors)

GENERAL CONSIDERATIONS

- Most common benign neoplasm of the female genital tract
- Tumor is discrete, round, firm, and often multiple, composed of smooth muscle and connective tissue
- The most convenient classification is by anatomic location
  - Intramural
  - Submucous
  - Subserous
  - Intraligamentous
  - Parasitic (ie, deriving its blood supply from an organ to which it becomes attached)
  - Cervical
- A submucous myoma may become pedunculated and descend through the cervix into the vagina

CLINICAL FINDINGS

SYMPTOMS AND SIGNS

- In nonpregnant women, myomas are frequently asymptomatic
- However, they can cause urinary frequency, dysmenorrhea, heavy bleeding (often with anemia), or other complications due to the presence of an abdominal mass
- Occasionally, degeneration occurs, causing intense pain

DIFFERENTIAL DIAGNOSIS

- Adenomyosis (uterine endometriosis)
- Pregnancy
- Ovarian tumor
- Endometrial polyp
- Endometrial cancer
- Leiomyosarcoma

DIAGNOSIS

LABORATORY TESTS

- Anemia from blood loss may occur
- Rarely, polycythemia is present, presumably as a result of the production of erythropoietin by the myomas

IMAGING STUDIES

- Ultrasonography
  - Confirms the presence of uterine myomas
  - Used to exclude ovarian masses when multiple subserous or pedunculated myomas are being monitored
- MRI can delineate intramural and submucous myomas accurately

DIAGNOSTIC PROCEDURES

- Saline infusion hysterography or hysteroscopy can confirm cervical or submucous myomas

TREATMENT

MEDICATIONS

- Depot medroxyprogesterone acetate (150 mg IM q28d) or danazol (400–800 mg PO once daily)
  - Used as preoperative treatment for marked anemia as a result of heavy menstrual periods
  - Slows or stops bleeding
- Because the risk of surgical complications increases with the increasing size of the myoma, preoperative reduction of myoma size is desirable
- Depot leuprolide (3.75 mg IM monthly) or nafarelin (0.2–0.4 mg intranasally BID)
  - Gonadotropin-releasing hormone analogs
  - Used preoperatively for 3- to 4-month periods to induce reversible hypogonadism, which temporarily reduces the size of myomas, suppresses their further growth, and reduces surrounding vascularity

SURGERY

- Emergency surgery is required for acute torsion of a pedunculated myoma
- The only emergency indication for myomectomy during pregnancy is torsion; abortion is not inevitable
- Surgical measures: available for treatment are myomectomy and total or subtotal abdominal, vaginal, or laparoscopy-assisted vaginal hysterectomy
- Myomectomy is the treatment of choice during the childbearing years
- Myomas do not require surgery on an urgent basis unless they cause significant pressure on the ureters, bladder, or bowel or severe bleeding leading to anemia or unless they are undergoing rapid growth
- Cervical myomas larger than 3–4 cm in diameter or pedunculated myomas that protrude through the cervix must be removed
- Submucous myomas can be removed using a hysteroscope and laser or resection instruments
- Recent alternatives to myomectomy include
  - Transcatheter bilateral uterine artery embolization
  - Myolysis with MRI-guided, high-frequency, focused ultrasound
  - Laser cauterization
- However, randomized trials to compare long-term outcomes of the methods with conventional therapy are needed

 OUTCOME

FOLLOW-UP

- Women who have small asymptomatic myomas should be examined at 6-month intervals
- Ultrasound can be used sequentially to monitor growth

COMPLICATIONS

- Infertility may be due to a myoma that significantly distorts the uterine cavity

PROGNOSIS

- Surgical therapy is curative
- Future pregnancies are not endangered by myomectomy, although cesarean delivery may be necessary after wide dissection with entry into the uterine cavity

WHEN TO REFER

- Refer to gynecologist for treatment of symptomatic leiomyomata

WHEN TO ADMIT

- For acute abdomen associated with an infarcted leiomyoma (rare)

 EVIDENCE

PRACTICE GUIDELINES

- Lefebvre G et al; Clinical Practice Gynaecology Committee, Society for Obstetricians and Gynaecologists of Canada. The management of uterine leiomyomas. J Obstet Gynaecol Can. 2003;25:396. [PMID: 12738981]

WEB SITE

- National Uterine Fibroids Foundation

INFORMATION FOR PATIENTS

- American Association of Family Physicians: Uterine Fibroid Embolization
- MedlinePlus: Uterine Fibroids
- MedlinePlus: Uterine Fibroids Interactive Tutorial
- National Institute of Child Health & Human Development: Uterine Fibroids

REFERENCES

- Spies JB et al. Recent advances in uterine fibroid embolization. Curr Opin Obstet Gynecol. 2005 Dec;17(6):562–7. [PMID: 16258335]
- Walker CL et al. Uterine fibroids: the elephant in the room. Science. 2005 Jun 10; 308(5728):1589–92. [PMID: 15947177]

Leptospirosis

 KEY FEATURES

ESSENTIALS OF DIAGNOSIS

- Leptospirosis is an acute and often severe infection caused by *Leptospira interrogans,* a diverse organism of 24 serogroups and over 200 serovars
- The three most common serovars
  - *Leptospira icterohaemorrhagiae* of rats
  - *Leptospira canicola* of dogs
  - *Leptospira pomona* of cattle and swine
- Leptospirosis
  - Occurs worldwide
  - Transmitted to humans by the ingestion of food and drink contaminated by the urine of the reservoir animal

- The organism may also enter through minor skin lesions and probably via the conjunctiva
- The incubation period is 2–20 days

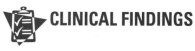 **CLINICAL FINDINGS**

SYMPTOMS AND SIGNS

- **Anicteric** leptospirosis is the more common and milder form of the disease and is often biphasic
- **Icteric** leptospirosis (Weil's syndrome) is characterized by
  - Impaired renal and hepatic function
  - Abnormal mental status
  - Hemorrhagic pneumonia
  - Hypotension
- Initial or "septicemic" phase
  - Abrupt fever to 39–40°C
  - Chills
  - Abdominal pain
  - Severe headache
  - Myalgias
  - Marked conjunctival suffusion
- Following a 1- to 3-day period of improvement, the second or "immune" phase begins
- Specific antibodies appear
- A recurrence of symptoms with the onset of meningitis
- Uveitis—unilateral or bilateral
- Rash and adenopathy
- Hemorrhagic pneumonia

DIFFERENTIAL DIAGNOSIS

- Bacterial meningitis
- Influenza
- Viral hepatitis
- Yellow fever
- Dengue
- Hemorrhagic fever, eg, hantavirus
- Relapsing fever

 DIAGNOSIS

LABORATORY TESTS

- Leptospires
  - Can be isolated from blood and cerebrospinal fluid (if meningitis present) early in the course of disease, but special medium (eg, Fletcher's EMJH) is required
  - Excreted in the urine, and urine cultures may be positive from 10 days to 6 weeks
- Cultures may take 1–6 weeks to become positive

- Dark field examination of the blood for spirochetes may be positive early in the disease
- Leukocyte count may be normal or as high as 50,000/mcL
- Urine bile, protein, casts, and red cells
- Uremia
- Elevated bilirubin and aminotransferases in 75%
- Elevated creatine kinase (> 1.5 mg/dL) in 50%
- Serum creatinine is usually elevated
- Diagnosis is usually made by serologic tests
- Agglutination tests show a fourfold or greater rise in titer
- Indirect hemagglutination, enzyme immunosorbent assay (EIA), and ELISA tests are also available. The IgM EIA is particularly useful (positive as early as 2 days into illness, extremely sensitive and specific [93%])
- Polymerase chain reaction methods are investigational but promising

IMAGING STUDIES

- Dictated by symptoms; hemorrhagic pneumonia has been described

DIAGNOSTIC PROCEDURES

- Lumbar puncture for CNS symptoms

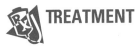

TREATMENT

MEDICATIONS

- **Mild to moderate** leptospirosis
  - Doxycycline, 100 mg PO BID for 7 days, is effective if started early
  - Penicillin, 500 mg PO QID for 7 days is effective for mild disease
  - Azithromycin is also active, but clinical experience is limited
- **Severe** leptospirosis
  - Drugs of choice: penicillin (1.5 million units q6h IV) or ceftriaxone (1 g/d IV)
  - Especially effective if started within the first 4 days of illness
  - Jarisch–Herxheimer reactions may occur

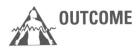

OUTCOME

FOLLOW-UP

- Routine

COMPLICATIONS

- Myocarditis, aseptic meningitis, renal failure, and pulmonary infiltrates with hemorrhage
- Iridocyclitis

PROGNOSIS

- Anicteric leptospirosis
  - Usually self-limited
  - Lasts 4–30 days
  - Almost never fatal
  - Complete recovery is the rule
- Icteric leptospirosis
  - Symptoms and signs are often continuous and not biphasic
  - Mortality rate for those under age 30 is 5%; for those over age 60, it is 30%

WHEN TO REFER

- Refer for supportive care such as dialysis

WHEN TO ADMIT

- Admit for severe liver or renal disease

PREVENTION

- Prophylaxis: doxycycline, 200 mg PO once weekly during the risk of exposure

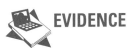

EVIDENCE

PRACTICE GUIDELINES

- Guidugli F et al. Antibiotics for preventing leptospirosis. Cochrane Database Syst Rev. 2000;(4):CD001305. [PMID: 11034711]
- Guidugli F et al. Antibiotics for treating leptospirosis. Cochrane Database Syst Rev. 2000;(2):CD001306. [PMID: 10796767]

WEB SITES

- Centers for Disease Control and Prevention Traveler's Information on Leptospirosis
- Centers for Disease Control and Prevention—Division of Bacterial and Mycotic Diseases

INFORMATION FOR PATIENTS

- Centers for Disease Control and Prevention Leptospirosis General Information

REFERENCES

- Ahmad SN et al. Laboratory diagnosis of leptospirosis. J Postgrad Med. 2005 Jul–Sep;51(3):195–200. [PMID: 16333192]
- Faucher JF et al. The management of leptospirosis. Expert Opin Pharmacother. 2004 Apr;5(4):819–27. [PMID: 15102566]
- Kobayashi Y. Human leptospirosis: Management and prognosis. J Postgrad Med. 2005 Jul–Sep;51(3):201–4. [PMID: 16333193]
- Ricaldi JN et al. Leptospirosis in the tropics and in travelers. Curr Infect Dis Rep. 2006 Jan;8(1):51–8. [PMID: 16448601]

Leukemia, Acute

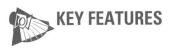

KEY FEATURES

ESSENTIALS OF DIAGNOSIS

- Short duration of symptoms, including fatigue, fever, and bleeding
- Cytopenias or pancytopenia
- Blasts in peripheral blood in 90% of cases
- > 20% blasts in bone marrow
- Classify as acute myelogenous leukemia (AML) or acute lymphoblastic leukemia (ALL)

GENERAL CONSIDERATIONS

- A malignancy of the hematopoietic progenitor cell; cells proliferate in uncontrolled fashion and replace normal bone marrow elements
- Most cases arise with no clear cause
- Radiation and some toxins (benzene) are leukemogenic; chemotherapeutic agents (cyclophosphamide, melphalan, other alkylating agents, and etoposide) may cause leukemia
- Acute promyelocytic leukemia (APL)
  - Characterized by chromosomal translocation t(15;17)
  - Has different biology and treatment
- AML is usually categorized by morphology and histochemistry
  - Acute undifferentiated leukemia (M0)
  - Acute myeloblastic leukemia (M1)
  - Acute myeloblastic leukemia with differentiation (M2)
  - Acute promyelocytic leukemia (M3)
  - Acute myelomonocytic leukemia (M4)
  - Acute monoblastic leukemia (M5)
  - Erythroleukemia (M6)
  - Megakaryoblastic leukemia (M7)

- ALL is classified by immunologic phenotype as B- or T-cell lineage
- Cytogenetics are single most important prognostic factor

DEMOGRAPHICS

- ALL comprises 80% of acute leukemias of childhood; peak incidence is between ages 3 and 7 years
- ALL is also seen in adults, causing ~20% of adult acute leukemias
- AML chiefly occurs in adults with median age at presentation of 60 years and increasing incidence with advanced age

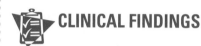 **CLINICAL FINDINGS**

SYMPTOMS AND SIGNS

- Clinical findings are due to replacement of normal bone marrow or infiltration of organs (skin, gastrointestinal tract, meninges)
- Gingival bleeding, epistaxis, or menorrhagia common
- Less commonly, widespread bleeding from disseminated intravascular coagulation (DIC) (in APL and monocytic leukemia)
- Increased susceptibility to infection when neutrophil count < 500/μL
  - Infection (eg, cellulitis, pneumonia, and perirectal infections) within days is the rule when neutrophil count < 100/μL
  - Death within a few hours may occur if treatment is delayed
  - Signs of infection may be absent
  - Gram-negative bacteria or fungi (*Candida, Aspergillus*) are the most common pathogens
- Gum hypertrophy
- Bone and joint pain
- Impaired circulation, causing headache, confusion, and dyspnea, with hyperleukocytosis (circulating blast count usually > 200,000/μL)
- Pallor, purpura, and petechiae common
- Hepatosplenomegaly and lymphadenopathy are variable
- Bone tenderness, particularly in the sternum, tibia

DIFFERENTIAL DIAGNOSIS

- AML
  - Chronic myelogenous leukemia
  - Myelodysplastic syndromes
  - Left-shifted bone marrow recovering from toxic insult
- ALL
  - Chronic lymphocytic leukemia
  - Lymphoma
  - Hairy cell leukemia
  - Atypical lymphocytosis of mononucleosis or pertussis

 DIAGNOSIS

LABORATORY TESTS

- Combination of pancytopenia with circulating blasts on peripheral smear
- Blasts absent from peripheral smear in up to 10% ("aleukemic leukemia")
- DIC
  - Serum fibrinogen low
  - Prothrombin time prolonged
  - Fibrin degradation products or fibrin D-dimers present
- Blasts in cerebrospinal fluid occur with meningeal leukemia in ~5% of cases at diagnosis
- Auer rod, an eosinophilic needle-like inclusion in cytoplasm of blasts, is pathognomonic of AML
- Lack of morphologic or histochemical evidence of myeloid or monocytic lineage suggests diagnosis of ALL
- Demonstration of characteristic surface markers by immunophenotype confirms diagnosis of ALL
- In ALL, Philadelphia chromosome t(9; 22) and t(4;11) has an unfavorable prognosis
- In AML, cytogenetic studies showing t(8;21), t(15;17), and inv(16)(p13;q22) have favorable prognosis; those showing monosomy 5 and 7 and complex abnormalities are unfavorable

IMAGING STUDIES

- Chest radiograph: mediastinal mass in ALL (especially T cell)

DIAGNOSTIC PROCEDURES

- Bone marrow is hypercellular, with > 20% blasts required for diagnosis

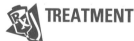 **TREATMENT**

MEDICATIONS

Remission induction therapy

- AML: combination of an anthracycline (daunorubicin or idarubicin) plus cytarabine, either alone or in combination with other agents

- APL
  - Treated differently from other forms of AML
  - Induction therapy should include an anthracycline plus all-*trans*-retinoic acid
  - For patients with high-risk APL based on an initial WBC > 10,000/mcL, the addition of arsenic trioxide may be beneficial
- ALL
  - Combination chemotherapy, including daunorubicin, vincristine, prednisone, and asparaginase
  - Those patients with Philadelphia chromsome-positive ALL (or bcr-abl + ALL) should have imatinib (or dasatinib) added to their initial chemotherapy
  - Less myelosuppressive than treatment for AML and does not necessarily produce marrow aplasia

Postremission therapy

- Once in remission, postremission therapy is given with curative intent
- AML
  - Standard chemotherapy and autologous and allogeneic transplantation
  - Optimal treatment strategy depends on the patient's age and clinical status and the risk factor profile of the leukemia
- APL
  - Chemotherapy plus retinoic acid
  - Arsenic trioxide has been approved for treatment of relapsed disease
- ALL
  - After achieving complete remission, patients receive CNS prophylaxis so that meningeal sequestration of leukemic cells does not develop
  - Chemotherapy or high-dose chemotherapy plus bone marrow transplantation
  - Treatment decisions are based on patient age and risk factors of the disease

THERAPEUTIC PROCEDURES

- AML: Allogeneic transplantation is treatment of choice for high-risk patients
- ALL
  - Allogeneic transplantation if adverse cytogenetics or poor responses to chemotherapy
  - Autologous transplantation is an option in patients without a suitable donor

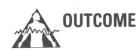

OUTCOME

FOLLOW-UP

- Repeat bone marrow

COMPLICATIONS

- Infection

PROGNOSIS

- AML
  - About 70–80% of adults under age 60 years achieve complete remission
  - Cure rates
    - 35–40% for postremission chemotherapy
    - 50% for autologous transplantation
    - 50–60% for allogeneic transplantation
  - About 50% of adults older than age 60 achieve complete remission
  - Cure rates for older patients has been very low (about 10–15%) even if they achieve remission and are able to receive post-remission chemotherapy
- ALL: Combination chemotherapy produces complete remissions in 80–90% of patients
- APL
  - Anthracycline plus all-*trans*-retinoic acid achieves complete remission in 90–95% of patients
  - Chemotherapy plus retinoic acid produces long-term remission in 70–80% of patients
  - Arsenic trioxide has been shown to increase the cure rate when added to primary therapy

WHEN TO REFER

- Refer all patients with acute leukemia to hematologist-oncologist

WHEN TO ADMIT

- Hyperleukocytosis (leukostasis syndrome)
- With initial diagnosis

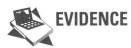

EVIDENCE

PRACTICE GUIDELINES

- O'Donnell MR et al. NCCN Acute Myeloid Leukemia Practice Guidelines Panel. National Comprehensive Cancer Network: Acute Myeloid Leukemia v.2.2005

WEB SITE

- National Cancer Institute: Leukemia

INFORMATION FOR PATIENTS

- American Cancer Society: Overview: Leukemia—Acute Lymphocytic
- American Cancer Society: Overview: Leukemia—Acute Myeloid
- Leukemia & Lymphoma Society: Leukemia
- MedlinePlus: Leukemia Interactive Tutorial

REFERENCES

- Berg SL et al; Children's Oncology Group. Phase II study of nelarabine (compound 506U78) in children and young adults with refractory T-cell malignancies: a report from the Children's Oncology Group. J Clin Oncol. 2005 May 20;23(15):3376–82. [PMID: 15908649]
- Breems DA et al. Prognostic index for adult patients with acute myeloid leukemia in first relapse. J Clin Oncol. 2005 Mar 20;23(9):1969–78. [PMID: 15632409]
- Farag S et al. Outcome of induction and postremission therapy in younger adults with acute myeloid leukemia with normal karyotype: a cancer and leukemia group B study. J Clin Oncol. 2005 Jan 20;23(3):482–93. [PMID: 15534356]
- Lee S et al. The effect of first-line imatinib interim therapy on the outcome of allogeneic stem cell transplantation in adults with newly diagnosed Philadelphia chromosome-positive acute lymphoblastic leukemia. Blood. 2005 May 1;105(9):3449–57. [PMID: 15657178]
- Mancini M et al. A comprehensive genetic classification of adult acute lymphoblastic leukemia (ALL): analysis of the GIMEMA 0496 protocol. Blood. 2005 May 1;105(9):3434–41. [PMID: 15650057]
- Pui CH et al. Treatment of acute lymphoblastic leukemia. N Engl J Med. 2006 Jan 12;354(2):166–78. [PMID: 16407512]
- Sanz MA et al. Tricks of the trade for the appropriate management of newly diagnosed acute promyelocytic leukemia. Blood. 2005 Apr 15;105(8):3019–25. [PMID: 15604216]

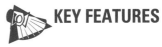

Leukemia, Chronic Lymphocytic

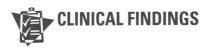

KEY FEATURES

ESSENTIALS OF DIAGNOSIS

- Most patients are asymptomatic at presentation
- Lymphocytosis > 5000/mcL
- Mature morphologic appearance of lymphocytes
- Coexpression of CD19, CD5

GENERAL CONSIDERATIONS

- A clonal malignancy of B lymphocytes
- The course is usually indolent, with slowly progressive accumulation of long-lived small lymphocytes that are immunoincompetent
- Results in immunosuppression, bone marrow failure, and organ infiltration with lymphocytes
- Immunodeficiency also related to inadequate antibody production by abnormal B cells
- Prognostically a useful staging system (Rai system)
  - Stage 0, lymphocytosis only
  - Stage I, lymphocytosis plus lymphadenopathy
  - Stage II, organomegaly
  - Stage III, anemia
  - Stage IV, thrombocytopenia

DEMOGRAPHICS

- Chronic lymphocytic leukemia (CLL) occurs mainly in older patients
  - 90% of cases occur in persons over age 50
  - Median age at presentation is 65

CLINICAL FINDINGS

SYMPTOMS AND SIGNS

- Incidentally discovered lymphocytosis in many patients
- Fatigue
- Lymphadenopathy in 80%
- Hepatomegaly or splenomegaly in 50%
- Occasionally, symptoms of hemolytic anemia or thrombocytopenia

DIFFERENTIAL DIAGNOSIS

- Atypical lymphocytosis of mononucleosis or pertussis
- Lymphoma in leukemic stage, especially mantle cell lymphoma
- Hairy cell leukemia

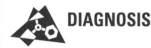

DIAGNOSIS

LABORATORY TESTS

- White blood cell count variable and may be several hundred thousand
- Differential: usually 75–98% of circulating cells are lymphocytes
- Hematocrit and platelet count usually normal at presentation
- Autoimmune hemolytic anemia or thrombocytopenia present in 5–10%
- On peripheral smear, lymphocytes are usually morphologically indistinguishable from normal small lymphocytes
- Larger and more immature cells in prolymphocytic leukemia (PLL)
- CLL is diagnosed by coexpression of B-lymphocyte lineage marker CD19 with T-lymphocyte marker CD5
- CLL is distinguished from mantle cell lymphoma by
  - Expression of CD23
  - Low expression of surface immunoglobulin and CD20
  - Absence of overexpression of cyclin D1
- High expression of CD38 or ZAP-70 is correlated with more aggressive course
- Fluorescence in-situ hybridization (FISH) assesses genomic changes
- Hypogammaglobulinemia in half, becomes more common with advanced disease
- Serum protein electrophoresis: IgM paraprotein may be present

DIAGNOSTIC PROCEDURES

- Bone marrow is variably infiltrated with small lymphocytes
- Lymph node biopsy shows same pathologic changes as in diffuse small cell lymphocytic lymphoma

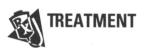

TREATMENT

MEDICATIONS

- Most patients with early stage disease do not require treatment for months or years
- Fludarabine plus rituximab
  - Treatment of choice

- Given monthly for 6 months and then stopped
- Fludarabine plus cyclophosphamide (and the three-drug combination adding rituximab)
  - Also produces high response rates
  - However, regimen produces somewhat more toxicity
- Chlorambucil, 0.6–1 mg/kg PO every 3 weeks for approximately 6 months is a convenient, well tolerated, and reasonable first choice for elderly patients
- Alemtuzumab
  - Has been approved for treatment of refractory CLL
  - However, it produces significant immunosuppresssion
- Associated autoimmune hemolytic anemia or immune thrombocytopenia
  - May require treatment with rituximab or prednisone
  - Avoid fludarabine in patients with autoimmune hemolytic anemia since it may exacerbate this condition
- Prophylactic infusions of gamma globulin 0.4 g/kg/month for patients with recurrent, severe bacterial infections and hypogammaglobulinemia

SURGERY

- Splenectomy for associated autoimmune hemolytic anemia or immune thrombocytopenia

THERAPEUTIC PROCEDURES

- Indications for treatment include
  - Progressive fatigue
  - Symptomatic lymphadenopathy
  - Anemia or thrombocytopenia (symptomatic and progressive stage II disease or stage III/IV disease)
- Allogeneic transplantation potentially curative, but used only if CLL cannot be controlled by standard therapies
- Nonmyeloablative allogeneic transplantation is newer technique; has expanded role of transplantation in CLL

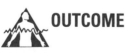

OUTCOME

COMPLICATIONS

- Autoimmune hemolytic anemia or autoimmune thrombocytopenia in 5–10%
- Isolated lymph node transformation into aggressive large cell lymphoma (Richter's syndrome) despite stable systemic disease in ~5% of cases

PROGNOSIS

- CLL often pursues an indolent course

- Treatment results are improving with new therapies, and long-term prognosis is very likely to improve
- In the past, median survival has been ~6 years, and 10-year survival is 25%
- Patients with stage 0 or stage I disease have median survival > 10 years
- Patients with stage III or stage IV disease have a 2-year survival rate > 90%
- Biologic markers (eg, gene mutation status, ZAP-70 expression, and cytogenetic abnormalities) useful in predicting outcomes of subsets of CLL patients
- Prolymphocytic leukemia, a variant of CLL, often pursues a more aggressive course
- FISH provides important prognostic information
  - Findings of deletions of chromosome 17p or 11q confers a poor prognosis
  - However, deletion of only 13q confers a very favorable outcome

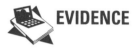

EVIDENCE

PRACTICE GUIDELINES

- Oscier D et al. Guidelines on the diagnosis and management of chronic lymphocytic leukaemia. Br J Haematol 2004;125:294. [PMID: 15086411]

WEB SITE

- National Cancer Institute: Chronic Lymphocytic Leukemia: Treatment

INFORMATION FOR PATIENTS

- American Cancer Society: Detailed Guide: Leukemia—Chronic Lymphocytic
- Leukemia & Lymphoma Society: Chronic Lymphocytic Leukemia
- MedlinePlus: Leukemia Interactive Tutorial
- National Cancer Institute: Chronic Lymphocytic Leukemia: Treatment

REFERENCES

- Byrd JC et al. Addition of rituximab to fludarabine may prolong progression-free survival and overall survival in patients with previously untreated chronic lymphocytic leukemia: an updated retrospective comparative analysis of CALGB 9712 and CALGB 9011. Blood. 2005 Jan 1;105(1):49–53. [PMID: 15138165]
- Chiorazzi N et al. Chronic lymphocytic leukemia. N Engl J Med. 2005 Feb 24; 352(8):804–15. [PMID: 15728813]

- Keating MJ et al. Early results of a chemoimmunotherapy regimen of fludarabine, cyclophosphamide, and rituximab as initial therapy for chronic lymphocytic leukemia. J Clin Oncol. 2005 Jun 20;23(18):4079–88. [PMID: 15767648]
- Montserrat E et al. How I treat refractory CLL. Blood. 2006 Feb 15; 107(4):1276–83. [PMID: 16204307]
- Moreno C et al. Allogeneic stem-cell transplantation may overcome the adverse prognosis of unmutated VH gene in patients with chronic lymphocytic leukemia. J Clin Oncol. 2005 May 20;23(15):3433–8. [PMID: 15809449]
- Moreton P et al. Eradication of minimal residual disease in B-cell chronic lymphocytic leukemia after alemtuzumab therapy is associated with prolonged survival. J Clin Oncol. 2005 May 1; 23(13):2971–9. [PMID: 15738539]

Leukemia, Chronic Myelogenous

 KEY FEATURES

ESSENTIALS OF DIAGNOSIS

- Elevated (often markedly) white blood cell count (WBC)
- Left-shifted myeloid series but low percentage of promyelocytes and blasts
- Presence of Philadelphia chromosome or *bcr/abl* gene

GENERAL CONSIDERATIONS

- Myeloproliferative disorder characterized by overproduction of myeloid cells
- Associated with characteristic chromosomal abnormality, the Philadelphia chromosome, a reciprocal translocation between long arms of chromosomes 9 and 22
- Translocated portion of 9q contains *abl*, a protooncogene, which is received on 22q, at the break point cluster (bcr) site
- The fusion gene *bcr/abl* produces a novel protein that possesses tyrosine kinase activity, leading to leukemia
- Disease may progress from chronic phase to accelerated phase and to blast crisis

- Progression often associated with added chromosomal defects superimposed on Philadelphia chromosome
- Blast crisis CML is morphologically indistinguishable from acute leukemia

DEMOGRAPHICS

- CML occurs mainly in middle age; median age at presentation is 50 years

 CLINICAL FINDINGS

SYMPTOMS AND SIGNS

- Fatigue, night sweats, and low-grade fever
- Abdominal fullness related to splenomegaly
- Uncommom leukostasis clinical syndrome with blurred vision, respiratory distress, or priapism (rare)
- Sternal tenderness
- Fever in absence of infection, bone pain, and splenomegaly may mark disease acceleration

DIFFERENTIAL DIAGNOSIS

- Reactive leukocytosis resulting from infection, inflammation, or cancer
- Other myeloproliferative disorder: essential thrombocytosis, polycythemia vera, or myelofibrosis

 DIAGNOSIS

LABORATORY TESTS

- Median WBC at diagnosis is 150,000/ mcL, although some cases are discovered when WBC is only modestly increased
- WBC usually > 500,000/mcL in rare cases of symptomatic leukostasis
- Hematocrit is usually normal at presentation
- Platelet count may be normal or elevated (sometimes strikingly elevated)
- Basophilia and eosinophilia may be present
- Peripheral blood smear
  - Myeloid series left-shifted with mature forms dominating
  - Blasts usually < 5%
  - Red blood cell (RBC) morphology normal; nucleated RBCs rarely seen
- The diagnosis is confirmed by finding *bcr/abl* gene in peripheral blood
- Progressive anemia and thrombocytopenia occur in accelerated and blast phases, and percentage of blasts in blood and bone marrow increases

DIAGNOSTIC PROCEDURES

- Bone marrow aspirate and biopsy: hypercellular, with left-shifted myelopoiesis is not diagnostic, but distinguishes chronic phase from more advanced disease
- Cytogenetics in bone marrow may show abnormalities in addition to Philadelphia chromosome
- When blasts comprise > 20% of bone marrow cells, blast phase of CML is diagnosed

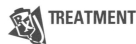 TREATMENT

MEDICATIONS

- Imatinib mesylate, 400 mg PO once daily
  - An inhibitor of tyrosine kinase activity of the *bcr/abl* oncogene
  - Treatment of choice for chronic phase CML
  - Well tolerated
  - Most common side effects are mild nausea, periorbital swelling, rash, and myalgia
- Higher doses of imatinib (600–800 mg daily)
  - May overcome some degree of resistance
  - May produce more rapid initial responses
  - Side effects are more prominent with these doses
- New investigatinal tyrosine kinase inhibitors (eg, dasatinib) are effective in most imatinib-resistant cases

THERAPEUTIC PROCEDURES

- Treatment usually not emergent even with WBC > 200,000/mcL
- Emergent leukapheresis is performed in conjunction with myelosuppressive therapy in rare instances of symptomatic leukostasis
- Allogeneic transplantation is recommended if there is suboptimal response, either lack of a complete cytogenetic response, a suboptimal molecular response, or an increasing level of *bcr/ abl* transcripts
- Allogeneic transplantation remains the only proven curative treatment

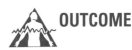 OUTCOME

FOLLOW-UP

- Response is assessed by
  - Hematologic complete remission, with normalization of blood counts

and splenomegaly, usually within several weeks to 3 months

- Cytogenetic responses within 6–12 months
- Quantitative assessment of the *bcr/abl* gene by polymerase chain reaction (PCR) assay

• Bone marrow cytogenetics after 6 months of imatinib treatment to assess hematologic and cytogenetic remission

COMPLICATIONS

• Leukostasis clinical syndrome

PROGNOSIS

• Patients with complete cytogenetic response and > 3 log reduction in *bcr/abl* appear to have excellent prognosis, with 100% remaining in control at > 4 years
• In the past, median survival was 3–4 years
• Allogeneic stem cell transplantation is only proven curative option
• Infusion of T lymphocytes from initial bone marrow donor in recurrent disease after allogeneic transplant can produce long-term remission in 50–70%

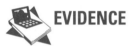 **EVIDENCE**

PRACTICE GUIDELINES

• O'Brien S et al. NCCN Chronic Myelogenous Leukemia Practice Guidelines Panel. National Comprehensive Cancer Network: Chronic myelogenous leukemia v.2.2005.

WEB SITE

• National Cancer Institute: Chronic Myelogenous Leukemia: Treatment

INFORMATION FOR PATIENTS

• American Cancer Society: Detailed Guide: Leukemia—Chronic Myeloid
• Leukemia & Lymphoma Society: Chronic Myelogenous Leukemia
• MedlinePlus: Leukemia Interactive Tutorial
• National Cancer Institute: Chronic Myelogenous Leukemia: Treatment

REFERENCES

• Crossman LC et al. Imatinib therapy in chronic myeloid leukemia. Hematol Oncol Clin North Am. 2004 Jun; 18(3):605–17. [PMID: 15271395]
• Deininger M et al. The development of imatinib as a therapeutic agent for chronic myeloid leukemia. Blood. 2005 Apr 1;105(7):2640–53. [PMID: 15618470]
• Kantarjian HM et al. Long-term survival benefit and improved complete cytogenetic and molecular response rates with imatinib mesylate in Philadelphia chromosome-positive chronic-phase chronic myeloid leukemia after failure of interferon-alpha. Blood. 2004 Oct 1;104(7):1979–88. [PMID: 15198956]
• Radich JP et al. HLA-matched related hematopoietic cell transplantation for chronic-phase CML using a targeted busulfan and cyclophosphamide preparative regimen. Blood. 2003 Jul 1; 102(1):31–5. [PMID: 12595317]
• Shah NP et al. Overriding imatinib resistance with a novel ABL kinase inhibitor. Science. 2004 Jul 16;305(5682):399–401. [PMID: 15256671]

Leukoplakia & Erythroplakia

KEY FEATURES

ESSENTIALS OF DIAGNOSIS

Leukoplakia
• A white lesion that, unlike oral candidiasis, cannot be removed by rubbing the mucosal surface

Hairy leukoplakia
• Found in patients with HIV infection
• Occurs on lateral border of tongue
• Develops quickly
• Appears as slightly raised leukoplakic areas with corrugated surface

Erythroplakia
• Similar to leukoplakia except that it has a definite erythematous component

Oral lichen planus
• Most commonly presents as lacy leukoplakia but may be erosive
• Definitive diagnosis requires biopsy

Oral cancer
• Early lesions appear as leukoplakia or erythroplakia
• More advanced lesions are larger, with invasion into tongue such that a mass lesion is palpable
• Ulceration may be present

GENERAL CONSIDERATIONS

Leukoplakia
• About 5% represent either dysplasia or early invasive squamous cell carcinoma (SCC)
• Histologically, there is often hyperkeratoses, occurring in response to chronic irritation

Hairy leukoplakia
• Seen in about 19% of HIV-positive patients with oral lesions
• May herald subsequent more ominous manifestations of AIDS

Erythroplakia
• About 90% of cases are either dysplasia or carcinoma, so distinction from leukoplakia is important

Oral lichen planus
• An inflammatory pruritic disease of the skin and mucous membranes
• Mucosal lichen planus must be differentiated from leukoplakia
• Erosive oral lesions require biopsy and often direct immunofluorescence for diagnosis because lichen planus may simulate other erosive diseases
• There is a low risk (1%) of SCC arising within lichen planus

DEMOGRAPHICS

• Alcohol and tobacco use are the major etiologic risk factors for oral carcinoma

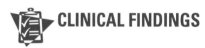 **CLINICAL FINDINGS**

SYMPTOMS AND SIGNS

• Intraoral examination (lateral tongue, floor of the mouth, gingiva, buccal area, palate, and tonsillar fossae) and palpation of the neck for enlarged lymph nodes in patients over 45 who smoke tobacco or drink immoderately

Leukoplakia
• Any white lesion that, unlike oral candidiasis, cannot be removed by rubbing the mucosal surface
• Usually small

Hairy leukoplakia
• Appears as slightly raised leukoplakic areas with corrugated or "hairy" surface
• Parakeratosis and koilocytes are seen with little or no underlying inflammation

Erythroplakia
• A white lesion with an erythematous component that cannot be removed by rubbing the mucosal surface

Oral lichen planus
• Lacy leukoplakia but may be erosive

- Reticular pattern mimics candidiasis
- Erosive pattern mimics carcinoma

Oral cancer

- Early lesions appear as leukoplakia or erythroplakia; advanced lesions larger
- Invasion into tongue leads to palpable mass; ulceration may be present
- Biopsy essential for diagnosis
- Metastases to submandibular and jugulodigastric neck nodes are common

DIFFERENTIAL DIAGNOSIS

Oral leukoplakia

- Hyperkeratosis resulting from irritation
- Dysplasia or carcinoma
- Lichen planus
- Oral candidiasis
- Oral hairy leukoplakia

Erythroplakia

- Dysplasia or carcinoma
- Necrotizing sialometaplasia (when on hard palate)
- Ulcerative lichen planus

Oral lichen planus

- Oral cancer
- Candidiasis
- Erythema multiforme
- Pemphigus vulgaris
- Bullous pemphigoid
- Inflammatory bowel disease

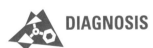 **DIAGNOSIS**

IMAGING STUDIES

- If SCC is suspected, then metastatic evaluation of neck and imaging deep extent in oral cavity is warranted
- Both PET scans and MRI are useful

DIAGNOSTIC PROCEDURES

- Oral lichen planus may be difficult to diagnose clinically. Exfoliative cytology or a small incisional or excisional biopsy is indicated, especially if SCC is suspected
- Any area of erythroplakia, enlarging area of leukoplakia, or a lesion that has submucosal depth on palpation should have an incisional biopsy or an exfoliative cytologic examination
- Intraoral staining with 1% toluidine blue may aid in selection of the most suspicious biopsy site
- Fine-needle aspiration biopsy may expedite the diagnosis if an enlarged lymph node is found

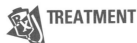 **TREATMENT**

MEDICATIONS

Lichen planus

- Therapy for confirmed diagnoses is management of pain
- Local and, if needed, systemic corticosteroids are widely used

Hairy leukoplakia

- May respond to zidovudine or acyclovir

SURGERY

Oral cancer

- Most patients in whom the tumor is detected before it is 2 cm in diameter are cured by local resection
- Larger tumors of the oral cavity are usually treated wth resection of the primary tumor, neck dissection, and postoperative irradiation
- Reconstruction, when needed, is done at the time of initial surgery
  - Vascularized free flaps, with bone if needed, are commonly used
  - Myocutaneous flaps may also be used

THERAPEUTIC PROCEDURES

- Radiation is an alternative to surgery but not generally used as first-line therapy for small lesions
- Tumors of the tonsillar fossa and base of tongue are usually best treated with radiation, often with concomitant chemotherapy, reserving surgery for salvage

 OUTCOME

FOLLOW-UP

- Leukoplakia, erythroplakia, lichen planus, and oral cancer require monitoring; early diagnosis of recurrent SCC or a new primary lesion is key to management
- Commonly a patient with a prior malignancy is examined
  - Every 4–6 weeks in the first year
  - Every 8–10 weeks in the second year
  - Every 3–4 months thereafter for several additional years
- The incidence of second tumors is about 3–4% annually, likely associated with prior use of tobacco or alcohol, or both
- Periodic PET scans and baseline posttreatment MRIs are frequently used in subsequent tumor surveillance

COMPLICATIONS

- Failure to recognize early tumors contributes to the need for more extensive intervention

PROGNOSIS

- SCC that invades < 4–5 mm into the tongue has a < 10% rate of nodal metastasis
- Floor of mouth and alveolar ridge are associated with neck metastases
- Base of tongue and tonsillar fossa are usually associated with nodal metastases; late distant metastases may occur in as many as 30%
- Early-stage tumors (< 2 cm without nodal involvement) have cure rates above 90%

WHEN TO REFER

- Specialty referral should be sought early for both diagnosis and treatment
- Consider indirect or fiberoptic examination of the nasopharynx, oropharynx, hypopharynx, and larynx by an otolaryngologist–head and neck surgeon when there is oral erythroplakia, unexplained throat or ear pain, or unexplained oral or nasal bleeding

PREVENTION

- Smoking cessation and alcohol abatement programs

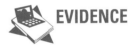 **EVIDENCE**

PRACTICE GUIDELINES

- Forastiere AA et al. NCCN Head and Neck Cancers Practice Guidelines Panel. National Comprehensive Cancer Network: Head and Neck Cancers v.1.2004.

WEB SITE

- Baylor College of Medicine Otolaryngology Resources

INFORMATION FOR PATIENTS

- Mayo Clinic: Leukoplakia
- MedlinePlus: Leukoplakia
- MedlinePlus: Lichen Planus
- National Cancer Institute: Oral Cancer

REFERENCES

- Eisen D et al. Number V. Oral lichen planus: clinical features and management. Oral Dis. 2005 Nov;11(6):338–49. [PMID: 16269024]

- Kujan O et al. Screening programmes for the early detection and prevention of oral cancer. Cochrane Database Syst Rev. 2006 Jul 19;3:CD004150. [PMID: 16856035]
- Rhodus NL. Oral cancer: leukoplakia and squamous cell carcinoma. Dent Clin North Am. 2005 Jan;49(1):143–65. [PMID: 15567366]

Lichen Planus

KEY FEATURES

ESSENTIALS OF DIAGNOSIS

- Pruritic, violaceous, flat-topped papules with fine white streaks and symmetric distribution
- Lacy lesions of the buccal mucosa
- Commonly seen along linear scratch marks (Koebner phenomenon) on anterior wrists, penis, legs
- Histopathologic examination is diagnostic

GENERAL CONSIDERATIONS

- An inflammatory pruritic disease of the skin and mucous membranes characterized by distinctive papules with a predilection for the flexor surfaces and trunk
- Three cardinal findings
  - Typical skin lesions
  - Mucosal lesions
  - Histopathologic features of band-like infiltration of lymphocytes and melanophages in the dermis

Oral lichen planus

- A relatively common (0.5–2.0% of the population) chronic inflammatory autoimmune disease
- May be difficult to diagnose clinically because of its numerous distinct phenotypic subtypes, eg, the reticular pattern may mimic candidiasis or hyperkeratosis, while the erosive pattern may mimic squamous cell carcinoma
- There is probably a low rate (1%) of squamous cell carcinoma arising within lichen planus (in addition to the possibility of clinical misdiagnosis)
- Most common drugs causing lichen planus–like reactions include
  - Gold
  - Sulfonamides
  - Tetracycline
  - Quinidine
  - Nonsteroidal anti-inflammatory drugs
  - Hydrochlorothiazide
- Hepatitis C infection is found with greater frequency in lichen planus patients than in controls in Europe and the United States
- A benign disease, but it may persist for months or years and may be recurrent

CLINICAL FINDINGS

SYMPTOMS AND SIGNS

- Itching is mild to severe
- The lesions are
  - Violaceous, flat-topped, angulated papules, 1–4 mm in diameter
  - Discrete or in clusters
  - Contain very fine white streaks (Wickham's striae) on the flexor surfaces of the wrists and on the penis, lips, tongue, and buccal and vaginal mucous membranes
- In the oral mucosa lichen planus may be confused with leukoplakia
- Mucosal lichen planus in the oral, genital, and anorectal areas may be erosive and painful
- The papules may become bullous
- The disease may be generalized
- The Koebner phenomenon (appearance of lesions in areas of trauma) may be seen

DIFFERENTIAL DIAGNOSIS

- Lichenoid drug eruption
- Psoriasis
- Lichen simplex chronicus
- Secondary syphilis
- Pityriasis rosea
- Discoid lupus erythematosus
- Graft-versus-host disease
- Mucosal lesions
  - Leukoplakia
  - Candidiasis
  - Erythema multiforme
  - Pemphigus vulgaris
  - Bullous pemphigoid
  - Lichen sclerosus
- Lichen planus on the mucous membranes must be differentiated from leukoplakia; erosive oral lesions require biopsy and often direct immunofluorescence for diagnosis since lichen planus may simulate other erosive diseases

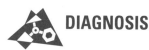

DIAGNOSIS

LABORATORY TESTS

- Confirmed by biopsy showing a band-like infiltration of lymphocytes and melanophages in the dermis

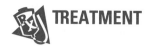

TREATMENT

MEDICATIONS

Topical therapy

- See Table 150
- Superpotent topical corticosteroid ointments
  - Examples are betamethasone dipropionate in optimized vehicle, diflorasone diacetate, clobetasol propionate, and halobetasol propionate
  - Apply twice daily for localized disease in nonflexural area
  - Alternatively, high-potency corticosteroid cream or ointment may be used nightly under thin pliable plastic film
- Tretinoin cream 0.05%, applied to mucosal lichen planus, followed by a corticosteroid ointment, may be helpful
- Topical tacrolimus
  - Appears effective in oral and vaginal erosive lichen planus, but long-term therapy is required to prevent relapse
  - Concern regarding absorption suggests monitoring blood counts when treating mucosal lesions

Systemic therapy

- Corticosteroids may be required in severe cases, or where the most rapid response to treatment is desired
- Unfortunately, relapse almost always occurs as the corticosteroids are tapered
- Psoralens plus long-wave ultraviolet light (PUVA)

OUTCOME

PROGNOSIS

- Benign disease, but it may persist for months or years
- May be recurrent
- Hypertrophic lichen planus and oral lesions tend to be especially persistent, and neoplastic degeneration has been described in chronically eroded lesions

WHEN TO REFER

- If there is a question about the diagnosis, if recommended therapy is ineffective, or specialized treatment is necessary

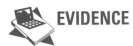

EVIDENCE

WEB SITE

- American Academy of Dermatology

INFORMATION FOR PATIENTS

- American Association of Family Physicians: Lichen Planus
- American Academy of Dermatology: Lichen Planus
- Mayo Clinic: Lichen Planus
- MedlinePlus: Lichen Planus

REFERENCE

- Cooper SM et al. Influence of treatment of erosive lichen planus of the vulva on its prognosis. Arch Dermatol. 2006 Mar; 142(3):289–94. [PMID: 16549703]

Lipid Abnormalities

KEY FEATURES

ESSENTIALS OF DIAGNOSIS

- Elevated serum total cholesterol or low-density lipoprotein (LDL) cholesterol, low serum high-density lipoprotein (HDL) cholesterol, or elevated serum triglycerides
- Usually asymptomatic
- In severe cases associated with metabolic abnormalities, superficial lipid deposition occurs

GENERAL CONSIDERATIONS

- Cholesterol and triglycerides are the two main circulating lipids
- Elevated levels of LDL cholesterol are associated with increased risk of atherosclerotic heart disease
- High levels of HDL cholesterol are associated with lower risk of atherosclerotic heart disease
- The exact mechanism by which LDL and HDL affect atherosclerosis is not fully delineated
- Familial genetic disorders are an uncommon, but often lethal, cause of elevated cholesterol
- Familial genetic disorders should be considered in patients who have onset of atherosclerosis in their 20s or 30s

DEMOGRAPHICS

- More common in men than women before age 50
- More common in women than men after age 50
- More common in whites and Hispanics than among blacks
- Up to 25% of Americans have the metabolic syndrome that consists of
  - A large waist circumference
  - Elevated blood pressure
  - Elevated triglycerides
  - Low HDL cholesterol
  - Elevated serum glucose

CLINICAL FINDINGS

SYMPTOMS AND SIGNS

- Usually asymptomatic
- Extremely high levels of chylomicrons or VLDL particles are associated with eruptive xanthomas
- Very high LDL levels are associated with tendinous xanthomas
- Very high triglycerides (> 2000 mg/dL) are associated with lipemia retinalis (cream-colored vessels in the fundus)

DIFFERENTIAL DIAGNOSIS

Hypercholesterolemia (cholesterol, elevated)

- Idiopathic
- Hypothyroidism
- Nephrotic syndrome
- Chronic renal insufficiency
- Obstructive liver disease
- Diabetes mellitus
- Anorexia nervosa
- Cushing's syndrome
- Familial, eg, familial hypercholesterolemia
- Drugs
  - Oral contraceptives
  - Thiazides (short-term effect)
  - β-Blockers (short-term effect)
  - Corticosteroids
  - Cyclosporine

Hypertriglyceridemia (triglycerides, elevated)

- Alcohol
- Obesity
- Metabolic syndrome (insulin resistance, low HDL)
- Diabetes mellitus
- Chronic renal insufficiency
- Lipodystrophy, eg, protease inhibitors
- Pregnancy

- Familial
- Drugs
  - Oral contraceptives
  - Isotretinoin
  - Thiazides (short-term effect)
  - β-Blockers (short-term effect)
  - Corticosteroids
  - Bile-acid binding resins

DIAGNOSIS

- Screen for lipid disorders in
  - Patients with coronary heart disease (CHD), diabetes, peripheral vascular disease, aortic aneurysm, cerebrovascular disease, chronic renal insufficiency, congestive heart failure, or a family history of premature coronary heart disease
  - Men older than 35 years and women older than 45 years if asymptomatic or no family history of premature heart disease
  - Obtain fasting serum total cholesterol, HDL cholesterol, and triglyceride levels
  - LDL cholesterol estimated by the following formula: LDL cholesterol = (Total cholesterol) − (HDL) − (Triglycerides/5)
- Serum thyroid-stimulating hormone to screen for hypothyroidism
- Other tests only as indicated by symptoms and signs suggestive of a secondary cause
- LDL cholesterol (mg/dL) is classified into 5 categories
  - Optimal, < 100
  - Near optimal, 100–129
  - Borderline high, 130–159
  - High, 160–189
  - Very high, ≥ 190

TREATMENT

MEDICATIONS

- See Table 89
- Choice of whether to initiate drug therapy should be based on overall risk profile and LDL cholesterol level
- LDL cholesterol threshold for treatment depends on absolute risk of CHD
- Most aggressive therapy required for
  - CHD
  - Diabetes
  - Cerebrovascular disease
  - Peripheral vascular disease
  - 10-year risk > 20%

- LDL ≥ 130 mg/dL plus presence of two or more of following risk factors requires treatment
  - Smoking
  - Hypertension
  - Older age
  - Family history of CHD
  - 10-year risk 10–20%
- LDL ≥ 160 mg/dL plus presence of two or more risk factors and 10-year risk < 10% requires treatment
- LDL ≥ 190 mg/dL plus presence of one or no risk factors requires treatment
- See Table 88
- **HMG-CoA reductase inhibitors** (statins eg, atorvastatin, fluvastatin, lovastatin, pravastatin, rosuvastatin, simvastatin)
  - Potent impact on LDL
  - Minimal impact on HDL
  - Best data for reducing coronary events, mortality
- **Niacin**
  - Moderate impact on LDL and HDL
  - Reduces triglycerides and has mortality benefit
  - High rates of intolerance, which can be improved with use of extended-release niacin and concomitant aspirin use
- **Bile acid binding resins** (eg, cholestyramine, colestipol, colesevelam)
  - Moderate impact on LDL
  - Minimal impact on HDL
  - Reduce coronary events but not mortality
  - Mainly gastrointestinal side effects and can block the absorption of fat-soluble vitamins
  - Safe in pregnancy
- **Fibric acid derivatives** (eg, gemfibrozil, fenofibrate)
  - Moderate impact on LDL and HDL
  - Reduce triglycerides
  - Reduce coronary events but not mortality
  - Side effects increased when taken with statins

THERAPEUTIC PROCEDURES

- For **hypercholesterolemia**, low-fat diets may produce a moderate (5–10%) decrease in LDL cholesterol
- More restricted, plant-based diets may lower LDL cholesterol substantially more
- Low-fat diet may also lower HDL cholesterol
- Substituting monounsaturated fats for saturated fats can lower LDL without affecting HDL

- In diabetics, control of hyperglycemia can improve lipid profile, particularly triglycerides
- Exercise and moderate alcohol consumption can increase HDL levels
- For **hypertriglyceridemia**, primary therapy is dietary, including reducing alcohol, reducing fatty foods and excess dietary carbohydrates, and controlling hyperglycemia in diabetics

 OUTCOME

- Fasting lipid panel 3–6 months after initiation of therapy
- Annual or biannual screening depending on risk factors
- Monitoring for side effects of therapy, such as liver enzyme elevation or myopathy in those on statins
- Atherosclerotic: myocardial infarction, stroke, and other vascular diseases
- Nonatherosclerotic: xanthomas and pancreatitis
- Metabolic syndrome patients are at increased risk for cardiovascular events
- Very high triglyceride levels (fasting triglyceride > 500 mg/dL) increase the risk of pancreatitis
- Refer patients with evidence of genetic disorders such as very high LDL or triglycerides to a lipid specialist
- Acute pancreatitis

 EVIDENCE

PRACTICE GUIDELINES

- Update (2004) of the Third Report of the National Cholesterol Education Program Expert Panel on Detection, Evaluation, and Treatment of High Blood Cholesterol in Adults (2001)
- Mosca L et al. Evidence-based guidelines for cardiovascular disease in women. Circulation. 2004 Feb 10; 109(5):672–93. [PMID: 14761900]

WEB SITE

- National Heart, Lung, and Blood Institute

INFORMATION FOR PATIENTS

- American Academy of Family Physicians: Cholesterol: What You Can Do to Lower Your Level
- American Heart Association: Cholesterol
- National Cholesterol Education Program: High Blood Cholesterol

REFERENCES

- Baigent C et al. Efficacy and safety of cholesterol-lowering treatment: prospective meta-analysis of data from 90,056 participants in 14 randomised trials. Lancet. 2005 Oct 8;366(9493):1267–78. [PMID: 16214597]
- Brunner E et al. Dietary advice for reducing cardiovascular risk. Cochrane Database Syst Rev. 2005 Oct 19; (4):CD002128. [PMID: 16235299]
- Dale KM et al. Statins and cancer risk: a meta-analysis. JAMA. 2006 Jan 4; 295(1):74–80. [PMID: 16391219]
- Szapary PO et al: The triglyceride-high-density lipoprotein axis: an important target of therapy? Am Heart J. 2004 Aug; 148(2):211–21. [PMID: 15308990]
- Whitney EJ et al. A randomized trial of a strategy for increasing high-density lipoprotein cholesterol levels: effects of progression of coronary heart disease and clinical events. Ann Intern Med. 2005 Jan 18;142(2):95–104. [PMID: 15657157]

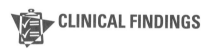

Livedo Reticularis

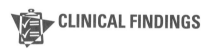 **KEY FEATURES**

- A benign condition that primarily affects the extremities
- Usually asymptomatic (apart from cosmetic concerns)
- Occurs in association with various diseases that cause vascular obstruction or inflammation
- Produces a mottled, purplish discoloration of the skin in a fishnet pattern with reticulated cyanotic areas surrounding paler central cores
- Can be idiopathic or a manifestation of a serious underlying condition

CLINICAL FINDINGS

- Spasm or obstruction of perpendicular arterioles combined with pooling of blood in surrounding venous plexuses
- Worsens with cold exposure
- Improves with warming
- Consider an underlying disease when
  - Systemic symptoms are present
  - Cutaneous ulcerations develop

- Presenting manifestation in 25% of patients with antiphospholipid antibody syndrome
- Other underlying causes include
  - Sneddon's syndrome (livedo reticularis and cerebrovascular events)
  - The vasculitides (particularly polyarteritis nodosa)
  - Cholesterol emboli syndrome
  - Thrombocythemia
  - Cryoglobulinemia
  - Cold agglutinin disease
  - Primary hyperoxaluria (due to vascular deposits of calcium oxalate)
  - Disseminated intravascular coagulation

 DIAGNOSIS

- Clinical diagnosis

 TREATMENT

- Protection from exposure to cold
- Vasodilators seldom indicated
- If ulcerations or gangrene, exclude an underlying systemic disease

Liver Disease, Alcoholic

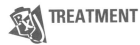 **KEY FEATURES**

ESSENTIALS OF DIAGNOSIS

- Excessive alcohol intake can lead to fatty liver, hepatitis, and cirrhosis
- Fatty liver is often asymptomatic
- Fever, right upper quadrant pain, tender hepatomegaly, and jaundice, or asymptomatic in hepatitis
- Aspartate aminotransferase (AST) is usually elevated but rarely above 300 units/L
- AST is greater than alanine aminotransferase (ALT), usually by a factor of 2 or more
- Often reversible, but it is the most common precursor of cirrhosis in the United States

GENERAL CONSIDERATIONS

- Generally, consumption of alcohol is > 80 g/day in men and 30–40 g/day in women

- Many of the adverse effects of alcohol are probably mediated by tumor necrosis factor α and by the oxidative metabolite acetaldehyde, which contributes to lipid peroxidation and induction of an immune response
- Alcoholic hepatitis is characterized by acute or chronic inflammation and parenchymal necrosis
- Deficiencies of vitamins and calories probably contribute to development of alcoholic hepatitis or its progression to cirrhosis

DEMOGRAPHICS

- Over 80% of patients have been drinking 5 years or more before developing any liver symptoms
- The longer the duration of drinking (10–15 or more years) and the larger the alcoholic consumption, the greater the probability of developing alcoholic hepatitis and cirrhosis

 CLINICAL FINDINGS

SYMPTOMS AND SIGNS

- Can vary from asymptomatic hepatomegaly to a rapidly fatal acute illness or end-stage cirrhosis
- Recent period of heavy drinking
- Anorexia and nausea
- Hepatomegaly and jaundice
- Abdominal pain and tenderness, splenomegaly, ascites, fever, and encephalopathy may be present

DIFFERENTIAL DIAGNOSIS

- Nonalcoholic fatty liver disease
- Viral hepatitis
- Drug-induced hepatitis
- Cirrhosis
- Biliary tract disease
- Pneumonia

 DIAGNOSIS

LABORATORY TESTS

Liver panel
- AST is usually elevated up to 300 units/L, but not higher
- AST is > ALT, usually by a factor of 2 or more
- Serum alkaline phosphatase is generally elevated, but seldom more than three times the normal value

- Serum bilirubin is increased in 60–90% of patients with alcoholic hepatitis

Complete blood cell count
- Anemia (usually macrocytic) may be present
- Leukocytosis with shift to the left is common with severe alcoholic hepatitis
- Leukopenia is occasionally seen and resolves after cessation of drinking
- About 10% of patients have thrombocytopenia related to a direct toxic effect of alcohol on megakaryocyte production or to hypersplenism

Other laboratory tests
- Serum γ-glutamyl transpeptidase, carbohydrate-deficient transferrin, and mitochondrial AST may be elevated, but these tests lack both sensitivity and specificity
- The serum albumin is depressed, and the γ-globulin level is elevated in 50–75% of persons with alcoholic hepatitis, even in the absence of cirrhosis
- Increased transferrin saturation, hepatic iron stores, and sideroblastic anemia are found in many alcoholic patients
- Folic acid deficiency may coexist

IMAGING STUDIES

- May show hepatic steatosis but are generally not helpful in the diagnosis of alcoholic hepatitis
- Ultrasound helps exclude biliary obstruction and identifies subclinical ascites
- CT scanning with IV contrast or MRI may be indicated in selected cases to evaluate patients for collateral vessels, space-occupying lesions of the liver, or concomitant disease of the pancreas

DIAGNOSTIC PROCEDURES

- Liver biopsy
  - If done, demonstrates various combinations of macrovesicular fat, polymorphonuclear neutrophil infiltration with hepatic necrosis, and Mallory bodies (alcoholic hyaline), and perivenular and perisinusoidal fibrosis
  - Micronodular cirrhosis may be present as well
  - The findings are identical to those of nonalcoholic steatohepatitis

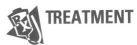 **TREATMENT**

MEDICATIONS

- Give **vitamins**, particularly folic acid and thiamine

- Glucose administration increases the vitamin B_1 requirement and can precipitate Wernicke-Korsakoff syndrome if thiamine is not coadministered
- Methylprednisolone, 32 mg/day PO for 1 month or the equivalent, may reduce short-term mortality and either encephalopathy or a discriminant function (defined by patient's prothrombin time minus the control prothrombin time times 4.6 plus the total bilirubin in mg/dL) > 32
- Pentoxifylline
  - A tumor necrosis factor inhibitor
  - Administer 400 mg PO TID for 4 weeks
  - May reduce 1-month mortality rates in severe disease, primarily by decreasing the risk of hepatorenal syndrome
- Other experimental therapies
  - Propylthiouracil
  - Oxandrolone
  - S-adenosyl-l-methionine

THERAPEUTIC PROCEDURES

- Abstinence from alcohol is essential; fatty liver is quickly reversible
- Provide sufficient carbohydrates and calories in anorectic patients to reduce endogenous protein catabolism, promote gluconeogenesis, and prevent hypoglycemia
- Nutritional support (40 kcal/kg with 1.5–2.0 g/kg as protein) improves survival in malnutrition
- Use of liquid formulas rich in branched-chain amino acids does not improve survival beyond that achieved with less expensive caloric supplementation

 OUTCOME

COMPLICATIONS

Alcoholic cirrhosis

- Occurs in about 10–15% of persons who consume over 50 g of alcohol (4 oz of 100-proof whiskey, 15 oz of wine, or four 12-oz cans of beer) daily for over 10 years (the risk may be lower for wine than for comparable intake of beer or spirits)
- The risk of cirrhosis is lower (5%) in the absence of other cofactors such as chronic viral hepatitis and obesity
- There are associations with polymorphisms of the genes encoding for tumor necrosis factor-α and cytochrome P450 2E1
- Women appear to be more susceptible than men, in part because of lower gastric mucosal alcohol dehydrogenase levels

PROGNOSIS

Short term

- A prothrombin time short enough to permit liver biopsy (< 3 s above control) has a 1-year mortality rate of 7%, rising to 20% if there is progressive prolongation of the prothrombin time during hospitalization
- If the prothrombin time prohibits liver biopsy, there is a 40% 1-year mortality rate
- Other unfavorable prognostic factors
  - Hepatic encephalopathy
  - Azotemia
  - Leukocytosis
  - Little steatosis on a liver biopsy specimen
  - Reversal of portal blood flow on Doppler ultrasound
- Serum bilirubin levels > 10 mg/dL and marked prolongation of the prothrombin time (≥ 6 s above control) indicate severe hepatitis with a mortality rate as high as 50%
- The Model for End-Stage Liver disease (MELD) score (used to prioritize patients with cirrhosis for liver transplantation, see Cirrhosis) also correlates with mortality from alcoholic hepatitis

Long term

- In the United States, the 3-year mortality rate after recovery from acute alcoholic hepatitis is 10 times that of controls
- Histologically severe disease is associated with continued excessive mortality rates after 3 years, whereas the death rate is not increased after the same period in those whose liver biopsies show only mild alcoholic hepatitis
- Poor prognosis suggested by
  - Complications of portal hypertension (ascites, variceal bleeding, hepatorenal syndrome)
  - Coagulopathy following recovery from acute alcoholic hepatitis
  - Continued excessive drinking (the most important prognostic indicator); a 6-month period of abstinence is generally required before liver transplantation can be considered

PREVENTION

- Abstinence from alcohol

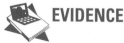 **EVIDENCE**

WEB SITES

- Diseases of the Liver
- Hepatic Ultrasound Images
- Pathology Index

INFORMATION FOR PATIENTS

- Alcoholics Anonymous
- Mayo Clinic

REFERENCES

- Ceccanti M et al. Acute alcoholic hepatitis. J Clin Gastroenterol. 2006 Oct; 40(9):833–41. [PMID: 17016141]
- Dunn W et al. Utility of a new model to diagnose an alcohol basis for steatohepatitis. Gastroenterology. 2006 Oct; 131(4):1057–63. [PMID: 17030176]
- Gramenzi A et al. Review article: alcoholic liver disease—pathophysiological aspects and risk factors. Aliment Pharmacol Ther. 2006 Oct 15;24(8):1151–61. [PMID: 17014574]
- Sass DA et al. Alcoholic hepatitis. Clin Liv Dis. 2006 May;10(2):219–37. [PMID: 16971259]

Low Back Pain

 KEY FEATURES

ESSENTIALS OF DIAGNOSIS

- A precise diagnosis cannot be made in the majority of cases
- Even when anatomic defects—such as vertebral osteophytes or a narrowed disk space—are present, causality cannot be assumed since such defects are common in asymptomatic patients
- The majority of patients will improve in 1–4 weeks and need no evaluation beyond the initial history and physical examination

GENERAL CONSIDERATIONS

- Exceedingly common, experienced at some time by up to 80% of the population

DEMOGRAPHICS

- Chronic low back pain from degenerative joint disease is rare before age 40

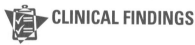 **CLINICAL FINDINGS**

SYMPTOMS AND SIGNS

- Pattern of pain
  - **Radiation down the buttock** and below the knee suggests nerve root irritation from a herniated disc

– **Pain that worsens with rest** and improves with activity is characteristic of ankylosing spondylitis or other seronegative spondyloarthropathies, especially when the onset begins before age 40

– Most degenerative back diseases produce precisely the opposite pattern, with rest alleviating and activity aggravating the pain

• **Low back pain at night,** unrelieved by rest or the supine position, suggests the possibility of malignancy

• Symptoms of **large or rapidly evolving neurologic** deficits identify patients who need urgent evaluation for possible cauda equina tumor, epidural abscess or, rarely, massive disk herniation

• **Bilateral leg weakness** (from multiple lumbar nerve root compressions) or saddle area anesthesia, bowel or bladder incontinence, or impotence (indicating sacral nerve root compressions) indicates a cauda equina process

• Positive straight leg raising test indicates nerve root irritation

– The examiner performs the test on the supine patient by passively raising the patient's leg

– The test is positive if radicular pain is produced with the leg raised 60 degrees or less

– The test has a specificity of 40% but is 95% sensitive with herniation at the L4–5 or L5–S1 level (the sites of 95% of disk herniations)

• The crossed straight leg sign has a sensitivity of 25% but is 90% specific for disk herniation and is positive when raising the contralateral leg reproduces the sciatica

• Disk herniation produces deficits predictable for the site involved (Table 125)

• Deficits of multiple nerve roots suggest a cauda equina tumor, an epidural abscess, or some other important process that requires urgent evaluation and treatment

• Palpation of the spine usually does not yield diagnostic information. Point tenderness over a vertebral body may suggest osteomyelitis

DIFFERENTIAL DIAGNOSIS

• Muscular strain
• Herniated disk
• Lumbar spinal stenosis
• Compression fracture
• Degenerative joint disease
• Infectious diseases (eg, osteomyelitis, epidural abscess, subacute bacterial endocarditis)

• Neoplastic disease (vertebral metastases)
• Seronegative spondylarthopathies, eg, ankylosing spondylitis
• Leaking abdominal aortic aneurysm
• Renal colic

 DIAGNOSIS

IMAGING STUDIES

• Radiographs are warranted promptly for suspected infection, cancer, fractures, or inflammation; selected other patients who do not improve after 2–4 weeks of conservative therapy are also candidates

• The Agency for Health Care Policy and Research guidelines for obtaining lumbar radiographs are summarized in Table 126

• MRI is needed urgently in any patient suspected of having an epidural mass or cauda equina tumor but not if a patient is felt to have a routine disk herniation, since most will improve over 4–6 weeks of conservative therapy

DIAGNOSTIC PROCEDURES

• If the history and physical examination do not suggest the presence of infection, cancer, inflammatory back disease, major neurologic deficits, or pain referred from abdominal or pelvic disease, further evaluation can be deferred while conservative therapy is tried

 TREATMENT

MEDICATIONS

• Nonsteroidal anti-inflammatory drugs (NSAIDs) for analgesia, but severe pain may require opioids

• Limited evidence supports the use of "muscle relaxants" such as

– Diazepam
– Cyclobenzaprine
– Carisoprodol
– Methocarbamol

• These drugs should be reserved for patients who do not respond to NSAIDs and should also be limited to courses of 1–2 weeks

SURGERY

• Surgical consultation is needed urgently for any patient with a large or evolving neurologic deficit

• Surgery for disk disease is indicated when there is documentation of herniation by some imaging procedure, a consistent

pain syndrome, and a consistent neurologic deficit that has failed to respond to 4–6 weeks of conservative therapy

THERAPEUTIC PROCEDURES

• All patients should be taught how to protect the back in daily activities

• Rest and back exercises, once thought to be cornerstones of conservative therapy, are now known to be ineffective for acute back pain

• Epidural corticosteroid injections can provide short-term relief of sciatica but do not improve functional status or reduce the need for surgery

• Corticosteroid injections into facet joints are ineffective for chronic low back pain

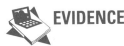 **OUTCOME**

PROGNOSIS

• The great majority of patients will spontaneously improve with conservative care over 1–4 weeks

WHEN TO REFER

• Refer to neurosurgeon or orthopedist if patient has disk herniation that does not respond after 4–6 weeks of conservative therapy or sooner if patient has important neurologic deficits

WHEN TO ADMIT

• Admit if symptoms and signs suggest epidural or spinal abscess, cauda equina syndrome, or new metastatic cancer

EVIDENCE

INFORMATION FOR PATIENTS

• American Academy of Family Physicians
• JAMA patient page. Low back pain. JAMA. 1998;279:1846. [PMID: 9628721]

REFERENCES

• Arden NK et al; WEST Study Group. A multicentre randomized controlled trial of epidural corticosteroid injections for sciatica: the WEST study. Rheumatology (Oxford). 2005 Nov;44(11):1399–406. [PMID: 16030082]

• Hagen K et al. Bed rest for acute low-back pain and sciatica. Cochrane Database Syst Rev. 2004 Oct 18; (4):CD001254. [PMID: 15495012]

- Speed C. Low back pain. BMJ. 2004 May 8;328(7448):1119–21. [PMID: 15130982]
- van Poppel MN et al. An update of a systematic review of controlled clinical trials on the primary prevention of back pain at the workplace. Occup Med (Lond). 2004 Aug;54(5):345–52. [PMID: 15289592]
- Weinstein JN et al. Surgical vs nonoperative treatment for lumbar disk herniation: the Spine Patient Outcomes Research Trial (SPORT): a randomized trial. JAMA. 2006 Nov 22; 296(20):2441–50. [PMID: 17119140]
- Weinstein JN et al Surgical vs nonoperative treatment for lumbar disk herniation: the Spine Patient Outcomes Research Trial (SPORT) observational cohort. JAMA. 2006 Nov 22; 296(20):2451–9. [PMID: 17119141]

Lupus Anticoagulant

KEY FEATURES

- IgM or IgG antibody that produces prolonged PTT by binding to phospholipid used in PTT assay
- A laboratory artifact that does not cause clinical bleeding
- Occurs in 5–10% of patients with systemic lupus erythematosus
- More common in patients without underlying disorder and in patients taking phenothiazines

CLINICAL FINDINGS

- No bleeding unless a second disorder is present (eg, thrombocytopenia, hypoprothrombinemia, prolonged bleeding time)
- Increased risk of thrombosis and recurrent spontaneous abortions

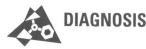

DIAGNOSIS

- PTT prolonged, fails to correct when patient's plasma is mixed in 1:1 dilution with normal plasma because lupus anticoagulant acts as inhibitor

---

- PT normal or slightly prolonged
- Serum fibrinogen level and thrombin time normal
- Russell viper venom test is a sensitive assay designed to demonstrate presence of lupus anticoagulant
- A related autoantibody, anticardiolipin, can be detected by separate assays

 TREATMENT

- No specific treatment necessary
- Anticoagulation in standard doses for patients with thromboses, aiming for INR of 2.0–3.0
- Because of artificially prolonged PTT, heparin therapy is difficult to monitor; thus, low-molecular-weight heparin is preferred
- Prophylaxis during pregnancy with low-molecular-weight heparin

Lyme Disease

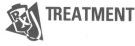

KEY FEATURES

ESSENTIALS OF DIAGNOSIS

- Erythema migrans, a flat or slightly raised red lesion that expands with central clearing
- Headache or stiff neck
- Arthralgias, arthritis, and myalgias; arthritis is often chronic and recurrent
- Wide geographic distribution, with most cases in the northeast, mid-Atlantic, upper midwest, and Pacific coastal regions of the United States

GENERAL CONSIDERATIONS

- Causative spirochete varies by geography
  - In the United States, it is *Borrelia burgdorferi*
  - In Europe and Asia, it is *Borrelia garinii* and *Borrelia afzelli*
- Incidence of disease is significantly higher when tick attachment is for longer than 72 h
- The percentage of ticks infected varies on a regional basis. In the northeast and midwest, 15–65%, in the west, only 2%
- Congenital infection has been documented

DEMOGRAPHICS

- Most cases (over 90%) were reported from the mid-Atlantic, northeastern, and north central regions of the country
- True incidence is unknown and overreporting continues to be a problem for following reasons:
  - Serologic tests are not standardized
  - Clinical manifestations are nonspecific
  - Serology tests are insensitive in early disease
  - Other as yet unidentified organisms may cause illnesses similar to Lyme disease (eg, the Lone Star tick [*Amblyomma americanum*], which is found in the midwest and south, can carry a spirochete that produces skin lesions indistinguishable from erythema migrans)
- Most infections occur in the spring and summer

 CLINICAL FINDINGS

SYMPTOMS AND SIGNS

- **Stage 1, early localized infection**
  - Erythema migrans (seen in ~50%)
    - A flat or slightly raised red lesion at the bite site ~1 week after the tick bite (range, 3–30 days)
    - Common in areas of tight clothing such as the groin, thigh, or axilla
    - The lesion expands over several days
    - Classic lesion progresses with central clearing ("bulls-eye" lesion); often there is a more homogeneous appearance or even central intensification
  - Concomitant viral-like illness develops in most patients and is characterized by
    - Myalgias, arthralgias
    - Headache, fatigue
    - Fever may or may not be present
- **Stage 2, early disseminated infection** (weeks to months later)
  - Bacteremia (in up to 50–60% of patients with erythema migrans)
  - Secondary skin lesions not associated with a tick bite
    - Develop within days to weeks of original infection in about 50% of patients
    - Lesions similar to primary lesion but smaller
  - Malaise, fatigue, fever, headache, neck pain generalized achiness common with skin lesions
  - Myopericarditis, with atrial or ventricular arrhythmias and heart block (4–10%)

- Neurologic manifestations (10–15%)
  - Aseptic meningitis with mild headache and neck stiffness
  - Cranial neuropathy (eg, Bell's palsy)
  - Sensory or motor radiculopathy and mononeuritis multiplex occur less frequently
- Conjunctivitis, keratitis
- Panophthalmitis (rare)
- **Stage 3, late persistent infection** (months to years later)
  - Musculoskeletal manifestations (up to 60%)
    - Monoarticular or oligoarticular arthritis of knee or other large weight-bearing joints
    - Chronic arthritis develops in about 10% of patients
  - Neurologic manifestations (rare)
    - Subacute encephalopathy (memory loss, mood changes, and sleep disturbance)
    - Intermittent paresthesias, often in stocking glove distribution, or radicular pain
    - Severe encephalomyelitis, seen more in Europe, presents with cognitive dysfunction, spastic paraparesis, ataxia, and bladder dysfunction
  - Acrodermatitis chronicum
    - Cutaneous manifestation
    - Usually bluish-red discoloration of distal extremity with associated swelling
    - Lesions atrophic and sclerotic, resemble localized scleroderma
- **Great overlap between stages;** the skin, CNS, and musculoskeletal system can be involved early or late

DIFFERENTIAL DIAGNOSIS

- Babesiosis, ehrlichiosis
- *A americanum* (Lone Star tick) bite-related illness
- Urticaria, reaction to arthropod bite, cellulitis, erythema multiforme, granuloma annulare
- Rocky Mountain spotted fever
- Primary HIV infection
- Parvovirus B19 infection
- Rheumatic fever, Still's disease, gonococcal arthritis, sarcoidosis, systemic lupus erythematosus
- Viral meningitis, Bell's palsy

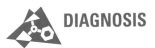 **DIAGNOSIS**

LABORATORY TESTS

- Elevated sedimentation rate of > 20 mm/h (50% of cases)

- Mildly abnormal liver function tests (30% of cases)
- Mild anemia, leukocytosis, and microscopic hematuria in 10% or less
- Detection of specific antibodies to *B burgdorferi* in serum, either by indirect immunofluorescence assay (IFA) or ELISA; both false-positive and false-negative reactions occur
- A Western blot assay that can detect both IgM and IgG antibodies is used as a confirmatory test if IFA or ELISA is positive
- A two-test approach is now recommended
- Polymerase chain reaction (PCR) test
  - Very specific for detecting *Borrelia* DNA
  - However, sensitivity is variable and depends on which body fluid is tested and which stage of disease
- Up to 85% of synovial fluid samples are PCR positive in active arthritis
- 38% of cerebrospinal fluid (CSF) samples are PCR positive in acute neuroborreliosis, but only 25% are positive in chronic neuroborreliosis
- Lyme urinary antigen, lymphocyte stimulation test, PCR on blood and urine
  - Have not been approved or standardized
  - Should not be used to support the diagnosis of Lyme disease

DIAGNOSTIC PROCEDURES

- A person who has been exposed to a potential tick habitat (within the 30 days just prior to developing erythema migrans) with the following fulfills the diagnostic criteria for Lyme disease
  - Erythema migrans diagnosed by a physician
  - At least one late manifestation of the disease
  - Laboratory confirmation
- Cultures for *B burgdorferi* can be performed but are not routine
  - Aspiration of erythema migrans lesions is positive in up to 30% of cases
  - 2-mm punch biopsy is positive in 50–70%
  - Blood cultures positive in up to 50%
  - CSF positive in 1–10%
- Peripheral neuropathy may be detected by electromyography

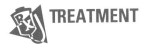 **TREATMENT**

MEDICATIONS

- See Table 78

- Erythema migrans
  - Doxycycline, 100 mg PO BID for 2–3 weeks, **or**
  - Amoxicillin, 500 mg PO TID for 2–3 weeks, **or**
  - Cefuroxime axetil, 500 mg PO BID for 2–3 weeks
- Bell's palsy
  - Doxycycline, 100 mg PO BID for 2–3 weeks, **or**
  - Amoxicillin, 500 mg PO TID for 2–3 weeks
  - Cefuroxime axetil, 500 mg PO BID for 2–3 week
- Other CNS disease
  - Ceftriaxone, 2 g IV once daily for 2–4 weeks, **or**
  - Penicillin G, 20 million units daily IV in six divided doses for 2–4 weeks, **or**
  - Cefotaxime, 2 g IV q8h for 2–4 weeks
- First-degree block (PR < 0.3 s)
  - Doxycycline, 100 mg PO BID for 3–4 weeks, **or**
  - Amoxicillin, 500 mg PO TID for 3–4 weeks
- High-degree atrioventricular block
  - Ceftriaxone, 2 g IV once daily for 2–4 weeks, **or**
  - Penicillin G, 20 million units daily IV in six divided doses for 2–4 weeks
- Arthritis
  - Oral: doxycycline, 100 mg BID for 4 weeks; or amoxicillin, 500 mg TID for 4 weeks; if this fails (persistent or recurrent joint swelling), re-treat with oral agent for 8 weeks or switch to IV agent for 2–4 weeks
  - Parenteral: ceftriaxone, 2 g IV once daily for 2–4 weeks; or penicillin G, 20 million units daily IV in six divided doses for 2–4 weeks
- Acrodermatitis chronicum atrophicans
  - Doxycycline, 100 mg PO BID for 3–4 weeks, **or**
  - Amoxicillin, 500 mg PO TID for 4 weeks

THERAPEUTIC PROCEDURES

- Tick bite: no treatment in most circumstances; observe
- If acute arthritis, need aspiration to rule out pyogenic arthritis
- If neurologic symptoms, need lumbar puncture because drug and duration of therapy are unique for neuroborreliosis
- If suspect peripheral neuropathy, perform nerve conduction studies

OUTCOME

FOLLOW-UP

- Routine follow-up
- Complete recovery in 4–6 weeks after therapy of early disease
- Fatigue, arthralgias, myalgias may persist for weeks or months but do not require antimicrobial therapy
- After treatment of arthritis, arthralgias may persist and be severe; if not resolved after 3 months, re-treat with antibiotics; if arthralgias still persist treat symptomatically

COMPLICATIONS

- Rarely, residual facial nerve palsy, synovitis or heart block requiring a pacemaker

PROGNOSIS

- With appropriate therapy, symptoms usually resolve within 4 weeks
- The long-term outcome of adult patients with Lyme disease is not clear
- Long-term sequelae are uncommon

WHEN TO REFER

- If persistent symptoms after initial appropriate therapy; usually continued symptoms are part of the natural history of the disease and not reinfection or indication for prolonged use of antibiotics

WHEN TO ADMIT

- For serious complications such as high-degree heart block

PREVENTION

- Avoiding tick-infested areas, covering exposed skin, using repellents, and inspecting for ticks after exposure
- Prophylactic antibiotics (eg, single 200 mg dose of doxycycline) is recommended in certain high risk situations if all of the following criteria are met
  - A tick identified as an adult or nymphal *Ixodes scapularis* has been attached for ≥ 36 h
  - Prophylaxis can be started within 72 h of tick removal
  - More than 20% of ticks in the area are known to be infected with *B burgdorferi*
  - There is no contraindication to the use of doxycycline (not pregnant, age > 8 years, not allergic)

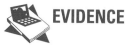 **EVIDENCE**

PRACTICE GUIDELINES

- Wormser GP et al. The clinical assessment, treatment, and prevention of Lyme disease, human granulocytic anaplasmosis, and babesiosis: clinical practice guidelines by the Infectious Diseases Society of America. Clin Infect Dis. 2006 Nov 1;43(9):1089–134. [PMID: 17029130]

WEB SITES

- American Lyme Disease Foundation
- Centers for Disease Control and Prevention: Lyme Disease Home Page
- Lyme Disease Network
- The Lyme Disease Foundation

INFORMATION FOR PATIENTS

- American College of Physicians: Lyme Disease, A Patient's Guide, Diagnosis
- American College of Physicians: Lyme Disease, A Patient's Guide, Treatment
- Centers for Disease Control and Prevention—Division of Vector Borne Infectious Diseases. Lyme Disease: A Public Information Guide

REFERENCES

- Aguero-Rosenfeld ME et al. Diagnosis of Lyme borreliosis. Clin Microbiol Rev. 2005 Jul;18(3):484–509. [PMID: 16020686]
- Depietropaolo DL et al. Diagnosis of Lyme disease. Am Fam Physician. 2005 Jul 15;72(2):297–304. [PMID: 16050454]
- Halperin JJ. Central nervous system Lyme disease. Curr Infect Dis Rep. 2004 Aug;6(4):298–304. [PMID: 15265459]
- Wormser GP. Clinical practice. Early Lyme disease. N Engl J Med. 2006 Jun 29;354(26):2794–801. [PMID: 16807416]

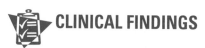
Lymphangitis & Lymphadenitis

 KEY FEATURES

ESSENTIALS OF DIAGNOSIS

- Red streak from wound or cellulitis toward enlarged, tender regional lymph nodes
- Chills, fever, and malaise

GENERAL CONSIDERATIONS

- Lymphangitis and lymphadenitis are common manifestations of a bacterial infection
  - Usually caused by hemolytic streptococci or staphylococci (or both)
  - Usually arises from an area of cellulitis, generally at the site of an infected wound
- Wound may be small or superficial, or an established abscess may be present
- Infection may progress rapidly, often in a matter of hours

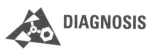 **CLINICAL FINDINGS**

SYMPTOMS AND SIGNS

- Throbbing pain usually present in area of cellulitis at the site of bacterial invasion
- Malaise
- Anorexia
- Sweating
- Chills
- Temperature of 37.8–40°C
- Rapid pulse
- Red streak may be definite or very faint and easily missed
- Regional lymph nodes may be significantly enlarged and tender

DIFFERENTIAL DIAGNOSIS

- Superficial thrombophlebitis
- Cat-scratch fever
- Acute streptococcal hemolytic gangrene
- Cellulitis
- Necrotizing fasciitis

DIAGNOSIS

LABORATORY TESTS

- Leukocytosis with a left shift
- Blood cultures often positive for *Staphylococcus* or *Streptococcus*

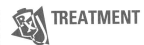

TREATMENT

MEDICATIONS

- Analgesics
- Antibiotics
  - Tables 62 and 63
  - Should be started when local infection becomes invasive
  - Cephalosporins or extended-spectrum penicillins commonly used
  - Consider coverage for methicillin-resistant *Staphylococcus aureus*

SURGERY

- Incision and drainage of abscess

THERAPEUTIC PROCEDURES

- Elevation (when feasible) and immobilization of infected area
- Heat (hot, moist compresses or heating pad)

OUTCOME

PROGNOSIS

- With proper therapy and effective antibiotic therapy, control of infection is achieved in a few days
- Delayed or inadequate therapy can lead to overwhelming infection with septicemia and even death

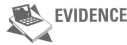

EVIDENCE

INFORMATION FOR PATIENTS

- Cleveland Clinic: Lymphedema
- Mayo Clinic: Swollen Lymph Glands (Lymphadenitis)
- MedlinePlus: Lymphadenitis and Lymphangitis

REFERENCES

- Falagas ME et al. Red streaks on the leg. Lymphangitis. Am Fam Physician. 2006 Mar 15;73(6):1061–2. [PMID: 16570742]
- Polesky A et al. Peripheral tuberculous lymphadenitis: epidemiology, diagnosis, treatment, and outcome. Medicine (Baltimore). 2005 Nov;84(6):350–62. [PMID: 16267410]

Lymphedema

KEY FEATURES

ESSENTIALS OF DIAGNOSIS

- Painless persistent edema of one or both lower extremities, primarily in young women
- Pitting edema, which rarely becomes brawny and non-pitting
- No ulceration, varicosities, or stasis pigmentation
- Episodes of lymphangitis and cellulitis

GENERAL CONSIDERATIONS

- Underlying mechanism in lymphedema is impaired lymph flow from an extremity
- Primary lymphedema
  - Due to congenital developmental abnormalities of lymphatics
  - Obstruction may be in the pelvic or lumbar lymph channels and nodes when the disease is extensive and progressive
- Secondary lymphedema involves inflammatory or mechanical lymphatic obstruction due to
  - Trauma
  - Regional lymph node resection or irradiation
  - Extensive involvement of regional nodes by malignant disease or filariasis
- Secondary dilation of the lymphatics occurs in both forms and leads to incompetence of the valve system, which
  - Disrupts the orderly flow along the lymph vessels
  - Results in progressive stasis of a protein-rich fluid, with secondary fibrosis

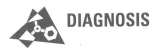

CLINICAL FINDINGS

SYMPTOMS AND SIGNS

- Episodes of acute and chronic inflammation
- Hypertrophy of the limb
- Markedly thickened and fibrotic skin and subcutaneous tissue

DIAGNOSIS

IMAGING STUDIES

- Lymphangiography and radioactive isotope studies may identify focal defects in lymph flow but are of little value in planning therapy

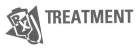

TREATMENT

MEDICATIONS

- No effective cure
- Antibiotic therapy for secondary infection
  - Should cover *Staphylococcus* and *Streptococcus* organisms
  - Dicloxacillin good choice for intermittent prophylactic therapy
- Diuretic therapy: intermittent courses can be helpful, especially in those with premenstrual or seasonal exacerbations

SURGERY

- Amputation for the rare complication of lymphangiosarcoma

THERAPEUTIC PROCEDURES

- Intermittent elevation of the extremity, especially during the sleeping hours (foot of bed elevated 15–20 degrees)
- Constant use of graduated elastic compression stockings
- Massage toward the trunk, either manually or pneumatic sequential pressure devices
- Good hygiene and treatment of any trichophytosis of toes to avoid secondary cellulitis

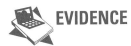

OUTCOME

COMPLICATIONS

- Secondary infection

PROGNOSIS

- Dictated by associated conditions and avoidance of recurrent cellulitis
- Good with aggressive treatment

EVIDENCE

PRACTICE GUIDELINES

- Harris SR et al. Clinical practice guidelines for the care and treatment of breast cancer: 11. Lymphedema. CMAJ 2001 Jan 23;164(2):191–9. [PMID: 11332311]
- Surgical management of early-stage invasive breast cancer. Practice Guidelines Initiative, 2003

INFORMATION FOR PATIENTS

- Cleveland Clinic: Lymphedema
- MedlinePlus: Lymphatic Obstruction

REFERENCES

- Karakousis CP. Surgical procedures and lymphedema of the upper and lower extremity. J Surg Oncol. 2006 Feb 1; 93(2):87–91. [PMID: 16425311]
- King B. Diagnosis and management of lymphoedema. Nurs Times. 2006 Mar 28–Apr 3;102(13):47, 49, 51. [PMID: 16605153]
- Kligman L et al. The treatment of lymphedema related to breast cancer: a systematic review and evidence summary. Support Care Cancer. 2004 Jun; 12(6):421–31. [PMID: 15095073]
- Mansel RE et al. Randomized multicenter trial of sentinel node biopsy versus standard axillary treatment in operable breast cancer: the ALMANAC Trial. J Natl Cancer Inst. 2006 May 3; 98(9):599–609. [PMID: 16670385]
- Ozaslan C et al. Lymphedema after treatment of breast cancer. Am J Surg. 2004 Jan;187(1):69–72. [PMID: 14706589]
- Rockson SG. Lymphedema. Curr Treat Options Cardiovasc Med. 2006 Apr; 8(2):129–36. [PMID: 16533487]
- Tiwari A et al. Differential diagnosis, investigation, and current treatment of lower limb lymphedema. Arch Surg. 2003 Feb;138(2):152–61. [PMID: 12578410]

Lymphoma, Gastric

KEY FEATURES

- Second most common gastric malignancy, 3–6% of gastric cancers
- More than 95% are non-Hodgkin's B-cell lymphomas
- May be primary (gastric mucosal lymphoma) or secondary (in patients with nodal lymphomas)
- ~60% of primary gastric lymphomas are mucosa-associated lymphoid tissue (MALT)
- B cells of nodal origin may be distinguished from B cells derived from MALT (CD19- and CD20-positive)
- Infection with *Helicobacter pylori* is an important risk factor for primary gastric lymphoma
- > 85% of low-grade primary gastric lymphomas and 40% of high-grade lymphomas are associated with *H pylori*

CLINICAL FINDINGS

- Abdominal pain
- Weight loss
- Upper GI bleeding

DIAGNOSIS

- Endoscopy with biopsy useful in diagnosis
- Abdominal and chest CT and endoscopic ultrasonography useful in staging

TREATMENT

- Primary low-grade gastric lymphomas
  - Usually localized to the stomach wall (stage IE) or adjacent lymph nodes (stage IIE)
  - Have an excellent prognosis
- Nodal lymphomas with secondary gastric involvement
  - Usually diagnosed at an advanced stage
  - Seldom curable
- Complete lymphoma regression occurs in 75% of cases of stage IE low-grade lymphoma after successful *H pylori* eradication
- Patients with stage IE or IIE low-grade lymphomas who are not infected with *H pylori* or do not respond to eradication therapy can be treated successfully with
  - Surgical resection
  - Local radiation therapy
  - Combination therapy
- Stage IE or IIE high-grade lymphomas are treated with resection and CHOP chemotherapy (cyclophosphamide, hydroxydaunomycin, Oncovin, prednisone)
- Stage III or IV primary lymphomas
  - Treated with combination chemotherapy
  - Surgical resection is no longer recommended
- Long-term survival of primary gastric lymphoma for stage I is > 85% and for stage II 35–65%

Macular Degeneration, Age-Related

KEY FEATURES

- Age-related macular degeneration is the leading cause of permanent visual loss in the older population
- Exact cause is unknown but a precursor is the development of age-related maculopathy, characterized by retinal drusen
- Two subtypes: atrophic and exudative

CLINICAL FINDINGS

- Loss of central vision
- Atrophic subtype is characterized by progressive, bilateral visual loss of moderate severity resulting from atrophy and degeneration of the outer retina
- Exudative subtype is characterized by rapid and severe unilateral visual loss, with a high risk of subsequent involvement of the fellow eye
- Older patients in whom sudden central visual loss develops, particularly paracentral distortion or scotoma with preservation of central acuity, should be referred urgently to an ophthalmologist for assessment

DIAGNOSIS

- On ophthalmoscopic examination, various abnormalities are visualized in the macula
- Fundal photography after IV fluorescein (fluorescein angiography) is often required

TREATMENT

- Conventional laser retinal photocoagulation continues to be suitable for well-defined ("classic") choroidal neovascular membranes away from or adjacent to the fovea (extrafoveal or juxtafoveal), but these are a relatively small proportion
- Photodynamic laser therapy (PDT) is particularly indicated for well-defined lesions lying under the fovea (subfoveal)
- Antiangiogenic agents

Malaria

KEY FEATURES

ESSENTIALS OF DIAGNOSIS

- Residence or exposure in a malaria-endemic area
- Intermittent attacks of chills, fever, and sweating
- Headache, malaise, myalgia, nausea, vomiting, splenomegaly; anemia, thrombocytopenia
- Intraerythrocytic parasites identified in thick or thin blood smears
- Severe complications of falciparum malaria, including
  - Cerebral malaria
  - Severe anemia
  - Hypotension
  - Noncardiogenic pulmonary edema
  - Renal failure
  - Hypoglycemia
  - Acidosis
  - Hemolysis

GENERAL CONSIDERATIONS

- Four species of the genus *Plasmodium* are responsible for human malaria
  - *P vivax*
  - *P malariae*
  - *P ovale*
  - *P falciparum*
- Mode of transmission
  - Bite of infected female anopheline mosquitoes
  - Can be transmitted congenitally and by blood transfusion (uncommon)
- *P falciparum* is responsible for nearly all severe disease
- *P vivax* seldom causes severe disease
- *P ovale* and *P malariae* generally do not cause severe illness
- For all plasmodial species, parasites may recrudesce following initial clinical improvement after suboptimal therapy
- Disease and response to therapy are dramatically affected by immune status

DEMOGRAPHICS

- Causes hundreds of millions of cases and probably over 1 million deaths each year
- Disease is endemic in most of the tropics, including
  - Central and South America
  - Africa
  - The Middle East
  - The Indian subcontinent
  - Southeast Asia
  - Oceania
- Transmission, morbidity, and mortality are greatest in Africa
- Disease also common in travelers from nonendemic areas
- Groups at particular risk for severe malaria
  - Children
  - Pregnant women
  - HIV-infected persons
  - Nonimmune travelers

CLINICAL FINDINGS

SYMPTOMS AND SIGNS

Acute malaria

- Typically begins with a prodrome of headache and fatigue, followed by fever (usually irregular)
- Without therapy, however, fevers may become regular, especially with non-falciparum disease
  - 48-hour cycles (for *P vivax* and *P ovale*)
  - 72-hour cycles (for *P malariae*)
- Headache, malaise
- Myalgias, arthralgias
- Cough
- Chest pain, abdominal pain
- Anorexia, nausea, vomiting, and diarrhea
- Seizures may represent simple febrile convulsions or evidence of severe neurologic disease
- Physical findings may be absent or include signs of
  - Anemia
  - Jaundice
  - Splenomegaly
  - Mild hepatomegaly

Severe malaria

- Principally a result of *P falciparum* infection
- Can include dysfunction of any system, including
  - Neurologic abnormalities progressing to alterations in consciousness, repeated seizures, and coma (cerebral malaria)
  - Severe anemia
  - Hypotension and shock
  - Noncardiogenic pulmonary edema and the acute respiratory distress syndrome
  - Renal failure (due to acute tubular necrosis or, less commonly, severe homolysis)
  - Hypoglycemia
  - Acidosis
  - Hemolysis with jaundice
  - Hepatic dysfunction

– Retinal hemorrhages and other fundoscopic abnormalities

– Bleeding abnormalities, including disseminated intravascular coagulation

– Secondary bacterial infections, including pneumonia and *Salmonella* bacteremia

Chronic malaria

• Massive splenomegaly

• Immune complex glomerulopathy with nephrotic syndrome (with *P malariae* infection)

• Although both these disorders are uncommon, they result from immunologic responses to chronic infection

DIFFERENTIAL DIAGNOSIS

• Influenza
• Typhoid fever
• Viral hepatitis
• Dengue
• Visceral leishmaniasis (kala azar)
• Amebic liver abscess
• Babesiosis
• Leptospirosis
• Relapsing fever

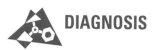 **DIAGNOSIS**

LABORATORY TESTS

• Giemsa-stained blood smears

– Mainstay of diagnosis, although other routine stains (eg, Wright stain) also demonstrate parasites

– Thick smears provide efficient evaluation of large volumes of blood, but thin smears are simpler and better for discrimination of parasite species

– Single smears are usually positive in infected individuals, although parasitemias may be very low in nonimmune individuals

– If illness is suspected, repeating smears in 8- to 24-hour intervals is appropriate

• Rapid diagnostic tests

– Can identify circulating plasmodial antigens with a simple "dipstick" format

– Not yet well standardized but are increasingly available around the world

– Offer sensitivity and specificity near that of high-quality blood smear analysis and are simpler to perform

• Serologic tests indicate history of disease but are not useful for diagnosis of acute infection

• Polymerase chain reaction (PCR) is highly sensitive but not available for routine diagnosis

• Liver function tests

• Complete blood count reveals thrombocytopenia, anemia, leukocytosis or leukopenia

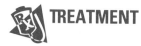 **TREATMENT**

MEDICATIONS

• Table 82 lists major antimalarial drugs

• See Table 80 for treatment recommendations established by the World Health Organization

• Table 83 outlines treatment options

• Table 84 has the CDC's guidelines for treatment of malaria in the United States

• Therapeutic decisions made based on infecting species and geography

• First-line drug for non-falciparum malaria is chloroquine

• Standard therapy for severe malaria

– IV quinine

– IV quinidine used in United States

– Patients taking these drugs should receive continuous cardiac monitoring

 OUTCOME

PROGNOSIS

• When treated appropriately, uncomplicated malaria responds well, with a mortality rate of about 0.1%

• With appropriate therapy and initial supportive care, rapid recoveries may be seen in even very ill persons

• Prognosis is poor if

– > 10–20% of erythrocytes are infected or > 200,000–500,000 parasites/mcL

– > 5% of neutrophils contain malarial pigment (a breakdown product of hemoglobin)

WHEN TO REFER

• All patients should be referred to a provider with expertise in this area

WHEN TO ADMIT

• Severe *P falciparum* malaria is a medical emergency that requires

– Hospitalization

– Intensive care with monitoring of electrolytes and acid-base balance

– Immediate treatment without waiting for all laboratory results to be available

PREVENTION

• Avoid mosquito bites (bed nets treated with permethrin insecticides, insect repellents)

• Chemoprophylaxis

– Recommended for all travelers from nonendemic regions to endemic areas, although risks vary greatly for different locations, and some tropical areas entail no risk

– See Table 81

– Specific recommendations for travel to different locales are available from the CDC

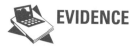 **EVIDENCE**

PRACTICE GUIDELINES

• World Health Organization: Guidelines for the treatment of Malaria. Geneva. 2006.

WEB SITES

• Centers for Disease Control and Prevention—Department of Health and Human Services

• Malaria Foundation International

INFORMATION FOR PATIENTS

• Centers for Disease Control and Prevention

• JAMA patient page. Malaria. JAMA. 2005;293:1542. [PMID: 15784878]

REFERENCES

• Baird JK. Effectiveness of antimalarial drugs. N Engl J Med. 2005 Apr 14; 352(15):1565–77. [PMID: 15829537]

• Franco-Paredes C et al. Problem pathogens: prevention of malaria in travellers. Lancet Infect Dis. 2006 Mar;6(3):139–49. [PMID: 16500595]

• Greenwood PM et al. Malaria. 2005 Apr 23–29;365(9469):1487–98. [PMID: 15850634]

• Prevention of malaria. Med Lett Drug Ther. 2005 Dec 5–19;47(1223–1224):100–2. [PMID: 16331244]

• Whitty CJ et al. Malaria: an update on treatment of adults in non-endemic countries. BMJ. 2006 Jul 29; 333(7561):241–5. [PMID: 16873859]

Mallory-Weiss Syndrome

 KEY FEATURES

ESSENTIALS OF DIAGNOSIS

- Nonpenetrating mucosal tear at the gastroesophageal junction
- Hematemesis; usually self-limited
- Prior history of vomiting, retching, straining, lifting in 50%
- Endoscopy establishes diagnosis

GENERAL CONSIDERATIONS

- Accounts for ~5% of upper gastrointestinal bleeding

DEMOGRAPHICS

- Hiatal hernia present in majority; with vomiting, increased risk of tear
- Heavy alcohol use with vomiting or retching in 50% of patients
- Other risk factors: age, hiccups

 CLINICAL FINDINGS

SYMPTOMS AND SIGNS

- History of vomiting, retching, straining, lifting in 50%
- Hematemesis with or without melena

DIFFERENTIAL DIAGNOSIS

Other causes of hematemesis
- Hemoptysis
- Erosive esophagitis
- Peptic ulcer disease
- Esophageal or gastric varices
- Erosive gastritis, eg, nonsteroidal anti-inflammatory drugs, alcohol, stress
- Portal hypertensive gastropathy
- Vascular ectasias (angiodysplasias)
- Gastric cancer

Rare causes
- Aortoenteric fistula
- Dieulafoy's lesion (aberrant gastric submucosal artery)
- Hemobilia (blood in biliary tree), eg, iatrogenic, malignancy
- Pancreatic cancer
- Hemosuccus pancreaticus (pancreatic pseudoaneurysm)

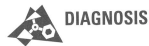 **DIAGNOSIS**

LABORATORY TESTS

- Complete blood cell count
- Platelet count
- Prothrombin time
- Partial thromboplastin time
- Serum creatinine
- Liver enzymes and serologies
- Type and cross-matching for 2–4 units or more of packed red blood cells
- Hematocrit is not a reliable indicator of the severity of acute bleeding

DIAGNOSTIC PROCEDURES

- Upper endoscopy
  – Diagnostic
  – Identifies a 0.5–4.0 cm linear mucosal tear usually located either at the gastroesophageal junction or, more commonly, just below the junction in the gastric mucosa of a hiatal hernia at the level of the diaphragm
- Assess volume (hemodynamic) status
  – Systolic blood pressure
  – Heart rate
  – Postural hypotension

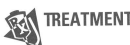 **TREATMENT**

MEDICATIONS

- Proton pump inhibitors to accelerate mucosal healing
  – Omeprazole or rabeprazole, 20 mg PO once daily
  – Esomeprazole or pantoprazole, 40 mg PO once daily

SURGERY

- Surgery with oversew of bleeding vessel rarely necessary

THERAPEUTIC PROCEDURES

- In patients without hemodynamic compromise or overt active bleeding, delay aggressive fluid repletion until extent of bleeding clarified
- For those with continuing active bleeding, insert two 18-gauge or larger IV lines
- Patients with hemodynamic compromise should be given 0.9% saline or lactated Ringer's injection and cross-matched blood
- Blood replacement to maintain a hematocrit of 25–28%
- In the absence of continued bleeding, the hematocrit should rise 3% for each unit of transfused packed red cells
- Transfuse blood in patients with brisk active bleeding regardless of the hematocrit
- Transfuse platelets if platelet count < 50,000/mcL or if impaired platelet function due to aspirin use
- Uremic patients with active bleeding should be given 1–2 doses of desmopressin (DDAVP), 0.3 mcg/kg IV at 12- to 24-h intervals
- Fresh frozen plasma should be given for actively bleeding patients with a coagulopathy and INR > 1.5
- In massive bleeding, give 1 unit of fresh frozen plasma for each 5 units of packed red blood cells transfused
- Endoscopic hemostatic therapy for those with continuing active bleeding
- Epinephrine 1:10,000 injection, cautery with a bipolar or heater probe coagulation device or application of metallic clip is effective in 90–95% of cases
- Angiographic arterial embolization or operative intervention is required in patients in whom endoscopic therapy fails

 OUTCOME

FOLLOW-UP

- None required

COMPLICATIONS

- Persistent bleeding

PROGNOSIS

- Most Mallory-Weiss bleeds stop spontaneously with rapid healing of mucosal tears
- Persistent or recurrent bleeding most likely in patients with concomitant portal hypertension or coagulopathy

WHEN TO ADMIT

- All patients with significant hematemesis
- Patients without active bleeding and without portal hypertension or coagulopathy may be discharged after 24 h
- Patients with active bleeding requiring hemostasis therapy should be observed in hospital at least 48 h

EVIDENCE

PRACTICE GUIDELINES

- Adler DG. ASGE Guideline: the role of endoscopy in acute non-variceal hemorrhage. Gastrointest Endosc. 2004; 60:497. [PMID: 14623622]
- Barkus A et al. A Canadian clinical practice algorithm for the management of patients with nonvariceal upper gastrointestinal bleeding. Can J Gastroenterol. 2004;18:605. [PMID: 15497000]

INFORMATION FOR PATIENTS

- MedlinePlus Medical Encyclopedia
- National Digestive Diseases Information Clearinghouse

REFERENCE

- Park CH et al. A prospective, randomized trial of endoscopic band ligation vs. epinephrine injection for actively bleeding Mallory-Weiss syndrome. Gastrointest Endosc. 2004 Jul;60(1):22–7. [PMID: 15229420]

Marfan Syndrome

KEY FEATURES

ESSENTIALS OF DIAGNOSIS

- Characterized by abnormalities of following systems
  - Musculoskeletal
  - Ocular
  - Pulmonary
  - Cardiovascular
- Disproportionately tall stature, thoracic deformity, and joint laxity or contractures
- Ectopia lentis and myopia
- Aortic dilation and dissection; mitral valve prolapse
- Autosomal dominant inheritance

GENERAL CONSIDERATIONS

- A systemic connective tissue disease
- Autosomal dominant pattern of inheritance
- Of most concern is disease of the ascending aorta, which is associated with a dilated aortic root
  - Histology of the aorta shows diffuse medial abnormalities

- – Aortic and mitral valve leaflets are also abnormal
- Mitral regurgitation may be present as well, often with elongated chordae tendineae, which on occasion may rupture

CLINICAL FINDINGS

SYMPTOMS AND SIGNS

- Wide variability in clinical presentation
- Affected patients typically are tall, with particularly long arms, legs, and digits (arachnodactyly)
- Commonly, joint dislocations and pectus excavatum
- Ectopia lentis, severe myopia, and retinal detachment
- Mitral valve regurgitation occur often from elongated chordae tendineae, which on occasion may rupture
- Mitral valve prolapse in about 85%
- Ascending aortic involvement produces a dilated aortic root, aortic regurgitation, and aortic dissection
- Spontaneous pneumothorax
- Dural ectasia
- Striae atrophicae

DIFFERENTIAL DIAGNOSIS

- Tall stature (normal)
- Homocystinuria (with lens dislocation) as a result of cystathionine synthase deficiency
- Aortic root disease resulting from other cause, eg, ankylosing spondylitis, syphilis, temporal (giant cell) arteritis, Takayasu's arteritis, familial aortic aneurysm, bicuspid aortic valve
- Ehlers-Danlos syndrome
- Loeys-Dietz syndrome
- MASS phenotype
- Idiopathic mitral valve prolapse

DIAGNOSIS

LABORATORY TESTS

- No simple laboratory test
- DNA analysis can detect mutations in the fibrillin gene (FBN1) on chromosome 15
- Clinical diagnosis based on family history, detailed ophthalmologic examination (including slit lamp), echocardiography, and physical examination

TREATMENT

MEDICATIONS

- Standard endocarditis prophylaxis
- Chronic β-adrenergic blockade (eg, atenolol, 1–2 mg/kg) retards the rate of aortic dilation
- Clinical trial of losartan will determine if this drug, which is effective in the mouse model of Marfan syndrome, treats or prevents specific features in humans

SURGERY

- Prophylactic replacement of the aortic root (and, if necessary, aortic valve) when the diameter reaches 45–50 mm (normal: < 40 mm) prolongs life
- Annual orthopedic consultation if moderately severe scoliosis present

THERAPEUTIC PROCEDURES

- Regular ophthalmologic surveillance to correct visual acuity and thus prevent amblyopia
- Restriction of vigorous physical exertion

OUTCOME

FOLLOW-UP

- Echocardiography at least annually to monitor aortic diameter and aortic and mitral valve function

PROGNOSIS

- Untreated, Marfan's syndrome patients commonly die in the fourth or fifth decade from aortic dissection or congestive heart failure secondary to aortic regurgitation

PREVENTION

- Prenatal and presymptomatic diagnosis for patients in whom a molecular defect in fibrillin has been found and for families in whom linkage analysis using polymorphic markers around the fibrillin gene can be performed

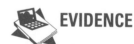

EVIDENCE

PRACTICE GUIDELINES

- European Society of Cardiology: Management of grown up congenital heart disease, 2003

WEB SITES

- National Center for Biotechnology Information: Online Mendelian Inheritance in Man
- National Marfan Foundation

INFORMATION FOR PATIENTS

- Dolan DNA Learning Center: Marfan Syndrome
- Mayo Clinic: Marfan Syndrome
- National Institute of Arthritis and Musculoskeletal and Skin Diseases: Questions and Answers About Marfan Syndrome
- National Library of Medicine: Marfan Syndrome

REFERENCES

- Judge DP et al. Marfan's syndrome. Lancet. 2005 Dec 3;366(9501):1965–76. [PMID: 16325700]
- Miller DC. Valve-sparing aortic root replacement in patients with Marfan syndrome. J Thorac Cardiovasc Surg. 2003 Apr;125(4):773–8. [PMID: 12698136]
- Pyeritz RE. Marfan syndrome and related disorders. In: *Emery and Rimoin's Principles and Practice of Medical Genetics*, 5th ed. Rimoin DL et al (editors). Churchill Livingstone, 2007.

Measles

KEY FEATURES

- Transmitted by inhalation of infected respiratory droplets
- Estimated 1 million deaths annually worldwide, mainly from gastroenteritis
- Declining US incidence because of widespread vaccine use

CLINICAL FINDINGS

- Initial prodrome of malaise and fever; rash 3–4 days later
- Fever persists through the early rash
- Koplik's spots, tiny "table crystals" on mucous membranes, are pathognomonic and appear 2 days before rash
- Rash begins as pin-sized papules on face and behind ears, spreading to trunk and then extremities
- Pulmonary involvement occurs in up to 5% of cases and is most common cause of death
- Encephalitis in up to 0.1% of cases
- Subacute sclerosing panencephalitis (SSPE) is a rare, late CNS complication, largely among rural boys

DIAGNOSIS

- Often difficult to differentiate clinical symptoms from other viral illnesses
- Koplik's spots clinch the diagnosis
- History of exposure to patients with measles helpful but not always present
- Leukopenia usually present
- Lymphocyte count < 2000/mcL associated with poor prognosis
- Detection of IgM measles antibodies with ELISA or fourfold rise in measles antibody titer is diagnostic

TREATMENT

- Supportive measures
- High-dose vitamin A recommended in children
- Antibiotics for bacterial pneumonia superinfection
- Prevention: measles vaccination of children and young adults (Tables 67 and 68)
- Postexposure prophylaxis: Live virus vaccine may be effective in prevention up to 5 days postexposure in susceptible individuals
- Pregnant women and immunocompromised individuals should avoid vaccination, although HIV-infected adults can be safely vaccinated

Melanoma, Malignant

KEY FEATURES

ESSENTIALS OF DIAGNOSIS

- ABCD mnemonic = Asymmetry, Border irregularity, Color variegation, and Diameter > 6 mm
- Should be suspected in any pigmented skin lesion with recent change in appearance
- Examination with good light may show varying colors, including red, white, black, and bluish

GENERAL CONSIDERATIONS

- Leading cause of death due to skin disease
- Favors fair-skinned whites with a history of significant (blistering) sun exposure before the age of 18
- 10% of melanomas occur in "melanoma prone kindreds," ie, familial

Classification

- **Superficial spreading malignant melanoma** (the most common type, occurring in two-thirds of individuals developing melanoma, largely a disease of whites)
- **Lentigo maligna melanoma** (arising on sun-exposed skin of older individuals)
- **Nodular malignant melanoma**
- **Acral lentiginous melanomas** (arising on palms, soles, and nail beds)
  – Occur in nonwhites primarily
  – May be difficult to diagnosis because benign pigmented lesions in these areas occur commonly in more darkly pigmented persons; clinicians may hesitate to biopsy the palms and especially the soles and nail beds
  – As a result, the diagnosis is often delayed until the tumor is clinically obvious and histologically thick
  – Clinicians should give special attention to new or changing lesions in these areas
- Malignant melanomas on mucous membranes
- **Miscellaneous forms** such as amelanotic (nonpigmented) melanoma and melanomas arising from blue nevi (rare) and congenital nevi

DEMOGRAPHICS

- One in four cases of melanoma occur before the age of 40
- In 2004, there were 55,000 cases of melanoma in the United States, with 7900 deaths
- Lifetime risk for white Americans is 1/65
- At least 10% of cases of melanoma are related to inherited genetic predisposition

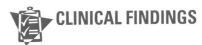

CLINICAL FINDINGS

SYMPTOMS AND SIGNS

- An irregular notched border where the pigment appears to be leaking into the normal surrounding skin

- Topography may be irregular, ie, partly raised and partly flat
- Color variegation, and colors such as pink, blue, gray, white, and black are indications for referral
- Bleeding and ulceration
- A mole that stands out from the patient's other moles (the "ugly duckling sign")
- A patient with a large number of moles is at increased risk for melanoma
- The history of a changing mole (evolution) is the single most important historical reason for close evaluation and possible referral
- Acral lentiginous melanomas: dark, sometimes irregularly shaped lesions on the palms and soles and new, often broad and solitary, darkly pigmented longitudinal streaks in the nails

DIFFERENTIAL DIAGNOSIS

- Acquired nevus (mole), eg, junctional nevus, compound nevus
- Seborrheic keratosis
- Lentigo, eg, solar lentigo
- Dermatofibroma
- Basal cell carcinoma (pigmented type)
- Congenital nevus
- Atypical (dysplastic) nevus
- Blue nevus
- Halo nevus
- Pyogenic granuloma
- Kaposi's sarcoma
- Pregnancy-associated darkening of nevi

 DIAGNOSIS

LABORATORY TESTS

- Skin biopsies

 TREATMENT

MEDICATIONS

- Alpha interferon and vaccine therapy may reduce recurrences in patients with high-risk melanomas

SURGERY

- Treatment consists of excision once a histologic diagnosis is made
- The area is usually excised with margins dictated by the thickness of the tumor
  – Large margins (radius ≥ 5 cm) are no longer indicated

– Thin low-risk and intermediate-risk tumors require only conservative margins of 1–3 cm
– More specifically, surgical margins of 0.5 cm for melanoma in situ and 1 cm for lesions < 1 mm in thickness are most often recommended
- Sentinel lymph node biopsy (selective lymphadenectomy) using preoperative lymphoscintigraphy and intraoperative lymphatic mapping
  – Effective for staging melanoma patients with intermediate risk without clinical adenopathy
  – Recommended for all patients with lesions over 1 mm in thickness or with high-risk histologic features

 OUTCOME

PROGNOSIS

- Tumor thickness is the single most important prognostic factor
- 10-year survival rates—related to thickness in millimeters—are as follows
  – < 1 mm, 95%
  – 1–2 mm, 80%
  – 2–4 mm, 55%
  – > 4 mm, 30%
- With lymph node involvement, the 5-year survival rate is 30%
- With distant metastases, it is < 10%
- More accurate prognoses can be made on the basis of thickness, site, histologic features, and sex of the patient
- Overall survival for melanomas in whites has risen from 60% in 1960–1963 to more than 85% currently, primarily due to earlier detection of lesions

WHEN TO REFER

- Any pigmented lesion with suspicious features should be referred to a dermatologist for possible biopsy

 EVIDENCE

PRACTICE GUIDELINES

- Houghton AN et al; NCCN Melanoma Practice Guidelines Panel. National Comprehensive Cancer Network: Melanoma v.1.2004

WEB SITES

- American Academy of Dermatology
- National Cancer Institute: Melanoma Information for Patients and Health Professionals

INFORMATION FOR PATIENTS

- American Academy of Family Physicians: Melanoma: A Kind of Skin Cancer
- American Cancer Society: Melanoma
- MedlinePlus: Melanoma Interactive Tutorial
- Skin Cancer Foundation: Melanoma

REFERENCES

- Miller AJ et al. Melanoma. N Engl J Med. 2006 Jul 6;355(1):51–65. [PMID: 16822996]
- Morton DL et al; MSLT Group. Sentinel-node biopsy or nodal observation in melanoma. N Engl J Med. 2006 Sep 28; 355(13):1307–17. [PMID: 17005948]
- Thompson JF et al. Case records of the Massachusetts General Hospital. Case 2-200 pigmented lesion on the arm. N Engl J Med. 2007 Jan 18:356(3):285–92. [PMID: 17229956]

Meningitis, Meningococcal

 KEY FEATURES

ESSENTIALS OF DIAGNOSIS

- Fever, headache, vomiting, confusion, delirium, convulsions
- Petechial rash of skin and mucous membranes
- Neck and back stiffness
- Purulent spinal fluid with gram-negative intracellular and extracellular diplococci
- Culture of cerebrospinal fluid, blood, or petechial aspiration confirms the diagnosis

GENERAL CONSIDERATIONS

- Caused by *Neisseria meningitidis* of groups A, B, C, Y, W-135, and others
- Infection is transmitted by droplets
- The clinical illness may take the form of meningococcemia (a fulminant form of septicemia) without meningitis, meningococcemia with meningitis, or predominantly meningitis
- Chronic recurrent meningococcemia with fever, rash, and arthritis can occur, particularly in those with terminal complement deficiencies

DEMOGRAPHICS

- College freshmen—particularly those living in dormitories—have been shown to have a modestly increased risk of invasive meningococcal disease

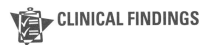 **CLINICAL FINDINGS**

SYMPTOMS AND SIGNS

- High fever, chills, and headache; back, abdominal, and extremity pains; and nausea and vomiting are typical
- In severe cases, rapidly developing confusion, delirium, seizures, and coma occur
- Nuchal and back rigidity are typical
- A petechial rash often first appearing in the lower extremities and at pressure points is found in most cases
- Petechiae may vary from pinhead sized to large ecchymoses or even areas of skin gangrene that may later slough if the patient survives

DIFFERENTIAL DIAGNOSIS

- Meningitis due to other causes, eg, pneumococcus, *Listeria*, aseptic
- Subarachnoid hemorrhage
- Encephalitis
- Petechial rash due to
  – Gonococcemia
  – Infective endocarditis
  – Thrombotic thrombocytopenic purpura
  – Rocky Mountain spotted fever
  – Viral exanthem
  – Rickettsial or echovirus infection
  – Other bacterial infections (eg, staphylococcal infections, scarlet fever)
- "Neighborhood reaction" causing abnormal cerebrospinal fluid, such as
  – Brain abscess
  – Epidural abscess
  – Vertebral osteomyelitis
  – Mastoiditis
  – Sinusitis
  – Brain tumor
- Dural sinus thrombosis
- Noninfectious meningeal irritation
  – Carcinomatous meningitis
  – Sarcoidosis
  – Systemic lupus erythematosus
  – Drugs (eg, nonsteroidal anti-inflammatory drugs, trimethoprim-sulfamethoxazole)
  – Pneumonia
  – Shigellosis

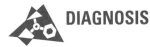 **DIAGNOSIS**

LABORATORY TESTS

- The organism is usually found by smear or culture of the cerebrospinal fluid, oropharynx, blood, or aspirated petechiae
- Prothrombin time and partial thromboplastin time are prolonged, fibrin dimers are elevated, fibrinogen is low, and the platelet count is depressed if disseminated intravascular coagulation is present

Cerebrospinal fluid analysis
- See Table 65
- Typically, a cloudy or purulent fluid, with elevated pressure, increased protein, and decreased glucose content
- Usually contains more than 1000 cells/mcL, with polymorphonuclear cells predominating and containing gram-negative intracellular diplococci
- The absence of organisms in a Gram stained smear does not rule out the diagnosis
- The capsular polysaccharide can often be demonstrated in cerebrospinal fluid or urine by latex agglutination; this is especially useful in partially treated patients, though sensitivity is only 60–80%

IMAGING STUDIES

- For neurologic defects or signs of elevated intracranial pressure, MRI or CT imaging can exclude mass lesions

DIAGNOSTIC PROCEDURES

- Lumbar puncture

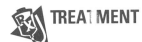 **TREATMENT**

MEDICATIONS

- See Tables 63 and 64
- Intravenous antimicrobial therapy should be started immediately after blood cultures are obtained in all acutely ill patients and before proceeding with imaging studies, if these are indicated
- Aqueous penicillin G is the antibiotic of choice (24 million units/24 h) in divided doses q4h
- In penicillin-allergic patients or those in whom pneumococcal or gram-negative meningitis is a consideration, ceftriaxone, 2 g IV BID, should be used
- Chloramphenicol, 1 g q6h, is an alternative in the severely penicillin- or cephalosporin-allergic patient
- In critically ill patients with evidence of increased intracranial pressure, administration of dexamethasone (0.6 mg/kg/day in four divided doses) may help
- Duration of therapy: 7 days

THERAPEUTIC PROCEDURES

- Lumbar puncture
  – Should be performed in all patients with suspected meningococcal meningitis
  – Obtain imaging studies before lumbar puncture to rule out mass lesions if papilledema, other evidence of increased intracranial pressure, or focal neurologic deficits are present

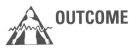 **OUTCOME**

COMPLICATIONS

- Obtundation or deterioration in mental status may result from cerebral edema and increased intracranial pressure
- Disseminated intravascular coagulation
- Ischemic necrosis of digits, distal extremities

PROGNOSIS

- Mortality < 5% with early therapy of patients with meningitis
- Meningococcemia associated with a 20% mortality

WHEN TO ADMIT

- All patients in whom meningococcal meningitis is suspected should be admitted for observation and empiric therapy

PREVENTION

- Effective polysaccharide vaccines for groups A, C, Y, and W-135 are available (Tables 67 and 68)
- The Advisory Committee on Immunization Practices recommends immunization with a single dose of polyvalent vaccine (active against meningococcal groups A, C, Y, and W-135) for adolescents at age 11–12 or upon entry into high school and for college freshmen
- Outbreaks in closed populations are best controlled by eliminating nasopharyngeal carriage of meningococci
  – Rifampin is the drug of choice, in a dosage of 600 mg PO BID for 2 days
  – A single 500-mg oral dose of ciprofloxacin or one intramuscular 250-mg dose of ceftriaxone in adults is also effective

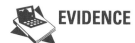
EVIDENCE

WEB SITES

- CDC—Division of Bacterial and Mycotic Diseases
- Meningococcemia Case Study

INFORMATION FOR PATIENTS

- CDC—Division of Bacterial and Mycotic Diseases
- JAMA Patient Page: meningitis. JAMA 1999;281:1560. [PMID: 10227329]
- Torpy JM: JAMA patient page: Lumbar puncture. JAMA 2002;288:2056. [PMID: 12387666]

REFERENCES

- Bilukha OO et al; National Center for Infectious Diseases, Centers for Disease Control and Prevention (CDC). Prevention and control of meningococcal disease. Recommendations of the Advisory Committee on Immunization Practices (ACIP). MMWR Recomm Rep. 2005 May 27;54(RR-7):1–21. [PMID: 15917737]
- Van de Beek D et al. Current concepts: community-acquired bacterial meningitis in adults. N Engl J Med. 2006 Jan 5; 354(1):44–53. [PMID: 16394301]

Meningitis, Pneumococcal

KEY FEATURES

ESSENTIALS OF DIAGNOSIS

- Fever, headache, altered mental status
- Meningismus
- Gram-positive diplococci on Gram stain of cerebrospinal fluid; counterimmunoelectrophoresis may be positive in partially treated cases

GENERAL CONSIDERATIONS

- *Streptococcus pneumoniae* is the most common cause of meningitis in adults and the second most common cause of meningitis in children over the age of 6 years
- Head trauma, with cerebrospinal fluid leaks, sinusitis, and pneumonia may precede it

- Penicillin-resistant strains may cause meningitis

DEMOGRAPHICS

- Until 2000, *S pneumoniae* infections caused 100,000–135,000 hospitalizations for pneumonia, 6 million cases of otitis media, and 60,000 cases of invasive disease, including 3300 cases of meningitis
- Disease figures are now changing due to conjugate vaccine introduction

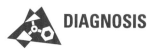
CLINICAL FINDINGS

SYMPTOMS AND SIGNS

- Rapid onset, with fever, headache, and altered mentation
- Pneumonia may be present
- Compared with meningitis caused by the meningococcus
  - Pneumococcal meningitis lacks a rash
  - Focal neurologic deficits, cranial nerve palsies, and obtundation are more prominent features

DIFFERENTIAL DIAGNOSIS

- Meningitis due to other causes, eg, meningococcus, *Listeria*, aseptic
- Subarachnoid hemorrhage
- Encephalitis
- "Neighborhood reaction" causing abnormal cerebrospinal fluid, such as
  - Brain abscess
  - Epidural abscess
  - Vertebral osteomyelitis
  - Mastoiditis
  - Sinusitis
  - Brain tumor
- Dural sinus thrombosis
- Noninfectious meningeal irritation
  - Carcinomatous meningitis
  - Sarcoidosis
  - Systemic lupus erythematosus
  - Drugs (eg, nonsteroidal anti-inflammatory drugs, trimethoprim-sulfamethoxazole)
  - Pneumonia
  - Shigellosis

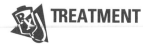
DIAGNOSIS

LABORATORY TESTS

- See Table 65
- Cerebrospinal fluid
  - Typically has more than 1000 white blood cells per microliter, over 60%

of which are polymorphonuclear leukocytes
  - Glucose concentration is less than 40 mg/dL, or less than 50% of the simultaneous serum concentration
  - Protein usually exceeds 150 mg/dL
  - Gram stain shows gram-positive cocci in up to 80–90% of cases
- In untreated cases, blood or cerebrospinal fluid cultures are almost always positive
- Fifty percent rate of bacteremia
- Antigen detection tests may occasionally be helpful in establishing the diagnosis in the patient who has been partially treated and in whom cultures and stains are negative

TREATMENT

MEDICATIONS

- See Tables 63 and 64
- Give antibiotics as soon as the diagnosis is suspected
- If lumbar puncture must be delayed (eg, while awaiting results of an imaging study to exclude a mass lesion), ceftriaxone, 4 g IV, should be given after blood cultures (positive in 50% of cases) have been obtained
- If gram-positive diplococci are present on the Gram stain, then vancomycin, 30 mg/kg/day IV in two divided doses, should be administered in addition to ceftriaxone until the isolate is confirmed not to be penicillin-resistant
- Once susceptibility to penicillin has been confirmed, penicillin, 24 million units IV daily in six divided doses, or ceftriaxone, 4 g/day as a single dose or as two divided doses, is recommended
- For severe penicillin allergy, chloramphenicol, 50 mg/kg q6h, is an alternative (failures have occurred with penicillin-resistant strains)
- Duration of therapy is 10–14 days in documented cases
- The best therapy for penicillin-resistant strains is not known. Susceptibility testing is essential
- If the minimum inhibitory concentration (MIC) of ceftriaxone or cefotaxime is ≤ 0.5 mcg/mL, single-drug therapy with either of these cephalosporins is likely to be effective
- When the MIC is ≥ 1 mcg/mL, treatment with a combination of ceftriaxone, 2 g q12h, plus vancomycin, 30 mg/kg/day in two divided doses, is recommended

- Give 10 mg of dexamethasone IV immediately prior to or concomitantly with the first dose of appropriate antibiotic and every 6 h thereafter for a total of 4 days

OUTCOME

FOLLOW-UP

- If a patient with a penicillin-resistant organism has not responded to a third-generation cephalosporin, repeat lumbar puncture is indicated to assess the bacteriologic response

COMPLICATIONS

- Hearing loss
- Residual neurologic deficit

PROGNOSIS

- Patients presenting with depressed levels of consciousness have a worse outcome
- Dexamethasone administered with antibiotic to adults with meningitis has been associated with a 60% reduction in mortality and a 50% reduction in unfavorable outcome, primarily in patients with pneumococcal meningitis

WHEN TO REFER

- Consider early referral to an infectious disease specialist

WHEN TO ADMIT

- All patients with suspected bacterial meningitis

PREVENTION

- Pneumococcal vaccine recommendations (Tables 67 and 68)

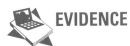

EVIDENCE

WEB SITES

- CDC—Division of Bacterial and Mycotic Diseases
- Karolinska Institute—Directory of Bacterial Infections and Mycoses

INFORMATION FOR PATIENTS

- CDC—Division of Bacterial and Mycotic Diseases
- JAMA Patient Page. meningitis. JAMA. 1999;281:1560. [PMID: 10227329]
- National Institutes of Health

- Torpy JM. JAMA patient page: Lumbar puncture. JAMA. 2002;288:2056. [PMID: 12387666]

REFERENCE

- Weisfelt M et al. Dexamethasone treatment in adults with pneumococcal meningitis: risk factors for death. Eur J Clin Microbiol Infect Dis. 2006 Feb; 25(2):73–8. [PMID: 16470361]

Menopausal Syndrome

KEY FEATURES

ESSENTIALS OF DIAGNOSIS

- Cessation of menses due to aging or to bilateral oophorectomy
- Elevation of follicle-stimulating hormone (FSH) and luteinizing hormone (LH) levels
- Hot flushes and night sweats (in 80% of women)
- Decreased vaginal lubrication; thinned vaginal mucosa with or without dyspareunia

GENERAL CONSIDERATIONS

- Menopause denotes a 1- to 3-year period during which a woman adjusts to a diminishing and then absent menstrual flow and the physiologic changes that may be associated—hot flushes, night sweats, and vaginal dryness
- Premature menopause is defined as ovarian failure and menstrual cessation before age 40; this often has a genetic or autoimmune basis
- Surgical menopause due to bilateral oophorectomy is common and can cause more severe symptoms owing to the sudden rapid drop in sex hormone levels
- Cessation of ovarian function is not associated with severe emotional disturbance or personality changes. The time of menopause often coincides with other major life changes, such as departure of children from the home, a midlife identity crisis, or divorce

DEMOGRAPHICS

- The average age at menopause in Western societies today is 51 years

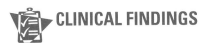

CLINICAL FINDINGS

SYMPTOMS AND SIGNS

- Menstrual cycles generally become irregular as menopause approaches
- Anovular cycles occur more often, with irregular cycle length and occasional menorrhagia
- Menstrual flow amount diminishes
- Finally, cycles become longer, with missed periods or episodes of spotting only
- When no bleeding has occurred for 1 year, the menopausal transition has occurred
- Hot flushes
  - Feelings of intense heat over the trunk and face, with flushing of the skin and sweating
  - Can begin before the cessation of menses and are more severe after surgical menopause
  - More pronounced late in the day, during hot weather, after ingestion of hot foods or drinks, or during periods of tension
  - When they occur at night, they often cause sweating and insomnia and result in fatigue on the following day
- Vaginal atrophy and decreased vaginal lubrication
- The introitus decreases in diameter
- Pelvic examination reveals pale, smooth vaginal mucosa and a small cervix and uterus
- The ovaries are not normally palpable after the menopause

DIFFERENTIAL DIAGNOSIS

- Pregnancy
- Premature ovarian failure
- Hypothyroidism or hyperthyroidism
- Hyperprolactinemia
- Polycystic ovary syndrome
- Hypothalamic amenorrhea, eg, stress, weight change, exercise
- Other endocrine causes
  - Cushing's syndrome
  - Addison's disease
  - Androgen-secreting tumor (adrenal, ovarian)
  - Congenital adrenal hyperplasia
  - Acromegaly
- Depression

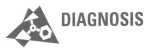

DIAGNOSIS

LABORATORY TESTS

- Serum FSH and LH levels are elevated

- Vaginal cytologic examination will show a low estrogen effect with predominantly parabasal cells

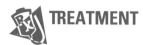 **TREATMENT**

MEDICATIONS

Natural menopause

- Oral conjugated estrogens, 0.3 mg or 0.625 mg; estradiol, 0.5 or 1 mg; or estrone sulfate, 0.625 mg; or estradiol can be given transdermally as skin patches that are changed once or twice weekly and secrete 0.05–0.1 mg of hormone daily
- When either form of estrogen is used, add a progestin (medroxyprogesterone acetate) to prevent endometrial hyperplasia or cancer; a patch containing estradiol and levonorgestrel is also available
  - Give estrogen on days 1–25 of each calendar month, with 5–10 mg of medroxyprogesterone acetate added on days 14–25. Withhold hormones from day 26 until the end of the month, which will produce a light, generally painless monthly period
  - Alternatively, give the estrogen along with 2.5 mg of medroxyprogesterone acetate daily, without stopping. This causes initial bleeding or spotting, but within a few months it produces an atrophic endometrium that will not bleed
- If the patient has had a hysterectomy, a progestin need not be used
- Explain that hot flushes will probably return if the hormone is discontinued
- Data from the Women's Health Initiative (WHI) study
  - Women should not use combination progestin-estrogen therapy for more than 3 or 4 years
  - The increased risk of cardiovascular disease, cerebrovascular disease, and breast cancer with this regimen outweighed the benefits
  - Women who cannot find relief with alternative approaches may wish to consider continuing use of combination therapy after a thorough discussion of the risks and benefits
  - Alternatives to hormone therapy for vasomotor symptoms include
    □ Selective serotonin reuptake inhibitors such as paroxetine 12.5 mg or 25 mg/day, or venlafaxine 75 mg/day
    □ Gabapentin, an antiseizure medication, is also effective at 900 mg/day
    □ Clonidine given orally or transdermally, 100–150 mcg daily, also may reduce the frequency of hot flushes,

but its use is limited by side effects, including dry mouth, drowsiness, and hypotension

- Estradiol vaginal ring, left in place for 3 months, is suitable for long-term use. Progestin therapy to protect the endometrium is unnecessary
- Short-term use of estrogen vaginal cream will relieve symptoms of atrophy, but because of variable absorption, therapy with either systemic hormone replacement or the vaginal ring is preferable
- Testosterone propionate, 1–2%, 0.5–1.0 g, in a vanishing cream base used in the same manner is also effective if estrogen is contraindicated
- A bland lubricant such as unscented cold cream or water-soluble gel can be helpful at the time of coitus
- Women should ingest at least 800 mg of calcium daily and 1 g of elemental calcium should be taken as a daily supplement at the time of the menopause and thereafter
  - Calcium supplements should be taken with meals to increase their absorption
  - Vitamin D, 400–800 international units/day from food, sunlight, or supplements, enhances calcium absorption and maintains bone mass
- Daily energetic walking and exercise help maintain bone mass
- The use of long-term hormone replacement therapy for prevention is no longer indicated. Clinicians should review with women and carefully consider the risks and benefits
- Current indications for hormone therapy (estrogen and progestin) are for treatment of vasomotor symptoms, which resolve within several months to a few years
- Postmenopausal women with decreased sexual desire may be treated successfully with testosterone along with estrogen or estrogen/progestin therapy
  - The transdermal route of testosterone delivery, rather than the IM or PO route, should be used to avoid first-pass effect
  - A compounded preparation of 1% testosterone gel, cream, or ointment, 0.5 g/day, will deliver the desired dose of 5 mg daily
  - Testosterone preparation formulated for men should not be used because the doses are far higher than are necessary for women

Surgical menopause

- Estrogen replacement is generally started immediately after surgery

- Conjugated estrogens 1.25 mg, estrone sulfate 1.25 mg, or estradiol, 2 mg is given for 25 days of each month
- After age 45–50 years, this dose can be tapered to 0.625 mg of conjugated estrogens or equivalent

 OUTCOME

FOLLOW-UP

- Annual visit to monitor symptoms and need for therapy
- Any bleeding after cessation of menses warrants investigation by endometrial curettage or aspiration to rule out endometrial cancer
- For women who are receiving hormone replacement therapy for vasomotor symptoms, an attempt should be made at least every 6 months to taper the dose and to discontinue therapy

COMPLICATIONS

- Dyspareunia from vaginal atrophy and decreased vaginal lubrication
- Overall health risks exceed benefits from use of both combined estrogen plus progestin and estrogen alone for an average of 5 years
  - For combination therapy, these risks include
    □ Coronary heart disease events
    □ Cerebral vascular accidents
    □ Pulmonary emboli
    □ Invasive breast cancer
    □ Gallbladder disease
    □ Mild cognitive impairment and dementia
  - For estrogen alone, the risks include
    □ Increased risk of stroke
    □ No evidence of protection from coronary heart disease
    □ Increase in the combined risk of mild cognitive impairment and dementia compared with placebo

PREVENTION

- Continued sexual activity will help prevent vaginal shrinkage

 EVIDENCE

PRACTICE GUIDELINES

- Institute for Clinical Systems Improvement. Menopause and Hormone Therapy: Collaborative Decision Making and Management, 2004.

WEB SITE

- North American Menopause Society

INFORMATION FOR PATIENTS

- American Academy of Family Physicians: Menopause
- MedlinePlus: Menopause Interactive Tutorial
- National Women's Health Information Center: Menopause

REFERENCES

- Blake J. Menopause: evidence-based practice. Best Pract Res Clin Obstet Gynaecol. 2006 Dec;20(6):799–839. [PMID: 17084674]
- Ettinger B et al. When is it appropriate to prescribe postmenopausal hormone therapy? Menopause. 2006 May–Jun; 13(3):404–10. [PMID: 16735937]
- National Institutes of Health: National Institutes of Health State-of-the-Science Conference statement: management of menopause-related symptoms. Ann Intern Med. 2005 Jun 21;142(12 Pt 1):1003–13. [PMID: 15968015]
- North American Menopause Society. The role of testosterone therapy in postmenopausal women: position statement of the North American Menopause Society. Menopause. 2005 Sep–Oct; 12(5):496–511. [PMID: 16145303]

Mesothelioma

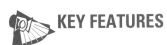

KEY FEATURES

ESSENTIALS OF DIAGNOSIS

- Chronic progressive chest pain and dyspnea
- Pleural effusion and/or pleural thickening on chest radiographs
- Malignant cells in pleural fluid or tissue
- History of asbestos exposure is common

GENERAL CONSIDERATIONS

- Primary tumors arising from the mesothelial surfaces of the pleura (80% of cases), peritoneum, pericardium, or tunica vaginalis
- 75% of pleural mesotheliomas are diffuse (usually malignant)
- Mean age at symptom onset is 60 years with usual time between exposure to asbestos and onset of symptoms 20–40 years

DEMOGRAPHICS

- Men outnumber women 3:1
- Malignant pleural mesothelioma is associated with asbestos exposure (70% of cases), with a lifetime risk to asbestos workers of 8%
- Cigarette smoking significantly increases the risk of bronchogenic carcinoma in asbestos workers and aggravates asbestosis, but there is no association between smoking and mesothelioma independent of asbestos
- Asbestos exposure occurs through
  - Mining
  - Milling
  - Manufacturing
  - Shipyard work
  - Insulation
  - Brake linings
  - Building construction and demolition
  - Roofing materials
  - Other asbestos-containing products

 ## CLINICAL FINDINGS

SYMPTOMS AND SIGNS

- Insidious onset of shortness of breath, nonpleuritic chest pain, and weight loss
- Physical findings include
  - Dullness to percussion
  - Diminished breath sounds
  - Finger clubbing in some cases
- Malignant pleural mesothelioma progresses rapidly as the tumor spreads along the pleural surface to involve the pericardium, mediastinum, and contralateral pleura
- Tumor may eventually extend beyond the thorax to involve abdominal lymph nodes and organs

DIFFERENTIAL DIAGNOSIS

- Chronic organized empyema
- Sarcoma
- Metastatic tumor to the pleura, especially adenocarcinoma
- Malignant fibrosing histiocytoma
- Other causes of pleural effusion (see Pleural Effusion)

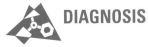 ## DIAGNOSIS

LABORATORY TESTS

- Pleural fluid analysis often reveals a hemorrhagic exudate

IMAGING STUDIES

- Radiographic findings
  - Nodular, irregular, unilateral pleural thickening
  - Varying degrees of unilateral pleural effusion
- CT helps determine the extent of pleural and extrapleural involvement

DIAGNOSTIC PROCEDURES

- Thoracentesis
- Closed pleural biopsy
- Open pleural biopsy may be necessary to obtain an adequate specimen for histologic diagnosis

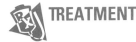 ## TREATMENT

SURGERY

- Some surgeons believe that extrapleural pneumonectomy is the preferred approach for patients with early-stage disease
- Resection may offer palliative benefit in some cases

THERAPEUTIC PROCEDURES

- Treatment with surgery, radiation, chemotherapy, or a combination of methods is generally unsuccessful
- Drainage of effusions, pleurodesis, and radiation therapy may offer palliative benefit

 ## OUTCOME

COMPLICATIONS

- Local invasion of thoracic structures with superior vena cava syndrome, hoarseness, Horner's syndrome, dysphagia
- Paraneoplastic syndrome
  - Thrombocytosis
  - Hemolytic anemia
  - Disseminated intravascular coagulopathy
  - Migratory thrombophlebitis
- Metastatic disease

PROGNOSIS

- Median survival from symptom onset ranges from 5 months in extensive disease to 16 months in localized disease
- 75% of patients are dead at 1 year following diagnosis
- Most patients die of respiratory failure and complications of local extension

WHEN TO REFER

- Upon diagnosis, refer to a pulmonologist, oncologist, or possibly a thoracic surgeon who can evaluate the patient for multidisciplinary treatment

WHEN TO ADMIT

- For pleural fluid drainage
- For severe dyspnea
- For pain management

PREVENTION

- Avoidance of tobacco smoke (primary or secondary) in those with a history of asbestos exposure

EVIDENCE

PRACTICE GUIDELINES

- Detterbeck FC et al. Lung cancer. Invasive staging: the guidelines. Chest. 2003;123(1 Suppl):167S. [PMID: 12527576]
- National Guideline Clearinghouse
- Rivera MP et al. Diagnosis of lung cancer: the guidelines. Chest. 2003;123(1 Suppl):129S. [PMID: 12527572]

INFORMATION FOR PATIENTS

- National Cancer Institute
- National Institutes of Health

REFERENCES

- Robinson BW et al. Advances in malignant mesothelioma. N Engl J Med. 2005 Oct 13;353(15):1591–603. [PMID: 16221782]
- West SD et al. Management of malignant pleural mesothelioma. Clin Chest Med. 2006 Jun;27(2):335–54. [PMID: 16716822]

Methanol and Ethylene Glycol Poisoning

KEY FEATURES

- The toxicity of both agents is caused by metabolism to toxic organic acids
  - Methanol to formic acid

  - Ethylene glycol to glycolic and oxalic acids

CLINICAL FINDINGS

- Shortly after ingestion of either agent, patients usually appear drunk
- After several hours, there is tachypnea, confusion, convulsions, and coma
- Methanol intoxication frequently causes visual disturbances
- Ethylene glycol often produces oxalate crystalluria and renal failure

DIAGNOSIS

- Initially, the serum osmolality (and osmolar gap) is usually increased
- After several hours, there is a severe anion gap metabolic acidosis
- Ethylene glycol often produces oxalate crystalluria
- Differential diagnosis: alcoholic ketoacidosis also can cause a combined anion gap acidosis and osmolar gap

TREATMENT

- Empty stomach by gastric lavage if recent ingestion
- Administer fomepizole or ethanol to block metabolism of methanol and ethylene glycol to their toxic metabolites; contact a regional poison control center for indications and dosing
- For significant toxicity (manifested by severe metabolic acidosis, altered mental status, markedly elevated osmolar gap), perform hemodialysis as soon as possible

Mitral Regurgitation

KEY FEATURES

- Mitral regurgitation results from
  - Displacement of papillary muscles (dilated cardiomyopathy)
  - Excessive length of chordae or myxomatous degeneration of leaflets (mitral prolapse)

  - Noncontraction of annulus (annular calcification)
  - Scarring (rheumatic fever, calcific invasion)
  - Infection (endocarditis)
- Places a volume load on heart (increased preload), but reduces afterload, resulting in enlarged left ventricle (LV) and initial increase in ejection fraction (EF)
- Over time, LV weakens and EF drops

CLINICAL FINDINGS

- Pansystolic murmur at the apex, radiating into the axilla in most patients
- Often associated with an S_3
- Hyperdynamic LV impulse
- Brisk carotid upstroke
- May be asymptomatic for many years (or life)
- When regurgitation develops acutely, left atrial pressure rises abruptly, leading to pulmonary edema if severe
- When regurgitation progresses more slowly, exertional dyspnea and fatigue worsen gradually over many years
- Left atrial enlargement may lead to atrial fibrillation and systemic embolization
- Predisposition to infective endocarditis

DIAGNOSIS

- ECG: left atrial abnormality or atrial fibrillation and LV hypertrophy
- Chest radiograph: left atrial and ventricular enlargement
- Doppler echocardiography
  - Confirms the diagnosis, etiology and estimates severity by a variety of methods
  - Used for measuring LV function and LV end-systolic and diastolic sizes
- Transesophageal echocardiography
  - May reveal the cause and better identify candidates for valvular repair
  - Important in endocarditis
- Coronary angiography is often indicated (especially after age 45) to determine the presence of coronary artery disease before valve surgery

TREATMENT

- Antibiotic prophylaxis for dental and other procedures
- ACE inhibitor therapy is used to reduce afterload, though little data to support

- Acute mitral regurgitation resulting from endocarditis, myocardial infarction, and ruptured chordae tendineae often requires emergency surgery
- Chronic regurgitation usually requires surgery when symptoms develop or in asymptomatic patients when the LV end-systolic dimension is > 4.0 cm or EF < 60%
- Surgical valve repair
  - Preferred in mitral prolapse and in some with endocarditis
  - Essentially all patients who undergo valve repair also get mitral annular rings placed
  - Also used in patients with cardiomyopathy
- Mitral valve replacement uses mechanical or bioprosthetic valves
- Novel percutaneous approaches to mitral valve repair include
  - Transseptal stitching of leaflets (Evalve procedure)
  - Coronary sinus crimping
  - Other measures to reduce annular size

Mitral Stenosis

 ## KEY FEATURES

- Underlying rheumatic heart disease in almost all patients (although history of rheumatic fever is often absent)

 ## CLINICAL FINDINGS

- An opening snap following S_2 due to stiff mitral valve
- Interval between opening snap and aortic closure sound is long when the left atrial pressure is low but shortens as left atrial pressure rises and approaches the aortic diastolic pressure
- Low-pitched rumble at apex with patient in left decubitus position, increased by brief exercise
- **Moderate stenosis** (valve area 1.8–1.3 cm^2): exertional dyspnea and fatigue common, especially with tachycardia
- **Severe stenosis** (valve area < 1.0 cm^2): pulmonary congestion at rest, with dyspnea, fatigue, right-sided heart failure, orthopnea, paroxysmal nocturnal dyspnea, and occasional hemoptysis

- Sudden increase in heart rate may precipitate pulmonary edema
- Paroxysmal or chronic atrial fibrillation develops in ~50–80%, may precipitate dyspnea or pulmonary edema

 ## DIAGNOSIS

- ECG typically shows left atrial abnormality and, often, atrial fibrillation
- Doppler echocardiography confirms diagnosis and quantifies severity by assigning 1–4 points to each of four observed parameters, with 1 being the least involvement and 4 the greatest
  - Mitral leaflet thickening
  - Mitral leaflet mobility
  - Submitral scarring
  - Commissural calcium
- Cardiac catheterization to detect valve, coronary, or myocardial disease, usually done only after a decision to intervene has been made

 ## TREATMENT

- Control heart rate
- Attempt conversion of atrial fibrillation
- Once atrial fibrillation occurs, provide lifelong anticoagulation with warfarin, even if sinus rhythm is restored
- Intervention to relieve stenosis indicated for symptoms (eg, pulmonary edema, decline in exercise capacity) or evidence of pulmonary hypertension
- Percutaneous balloon valvuloplasty can be done when there is minimal mitral regurgitation
- Surgical valve replacement is done in combined stenosis and regurgitation or when the mitral valve is significantly distorted and calcified
- Operative mortality rate is ~1–3%

Mitral Valve Prolapse

 ## KEY FEATURES

- Usually asymptomatic
- When symptoms are present, they include
  - Nonspecific chest pain

  - Dyspnea
  - Fatigue
  - Ventricular or supraventricular arrhythmias
- Most patients are female, many are thin, and some have minor chest wall deformities
- The significance of mitral valve prolapse (MVP) is disputed because it is diagnosed frequently in healthy young women (up to 10%)
- In occasional patients, MVP is not benign
- Infective endocarditis may occur, chiefly in patients with murmurs

 ## CLINICAL FINDINGS

- One or more characteristic midsystolic clicks often—but not always—followed by a late systolic murmur
- Findings are accentuated in the standing position
- A single midsystolic click is usually benign
- The late or pansystolic murmur may presage significant mitral regurgitation, often resulting from rupture of chordae tendineae

 ## DIAGNOSIS

- The diagnosis is primarily clinical but can be confirmed by Doppler echocardiography
- Echocardiography: Marked thickening or redundancy of the valve is associated with a higher incidence of complications

 ## TREATMENT

- Usually, no treatment is indicated
- In asymptomatic patients, serial clinical examinations to rule out progression to mitral regurgitation
- In patients with murmurs, antibiotic prophylaxis before dental work and other procedures
- β-Blockers for supraventricular arrhythmias
- A cardioverter-defibrillator for symptomatic ventricular tachycardia
- If regurgitation evolves, treat as indicated for mitral regurgitation (see Mitral Regurgitation)

Molluscum Contagiosum

 KEY FEATURES

- Caused by a poxvirus
- The lesions are autoinoculable and spread by wet skin-to-skin contact
- In sexually active individuals, lesions may be confined to the penis, pubis, and inner thighs and are considered a sexually transmitted infection
- Common in AIDS patients
  - Usually with a helper T cell count < 100/mcL
  - Extensive lesions tend to develop over the face and neck as well as in the genital area
  - Lesions are difficult to eradicate unless immunity improves, in which case spontaneous clearing may occur

 CLINICAL FINDINGS

- Presents as single or multiple rounded, dome-shaped, waxy papules 2–5 mm in diameter that are umbilicated
- Lesions at first are firm, solid, and flesh colored but on reaching maturity become softened, whitish, or pearly gray and may suppurate
- The principal sites are the face, lower abdomen, and genitals
- Individual lesions persist for ~2 mo

 DIAGNOSIS

- Clinical; based on the distinctive central umbilication of the dome-shaped lesion
- Differential diagnosis
  - Warts
  - Varicella (chickenpox)
  - Basal cell carcinoma
  - Lichen planus
  - Smallpox
  - Cutaneous cryptococcosis (in AIDS)

 TREATMENT

- The best treatment is by curettage or applications of liquid nitrogen as for warts but more briefly

- When lesions are frozen, the central umbilication often becomes more apparent
- Light electrosurgery with a fine needle is also effective

Monoclonal Gammopathy of Uncertain Significance (MGUS)

 KEY FEATURES

- Stable quantity of M protein in the serum without symptoms or signs of multiple myeloma, macroglobulinemia, amyloidosis, or lymphoma
- MGUS increases with age and is seen in 5% in persons aged 70 years of age or older
- Lymphoid malignancies, amyloidosis, macroglobulinemia, or multiple myeloma will develop in as many as one-third of patients with apparently benign monoclonal gammopathies

 CLINICAL FINDINGS

- Asymptomatic
- No lymphadenopathy, splenomegaly, or bony lesions of multiple myeloma

 DIAGNOSIS

- Monoclonal spike on serum protein electrophoresis, confirmed by immuno-electrophoresis to be a homogeneous immunoglobulin with either κ or γ light chains
- Parameters that suggest a favorable prognosis include
  - Concentrations of homogeneous immunoglobulin < 2 g/dL
  - No increase in concentration of the immunoglobulin from the time of diagnosis
  - No decrease in the concentration of normal immunoglobulins

- Absence of a homogeneous light chain in the urine, and normal hematocrit and serum albumin

 TREATMENT

- No specific treatment
- Monitor periodically for changes in serum M proteins, urinary Bence Jones proteins, evidence of renal failure, anemia, hypercalcemia, lytic bone lesions, or bone marrow plasmacytoses

Mononucleosis

 KEY FEATURES

- Acute infection can occur at any age but is most common at age 10–35 years
- Epstein-Barr virus (EBV) is the causative agent
- Similar syndromes are caused by
  - Cytomegalovirus (CMV)
  - Acute HIV infection
  - Toxoplasmosis
- EBV shows a strong serologic association with
  - HIV-related lymphomas
  - Nasopharyngeal carcinoma
  - Burkitt's lymphoma
  - Oral hairy leukoplakia
  - Posttransplant lymphoproliferative disorder

 CLINICAL FINDINGS

- Fever, sore throat common
- Lymphadenopathy very common
- Splenomegaly (50%)
- Maculopapular rash uncommon (15%), except in patients receiving ampicillin (90%)
- Exudative pharyngitis common
- Hepatitis, mononeuropathy, aseptic meningitis, hemolytic anemia, thrombocytopenia uncommon
- Secondary bacterial infections of the throat
- Splenic rupture is rare but dramatic
- Nonspecific ECG changes (5%)

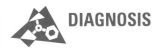
DIAGNOSIS

- Combination of sore throat, fever, fatigue, adenopathy, and splenomegaly suggests the diagnosis
- Chronicity of pharyngitis makes infectious mononucleosis more likely than bacterial pharyngitis
- Granulocytopenia with lymphocytosis, especially large, atypical lymphocytes
- Hemolytic anemia and thrombocytopenia
- Heterophil antibody and Monospot tests usually positive
- Antibody (IgM) titers to early antigens including viral capsid antigen can be useful early in disease

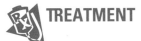
TREATMENT

- 95% of patients recover without antiviral therapy
- Acyclovir and other antiviral drugs are without verified clinical benefit
- Chronic EBV syndromes are increasingly recognized, especially in immunodeficient persons (Duncan's syndrome)

Motor Neuron Disease, Degenerative

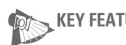
KEY FEATURES

ESSENTIALS OF DIAGNOSIS

- Variable weakness and wasting of muscles without sensory changes
- Progressive course
- No identifiable underlying cause other than genetic basis in familial cases

GENERAL CONSIDERATIONS

- There is degeneration of the
  - Anterior horn cells in the spinal cord
  - Motor nuclei of the lower cranial nerves
  - Corticospinal and corticobulbar pathways
- Five varieties have been characterized on clinical grounds

Progressive bulbar palsy
- Bulbar involvement predominates

- Disease processes affect primarily the motor nuclei of the cranial nerves

Pseudobulbar palsy
- Bulbar involvement predominates
- Due to bilateral corticobulbar disease and thus reflects upper motor neuron dysfunction

Progressive spinal muscular atrophy
- A lower motor neuron deficit in the limbs
- Due to degeneration of the anterior horn cells in the spinal cord

Primary lateral sclerosis
- There is a purely upper motor neuron deficit in the limbs

Amyotrophic lateral sclerosis
- A mixed upper and lower motor neuron deficit is found in the limbs and bulbar muscles
- This disorder is sometimes associated with cognitive decline (in a pattern consistent with frontotemporal dementia) or parkinsonism

DEMOGRAPHICS

- Symptoms generally begin between 30 and 60 years of age
- The disease is usually sporadic, but familial cases may occur

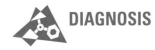
CLINICAL FINDINGS

SYMPTOMS AND SIGNS

- Difficulty in swallowing, chewing, coughing, breathing, and talking (dysarthria) occur with bulbar involvement
- In **progressive bulbar palsy**, there is
  - Drooping of the palate
  - A depressed gag reflex
  - Pooling of saliva in the pharynx
  - A weak cough
  - A wasted, fasciculating tongue
- In **pseudobulbar palsy**, the tongue is contracted and spastic and cannot be moved rapidly from side to side
- Limb involvement is characterized by motor disturbances (weakness, stiffness, wasting, fasciculations) reflecting lower or upper motor neuron dysfunction
- There are no objective changes on sensory examination, though there may be vague sensory complaints
- The sphincters are generally spared

DIFFERENTIAL DIAGNOSIS

Upper motor neuron disease
- Stroke
- Space-occupying lesion

- Compressive spinal cord lesion
- Multiple sclerosis

Lower motor neuron disease
- Infections of anterior horn cells (eg, poliovirus or West Nile virus)
- Radiculopathy, plexopathy, peripheral neuropathy, and myopathy are distinguished by clinical examination
- Pure motor syndromes resembling motor neuron disease may occur in association with
  - Monoclonal gammopathy
  - Multifocal motor neuropathies with conduction block, which can be distinguished by electrodiagnostic studies
- A motor neuronopathy may develop in Hodgkin's disease and has a relatively benign prognosis

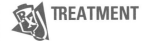
DIAGNOSIS

LABORATORY TESTS

- The serum creatine kinase may be slightly elevated but never reaches the extremely high values seen in some of the muscular dystrophies
- The cerebrospinal fluid is normal

DIAGNOSTIC PROCEDURES

- Electromyography may show changes of chronic partial denervation and reinnervation, with abnormal spontaneous activity in the resting muscle and a reduction in the number of motor units under voluntary control
- In patients with suspected spinal muscular atrophy or amyotrophic lateral sclerosis, the diagnosis should not be made with confidence unless such changes are found in three spinal regions (cervical, thoracic, lumbosacral) or two spinal regions and the bulbar muscles
- Motor conduction velocity is usually normal but may be slightly reduced
- Sensory conduction studies are also normal
- Biopsy of a wasted muscle shows the histologic changes of denervation

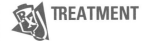
TREATMENT

MEDICATIONS

- Riluzole, 100 mg PO once daily
  - Reduces the presynaptic release of glutamate
  - May slow progression of amyotrophic lateral sclerosis

- Otherwise, no specific treatment except in patients with gammopathy, in whom plasmapheresis and immunosuppression may lead to improvement
- Multifocal motor neuropathy is treated with
  - Intravenous immunoglobulin
  - Cyclophosphamide
- Symptomatic and supportive measures
  - Anticholinergic drugs (such as trihexyphenidyl, amitriptyline, or atropine) if drooling is troublesome
  - Braces or a walker improve mobility
  - Physical therapy prevents contractures
- Spasticity may be helped by baclofen or diazepam

SURGERY

- In extreme cases of predominant bulbar involvement
  - Gastrostomy or cricopharyngomyotomy sometimes performed
  - Tracheostomy may be necessary if respiratory muscles are severely affected
- However, in the terminal stages of these disorders, the aim of treatment should be to keep patients as comfortable as possible

THERAPEUTIC PROCEDURES

- A semiliquid diet or nasogastric tube feeding may be needed if dysphagia is severe

 ## OUTCOME

PROGNOSIS

- The disorder is progressive
- Amyotrophic lateral sclerosis is usually fatal within 3–5 years
- Death usually results from pulmonary infections
- Patients with bulbar involvement generally have the poorest prognosis

WHEN TO REFER

- All patients should be referred to a physician with expertise in the diagnosis and treatment of these disorders

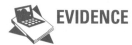 ## EVIDENCE

PRACTICE GUIDELINES

- Brooks BR et al; World Federation of Neurology Research Group on Motor Neuron Diseases. El Escorial revisited: revised criteria for the diagnosis of amy-

otrophic lateral sclerosis. Amyotroph Lateral Scler Other Motor Neuron Disord. 2000;1:293. [PMID: 11464847]

WEB SITE

- Neuromuscular Disease Center

INFORMATION FOR PATIENTS

- National Institute of Neurological Disorders and Stroke

REFERENCES

- McGeer EG et al. Pharmacologic approaches to the treatment of amyotrophic lateral sclerosis. BioDrugs. 2005;19(1):31–7. [PMID: 15691215]
- Mitsumoto H, Rabkin JG. Palliative care for patients with amyotrophic lateral sclerosis: "prepare for the worst and hope for the best". JAMA. 2007 Jul 11; 298(2):207–16. [PMID: 17622602]
- Rippon GA et al. An observational study of cognitive impairment in amyotrophic lateral sclerosis. Arch Neurol. 2006 Mar;63(3):345–52. [PMID: 16533961]
- Winhammar JM et al. Assessment of disease progression in motor neuron disease. Lancet Neurol. 2005 Apr; 4(4):229–38. [PMID: 15778102]

Multiple Endocrine Neoplasia, Types 1 & 2

 ## KEY FEATURES

ESSENTIALS OF DIAGNOSIS

- Rare familial autosomal dominant multiglandular syndromes

GENERAL CONSIDERATIONS

Multiple endocrine neoplasia (MEN) 1 (Wermer's syndrome)

- Parathyroid, enteropancreatic, and pituitary tumors
- Nonendocrine tumors
  - Subcutaneous lipomas
  - Facial angiofibromas
  - Collagenomas
- Mutations in 1 of the 10 exons of the *menin* gene (11q13) detectable in 60–95%

- Variants of MEN 1 occur, eg, kindreds with MEN 1 Burin have a high prevalence of prolactinomas, late-onset hyperparathyroidism, and carcinoid tumors, but rarely enteropancreatic tumors
- In patients with MEN 1 gastrinomas, depending on the kindred, hepatic metastases tend to be less aggressive than sporadic gastrinomas

MEN 2A (Sipple's syndrome)

- Medullary thyroid carcinoma, hyperparathyroidism, pheochromocytomas
- Nonendocrine: Hirschsprung's disease
- Caused by a mutation of the *ret* proto-oncogene (*RET*) on chromosome 10 (95%)
- Each kindred has a certain *ret* codon mutation that correlates with the particular variation in the MEN 2 syndrome, such as the age of onset and aggressiveness of medullary thyroid cancer

MEN 2B

- Adrenal pheochromocytomas, medullary thyroid carcinoma, mucosal neuromas
- Nonendocrine manifestations
  - Intestinal ganglioneuromas
  - Marfan-like habitus
  - Skeletal abnormalities
  - Delayed puberty

DEMOGRAPHICS

- MEN 1 has a prevalence of 2–10 per 100,000

 ## CLINICAL FINDINGS

SYMPTOMS AND SIGNS

MEN 1

- Tumors may develop in childhood or adulthood; presentation variable, even in same kindred
- Hyperparathyroidism in > 90%; initial presentation in two-thirds of patients
- Enteropancreatic tumors in ~75%
  - Gastrinomas in 35% (Zollinger-Ellison syndrome)
  - Gastrinomas tend to be small, multiple and ectopic
    - Frequently in the duodenum
    - Can metastasize to the liver
  - Concurrent hyperparathyroidism stimulates gastrin and gastric acid secretion
- Insulinomas in ~15% of patients cause fasting hypoglycemia
- Glucagonomas (2%) cause diabetes mellitus and migratory necrolytic erythema

- VIPomas (1%) cause profuse watery diarrhea, hypokalemia, and achorhydria (WDHA, Verner-Morrison syndrome)
- Somatostatinomas (1%) can cause diabetes mellitus, steatorrhea, and cholelithiasis
- Pituitary adenomas in 42%; presenting tumor in 17%
- Adrenal adenomas or hyperplasia in ~37%; bilateral in 50%; generally benign and nonfunctional
- Nonendocrine tumors are common
  – Small facial angiofibromas and subcutaneous lipomas
  – Collagenomas (firm skin nodules)
  – Malignant melanomas can occur

MEN 2A
- Pheochromocytomas (often bilateral)
- Calcitonin levels in medullary thyroid carcinoma are usually > 80 pg/mL in women or > 190 pg/mL in men

MEN 2B
- Medullary thyroid carcinoma is aggressive and presents early in life
- Mucosal neuromas (> 90%) with bumpy and enlarged lips and tongue
- Marfan-like habitus (75%)
- Adrenal pheochromocytomas (60%), often bilateral and rarely malignant
- Medullary thyroid carcinoma (80%)
- Intestinal abnormalities, eg, ganglioneuromas, in 75%
- Skeletal abnormalities (87%)
- Delayed puberty (43%)

DIFFERENTIAL DIAGNOSIS
- Tumors of pituitary, parathyroids, or pancreatic islets
- Other causes of hypercalcemia may increase gastrin levels, simulating gastrinoma

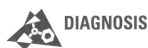 DIAGNOSIS

LABORATORY TESTS
MEN 1
- Genetic linkage analysis can be done if there are several affected members in the kindred
- *Menin* mutation genetic testing permits the rest of the kindred to be tested for the specific gene defect and allows informed genetic counseling

MEN 2A
- *RET* mutation genetic testing permits first-degree relatives to be tested for the specific gene defect and allows informed genetic counseling

- Serum calcitonin level drawn after 3 days of omeprazole, 20 mg PO BID, enables screening for medullary thyroid carcinoma

MEN 2B
- Genetic testing of infants who have a parent with MEN 2B is possible

TREATMENT

MEDICATIONS
MEN 1
- Cinacalcet orally is effective for hyperparathyroidism
- Conservative treatment for patients with gastrinomas in MEN 1
  – High-dose proton pump inhibitor therapy
  – Control of hypercalcemia

SURGERY
MEN 1
- Parathyroidectomy (3½ glands resected, along with thymectomy) for patients with hyperparathyroidism is effective in 62%
- Surgery for gastrinomas is palliative and usually reserved for aggressive gastrinomas and those tumors arising in the duodenum
- Surgical resection is usually attempted for insulinomas, but the tumors can be small, multiple, and difficult to detect

MEN 2A
- Prophylactic total thyroidectomy for children with a MEN 2A *RET* gene mutation, usually by age 6, though ~30% never manifest endocrine tumors
- Screen MEN 2 mutation carriers for pheochromocytoma before any surgical procedure

OUTCOME

COMPLICATIONS
MEN 1
- Aggressive parathyroid resection can cause permanent hypoparathyroidism
- Control of the hypercalcemia can reduce serum gastrin levels, gastric acidity, and frequency of peptic ulcer disease

PROGNOSIS
MEN 1
- Hyperparathyroidism recurrence rate is 16%, with hypercalcemia often recurring many years after neck surgery

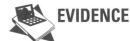 EVIDENCE

PRACTICE GUIDELINES
- Brandi ML et al. Guidelines for diagnosis and therapy of MEN type 1 and type 2. J Clin Endocrinol Metab. 2001; 86:5658. [PMID: 11739416]
- Lips CJ et al. Counselling in multiple endocrine neoplasia syndromes: from individual experience to general guidelines. J Intern Med. 2005;257:69. [PMID: 15606378]

WEB SITES
- National Cancer Institute
- National Institute of Diabetes and Digestive and Kidney Diseases

INFORMATION FOR PATIENTS
- MedlinePlus: Multiple Endocrine Neoplasia
- NIDDK MEN 1

REFERENCES
- Gertner ME et al. Multiple endocrine neoplasia type 2. Curr Treat Options Oncol. 2004 Aug;5(4):315–25. [PMID: 15233908]
- Lambert LA et al. Surgical treatment of hyperparathyroidism in patients with multiple endocrine neoplasia type 1. Arch Surg. 2005 Apr;140(4):374–82. [PMID: 15841561]
- Skinner MA et al. Prophylactic thyroidectomy in multiple endocrine neoplasia type 2A. N Engl J Med. 2005 Sep 15; 353(11):1105–13. [PMID: 16162881]
- Waldmann J et al. Adrenal involvement in multiple endocrine neoplasia type 1: results of 7 years of prospective screening. Langenbecks Arch Surg. 2007 Jul; 392(4):437–43. [PMID: 17235589]

Multiple Myeloma

KEY FEATURES

ESSENTIALS OF DIAGNOSIS
- Monoclonal paraprotein in serum or urine by protein electrophoresis or immunoelectrophoresis
- Malignant plasma cells in bone marrow

- Bone pain, especially back pain, is common

GENERAL CONSIDERATIONS

- Malignancy of plasma cells characterized by replacement of bone marrow, bone destruction, and paraprotein formation
- Replacement of bone marrow initially causes anemia and later general bone marrow failure
- Malignant plasma cells can form tumors (plasmacytomas) that may cause spinal cord compression
- Bone involvement causes bone pain, osteoporosis, lytic lesions, pathologic fractures, and hypercalcemia
- Light chain component of immunoglobulin often leads to renal failure
- Light chain components may be deposited in tissues as amyloid, worsening renal failure and causing systemic symptoms
- Failure of antibody production in response to antigen challenge makes myeloma patients especially prone to infections with encapsulated organisms, eg, *Streptococcus pneumoniae* and *Haemophilus influenzae*
- Salmon-Durie staging system
  - Standard for multiple myeloma
  - Based on level of paraprotein, blood counts, bone radiographs, and serum calcium
  - A new International Staging System based on serum albumin and β_2-microglobulin has come into use

DEMOGRAPHICS

- Occurs most commonly in older adults: median age at presentation is 65 years

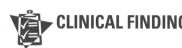 **CLINICAL FINDINGS**

SYMPTOMS AND SIGNS

- Symptoms of anemia
- Increased susceptibility to infection
- Bone pain most common in back or ribs or may present as pathologic fracture
- Symptoms of renal failure
- Neuropathy or spinal cord compression
- Soft tissue masses

DIFFERENTIAL DIAGNOSIS

- Monoclonal gammopathy of uncertain significance (MGUS)
- Reactive polyclonal hypergammaglobulinemia
- Waldenström's macroglobulinemia
- Metastatic cancer
- Primary hyperparathyroidism
- Lymphoma or leukemia
- Primary amyloidosis

 DIAGNOSIS

LABORATORY TESTS

- Anemia is nearly universal
- Red blood cell morphology is normal, but rouleau formation is common and may be marked
- Hypercalcemia
- Proteinuria
- Peripheral blood smear: plasma cells rarely visible (plasma cell leukemia)
- Serum protein electrophoresis (SPEP) usually demonstrates paraprotein, in the majority demonstrable as a monoclonal spike in β- or γ-globulin region
- Immunoelectrophoresis (IEP) reveals this to be monoclonal protein; 60% are IgG, 25% IgA, and 15% light chains only
- When myeloma is suspected and there is no serum paraprotein, test urine with protein electrophoresis and IEP
- Serum albumin < 3.5 mg/dL and serum β_2-microglobulin level > 3.5 mg/L (and especially > 5.5 mg/L) associated with decreased survival

IMAGING STUDIES

- Bone radiographs: lytic lesions, especially in axial skeleton (skull, spine, proximal long bones, and ribs); or generalized osteoporosis
- Radionuclide bone scan: not useful in detecting bone lesions in myeloma, since usually no osteoblastic component
- MRI scans may be helpful in demonstrating the extent of bone and bone marrow disease, but are not currently standard practice

DIAGNOSTIC PROCEDURES

- Bone marrow biopsy: infiltration by > 20% plasma cells
- Poor outcome if bone marrow cytogenetic analysis shows deletions of chromosome 13q

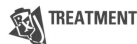 **TREATMENT**

MEDICATIONS

- Thalidomide plus dexamethasone is most commonly used initial treatment
- Bortezomib
  - A proteosome inhibitor
  - Available only intravenously
  - Has significant activity in myeloma either alone or in combination
  - Extremely expensive
- Lenolidomide
  - A derivative of thalidomide
  - Available orally
  - Has both improved efficacy and greatly reduced toxicity
  - Extremely expensive
- Mobilization, hydration, and bisphosphonates for hypercalcemia
- Bisphosphonates (eg, pamidronate, 90 mg, or zoledronic acid, 4 mg IV every month) to reduce pathologic fractures in patients with significant bony disease
- See Table 7

THERAPEUTIC PROCEDURES

- Observe without therapy if minimal disease or unclear whether paraproteinemia is benign (MGUS) or malignant, since no advantage to early treatment of asymptomatic multiple myeloma
- Autologous stem cell transplantation is part of overall treatment plan for most patients, and improves survival
- Allogeneic transplantation potentially curative, but role limited by high mortality rate in myeloma patients
- Reduced-intensity allogeneic transplant regimens have produced encouraging results

 OUTCOME

FOLLOW-UP

- Follow height of paraprotein spike on SPEP as a useful marker for monitoring response to therapy

COMPLICATIONS

- Bony fractures
- Hypercalcemia

PROGNOSIS

- Median survival for myeloma has been 3 years but is improving with new treatments
- Median survival is 5–6 years if low tumor burden (IgG spike < 5 g/dL, no more than one lytic bone lesion, and no hypercalcemia or renal failure)
- Median survival was 1–2 years if high tumor burden (IgG spike > 7 g/dL,

hematocrit < 25%, calcium > 12 mg/dL, or > 3 lytic bone lesions)
  – However, survival is now 5–6 years with early autologous stem cell transplantation
  – Immunotherapy with allogeneic transplantation and new agents bortezomib and lenolidomide may further improve results

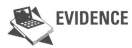

EVIDENCE

PRACTICE GUIDELINES

- Anderson KC et al; NCCN Multiple Myeloma Practice Guidelines Panel. National Comprehensive Cancer Network: Multiple Myeloma v.1.2005.
- Durie BG et al; Scientific Advisors of the International Myeloma Foundation. Myeloma management guidelines: a consensus report from the Scientific Advisors of the International Myeloma Foundation. Hematol J. 2003;4:379. Erratum in: Hematol J. 2004;5:285. [PMID: 14671610]

WEB SITES

- International Myeloma Foundation
- Multiple Myeloma Research Foundation
- National Cancer Institute: Multiple Myeloma Treatment

INFORMATION FOR PATIENTS

- American Cancer Society: Multiple Myeloma
- MedlinePlus: Multiple Myeloma Interactive Tutorial
- National Cancer Institute: Multiple Myeloma

REFERENCES

- Cavo M et al; Bologna 2002 Study. Superiority of thalidomide and dexamethasone over vincristine-doxorubicin-dexamethasone (VAD) as primary therapy in preparation for autologous transplantation for multiple myeloma. Blood. 2005 Jul 1;106(1):35–9. [PMID: 15761019]
- Crawley C et al. Outcome for reduced-intensity allogeneic transplantation for multiple myeloma: an analysis of prognostic factors from the Chronic Leukaemia Working Party of the EBMT. Blood. 2005 Jun 1;105(11):4532–9. [PMID: 15731182]
- Greipp PR et al. International staging system for multiple myeloma. J Clin Oncol. 2005 May 20;23(15):3412–20. [PMID: 15809451]
- Rajkumar SV et al. Combination therapy with lenalidomide plus dexamethasone (Rev/Dex) for newly diagnosed myeloma. Blood. 2005 Dec 15; 106(13):4050–3. [PMID: 16118317]
- Richardson PG et al. Bortezomib or high-dose dexamethasone for relapsed multiple myeloma. N Engl J Med. 2005 Jun 16;352(24):2487–98. [PMID: 15958804]

Multiple Sclerosis

 ## KEY FEATURES

ESSENTIALS OF DIAGNOSIS

- Episodic neurologic symptoms
- Usually under 55 years of age at onset
- Single pathologic lesion cannot explain clinical findings
- Multiple foci best visualized by MRI

GENERAL CONSIDERATIONS

- Should not be diagnosed unless there is evidence that two or more different regions of the central white matter have been affected at different times
- A diagnosis of clinically definite disease can be made
  – In patients with a relapsing-remitting course
  – When there is evidence of at least two lesions involving different regions of the central white matter
- The diagnosis is probable
  – In patients with multifocal white matter disease but only one clinical attack
  – In patients with a history of at least two clinical attacks but signs of only a single lesion

DEMOGRAPHICS

- Common disorder, probably an autoimmune basis, with its greatest incidence in young adults
- Much more common in persons of western European lineage who live in temperate zones
- No population with a high risk for multiple sclerosis exists between latitudes 40 °N and 40 °S
- Genetic, dietary, and climatic factors cannot account for these differences
- Nevertheless, a genetic susceptibility to the disease is likely, based on twin studies, familial cases, and an association with specific HLA antigens (HLA-DR2)

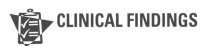 ## CLINICAL FINDINGS

SYMPTOMS AND SIGNS

- Common **initial presentation**
  – Weakness, numbness, tingling, or unsteadiness in a limb
  – Spastic paraparesis
  – Retrobulbar neuritis
  – Diplopia
  – Dysequilibrium
  – Sphincter disturbance, such as urinary urgency or hesitancy
- Symptoms may disappear after a few days or weeks, although examination often reveals a residual deficit

Relapsing-remitting disease
- Symptoms occur months or years after initial presentation
- Eventually relapses and usually incomplete remissions lead to increasing disability, with weakness, spasticity, and ataxia of the limbs, impaired vision, and urinary incontinence
- Findings on examination commonly include
  – Optic atrophy
  – Nystagmus
  – Dysarthria
  – Pyramidal, sensory, or cerebellar deficits in some or all of the limbs

Secondary progressive disease
- In some of the relapsing-remitting patients, the clinical course changes to steady deterioration, unrelated to acute relapses

Primary progressive disease
- Less common
- Symptoms steadily progress from their onset, and disability develops at a relatively early stage
- The diagnosis cannot be made unless the total clinical picture indicates involvement of different parts of the CNS at different times
- A number of factors (eg, infection, trauma) may precipitate or trigger exacerbations
- Relapses are also more likely during the 2 or 3 months following pregnancy

DIFFERENTIAL DIAGNOSIS

- Acute disseminated encephalomyelitis
- Foramen magnum lesion (Arnold-Chiari malformation)
- Progressive multifocal leukoencephalopathy

- Subacute combined degeneration of the spinal cord (B_{12} deficiency)
- Spinal cord tumor
- Vasculitis
- Neurosyphilis
- Lyme disease
- Syringomyelia
- HIV-associated myelopathy
- Human T cell lymphotropic virus-I myelopathy

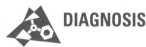 **DIAGNOSIS**

LABORATORY TESTS

- A definitive diagnosis can never be based solely on the laboratory findings
- Cerebrospinal fluid may reveal
  - Mild lymphocytosis or a slightly increased protein concentration, especially after an acute relapse
  - Elevated IgG and discrete bands of IgG (oligoclonal bands), which are not specific, having been found in a variety of inflammatory neurologic disorders and occasionally in patients with vascular or neoplastic disorders of the nervous system

IMAGING STUDIES

- MRI of the brain or cervical cord is often helpful in demonstrating the presence of a multiplicity of lesions
- Myelography or MRI
  - May be necessary in patients presenting with myelopathy alone and in whom there is no clinical or laboratory evidence of more widespread disease to exclude a congenital or acquired surgically treatable lesion
  - The foramen magnum region must be visualized to exclude the possibility of Arnold-Chiari malformation, in which part of the cerebellum and the lower brainstem are displaced into the cervical canal, producing mixed pyramidal and cerebellar deficits in the limbs

DIAGNOSTIC PROCEDURES

- Monocular visual stimulation with a checkerboard pattern stimulus detects subclinical involvement of visual pathway
- Monaural click stimulation detects subclinical involvement of brainstem auditory pathway
- Electrical stimulation of a sensory or mixed peripheral nerve detects subclinical involvement of the somatosensory pathway

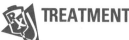 **TREATMENT**

MEDICATIONS

- Recovery from acute relapses may be hastened by corticosteroids
  - A high dose (eg, prednisone, 60 or 80 mg PO) is given daily for 1 week
  - Medication is then tapered over the following 2 or 3 weeks
  - Such a regimen is often preceded by methylprednisolone, 1 g IV for 3 days
  - However, extent of recovery is unchanged
- Long-term treatment with corticosteroids
  - Provides no benefit
  - Does not prevent further relapses
- Frequency of exacerbations can be reduced in patients with relapsing-remitting or secondary progressive disease with
  - β-Interferon therapy
  - Glatiramer acetate, given daily subcutaneously
- Immunosuppressive therapy
  - Examples include cyclophosphamide, azathioprine, methotrexate, cladribine, or mitoxantrone
  - May help arrest the course of secondary progressive multiple sclerosis
  - However, the evidence of benefit is incomplete
- Natalizumab
  - An alpha4 integrin antagonist that reduces the development of brain lesions in experimental models
  - Shown to reduce the relapse rate
  - Can only be prescribed under a risk management plan because of rare reports of progressive multifocal leukoencephalopathy developing in patients while receiving this drug
- There is little evidence that plasmapheresis enhances any beneficial effects of immunosuppression
- Intravenous immunoglobulins
  - May reduce the clinical attack rate in relapsing-remitting disease
  - However, available studies are inadequate to permit treatment recommendations

THERAPEUTIC PROCEDURES

- Treatment for spasticity and for neurogenic bladder may be needed in advanced cases
- Excessive fatigue must be avoided, and patients should rest during periods of acute relapse

 OUTCOME

PROGNOSIS

- At least partial recovery from acute exacerbations can reasonably be expected
- Relapses may occur without warning
- There is no means of preventing progression of the disorder
- Some disability is likely to result eventually
- About half of all patients are without significant disability even 10 years after onset of symptoms

WHEN TO REFER

- If confirmation of the diagnosis is needed, or if the disease is progressive despite standard therapy
- For expertise in the use of immunotherapy

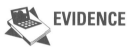 **EVIDENCE**

PRACTICE GUIDELINES

- American Academy of Neurology

WEB SITE

- National Institute of Neurological Disorders and Stroke

INFORMATION FOR PATIENTS

- The Mayo Clinic
- National Multiple Sclerosis Society

REFERENCES

- Fox EJ. Management of worsening multiple sclerosis with mitoxantrone: a review. Clin Ther. 2006 Apr;28(4):461–74. [PMID: 16750460]
- Goodin DS. Magnetic resonance imaging as a surrogate outcome measure of disability in multiple sclerosis: have we been overly harsh in our assessment? Ann Neurol. 2006 Apr;59(4):597–605. [PMID: 16566022]
- Polman CH et al. A randomized, placebo-controlled trial of natalizumab for relapsing multiple sclerosis. N Engl J Med. 2006 Mar 2;354(9):899–910. [PMID: 16510744]

Muscle Cramps

 KEY FEATURES

- Usually caused by sports or occupational muscle injury
- Noctural leg cramps
  - Idiopathic (most common)
  - Systemic diseases
    □ Diabetes mellitus
    □ Parkinson's disease
    □ CNS or spinal cord lesions
    □ Peripheral neuropathy
    □ Hemodialysis
- Drugs
  - Cisplatin
  - Vincristine
  - Cholinesterase inhibitors
  - Bisphosphonates
  - Chemotherapy (eg, imatinib)
- Electrolyte disorders
  - Hypocalcemia
  - Hypokalemia
  - Hyponatremia
  - Hypoglycemia
  - Hyperkalemia
  - Hypermagnesemia
  - Alkalosis (decreases ionized calcium)
- Leg cramps during walking
  - Peripheral vascular disease
  - Hyperthyroidism
  - Hypothyroidism
- Pregnancy
- Arsenic intoxication
- Causes of muscle pain, though usually not with cramping
  - HMGCoA reductase inhibitor (statin)
  - Dermatomyositis and polymyositis
  - Fibromyalgia, especially with "trigger points"

 CLINICAL FINDINGS

- Physical examination usually normal or shows signs of associated conditions listed above
- Exertional claudication and reduced pedal pulses suggest lower extremity arterial occlusive disease

 DIAGNOSIS

- Obtain serum electrolytes, glucose, calcium, magnesium levels
- If leg cramps occur during walking, serum TSH or Doppler ankle–brachial index evaluation for peripheral vascular disease
- Serum CK level is elevated in enzyme deficiencies, such as McArdle's disease

 TREATMENT

- Correct electrolyte disorders
- Gabapentin, 600–1200 mg/day divided PO BID–TID
  - For recurrent, severe, or prolonged muscle cramping
  - May cause leukopenia or CNS effects
- Calcium or magnesium citrate supplementation for pregnancy-associated leg cramps
- See (Vascular Disease, Peripheral)
- Botulinum toxin injections for recurrent cervicofacial dystonias, laryngeal dystonias, and hand cramps
- FDA has prohibited the marketing of quinine for leg cramps because of side effects

Muscular Dystrophies

 KEY FEATURES

- Inherited myopathic disorders
  - Characterized by progressive muscle weakness and wasting
  - Subdivided by mode of inheritance, age at onset, and clinical features (Table 137)
- Duchenne muscular dystrophy
  - Due to a genetic defect on the short arm of the X chromosome
  - Affected gene codes for the protein dystrophin, which is almost absent from diseased muscles
  - Genetic defect is detectable in pregnancy
- Becker muscular dystrophy
  - Dystrophin levels are generally normal
  - Protein is qualitatively altered

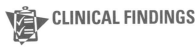 **CLINICAL FINDINGS**

- Muscle weakness, often in a characteristic distribution
- Age at onset and inheritance pattern depend on specific dystrophy
- Duchenne dystrophy
  - Pseudohypertrophy of muscles
  - Intellectual retardation
  - Skeletal deformities, muscle contractures, and cardiac involvement

 DIAGNOSIS

- Serum creatine kinase level
  - Increased, especially in the Duchenne and Becker varieties
  - Mildly increased in limb-girdle dystrophy
- Electromyography may confirm myopathic, rather than neurogenic, weakness
- Histopathologic examination of muscle biopsy specimen can distinguish between various muscle diseases

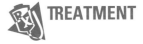 **TREATMENT**

- No specific treatment
- Prednisone (0.75 mg/kg daily) improves muscle strength and function in boys with Duchenne dystrophy but side effects need to be monitored
- Important to encourage patients to lead as normal lives as possible
- Prolonged bed rest must be avoided; inactivity often leads to worsening of the underlying muscle disease
- Physical therapy and orthopedic procedures may help counteract deformities or contractures

Mushroom Poisoning

 KEY FEATURES

ESSENTIALS OF DIAGNOSIS

- Vomiting, diarrhea, and abdominal cramps after ingestion of many different toxic mushrooms
- Amatoxin-type
  - Delayed-onset severe gastroenteritis, followed by severe hepatic injury

GENERAL CONSIDERATIONS

- There are thousands of toxic mushroom species
- Ingestion of even a portion of an amatoxin-containing mushroom may be sufficient to cause death
- Cooking amatoxin-type cyclopeptides does not prevent the poisoning

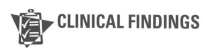 **CLINICAL FINDINGS**

SYMPTOMS AND SIGNS

- **Amatoxin-type** cyclopeptides (*Amanita phalloides, Amanita verna, Amanita virosa,* and *Galerina* species)
  - After a latent interval of 8–12 h, severe abdominal cramps and vomiting begin and progress to profuse diarrhea Hepatic necrosis, hepatic encephalopathy, and frequently renal failure occur in 1–2 days
- **Gyromitrin** type (*Gyromitra* and *Helvella* species)
  - Toxicity is more common following ingestion of uncooked mushrooms
  - Vomiting, diarrhea, hepatic necrosis, convulsions, coma, and hemolysis may occur after a latent period of 8–12 h
- **Muscarinic** type (*Inocybe* and *Clitocybe* species)
  - Vomiting, diarrhea, bradycardia, hypotension, salivation, miosis, bronchospasm, and lacrimation occur shortly after ingestion
- **Anticholinergic** type (*Amanita muscaria, Amanita pantherina*)
  - Excitement
  - Delirium
  - Flushed skin
  - Dilated pupils
  - Muscular jerking tremors
- **Gastrointestinal irritant** type (*Boletus, Cantharellus*)
  - Nausea, vomiting, and diarrhea occur shortly after ingestion
- **Disulfiram** type (*Coprinus* species)
  - Disulfiram-like sensitivity to alcohol may persist for several days
  - Toxicity is characterized by flushing, hypotension, and vomiting after co-ingestion of alcohol
- **Hallucinogenic** (*Psilocybe* and *Panaeolus* species)
  - Mydriasis, nausea and vomiting, and intense visual hallucinations occur 1–2 h after ingestion
- **Cortinarius orellanus**
  - May cause acute renal failure due to tubulointerstitial nephritis

DIFFERENTIAL DIAGNOSIS

- Differential diagnosis of Amatoxin-type mushroom poisoning
  - Acetaminophen poisoning
  - Acute viral hepatitis

 DIAGNOSIS

DIAGNOSTIC PROCEDURES

- There are no readily available laboratory tests for mushroom toxins
- Local mycologist may help identify suspect fungi
- Amatoxin-type mushrooms
  - Typical delay of 8–12 hours before gastrointestinal symptoms occur
  - Hepatic transaminases elevated after 24 hours
  - Necrosis of the liver, massive and acute
  - Metabolic acidosis, hypoglycemia, elevated ammonia suggest severe hepatic failure

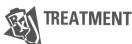 **TREATMENT**

MEDICATIONS

Emergency measures

- Administer activated charcoal (60–100 g PO or via gastric tube, mixed in aqueous slurry) for any recent ingestion
- Give intravenous fluids to replace losses from vomiting and diarrhea
- After the onset of symptoms, efforts to remove the toxic agent are probably useless, especially in cases of amatoxin or gyromitrin poisoning, in which there is usually a delay of 12 h or more before symptoms occur

Specific measures

- **Amatoxin-type** cyclopeptides
  - Aggressive fluid replacement for diarrhea and intensive supportive care for hepatic failure (including liver transplant if needed) are the mainstays of treatment
  - Antidote efficacy (eg, penicillin, corticosteroids, silymarin) is uncertain although often used in Europe
- **Gyromitrin type:** pyridoxine, 25 mg/kg IV
- **Muscarinic type**
  - Give atropine, 0.005–0.01 mg/kg IV
  - Repeat as needed
- **Anticholinergic type**
  - Physostigmine, 0.5–1.0 mg IV
  - May calm extreme agitation and reverse peripheral anticholinergic manifestations

  - However, may also cause bradycardia, asystole, and seizures
- **Gastrointestinal irritant type:** treat with antiemetics and IV or oral fluid
- **Disulfiram type:** avoid alcohol and treat alcohol reaction with fluids and supine position
- **Hallucinogenic type**
  - Provide a quiet, supportive atmosphere
  - Diazepam or haloperidol may be used for sedation
- **Cortinarius**
  - Provide supportive care
  - Hemodialysis as needed for renal failure

 OUTCOME

PROGNOSIS

- The fatality rate of amatoxin-type cyclopeptides is about 10–20% without liver transplant
- The fatality rate of gyromitrin-type mushrooms is < 10%
- Fatalities are rare with
  - Muscarinic type
  - Anticholingeric type
  - Gastrointestinal irritant type
  - Hallucinogenic mushrooms

WHEN TO REFER

- Liver transplant may be necessary, particularly for amatoxin-type cyclopeptides
- Contact a transplant center early

 EVIDENCE

WEB SITES

- eMedicine: Toxicology Articles
- Karolinska Institute: Diseases and Disorders: Links Pertaining to Poisoning
- North American Mycological Association: Mushroom Poisoning Case Registry
- U.S. Food and Drug Administration: Mushroom Toxins

INFORMATION FOR PATIENTS

- American Academy of Family Physicians: Mushroom Poisoning in Children
- California Poison Control System: Mushrooms
- MedlinePlus: Poisoning First Aid

REFERENCES

- Bickel M et al. Severe rhabdomyolysis, acute renal failure and posterior encephalopathy after 'magic mushroom' abuse. Eur J Emerg Med. 2005 Dec; 12(6):306–8. [PMID: 16276262]

- Diaz JH. Evolving global epidemiology, syndromic classification, general management, and prevention of unknown mushroom poisonings. Crit Care Med. 2005 Feb;33(2):419–26. [PMID: 15699848]

- Diaz JH. Syndromic diagnosis and management of confirmed mushroom poisonings. Crit Care Med. 2005 Feb; 33(2):427–36. [PMID: 15699849]

- Nieminen P et al. Suspected myotoxicity of edible wild mushrooms. Exp Biol Med (Maywood). 2006 Feb; 231(2):221–8. [PMID: 16446499]

- Panaro F et al. Liver transplantation represents the optimal treatment for fulminant hepatic failure from *Amanita phalloides* poisoning. Transpl Int. 2006 Apr;19(4):344–5. [PMID: 16573553]

- Yang WS et al. Acute renal failure caused by mushroom poisoning. J Formos Med Assoc. 2006 Mar;105(3):263–7. [PMID: 16520846]

Myasthenia Gravis

 KEY FEATURES

ESSENTIALS OF DIAGNOSIS

- Fluctuating weakness of voluntary muscles, producing symptoms such as
  - Diplopia
  - Ptosis
  - Difficulty in swallowing
- Activity increases weakness of affected muscles
- Short-acting anticholinesterases transiently improve the weakness

GENERAL CONSIDERATIONS

- Occurs at all ages, sometimes in association with
  - Thymic tumor
  - Thyrotoxicosis
  - Rheumatoid arthritis
  - Lupus erythematosus
- Onset is usually insidious, but the disorder is sometimes unmasked by a coincidental infection
- Exacerbations may occur before the menstrual period and during or shortly after pregnancy

- Symptoms are due to blocks of neuromuscular transmission caused by autoantibodies binding to acetylcholine receptors
- The external ocular muscles and certain other cranial muscles, including the masticatory, facial, and pharyngeal muscles, are especially likely to be affected
- The respiratory and limb muscles may also be involved

DEMOGRAPHICS

- Most common in young women with HLA-DR3
- If thymoma is associated, older men are more commonly affected

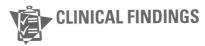 **CLINICAL FINDINGS**

SYMPTOMS AND SIGNS

- Initial symptoms
  - Ptosis
  - Diplopia
  - Difficulty in chewing or swallowing
  - Respiratory difficulties
  - Limb weakness
  - Some combination of these problems
- Weakness
  - May remain localized to a few muscle groups, especially the ocular muscles
  - May become generalized
- Symptoms often fluctuate in intensity during the day
- This diurnal variation is superimposed on a tendency to longer-term spontaneous relapses and remissions that may last for weeks
- Clinical examination confirms the weakness and fatigability of affected muscles
- Extraocular palsies and ptosis, often asymmetric, are common
- Pupillary responses are normal
- The bulbar and limb muscles are often weak, but the pattern of involvement is variable
- Sustained activity of affected muscles increases the weakness, which improves after a brief rest
- Sensation is normal
- Usually no reflex changes

DIFFERENTIAL DIAGNOSIS

- Lambert-Eaton myasthenic syndrome (usually paraneoplastic)
- Botulism
- Aminoglycoside-induced neuromuscular weakness

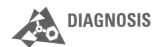 **DIAGNOSIS**

LABORATORY TESTS

- Elevated level of serum acetylcholine receptor antibodies has a sensitivity of 80–90%
- Certain patients have serum antibodies to muscle-specific tyrosine kinase (MuSK), which should be determined
  - These patients are more likely to have facial, respiratory and proximal muscle weakness than those with antibodies to acetylcholine receptors

IMAGING STUDIES

- Lateral and anteroposterior radiographs and CT scan of the chest
  - Should be obtained to demonstrate a coexisting thymoma
  - However, normal studies do not exclude this possibility

DIAGNOSTIC PROCEDURES

- Response to **short-acting anticholinesterase** can confirm diagnosis
  - Edrophonium can be given IV in a dose of 10 mg (1 mL), 2 mg being given initially and the remaining 8 mg about 30 s later if the test dose is well tolerated
  - In myasthenic patients, there is an obvious improvement in strength of weak muscles lasting for about 5 min
  - Alternatively, 1.5 mg of neostigmine can be given IM, and the response then lasts for about 2 h
  - Atropine sulfate (0.6 mg) should be available to reverse muscarinic side effects
- **Electrophysiology**
  - Demonstration of a decrementing muscle response to repetitive 2- or 3-Hz stimulation of motor nerves indicates a disturbance of neuromuscular transmission
  - Such an abnormality may even be detected in clinically strong muscles with certain provocative procedures
- **Needle electromyography**
  - Shows a marked variation in configuration and size of individual motor unit potentials in affected muscles
  - Single-fiber electromyography reveals an increased jitter, or variability, in the time interval between two muscle fiber action potentials from the same motor unit

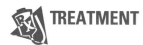 **TREATMENT**

MEDICATIONS

- Drugs, such as aminoglycosides, that may exacerbate myasthenia gravis should be avoided
- Anticholinesterase drugs provide symptomatic benefit without influencing the course of the disease
- Neostigmine, pyridostigmine, or both can be used
  - Dose is determined on an individual basis
  - Usual dose of neostigmine, 7.5–30.0 mg PO QID (average, 15 mg)
  - Usual dose of pyridostigmine, 30–180 mg PO QID (average, 60 mg)
  - Overmedication may temporarily increase weakness, which is then unaffected or enhanced by IV edrophonium
- Corticosteroids
  - Indicated if there has been a poor response to anticholinesterase drugs and the patient has had thymectomy
  - Start while the patient is in the hospital, since weakness may initially be aggravated
  - Dose is determined on an individual basis
- Azathioprine
  - May also be effective
  - Usual dose, 2–3 mg/kg PO daily after a lower initial dose
- Mycophenolate mofetil
  - May provide symptomatic relief
  - May allow for dose reduction of corticosteroid
- Plasmapheresis or intravenous immunoglobulin therapy
  - May be helpful in patients with major disability
  - May also be useful for stabilizing patients before thymectomy and for managing acute crisis

SURGERY

- Thymectomy
  - Usually leads to symptomatic benefit or remission
  - Should be considered in all patients younger than age 60, unless weakness is restricted to the extraocular muscles
- If the disease is of recent onset and only slowly progressive, operation is sometimes delayed for a year or so, in the hope that spontaneous remission will occur

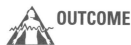 **OUTCOME**

COMPLICATIONS

- Aspiration pneumonia

PROGNOSIS

- The disorder follows a slowly progressive course and may have a fatal outcome owing to respiratory complications such as aspiration pneumonia

WHEN TO REFER

- Most patients with a suspected or proven diagnosis should be referred to a clinician with expertise in managing this disorder

 EVIDENCE

PRACTICE GUIDELINES

- National Guideline Clearinghouse

INFORMATION FOR PATIENTS

- National Institute of Neurological Disorders and Stroke

REFERENCES

- Keesey JC. Clinical evaluation and management of myasthenia gravis. Muscle Nerve. 2004 Apr;29(4):484–505. [PMID: 15052614]
- Schneider-Gold C et al. Mycophenolate mofetil and tacrolimus: new therapeutic options in neuroimmunological diseases. Muscle Nerve. 2006 Sep; 34(3):284–91. [PMID: 16583368]

Myasthenic Syndrome

 KEY FEATURES

- Clinical similarity to myasthenia gravis, but myasthenic syndrome occurs mainly as a paraneoplastic syndrome (Table 10)
- There is defective release of acetylcholine in response to a nerve impulse, leading to weakness, especially of the proximal muscles of the limbs
- May be associated with small cell lung carcinoma, sometimes developing before the tumor is diagnosed, and

occasionally occurs with certain autoimmune diseases

 CLINICAL FINDINGS

- Variable weakness, typically improving with activity
- Dysautonomic symptoms may also be present
- A history of malignant disease may be obtained
- Unlike myasthenia gravis, power steadily increases with sustained contraction

 DIAGNOSIS

- Electrophysiologic diagnosis: the muscle response to stimulation of its motor nerve increases remarkably if the nerve is stimulated repetitively at high rates, even in muscles that are not clinically weak

 TREATMENT

- Plasmapheresis and immunosuppressive drug therapy (prednisone and azathioprine), in addition to therapy directed at a tumor
- Prednisone is usually initiated in a daily dose of 60–80 mg and azathioprine in a daily dose of 2 mg/kg
- Guanidine hydrochloride (25–50 mg/kg/day in divided doses) is occasionally helpful in seriously disabled patients, but adverse effects of the drug include marrow suppression
- Anticholinesterase drugs, such as pyridostigmine or neostigmine, either alone or in combination with guanidine, yield variable treatment responses

Myelodysplastic Syndromes

 KEY FEATURES

ESSENTIALS OF DIAGNOSIS

- Cytopenias
- Morphologic abnormalities in two or more hematopoietic cell lines

GENERAL CONSIDERATIONS

- Group of acquired clonal disorders of the hematopoietic stem cell, characterized by cytopenias, usually hypercellular marrow, and morphologic and cytogenetic abnormalities
- No specific chromosomal abnormality is seen, but abnormalities in chromosomes 5 and 7 are common
- Causes
  - Idiopathic (most common)
  - Postcytotoxic chemotherapy, either alkylating agents (cyclophosphamide) or topoisomerase inhibitors (etoposide, doxorubicin)
- May evolve into acute myelogenous leukemia (AML); had been termed "preleukemia" in the past
- Myelodysplasia encompasses several heterogeneous syndromes
  - Refractory anemia (with or without ringed sideroblasts): no excess bone marrow blasts
  - Refractory anemia with excess blasts (RAEB): 5–19% blasts
  - Chronic myelomonocytic leukemia (CMML): a proliferative syndrome, including peripheral blood monocytosis > 1000/mcL

DEMOGRAPHICS

- Occurs most often in patients aged > 60

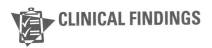 **CLINICAL FINDINGS**

SYMPTOMS AND SIGNS

- Asymptomatic, with incidentally found cytopenias
- Fatigue, infection, or bleeding is related to bone marrow failure
- Wasting, fever, weight loss
- Pallor
- Bleeding
- Signs of infection

DIFFERENTIAL DIAGNOSIS

- AML (≥ 20% blasts)
- Aplastic anemia
- Anemic of chronic disease
- Vitamin B_{12} or folate deficiency

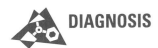 **DIAGNOSIS**

LABORATORY TESTS

- Anemia may be marked
- Mean cell volume is normal or increased
- Peripheral blood smear may show macro-ovalocytes
- White blood cell count usually normal or reduced; neutropenia is common
- Neutrophils may exhibit morphologic abnormalities, including deficient numbers of granules, or bilobed nucleus (Pelger-Huet anomaly)
- Myeloid series may be left shifted with small numbers of promyelocytes or blasts
- Platelet count is normal or reduced; hypogranular platelets may be present

DIAGNOSTIC PROCEDURES

- Bone marrow aspirate and biopsy are characteristically hypercellular, but it may be hypocellular
- Signs of abnormal erythropoiesis include
  - Megaloblastic features
  - Nuclear budding
  - Multinucleated erythroid precursors
- Prussian blue stain may demonstrate ringed sideroblasts
- Myeloid series is often left shifted with variable increases in blasts
- Deficient or abnormal myeloid granules may be seen
- A characteristic abnormality is dwarf megakaryocytes with unilobed nucleus
- Cytogenetics may be abnormal

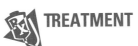 **TREATMENT**

MEDICATIONS

- Erythropoietin, 30,000 U SQ weekly, reduces red blood cell transfusion requirement in 20%
- The combination of high-dose erythropoietin and myeloid growth factors produces higher response rate, but the cost is very high
- Lenolidomide
  - Recommended initial dose is 10 mg/day
  - Approved for treatment of transfusion-dependent anemia due to myelodysplasia
  - Effective in patients with the 5q-cytogenetic abnormality
  - Most common side effects are neutropenia and thrombocytopenia, but venous thrombosis are also seen
  - Cost is extremely high, and it is not effective either for cell lines other than red blood cells or for patients with increased blasts
- Patients affected primarily with severe neutropenia may benefit from the use of myeloid growth factors such as G-CSF
- Azacitidine (5-azacytidine) improves both symptoms and blood counts and prolongs time to conversion to acute leukemia
- Decitabine can produce similar responses

THERAPEUTIC PROCEDURES

- Red blood cell transfusions are indicated for severe anemia
- Allogeneic stem cell transplantation
  - Only curative therapy for myelodysplasia
  - Role is limited by advanced age of many patients and indolent course of disease

 OUTCOME

COMPLICATIONS

- Infection and bleeding

PROGNOSIS

- Myelodysplasia is ultimately fatal, most commonly because of infections or bleeding
- Risk of transformation to AML depends on the percentage of blasts in bone marrow
- Patients with refractory anemia without excess blasts may survive many years, with low risk of leukemia (< 10%)
- Patients with excess blasts or CMML have short survivals (usually < 2 years) and higher (20–50%) risk of developing acute leukemia
- Deletions of chromosomes 5 and 7 associated with poor prognosis
- Cure rates of allogeneic transplantation are 30–60%, depending on risk status of disease
- International Prognostic Scoring System (IPSS) classifies patients by risk status based on
  - Percentage of bone marrow blasts
  - Cytogenetics
  - Severity of cytopenias

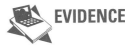 **EVIDENCE**

PRACTICE GUIDELINES

- Bowen D et al. Guidelines for the diagnosis and therapy of adult myelodysplastic syndromes. Br J Haematol. 2003;120:187. [PMID: 12542475]
- Greenberg PL et al. NCCN Myelodysplastic Syndromes Practice Guidelines

Panel. National Comprehensive Cancer Network: Myelodysplastic Syndromes v.1.2005

WEB SITE

- National Cancer Institute: Myelodysplastic Syndromes: Treatment

INFORMATION FOR PATIENTS

- American Cancer Society: Myelodysplastic Syndrome
- Leukemia & Lymphoma Society: Detailed Guide: Myelodysplastic Syndrome
- National Cancer Institute: Myelodysplastic Syndromes: Treatment

REFERENCES

- Cortes J et al. Phase I study of BMS-214662, a farnesyl transferase inhibitor in patients with acute leukemias and high-risk myelodysplastic syndromes. J Clin Oncol. 2005 Apr 20;23(12):2805–12. [PMID: 15728224]
- Ho AY et al. Reduced-intensity allogeneic hematopoietic stem cell transplantation for myelodysplastic syndrome and acute myeloid leukemia with multilineage dysplasia using fludarabine, busulphan, and alemtuzumab (FBC) conditioning. Blood. 2004 Sep 15; 104(6):1616–23. [PMID: 15059843]
- Jädersten M et al. Long-term outcome of treatment of anemia in MDS with erythropoietin and G-CSF. Blood. 2005 Aug 1;106(3):803–11. [PMID: 15840690]
- List A et al. Efficacy of lenalidomide in myelodysplastic syndromes. N Engl J Med. 2005 Feb 10;352(6):549–57. [PMID: 15703420]
- Schiffer CA. Clinical issues in the management of patients with myelodysplasia. Hematology Am Soc Hematol Educ Program. 2006:205–10. [PMID: 17124062]

Myocarditis

KEY FEATURES

- Focal or diffuse inflammation of the myocardium
- Primary causes: acute viral infection or postviral immune response
- Secondary causes
  - Nonviral pathogens, such as bacterial, rickettsial, spirochetal, fungal, or parasitic
  - Toxins, drugs (especially cocaine)
  - Immunologic disorders (eg, systemic lupus erythematosus)
- Many cases resolve spontaneously
- In other cases, cardiac function deteriorates progressively and may lead to dilated cardiomyopathy

CLINICAL FINDINGS

- Onset: several days to a few weeks after onset of an acute febrile illness or respiratory infection
- Congestive heart failure: gradual or abrupt and fulminant
- Symptoms: chest pain (pleuritic or nonspecific), dyspnea
- Physical examination
  - Tachycardia
  - Gallop rhythm
  - Edema
  - Conduction defect
- Emboli due to procoagulant effect of cytokines, decreased myocardial contractility, and blood pooling

DIAGNOSIS

- Elevated white blood count, erythrocyte sedimentation rate, troponin I (in 33%), CK-MB (in 10%)
- ECG
  - Sinus tachycardia
  - Ventricular ectopy
  - Nonspecific repolarization changes
  - Intraventricular conduction delay
  - Occasionally, ST-T changes may mimic acute myocardial infarction
- Chest radiograph: nonspecific, cardiomegaly is common, pulmonary venous hypertension, even pulmonary edema
- Echocardiogram: cardiomegaly and contractile dysfunction
- Myocardial biopsy, although not sensitive, may reveal a characteristic inflammatory pattern

TREATMENT

- Specific antimicrobial therapy for any identified infectious agent
- Immunosuppressive agents for acute (< 6 mo) myocarditis only if myocardial

biopsy suggests ongoing inflammation; however, most agents are ineffective
- Supportive care is important (including the use of left ventricular assist devices)
- Otherwise, treat heart failure and arrhythmias
- Evaluation for cardiac transplantation

Myopathies Dermatomyositis & Polymyositis

KEY FEATURES

ESSENTIALS OF DIAGNOSIS

- Bilateral proximal muscle weakness
- Characteristic cutaneous manifestations in dermatomyositis (Gottron's papules, heliotrope rash)
- Diagnostic tests: elevated creatine kinase, muscle biopsy, electromyography
- Increased risk of malignancy, particularly in dermatomyositis

GENERAL CONSIDERATIONS

- An autoimmune disease of unknown cause characterized primarily by inflammation of muscles
- Five clinically defined subsets
  - Juvenile dermatomyositis
  - Dermatomyositis
  - Polymyositis
  - Myositis associated with malignancy
  - Myositis associated with another connective tissue disease (especially systemic lupus erythematosus [SLE])
- Disorders of the peripheral and central nervous systems (eg, chronic inflammatory polyneuropathy, multiple sclerosis, myasthenia gravis, Eaton-Lambert disease, and amyotrophic lateral sclerosis)
  - Can produce weakness
  - However, they are distinguished from inflammatory myopathies by characteristic symptoms and neurologic signs and often by distinctive electromyographic abnormalities
- Inclusion body myositis can mimic polymyositis but is less responsive to treatment and has different epidemiologic features
- Patients with polymyalgia rheumatica are over the age of 50 and—in contrast

to patients with polymyositis—have pain but no objective weakness

- Malignancies most commonly associated with dermatomyositis in descending order of frequency
  – Ovarian
  – Lung
  – Pancreatic
  – Stomach
  – Colorectal
  – Non-Hodgkins lymphoma

DEMOGRAPHICS

- Peak incidence: fifth and sixth decades
- Women are affected twice as commonly as men
- The typical inclusion body myositis patient is white, male, and over age 50

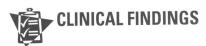 **CLINICAL FINDINGS**

SYMPTOMS AND SIGNS

- Gradual and progressive muscle weakness of the proximal muscle groups of the upper and lower extremities
- Leg weakness (eg, difficulty in rising from a chair or climbing stairs) typically precedes arm symptoms
- No facial or ocular muscle weakness
- Pain and tenderness of affected muscles (25%)

In dermatomyositis

- The characteristic rash is dusky red and may appear in malar distribution mimicking the classic rash of SLE
- Erythema also occurs over other areas of the face, neck, shoulders, and upper chest and back ("shawl sign")
- Periorbital edema and a purplish (heliotrope) suffusion over the eyelids are typical signs
- Periungual erythema, dilations of nail-bed capillaries, and scaly patches over the dorsum of proximal interphalangeal and metacarpophalangeal joints (Gottron's sign) are highly suggestive
- A subset of patients with polymyositis and dermatomyositis develops the "anti-synthetase syndrome," a group of findings including
  – Inflammatory arthritis
  – Raynaud's phenomenon
  – Interstitial lung disease
  – Often, severe muscle disease associated with certain autoantibodies (eg, anti-Jo-1 antibodies)

DIFFERENTIAL DIAGNOSIS

Muscle inflammation

- Polymyositis
- Dermatomyositis
- SLE
- Scleroderma
- Sjögren's syndrome
- Inclusion body myositis
- Trichinosis

Other causes of proximal muscle weakness

- Polymyalgia rheumatica
- Endocrine
  – Hypothyroidism
  – Hyperthyroidism
  – Cushing's syndrome
- Alcoholism
- Drugs
  – Corticosteroids
  – Statins
  – Clofibrate
  – Colchicine
  – Chloroquine
  – Emetine
  – Aminocaproic acid
  – Bretylium
  – Penicillamine
  – Drugs causing hypokalemia
- HIV myopathy
- Hyperparathyroidism
- Spinal stenosis
- Osteomalacia
- Mitochondrial myopathy

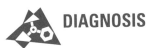 **DIAGNOSIS**

LABORATORY TESTS

- Serum levels of muscle enzymes, especially creatine kinase and aldolase, are elevated
- Antinuclear antibodies are present in many patients, and anti-Jo-1 antibodies are seen in the subset of patients that has associated interstitial lung disease
- CA-125 levels (and pelvic ultrasonography) may be useful in women, given the strong association of ovarian carcinoma and dermatomyositis

DIAGNOSTIC PROCEDURES

- Biopsy of clinically involved muscle is the only specific diagnostic test
- The pathologic findings in polymyositis and dermatomyositis are distinct, although both include lymphoid inflammatory infiltrates
- Electromyographic abnormalities consisting of polyphasic potentials, fibrillations,

and high-frequency action potentials are helpful in establishing the diagnosis. None of the studies is specific

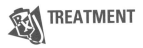 **TREATMENT**

MEDICATIONS

- Most patients respond to corticosteroids
  – 40–60 mg or more of oral prednisone is required initially daily
  – The dose is then adjusted downward according to the response of sequentially observed serum levels of muscle enzymes
- In patients resistant or intolerant to corticosteroids, therapy with methotrexate or azathioprine may be helpful
- Hydroxychloroquine (200–400 mg/day orally not to exceed 6.5 mg/kg) can help ameliorate skin disease

THERAPEUTIC PROCEDURES

- Limit sun exposure for patients with rash of dermatomyositis

 OUTCOME

FOLLOW-UP

- Up to one patient in four with dermatomyositis has an occult malignancy that may not be detected until months afterward in some cases
- Search for an occult malignancy should include age- and risk-appropriate cancer screening tests
- If these evaluations are unrevealing, then a more invasive or extensive laboratory evaluation is probably not cost effective

COMPLICATIONS

- Hypercapnea and respiratory failure can develop from weakness of respiratory muscles
- Rhabdomyolysis with renal failure can complicate very severe muscle inflammation

PROGNOSIS

- Patients with an associated neoplasm have a poor prognosis
  – However, remission may follow treatment of the tumor
  – Corticosteroids may or may not be effective in these patients

WHEN TO REFER

- Refer to a rheumatologist if respiratory weakness or rhabdomyolysis develops

WHEN TO ADMIT

- Admit for airway protection and urgent treatment if weakness of respiratory muscles develops
- Admit for rhabdomyolysis

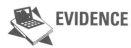

EVIDENCE

WEB SITE

- The Myositis Association

INFORMATION FOR PATIENTS

- American Academy of Orthopaedic Surgeons
- Arthritis Foundation

REFERENCES

- Callen JP et al. Dermatomyositis. Clin Dermatol. 2006 Sep–Oct;24(5):363–73. [PMID: 16966018]
- Troyanov Y et al. Novel classification of idiopathic inflammatory myopathies based on overlap syndrome features and autoantibodies: analysis of 100 French Canadian patients. Medicine (Baltimore). 2005 Jul;84(4):231–49. [PMID: 16010208]
- Ytterberg SR. Treatment of refractory polymyositis and dermatomyositis. Curr Rheumatol Rep. 2006 Jun;8(3):167–73. [PMID: 16901073]

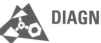

Myotonic Dystrophy

KEY FEATURES

- A slowly progressive, dominantly inherited myopathic disorder
- Usually manifests itself in the third or fourth decade but occasionally appears early in childhood
- The genetic defect has been localized to the long arm of chromosome 19 in the type-1 disorder

CLINICAL FINDINGS

- Complaints of muscle stiffness
- Marked delay occurs before affected muscles can relax after a contraction; this can often be demonstrated clinically by delayed relaxation of the hand after sustained grip or by percussion of the belly of a muscle
- Weakness and wasting of the facial, sternocleidomastoid, and distal limb muscles
- Cataracts
- Frontal baldness
- Testicular atrophy
- Diabetes mellitus
- Cardiac abnormalities
- Intellectual changes

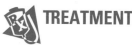

DIAGNOSIS

- Electromyography of affected muscles reveals myotonic discharges in addition to changes suggestive of myopathy

TREATMENT

- Phenytoin, 100 mg PO TID; quinine sulfate, 300–400 mg PO TID; or procainamide, 0.5–1.0 g PO QID
- Phenytoin is preferred because the other drugs may have undesirable effects on cardiac conduction
- Tocainide and mexiletine have also been used
- Neither the weakness nor the course of the disorder is influenced by treatment

Nausea & Vomiting

KEY FEATURES

ESSENTIALS OF DIAGNOSIS

- Nausea is a vague, intensely disagreeable sensation of sickness or "queasiness"
- Distinguished from anorexia
- Retching (spasmodic respiratory and abdominal movements) often follows
- Vomiting may or may not follow
- Vomiting should be distinguished from regurgitation, the effortless reflux of liquid or solid (food) stomach contents

GENERAL CONSIDERATIONS

- May be caused by wide variety of conditions that stimulate the vagal afferent receptors, the brainstem vomiting center, or the chemoreceptor trigger zone (Table 36)
- May lead to serious complications, including electrolyte disturbances (hypokalemia, metabolic alkalosis), dehydration, aspiration pneumonia, Mallory-Weiss tear, and esophageal rupture

CLINICAL FINDINGS

SYMPTOMS AND SIGNS

- Acute symptoms without abdominal pain suggest food poisoning, infectious gastroenteritis, or drugs
- Acute pain with vomiting suggests peritoneal irritation, acute gastric or intestinal obstruction, or pancreaticobiliary disease
- Persistent vomiting suggests pregnancy, gastric outlet obstruction, gastroparesis, intestinal dysmotility, psychogenic disorders, and CNS or systemic disorders
- Vomiting immediately after meals suggests bulimia or psychogenic causes
- Vomiting of undigested food suggests gastroparesis or a gastric outlet obstruction; physical examination reveals a succussion splash
- Inquire about neurologic symptoms such as
  - Headaches
  - Stiff neck
  - Vertigo
  - Focal paresthesias or weakness

DIFFERENTIAL DIAGNOSIS

- Visceral afferent stimulation (Table 36)
  - Infections
  - Mechanical obstruction

- Dysmotility
- Peritoneal irritation
- Hepatobiliary or pancreatic disorders
- Topical GI irritants
- Postoperative
- CNS disorders
  - Vestibular disorders
  - Increased intracranial pressure
  - Migraine
  - Infections
  - Psychogenic
- Irritation of chemoreceptor trigger zone
  - Antitumor chemotherapy
  - Drugs and medications
  - Radiation therapy
  - Systemic disorders

DIAGNOSIS

LABORATORY TESTS

- Serum electrolytes
- Serum glucose
- Serum creatinine
- Serum calcium
- Serum amylase
- Liver enzymes
- Thyroid-stimulating hormone
- Urine or serum pregnancy test

IMAGING STUDIES

- Flat and upright abdominal radiographs
- Ultrasound or CT scan of abdomen
- Barium upper GI series
- Nuclear scintigraphic study for gastroparesis

DIAGNOSTIC PROCEDURES

- Nasogastric tube suction for patients with vomiting due to
  - GI obstruction
  - Gastroparesis
  - Ileus
  - Peritonitis
- Saline load test
  - Formerly used to distinguish gastric outlet obstruction from delayed gastric emptying
  - Seldom used in era of endoscopy
- Upper endoscopy

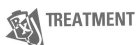

TREATMENT

MEDICATIONS

- Antiemetic medications (Table 37) given to control vomiting
- Combinations of drugs from different classes may provide better control

- Avoid antiemetic medications in pregnancy

THERAPEUTIC PROCEDURES

- For mild, self-limited, acute vomiting
  - No specific treatment
  - Clear liquids and small quantities of dry foods
- For moderate to severe vomiting
  - Nothing by mouth
  - Give IV saline 0.45% solution with 20 mEq/L of potassium chloride
- Nasogastric suction for gastric decompression in patients with
  - GI obstruction
  - Ileus or gastroparesis
  - Peritonitis

OUTCOME

COMPLICATIONS

- Dehydration
- Hypokalemia
- Metabolic alkalosis
- Aspiration
- Rupture of the esophagus (Boerhaave's syndrome)
- Bleeding secondary to a mucosal tear at the gastroesophageal junction (Mallory-Weiss syndrome)

WHEN TO ADMIT

- Hospitalize patient who has severe acute vomiting for rehydration, evaluation, and specific therapy

PREVENTION

- Antiemetic medications (especially 5-HT$_3$ antagonists) can be given to prevent vomiting in patients undergoing chemotherapy and abdominal surgery

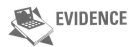

EVIDENCE

INFORMATION FOR PATIENTS

- American Academy of Family Physicians
- National Digestive Diseases Information Clearinghouse

REFERENCES

- Carlisle JB et al. Drugs for preventing postoperative nausea and vomiting. Cochrane Database Syst Rev. 2006 Jul 19;3:CD004125. [PMID: 16856030]
- Kris MG et al. American Society of Clinical Oncology guideline for chemo-

therapy-induced nausea or vomiting. J Clin Oncol. 2006 Jun 20;24(18):2932–47. [PMID: 16717289]

- Sharma R et al. Management of chemotherapy-induced nausea, vomiting, oral mucositis, and diarrhoea. Lancet Oncol. 2005 Feb;6(2):93–102. [PMID: 15683818]

Neck Masses

KEY FEATURES

ESSENTIALS OF DIAGNOSIS

- Rapid growth and tenderness suggest an inflammatory process
- Firm, painless, and slowly enlarging masses are often neoplastic

GENERAL CONSIDERATIONS

- **Neck masses in young adults**
  - Most neck masses are benign
    □ Branchial cleft cyst
    □ Thyroglossal duct cyst
    □ Reactive lymphadenitis
  - However, malignancy should always be considered
    □ Lymphoma
    □ Metastatic thyroid carcinoma
- Lymphadenopathy is common in HIV-positive individuals, but a growing or dominant mass may well represent lymphoma
- **Neck masses in adults over 40**
  - Cancer is the most common cause of persistent neck mass
  - A metastasis from squamous cell carcinoma (SCC) arising within the mouth, pharynx, larynx, or upper esophagus should be suspected, especially if there is a history of tobacco or significant alcohol use
- An enlarged node unassociated with an obvious infection should be further evaluated, especially if the patient has a history of smoking or alcohol use or a history of cancer

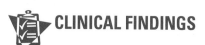

CLINICAL FINDINGS

SYMPTOMS AND SIGNS

Congenital lesions

- Branchial cleft cysts
  - Soft cystic mass on anterior border of sternocleidomastoid muscle; present with sudden swelling or infection at age 10–30
  - First branchial cleft cysts present just below ear; fistulous connection with external auditory canal floor may occur
  - Second branchial cleft cysts more common; may communicate with tonsillar fossa
  - Third branchial cleft cysts rare; may communicate with piriform sinus
- Thyroglossal duct cysts
  - Most common at age < 20
  - Midline neck mass, often just below hyoid bone, that moves on swallowing

Reactive lymphadenopathy

- Tender enlargement of neck nodes caused by pharynx, salivary gland, and scalp or HIV infection

Tuberculous and nontuberculous mycobacterial lymphadenitis

- Single or matted nodes
- Can drain externally (scrofula)

Neoplastic

- In older adults, 80% of firm, persistent, enlarging neck masses are metastases
- Most metastases arise from SCC of upper aerodigestive tract
- Complete head and neck examination indicated
- Other than thyroid carcinoma, non-squamous cell metastases to neck are infrequent
- Except for lung and breast tumors, non-head and neck tumors seldom metastasize to middle or upper neck
- Except for renal cell carcinoma, infradiaphragmatic tumors rarely metastasize to neck

Lymphoma

- About 10% present in head and neck
- A growing concern in AIDS patients
- Multiple rubbery nodes, especially in young adults

DIFFERENTIAL DIAGNOSIS

- Reactive lymphadenopathy
- Lymphoma
- Skin abscess
- Parotitis
- Goiter
- Thyroiditis, thyroid carcinoma
- Branchial cleft or thyroglossal duct cyst
- SCC of upper aerodigestive tract
- Sarcoidosis
- Autoimmune adenopathy
- Kikuchi's disease

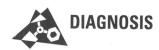

DIAGNOSIS

IMAGING STUDIES

- An MRI or PET scan before open biopsy may yield valuable information about a possible presumed primary site or another site for fine-needle aspiration (FNA) biopsy

DIAGNOSTIC PROCEDURES

- Common indications for FNA biopsy of a node include persistence or continued enlargement, particularly if an obvious primary tumor is not obvious on physical examination

Tuberculous and nontuberculous mycobacterial lymphadenitis

- FNA is usually the best initial diagnostic approach: send specimens for cytology, smear for acid-fast bacilli, culture and sensitivity, and polymerase chain reaction (PCR), as indicated

Infectious, inflammatory, and neoplastic neck masses

- Examination under anesthesia with direct laryngoscopy, esophagoscopy, or bronchoscopy is usually required to fully evaluate the tumor and exclude second primaries

Lymphoma

- FNA may be diagnostic, but open biopsy is often required

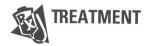

TREATMENT

SURGERY

Branchial cleft cysts

- To prevent recurrent infection and possible carcinoma, branchial cleft cysts should be completely excised, along with their fistulous tracts

Thyroglossal duct cysts

- Surgical excision is recommended to prevent recurrent infection

Reactive cervical lymphadenopathy

- Except for the occasional node that suppurates and requires incision and drainage, treatment is directed against the underlying infection

Infectious, inflammatory, and neoplastic neck masses

- Treat the underlying pathology

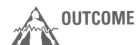

OUTCOME

PROGNOSIS

- Prognosis is that of the underlying pathology

WHEN TO REFER

- When the diagnosis is in question or for specialized treatment, particularly for a malignancy

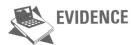

EVIDENCE

PRACTICE GUIDELINES

- Forastiere AA et al. NCCN Head and Neck Cancers Practice Guidelines Panel. National Comprehensive Cancer Network: Head and Neck Cancers v.1.2005.
- Sherman SI et al. NCCN Thyroid Carcinoma Practice Guidelines Panel. National Comprehensive Cancer Network: Thyroid Carcinoma v.1.2005.

WEB SITES

- Baylor College of Medicine Otolaryngology Resources
- Lymphoma of the Head and Neck Demonstration Case

INFORMATION FOR PATIENTS

- Mayo Clinic: Swollen Lymph Glands
- MedlinePlus: Branchial Cleft Cyst
- MedlinePlus: Neck Lump
- National Cancer Institute: Head and Neck Cancer: Q & A

REFERENCES

- Briggs RD. Cystic metastasis versus branchial cleft carcinoma: a diagnostic challenge. Laryngoscope. 2002 Jun; 112(6):1010–4. [PMID: 12160265]
- Enepekides DJ. Management of congenital anomalies of the neck. Facial Plast Surg Clin North Am. 2001 Feb; 9(1):131–45. [PMID: 11465000]
- Schwetschenau E et al. The adult neck mass. Am Fam Physician. 2002 Sep 1; 66(5):831–8. [PMID: 12322776]

Neck Pain

KEY FEATURES

ESSENTIALS OF DIAGNOSIS

- Most chronic neck pain is caused by degenerative joint disease and responds to conservative approaches

GENERAL CONSIDERATIONS

- A large group of articular and extra-articular disorders is characterized by pain that may involve simultaneously the neck, shoulder girdle, and upper extremity
- Diagnostic differentiation among these disorders may be difficult

Etiology

- Cervical strain is generally caused by mechanical postural disorders, overexertion, or injury (eg, whiplash)
- Cervical spondylosis (degenerative arthritis) is a collective term describing degenerative changes that occur in the apophysial joints and intervertebral disk joints, with or without neurologic signs

DEMOGRAPHICS

- Degeneration of cervical disks and joints may occur in adolescents but is more common after age 40

CLINICAL FINDINGS

SYMPTOMS AND SIGNS

- Pain may be limited to the posterior neck region or, depending on the level of the symptomatic joint, may radiate segmentally to the occiput, anterior chest, shoulder girdle, arm, forearm, and hand
- Radiating pain in the upper extremity is often intensified by hyperextension of the neck and deviation of the head to the involved side
- Limitation of cervical movements is the most common objective finding
- Neurologic signs depend on the extent of compression of nerve roots or the spinal cord
- Compression of the spinal cord may cause long-tract involvement resulting in paraparesis or paraplegia

Acute or chronic cervical musculotendinous strain

- Acute episodes are associated with pain, decreased cervical spine motion, and paraspinal muscle spasm, resulting in stiffness of the neck and loss of motion
- Local tenderness is often present in acute but not chronic strain

Herniated nucleus pulposus

- Rupture or prolapse of the nucleus pulposus of the cervical disks into the spinal canal causes pain that radiates to the arms at the level of C6–C7
- When intra-abdominal pressure is increased by coughing, sneezing, or other movements, symptoms are aggravated, and cervical muscle spasm may often occur
- Neurologic abnormalities may include decreased reflexes of the deep tendons of the biceps and triceps and decreased sensation and muscle atrophy or weakness in the forearm or hand

Arthritic disorders

- Osteoarthritis of the cervical spine is often asymptomatic but may cause diffuse neck pain, radicular pain, or myelopathy
- Myelopathy develops insidiously and is manifested by numb, clumsy hands
- Some patients also complain of unsteady walking, urinary frequency and urgency, or electrical shock sensations with neck flexion or extension (Lhermitte's sign)
- Weakness, sensory loss, and spasticity with exaggerated reflexes develop below the level of spinal cord compression

DIFFERENTIAL DIAGNOSIS

- Acute or chronic cervical musculotendinous strain
- Herniated nucleus pulposus
- Degenerative arthritides (eg, osteoarthritis)
- Inflammatory arthritides (eg, rheumatoid arthritis, ankylosing spondylitis)
- Infections (eg, meningitis, osteomyelitis)
- Cancer (eg, cervical spine metastases)
- Fibromyalgia

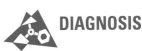

DIAGNOSIS

IMAGING STUDIES

- Radiographs are often normal in an acute cervical strain
- In osteoarthritis, comparative reduction in height of the involved disk space is a frequent finding. The most common late radiographic finding is osteophyte formation
- Use of MRI or CT is indicated in the patient who has severe pain of unknown cause that fails to respond to conserva-

tive therapy or in the patient who has evidence of myelopathy

- MRI is more sensitive than CT in detecting disk disease, extradural compression, and intramedullary cord disease
- CT is more sensitive for demonstration of fractures

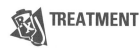 **TREATMENT**

MEDICATIONS

Acute or chronic cervical musculotendinous strain

- Analgesics and early mobilization (including whiplash)

Herniated nucleus pulposus

- Cervical traction, bed rest, and analgesics are usually successful for pain and radicular symptoms
- Cervical epidural corticosteroid injections may help those who fail to improve

SURGERY

- Surgery is indicated for unremitting pain and progressive weakness from a herniated nucleus pulposus despite a full trial of conservative therapy and if a surgically correctable abnormality is identified by MRI or CT myelography. Surgical decompression achieves excellent results in 70–80% of such patients
- Surgical treatment may involve stabilization of the cervical spine when atlanto-axial subluxation occurs in patients with rheumatoid arthritis

THERAPEUTIC PROCEDURES

- Chronic pain in the zygapophysial joints resulting from whiplash injuries may benefit from percutaneous radiofrequency neurotomy

 OUTCOME

COMPLICATIONS

- Progressive degenerative disease of the cervical spine can cause cervical myelopathy with weakness and spasticity of the legs
- Serious erosive disease of joints may lead to neurologic complications as sometimes occurs in rheumatoid arthritis and occasionally in ankylosing spondylitis; the usual joint involved in these disorders is the atlantoaxial joint (C1–C2)

WHEN TO REFER

- Refer to a neurosurgeon for indications described under Surgery

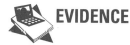 **EVIDENCE**

PRACTICE GUIDELINES

- Gross AR et al. Clinical practice guideline on the use of manipulation or mobilization in the treatment of adults with mechanical neck disorders. Man Ther. 2002;7:193. [PMID: 12419654]

INFORMATION FOR PATIENTS

- American Academy of Orthopedic Surgeons
- American Physical Therapy Association

REFERENCES

- Hendriks EJ et al. Prognostic factors for poor recovery in acute whiplash patients. Pain. 2005 Apr;114(3):408–16. [PMID: 15777866]
- Kaiser MG. Multilevel cervical spondylosis. Neurosurg Clin N Am. 2006 Jul;17(3):263–75. [PMID: 16876027]
- Peloso PM et al. Medicinal and injection therapies for mechanical neck disorders: a Cochrane systematic review. J Rheumatol. 2006 May;33(5):957–67. [PMID: 16652427]

Neck Pain, Discogenic

 KEY FEATURES

ESSENTIALS OF DIAGNOSIS

- Neck pain, sometimes radiating to one or both arms
- Restricted neck movements
- Motor, sensory, or reflex changes in in one or both arms with root involvement
- Neurologic deficit in legs, gait disorder, or sphincter disturbance with cord involvement

GENERAL CONSIDERATIONS

Acute cervical disk protrusion

- Acute cervical disk protrusion leads to pain in the neck and radicular pain in the arm, exacerbated by head movement

Cervical spondylosis

- Results from
  - Chronic cervical disk degeneration, with herniation of disk material

- Secondary calcification
- Associated osteophytic outgrowths
- One or more of the cervical nerve roots may be compressed, stretched, or angulated
- Myelopathy may also develop as a result of
  - Compression
  - Vascular insufficiency
  - Recurrent minor trauma to the cord

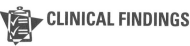 **CLINICAL FINDINGS**

SYMPTOMS AND SIGNS

Acute cervical disk protrusion

- With lateral disk herniation, motor, sensory, or reflex changes are in a radicular (usually C6 or C7) distribution on the affected side (Figure 9)
- With more centrally directed herniations, the spinal cord may also be involved, leading to spastic paraparesis and sensory disturbances in the legs, sometimes accompanied by impaired sphincter function

Cervical spondylosis

- Neck pain and restricted head movement, occipital headaches, radicular pain and other sensory disturbances in the arms, weakness of the arms or legs, or some combination of these symptoms
- Examination generally reveals that lateral flexion and rotation of the neck are limited
- A segmental pattern of weakness or dermatomal sensory loss (or both) may be found unilaterally or bilaterally in the upper limbs, and tendon reflexes mediated by the affected root or roots are depressed
- The C5 and C6 nerve roots are most commonly involved; then, examination frequently reveals
  - Weakness of muscles supplied by these roots (eg, deltoids, supraspinatus and infraspinatus, biceps, brachioradialis)
  - Pain or sensory loss about the shoulder and outer border of the arm and forearm
  - Depressed biceps and brachioradialis reflexes
- Spastic paraparesis may also be present if there is an associated myelopathy, sometimes accompanied by posterior column or spinothalamic sensory deficits in the legs

DIFFERENTIAL DIAGNOSIS

- Congenital abnormalities may involve the cervical spine and lead to neck pain

(eg, hemivertebrae, fused vertebrae, basilar impression, instability of the atlantoaxial joint)
- Traumatic, degenerative, infective, and neoplastic disorders may also lead to pain in the neck
- Spinal rheumatoid arthritis tends to affect especially the cervical region, leading to pain, stiffness, and reduced mobility; displacement of vertebrae or atlantoaxial subluxation may lead to cord compression that can be life-threatening if not treated by fixation

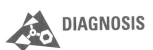 **DIAGNOSIS**

IMAGING STUDIES

Acute cervical disk protrusion
- The diagnosis is confirmed by MRI or CT myelography

Cervical spondylosis
- Plain radiographs of the cervical spine show
  - Osteophyte formation
  - Narrowing of disk spaces
  - Encroachment on the intervertebral foramina
- However, such changes are common in middle-aged persons and may be unrelated to the presenting complaint
- CT or MRI helps confirm the diagnosis and exclude other structural causes of the myelopathy

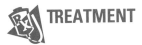 **TREATMENT**

SURGERY

Acute cervical disk protrusion
- If other measures are unsuccessful or the patient has a significant neurologic deficit, surgical removal of the protruding disk may be necessary

Cervical spondylosis
- Operative treatment may be necessary to prevent further progression if there is a significant neurologic deficit or if root pain is severe, persistent, and unresponsive to conservative measures

THERAPEUTIC PROCEDURES

Acute cervical disk protrusion
- In mild cases, bed rest or intermittent neck traction may help, followed by immobilization of the neck in a collar for several weeks

Cervical spondylosis
- Restriction of neck movements by a cervical collar may relieve pain

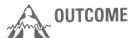 **OUTCOME**

PROGNOSIS
- Self-limited

WHEN TO REFER
- Ergonomic consultation may improve symptoms

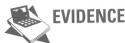 **EVIDENCE**

PRACTICE GUIDELINES
- Philadelphia Panel evidence-based clinical practice guidelines on selected rehabilitation interventions for neck pain. Phys Ther. 2001;81:1701. [PMID: 11589644]

INFORMATION FOR PATIENTS
- JAMA patient page. Neck injuries. JAMA. 2001;286:1928. [PMID: 11680473]
- American Academy of Orthopaedic Surgeons

REFERENCES
- Ahmed M et al. Neck and low back pain: neuroimaging. Neurol Clin. 2007 May; 25(2):439–71. [PMID: 17445738]
- Harris G. Managing musculoskeletal complaints with rehabilitation therapy: summary of the Philadelphia Panel evidence-based clinical practice guidelines on musculoskeletal rehabilitation interventions. J Fam Pract. 2002;51:1042. [PMID: 12540330]
- Jensen I et al. Strategies for prevention and management of musculoskeletal conditions. Neck pain. Best Pract Res Clin Rheumatol. 2007 Feb;21(1):93–108. [PMID: 17350546]
- Meleger AL et al. Neck and back pain: musculoskeletal disorders. Neurol Clin. 2007 May;25(2):419–38. [PMID: 17445737]
- Niemisto L. Radiofrequency denervation for neck and back pain. A systematic review of randomized controlled trials. Cochrane Database Syst Rev. 2003;CD004058. [PMID: 12535508]
- Peloso P et al; Cervical Overview Group. Medicinal and injection therapies for mechanical neck disorders. Cochrane Database Syst Rev. 2007 Jul 18;(3):CD000319. [PMID: 17636629]
- Polston DW. Cervical radiculopathy. Neurol Clin. 2007 May;25(2):373–85. [PMID: 17445734]

- Schonstein E. Work conditioning, work hardening and functional restoration for workers with back and neck pain. Cochrane Database Syst Rev. 2003; CD001822. [PMID: 12535416]
- Wieser ES et al. Surgery for neck pain. Neurosurgery. 2007 Jan;60(1 Suppl 1):S51-6. [PMID: 17204886]

Nephritis, Lupus

 KEY FEATURES

- Renal involvement is common in systemic lupus erythematosus (SLE), occurring in 35–90% of SLE patients

 CLINICAL FINDINGS

- History and physical examination consistent with SLE
- Urinalysis: hematuria and proteinuria

 DIAGNOSIS

- Renal biopsy shows one of five histologic patterns
  - Type I: normal
  - Type II: mesangial proliferative
  - Type III: focal and segmental proliferative
  - Type IV: diffuse proliferative
  - Type V: membranous nephropathy
- These are further classified as acute or chronic and global or segmental, both of which seem to have prognostic value

TREATMENT

- No treatment required for types I and II
- Immunosuppressive therapy with corticosteroids and cytotoxic agents for extensive type III lesions and all type IV lesions
- Indications for treatment of type V disease are unclear
- Corticosteroids: methylprednisolone, 1 g IV once daily for 3 days, followed by prednisone, 60 mg PO once daily for 4–6 weeks
- Cytotoxic agents: cyclophosphamide, IV every month for 6 doses and then every 3 mo for 6 doses

- Cyclosporine useful
- Mycophenolate mofetil may be helpful
- Monitoring serum creatinine; dsDNA antibodies; C3, C4, and CH50; urinary protein; and sediment can be useful during treatment
- Renal transplantation, but recurrent renal disease occurs in 8% of cases

Nephropathy, Diabetic

 KEY FEATURES

- Most common cause of end-stage renal disease in United States
- Type 1 diabetes mellitus imposes a 30–40% risk of nephropathy after 20 years
- Type 2 imposes a 15–20% risk after 20 years
- Males, African Americans, and Native Americans are at higher risk

 CLINICAL FINDINGS

- Diabetic retinopathy is often present
- Microalbuminuria develops within 10–15 years after onset of diabetes and progresses over the next 3–7 years to overt proteinuria
- Kidney size usually normal to large on renal ultrasound

 DIAGNOSIS

- Increase in glomerular filtration rate (GFR) at onset
- With the development of macroalbuminuria, GFR returns to normal and then to subnormal as nephropathy progresses
- Renal biopsy: most common lesion is diffuse glomerulosclerosis, but nodular glomerulosclerosis (Kimmelstiel-Wilson nodules) is pathognomonic

 TREATMENT

- Strict glycemic control and treatment of hypertension slow progression of diabetic nephropathy
- Angiotensin-converting enzyme inhibitors and angiotensin II receptor antagonists lower the rate of progression to clinical proteinuria and overt renal failure

Nephropathy, Immunoglobulin A

 KEY FEATURES

- Primary renal disease of IgA deposition in the glomerular mesangium
- Inciting cause unknown
- Associated with
  - Hepatic cirrhosis
  - Celiac disease
  - HIV infection
  - Cytomegalovirus infection
- Most common form of acute glomerulonephritis in United States
- Usually occurs in children and young adults
- Males affected 2–3 times more often than females

 CLINICAL FINDINGS

- Gross hematuria, frequently associated with an upper respiratory tract infection (50%), gastrointestinal symptoms (10%), or flu-like illness (15%)
- Urine becomes red or cola-colored 1–2 days after illness onset
- Asymptomatic microscopic hematuria may be found incidentally
- Hypertension
- Nephrotic syndrome possible

 DIAGNOSIS

- Persistent microscopic hematuria and proteinuria
- Serum creatinine and blood urea nitrogen sometimes elevated
- Serum IgA level is increased in < 50% of patients
- Serum complement levels usually normal
- Renal biopsy
  - Light microscopy shows focal glomerulonephritis with proliferation of mesangial cells
  - Immunofluorescence shows diffuse mesangial IgA, IgG, and C3 deposits
- Skin biopsy: granular deposits of IgA in dermal capillaries

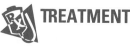 **TREATMENT**

- ~33% of patients experience spontaneous remission
- Chronic microscopic hematuria and stable serum creatinine in 50–60%; progressive renal insufficiency in 40–50%
- Prognosis worse if proteinuria > 1 g/day
- Angiotensin-converting enzyme inhibitors or angiotensin II receptor-blocking drugs to reduce blood pressure and proteinuria (Table 18)
- Methylprednisolone, 1 g/day IV for 3 days during months 1, 3, and 5, plus prednisone, 0.5 mg/kg every other day for 6 mo in nephrotic patients with glomerular filtration rate > 60–70 mL/min
- Fish oil, 2–5 g/day, debatable
- Renal transplantation

Nephrotic Syndrome

 KEY FEATURES

- Proteinuria > 3 g/day
- Albumin < 3 g/dL
- Edema
- Typically hyperlipidemia

 CLINICAL FINDINGS

- Peripheral edema with serum albumin < 3 g/dL
- Edema can become generalized
- Dyspnea caused by pulmonary edema, pleural effusions, and diaphragmatic compromise with ascites
- Abdominal distention from ascites
- Increased susceptibility to infection because of urinary loss of immunoglobulins and complement
- Hypercoagulable state, with renal vein thrombosis and venous thromboemboli, particularly in membranous nephropathy

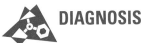

DIAGNOSIS

- Urinalysis: proteinuria; few cellular elements or casts
- Oval fat bodies appear as "grape clusters" under light microscopy and "Maltese crosses" under polarized light
- Serum albumin < 3 g/dL, serum protein < 6 g/dL
- Hyperlipidemia
- Elevated erythrocyte sedimentation rate
- Send serum complement levels, serum and urine protein electrophoresis, antinuclear antibodies, and serologic tests for hepatitis as indicated
- Renal biopsy indicated in adults with new-onset idiopathic nephrotic syndrome if a primary renal disease is suspected
- Renal biopsy useful for prognosis and treatment decisions
- Four most common lesions (Table 87)
  - Minimal change disease
  - Focal glomerular sclerosis
  - Membranous nephropathy
  - Membranoproliferative glomerulonephritis

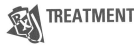

TREATMENT

- Protein intake should replace total daily urinary protein losses
- Salt and water restriction for edema
- Loop and thiazide diuretics in combination
- Antilipidemic agents
- Corticosteroids, cytotoxic agents as indicated for primary renal lesion
- Warfarin in patients with thrombosis for at least 3–6 mo

Neuroleptic Malignant Syndrome

KEY FEATURES

- A catatonia-like state manifested by
  - Extrapyramidal signs
  - Blood pressure changes
  - Altered consciousness
  - Hyperpyrexia
- Uncommon complication of neuroleptic treatment
- Comorbid affective disorder as well as concomitant lithium use may increase risk
- In most cases, occurs within 2 weeks of starting neuroleptic agent

CLINICAL FINDINGS

- Muscle rigidity, involuntary movements, confusion, dysarthria, dysphagia
- Pallor, cardiovascular instability, pulmonary congestion, diaphoresis
- Can result in stupor, coma, death

DIAGNOSIS

- Elevated creatinine kinase and leukocytosis with left shift in 50% of cases

TREATMENT

- Control of fever and IV fluid support
- Bromocriptine, 2.5–10.0 mg TID, and amantadine, 100–200 mg BID, are useful
- Dantrolene, 50 mg IV PRN to maximum of 10 mg/kg/day, can alleviate rigidity
- Electroconvulsive therapy has been used in resistant cases
- Clozapine has been used safely in patients with a history of neuroleptic malignant syndrome

Nipple Discharge

KEY FEATURES

- Common causes in the nonlactating breast
  - Duct ectasia
  - Intraductal papilloma
  - Carcinoma
- Factors to be assessed by history and physical examination
  - Nature of discharge (serous, bloody, or other)
  - Discharge associated with a mass
  - Unilateral or bilateral discharge
  - Single or multiple duct discharge
  - Discharge is spontaneous (persistent or intermittent) or must be expressed
  - Discharge is produced by pressure at a single site or by general pressure on breast
  - Relationship of discharge to menses
  - Premenopausal or postmenopausal patient
  - Patient taking oral contraceptives or estrogen

CLINICAL FINDINGS

- Unilateral, spontaneous serous, or serosanguineous discharge from a single duct caused by
  - Intraductal papilloma (usually)
  - Intraductal cancer (rarely)
- Bloody discharge is worrisome for malignancy
- Fibrocystic condition in premenopausal women characterized by
  - Spontaneous, brown or green discharge
  - From multiple ducts
  - Unilateral or bilateral
  - Most marked just before menstruation
- Milky discharge from multiple ducts occurs from
  - Hyperprolactinemia
  - Certain drugs (antipsychotics)
  - Fibrocystic condition
- A clear, serous, or milky discharge from single or multiple ducts
  - Can occur with oral contraceptives or estrogen replacement therapy
  - Disappears when patient stops taking drugs
  - Can be due to fibrocystic condition
  - More evident just before menstruation
- Purulent discharge may originate in a subareolar abscess

DIAGNOSIS

- If unilateral discharge from single duct, involved duct can be identified by pressure at different sites around nipple at margin of areola
- Cytologic examination of discharge for exfoliated cancer cells may rarely be helpful in determining diagnosis
- Check serum prolactin and thyroid-stimulating hormone levels if discharge is milky
- Mammography and ultrasound may be helpful if localization of lesion is not possible

- Differential diagnosis
  - Galactorrhea (eg, pregnancy, post-partum, hyperprolactinemia)
  - Mammary duct ectasia
  - Intraductal papilloma
  - Breast cancer
  - Oral contraceptives or estrogen replacement therapy
  - Fibrocystic condition
  - Subareolar abscess

 TREATMENT

- Any mass or, in the case of duct ectasia or intraductal papilloma, any involved duct should be excised
- Abscesses require drainage or removal along with the related lactiferous sinus
- When localization is not possible, no mass is palpable, and discharge is non-bloody, the patient should be reexamined every 6 mo for 1 yr, and mammography performed

Non-Hodgkin's Lymphoma

 KEY FEATURES

GENERAL CONSIDERATIONS

- Heterogeneous group of cancers of lymphocytes
- Clinical presentation and course vary from indolent to rapidly progressive
- Indolent lymphomas are often disseminated at diagnosis, and bone marrow involvement is frequent
- In Burkitt's lymphoma, a protoonco-gene c-*myc* is translocated from chromosome 8 to heavy chain locus on chromosome 14, where c-*myc* overexpression is likely related to malignant transformation
- In follicular lymphomas, the t(14,18) translocation is characteristic and results in overexpression of *bcl-2*, resulting in protection against apoptosis, the usual mechanism of cell death

REAL/WHO proposed classification of lymphomas

- B cell lymphomas
  - Precursor B cell lymphoblastic lymphoma
  - Small lymphocytic lymphoma/chronic lymphocytic leukemia
  - Marginal zone lymphomas: nodal marginal zone lymphoma, extranodal MALT, splenic
  - Hairy cell leukemia
  - Follicular lymphoma
  - Mantle cell lymphoma
  - Diffuse large B cell lymphoma
  - Burkitt's lymphoma
- T cell lymphomas
  - Anaplastic large cell lymphoma
  - Peripheral T cell lymphoma
  - Mycosis fungoides

 CLINICAL FINDINGS

SYMPTOMS AND SIGNS

- Painless lymphadenopathy, isolated or widespread (retroperitoneal, mesenteric, and pelvic)
- Constitutional symptoms, eg, fever, drenching night sweats, or weight loss
- Extranodal sites of disease (skin, gastrointestinal tract) sometimes found on examination
- Abdominal pain or abdominal fullness in Burkitt's lymphoma because of predilection for abdomen

DIFFERENTIAL DIAGNOSIS

- Hodgkin's disease
- Metastatic cancer
- Infectious mononucleosis
- Cat-scratch disease
- Sarcoidosis
- Drug-induced pseudolymphoma (eg, phenytoin)

DIAGNOSIS

LABORATORY TESTS

- Peripheral blood is usually normal, but some lymphomas may present in leukemic phase
- Cerebrospinal fluid cytology shows malignant cells in some high-grade lymphomas with meningeal involvement
- Serum lactate dehydrogenase (LDH) is a useful prognostic marker and is incorporated in risk stratification of treatment

IMAGING STUDIES

- Chest radiograph: mediastinal mass in lymphoblastic lymphoma, others
- CT scan of chest, abdomen, pelvis

DIAGNOSTIC PROCEDURES

- Needle aspiration biopsy may yield suspicious results, but lymph node biopsy (or biopsy of involved extranodal tissue) is required for diagnosis and staging
- Bone marrow involvement is manifested as paratrabecular lymphoid aggregates
- Staging after pathologic diagnosis involves
  - Chest radiograph and CT of abdomen and pelvis
  - Bone marrow biopsy
  - Lumbar puncture in selected cases with high-risk morphology

 TREATMENT

MEDICATIONS

- Follicular lymphoma may be initially treated in many ways, including
  - Rituximab
  - Rituximab plus fludarabine
  - Rituximab plus cyclophosphamide, vincristine and prednisone (R-CVP)
- Anti-idiotype vaccines are being studied as part of initial therapy
- Treatment for recurrent follicular lymphomas includes repeat of any of the initial strategies or radio-immunotherapy
- Intermediate-grade lymphoma (eg, diffuse large B cell) is treated initially with rituximab plus cyclophosphamide, doxorubicin, vincristine, and prednisone (R-CHOP)
- Localized diffuse large cell lymphoma is treated with short-course chemoimmunotherapy and local irradiation
- See Table 7

THERAPEUTIC PROCEDURES

- Most indolent lymphomas are disseminated at diagnosis
  - If lymphoma is not bulky and the patient is asymptomatic, no initial therapy is required
  - Spontaneous remission occurs in some
- Localized radiation therapy for patients who have localized follicular lymphoma (uncommon)
- Radioimmunoconjugates, eg, yttrium-90 ibritumomab, which fuse anti-B cell antibodies with radiation, may produce improved results compared with antibody alone
- Special forms of lymphoma require individualized therapy
  - Burkitt's lymphoma—very intensive chemotherapy
  - Lymphoblastic lymphoma—treated like acute lymphoblastic leukemia

– Mantle cell lymphoma—autologous stem cell transplantation in first remission

- Intensive initial therapy with autologous stem cell transplantation is the standard of care for relapsed large cell lymphoma
- Allogeneic transplantation for patients with clinically aggressive low-grade lymphomas
- Autologous stem cell transplantation early in course for high-risk lymphoma

OUTCOME

PROGNOSIS

- Median survival with follicular lymphomas has been 6–8 years; this appears to be improving
- For intermediate-grade lymphoma, the International Prognostic Index is widely used to categorize patients into prognostic groups
- Worse prognosis if age over 60, elevated serum LDH, stage III or stage IV disease, or poor performance status
- **0–1 risk factor**
  – 80% complete response rate to standard chemotherapy
  – Most responses (80%) durable
- **2 risk factors**
  – 70% complete response rate
  – 70% durable
- **> 2 risk factors**
  – Lower response rates and poor survival with standard regimens

– Early treatment with high-dose therapy and autologous stem cell transplantation may improve outcome

- With relapse after initial chemotherapy, if lymphoma still partially sensitive to chemotherapy, autologous transplantation offers 50% chance of long-term salvage

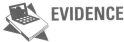

PRACTICE GUIDELINES

- Zelenetz AD et al; NCCN Non-Hodgkin's Lymphoma Practice Guidelines Panel. National Comprehensive Cancer Network: Non-Hodgkin's Lymphoma v.1.2005.

WEB SITE

- National Cancer Institute: Adult Non-Hodgkin's Lymphoma Treatment

INFORMATION FOR PATIENTS

- American Cancer Society
- Leukemia & Lymphoma Society
- National Cancer Institute

REFERENCES

- Abramson JS et al. Advances in the biology and therapy of diffuse large B-cell lymphoma: moving toward a molecularly targeted approach. Blood. 2005 Aug 15;106(4):1164–74. [PMID: 15855278]
- Dreyling M et al. Early consolidation by myeloablative radiochemotherapy followed by autologous stem cell transplantation in first remission significantly prolongs progression-free survival in mantle-cell lymphoma: results of a prospective randomized trial of the European MCL Network. Blood. 2005 Apr 1;105(7):2677–84. [PMID: 15591112]
- Feugier P et al. Long-term results of the R-CHOP study in the treatment of elderly patients with diffuse large B-cell lymphoma: a study by the Groupe d'Etude des Lymphomes de l'Adulte. J Clin Oncol. 2005 Jun 20;23(18):4117–26. [PMID: 15867204]
- Fisher RI et al. New treatment options have changed the survival of patients with follicular lymphoma. J Clin Oncol. 2005 Nov 20;23(33):8447–52. [PMID: 16230674]
- Marcus R et al. CVP chemotherapy plus rituximab compared with CVP as first-line treatment for advanced follicular lymphoma. Blood. 2005 Feb 15; 105(4):1417–23. [PMID: 15494430]
- Milpied N et al. Initial treatment of aggressive lymphoma with high-dose chemotherapy and autologous stem-cell support. N Engl J Med. 2004 Mar 25; 350(13):1287–95. [PMID: 15044639]
- Sehn LH et al. Introduction of combined CHOP plus rituximab therapy dramatically improved outcome of diffuse large B-cell lymphoma in British Columbia. J Clin Oncol. 2005 Aug 1; 23(22):5027–33. [PMID: 15955905]

Obesity

KEY FEATURES

ESSENTIALS OF DIAGNOSIS

- Excess adipose tissue, resulting in body mass index (BMI) > 30
- Upper body obesity (abdomen and flank) of greater health consequence than lower body obesity (buttocks and thighs)

GENERAL CONSIDERATIONS

- Quantitative evaluation involves determination of BMI
- BMI accurately reflects the presence of excess adipose tissue; it is calculated by dividing measured body weight in kilograms by the height in meters squared
  - Normal: BMI = 18.5–24.9
  - Overweight: BMI = 25–29.9
  - Class I obesity: BMI = 30–34.9
  - Class II obesity: BMI = 35–39.9
  - Class III (extreme) obesity: BMI > 40
- Increased abdominal circumference (> 102 cm in men and > 88 cm in women) or high waist/hip ratios (> 1.0 in men and > 0.85 in women) confers greater risk of
  - Diabetes mellitus
  - Stroke
  - Coronary artery disease
  - Early death
- Associated with significant increases in morbidity and mortality
- Surgical and obstetric risks greater
- The relative risk associated with obesity decreases with age, and excess weight is no longer a risk factor in adults aged > 75

DEMOGRAPHICS

- 65% of Americans are overweight
- 30.4% of Americans are obese
- As much as 50% of obesity may be explained by genetic influences

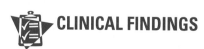

CLINICAL FINDINGS

SYMPTOMS AND SIGNS

- Assess degree and distribution of body fat
- Assess overall nutritional status
- Signs of secondary causes of obesity (hypothyroidism and Cushing's syndrome) are found in < 1%

DIFFERENTIAL DIAGNOSIS

- Increased caloric intake
- Fluid retention: congestive heart failure, cirrhosis, nephrotic syndrome
- Cushing's syndrome
- Hypothyroidism
- Diabetes mellitus (type 2)
- Drugs, eg, antipsychotics, antidepressants, corticosteroids
- Insulinoma
- Depression
- Binge eating disorder

DIAGNOSIS

LABORATORY TESTS

- Endocrinologic evaluation, including serum thyroid-stimulating hormone and dexamethasone suppression test in obese patients with unexplained recent weight gain or clinical features of endocrinopathy, or both
- Assessment for medical consequences and metabolic syndrome
  - Blood pressure
  - Fasting glucose
  - Low-density (LDL) and high-density cholesterol (HDL)
  - Triglyceride levels

DIAGNOSTIC PROCEDURES

- Calculation of BMI
- Measurement of abdominal circumference

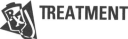

TREATMENT

MEDICATIONS

- Catecholaminergic or serotonergic medications
  - Sometimes used in patients with BMI > 30 or patients with BMI > 27 who have obesity-related health risks
  - Average weight loss approximately 3–5 kg more than placebo
  - No evidence of long-term benefit
- Catecholaminergic medications
  - Amphetamines (high abuse potential)
  - Nonamphetamine schedule IV appetite suppressants (phentermine, diethylpropion, and mazindol) are approved for short-term use only and have limited utility
- Sibutramine (10 mg PO once daily)
  - Blocks uptake of both serotonin and norepinephrine in the CNS
  - Side effects include dry mouth, anorexia, constipation, insomnia, dizzi-

ness, and increased blood pressure (< 5%)
- Orlistat (120 mg PO TID with meals)
  - Reduces fat absorption in the gastrointestinal tract by inhibiting intestinal lipase
  - Side effects include diarrhea, gas, and cramping and perhaps reduced absorption of fat-soluble vitamins
- Rimonabant
  - New drug under investigation
  - Initial studies showed 20 mg resulted in 5 kg greater weight loss than placebo
  - Drug has more adverse affects than placebo, including nervous system, psychiatric, and gastrointestinal symptoms
  - Attrition rates at 1 year were approximately 40%

SURGERY

- Consider for patients with BMI > 40, or BMI > 35 if obesity-related comorbidities are present
- Effective surgical procedures (each can be done laparoscopically)
  - Roux-en-Y gastric bypass
  - Vertical banded gastroplasty
  - Gastric banding
- Surgical complications are common and include
  - Peritonitis due to anastomotic leak
  - Abdominal wall hernias
  - Staple line disruption
  - Gallstones
  - Marginal ulcers
  - Stomal stenosis
  - Wound infections
  - Thromboembolic disease
  - Nutritional deficiencies
  - Gastrointestinal symptoms
- Surgical mortality (30 day) ranges from 0.1% to 1.1%; 1-year mortality is higher, especially in high-risk and older patients

THERAPEUTIC PROCEDURES

- Multidisciplinary approach
  - Hypocaloric diets
  - Behavior modification
  - Exercise
  - Social support
- Limit foods that provide large amounts of calories without other nutrients, ie, fat, sucrose, and alcohol
- No special advantage to carbohydrate-restricted or high-protein diets, nor to ingestion of foods one at a time
- Plan and keep records of menus and exercise sessions

- Aerobic exercise useful for long-term weight maintenance
- For BMI > 35
  - Consider very low-calorie diets (< 800 kcal/day) for 4–6 months
  - Side effects include fatigue, orthostatic hypotension, cold intolerance, and fluid and electrolyte disorders
  - Less common complications include gout, gallbladder disease, and cardiac arrhythmias

 OUTCOME

COMPLICATIONS

- Hypertension
- Type 2 diabetes mellitus
- Hyperlipidemia
- Coronary artery disease
- Degenerative joint disease
- Psychosocial disability
- Cancers (colon, rectum, prostate, uterus, biliary tract, breast, ovary)
- Thromboembolic disorders
- Digestive tract diseases (gallstones, reflux esophagitis)
- Skin disorders

PROGNOSIS

- Only 20% of patients will lose 20 lb and maintain the loss for > 2 years; only 5% will maintain a 40-lb loss
- With very low-calorie diets, patients lose an average of 2 lb per week; long-term weight maintenance is less predictable and requires concurrent behavior modification and exercise
- Sibutramine, 10 mg PO QD, for 6–12 months results in average weight losses of 3–5 kg more than placebo
- Orlistat, 120 mg PO TID with meals, for up to 2 years results in 2–4 kg greater weight loss than placebo
- Surgical procedures lead to substantial weight loss—20–40% of initial body weight

WHEN TO REFER

- Refer for bariatric surgery for BMI > 40 or > 35 with comorbid conditions

WHEN TO ADMIT

- For bariatric surgery

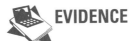 **EVIDENCE**

PRACTICE GUIDELINES

- Cummings S et al. Position of the American Dietetic Association: weight management. J Am Diet Assoc. 2002; 102:1145. [PMID: 12171464]
- American Medical Association. Assessment and Management of Adult Obesity: A Primer for Physicians, 2003.

WEB SITE

- American Obesity Association

INFORMATION FOR PATIENTS

- American Obesity Association
- Cleveland Clinic—Obesity

REFERENCES

- Dansinger ML et al. Comparison of the Atkins, Ornish, Weight Watchers, and Zone diets for weight loss and heart disease risk reduction: a randomized trial. JAMA. 2005 Jan 5;293(1):43–53. [PMID: 15632335]
- Flum DR et al. Early mortality among Medicare beneficiaries undergoing bariatric surgical procedures. JAMA. 2005 Oct 19;294(15):1903–8. [PMID: 16234496]
- Heilbronn LK et al. Effect of 6-month calorie restriction on biomarkers of longevity, metabolic adaptation, and oxidative stress in overweight individuals: a randomized controlled trial. JAMA. 2006 Apr 5;295(13):1539–48. [PMID: 16595757]
- Howard BV et al. Low-fat dietary pattern and weight change over 7 years: the Women's Health Initiative Dietary Modification Trial. JAMA. 2006 Jan 4; 295(1):39–49. [PMID: 16391215]
- O'Brien PE et al. Treatment of mild to moderate obesity with laparoscopic adjustable gastric banding or an intensive medical program: a randomized trial. Ann Intern Med. 2006 May 2; 144(9):625–33. [PMID: 16670131]
- Shaw K et al. Exercise for overweight or obesity. Cochrane Database Syst Rev. 2006 Oct 18;(4):CD003817. [PMID: 17054187]
- Sjostrom L et al; Swedish Obese Subjects Study Scientific Group. Lifestyle, diabetes, and cardiovascular risk factors 10 years after bariatric surgery. N Engl J Med. 2004 Dec 23;351(26):2683–93. [PMID: 15616203]

Occlusive Disease: Aorta & Iliac Arteries

 KEY FEATURES

ESSENTIALS OF DIAGNOSIS

- Cramping; pain or tiredness in the calf, leg, or hip while walking (claudication)
- Diminished femoral pulses
- Tissue loss (ulceration, gangrene) unusual

GENERAL CONSIDERATIONS

- Patients are typically male smokers aged 50–60 years
- Begins most frequently at the bifurcation of the aorta in the proximal common iliac arteries
- Lesions affecting the external iliac arteries are less common
- Disease progression may lead to complete occlusion of one or both common iliac arteries, which can precipitate occlusion of the entire abdominal aorta to the level of the renal arteries
- Pathologic changes of atherosclerosis may be diffuse, but flow-limiting stenoses occur segmentally
- This is particularly true of the aortoiliac segment where patients may have limited or no narrowing of the vessels in the more distal vessels

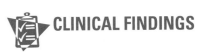 **CLINICAL FINDINGS**

SYMPTOMS AND SIGNS

- Intermittent claudication
  - Occurs as cramping pain brought on by exercise
  - Usually located in the calf muscles
- Pain
  - May extend into thigh and buttocks with continued exercise
  - May be unilateral or bilateral
- Weakness in the legs when walking or simply extreme limb fatigue
- Symptoms relieved with rest
- Impotence common with bilateral symptoms
- Femoral and distal pulses are absent or very weak
- A bruit may be heard over the aorta, iliac, and femoral arteries

DIFFERENTIAL DIAGNOSIS

- Vascular disease of the femoral or popliteal arteries
- Lumbar spinal stenosis
- Degenerative joint disease of the hips

DIAGNOSIS

IMAGING STUDIES

- CT angiography and magnetic resonance angiography have replaced traditional invasive angiography
- Imaging only required when intervention is contemplated, since a segmental wave-form analysis should identify the involved levels of the arterial tree

DIAGNOSTIC PROCEDURES

- Doppler examination
  - Ratio of systolic blood pressure at ankle compared with brachial artery of upper arm is reduced to below 0.9 (normal ratio is 1.0–1.2)
  - This difference is exaggerated by exercise
- Segmental wave-forms or pulse volume recordings
  - Obtained by strain gaze technology through blood pressure cuffs
  - Demonstrate blunting of the arterial inflow throughout the leg

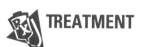

TREATMENT

MEDICATIONS

- Phosphodiesterase inhibitors, such as cilostazol 100 mg PO BID, may be beneficial in about two-thirds of patients

SURGERY

- Consider intervention to relieve obstruction if claudication interferes appreciably with patient's essential activities or employment
- Aorto-femoral bypass graft
  - Highly effective and durable
  - Prosthetic graft extends from the infrarenal abdominal aorta to the common femoral arteries
  - Mortality is low, in range of 2–3%
  - Morbidity is higher with a 5–10% rate of myocardial infarction
- High-risk patients may also be treated with a graft from axillary artery to femoral arteries (axillo-femoral bypass graft)
- In the unusual case of iliac disease limited to one side, a graft from the contra-

lateral femoral artery (fem-fem bypass) may be done
- The less extensive operations have lower operative risk, but they are less durable

THERAPEUTIC PROCEDURES

- Smoking cessation, risk factor reduction, weight loss, and walking will substantially improve exercise tolerance
- Angioplasty and stenting effectively treat occlusive lesions of the aortoiliac segment

OUTCOME

COMPLICATIONS

- Aorto-femoral bypass
  - Similar to those of any major abdominal reconstruction in a patient population with high penetrance of cardiovascular disease
  - Total complication rate may be > 10%
- Endovascular repair
  - Embolization and vessel dissection (relatively uncommon)
  - Total complication rate should be < 5%

PROGNOSIS

- Without intervention, the prognosis for patients with aorto-iliac disease include reduction in walking distance but rarely include rest pain or threatened limb loss
- Life expectancy is related to attendant cardiac disease, with a mortality rate of 25–40% at 5 years
- Symptomatic relief is generally excellent after intervention
- After aorto-femoral bypass, a patency rate of 90% at 5 years is common
- Patency rates and symptom relief for less extensive procedures are also good with 20–30% symptom return at 3 years

EVIDENCE

PRACTICE GUIDELINES

- Hirsch AT et al. ACC/AHA 2005 Practice Guidelines for the management of patients with peripheral arterial disease (lower extremity, renal, mesenteric, and abdominal aortic): a collaborative report from the American Association for Vascular Surgery/Society for Vascular Surgery, Society for Cardiovascular Angiography and Interventions, Society for Vascular Medicine and Biology, Society of Interventional Radiology, and the

ACC/AHA Task Force on Practice Guidelines (Writing Committee to Develop Guidelines for the Management of Patients With Peripheral Arterial Disease): endorsed by the American Association of Cardiovascular and Pulmonary Rehabilitation; National Heart, Lung, and Blood Institute; Society for Vascular Nursing; TransAtlantic Inter-Society Consensus; and Vascular Disease Foundation. Circulation. 2006 Mar 21; 113(11):e463–654. [PMID: 16549646]

REFERENCES

- Sontheimer DL. Peripheral vascular disease: diagnosis and treatment. Am Fam Physician. 2006 Jun 1;73(11):1971–6. [PMID: 16770929]
- WAVE Investigators. The effects of oral anticoagulants in patients with peripheral arterial disease: rationale, design, and baseline characteristics of the Warfarin and Antiplatelet Vascular Evaluation (WAVE) trial, including a meta-analysis of trials. Am Heart J. 2006 Jan; 151(1):1–9. [PMID: 16368284]

Occlusive Disease: Femoral & Popliteal Arteries

 KEY FEATURES

ESSENTIALS OF DIAGNOSIS

- Cramping; pain or tiredness in the calf only with exercise
- Reduced popliteal or pedal pulses
- Foot pain at rest, relieved by dependency
- Foot gangrene or ulceration

GENERAL CONSIDERATIONS

- The superficial femoral artery (SFA) is the artery most commonly occluded by atherosclerosis
- The lesions frequently occur where the SFA passes through the abductor magnis tendon in the distal thigh
- The profunda femoris artery and the popliteal artery are relatively spared occlusive lesions except in diabetics
- As with atherosclerosis of the aorto-iliac segment, these lesions are closely associated with a history of smoking

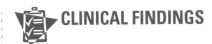 **CLINICAL FINDINGS**

SYMPTOMS AND SIGNS

- Intermittent claudication is confined to the calf
- Claudication at about 2–4 blocks when SFA is occluded at the abductor canal and good collaterals from profunda femoris are present
- Concomitant disease of the profunda femoris or the popliteal artery may trigger symptoms at much shorter distances
- Dependent rubor of the foot with blanching on elevation may be present with short-distance claudication
- Chronic low blood flow states cause atrophic changes in the lower leg and foot with
  - Loss of hair
  - Thinning of the skin and subcutaneous tissues
  - Disuse atrophy of the muscles
- Popliteal and pedal pulses are reduced

DIFFERENTIAL DIAGNOSIS

- Occlusive disease of the iliac arteries
- Lumbar spinal stenosis

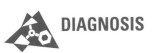 **DIAGNOSIS**

IMAGING STUDIES

- Angiography, CT angiography, or magnetic resonance angiography
  - All adequately show the anatomic location of the obstructive lesions
  - These studies are only done if revascularization is planned

DIAGNOSTIC PROCEDURES

- The ankle-brachial index (ABI) is reduced; levels below 0.5 suggest severe reduction in flow
- ABIs must be accompanied by wave-form analysis in diabetic patients and the elderly
- Pulse volume recordings with cuffs placed at the high thigh, mid thigh, calf, and ankle will delineate the levels of obstruction with reduced pressures and blunted wave-forms

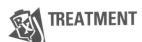 **TREATMENT**

MEDICATIONS

- After any procedure, patient generally receives lifelong antiplatelet medication
  - Periprocedural treatment with clopidogrel (75 mg/day)
  - Long-term maintenance therapy with aspirin

SURGERY

- Indications
  - Intermittent claudication that is progressive, incapacitating or interferes significantly with essential daily activities
  - Presence of rest pain
  - Threatened tissue loss of the foot
- Femoral-popliteal bypass with autogenous saphenous vein is most effective and durable treatment for lesions of the SFA
- Synthetic material, polytetrafluoroethylene (PTFE) can be done with relatively short bypasses with excellent distal vessels
- Removal of the atherosclerotic plaque is now limited to the lesions of the common femoral and profunda femoris artery where bypass grafts and endovascular techniques have no role
- Endovascular techniques
  - Have increased in popularity for lesions of the SFA
  - Several alternatives include angioplasty combined with stenting, cyroplasty, angioplasty with balloon cooled to a −20 °C, and endoluminal atherectomy
  - These techniques have lower morbidity than bypass but also have a lower rate of success and durability
  - Most effective for lesions that are < 10 cm long and in patients who are undergoing aggressive risk factor modification

THERAPEUTIC PROCEDURES

- Conservative management has an important role for patients with SFA occlusion and good profunda femoris collaterals

 OUTCOME

FOLLOW-UP

- Ultrasound surveillance after all interventions so that any recurrent narrowing can be treated promptly

COMPLICATIONS

- Leg infection or seroma can occur in as many as 15–20% of cases
- Myocardial infarction rates after open surgery are 5–10%, with a 1–4% mortality
- Complication rates of endovascular therapy are 1–5%

PROGNOSIS

- Excellent for motivated patients with isolated SFA disease
- Patency rate of bypass grafts of the femoral artery, SFA, and popliteal artery may be as high as 70% at 3 years with patency for endovascular procedures somewhat lower
- 5-year survival among patients with lower extremity disease associated with coronary disease is about 50%

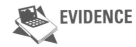 **EVIDENCE**

REFERENCE

- McDermott MM et al. Lower extremity nerve function in patients with lower extremity ischemia. Arch Intern Med. 2006 Oct 9;166(18):1986–92. [PMID: 17030832]

Occlusive Disease: Limb Arteries

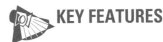 **KEY FEATURES**

ESSENTIALS OF DIAGNOSIS

- Sudden pain in an extremity
- Neurologic dysfunction (eg, numbness, weakness, or complete paralysis)
- Absent extremity pulses

GENERAL CONSIDERATIONS

- May be due to an embolus or to thrombosis of a diseased atherosclerotic segment
- Destinations of emboli from cardiac sources
  - Lower extremities (50%)
  - Cerebrovascular circulation (20%)
  - Upper extremities and mesenteric and renal circulation (30%)
- Emboli from arterial sources, such as arterial ulcerations or calcified excrescences, are usually small and go to the distal arterial tree (toes)
- Causes of the thrombus
  - Atrial fibrillation (most common)
  - Valvular disease
  - Ischemic heart disease
- Patients with primary thrombosis have a history of claudication

- If stenosis developed over time, collateral blood vessels develop and resulting occlusion may only reduce walking distance or cause minimal increase in symptoms

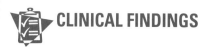

CLINICAL FINDINGS

SYMPTOMS AND SIGNS

- Sudden onset of extremity pain
- Neurologic dysfunction (eg, numbness or paralysis)
- With popliteal occlusion, only the foot may be affected
- With proximal occlusions, the whole leg may be affected
- Absent pulses in the arteries distal to the occlusion
- Signs of severe arterial ischemia
  - Pallor on elevation
  - Coolness of the extremity
  - Mottling
  - Impaired neurologic function with hyperesthesia progressing to anesthesia accompanied with paralysis

DIFFERENTIAL DIAGNOSIS

- Deep venous thrombosis
- Cerebrovascular accident

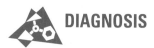

DIAGNOSIS

LABORATORY FINDINGS

- Blood work may indicate systemic acidosis

IMAGING STUDIES

- May be helpful in expediting revascularization procedure by
  - Identifying exact areas of occlusion
  - Delineating distal vessel patency
- Show an abrupt cutoff of the vessel involved
- When possible, should be done in the operating room because a delay in obtaining angiography, magnetic resonance angiography, or CT angiography may jeopardize the viability of the tissue at risk

DIAGNOSTIC PROCEDURES

- Doppler examination shows little or no flow in the distal vessels

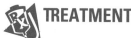

TREATMENT

MEDICATIONS

- IV heparin
  - Start as soon as the diagnosis is made
  - Dose: 5000–10,000 units
  - Helps prevent propagation of the clot
  - May also help relieve associated spasm of the vessels

SURGERY

- General anesthesia is usually indicated
- Local anesthesia may be used in extremely high-risk patients if the exploration is limited to the common femoral artery
- Revascularization
  - Treatment of choice in all cases of symptomatic acute arterial thrombosis
  - Embolectomy from femoral popliteal and even pedal vessels in extreme cases
  - Should be accomplished within 3 hours if evidence of neurologic injury is present
  - Longer delays carry significant risk of irreversible tissue damage
  - Risk approaches 100% at 6 hours

THERAPEUTIC PROCEDURES

- Chemical thrombolysis with tissue plasminogen activator (TPA)
  - May be done but often requires ≥ 24 hours to fully lyse the thrombus
  - This approach can be taken only in patients with an intact neurologic examination
  - An additional clot in atrium is a relative contraindication. Obtain echocardiogram before chemical thrombolysis to rule out clot
- Catheter-based mechanical thrombolysis may be an excellent alternative

OUTCOME

COMPLICATIONS

- Severe acidosis
- Myocardial arrest
- Postoperative wound hematoma

PROGNOSIS

- Acute arterial occlusion
  - 10–25% risk of amputation
  - 25% or higher in-hospital mortality rate
  - Prognosis is dismal in high-risk patients

- Better for acute occlusion of an atherosclerotic segment because collateral flow can maintain extremity viability

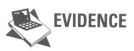

EVIDENCE

REFERENCES

- Collins R et al. Duplex ultrasonography, magnetic resonance angiography, and computed tomography angiography for diagnosis and assessment of symptomatic, lower limb peripheralarterial disease: systematic review. BMJ. 2007 Jun 16;334(7606):1257. [PMID: 17548364]
- Rogers JH et al. Overview of new technologies for lower extremity revascularization. Circulation. 2007 Oct 30; 116(18):2072–85. [PMID: 17967988]
- Vouyouka AG et al. Arterial vascular disease in women. J Vasc Surg. 2007 Dec;46(6):1295–302. [PMID: 17950570]

Occlusive Disease: Lower Leg & Foot Arteries

KEY FEATURES

ESSENTIALS OF DIAGNOSIS

- Rest pain of forefoot relieved by dependency
- Pain or numbness of foot with walking
- Ulceration or gangrene of foot or toes
- Pallor when foot is elevated

GENERAL CONSIDERATIONS

- Primarily involves tibial vessels
- Only extensive disease involves arteries of the foot
- Extensive calcification of the vessel wall often present
- This distribution of atherosclerosis is primarily seen in patients with diabetes mellitus
- Claudication may not be evident unless associated lesions are present in aorto-iliac or femoral-superficial femoral artery segments

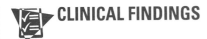

CLINICAL FINDINGS

SYMPTOMS AND SIGNS

- Foot ischemia without attendant claudication and rest pain
- Characteristics of rest pain
  - Severe, usually burning
  - Awakens patient
  - Confined to the dorsum of the foot at the area of the metatarsal heads
  - Relieved with dependency
- Pedal pulses are absent
- Dependent rubor with pallor on elevation
- Skin of the foot is generally cool, atrophic, and hairless

DIFFERENTIAL DIAGNOSIS

- Neuropathic dysesthesia

DIAGNOSIS

IMAGING STUDIES

- CT angiography, magnetic resonance angiography, or angiography is often needed to delineate the anatomy of the tibial-popliteal segment

DIAGNOSTIC PROCEDURES

- Dangling foot over edge of bed relieves rest pain, indicating vascular insufficiency
- Ankle-brachial index
  - May be quite low (in the range of 0.3)
  - May be falsely elevated because of the noncompressability of the calcified tibial vessels
- Wave-form analysis is important in these patients with a monophasic flow pattern denoting critically low flow
- Segmental pulse volume recordings
  - Show a fall-off in blood pressure between the calf and ankle
  - However, may also be affected by tibial vessel calcification

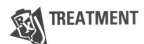

TREATMENT

SURGERY

Bypass and endovascular techniques

- Bypass with vein to the distal tibial arteries or foot effective in
  - Treating rest pain
  - Healing gangrene
  - Healing ischemic ulcerations of the foot
- These bypasses have good patency rates (70% at 3 years)

- In nearly all series, limb salvage rates are much higher than patency rates
- Endovascular techniques are beginning to be used in tibial vessels with modest results, but bypass grafting remains primary technique of revascularization

Amputation

- Reserved for cases when
  - Revascularization cannot be done
  - Debridement of necrotic or severely infected tissue is necessary
- Toe amputations, even of the first toe, have little or no affect on mechanics of walking
- A transmetatarsal amputation is durable but increases the energy required of walking by 5–10%
- Below knee amputation increases energy expenditure of walking by 50%
- Above knee amputation increases energy expenditure of walking by 100%

THERAPEUTIC PROCEDURES

- Indications for revascularization
  - Presence of ulcerations with no significant healing within 2–3 weeks
  - Occurrence of nightly rest pain with monophasic wave forms
- Infrequent rest pain is not an absolute indication for revascularization

OUTCOME

PROGNOSIS

- Good foot care may avoid ulceration
- Most diabetic patients do well with a conservative regimen

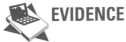

EVIDENCE

REFERENCES

- Cunningham LD et al. Lower-extremity arterial disease. Perspect Vasc Surg Endovasc Ther. 2005 Dec;17(4):351–61. [PMID: 16389429]
- Diehm C et al. Association of low ankle brachial index with high mortality in primary care. Eur Heart J. 2006 Jul;27(14):1743–9. [PMID: 16782720]
- Faries PL et al. The role of surgical revascularization in the management of diabetic foot wounds. Am J Surg. 2004 May;187(5A):34S–37S. [PMID: 15147990]
- Laird JR et al; LACI Investigators. Limb salvage following laser-assisted angioplasty for critical limb ischemia: results of the LACI multicenter trial. J Endovasc Ther. 2006 Feb;13(1):1–11. [PMID: 16445313]

Onychomycosis

KEY FEATURES

ESSENTIALS OF DIAGNOSIS

- A trichophyton infection of one or more fingernails or toenails
- Yellowish discoloration with heaping of keratin
- Separation of the nail bed

GENERAL CONSIDERATIONS

- The species most commonly found is *Trichophyton rubrum*
- "Saprophytic" fungi may rarely (< 5%) cause onychomycosis
- Onycholysis (distal separation of the nail plate from the nail bed, usually of the fingers) is caused by excessive exposure to water, soaps, detergents, alkalies, and industrial cleaning agents
- Candidal infection of the nail folds and subungual area, nail hardeners, and drug-induced photosensitivity may cause onycholysis, as may hyperthyroidism and hypothyroidism and psoriasis

CLINICAL FINDINGS

SYMPTOMS AND SIGNS

- The nails are lusterless, brittle, and hypertrophic
- The substance of the nail is friable

DIFFERENTIAL DIAGNOSIS

- Psoriasis
- Candidal onychomycosis
- Lichen planus
- Allergy to nail polish or nail glue

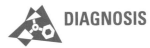

DIAGNOSIS

LABORATORY TESTS

- Laboratory diagnosis is mandatory since only 50% of dystrophic nails are due to dermatophytosis

- Portions of the nail should be cleared with 10% KOH and examined under the microscope for hyphae
- Fungi may also be cultured

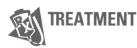 **TREATMENT**

MEDICATIONS

- Difficult to treat because of the long duration of therapy required and the frequency of recurrences
- Fingernails respond more readily than toenails
- For toenails, it is in some situations best to discourage therapy and to control discomfort by paring the thickened nail plate

Topical treatment

- Has relatively low efficacy (10% or less), but in well-motivated patients with minimally thickened nails it can be useful
- Naftifine gel 1% or ciclopirox nail lacquer (Penlac) 8% applied twice daily may rarely clear fingernails in 4–6 months and toenails in 12–18 months

Systemic therapy

- Is generally required for the treatment of nail onychomycosis; fingernails can virtually always be cleared, whereas toenails can be cured 35–50% of the time and improved in about 75% of cases
- Fingernails
  - Ultramicrosize griseofulvin, 250 mg PO TID for 6 months, is often effective
  - Treatment alternatives, in order of preference, are terbinafine, 250 mg PO once daily for 6 weeks, itraconazole, 400 mg/day PO for 7 days each month for 2 months, and itraconazole, 200 mg/day PO for 2 months
- Toenails
  - Neither griseofulvin nor ketoconazole are recommended
  - Terbinafine, 250 mg PO once daily for 12 weeks, is best treatment
  - If terbinafine cannot be used, itraconazole 200 mg PO BID for 1 week per month for 3 months is an inferior but acceptable alternative

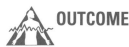 **OUTCOME**

FOLLOW-UP

- No matter which therapy is used, constant topical treatment for any coexisting tinea pedis is mandatory and should probably be continued for life to attempt to prevent recurrence
- Monitoring of liver ezymes and CBC is recommended monthly during terbinafine treatment

PROGNOSIS

- Once clear, fingernails often remain free of disease for years
- About 75% of patients will have substantial improvement with systemic therapy, and 35–50% will be mycologically and clinically cured at 1 year
- Relapses are more common with itraconazole than terbinafine in toenail onychomycosis

WHEN TO REFER

- If there is a question about the diagnosis, if recommended therapy is ineffective, or if specialized treatment is necessary

 EVIDENCE

PRACTICE GUIDELINES

- Roberts DT et al; British Association of Dermatologists. Guidelines for treatment of onychomycosis. Br J Dermatol. 2003;148:402. [PMID: 12653730]
- University of Texas at Austin: Recommendations for the management of onychomycosis in adults. 2003

INFORMATION FOR PATIENTS

- American Academy of Family Physicians: Fungal Infections of Fingernails and Toenails
- American Osteopathic College of Dermatology: Fungus Infections: Preventing Recurrence
- Mayo Clinic: Nail Fungal Infection
- MedlinePlus: Fungal Nail Infection

REFERENCES

- Hay R. Literature: Onychomycosis. J Eur Acad Dermatol Venereol. 2005 Sep; 19 Suppl 1:1–7. [PMID: 16120198]
- Heikkila H et al. Long-term results in patients with onychomycosis treated with terbinafine or itraconazole. Br J Dermatol. 2002 Feb;146(2):250–3. [PMID: 11903235]

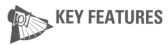
Opioid Dependency

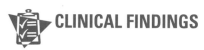 **KEY FEATURES**

ESSENTIALS OF DIAGNOSIS

- Dependency is a major concern when continued use of opioids occurs
- Withdrawal causes only moderate morbidity (similar in severity to a bout of "flu")
- Addicted patients sometimes consider themselves more addicted than they really are and may not require a withdrawal program

GENERAL CONSIDERATIONS

- The terms "opioids" and "narcotics" have been used interchangeably, but now, "opioids" is preferred
  - "Opioids" include a group of drugs with actions that mimic those of morphine
  - Natural derivatives of opium (opiates)
  - Synthetic surrogates (opioids)
  - A number of polypeptides, some of which have been discovered to be natural neurotransmitters
- The principal opioid of abuse is heroin (metabolized to morphine), which is not used as a legitimate medication
- Other common opioids are prescription drugs, which differ in milligram potency, duration of action, and agonist and antagonist capabilities (Table 2)
- The incidence of snorting and inhaling heroin ("smoking") is increasing, particularly among cocaine users

DEMOGRAPHICS

- In the United States, lifetime prevalence for heroin abuse in people age 12 and over is approximately 1.4%

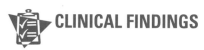 **CLINICAL FINDINGS**

SYMPTOMS AND SIGNS

- Mild opioid intoxication
  - Changes in mood
  - Feelings of euphoria
  - Drowsiness
  - Nausea with occasional emesis
  - Needle tracks
  - Miosis
- Overdosage
  - Respiratory depression

- Peripheral vasodilation
- Pinpoint pupils
- Pulmonary edema
- Coma
- Death
- Grades of withdrawal
  - Grade 0—craving and anxiety
  - Grade 1—yawning, lacrimation, rhinorrhea, and perspiration
  - Grade 2—previous symptoms plus mydriasis, piloerection, anorexia, tremors, and hot and cold flashes with generalized aching
  - Grades 3 and 4—increased intensity of previous symptoms and signs, with increased temperature, blood pressure, pulse, and respiratory rate and depth
  - In withdrawal from the most severe addiction, vomiting, diarrhea, weight loss, hemoconcentration, and spontaneous ejaculation or orgasm commonly occur

DIFFERENTIAL DIAGNOSIS

- Other drug dependence, eg, alcohol, amphetamines
- Underlying psychiatric disease, eg, depression, personality disorder
- Other drug withdrawal, eg, alcohol, benzodiazepines, amphetamines, cocaine
- Nausea or vomiting due to other cause
- Influenza or other viral syndrome

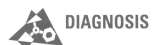 **DIAGNOSIS**

LABORATORY TESTS

- Serum or urine toxicology

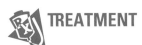 **TREATMENT**

MEDICATIONS

- Treatment for withdrawal begins if grade 2 signs develop
- Methadone
  - If a withdrawal program is necessary, use methadone, 10 mg PO (use parenteral administration if the patient is vomiting), and observe
  - If signs (piloerection, mydriasis, cardiovascular changes) persist for more than 4–6 hours, give another 10 mg
  - Continue to administer methadone at 4- to 6-hour intervals until signs are not present (rarely more than 40 mg of methadone in 24 hours)
  - Divide the total amount of drug required over the first 24-hour period by 2 and give that amount q12h
  - Each day reduce the total 24-hour dose by 5–10 mg
  - Thus, a patient who was moderately addicted and initially required 30–40 mg of methadone could complete the withdrawal process over 4–8 days
- Clonidine
  - 0.1 mg PO several times daily over 10–14 days
  - Is an alternative and an adjunct to methadone detoxification
  - It is not necessary to taper the dose
  - Helpful in alleviating cardiovascular symptoms
  - Does not significantly relieve anxiety, insomnia, or generalized aching
- Opioid antagonists (eg, naltrexone)
  - Can be used for treatment of the patient who has been free of opioids for 7–10 days
  - Blocks the opioid "high" of heroin when 50 mg is given PO q24h initially for several days and then 100 mg is given q48–72h
  - Liver disorders are a major contraindication
  - Compliance tends to be poor, partly because of the dysphoria that can persist long after opioid discontinuance

THERAPEUTIC PROCEDURES

- The use of rapid and ultrarapid detoxification is not supported by current evidence

 OUTCOME

FOLLOW-UP

- Methadone maintenance programs are of some value in chronic recidivism
- Under carefully controlled supervision, the opioid addict is maintained on fairly high doses of methadone (40–120 mg/day) that satisfy craving and block the effects of heroin to a great degree

COMPLICATIONS

- Treatment for overdosage (or suspected overdosage) is naloxone, 2 mg IV
- Complications of heroin administration
  - Infections (eg, pneumonia, septic emboli, hepatitis)
  - HIV infection from using nonsterile needles, traumatic insults (eg, arterial spasm due to drug injection, gangrene)
  - Pulmonary edema

PROGNOSIS

- There is a protracted abstinence syndrome of metabolic, respiratory, and blood pressure changes over 3–6 months
- The research on the impact of rapid detoxification on relapse rates, compared with more traditional methods, is limited at this time

WHEN TO REFER

- All opioid-dependent patients should be referred to an addiction specialist unless the primary caregiver has sufficient experience with this population

WHEN TO ADMIT

- For some patients, residential treatment offers the best chance for recovery
- Some patients are able to enter recovery in a structured, supportive outpatient program

 EVIDENCE

PRACTICE GUIDELINES

- American Academy of Family Physicians: Identification and Mangement of the Drug-Seeking Patient
- National Guideline Clearinghouse: VHA/DOD substance disorder guidelines, 2001
- National Guideline Clearinghouse: Washington State Department of Labor and Industries: opioid prescription guidelines, 2002

WEB SITES

- American Psychiatric Association
- National Institutes of Health—National Institute of Drug Abuse

INFORMATION FOR PATIENTS

- JAMA patient page. Treating drug dependency. JAMA. 2000;283:1378. [PMID: 10714739]
- JAMA patient page. Opioid abuse. JAMA. 2004;292:1394. [PMID: 15367561]
- National Institute of Drug Abuse

REFERENCES

- Fudala PJ et al. Office-based treatment of opiate addiction with sublingual-tablet formulation of buprenorphine and naloxone. N Engl J Med. 2003 Sep 4; 349(10):949–58. [PMID: 12954743]
- Hamilton RJ et al. Complications of ultrarapid opioid detoxification with subcutaneous naltrexone pellets. Acad Emerg Med. 2002;9:63. [PMID: 11772672]

Osmolar Gap

 KEY FEATURES

- Alcohol quickly equilibrates between intracellular and extracellular water, adding 22 mosm/L for every 1000 mg/L
- When measured osmolality exceeds that calculated from values of serum Na^+ and glucose and blood urea nitrogen, consider ethanol intoxication as an explanation of the discrepancy (osmolar gap)
- Toxic alcohol ingestion, particularly methanol or ethylene glycol, can produce an osmolar gap with an anion gap metabolic acidosis
- However, the combination of anion gap metabolic acidosis and an osmolar gap exceeding 10 mosm/kg is not specific for toxic alcohol ingestion
- Nearly half of patients with alcoholic ketoacidosis or lactic acidosis have similar findings, caused in part by elevations of endogenous glycerol, acetone, and acetone metabolites

 DIAGNOSIS

- The following substances can produce an osmolar gap:
  - Methanol
  - Ethylene glycol
  - Isopropyl alcohol
  - Ethanol toxicity
  - Acetone
  - Propylene glycol
  - Severe alcoholic or diabetic ketoacidosis
  - Lactic acidosis

Osteoarthritis

 KEY FEATURES

ESSENTIALS OF DIAGNOSIS

- A degenerative disorder; no systemic symptoms
- Pain relieved by rest; morning stiffness brief; articular inflammation minimal
- Radiographic findings
  - Narrowed joint space
  - Osteophytes
  - Increased density of subchondral bone
  - Bony cysts

GENERAL CONSIDERATIONS

- Degeneration of cartilage and hypertrophy of bone at the articular margins
- Inflammation is usually minimal

Primary

- Most commonly affects some or all of the following
  - Distal interphalangeal (DIP) joints and, less commonly, the proximal interphalangeal (PIP) joints
  - Carpometacarpal joints of the thumb
  - Hip
  - Knee
  - Metatarsophalangeal joint of the big toe
  - Cervical and lumbar spine

Secondary

- May occur in any joint as a sequela to articular injury resulting from either intra-articular or extra-articular causes
- Causes of articular injury that lead to secondary degenerative arthritis include
  - Trauma
  - Gout
  - Rheumatoid arthritis
  - Hyperparathyroidism
  - Hemochromatosis
  - Charcot joint

DEMOGRAPHICS

- The most common form of joint disease
- 90% of all people have radiographic features of osteoarthritis in weight-bearing joints by age 40
- Obesity is a risk factor for knee osteoarthritis and probably for the hip

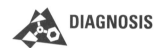 **CLINICAL FINDINGS**

SYMPTOMS AND SIGNS

- Insidious onset
- Pain is made worse by activity or weight bearing and relieved by rest
- Bony enlargement of the interphalangeal joints is occasionally prominent
  - DIP (Heberden's nodes)
  - PIP (Bouchard's nodes)
- Coarse crepitus may often be felt in the joint
- Joint effusion and other articular signs of inflammation are mild
- Because articular inflammation is minimal and systemic manifestations are absent, degenerative joint disease should seldom be confused with other arthritides

- The distribution of joint involvement in the hands also helps distinguish osteoarthritis from rheumatoid arthritis
  - Osteoarthritis primarily affects the DIP and PIP joints and spares the wrist and metacarpophalangeal joints (except at the thumb)
  - Rheumatoid arthritis involves the wrists and metacarpophalangeal joints and spares the DIP joints
- No systemic manifestations

DIFFERENTIAL DIAGNOSIS

- Rheumatoid arthritis
- Seronegative spondyloarthropathy, eg, psoriatic arthritis
- Gout
- Chondrocalcinosis, eg, pseudogout, Wilson's disease
- Other bone disease, eg, osteoporosis, metastatic cancer, multiple myeloma

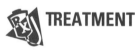 **DIAGNOSIS**

LABORATORY TESTS

- No laboratory evidence of inflammation such as elevated erythrocyte sedimentation rate

IMAGING STUDIES

- Radiographs may reveal
  - Narrowing of the joint space
  - Sharpened articular margins
  - Osteophyte formation and lipping of marginal bone
  - Thickened, dense subchondral bone
  - Bone cysts
- The correlation between radiographic findings and symptoms is poor

DIAGNOSTIC PROCEDURES

- Aspiration of effusions for pain relief
- Corticosteroid injections for pain relief

TREATMENT

MEDICATIONS

- Patients with mild disease should start with acetaminophen (2.4–4 g/day)
- Nonsteroidal anti-inflammatory drugs (NSAIDs) should be considered for patients who do not respond to acetaminophen, chondroitin sulfate, and glucosamine
- High doses of NSAIDs, as used in more inflammatory arthritides, are unnecessary

SURGERY

- Total hip and knee replacement provides excellent symptomatic and functional improvement when involvement of that severely restricts walking or causes pain at rest, particularly at night
- Although arthroscopic surgery for knee osteoarthritis is commonly performed, its long-term efficacy is unestablished

THERAPEUTIC PROCEDURES

- For patients with mild to moderate osteoarthritis of weight-bearing joints, a supervised walking program may result in clinical improvement of functional status without aggravating the joint pain. Weight loss can also improve the symptoms
- For patients with knee osteoarthritis and effusion, intra-articular injection of triamcinolone (20–40 mg) may obviate the need for analgesics or NSAIDs but should not be repeated more than two or three times in a year

 OUTCOME

WHEN TO REFER

- When other inflammatory arthritides cannot be confidently excluded
- For joint replacement

PROGNOSIS

- Symptoms may be quite severe and limit activity considerably (especially with involvement of the hips, knees, and cervical spine)

PREVENTION

- Weight reduction in women reduces the risk of developing symptomatic knee osteoarthritis

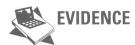 **EVIDENCE**

WEB SITE

- Arthritis Foundation

INFORMATION FOR PATIENTS

- Arthritis Foundation
- National Institute of Arthritis and Musculoskeletal and Skin Diseases

REFERENCES

- Bjordal JM et al. Non-steroidal anti-inflammatory drugs, including cyclo-oxygenase-2 inhibitors in osteoarthritis knee pain: meta-analysis of randomised placebo controlled trials. BMJ. 2004 Dec 4;329(7478):1317. [PMID: 15561731]
- Clegg DO et al. Glucosamine, chondroitin sulfate, and the two in combination for painful knee osteoarthritis. N Engl J Med. 2006 Feb 23;354(8):795–808. [PMID: 16495392]
- Felson DT. Clinical practice. Osteoarthritis of the knee. N Engl J Med. 2006 Feb 23;354(8):841–8. [PMID: 16495396]
- Fransen M. Dietary weight loss and exercise for obese adults with knee osteoarthritis: modest weight loss targets, mild exercise, modest effects. Arthritis Rheum. 2004 May; 50(5):1366–9. [PMID: 15146405]
- Schumacher HR et al. Injectable corticosteroids in treatment of arthritis of the knee. Am J Med. 2005 Nov; 118(11):1208–14. [PMID: 16271901]

Osteomalacia

 KEY FEATURES

ESSENTIALS OF DIAGNOSIS

- Bone pain and tenderness
- Decreased bone density
- Increased alkaline phosphatase, decreased 25-hydroxyvitamin D [25(OH)D$_3$]

GENERAL CONSIDERATIONS

- **Rickets:** Defective mineralization of growing skeleton in children
- **Osteomalacia:** Defective skeletal mineralization in adults
- Causes of osteomalacia
  - Vitamin D deficiency
    - Most common cause
    - ~25% of postmenopausal women have some vitamin D deficiency
    - 60% of the institutionalized elderly not receiving vitamin D supplementation
    - Incidence varies among regions: < 1% in Southeast Asia, 29% in the United States
    - Incidence of severe vitamin D deficiency (serum 25[OH]D < 25 nmol/L or < 10 ng/mL) is 3.5% in the United States
    - May arise from insufficient sun exposure, malnutrition, malabsorption, nephrotic syndrome
    - Cholestyramine, orlistat, and anticonvulsants decrease vitamin D levels
  - Dietary calcium deficiency, eg, in malnourished, elderly patients
    - Milk, especially skim milk, is a poor source of vitamin D
  - Phosphate deficiency, eg, due to
    - Nutritional deficiency
    - Malabsorption
    - Phosphate-binding antacids
    - Genetic disorders (vitamin D–resistant rickets)
    - Renal tubular acidosis
    - Fanconi's syndrome
  - Aluminum toxicity due to chronic hemodialysis with tap water dialysate or from aluminum-containing phosphate binders
  - Oncogenic osteomalacia
    - Caused by excessive production of phosphatonin by soft tissue tumors
    - Hypophosphatemia, excessive phosphaturia, reduced serum 1,25(OH)$_2$D$_3$ concentrations, osteomalacia
  - Disorders of bone matrix, eg, hypophosphatasia (deficient alkaline phosphatase)
  - Fibrogenesis imperfecta

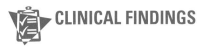 **CLINICAL FINDINGS**

SYMPTOMS AND SIGNS

- Initially asymptomatic
- Eventually, bone pain, simulating fibromyalgia
- Painful proximal muscle weakness (especially pelvic girdle) due to calcium deficiency
- Fractures with little or no trauma

DIFFERENTIAL DIAGNOSIS

- Osteoporosis
- Hypophosphatemia due to hyperparathyroidism
- Renal osteodystrophy
- Multiple myeloma, metastatic cancer
- Chronic hyperthyroidism
- Hypophosphatasia
  - A rare genetic cause of osteomalacia that is commonly misdiagnosed as osteoporosis
  - Incidence in the United States is about 1:100,000 live births; about 1:300 adults is a carrier

– Transmission can be autosomal recessive or dominant. Phenotypic presentation of hypophosphatasia is variable
– At its worst, it can present as a stillborn without dentition or calcified bones
– At its mildest, it can present in middle age with premature loss of teeth, foot pain (due to metatarsal stress fractures), thigh pain (due to femoral pseudofractures), or arthritis (due to chondrocalcinosis)

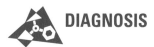

DIAGNOSIS

LABORATORY TESTS

- Alkaline phosphatase (age-adjusted) may be elevated
- $25(OH)D_3$ typically low < 20 ng/mL (< 50 nmol/L)
- Calcium or phosphate (age-adjusted) may be low
- Phosphate low in 47%
- Parathyroid hormone may be increased due to secondary hyperparathyroidism
- Urinary calcium may be low
- $1,25(OH)_2D_3$ may be low even when $25(OH)D_2$ levels are normal
- Screen for hypophosphatasia
  - Serum alkaline phosphatase is low for age
  - Confirm diagnosis with a 24-h urine assayed for phosphoethanolamine, a substrate for alkaline phosphatase, whose excretion is always elevated in patients with hypophosphatasia

IMAGING STUDIES

- Bone densitometry
- Radiographs may show diagnostic features
  - Cortical bone thinning
  - Looser lines
  - Stress or pathologic fractures
- Whole-body MRI may be required to search for occult tumors in sporadic adult-onset hypophosphatemia, hyperphosphaturia, and low serum $1,25(OH)_2D$ levels

DIAGNOSTIC PROCEDURES

- Bone biopsy not usually necessary but is diagnostic of osteomalacia if it shows significant unmineralized osteoid

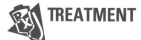 **TREATMENT**

MEDICATIONS

- Vitamin D deficiency
  - Ergocalciferol (D_2), 50,000 IU PO once weekly for 6–12 months, followed by at least 1000 IU PO once daily
  - May also be given 50,000 IU PO every 1–2 months
  - In intestinal malabsorption
    - 25,000–100,000 IU of vitamin D_2 may be required daily
    - Some patients with steatorrhea respond better to $25(OH)D$ (calcifediol), 50–100 mcg PO once daily or calcitriol 0.25–0.5 mcg once daily
- Oral calcium supplements with meals: calcium citrate (eg, Citracal) to provide 0.4–0.6 g elemental calcium per day; or calcium carbonate (eg, OsCal, Tums), 1–1.5 g elemental calcium per day
- Correct nutritional deficiencies in hypophosphatemic osteomalacia
  - Discontinue aluminum-containing antacids
  - Give bicarbonate therapy to patients with renal tubular acidosis
- Oral phosphate supplements given long-term for X-linked or idiopathic hypophosphatemia and hyperphosphaturia, along with calcitriol, 0.25–0.5 mcg PO once daily, to improve impaired calcium absorption caused by oral phosphate
  - Consider addition of human recombinant growth hormone to reduce phosphaturia
- Hypophosphatasia
  - No proven therapy except for supportive care
  - Teriparatide, a useful therapy for osteoporosis, has been tried, but its long-term efficacy is unknown

THERAPEUTIC PROCEDURES

- Sun exposure, without SPF, stimulates vitamin D_3 production in skin, except in very dark-skinned persons

 OUTCOME

COMPLICATIONS

- Fractures

PREVENTION

- Prevention of vitamin D deficiency by adequate sunlight exposure and vitamin D supplements

- US recommended daily allowance (RDA) of vitamin D is at least 10 mcg (400 IU) daily
  - In sunlight-deprived individuals (eg, veiled women, confined patients, or residents of higher latitudes during winter), RDA should be 25 mcg (1000 IU) daily
- Patients receiving long-term phenytoin therapy may be treated prophylactically with vitamin D, 50,000 IU PO every 2–4 weeks

 EVIDENCE

PRACTICE GUIDELINES

- Hanley DA et al. Vitamin D insufficiency in North America. J Nutr. 2005; 135:332. [PMID: 15671237]
- Mawer EB et al. Vitamin D nutrition and bone disease in adults. Rev Endocr Metab Disord. 2001;2:153. [PMID: 11705321]
- National Kidney Foundation

INFORMATION FOR PATIENTS

- The Magic Foundation
- MedlinePlus—Malacia
- MedlinePlus—Rickets
- Tayside University Hospitals—Osteomalacia and rickets

REFERENCES

- Armas LA et al. Vitamin D_2 is much less effective than vitamin D_3 in humans. J Clin Endocrinol Metab. 2004 Nov; 89(11):5387–91. [PMID: 15531486]
- Bielesz B et al. Renal phosphate loss in hereditary and acquired disorders of bone mineralization. Bone. 2004 Dec; 35(6):1229–39. [PMID: 15589204]
- Hanley DA et al. Vitamin D insufficiency in North America. J Nutr. 2005 Feb;135(2):332–7. [PMID: 15671237]
- Jan de Beur SM. Tumor-induced osteomalacia. JAMA. 2005 Sep 14; 294(10):1260–7. [PMID: 16160135]
- Lyman D. Undiagnosed vitamin D deficiency in the hospitalized patient. Am Fam Physician. 2005 Jan 15;71(2):299–304. [PMID: 15686300]
- Whyte MP et al. Adult hypophosphatasia treated with teriparatide. J Clin Endocrinol Metab. 2007 Apr; 92(4):1203–8. [PMID: 17213282]

Osteoporosis

KEY FEATURES

ESSENTIALS OF DIAGNOSIS

- Asymptomatic to severe pain from vertebral fractures
- Osteoporosis: bone densitometry T score (standard deviations below young normal mean) ≤ –2.5
- Osteopenia (at risk for osteoporosis): bone densitometry T score –1.5 to –2.4
- Serum parathyroid hormone (PTH), calcium, phosphorus, and alkaline phosphatase usually normal
- Serum 25-hydroxyvitamin D levels often low

GENERAL CONSIDERATIONS

- Causes approximately 1.5 million fractures annually in the United States, mainly of the spine and hip
- Morbidity and indirect mortality rates very high
- Rate of bone formation often normal, but bone resorption rate is increased
- Causes of osteoporosis include
  - Estrogen (women) or androgen (men) deficiency
  - Cushing's syndrome (eg, corticosteroid administration)
  - Hyperthyroidism
  - Hyperparathyroidism
  - Drugs (eg, alcohol, tobacco, excessive vitamin D or A, heparin)
  - Immobilization
  - Genetic disorders (eg, aromatase deficiency, type I collagen mutations)
  - Malignancy, especially multiple myeloma
  - Liver disease
  - Osteogenesis imperfecta
    □ Due to major mutation in type I collagen, results in severe osteoporosis
    □ Spontaneous fractures occur in utero or during childhood
  - Celiac disease

DEMOGRAPHICS

- Clinically evident in middle life and beyond
- Women more frequently affected than men

CLINICAL FINDINGS

SYMPTOMS AND SIGNS

- Usually asymptomatic until fractures occur
- May present as back pain of varying degrees of severity or as spontaneous fracture or collapse of a vertebra
- Loss of height common
- Fractures of femoral neck and distal radius also common
- Once osteoporosis is identified, careful history and physical examination are required to determine its cause

DIFFERENTIAL DIAGNOSIS

- Osteomalacia or rickets
- Inadequate mineralization of existing bone matrix (osteoid)
- Multiple myeloma
- Metastatic cancer
- Paget's disease of bone
- Renal osteodystrophy

DIAGNOSIS

LABORATORY TESTS

- Serum calcium, phosphate, and PTH: normal
- Alkaline phosphatase: usually normal but may be slightly elevated, especially following fracture
- Obtain serum thyroid-stimulating hormone, luteinizing hormone/follicle-stimulating hormone, testosterone (men), and 25(OH)D₃ level
- When appropriate, screen for hypogonadism in men and women
- Screen for celiac disease with serum IgA anti-tissue transglutaminase and IgA anti-endomysial antibodies

IMAGING STUDIES

- Radiographs of spine and pelvis may show demineralization; in skull and extremities, demineralization is less marked
- Radiographs of spine may show compression of vertebrae
- Dual-energy x-ray absorptiometry (DEXA) is quite accurate and delivers negligible radiation
- Osteoporosis: bone densitometry T score ≤ –2.5; osteopenia: T score ≤ –1.5 to –2.4
- DEXA screening recommended for
  - All white and Asian women ≥ 55 years
  - All patients taking prednisone long-term
  - All patients with neurologic disorder (eg, paraplegia); prior pathologic fractures; family history of osteoporosis, alcoholism, anorexia, or malnutrition
- CT bone densitometry: highly accurate and reproducible
  - More costly than DEXA
  - Reserved for assessing spinal bone density in patients with severe osteoporosis and compression fractures

TREATMENT

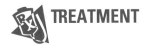

MEDICATIONS

- Calcium and vitamin D to prevent or treat osteoporosis
  - Calcium citrate (0.4–0.7 g elemental calcium PO once daily) or calcium carbonate (1.0–1.5 g elemental calcium PO once daily); calcium citrate causes less gastrointestinal intolerance
  - Vitamin D₂ 800–1000 IU PO once daily
- Bisphosphonates
  - Increase bone density, reduce fracture risk
  - Prevent corticosteroid-induced osteoporosis
  - Take in morning with ≥ 8 oz water, 30–60 minutes before any other food or liquid
  - Must remain upright for 30 minutes after taking to reduce risk of pill-induced esophagitis
  - Alendronate, 70 mg PO every week
  - Risedronate, 35 mg PO every week
  - Ibandronate sodium, 150 mg PO once monthly
  - Pamidronate or zoledronic acid IV if cannot tolerate oral bisphosphonates
  - All patients taking bisphosphonates should receive oral calcium with evening meal and vitamin D
- Consider estrogen or raloxifene for women with hypogonadism (see Menopausal Syndrome)
  - Raloxifene, 60 mg PO once daily decreases risk of vertebral, but not nonvertebral, fractures
- Nasal calcitonin-salmon (Miacalcin) if unable to tolerate bisphosphonates
- Consider teriparatide (Forteo, PTH analog) 20 mcg SQ once daily for ≤ 2 years for severe osteoporosis

THERAPEUTIC PROCEDURES

- Diet adequate in protein, total calories, calcium, and vitamin D
- Discontinue or reduce doses of corticosteroids, if possible
- High-impact physical activity (eg, jogging), stair-climbing, and weight training increase bone density
- Fall-avoidance measures
- Avoid alcohol and smoking
- Verterobroplasty, kyphoplasty are investigational procedures for pain relief following vertebral compression fractures

 OUTCOME

FOLLOW-UP

- DEXA bone densitometry every 2–3 years
- Monitor patients taking corticosteroids or thiazides or in renal failure for development of hypercalcemia when given calcium supplements
- Reduce bisphosphonate dosage in renal insufficiency, and monitor serum phosphate

COMPLICATIONS

- Fractures common, especially femur, vertebrae, and distal radius
- Bisphosphonates
  - Oral can cause esophagitis, gastritis, and abdominal pain
  - Oral and IV can cause fatigue, bone, joint, or muscle pain
    - Pains can be migratory or diffuse, mild to incapacitating
    - Onset of pain occurs 1 day to 1 year after therapy is initiated, with a mean of 14 days
    - Pain can be transient, lasting several days and resolving spontaneously, but typically recurs with subsequent doses
    - Most experience gradual pain relief when medication is stopped
- Raloxifene
  - Increases the risk for thromboembolism
  - Aggravates hot flashes
  - Nausea
  - Weight gain
  - Depression
  - Insomnia
  - Leg cramps
  - Rash
- Teriparitide
  - Orthostatic hypotension
  - Asthenia
  - Nausea

  - Leg cramps
  - Must not be given to patients with Paget's disease or a history of osteosarcoma or chondrosarcoma
- Nasal calcitonin-salmon can cause
  - Bronchospasm and allergic reactions
  - Rhinitis
  - Epistaxis
  - Back pain
  - Arthralgias
- Estrogen replacement
  - Increases risk of thromboembolism and myocardial infarction, breast and endometrial cancer
  - Cholestatic jaundice, hypertriglyceridemia, pancreatitis
  - Enlargement of uterine fibroids, migraines, edema

PROGNOSIS

- Bisphosphonates and raloxifene
  - Can reverse progressive osteopenia and osteoporosis
  - Can decrease fracture risk
- Give calcium supplements with meals to reduce risk of calcium oxalate nephrolithiasis
- Bone pain reduction may be noted within 2–4 weeks on nasal calcitonin

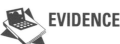 **EVIDENCE**

PRACTICE GUIDELINES

- AACE Practice Guidelines for osteoporosis
- NIH Current Bibliographies in Medicine

WEB SITE

- National Osteoporosis Foundation

INFORMATION FOR PATIENTS

- JAMA patient page. Osteoporosis. JAMA. 1999;282:1396. [PMID: 10527188]
- NIH Osteoporosis Resource Center

REFERENCES

- Black DM et al. Effects of continuing or stopping alendronate after 5 years of treatment: The Fracture Intervention Trial Long-term Extension (FLEX): a randomized trial. JAMA. 2006 Dec 27; 296(24):2927–38. [PMID: 17190893]
- Cosman F et al. Daily and cyclic parathyroid hormone in women receiving alendronate. N Engl J Med. 2005 Aug 11;353(6):566–75. [PMID: 16093465]
- Grant AM et al; RECORD Trial Group. Oral vitamin D3 and calcium for sec-

---

ondary prevention of low-trauma fractures in elderly people (Randomised Evaluation of Calcium Or vitamin D, RECORD): a randomised placebo-controlled trial. Lancet. 2005 May 7–13; 365(9471):1621–8. [PMID: 15885294]
- Jackson RD et al; Women's Health Initiative Investigators. Calcium plus vitamin D supplementation and the risk of fractures. N Engl J Med. 2006 Feb 16; 354(7):669–83. [PMID: 16481635]
- McClung MR et al. Opposite bone remodeling effects of teriparatide and alendronate in increasing bone mass. Arch Intern Med. 2005 Aug 8–22; 165(15):1762–8. [PMID: 16087825]
- Stenson WF et al. Increased prevalence of celiac disease and need for routine screening among patients with osteoporosis. Arch Intern Med. 2005 Feb 28; 165(4):393–9. [PMID: 15738367]

Otitis Media, Acute

 KEY FEATURES

ESSENTIALS OF DIAGNOSIS

- Otalgia, often with an upper respiratory tract infection
- Erythema and hypomobility of tympanic membrane

GENERAL CONSIDERATIONS

- Bacterial infection of the mucosally lined air-containing spaces of the temporal bone
- Purulent material forms within the middle ear cleft but also within the mastoid air cells and petrous apex when they are pneumatized
- Usually precipitated by a viral upper respiratory tract infection that causes eustachian tube edema, resulting in accumulation of fluid and mucus, which become secondarily infected by bacteria
- Nasotracheal intubation can cause otitis media
- Most common pathogens
  - *Streptococcus pneumoniae*
  - *Haemophilus influenzae*
  - *Streptococcus pyogenes*
- Chronic otitis media is usually not painful except during acute exacerbations

DEMOGRAPHICS

- Most common in infants and children, although it may occur at any age
- External otitis and acute otitis media are the most common causes of earache

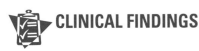 **CLINICAL FINDINGS**

SYMPTOMS AND SIGNS

- Otalgia, aural pressure, decreased hearing, and often fever
- Typically, erythema and decreased mobility of the tympanic membrane
- Occasionally, bullae will be seen on the tympanic membrane, but these rarely indicate *Mycoplasma* infection
- When middle ear empyema is severe, the tympanic membrane can be seen to bulge outward
- In external otitis the ear canal skin is erythematous, whereas in acute otitis media this generally occurs only if the tympanic membrane has ruptured, spilling purulent material into the ear canal
- Persistent otorrhea despite topical and systemic antibiotic therapy

DIFFERENTIAL DIAGNOSIS

- Otitis externa
- Eustachian tube dysfunction
- Mastoiditis
- Tympanosclerosis (scarred tympanic membrane)
- Referred pain: pharyngitis, sinusitis, tooth pain
- Glossopharyngeal neuralgia
- Temporomandibular joint syndrome
- Foreign body
- Cholesteatoma
- Bullous myringitis
- Herpes zoster oticus, especially when vesicles appear in the ear canal or concha

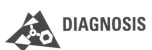 **DIAGNOSIS**

LABORATORY TESTS

- Bacterial (aerobic and anaerobic) and fungal culture of middle ear fluid obtained from tympanocentesis

DIAGNOSTIC PROCEDURES

- Clinical diagnosis

 TREATMENT

MEDICATIONS

- Oral antibiotic therapy
  - Amoxicillin (20–40 mg/kg/day) or erythromycin (50 mg/kg/day) plus sulfonamide (150 mg/kg/day) for 10 days
  - Alternatives useful in resistant cases are cefaclor (20–40 mg/kg/day) or amoxicillin-clavulanate (20–40 mg/kg/day) combinations
- Nasal decongestants, particularly if symptomatic
- Recurrent acute otitis media
  - Use long-term antibiotic prophylaxis: single oral daily doses of sulfamethoxazole (500 mg) or amoxicillin (250 or 500 mg) for 1–3 months

SURGERY

- Surgical drainage of the middle ear (myringotomy) is reserved for patients with severe otalgia or when complications of otitis (eg, mastoiditis, meningitis) have occurred
- Failure of the regimen for recurrent acute otitis media is an indication for insertion of ventilating tubes

THERAPEUTIC PROCEDURES

- Tympanocentesis is useful for otitis media in immunocompromised patients and when infection persists or recurs despite multiple courses of antibiotics

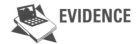 **OUTCOME**

COMPLICATIONS

- Tympanic membrane rupture
- Chronic otitis media
  - Medical treatment includes regular removal of infected debris, use of earplugs to protect against water exposure, and topical antibiotic drops for exacerbations
  - Ciprofloxacin may help to dry a chronically discharging ear when given in a dosage of 500 mg PO BID for 1–6 weeks
  - Definitive management is surgical in most cases
- Mastoiditis
- Meningitis
  - The most common intracranial complication of ear infection
  - In acute otitis media, it arises from hematogenous spread of bacteria, most commonly *H influenzae* and *S pneumoniae*
  - In chronic otitis media, it results either from passage of infections along preformed pathways or from direct extension
- Epidural or brain abscess (temporal lobe or cerebellum)
- Facial palsy
- Sigmoid sinus thrombosis

WHEN TO REFER

- Persistent earache demands specialty referral to exclude cancer of the upper aerodigestive tract

EVIDENCE

PRACTICE GUIDELINES

- American Academy of Pediatrics, American Academy of Family Physicians: Diagnosis and Management of Acute Otitis Media, 2004.

WEB SITE

- Baylor College of Medicine Otolaryngology Resources on the Internet

INFORMATION FOR PATIENTS

- MedlinePlus: Otitis Media Interactive Tutorial
- National Institute on Deafness and Other Communication Disorders: Otitis Media
- Nemours Foundation: Middle Ear Infections (Otitis Media)
- Parmet S et al. Patient page: acute otitis media. JAMA. 2003;290:1666. [PMID: 14506125]

REFERENCES

- Agrawal S et al. Complications of otitis media: an evolving state. J Otolaryngol. 2005 Jun;34(Suppl 1):S33–9. [PMID: 16089238]
- Bance M et al. Topical treatment for otorrhea: issues and controversies. J Otolaryngol. 2005 Aug;34(Suppl 2):S52–5. [PMID: 16076416]
- Hafidh MA et al. Otogenic intracranial complications. a 7-year retrospective review. Am J Otolaryngol. 2006 Nov–Dec;27(6):390–5. [PMID: 17084222]
- Leskinen K et al. Acute complications of otitis media in adults. Clin Otolaryngol. 2005 Dec;30(6):511–6. [PMID: 16402975]

• Rovers MM et al. Otitis media. Lancet. 2004 Feb 7;363(9407):465–73. [PMID: 14962529]

Otitis, External

KEY FEATURES

ESSENTIALS OF DIAGNOSIS

• Erythema and edema of the ear canal skin
• Often with a purulent exudate
• Persistent external otitis in the diabetic or immunocompromised patient may evolve into osteomyelitis of the skull base, often called malignant external otitis

GENERAL CONSIDERATIONS

External otitis

• There is often a history of recent water exposure ("swimmer's ear") or mechanical trauma (eg, scratching, cotton applicators)
• Otitis externa is usually caused by gram-negative rods (eg, *Pseudomonas, Proteus*) or fungi (eg, *Aspergillus*), which grow in the presence of excessive moisture

Malignant external otitis

• Usually caused by *Pseudomonas aeruginosa*
• Osteomyelitis begins in the floor of the ear canal and may extend into the middle fossa floor, the clivus, and even the contralateral skull base

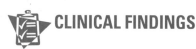

CLINICAL FINDINGS

SYMPTOMS AND SIGNS

External otitis

• Otalgia, frequently accompanied by pruritus and purulent discharge
• Erythema and edema of the ear canal skin, often with a purulent exudate
• Manipulation of the auricle often elicits pain
• Because the lateral surface of the tympanic membrane is ear canal skin, it is often erythematous
• In contrast to acute otitis media, the tympanic membrane in otitis externa moves normally with pneumatic otoscopy
• When the canal skin is very edematous, it may be impossible to visualize the tympanic membrane

Malignant external otitis

• Presents with persistent, refractory otalgia
• Granulation tissue in ear canal
• Cranial neuropathies (especially VII, IX, X)

DIFFERENTIAL DIAGNOSIS

• Otitis media
• Skin cancer
• Traumatic auricular hematoma
• Cellulitis
• Chondritis or perichondritis
• Relapsing polychondritis
• Chondrodermatitis nodularis helicis

DIAGNOSIS

LABORATORY TESTS

• Persistent discharge unresponsive to treatment should be cultured

IMAGING STUDIES

• Diagnosis of malignant otitis externa is confirmed by demonstration of osseous erosion on CT and radioisotope scanning

TREATMENT

MEDICATIONS

External otitis

• Otic drops containing a mixture of aminoglycoside antibiotic and anti-inflammatory corticosteroid in an acid vehicle are generally very effective (eg, neomycin sulfate, polymyxin B sulfate, and hydrocortisone)
• Drops should be used abundantly (5 or more drops three or four times a day) to penetrate the depths of the canal
• In recalcitrant cases, particularly when cellulitis of the periauricular tissue has developed, oral fluoroquinolones (eg, ciprofloxacin, 500 mg PO twice daily for 1 week) are the drugs of choice because of their effectiveness against *Pseudomonas* species

Malignant external otitis

• Prolonged antipseudomonal antibiotic administration, often for several months

SURGERY

• Surgical débridement of infected bone is reserved for cases of malignant external otitis that have worsened despite medical therapy or when material is needed for culture

THERAPEUTIC PROCEDURES

• Fundamental to the treatment of external otitis is protection of the ear from additional moisture and avoidance of further mechanical injury by scratching
• Purulent debris filling the ear canal should be gently removed to permit entry of the topical medication
• When substantial edema of the canal wall prevents entry of drops into the ear canal, a wick is placed to facilitate entry of the medication

OUTCOME

FOLLOW-UP

Malignant external otitis

• To avoid relapse, antibiotic therapy should be continued, even in the asymptomatic patient, until gallium scanning indicates a marked reduction in the inflammatory process

WHEN TO REFER

• Any cases of suspected malignant external otitis should be referred to an otolaryngologist

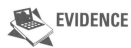

EVIDENCE

WEB SITE

• Baylor College of Medicine Otolaryngology Resources on the Internet

INFORMATION FOR PATIENTS

• American Academy of Family Physicians: Otitis Externa
• Centers for Disease Control and Prevention: Swimmer's Ear
• MedlinePlus: Malignant Otitis Externa

REFERENCES

• Block SL. Otitis externa: providing relief while avoiding complications. J Fam Pract. 2005 Aug;54(8):669–76. [PMID: 16061052]
• Roland PS et al; Ciprodex Otic AOE Study Group. Efficacy and safety of topical ciprofloxacin/dexamethasone versus neomycin/polymyxin B/hydrocortisone for otitis externa. Curr Med Res Opin. 2004 Aug;20(8):1175–83. [PMID: 15324520]

Ovarian Tumors
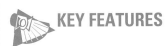

KEY FEATURES

ESSENTIALS OF DIAGNOSIS

- Vague gastrointestinal discomfort
- Pelvic pressure and pain
- Many cases of early-stage cancer are asymptomatic
- Pelvic examination, serum CA 125, and ultrasound are mainstays of diagnosis

GENERAL CONSIDERATIONS

- Ovarian tumors are common
- Most are benign, but malignant ovarian tumors are the leading cause of death from reproductive tract cancer
- The wide range of types and patterns of ovarian tumors is due to the complexity of ovarian embryology and differences in tissues of origin (Table 47)

DEMOGRAPHICS

- In women with no family history of ovarian cancer, the lifetime risk is 1.6%, whereas a woman with one affected first-degree relative has a 5% lifetime risk. With two or more affected first-degree relatives, the risk is 7%
- Approximately 3% of women with two or more affected first-degree relatives will have a hereditary ovarian cancer syndrome with a lifetime risk of 40%
- Women with a *BRCA1* gene mutation have a 45% lifetime risk of ovarian cancer and those with a *BRAC2* mutation have a 25% risk

CLINICAL FINDINGS
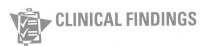

SYMPTOMS AND SIGNS

- Both benign and malignant ovarian neoplasms are either asymptomatic or experience only mild nonspecific gastrointestinal symptoms or pelvic pressure
- Early disease is typically detected on routine pelvic examination
- In advanced malignant disease, women may experience abdominal pain and bloating, and a palpable abdominal mass with ascites is often present

DIFFERENTIAL DIAGNOSIS

- Benign ovarian tumor, eg, follicle cyst, corpus luteum cyst
- Malignant ovarian tumor
- Teratoma (usually benign)
- Tuboovarian abscess
- Endometriosis
- Colon cancer
- Ectopic pregnancy
- Metastases to ovary, eg, gastrointestinal, breast

DIAGNOSIS
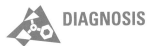

LABORATORY TESTS

- An elevated serum CA 125 (> 35 units) indicates a greater likelihood that an ovarian tumor is malignant
- Serum CA 125 is elevated in 80% of women with epithelial ovarian cancer overall but in only 50% of women with early disease
- Serum CA 125 may be elevated in premenopausal women with benign disease such as endometriosis

IMAGING STUDIES

- Transvaginal sonography (TVS) is useful for screening high-risk women but has inadequate sensitivity for screening low-risk women
- Ultrasound is helpful in differentiating ovarian masses that are benign and likely to resolve spontaneously from those with malignant potential
- Color Doppler imaging may further enhance the specificity of ultrasound diagnosis

TREATMENT
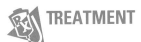

MEDICATIONS

- Except for women with low-grade ovarian cancer in an early stage, postoperative chemotherapy is indicated
- Several chemotherapy regimens are effective, such as the combination of cisplatin or carboplatin with paclitaxel, with clinical response rates of up to 60–70% (Table 7)

SURGERY

- Most ovarian masses in postmenopausal women require surgical evaluation
- However, a postmenopausal woman with an asymptomatic unilateral simple cyst < 5 cm in diameter and a normal serum CA 125 level may be monitored closely with TVS. All others require surgical evaluation
- Exploratory laparotomy has been the standard approach in postmenopausal women
- For ovarian cancer in an early stage, the standard therapy is complete surgical staging followed by abdominal hysterectomy and bilateral salpingo-oophorectomy with omentectomy and selective lymphadenectomy
- With more advanced disease, removal of all visible tumor improves survival
- For benign neoplasms, tumor removal or unilateral oophorectomy is usually performed

THERAPEUTIC PROCEDURES

- In a premenopausal woman, an asymptomatic, mobile, unilateral, simple cystic mass < 8–10 cm may be observed for 4–6 weeks
  - Most will resolve spontaneously
  - If the mass is larger or unchanged on repeat pelvic examination and TVS, surgical evaluation is required
- Laparoscopy may be considered for a small ovarian mass in a premenopausal woman
- If malignancy is suspected in a premenopausal woman, preoperative work-up should include chest radiograph, evaluation of liver and kidney function, and hematologic indices

OUTCOME
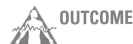

PROGNOSIS

- Approximately 75% of women with ovarian cancer are diagnosed with advanced disease after regional or distant metastases have become established
- The overall 5-year survival is approximately 17% with distant metastases, 36% with local spread, and 89% with early disease

WHEN TO REFER

- If a malignant ovarian mass is suspected, surgical evaluation should be performed by a gynecologic oncologist

PREVENTION

- Women with a *BRCA1* gene mutation should be screened annually with TVS and serum CA 125 testing, and prophylactic oophorectomy is recommended by age 35 or whenever childbearing is completed because of the high risk of disease
- The benefits of such screening for women with one or no affected first-degree relatives are unproved, and the

risks associated with unnecessary surgical procedures may outweigh the benefits in low-risk women

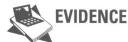 **EVIDENCE**

PRACTICE GUIDELINES

- Morgan R et al; NCCN Ovarian Cancer Practice Guidelines Panel. National Comprehensive Cancer Network: Ovarian Cancer v.1.2005.
- US Preventive Services Task Force. Screening for ovarian cancer: recommendation statement. 2004

WEB SITES

- Cystic Teratoma Demonstration Case
- Hemorrhagic Corpus Luteum Demonstration Case
- National Cancer Institute: Ovarian Cancer Information for Patients and Health Professionals

INFORMATION FOR PATIENTS

- American Academy of Family Physicians: Ovarian Cyst
- American Cancer Society: Ovarian Cancer
- MedlinePlus: Ovarian Cancer Interactive Tutorial
- MedlinePlus: Ovarian Cancer
- National Women's Health Information Center: Ovarian Cysts

REFERENCES

- Bhoola S et al. Diagnosis and management of epithelial ovarian cancer. Obstet Gynecol. 2006 Jun; 107(6):1399–410. [PMID: 16738170]
- Guppy AE et al. Epithelial ovarian cancer: a review of current management. Clin Oncol (R Coll Radiol). 2005 Sep; 17(6):399–411. [PMID: 16149282]

Paget's Disease of Bone

KEY FEATURES

ESSENTIALS OF DIAGNOSIS

- Often asymptomatic
- Bone pain may be first symptom
- Kyphosis, bowed tibias, large head, deafness
- Frequent fractures
- Serum calcium and phosphate normal; alkaline phosphatase elevated; urinary hydroxyproline elevated
- Dense, expanded bones on radiograph

GENERAL CONSIDERATIONS

- Common condition manifested by one or more bony lesions having high bone turnover and disorganized osteoid formation
- Involved bones become vascular, weak, and deformed
- Usually discovered incidentally during radiographic imaging or evaluation of serum alkaline phosphatase elevation
- Familial Paget's disease is unusual but generally more severe

DEMOGRAPHICS

- Present in 1–2% of US adults, especially those of northern European ancestry
  - Highest prevalence in northeastern United States (1.5%)
  - Lowest in the South (0.3%)
- Usually diagnosed in patients age > 40; highest prevalence is among persons aged 65–75 (2.3%); a rare form occurs in young people
- More common in elderly
- Slightly more common in men, with near-equal racial distribution

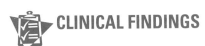

CLINICAL FINDINGS

SYMPTOMS AND SIGNS

- Often mild and asymptomatic; only 27% symptomatic at diagnosis
- Can involve just one bone (monostotic) or multiple bones (polyostotic), particularly skull, femur, tibia, pelvis, and humerus
- Pain is usual first symptom
- Bones become soft, leading to bowed tibias, kyphosis, and frequent fractures with slight trauma
- If skull is involved, patient may report headaches, increased hat size, and deafness
- Increased vascularity over involved bones causes increased warmth
- Sarcomatous change suggested by marked increase in bone pain

DIFFERENTIAL DIAGNOSIS

- Bone tumor, eg, osteosarcoma
- Multiple myeloma
- Metastatic cancer
- Fibrous dysplasia
- Osteitis fibrosa cystica (hyperparathyroidism)
- Fibrogenesis imperfecta ossium

DIAGNOSIS

LABORATORY TESTS

- Serum alkaline phosphatase markedly elevated
- Serum calcium and phosphorus typically normal
- Serum calcium may be elevated, particularly if patient is at bed rest
- Urinary hydroxyproline elevated in active disease
- Sarcomatous change suggested by sudden rise in serum alkaline phosphatase

IMAGING STUDIES

- Bone radiographs show involved bones as expanded and denser than normal
- Multiple fissure fractures in long bones
- Initial lesion may be destructive and radiolucent, especially in skull ("osteoporosis circumscripta")
- Sarcomatous change suggested by appearance of new lytic lesion
- Technetium pyrophosphate bone scans helpful in delineating activity of bone lesions even before radiographic changes are apparent

DIAGNOSTIC PROCEDURES

- Bone biopsy in suspected sarcomatous change

TREATMENT

MEDICATIONS

- **Oral bisphosphonates**
  - May be taken in evening or day
  - Should not be taken within 2 hours of meals, aspirin, indomethacin, calcium, magnesium, or aluminum-containing antacids
  - Esophagitis is uncommon (avoidance of recumbency after dosing not required)
  - Abdominal pain and nausea are common
  - Therapeutic response is evidenced by normalization of serum alkaline phosphatase. Therapy is then discontinued for ~3 months or until alkaline phosphatase rises; then another cycle commenced
  - Alendronate, 20–40 mg PO every morning (or 70 mg PO every week) for 3-month cycles
  - Risedronate, 30 mg PO every morning for 3-month cycles
  - Patient must remain upright after taking alendronate and risedronate to reduce risk of pill-induced esophagitis. Taken in morning with ≥ 8 oz water, at least 30–60 min before any other food or liquid
  - Tiludronate, 400 mg PO once daily for 3 months, is effective in reducing activity of bone lesions
- **Intravenous bisphosphonates**
  - If cannot tolerate oral biphosphonates
  - Zoledronic acid 4 mg IV over 20–30 minutes every 6 months
  - Pamidronate, 60–120 mg IV over 2–4 hours every 6 months
- Nasal calcitonin-salmon (Miacalcin), 200 IU one spray once daily, alternating nostrils. Used less often than bisphosphonates

THERAPEUTIC PROCEDURES

- Asymptomatic patients require no treatment unless there is extensive skull involvement, in which prophylactic treatment may prevent deafness and stroke

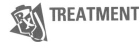

OUTCOME

FOLLOW-UP

- Monitor alkaline phosphatase

COMPLICATIONS

- Fractures frequently occur with minimal trauma
- If patient is immobilized and has excessive calcium intake, hypercalcemia and kidney stones may develop
- Vertebral collapse may lead to spinal cord compression
- Osteosarcoma may develop in long-standing lesions (rare)
- Increased vascularity may cause high-output congestive heart failure

- Arthritis frequently develops in joints adjacent to involved bone
- Extensive skull involvement may cause cranial nerve palsies
  - Deafness may result from entrapment of cranial nerve VIII (and from conductive hearing loss)
  - Tinnitus and vertigo occasionally occur
- Ischemic neurologic events may result form vascular "steal" phenomenon
- In severe forms, marked deformity, intractable pain, and congestive heart failure occur
- After bisphosphonates therapy, patients commonly experience fatigue, myalgia, and bone pain
  - Symptom onset may be anywhere from 1 day to months after institution of therapy and usually improve with discontinuation of therapy or with time after intermittent intravenous therapy
  - Symptoms can vary from nonexistent to incapacitation
  - Potent intravenous bisphosphonates, such as zoledronate, can cause fever

PROGNOSIS

- Prognosis generally good but prognosis is worse the earlier in life the disease starts
- Most patients treated with bisphosphonates have normalization of serum alkaline phosphatase within 6 months, most maintaining this biochemical remission for several years
- Fractures usually heal well

PREVENTION

- Prompt bisphosphonate treatment markedly reduces occurrence of complications of severe Paget's disease

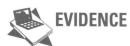

EVIDENCE

PRACTICE GUIDELINES

- Lyles KW et al. A clinical approach to diagnosis and management of Paget's disease of bone. J Bone Miner Res. 2001;16:1379. [PMID: 11499860]

WEB SITES

- National Osteoporosis Foundation
- The Paget Foundation

INFORMATION FOR PATIENTS

- MedlinePlus—Paget's Disease
- The National Institutes of Health Osteoporosis and Related Bone Diseases—National Resource Center—Information for patients about Paget's disease of bone

REFERENCES

- Langston AL et al. Management of Paget's disease of bone. Rheumatology (Oxford). 2004 Aug;43(8):955–9. [PMID: 15187244]
- Reid IR et al. Comparison of a single infusion of zoledronic acid with risedronate for Paget's disease. N Engl J Med. 2005 Sep 1;353(9):898–908. [PMID: 16135834]
- Walsh JP et al. A randomized clinical trial comparing oral alendronate and intravenous pamidronate for the treatment of Paget's disease of bone. Bone. 2004 Apr;34(4):747–54. [PMID: 15050907]
- Whyte MP. Clinical practice: Paget's disease of bone. N Engl J Med. 2006 Aug 10;355(6):593–600. [PMID: 16899779]

Pancreatic Cancer

 KEY FEATURES

ESSENTIALS OF DIAGNOSIS

- Obstructive jaundice (may be painless)
- Enlarged gallbladder (may be painful)
- Upper abdominal pain with radiation to back, weight loss, and thrombophlebitis are usually late manifestations

GENERAL CONSIDERATIONS

- Carcinomas
  - Most common pancreatic neoplasm
  - About 75% are in the head and 25% in the body and tail
  - Those involving the head of the pancreas, the ampulla of Vater, the distal common bile duct, and the duodenum are usually indistinguishable clinically
  - Of these, carcinomas of the pancreas constitute over 90%; they comprise 2% of all cancers and 5% of cancer deaths
- Neuroendocrine tumors account for 2–5% of pancreatic neoplasms
- Cystic neoplasms
  - Only 1% of pancreatic cancers
  - Often mistaken for pseudocysts
  - Should be suspected when a cystic lesion in the pancreas is found in the absence of a history of pancreatitis
  - Whereas serous cystadenomas are benign, mucinous cystadenomas, intraductal papillary mucinous tumors, papillary cystic neoplasms, and cystic islet cell tumors are premalignant
- Staging by the TNM classification
  - Tis: carcinoma in situ
  - T1: tumor limited to the pancreas, ≤ 2 cm in greatest dimension
  - T2: tumor limited to the pancreas, > 2 cm in greatest dimension
  - T3: tumor extends beyond the pancreas but without involvement of the celiac axis or the superior mesenteric artery
  - T4: tumor involves the celiac axis or the superior mesenteric artery

DEMOGRAPHICS

- Risk factors
  - Age
  - Obesity
  - Tobacco use
  - Chronic pancreatitis
  - Prior abdominal radiation
  - Family history
- About 7–8% of pancreatic cancer patients have a first-degree relative with pancreatic cancer, compared with 0.6% of control subjects

 CLINICAL FINDINGS

SYMPTOMS AND SIGNS

- Pain
  - Present in over 70%
  - Often vague and diffuse
  - Located in the epigastrium or left upper quadrant when the lesion is in the tail
  - Radiation into the back is common and sometimes predominates
  - Sitting up and leaning forward may afford some relief, which usually indicates extrapancreatic spread and inoperability
- Diarrhea, perhaps from maldigestion, is an occasional early symptom
- Weight loss commonly occurs late and may be associated with depression
- Occasionally, acute pancreatitis or new-onset diabetes mellitus is the presentation
- Jaundice is usually due to biliary obstruction in the pancreatic head
- A palpable gallbladder is indicative of obstruction by neoplasm (Courvoisier's law), but there are frequent exceptions

- A hard, fixed, occasionally tender mass may be present
- In advanced cases, a hard periumbilical (Sister Mary Joseph's) nodule may be palpable
- Migratory thrombophlebitis is a rare sign

DIFFERENTIAL DIAGNOSIS

- Choledocholithiasis
- Pancreatic pseudocyst or cystic neoplasm
- Carcinoma of the biliary tract
- Biliary stricture
- Hepatocellular carcinoma
- Primary sclerosing cholangitis
- Primary biliary cirrhosis

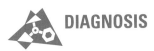 **DIAGNOSIS**

LABORATORY TESTS

- There may be mild anemia
- Glycosuria, hyperglycemia, and impaired glucose tolerance or true diabetes mellitus (10–20% of cases)
- The serum amylase or lipase level is occasionally elevated
- Liver biochemical tests may suggest obstructive jaundice
- Steatorrhea in the absence of jaundice is uncommon
- Occult blood in the stool is suggestive of ampulla of Vater carcinoma (the combination of biliary obstruction and bleeding may give the stools a distinctive silver appearance)
- CA 19-9, with a sensitivity of 70% and a specificity of 87%, is not sensitive enough for early detection; increased values are also found in acute and chronic pancreatitis and cholangitis

IMAGING STUDIES

- With carcinoma of the head of the pancreas, an upper gastrointestinal series may show
  - A widened duodenal loop
  - Mucosal abnormalities in the duodenum ranging from edema to invasion
  - Spasm or compression
- Ultrasonography is not reliable because of interference by intestinal gas
- Multiphase thin-cut helical CT
  - Detects a mass in over 80% of cases
  - Can delineate the extent of the tumor and allow for percutaneous fine-needle aspiration for cytologic studies
- MRI is an alternative to CT

- Positron emission tomography appears to be a sensitive technique for detecting pancreatic cancer and metastases

DIAGNOSTIC PROCEDURES

- Endoscopic ultrasonography
  - More sensitive than CT in diagnosing pancreatic cancer and is equivalent for determining nodal involvement and resectability
  - Can guide fine-needle aspiration for tissue diagnosis and tumor markers
- Endoscopic retrograde cholangiopancreatography (ERCP)
  - May clarify an ambiguous CT or MRI scan by delineating the pancreatic duct system or confirming an ampullary or biliary neoplasm
  - Facilitates decompression of an obstructed biliary tree
- Magnetic resonance cholangiopancreatography (MRCP) is as sensitive as ERCP in diagnosing pancreatic cancer
- Pancreatoscopy or intraductal ultrasonography
  - Can evaluate filling defects in the pancreatic duct
  - Can assess resectability of intraductal papillary mucinous tumors
- With obstruction of the splenic vein, splenomegaly or gastric varices are present; the latter delineated by endoscopy, endoscopic ultrasonography, or angiography
- Selective mesenteric arteriography
  - May demonstrate vessel invasion by a tumor, thus inoperable
  - In general, has been replaced by multiphase helical CT
- Cystic neoplasms can be distinguished by their appearance on CT, endoscopic ultrasonography, and ERCP and features of the cyst fluid on gross and cytologic analysis

 TREATMENT

MEDICATIONS

- Combined irradiation and chemotherapy may be used for palliation of unresectable cancer confined to the pancreas
- Chemotherapy with fluorouracil and gemcitabine has been disappointing in metastatic pancreatic cancer, though improved response rates have been reported with gemcitabine
- Adjuvant or neoadjuvant gemcitabine-based chemotherapy has some benefit, possibly in combination with irradiation

SURGERY

- In about 30% of cases, abdominal exploration is necessary when cytologic diagnosis cannot be made or if resection is attempted
- If a mass is localized in the head of the pancreas and there is no jaundice, laparoscopy may detect tiny peritoneal or liver metastases and thereby avoid resection in about 10% of patients
- Radical pancreaticoduodenal (Whipple) resection is indicated for lesions strictly limited to the head of the pancreas, periampullary zone, and duodenum
- Surgical resection is indicated for all mucinous cystic neoplasms, symptomatic serous cystadenomas, and cystic tumors that remain undefined after helical CT, endoscopic ultrasound, and diagnostic aspiration

THERAPEUTIC PROCEDURES

- When resection is not feasible, endoscopic stenting of the bile duct, or surgical biliary bypass, is performed to relieve jaundice
- A gastrojejunostomy is also done if duodenal obstruction is expected to develop later
- Alternatively, endoscopic placement of a self-expandable duodenal stent may be feasible
- Celiac plexus nerve block or thoracoscopic splanchnicectomy may improve pain control
- Photodynamic therapy is under study

 OUTCOME

PROGNOSIS

- Carcinoma of the pancreas, especially in the body or tail, has a poor prognosis. Reported 5-year survival rates range from 2% to 5%
- Jaundice and lymph node involvement are adverse prognostic factors
- Lesions of the ampulla have a better prognosis, with reported 5-year survival rates of 20–40% after resection
- Pancreatic cystic neoplasms have a better prognosis than pancreatic adenocarcinoma
- In carefully selected patients, resection of cancer of the pancreatic head is feasible and results in reasonable survival
- In a person whose disease progresses with treatment, meticulous efforts at palliative care are essential

PREVENTION

- In persons with a family history of pancreatic cancer, screening with spiral CT and endoscopic ultrasonography should be considered beginning 10 years before the age at which pancreatic cancer was diagnosed in a family member

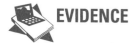

EVIDENCE

PRACTICE GUIDELINES

- Earle CC et al. Cancer Care Ontario Practice Guidelines Initiative's Gastrointestinal Cancer Disease Site Group. The treatment of locally advanced pancreatic cancer: a practice guideline. Can J Gastroenterol. 2003;17:161. [PMID: 12677264]
- Guidelines for the management of patients with pancreatic cancer periampullary and ampullary carcinomas. Gut. 2005;54 (Suppl V):v1. [PMID: 15888770]
- National Guideline Clearinghouse

WEB SITE

- Cystic and Papillary Epithelial Neoplasm of the Pancreas Demonstration Case

INFORMATION FOR PATIENTS

- National Cancer Institute

REFERENCES

- Canto MI et al. Screening for early pancreatic neoplasia in high-risk individuals: a prospective controlled study. Clin Gastroenterol Hepatol. 2006 Jun; 4(6):766–81. [PMID: 16682259]
- Gupta S et al. New-onset diabetes and pancreatic cancer. Clin Gastroenterol Hepatol. 2006 Nov;4(11):1366–72. [PMID: 16945591]
- Maire F et al. Long-term outcome of biliary and duodenal stents in palliative treatment of patients with unresectable adenocarcinoma of the head of pancreas. Am J Gastroenterol. 2006 Apr; 101(4):735–42. [PMID: 16635221]
- Newman EA et al. Adjuvant treatment strategies for pancreatic cancer. J Gastrointest Surg. 2006 Jun;10(6):916–26. [PMID: 16769552]
- Oettle H et al. Adjuvant chemotherapy with gemcitabine vs observation in patients undergoing curative-intent resection of pancreatic cancer: a randomized controlled trial. JAMA. 2007 Jan 17; 297(3):267–77. [PMID: 17227978]
- Shaib YH et al. The epidemiology of pancreatic cancer in the United States: changes below the surface. Aliment Pharmacol Ther. 2006 Jul 1;24(1):87–94. [PMID: 16803606]

Pancreatitis, Acute

KEY FEATURES

ESSENTIALS OF DIAGNOSIS

- Abrupt onset of deep epigastric pain, often with radiation to the back
- Nausea, vomiting, sweating, weakness, fever
- Leukocytosis, elevated serum amylase
- History of previous episodes, often related to alcohol intake

GENERAL CONSIDERATIONS

- Most often due to passed gallstone, usually < 5 mm in diameter, or heavy alcohol intake
- Rarely, may be the initial manifestation of a pancreatic neoplasm
- The pathogenesis may include edema or obstruction of the ampulla of Vater, bile reflux into pancreatic ducts, and direct injury of the pancreatic acinar cells

CLINICAL FINDINGS

SYMPTOMS AND SIGNS

- There may be a history of alcohol intake or a heavy meal immediately preceding the attack, or a history of milder similar episodes or biliary pain in the past

Pain

- Severe, steady, boring epigastric pain, generally abrupt in onset. Usually radiates into the back but may radiate to the right or left
- Often made worse by walking and lying and better by sitting and leaning forward
- The upper abdomen is tender, most often without guarding, rigidity, or rebound
- There may be distention and absent bowel sounds from paralytic ileus
- Nausea and vomiting
- Weakness, sweating, and anxiety in severe attacks

- Fever of 38.4–39.0°C, tachycardia, hypotension (even true shock), pallor, and cool clammy skin are often present
- Mild jaundice is common
- Occasionally, an upper abdominal mass may be palpated
- Acute renal failure (usually prerenal) may occur early in the course

DIFFERENTIAL DIAGNOSIS

- Acute cholecystitis or cholangitis
- Penetrating duodenal ulcer
- Pancreatic pseudocyst
- Ischemic bowel
- Small bowel obstruction
- Abdominal aortic aneurysm
- Kidney stone

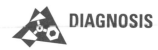

DIAGNOSIS

LABORATORY TESTS

- Serum amylase and lipase increase, usually > 3 times normal, within 24 h in 90% of cases; lipase remains elevated longer than amylase and is slightly more accurate for diagnosis
- Leukocytosis (10,000–30,000/mcL), proteinuria, granular casts, glycosuria (10–20% of cases), hyperglycemia, and elevated serum bilirubin may be present
- Blood urea nitrogen (BUN) and serum alkaline phosphatase may be elevated and coagulation tests abnormal
- A serum alanine aminotransferase level of more than 150 units/L suggests biliary pancreatitis
- Hypocalcemia correlates with severity of disease. Levels < 7 mg/dL (when serum albumin is normal) are associated with tetany
- Early hemoconcentration, hematocrit value above 44%, predicts pancreatic necrosis
- An elevated C-reactive protein concentration (> 150 mg/L) after 48 h suggests the development of pancreatic necrosis
- The fluid amylase content is high in ascites or left pleural effusions

IMAGING STUDIES

- Plain abdominal radiographs may show
  - Gallstones
  - A "sentinel loop" (a segment of air-filled left upper quadrant small intestine)
  - The "colon cutoff sign" (a gas-filled segment of transverse colon abruptly ending at the pancreatic inflammation)

- Linear focal atelectasis of the lower lobe of the lungs with or without pleural effusion
- Ultrasound
  - Often unhelpful for the diagnosis of acute pancreatitis
  - However, it may identify gallstones
- CT scan
  - Can demonstrate an enlarged pancreas and pseudocysts
  - Can differentiate pancreatitis from other possible intra-abdominal catastrophes
- Dynamic IV contrast-enhanced CT
  - Of particular value after the first 3 days of severe disease to identify necrotizing pancreatitis and assess prognosis (Table 94)
  - Avoid IV contrast when the serum creatinine level is > 1.5 mg/dL; order MRI instead
- Endoscopic ultrasonography is useful for occult biliary disease (eg, small stones, sludge)

DIAGNOSTIC PROCEDURES

- CT-guided needle aspiration of necrotizing pancreatitis may diagnose infection
- Endoscopic retrograde cholangiopancreatography (ERCP) is generally not indicated after a first attack unless there is associated cholangitis or jaundice
- However, aspiration of bile for crystal analysis may demonstrate microlithiasis in apparently idiopathic acute pancreatitis

℞ TREATMENT

MEDICATIONS

- Treat pain with meperidine, up to 100–150 mg IM q3–4h as necessary; reduce dose for severe hepatic or renal dysfunction
- Keep NPO until the patient is largely free of pain and has bowel sounds
- Begin with clear liquids and gradually advance to a low-fat diet, guided by the patient's tolerance and by absence of pain
- For **severe pancreatitis**, large amounts of IV fluids are needed to maintain intravascular volume
- Give calcium gluconate intravenously for hypocalcemia with tetany
- Infusions of fresh frozen plasma or serum albumin may be needed for coagulopathy or hypoalbuminemia
- If shock persists after adequate volume replacement (including packed red cells), pressors may be required

- Consider parenteral nutrition (including lipids) for ileus when there will be no nutrition for at least a week
- Enteral nutrition via a nasogastric or nasojejunal tube is preferable if tolerated
- Imipenem (500 mg IV q8h), the combination of ciprofloxacin (750 mg IV BID) and metronidazole (500 mg PO IV TID), or possibly cefuroxime (1.5 g IV TID, then 250 mg PO BID), given for 14 days for sterile pancreatic necrosis, may reduce the risk of pancreatic infection
- The role of IV somatostatin is uncertain, but octreotide is not beneficial

SURGERY

- For mild pancreatitis with cholelithiasis, cholecystectomy or cholecystotomy may be justified
- Infected pancreatic necrosis is an absolute indication for surgery
- Operation may improve survival of necrotizing pancreatitis and clinical deterioration with multiorgan failure or lack of resolution by 4–6 weeks

THERAPEUTIC PROCEDURES

- The pancreatic rest program includes
  - Nothing by mouth
  - Bed rest
  - Nasogastric suction for moderately severe pain, vomiting, or abdominal distention
- ERCP with endoscopic sphincterotomy and stone extraction is indicated when severe pancreatitis results from choledocholithiasis, particularly if jaundice (serum total bilirubin > 5 mg/dL) or cholangitis is present

⛰ OUTCOME

FOLLOW-UP

- Monitor severely ill patients closely
  - White blood cell count
  - Hematocrit
  - Serum electrolytes
  - Serum calcium
  - Serum creatinine
  - BUN
  - Serum aspartate aminotransferase and lactate dehydrogenase (LDH)
  - Arterial blood gases
- Cultures of blood, urine, sputum, and pleural effusion (if present) and needle aspirations of pancreatic necrosis (with CT guidance) should be obtained
- Following recovery from acute biliary pancreatitis, laparoscopic cholecystec-

tomy is generally performed, although endoscopic sphincterotomy alone may be done

COMPLICATIONS

- Acute tubular necrosis
- Necrotizing pancreatitis and infected pancreatic necrosis
- Acute respiratory distress syndrome (ARDS); cardiac dysfunction may be superimposed
- Pancreatic abscess may develop after 6 or more weeks; it requires prompt percutaneous or surgical drainage
- Treat pancreatic infections with imipenem, 500 mg q8h IV
- Pseudocysts < 6 cm in diameter often resolve spontaneously
  - They are multiple in 14% of cases
  - They may become secondarily infected and need drainage
  - Drainage may also help persisting pain or pancreatitis
  - Erosion into a blood vessel can result in a major hemorrhage into the cyst
- Pancreatic ascites may present after recovery from acute pancreatitis with absence of frank abdominal pain. Marked elevations in the ascitic protein (> 3 g/dL) and amylase (> 1000 units/L) levels are typical
- Chronic pancreatitis develops in about 10% of cases
- Permanent diabetes mellitus and exocrine pancreatic insufficiency occur uncommonly after a single acute episode

PROGNOSIS

Ranson's criteria

- Helps assess disease severity
- When three or more of the following are present on admission, a severe course complicated by pancreatic necrosis can be predicted with a sensitivity of 60–80%
  - Age over 55 years
  - White blood cell count > 16,000/mcL
  - Blood glucose > 200 mg/dL
  - Serum LDH > 350 units/L
  - AST > 250 units/L
- Development of the following in the first 48 h indicates a worsening prognosis
  - Hematocrit drop of more than 10 percentage points
  - BUN rise > 5 mg/dL
  - Arterial Po$_2$ of < 60 mm Hg
  - Serum calcium of < 8 mg/dL
  - Base deficit > 4 mEq/L
  - Estimated fluid sequestration of > 6 L

- Mortality rates correlate with the number of criteria present on admission and within the first 48 h
  - 0–2, 1%
  - 3–4, 16%
  - 5–6, 40%
  - 7–8, 100%
- Severity can also be assessed using the Acute Physiology and Chronic Health (APACHE) II or III scoring system as well as the CT scan index (Table 94)
- Multiorgan failure that persists beyond the first 48 hours is associated with a mortality rate over 50%

WHEN TO REFER

- A surgeon should be consulted in all cases of severe acute pancreatitis

WHEN TO ADMIT

- The patient with severe pancreatitis requires treatment in an intensive care unit

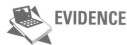 **EVIDENCE**

PRACTICE GUIDELINES

- Toouli J et al. Working Party of the Program Committee of the Bangkok World Congress of Gastroenterology 2002. Guidelines for the management of acute pancreatitis. J Gastroenterol Hepatol 2002;17(Suppl):S15. [PMID: 12000591]
- Uhl W et al. International Association of Pancreatology. IAP guidelines for the surgical management of acute pancreatitis. Pancreatology. 2002;2:565. [PMID: 12435871]

INFORMATION FOR PATIENTS

- National Digestive Diseases Information Clearinghouse
- National Pancreas Association

REFERENCES

- Banks PA et al. Practice guidelines in acute pancreatitis. Am J Gastroenterol. 2006 Oct;101(10):2379–400. [PMID: 17032204]
- Mazaki T et al. Meta-analysis of prophylactic antibiotic use in acute necrotizing pancreatitis. Br J Surg. 2006 Jun; 93(6):674–84. [PMID: 16703633]
- Whitcomb DC. Clinical practice. Acute pancreatitis. N Engl J Med. 2006 May 18;354(20):2142–50. [PMID: 16707751]
- Wilcox CM et al. Role of endoscopic evaluation in idiopathic pancreatitis: a systematic review. Gastrointest Endosc. 2006 Jun;63(7):1037–45. [PMID: 16733122]

Pancreatitis, Chronic

 KEY FEATURES

ESSENTIALS OF DIAGNOSIS

- Epigastric pain
- Steatorrhea
- Weight loss
- Abnormal pancreatic imaging
- A mnemonic for predisposing factors is TIGAR-O
  - Toxic-metabolic
  - Idiopathic
  - Genetic
  - Autoimmune
  - Recurrent and severe acute pancreatitis
  - Obstructive

GENERAL CONSIDERATIONS

- Occurs most often with alcoholism (70–80% of all cases)
- Risk of chronic pancreatitis increases with duration and amount of alcohol consumed, but it develops in only 5–10% of heavy drinkers
- Tobacco smoking may accelerate progression of alcoholic chronic pancreatitis
- Pancreatitis develops in about 2% of patients with hyperparathyroidism
- In tropical Africa and Asia, tropical pancreatitis, related in part to malnutrition, is most common cause of chronic pancreatitis
- A stricture, stone, or tumor obstructing the pancreas can lead to obstructive chronic pancreatitis
- Autoimmune pancreatitis is associated with hypergammaglobulinemia and is responsive to corticosteroids
- About 10–20% of cases are idiopathic
- The pathogenesis of chronic pancreatitis may be explained by the SAPE (sentinel acute pancreatitis event) hypothesis; a first episode of acute pancreatitis initiates an inflammatory process that results in injury fibrosis

DEMOGRAPHICS

- Genetic factors may predispose to chronic pancreatitis in some cases
  - For example, mutations of the cystic fibrosis transmembrane conductance regulator *(CFTR)* gene, the pancreatic secretory trypsin inhibitor gene (*PSTI*, serine protease inhibitor, *SPINK 1*), and possibly the gene for uridine 5'-diphosphate glucuronosyltransferase

 CLINICAL FINDINGS

SYMPTOMS AND SIGNS

- Persistent or recurrent episodes of epigastric and left upper quadrant pain with referral to the upper left lumbar region are typical
- Anorexia, nausea, vomiting, constipation, flatulence, and weight loss are common
- During attacks tenderness over the pancreas, mild muscle guarding, and ileus may be noted
- Attacks may last only a few hours or as long as 2 weeks; pain may eventually be almost continuous
- Steatorrhea (as indicated by bulky, foul, fatty stools) may occur late in the course

DIFFERENTIAL DIAGNOSIS

- Cholelithiasis
- Diabetes mellitus
- Malabsorption due to other causes
- Intractable duodenal ulcer
- Pancreatic cancer
- Irritable bowel syndrome

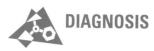 **DIAGNOSIS**

LABORATORY TESTS

- Serum amylase and lipase may be elevated during acute attacks; normal amylase does not exclude the diagnosis
- Serum alkaline phosphatase and bilirubin may be elevated owing to compression of the common duct
- Glycosuria may be present
- Excess fecal fat may be demonstrated in the stool
- Pancreatic insufficiency
  - May be confirmed by response to therapy with pancreatic enzyme supplements or a secretin stimulation test if available

- May be diagnosed by detection of decreased fecal chymotrypsin or elastase levels (if test available), though the tests lack sensitivity and specificity
- Vitamin B_{12} malabsorption is detectable in about 40% of patients, but clinical deficiency of vitamin B_{12} and fat-soluble vitamins is rare
- Accurate genetic tests are available for the major trypsinogen gene mutations
- Elevated IgG_4 levels, ANA, and antibodies to lactoferrin and carbonic anhydrase II often seen in cases of autoimmune pancreatitis

IMAGING STUDIES

- Plain radiographs show calcifications due to pancreaticolithiasis in 30% of patients
- CT may show calcifications not seen on plain radiographs as well as ductal dilation and heterogeneity or atrophy of the gland
- Magnetic resonance cholangiopancreatography (MRCP) and endoscopic ultrasonography (with pancreatic tissue sampling) are less invasive diagnostic tools than endoscopic retrograde cholangiopancreatography (ERCP)
- In autoimmune chronic pancreatitis imaging shows diffuse enlargement of the pancreas, peripheral rim hypoattenuation, and irregular narrowing of the main pancreatic duct

DIAGNOSTIC PROCEDURES

- ERCP
  - Most sensitive study for chronic pancreatitis
  - May show dilated ducts, intraductal stones, strictures, or pseudocysts
  - However, results may be normal in patients with so-called minimal change pancreatitis
- Endoscopic ultrasonography with pancreatic tissue sampling can detect changes of chronic pancreatitis

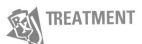 **TREATMENT**

MEDICATIONS

- Steatorrhea
  - Treat with pancreatic supplements, total dose of 30,000 units of lipase (Table 95)
  - Tablets should be taken at the start of, during, and at the end of a meal
  - Higher doses may be required in some cases
  - Concurrent administration of H_2-receptor antagonists (eg, ranitidine,

150 mg PO twice daily), or a proton pump inhibitor (eg, omeprazole, 20–60 mg PO daily), or sodium bicarbonate, 650 mg PO before and after meals, may thereby further decrease steatorrhea
- In selected cases of alcoholic pancreatitis and in cystic fibrosis, enteric-coated microencapsulated preparations may help
- However, in cystic fibrosis, high-dose pancreatic enzyme therapy has been associated with strictures of the ascending colon
- Pain secondary to idiopathic chronic pancreatitis may be alleviated by the use of pancreatic enzymes (not enteric-coated) or octreotide, 200 mcg SQ three times daily
- Associated diabetes should be treated
- Autoimmune pancreatitis is treated with prednisone 40 mg/day PO for 1–2 months, followed by a taper of 5 mg q2–4wks

SURGERY

- Correctable coexistent biliary tract disease should be treated surgically
- Surgery may be indicated to drain persistent pseudocysts, treat other complications, or relieve pain
- When the pancreatic duct is diffusely dilated, anastomosis between the duct after it is split longitudinally and a defunctionalized limb of jejunum (modified Puestow procedure), in some cases combined with local resection of the head of the pancreas, is associated with relief of pain in 80% of cases
- In advanced cases, subtotal or total pancreatectomy may be considered as a last resort but has variable efficacy and is associated with a high rate of pancreatic insufficiency and diabetes
- Endoscopic or surgical drainage is indicated for symptomatic pseudocysts and those over 6 cm in diameter

THERAPEUTIC PROCEDURES

- A low-fat diet should be prescribed
- Alcohol is forbidden because it frequently precipitates attacks
- Narcotics should be avoided if possible
- When obstruction of the duodenal end of the duct can be demonstrated by ERCP, dilation of the duct or surgical resection of the tail of the pancreas with implantation of the duct may be successful
- Pancreatic ascites or pancreaticopleural fistulas due to a disrupted pancreatic

duct can be treated with endoscopic placement of a stent across the duct
- Fragmentation of pancreatic duct stones by lithotripsy and endoscopic removal of stones from the duct, pancreatic sphincterotomy, or pseudocyst drainage may relieve pain in selected patients
- For patients with chronic pain and non-dilated ducts, a percutaneous celiac plexus nerve block may be considered under either CT or endoscopic ultrasound guidance, with pain relief (often short-lived) in approximately 50% of patients

 OUTCOME

COMPLICATIONS

- Opioid addiction is common
- Brittle diabetes mellitus, pancreatic pseudocyst or abscess, cholestatic liver enzymes with or without jaundice, common bile duct stricture, steatorrhea, malnutrition, and peptic ulcer
- Pancreatic cancer develops in 4% of patients after 20 years; the risk may relate to tobacco and alcohol use

PROGNOSIS

- In many cases, it is a self-perpetuating disease characterized by chronic pain or recurrent episodes of acute pancreatitis and ultimately by pancreatic exocrine or endocrine insufficiency
- After many years, chronic pain may resolve spontaneously or as a result of surgery tailored to the cause of pain
- Diabetes develops in over 80% of adults 25 years after the clinical onset of chronic pancreatitis
- Prognosis is best with recurrent acute pancreatitis caused by a remediable condition such as cholelithiasis, choledocholithiasis, stenosis of the sphincter of Oddi, or hyperparathyroidism
- In alcoholic pancreatitis, pain relief is most likely when a dilated pancreatic duct can be decompressed
- In patients with disease not amenable to decompressive surgery, addiction to narcotics is a frequent outcome

PREVENTION

- Abstinence from alcohol
- Medical management of the hyperlipidemia frequently associated with the condition may prevent recurrent attacks of pancreatitis

EVIDENCE

WEB SITE

- Collaborative Hypertext of Radiology (CHORUS)

INFORMATION FOR PATIENTS

- National Digestive Diseases Clearinghouse
- National Pancreas Foundation

REFERENCES

- Adler DG et al. The role of endoscopy in patients with chronic pancreatitis. Gastrointest Endosc. 2006 Jun; 63(7):933–7. [PMID: 16733106]
- Chari ST et al. Diagnosis of autoimmune pancreatitis: the Mayo Clinic experience. Clin Gastroenterol Hepatol. 2006 Aug;4(8):1010–6. [PMID: 16843735]
- Finkleberg DL et al. Autoimmune pancreatitis. N Engl J Med. 2006 Dec 21; 355(25):2670–6. [PMID: 17182992]

Paraneoplastic Syndromes

KEY FEATURES

- Occur in ≤ 15% of patients with cancer
- Small cell lung cancer is most common tumor association
- Can occur despite relatively limited neoplastic growth
- May provide an early clue to presence of certain types of cancer
- Course usually parallels course of the cancer
  - Effective cancer treatment should be accompanied by resolution of the syndrome
  - Conversely, recurrence of the cancer is sometimes heralded by return of syndrome
- Metabolic or toxic effects of the syndrome (eg, hypercalcemia, hyponatremia) may be a more urgent hazard to life than the underlying cancer
- Caused by
  - Tumor product such as ectopic hormone production
    - Serotonin in carcinoid syndrome
    - PTH-related peptide in hypercalcemia
    - ACTH in Cushing's syndrome
    - ADH in the syndrome of inappropriate antidiuretic hormone secretion (SIADH)
  - Destruction of normal tissues by tumor products (local secretion of cytokines leading to hypercalcemia)
  - Unknown mechanisms such as circulating immune complexes stimulated by the tumor or unidentified tumor products (eg, certain neurologic syndromes or osteoarthropathy resulting from bronchogenic carcinoma)

CLINICAL FINDINGS

- Hypercalcemia, hyponatremia
- Cushing's syndrome, SIADH
- Neuropathy, encephalitis, cerebellar degeneration
- Dermatomyositis, Sweet's syndrome
- Polycythemia, thrombocytosis
- Renal disease
- Diarrhea
- Arthropathy

DIAGNOSIS

- See Table 10

TREATMENT

- Treatment of underlying malignancy
- Bisphosphonates, corticosteroids (depending on tumor type) for hypercalcemia
- Symptomatic measures

Parkinsonism

KEY FEATURES

ESSENTIALS OF DIAGNOSIS

- Any combination of tremor, rigidity, bradykinesia, progressive postural instability
- Mild intellectual deterioration may occur

GENERAL CONSIDERATIONS

- Dopamine depletion due to degeneration of the dopaminergic nigrostriatal system leads to an imbalance of dopamine and acetylcholine
- Exposure to toxins can lead to parkinsonism
  - Manganese dust
  - Carbon disulfide
  - Severe carbon monoxide poisoning
  - 1-methyl-4-phenyl-1,2,5,6-tetrahydropyridine (MPTP) for recreational purposes
  - Neuroleptic drugs
  - Reserpine
  - Metoclopramide
- Postencephalitic parkinsonism is becoming increasingly rare
- Only rarely is hemiparkinsonism the presenting feature of a space-occupying lesion

DEMOGRAPHICS

- Common disorder that occurs in all ethnic groups, with an approximately equal sex distribution
- The most common variety, idiopathic Parkinson's disease (paralysis agitans), begins most often in people between ages 45 and 65 years
- May rarely occur on a familial basis

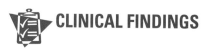

CLINICAL FINDINGS

SYMPTOMS AND SIGNS

- Cardinal features
  - Tremor
  - Rigidity
  - Bradykinesia
  - Postural instability
- Mild decline in intellectual function
- Tremor
  - Four to six cycles per second
  - Most conspicuous at rest
  - Enhanced by stress
  - Often less severe during voluntary activity
  - Commonly confined to one limb or to one side for months or years before becoming more generalized
  - Occasionally involves the lower jaw
- Rigidity causes the flexed posture
- Bradykinesia is the most disabling symptom, ie, a slowness of voluntary movement and a reduction in automatic movements such as swinging of the arms while walking
- The face
  - Relatively immobile with widened palpebral fissures

- Infrequent blinking
- Fixity of facial expression
- Mild blepharoclonus
- Repetitive tapping (about twice per second) over the bridge of the nose producing a sustained blink response (Myerson's sign)
- Other findings
  - Saliva drooling from the mouth
  - Soft and poorly modulated voice
  - Micrographia
- Typically no muscle weakness and no alteration in the tendon reflexes or plantar responses
- Difficulty rising from a sitting position and beginning to walk
- Gait
  - Small shuffling steps and a loss of the normal automatic arm swing
  - There may be unsteadiness on turning, difficulty in stopping, and a tendency to fall

DIFFERENTIAL DIAGNOSIS

- Different causes of parkinsonism
- Essential tremor
- Depression
- Wilson's disease
- Huntington's disease
- Normal-pressure hydrocephalus
- Shy-Drager syndrome or multisystem atrophy
- Progressive supranuclear palsy
- Cortical-basal ganglionic degeneration
- Creutzfeldt-Jakob disease
- Drugs causing parkinsonism
  - Antipsychotic agents
  - Reserpine
  - Metoclopramide

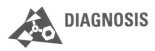 **DIAGNOSIS**

DIAGNOSTIC PROCEDURES

- Primarily a clinical diagnosis

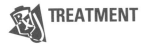 **TREATMENT**

MEDICATIONS

- **Amantadine** (100 mg PO BID) may improve all of the clinical features of parkinsonism
- **Anticholinergics** are more helpful for tremor and rigidity than bradykinesia
  - Start with a small dose (Table 135)
  - Contraindicated in patients with prostatic hypertrophy, narrow-angle

glaucoma, or obstructive intestinal disease
  - Often tolerated poorly by the elderly
- **Sinemet**
  - A combination of carbidopa and levodopa in a fixed ratio (1:10 or 1:4)
  - Start with small dose, eg, 1 tablet of Sinemet 25/100 (containing 25 mg of carbidopa and 100 mg of levodopa) PO TID, and gradually increase depending on the response
- **Sinemet CR**
  - A controlled-release formulation (containing 25 or 50 mg of carbidopa and 100 or 200 mg of levodopa)
  - Sometimes helpful in reducing fluctuations in clinical response and in reducing the frequency with which medication must be taken
- **Stalevo** is a commercial preparation of levodopa combined with both carbidopa and entacapone
  - Stalevo 50 (12.5 mg of carbidopa, 50 mg of levodopa, and 200 mg of entacapone)
  - Stalevo 100 (25 mg of carbidopa, 100 mg of levodopa, and 200 mg of entacapone)
  - Stalevo 150 (37.5 mg of carbidopa, 150 mg of levodopa, and 200 mg of entacapone)
- **Pramipexole**
  - Newer dopamine agonist that is not an ergot derivative
  - Start with 0.125 mg PO TID, doubled after 1 week, and again after another week
  - Daily dose is then increased by 0.75 mg at weekly intervals depending on response and tolerance
  - Most patients require between 0.5 and 1.5 mg PO TID
- **Ropinirole**
  - Newer dopamine agonist that is not an ergot derivative
  - Start with 0.25 mg PO TID
  - Total daily dose is increased at weekly intervals by 0.75 mg until the fourth week and increased by 1.5 mg thereafter
  - Most patients require between 2 and 8 mg PO TID
- **Rasagiline** and **selegiline**
  - Selective monoamine oxidase B inhibitors
  - Rasagiline (1 mg/day PO taken in morning) has a clear symptomatic benefit
  - Selegiline (5 mg PO with breakfast and lunch) is sometimes used as adjunctive treatment; improves fluctuations or declining response to levodopa

  - Tyramine-rich foods are best avoided when either of these agents are taken because of the theoretical possibility of a hypertensive ("cheese") effect
- **Entacapone** and **tolcapone**, two catecholamine-*O*-methyltransferase inhibitors, may be used as an adjunct to Sinemet when there are response fluctuations or inadequate responses
  - Entacapone is given as 200 mg PO with each dose of Sinemet
  - Entacapone is generally preferred over tolcapone because acute hepatic failure has occurred with tolcapone
  - Tolcapone is given in a dosage of 100 mg or 200 mg PO TID
  - With either preparation, the dose of Sinemet taken concurrently may have to be reduced by up to one-third to avoid side effects
- Confusion and psychotic symptoms often respond to atypical antipsychotic agents
  - Olanzapine
  - Quetiapine
  - Risperidone
  - Clozapine
- **Clozapine** may rarely cause marrow suppression, and weekly blood cell counts are therefore necessary
  - Starting dose, 6.25 mg PO HS
  - Dose is increased to 25–100 mg/day as needed
  - In low doses, clozapine may also improve iatrogenic dyskinesias
- **Bromocriptine** and **pergolide** not widely used in the United States because of side effects

SURGERY

- High-frequency bilateral stimulation of the subthalamic nuclei or globus pallidus internus may benefit all the major features of the disease, and it has a lower morbidity than lesion surgery

THERAPEUTIC PROCEDURES

- Drug therapy may not be required early
- Physical and speech therapy and simple aids to daily living may help
  - Rails or banisters placed strategically about the home
  - Special table cutlery with large handles
  - Nonslip rubber table mats
  - Devices to amplify the voice

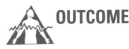 **OUTCOME**

COMPLICATIONS

- Levodopa-induced dyskinesias may take any form

– Chorea
– Athetosis
– Dystonia
– Tremor
– Tics
– Myoclonus

- Later complications of the drug include the "on-off phenomenon"

  – Abrupt but transient fluctuations in the severity of parkinsonism occur unpredictably but frequently during the day
  – The "off" period of marked bradykinesia has been shown to relate in some instances to falling plasma levels of levodopa
  – During the "on" phase, dyskinesias are often conspicuous but mobility is increased
  – Because of this complication, levodopa therapy should be postponed and dopamine agonists used instead, except in the elderly

WHEN TO REFER

- When expertise is needed to determine when to begin therapy
- Consultation with a practitioner with expertise in management may help when there is progressive disease despite appropriate therapy
- For physical and speech therapy

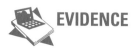

EVIDENCE

PRACTICE GUIDELINES

- Miyasaki JM et al. Practice parameter: initiation of treatment for Parkinson's disease: an evidence-based review: report of the Quality Standards Subcommittee of the American Academy of Neurology. Neurology. 2002;58(1):11. [PMID: 11781398]

INFORMATION FOR PATIENTS

- Torpy JM et al. JAMA patient page. Parkinson disease. JAMA. 2004;291:390. [PMID: 14734603]
- National Institute of Neurological Disorders and Stroke

REFERENCES

- Pahwa R et al. Practice Parameter: Treatment of Parkinson disease with motor fluctuations and dyskinesia (an evidence-based review). Report of the Quality Standards Subcommittee of the American Academy of Neurology. Neurology. 2006 Apr 11;66(7):983–95. [PMID: 16606909]

- Samii A et al. Parkinson's disease. Lancet. 2004 May 29;363(9423):1783–93. [PMID: 15172778]
- Suchowersky O et al. Practice Parameter: Neuroprotective strategies and alternative therapies for Parkinson disease (an evidence-based review). Report of the Quality Standards Subcommittee of the American Academy of Neurology. Neurology. 2006 Apr 11;66(7):976–82. [PMID: 16606908]
- Tolosa E et al. The diagnosis of Parkinson's disease. Lancet Neurol. 2006 Jan; 5(1):75–86. [PMID: 16361025]
- Wu SS et al. Treatment of Parkinson's disease: what's on the horizon? CNS Drugs. 2005;19(9):723–43. [PMID: 16142989]

Patent Ductus Arteriosus

KEY FEATURES

- Embryonic ductus arteriosus fails to close, resulting in continuous (systolic and diastolic) shunt of blood from aorta to left pulmonary artery (PA)
- Usually located near the origin of the left subclavian artery
- Effect of persistent left-to-right shunt on PA pressure depends on size of ductus
- Small or moderate size patent ductus usually asymptomatic until middle age
- Large patent ductus causes pulmonary hypertension, and Eisenmenger's physiology may result

CLINICAL FINDINGS

- Symptoms only if left ventricular (LV) failure or pulmonary hypertension develops
- Heart size is typically normal or slightly enlarged
- Hyperdynamic apical impulse
- Wide pulse pressure and low diastolic pressure
- Continuous rough "machinery" murmur
- Thrill is common in upper right chest
- Advanced disease: cyanotic lower legs (especially toes) in contrast to normally pink fingers due to reversal of shunt when pulmonary hypertension is present

DIAGNOSIS

- ECG: Normal tracing or LV hypertrophy
- Chest radiograph
  – Normal-sized heart or LV and left atrial enlargement
  – Prominent PA, aorta, and left atrium
- Doppler echocardiography is helpful, but lesion is best visualized by MRI, CT, or contrast angiography
- Cardiac catheterization can assess ductus and shunt size and direction and PA pressure

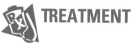

TREATMENT

- Large shunts: high mortality early in life
- Smaller shunts: compatible with long survival; congestive heart failure most common complication
- Antibiotic prophylaxis mandatory to prevent endocarditis
- Surgical ligation or, if ductus size is small enough, transcatheter closure using either coils or occluder devices
- Ductus closure is usually attempted unless pulmonary hypertension and right-to-left shunting is present

Pelvic Inflammatory Disease (PID)

KEY FEATURES

ESSENTIALS OF DIAGNOSIS

- Lower abdominal, adnexal, or cervical motion tenderness
- Absence of a competing diagnosis

GENERAL CONSIDERATIONS

- A polymicrobial infection of the upper genital tract associated with
  – The sexually transmitted organisms *Neisseria gonorrhoeae* and *Chlamydia trachomatis*
  – Endogenous organisms, including anaerobes, *Haemophilus influenzae*, enteric gram-negative rods, and streptococci

- Tuberculous salpingitis is rare in the United States but more common in developing countries
  - It is characterized by pelvic pain and irregular pelvic masses not responsive to antibiotic therapy
  - It is not sexually transmitted

DEMOGRAPHICS

- Most common in young, nulliparous, sexually active women with multiple partners
- Other risk markers include nonwhite race, douching, and smoking
- The use of oral contraceptives or barrier methods of contraception may provide significant protection

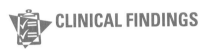 **CLINICAL FINDINGS**

SYMPTOMS AND SIGNS

- Symptoms may include
  - Lower abdominal pain
  - Chills and fever
  - Menstrual disturbances
  - Purulent cervical discharge
  - Cervical and adnexal tenderness
- Right upper quadrant pain (Fitz-Hugh and Curtis syndrome) may indicate an associated perihepatitis
- Diagnosis is complicated by the fact that many women have mild symptoms, not readily recognized as PID

Minimum diagnostic criteria

- Lower abdominal, adnexal, or cervical motion tenderness should be treated as PID with antibiotics unless there is a competing diagnosis such as ectopic pregnancy or appendicitis
- The following criteria may be used to enhance the specificity of the diagnosis
  - Oral temperature > 38.3°C
  - Abnormal cervical or vaginal discharge with white cells on saline microscopy
  - Elevated erythrocyte sedimentation rate
  - Elevated C-reactive protein
  - Laboratory documentation of cervical infection with *N gonorrhoeae* or *C trachomatis* awaiting results

Definitive criteria

- When the clinical or laboratory evidence is uncertain, the following criteria may be used
  - Histopathologic evidence of endometritis on endometrial biopsy
  - Transvaginal sonography or other imaging techniques showing thickened fluid-filled tubes with or without free pelvic fluid or tuboovarian complex
  - Laparoscopic abnormalities consistent with PID

DIFFERENTIAL DIAGNOSIS

- Ectopic pregnancy
- Appendicitis
- Septic abortion
- Ruptured ovarian cyst or tumor
- Ovarian torsion
- Tuboovarian abscess
- Degeneration of leiomyoma (fibroid)
- Diverticulitis
- Cystitis
- Tuberculous salpingitis
- Actinomycosis with prolonged intrauterine device use

 DIAGNOSIS

LABORATORY TESTS

- Abnormal cervical or vaginal discharge may show white blood cells on saline microscopy
- Endocervical culture for *N gonorrhoeae* and saline wet mount for *C trachomatis*
- Erythrocyte sedimentation rate and C-reactive protein may be elevated

IMAGING STUDIES

- Pelvic and vaginal ultrasound can differentiate ectopic pregnancy of over 6 weeks

DIAGNOSTIC PROCEDURES

- Culdocentesis will differentiate hemoperitoneum (ruptured ectopic pregnancy or hemorrhagic cyst) from pelvic sepsis (salpingitis, ruptured pelvic abscess, or ruptured appendix)
- Laparoscopy
  - Can diagnose PID
  - It is imperative if the diagnosis is not certain or if the patient has not responded to antibiotic therapy after 48 h
  - The appendix should be visualized at laparoscopy to rule out appendicitis
  - Cultures obtained at the time of laparoscopy are often helpful

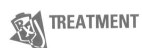 **TREATMENT**

MEDICATIONS

- Antibiotic treatment should not be delayed while awaiting culture results
- The sexual partner should be examined and treated appropriately

Inpatient regimens

- Cefoxitin, 2 g IV q6h, or cefotetan, 2 g IV q12h, plus doxycycline, 100 mg IV or PO q12h
  - This regimen is continued for at least 24 h after there is significant clinical improvement
  - Doxycycline, 100 mg PO BID, should be continued to complete a total of 14 days of therapy
- Clindamycin, 900 mg IV q8h, plus gentamicin IV in a loading dose of 2 mg/kg followed by 1.5 mg/kg q8h
  - This regimen is continued for at least 24 h after there is significant clinical improvement
  - It is followed by either clindamycin, 450 mg PO QID, or doxycycline, 100 mg PO BID, to complete a total of 14 days of therapy
- Ofloxacin, 400 mg IV q12h, or levofloxacin, 500 mg IV once daily with or without metronidazole 500 mg IV q8h
- Ampicillin-sulbactam, 3 g IV q6h, plus doxycycline, 100 mg IV or PO q12h

Outpatient regimens

- Ofloxacin, 400 mg PO BID for 14 days or levofloxacin, 500 mg PO once daily for 14 days, with or without metronidazole, 500 mg PO BID, for 14 days
- Either a single dose of cefoxitin, 2 g IM, with probenecid, 1 g PO or ceftriaxone, 250 mg IM, plus doxycycline, 100 mg PO BID, for 14 days with or without metronidazole, 500 mg PO BID for 14 days

SURGERY

- Tuboovarian abscesses may require surgical excision or transcutaneous or transvaginal aspiration
- Unilateral adnexectomy is acceptable for unilateral abscess
- Hysterectomy and bilateral salpingo-oophorectomy may be necessary for overwhelming infection or in cases of chronic disease with intractable pelvic pain

 OUTCOME

FOLLOW-UP

- Inpatient therapy for tuboovarian abscess should be monitored by ultrasound

COMPLICATIONS

- In spite of treatment, one-fourth of women with acute disease develop long-term sequelae, including
  - Repeated episodes of infection

– Chronic pelvic pain
– Dyspareunia
– Ectopic pregnancy
– Infertility
- The risk of infertility increases with repeated episodes of salpingitis: it is estimated at 10% after the first episode, 25% after a second episode, and 50% after a third episode

PROGNOSIS

- Early treatment with effective antibiotics is essential to prevent long-term sequelae
- For tuboovarian abscess, unless rupture is suspected, high-dose antibiotic therapy in the hospital is effective in 70% of cases. In 30%, there is inadequate response in 48–72 h, and surgical intervention is required

WHEN TO ADMIT

- Admit for IV antibiotic therapy if
  – Patient has a tuboovarian abscess
  – Patient is pregnant
  – Patient is unable to follow or tolerate an outpatient regimen
  – Patient has not responded clinically to outpatient therapy
  – Patient has severe illness, nausea and vomiting, or high fever
  – Patient is immunodeficient (ie, has HIV infection with low CD4 counts, is taking immunosuppressive therapy, or has another immunosuppressing disease)
  – Surgical emergencies, such as appendicitis, cannot be ruled out
- Outpatient parenteral therapy is available in some settings and may be an acceptable alternative
- Patients with tuboovarian abscesses should have direct inpatient observation for at least 24 h prior to switching to outpatient parenteral therapy

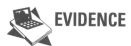 **EVIDENCE**

PRACTICE GUIDELINES

- Centers for Disease Control and Prevention. Pelvic inflammatory disease. Sexually transmitted diseases treatment guidelines. MMWR Recomm Rep 2006;55:1.

INFORMATION FOR PATIENTS

- American Academy of Family Physicians: Pelvic Inflammatory Disease
- American College of Obstetricians and Gynecologists: Pelvic Inflammatory Disease

- MedlinePlus: Pelvic Inflammatory Disease
- National Women's Health Information Center: Pelvic Inflammatory Disease

REFERENCES

- Centers for Disease Control and Prevention; Workowski KA et al. Sexually transmitted disease treatment guidelines 2006. Centers for Disease Control and Prevention. MMWR Recomm Rep. 2006 Aug 4;55(RR-11):1–94. [PMID: 16888612]
- Crossman SH. The challenge of pelvic inflammatory disease. Am Fam Physician. 2006 Mar 1;73(5):859–64. [PMID: 16529095]

Peptic Ulcer Disease

 KEY FEATURES

ESSENTIALS OF DIAGNOSIS

- Peptic ulcer is a break in the gastric or duodenal mucosa, extending through the muscularis mucosae, and usually > 5 mm in diameter
- Nonspecific epigastric pain in 80–90% with variable relationship to meals
- Ulcer symptoms characterized by rhythmicity and periodicity
- Ulcer complications without antecedent symptoms in 10–20%
- Most nonsteroidal anti-inflammatory drug (NSAID)-induced ulcers are asymptomatic
- Upper endoscopy with antral biopsy for *Helicobacter pylori* is diagnostic
- Gastric ulcer biopsy or documentation of complete healing is necessary to exclude gastric malignancy

GENERAL CONSIDERATIONS

- Ulcers are five times more common in the duodenum than in the stomach
- In the stomach, benign ulcers are most common
  – In the antrum (60%)
  – At the junction of the antrum and body on the lesser curvature (25%)
- Major causes of peptic ulcer disease
  – NSAIDs
  – Chronic *H pylori* infection

– Acid hypersecretory states, such as Zollinger-Ellison syndrome
- Up to 10% of ulcers are idiopathic
- Prevalence of *H pylori* infection in duodenal ulcer patients is ~75–90%; however, ulcer develops in only about one of six chronically infected persons
- Prevalence of gastric ulcers is 10–20% and duodenal ulcers is 2–5% in persons who take NSAIDs long-term
- *H pylori* infection increases risk of NSAID-induced ulcers and complications

DEMOGRAPHICS

- In the United States, ~500,000 new cases and 4 million ulcer recurrences per year
- Incidence of duodenal ulcers is declining, while that of gastric ulcers is increasing
- Lifetime prevalence of ulcers in adults is ~10%
- Gastric ulcers are slightly more common in men than in women (1.3:1)
- Duodenal ulcers are most common between the ages of 30 and 55
- Gastric ulcers are most common between the ages of 55 and 70
- Peptic ulcers are more common in smokers

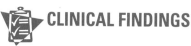 **CLINICAL FINDINGS**

SYMPTOMS AND SIGNS

- Epigastric pain (dyspepsia)
  – Present in 80–90% of persons, but not sensitive or specific enough to serve as reliable diagnostic criterion
  – Typically well localized to epigastrium and not severe
  – Described as gnawing, dull, aching, or "hunger-like"
  – Relieved by food or antacids in about 50%
- Ulcer complications, such as bleeding, in 20% with no antecedent symptoms ("silent ulcers")
- Nocturnal pain awakens two-thirds of patients with duodenal ulcers and one-third of patients with gastric ulcers
- Most patients have symptomatic periods lasting several weeks with intervals of months to years in which they are pain free (periodicity)
- Nausea and anorexia
- Significant vomiting and weight loss suggest gastric outlet obstruction or gastric malignancy
- Physical examination often normal
- Mild, localized epigastric tenderness to deep palpation

DIFFERENTIAL DIAGNOSIS

- Functional dyspepsia
- Gastritis, eg, NSAIDs, alcohol, stress, *H pylori*
- Biliary disease or pancreatitis
- Gastroesophageal reflux disease
- "Indigestion" from overeating, high-fat foods, coffee
- Gastric or pancreatic cancer
- Angina pectoris
- Severe pain
  - Esophageal rupture
  - Gastric volvulus
  - Ruptured aortic aneurysm

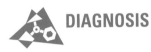 **DIAGNOSIS**

LABORATORY TESTS

- Anemia from acute blood loss with bleeding ulcer
- Leukocytosis suggests ulcer penetration or perforation
- Elevated serum amylase suggests ulcer penetration into the pancreas
- Obtain fasting serum gastrin level to screen for Zollinger-Ellison syndrome, when suspected

Noninvasive testing for **H pylori**

- Serologic, fecal antigen, or urea breath tests
- Rapid, office-based serologic tests
  - Have lower sensitivity (75%) than laboratory-based serologic ELISA test (sensitivity 90%; overall accuracy 80%)
  - Positive test does not necessarily indicate active infection
  - After eradication with antibiotics, ELISA antibody levels decline to undetectable in 50% of patients by 12–18 months
- Fecal antigen immunoassay or ^{13}C-urea breath test
  - Sensitivity and specificity of 90%
  - Positive test indicates active infection
  - Although more expensive than serologic tests, these tests may be more cost-effective because they reduce unnecessary treatment of patients without active infection
  - Proton pump inhibitors significantly reduce the sensitivity of fecal antigen and urea breath tests (but not serologic tests); discontinue 14 days prior to testing

Endoscopic testing for **H pylori**

- Gastric biopsy specimens can detect active *H pylori* infection by histology or by urease production

- Urease test has sensitivity and specificity of 90%

IMAGING STUDIES

- Obtain abdominal CT scan when complications of peptic ulcer disease (perforation, penetration, or obstruction) are suspected

DIAGNOSTIC PROCEDURES

- Upper endoscopy is procedure of choice
- Biopsy indicated for the presence of *H pylori* infection and malignancy
- With benign-appearing gastric ulcers, cytologic brushings and biopsies of the ulcer margin reveal that 3–5% are malignant
- Nonhealing gastric ulcers may be malignant
- Duodenal ulcers are rarely malignant and do not require biopsy

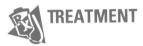 **TREATMENT**

MEDICATIONS

- See Table 39

Peptic ulcers with active **H pylori** *infection*

- Initial treatment for 7–14 days with one of the following
  - Triple-therapy regimen
    - Proton pump inhibitor before meals: omeprazole, 20 mg PO BID; rabeprazole, 20 mg PO BID; lansoprazole, 30 mg PO BID; pantoprazole, 40 mg PO BID; or esomeprazole, 40 mg PO once daily; **plus** clarithromycin, 500 mg PO BID; and amoxicillin, 1 g PO BID; **or** metronidazole, 500 mg PO BID (in penicillin-allergic patients) for 7–10 days
  - Quadruple-therapy regimen
    - Proton pump inhibitor before meals: omeprazole, 20 mg PO BID; rabeprazole, 20 mg PO BID; lansoprazole, 30 mg PO BID; pantoprazole, 40 mg PO BID; or esomeprazole 40 mg once daily; **plus** bismuth subsalicylate, 2 tablets PO QID; **plus** tetracycline, 500 mg PO QID; **plus** metronidazole, 250 mg PO QID for 14 days
    - Recommended for patients in whom an initial attempt at eradication with triple therapy fails
- Continue treatment for 4–8 weeks with omeprazole, 20 mg PO once daily; rabeprazole, 20 mg PO once daily; lansoprazole, 30 mg PO once daily; panto-

prazole, 40 mg PO once daily; or esomeprazole, 40 mg once daily

Peptic ulcers with no **H pylori** *infection*

- Proton pump inhibitors
  - Omeprazole or rabeprazole, 20 mg PO once daily; lansoprazole, 15–30 mg PO once daily; pantoprazole, 40 mg PO once daily; or esomeprazole, 40 mg once daily given 30 min before breakfast heals > 90% of duodenal ulcers after 4 weeks and 90% of gastric ulcers after 8 weeks
- H$_2$-receptor antagonists
  - May be used as a less expensive alternative to proton pump inhibitors
  - Ranitidine, 300 mg PO at bedtime; nizatidine, 300 mg PO at bedtime; famotidine, 40 mg PO at bedtime; or cimetidine, 800 mg PO at bedtime heals 85–90% of duodenal and gastric ulcers within 6–8 weeks
- Maintenance therapy
  - Indicated in patients with recurrent ulcers who are *H pylori* negative, who have failed attempts at eradication therapy, or who require long-term therapy with NSAID or low-dose aspirin
  - Omeprazole, 20 mg PO once daily; rabeprazole, 20 mg PO once daily; lansoprazole, 30 mg PO once daily; esomeprazole, 40 mg PO once daily; pantoprazole, 40 mg PO once daily
  - Cimetidine, 400–800 mg PO at bedtime; nizatidine or ranitidine, 150–300 mg PO at bedtime; famotidine, 20–40 mg PO at bedtime

SURGERY

- For complications of peptic ulcer disease—including perforation, penetration, gastric outlet obstruction, and bleeding—that cannot be controlled with endoscopic therapy

THERAPEUTIC PROCEDURES

- Moderate alcohol intake
- Discontinue smoking
- Discontinue NSAIDs when possible

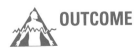 **OUTCOME**

FOLLOW-UP

- For gastric ulcers repeat endoscopy after 2–3 months of therapy to verify complete healing; biopsy if gastric ulcer unhealed to exclude malignancy

COMPLICATIONS

- See Peptic Ulcer Disease, Complications

PROGNOSIS

- If *H pylori* is not eradicated, 85% of patients will have ulcer recurrence within 1 year, half symptomatic; if successfully eradicated, recurrence rates are reduced dramatically to 5–20% at 1 year

WHEN TO REFER

- Patients with persistent dyspepsia after 1–2 weeks of medical treatment
- Complications of peptic ulcer disease

WHEN TO ADMIT

- Complications of peptic ulcer disease

PREVENTION

- To prevent NSAID-induced ulcers: consider the following options
  - Co-therapy with proton pump inhibitors: omeprazole or rabeprazole 20 mg PO once daily; lansoprazole, 30 mg PO once daily; pantoprazole or esomeprazole 20–40 mg PO once daily
  - Co-therapy with misoprostol, 100–200 mcg PO QID; use is limited by side effect profile and frequency of dosing
  - For patients at low risk for cardiovascular disease, consider celecoxib or one of the "safer" nonselective NSAIDs (etodolac, meloxicam, ibuprofen)

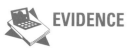

EVIDENCE

PRACTICE GUIDELINES

- Dubois RW et al. Guidelines for the appropriate use of non-steroidal anti-inflammatory drugs, cyclo-oxygenase-2-specific inhibitors and proton pump inhibitors in patients requiring chronic anti-inflammatory therapy. Aliment Pharmacol Ther. 2004;20:1. [PMID: 14723611]

WEB SITES

- National Digestive Diseases Information Clearinghouse
- WebPath Gastrointestinal Pathology Index

INFORMATION FOR PATIENTS

- JAMA patient page. Peptic ulcers. JAMA. 2001;286:2052. [PMID: 11693148]
- MedlinePlus Medical Encyclopedia

REFERENCES

- Papathcodoridis GV et al. Effects of *Helicobacter pylori* and nonsteroidal anti-inflammatory drugs on peptic ulcer disease: a systematic review. Clin Gastroenterol Hepatol. 2006 Feb;4(2):130–42. [PMID: 16469671]
- Saad RJ et al. Levofloxacin-based triple therapy versus bismuth-based quadruple therapy for persistent *Helicobacter pylori* infection: a meta-analysis. Am J Gastroenterol. 2006 Mar;101(3):488–96. [PMID: 16542284]
- Scheiman JM et al. Prevention of ulcers by esomeprazole in at-risk patients using non-selective NSAIDs and COX-2 inhibitors. Am J Gastroenterol. 2006 Apr;101(4):701–10. [PMID: 16494585]
- Vakil N. Primary and secondary treatment for *Helicobacter pylori* in the United States. Rev Gastroenterol Disord. 2005 Spring;5(2):67–72. [PMID: 15976737]
- Vergara M et al. Meta-analysis: role of *Helicobacter pylori* eradication in the prevention of peptic ulcer in NSAID users. Aliment Pharmacol Ther. 2005 Jun 15;21(12):1411–8. [PMID: 15948807]

Peptic Ulcer Disease, Complications

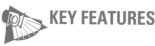

KEY FEATURES

ESSENTIALS OF DIAGNOSIS

- Upper gastrointestinal (GI) hemorrhage, with "coffee grounds" emesis, hematemesis, melena, or hematochezia
- Perforation, with severe pain and peritonitis
- Penetration, with severe pain and pancreatitis
- Gastric outlet obstruction, with vomiting
- Emergent upper endoscopy is usually diagnostic and sometimes therapeutic

GENERAL CONSIDERATIONS

Upper GI hemorrhage

- ~50% of upper GI bleeding is due to peptic ulcer disease

- Bleeding occurs in 10% of patients with an ulcer
- Bleeding stops spontaneously in about 80% of patients; the remainder have severe bleeding
- Overall mortality rate for ulcer bleeding is 6–10%
- Mortality rate is higher in
  - The elderly
  - Those with comorbid medical problems
  - Those with nosocomial bleeding, persistent hypotension, or shock
  - Those with bright red blood in the vomitus or nasogastric lavage fluid
  - Those with severe coagulopathy

Ulcer perforation

- Perforations develop in < 5%
- May be increasing due to use of nonsteroidal anti-inflammatory drugs and cocaine
- Consider Zollinger-Ellison syndrome

Ulcer penetration

- Penetration occurs into contiguous structures such as the pancreas, liver, or biliary tree

Gastric outlet obstruction

- Occurs in 2% of patients with ulcer disease causing obstruction of pylorus or duodenum by scarring and inflammation

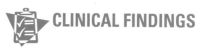

CLINICAL FINDINGS

SYMPTOMS AND SIGNS

Upper GI hemorrhage

- Up to 20% have no antecedent symptoms of pain
- "Coffee grounds" emesis, hematemesis, melena, or hematochezia

Ulcer perforation

- Sudden, severe abdominal pain
- Elderly or debilitated patients and those receiving long-term corticosteroid therapy may have minimal initial symptoms; bacterial peritonitis, sepsis, and shock may present later and then patients appear ill, with a rigid, quiet abdomen and rebound tenderness, hypotension

Ulcer penetration

- Pain is severe and constant, may radiate to the back, and is unresponsive to antacids or food
- Physical examination nonspecific

Gastric outlet obstruction

- Early satiety, vomiting, and weight loss
- Early symptoms: epigastric fullness or heaviness after meals

- Later symptoms: vomiting after eating of partially digested food contents
- Chronic obstruction may result in a grossly dilated, atonic stomach, severe weight loss, and malnutrition, dehydration
- Succussion splash in the epigastrium

DIFFERENTIAL DIAGNOSIS

- Upper GI bleeding
  - Bleeding esophageal varices
  - Mallory-Weiss tear
  - Vascular ectasias
  - Dieulafoy's lesion
  - Malignancy
  - Aortoenteric fistula
  - Hepatic or pancreatic lesions bleeding into pancreatobiliary system
- Severe epigastric pain
  - Esophageal rupture
  - Gastric volvulus
  - Cholecystitis
  - Acute pancreatitis
  - Small bowel obstruction
  - Appendicitis
  - Ureteral colic
  - Splenic rupture

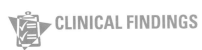 **CLINICAL FINDINGS**

LABORATORY TESTS

Upper GI hemorrhage
- Anemia
- Positive fecal occult blood test

Ulcer perforation
- Leukocytosis
- Mildly elevated serum amylase

Ulcer penetration
- Laboratory tests are nonspecific
- Elevated serum amylase

Gastric outlet obstruction
- Metabolic alkalosis
- Hypokalemia

IMAGING STUDIES

Ulcer perforation
- Upright or decubitus films of the abdomen reveal free intraperitoneal air in 75%
- Upper GI radiography with water-soluble contrast useful
- Abdominal CT increasingly used to establish diagnosis and exclude other causes of abdominal pain

Ulcer penetration
- Barium x-ray studies and endoscopy confirm ulceration but are not diagnostic of an actual penetration

Gastric outlet obstruction
- Endoscopy is preferred diagnostic study

DIAGNOSTIC PROCEDURES

Upper GI hemorrhage
- Nasogastric lavage demonstrates "coffee grounds" or bright red blood; lavage fluid negative for blood does not exclude active bleeding from a duodenal ulcer
- Endoscopy should be performed within 12–24 h in most cases
- It is possible to predict which patients are at a higher risk for rebleeding (see When to Admit)

Gastric outlet obstruction
- Nasogastric aspiration evacuation of a large amount (> 200 mL) of foul-smelling fluid establishes the diagnosis
- Saline load test seldom used

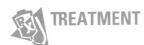 **TREATMENT**

MEDICATIONS

Upper GI hemorrhage
- Antisecretory agents: intravenous or oral proton pump inhibitors, with or without endoscopic therapy, reduce rebleeding, transfusions, and the need for further endoscopic therapy
- For ulcers documented at endoscopy to have active bleeding, adherent clot, or a visible vessel, treat with
  - IV proton pump inhibitor infusion for 3 days (esomeprazole or pantoprazole, 80 mg IV bolus, then 8 mg/h IV) **or**
  - High-dose oral therapy (omeprazole, rabeprazole, esomeprazole, or pantoprazole 40 mg PO BID; or lansoprazole, 60 mg PO BID)

Ulcer perforation
- Initial nonoperative management may be appropriate for selected patients, especially those
  - Who are poor operative candidates
  - Whose onset of symptoms is < 12 h
  - Whose upper GI series or abdominal CT scan with water-soluble contrast medium does not demonstrate leakage
- Nonoperative management
  - Fluids
  - Nasogastric suction
  - IV proton pump inhibitor infusion (esomeprazole or pantoprazole 80 mg IV bolus, then 8 mg/h IV)
  - Broad-spectrum antibiotics
- Up to 40% of ulcer perforations seal spontaneously

- For all others, emergency laparotomy or laparoscopy
- Postoperative treatment of *Helicobacter pylori*

Ulcer penetration
- IV esomeprazole or pantoprazole (80 mg IV bolus; 8 mg/h IV) until able to take oral proton pump inhibitor

Gastric outlet obstruction
- IV isotonic saline and KCl
- IV esomeprazole or pantoprazole (80 mg IV bolus; 8 mg/h IV) continuous infusion
- Nasogastric decompression of the stomach
- Severely malnourished patients should receive total parenteral nutrition

SURGERY

Upper GI hemorrhage
- Patients with high-risk endoscopic lesions or in whom bleeding cannot be controlled with endoscopic treatment should be evaluated by a surgeon
- < 5% of patients treated with hemostatic therapy require surgery

Ulcer perforation
- Closure of the perforation with an omental ("Graham") patch, at emergency laparotomy or laparoscopy

Gastric outlet obstruction
- Vagotomy and either pyloroplasty or antrectomy

THERAPEUTIC PROCEDURES

Gastric outlet obstruction
- Upper endoscopy with dilation by hydrostatic balloons achieves success in two-thirds of patients
- For those who do not respond, consider surgery

 OUTCOME

PROGNOSIS

Upper GI hemorrhage
- The risk of rebleeding or continued bleeding in ulcers with a nonbleeding visible vessel is 50%, and with active bleeding it is 80–90%
- Endoscopic therapy with injection thermocoagulation or application of metallic clip for such lesions reduces the
  - Risk of rebleeding
  - Number of transfusions
  - Need for subsequent surgery
- Surgical mortality for emergency ulcer bleeding is < 6%

Ulcer perforation
- Surgical mortality for emergency ulcer perforation is 5%

WHEN TO ADMIT

Upper GI hemorrhage
- Nonbleeding ulcers < 2 cm in size with a base that is clean have a < 5% chance of rebleeding
  - Young (under age 60), otherwise healthy patients who are stable hemodynamically may be discharged from the hospital or emergency department after endoscopy
  - Others may be observed for 24 h
- Ulcers that have only a flat red or black spot have a < 10% chance of significant rebleeding; hospitalization for 24–72 h usually recommended
- Patients with high-risk ulcers requiring endoscopic therapy (active bleeding, visible vessel, adherent clot) should be monitored in an ICU setting for at least 24 h and in hospital for 72 h; rebleeding occurs in 10–20%

PREVENTION

Upper GI hemorrhage
- Long-term prevention of rebleeding
  - *H pylori* eradication
  - In those with non–*H pylori*-associated ulcers, long-term therapy with H_2-antagonist at bedtime or once daily dose of a proton pump inhibitor

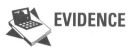

EVIDENCE

PRACTICE GUIDELINES
- Adler DG et al; ASGE. ASGE guideline: the role of endoscopy in acute non-variceal upper-GI hemorrhage. Gastrointest Endosc. 2004 Oct;60(4):497–504. [PMID: 15472669]
- Barkun A et al. Consensus guidelines for managing patients with nonvariceal upper gastrointestinal bleeding. Ann Intern Med. 2003 Nov 18; 139(10):843–57. [PMID: 14623622]

INFORMATION FOR PATIENTS
- American Gastroenterological Association Patient Information Resources
- JAMA patient page: Peptic ulcers. JAMA. 2001;286:2052. [PMID: 11693148]
- MedlinePlus Medical Encyclopedia
- National Digestive Diseases Information Clearinghouse

REFERENCES
- Bardou M et al. Meta-analysis: proton-pump inhibition in high-risk patients with acute peptic ulcer bleeding. Aliment Pharmacol Ther. 2005 Mar 15; 21(6):677–86. [PMID: 15771753]
- Calvet X et al. Addition of a second endoscopic treatment following epinephrine injection improves outcome in high-risk bleeding ulcers. Gastroenterology. 2004 Feb;126(2):441–50. [PMID: 14762781]
- Hung LC et al. Long-term outcome of *Helicobacter pylori*–negative idiopathic bleeding ulcers: a prospective cohort study. Gastroenterology. 2005 Jun; 128(7):1845–50. [PMID: 15940620]
- Julapalli VR et al. Appropriate use of intravenous proton pump inhibitors in the management of bleeding peptic ulcer. Dig Dis Sci. 2005 Jul; 50(7):1185–93. [PMID: 16047458]
- Lanas A et al. A nationwide study of mortality associated with hospital admission due to severe gastrointestinal events and those associated with nonsteroidal antiinflammatory drug use. Am J Gastroenterol. 2005 Aug; 100(8):1685–93. [PMID: 16086703]

Perianal Abscess & Fistula

 KEY FEATURES

- Infection of anal glands located at the base of the anal crypts at the dentate line, leading to abscess formation
- Causes include
  - Anal fissure
  - Crohn's disease
- Fistula in ano arises in an anal crypt and is usually preceded by an anal abscess
- Causes of fistulas that connect to the rectum include
  - Crohn's disease
  - Lymphogranuloma venereum
  - Rectal tuberculosis
  - Cancer

 CLINICAL FINDINGS

- Perianal abscess: throbbing, continuous perianal pain
  - Erythema, fluctuance, and swelling in the perianal region on external examination
  - Swelling in the ischiorectal fossa on digital rectal examination
- Fistula in ano: purulent discharge, itching, tenderness, and pain

 DIAGNOSIS

- Anorectal examination, anoscopy
- Fistulogram
- Pelvic MRI

 TREATMENT

- Perianal abscess is treated by surgical incision under local anesthesia
- Ischiorectal abscess is treated by surgical drainage in the operating room
- Fistula in ano is treated by surgical excision under anesthesia
- Fistulas caused by Crohn's disease are frequently asymptomatic
- Treatment of symptomatic fistulas includes
  - Antibiotics (metronidazole, 250 mg PO TID, or ciprofloxacin, 500 mg PO BID)
  - Immunomodulators (6-mercaptopurine, 1.0–1.5 mg/kg/day PO)
  - Anti-TNF antibody infliximab (5 mg/kg IV at 0, 2, and 6 weeks; then every 8 weeks)
  - Non-cutting Seton drains

Pericardial Effusion

 KEY FEATURES

- Can develop from any form of pericarditis
- Slow development of large effusions may produce no hemodynamic effects
- Rapid appearance of smaller effusions can cause cardiac tamponade (elevated intrapericardial pressure that restricts

venous return and ventricular filling), leading to shock and death

CLINICAL FINDINGS

- Pain in acute inflammatory pericarditis; neoplastic and uremic effusions are often painless
- Dyspnea and cough, especially with tamponade
- Other symptoms reflect primary disease
- Pericardial friction rub may be present (even with large effusions)
- Pulsus paradoxus (> 10 mm Hg decline in systolic pressure during inspiration) is common
- Characteristic features of tamponade
  - Tachycardia
  - Tachypnea
  - Narrow pulse pressure
  - Preserved systolic pressure
- Elevation of central venous pressure, edema, or ascites in chronic processes
- Hypotension, paradoxical pulse and an elevated jugular venous pressure all important signs

DIAGNOSIS

- ECG
  - Often reveals nonspecific T wave changes and low QRS voltage
  - Electrical alternans is pathognomonic but uncommon
- Chest radiograph: normal or enlarged cardiac silhouette with a globular configuration
- Echocardiography
  - Primary mode of diagnosis
  - Can distinguish effusion from congestive heart failure
- Diagnostic pericardiocentesis or biopsy is often indicated for microbiologic and cytologic studies
- Yield of diagnostic pericardial tap is low

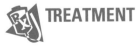

TREATMENT

- Small effusions can be followed clinically and by echocardiogram
- Urgent pericardiocentesis is required for tamponade
- Partial pericardiectomy may be required for recurrent effusion in neoplastic disease and uremia, either by video-assisted thoracic surgery (VATS) or thoracotomy

- Additional therapy (eg, dialysis) for the primary disease

Pericarditis, Acute

KEY FEATURES

- Acute inflammation of the pericardium
- Causes
  - Infections
  - Autoimmune diseases
  - Uremia
  - Neoplasms
  - Radiation
  - Drug toxicity
  - Hemopericardium
  - Postcardiac surgery
  - Contiguous inflammatory processes of the heart or lung (eg, myocardial infarction [MI], Dressler's syndrome, idiopathic)
- Viral infections are the most common cause; acute pericarditis often follows upper respiratory tract infection
- Males, usually younger than age 50, are most commonly affected

CLINICAL FINDINGS

- Often associated with pleuritic chest pain, relieved by sitting, that radiates to the neck, shoulders, back, or epigastrium
- Dyspnea and fever
- Pericardial friction rub with or without evidence of pericardial effusion or constriction
- Pericardial involvement
- Tuberculous pericarditis: subacute; symptoms may be present for days to months
- Bacterial pericarditis: rare; patients appear toxic and are often critically ill
- Uremic pericarditis: symptoms may or may not be present; fever is absent
- Neoplastic pericarditis: often painless, hemodynamic compromise
- Dressler's syndrome (post-MI pericarditis)
  - Occurs within days to 3 months post-MI
  - Usually self-limited

DIAGNOSIS

- Usually clinical
- Leukocytosis
- ECG
  - Generalized ST-T wave changes, characteristic progression beginning with diffuse ST elevations, followed by a return to baseline, then T wave inversions
  - PR depression indicates atrial injury
- Chest radiograph
  - Frequently normal
  - Cardiac enlargement if pericardial effusion
  - Signs of related pulmonary disease
- Echocardiogram
  - Often normal in inflammatory pericarditis
  - Otherwise, can demonstrate pericardial effusion, tamponade
- Rising titers in paired sera may confirm viral infection
- Cardiac enzymes slightly elevated if a myocarditic component
- Cytology of pericardial effusion or pericardial biopsy may be helpful
- Usually data from a diagnostic pericardial tap is unhelpful in diagnosis
- MRI and CT scan can visualize adjacent tumor when present

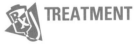

TREATMENT

- Treat underlying causes (eg, antibiotics for bacterial infection, dialysis for uremia)
- Symptomatic treatment with aspirin or nonsteroidal anti-inflammatory drugs (NSAIDs) for pain
- Corticosteroids for unresponsive cases and Dressler's syndrome
- Symptoms usually subside in several days to weeks
- Constrictive pericarditis develops rarely but may require pericardial resection
- Partial pericardiectomy for tamponade; usually done via video-assisted thoracic surgery (VATS)
- Drainage of malignant effusion, instillation of chemotherapeutic agents or tetracycline to prevent recurrence

Pericarditis, Constrictive

KEY FEATURES

- Generally caused by inflammation leading to a thickened, fibrotic, adherent pericardium that restricts diastolic filling and produces chronically elevated venous pressures
- Most common causes
  - Radiation therapy
  - Cardiac surgery
  - Viral pericarditis
- Less common causes
  - Tuberculosis (TB)
  - Histoplasmosis

CLINICAL FINDINGS

- Slowly progressive dyspnea, fatigue, and weakness
- Chronic edema, hepatic congestion, and ascites out of proportion to degree of peripheral edema
- Elevated jugular venous pressure with a rapid *y* descent
- Failure of jugular venous pressure to fall during inspiration (Kussmaul's sign)
- Pericardial knock in early diastole
- Atrial fibrillation is common
- Pulsus paradoxus is unusual

DIAGNOSIS

- Chest radiograph
  - Normal heart size or cardiomegaly
  - Pericardial calcification is rare since TB is cause less often; best seen on lateral view
- Echocardiography
  - Pericardium difficult to see
  - Septal bounce, respiratory fall in mitral Doppler filling pattern useful
  - Normal heart size
- CT and MRI may be more sensitive than echocardiography, but can only identify a thickened pericardium when it is > 4 mm
- Cardiac catheterization: Right atrium (RA)
  - Elevated pressure with *y* descent > *x* descent
  - Kussmaul's sign (lack of fall of RA pressure with inspiration)
- "Square root" diastolic pressures in both RV and LV
  - Equalization of diastolic pressures
  - RV end-diastolic pressure > one-third of RV systolic pressure
  - Evidence of RV-LV interaction (discordance in RV-LV systolic pressures with inspiration)

TREATMENT

- Diuretic agents (Table 16)
  - Right heart failure may respond best to torsemide (better bowel absorption)
  - Add spironolactone
- Complete surgical pericardiectomy
  - Usually required in symptomatic patients
    However, it carries relatively high mortality rate (up to 15%)
- Pericardium can only be removed from phrenic nerve to phrenic nerve

Peritonitis, Spontaneous Bacterial

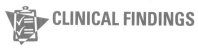

KEY FEATURES

ESSENTIALS OF DIAGNOSIS

- Spontaneous bacterial infection of ascitic fluid in the absence of an apparent intra-abdominal source of infection
- A history of chronic liver disease and ascites
- Fever and abdominal pain
- Neutrocytic ascites [> 250 white blood cells (WBCs)/mcL] with neutrophilic predominance

GENERAL CONSIDERATIONS

- Occurs with few exceptions in patients with chronic liver disease
- Affects ~20–30% of cirrhotic patients
- Most common pathogens are enteric gram-negative bacteria (*Escherichia coli*, *Klebsiella pneumoniae*, *Enterococcus*) or gram-positive bacteria (*Streptococcus pneumoniae*, viridans streptococci)

DEMOGRAPHICS

- Occurs in patients with ascites secondary to portal hypertension, usually with chronic liver disease
- Patients with serum ascites total protein of < 1 g/dL at increased risk

CLINICAL FINDINGS

SYMPTOMS AND SIGNS

- Symptoms in 80–90%; asymptomatic in 10–20%
- Fever and abdominal pain present in two-thirds
- Change in mental status due to exacerbation or precipitation of hepatic encephalopathy
- Signs of chronic liver disease with ascites
- Abdominal tenderness in < 50%

DIFFERENTIAL DIAGNOSIS

- Secondary bacterial peritonitis, eg, appendicitis, diverticulitis, perforated peptic ulcer, perforated gallbladder
- Peritoneal carcinomatosis
- Pancreatic ascites
- Tuberculous ascites

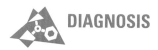

DIAGNOSIS

LABORATORY TESTS

- Renal dysfunction, abrupt worsening of renal function
- Ascitic fluid polymorphonuclear neutrophil (PMN) count of > 250 cells/mcL (neutrocytic ascites) or percentage of PMNs > 50–70% of the ascitic fluid WBC count is presumptive evidence of bacterial peritonitis
- Ascitic fluid Gram stain is insensitive
- Ascitic fluid cultures should be obtained by inoculating count blood culture bottles at the bedside
- 10–30% of patients with neutrocytic ascites have negative ascitic bacterial cultures ("culture-negative neutrocytic ascites"), but are presumed nonetheless to have bacterial peritonitis and treated empirically
- Blood cultures occasionally are positive, which helps identify the organism when ascitic fluid culture is negative

IMAGING STUDIES

- Abdominal ultrasound helpful in locating optimal site for paracentesis

DIAGNOSTIC PROCEDURES

- Abdominal paracentesis

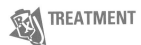

TREATMENT

MEDICATIONS

- Patients with neutrocytic ascites are presumed infected and should be started—regardless of symptoms—on antibiotics
- Empiric therapy usually uses a third-generation cephalosporin, such as cefotaxime, 2 g IV q8–12h (depending on renal function)
- If enterococcus infection is suspected, ampicillin is added
- Recommended duration of antibiotic is 5–10 days or until the ascites fluid PMN count decreases to < 250 cells/mcL
- IV albumin, 1.5 g/kg on day 1 and day 3, is recommended to reduce the development of renal failure and mortality

SURGERY

- Liver transplant is the most effective treatment for spontaneous bacterial peritonitis

OUTCOME

FOLLOW-UP

- Repeat paracentesis at 5 days after start of antibiotic therapy if there is persistent fever, pain, or clinical deterioration

COMPLICATIONS

- Renal failure develops in up to 40% of patients and is a major cause of death

PROGNOSIS

- Mortality of spontaneous bacterial peritonitis exceeds 30%, but if recognized and treated early, mortality is < 10%
- Causes of death include liver failure, hepatorenal syndrome, or bleeding complications

WHEN TO REFER

- Patients failing to improve within 3–5 days of initial therapy
- Patients with possible secondary peritonitis, ie, ascites infected by an intra-abdominal infection (appendicitis, diverticulitis)
- Consider secondary peritonitis in patients with
  - Ascites total protein < 1 g/dL, glucose < 50 mg/dL, or lactate dehydrogenase

(LDH) > upper limit of normal for serum
  - Polymicrobial infection
  - High ascitic neutrophil counts (> 10,000/mcL)

WHEN TO ADMIT

- Symptomatic patients require admission for IV antibiotics
- Selected asymptomatic patients may be treated with oral antibiotics with close follow-up

PREVENTION

- Up to 70% of patients who survive an episode of spontaneous bacterial peritonitis will have another episode within 1 year
- Secondary prophylaxis is recommended with norfloxacin, 400 mg PO once daily; ciprofloxacin, 750 mg PO once weekly; or trimethoprim-sulfamethoxazole, 1 double-strength tablet PO once daily
- Secondary prophylaxis reduces the rate of recurrent infections to < 20%
- Primary prophylaxis is recommended in patients with no history of spontaneous bacterial peritonitis but who are at increased risk for infection due to low-protein ascites (total ascitic protein < 1 g/dL); antibiotics as above

EVIDENCE

PRACTICE GUIDELINES

- American Association for the Study of Liver Diseases (AASLD) Practice Guideline: management of adult patients with ascites due to cirrhosis. Hepatology. 2004;39:841. [PMID: 14999706]
- Mowat C et al. Review article: spontaneous bacterial peritonitis—diagnosis, treatment and prevention. Aliment Pharmacol Ther. 2001;15:1851. [PMID: 11736714]

WEB SITE

- American Association for the Study of Liver Diseases (AASLD): Practice Guidelines: portal hypertension

INFORMATION FOR PATIENTS

- MedlinePlus—Peritonitis, spontaneous

REFERENCES

- Caruntu FA et al. Spontaneous bacterial peritonitis: pathogenesis, diagnosis, treatment. J Gastrointest Liver Dis.

2006 Mar;15(1):51–6. [PMID: 16680233]
- Ghassemi S et al. Prevention and treatment of infections in patients with cirrhosis. Best Pract Res Clin Gastroenterol. 2007;21(1):77–93. [PMID: 17223498]
- Planas R et al. Natural history of patients hospitalized for management of cirrhotic ascites. Clin Gastroenterol Hepatol. 2006 Nov;4(11):1385–94. [PMID: 17081806]
- Sheer TA et al. Spontaneous bacterial peritonitis. Dig Dis. 2005;23(1):39–46. [PMID: 15920324]

Pharyngitis & Tonsillitis

KEY FEATURES

ESSENTIALS OF DIAGNOSIS

- Sore throat
- Fever
- Anterior cervical adenopathy
- Tonsillar exudate
- Focus is to treat group A β-hemolytic streptococcus infection to prevent rheumatic sequelae

GENERAL CONSIDERATIONS

- Group A β-hemolytic streptococci (*Streptococcus pyogenes*) are the most common bacterial cause of exudative pharyngitis
- The main concern is to determine whether the cause is group A β-hemolytic streptococcal infection (GABHS), because of the complications of rheumatic fever and glomerular nephritis
- A second public health policy concern is to reduce the extraordinary cost (in both dollars and the development of antibiotic-resistant *Streptococcus pneumoniae* in the United States associated with unnecessary and unrecommended antibiotic use)
- Group A streptococci which produce erythrogenic toxin may cause scarlet fever rashes in susceptible persons
- About one-third of patients with infectious mononucleosis have secondary streptococcal tonsillitis, requiring treatment

- Ampicillin should routinely be avoided if mononucleosis is suspected because it induces a rash

DEMOGRAPHICS

- Pharyngitis and tonsillitis account for more than 10% of all office visits to primary care clinicians and 50% of outpatient antibiotic use

 CLINICAL FINDINGS

SYMPTOMS AND SIGNS

- Centor diagnostic criteria
  - Fever > 38°C
  - Tender anterior cervical adenopathy
  - Lack of cough
  - Pharyngotonsillar exudate
- Sore throat may be severe, with odynophagia, tender adenopathy, and a scarlatiniform rash
- Hoarseness, cough, and coryza are not suggestive of this disease
- Marked lymphadenopathy and a shaggy white-purple tonsillar exudate, often extending into the nasopharynx, suggest mononucleosis, especially if present in a young adult

DIFFERENTIAL DIAGNOSIS

- Viral pharyngitis
- Epstein-Barr virus (EBV)/infectious mononucleosis
- Primary HIV infection
- Candidiasis
- Necrotizing ulcerative gingivostomatitis (Vincent's fusospirochetal disease)
- Retropharyngeal abscess
- Diphtheria
- *Neisseria gonorrhoeae*
- Mycoplasma
- Anaerobic streptococci
- *Corynebacterium haemolyticum*
- Epiglottitis

 DIAGNOSIS

LABORATORY TESTS

- The presence of the four Centor diagnostic criteria strongly suggests GABHS, and some would treat regardless of laboratory results
- When three of the four Centor criteria are present, laboratory sensitivity of GABHS rapid antigen testing exceeds 90%
- When only one Centor criterion is present, GABHS is unlikely

- Routine throat cultures are not needed
- Leukocytosis with neutrophil predominance is common
- Lymphocyte-white blood cell count ratio differentiates tonsillitis from infectious mononucleosis; with about 90% sensitivity, ratios > 35% suggest EBV infection

 TREATMENT

MEDICATIONS

- Benzathine penicillin or procaine penicillin injection, 1.2 million U, once is optimal, but painful; use for noncompliant patients
- Analgesic, anti-inflammatory drugs (aspirin, acetaminophen)
- Oral antibiotics
  - Penicillin V potassium (250 mg TID or 500 mg PO BID for 10 days) or cefuroxime axetil (250 mg PO BID, 5–10 days)
  - Efficacy of 5-day penicillin V similar to 10-day course: 94% clinical response, 84% eradication
  - Erythromycin (500 mg PO QID) or azithromycin (500 mg PO once daily for 3 days) for penicillin-allergic patients
  - Macrolides not as effective as penicillins
    □ Macrolide resistance in group A streptococci strains as high as 25–40%
    □ Macrolides are second-line agents because of treatment failure risk
  - Macrolide-resistant strains susceptible to clindamycin (10-day course of 300 mg PO TID)
  - Cephalosporins more effective than penicillin for bacterial cure (eg, cefpodoxime and cefuroxime for 5 days)
- Treatment failure
  - Second course with same drug
  - Penicillin alternatives: cephalosporins (eg, cefuroxime), dicloxacillin, amoxicillin-clavulanate
  - Erythromycin resistance (failure rates of ~25%) increasing
  - With severe penicillin allergy, avoid cephalosporins; cross-reaction common (≥ 8%)

SURGERY

- Remove tonsils in cases of recurrent abscess

THERAPEUTIC PROCEDURES

- Salt-water gargling may be soothing

- Anesthetic gargles and lozenges (eg, benzocaine) for additional symptomatic relief

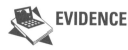 **OUTCOME**

FOLLOW-UP

- Patients who have had rheumatic fever should be treated with a continuous course of antimicrobial prophylaxis (erythromycin, 250 mg PO BID, or penicillin G, 500 mg PO once daily) for at least 5 years

COMPLICATIONS

- Low (10–20%) incidence of treatment failures (positive culture after treatment despite symptomatic resolution) and recurrences

Suppurative

- Sinusitis, otitis media, mastoiditis, peritonsillar abscess, suppuration of cervical lymph nodes

Nonsuppurative

- Rheumatic fever may follow recurrent episodes of pharyngitis 1–4 weeks after onset of symptoms
- Glomerulonephritis follows a single infection with a nephritogenic strain of streptococcus group A (eg, types 4, 12, 2, 49, and 60), more commonly on the skin than in the throat, and begins 1–3 weeks after onset of infection
- Toxic shock syndrome
- Scarlet fever

PROGNOSIS

- Streptococcal pharyngitis usually resolves after 1 week
- Spontaneous resolution of symptoms without treatment still leaves the risk of rheumatic complications

WHEN TO REFER

- Peritonsillar abscess

WHEN TO ADMIT

- Occasionally, odynophagia is so intense that hospitalization for intravenous hydration and antibiotics is necessary
- Suspected or known epiglottitis

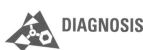 **EVIDENCE**

PRACTICE GUIDELINES

- Bisno AL et al. Practice guidelines for the diagnosis and management of group

MIBG). Ann N Y Acad Sci. 2006 Aug; 1073:465–90. [PMID: 17102115]

- Kercher KW et al. Laparoscopic curative resection of pheochromocytomas. Ann Surg. 2005 Jun;241(6):919–26. [PMID: 15912041]
- Lenders JW et al. Phaeochromocytoma. Lancet. 2005 Aug 20–26;366(9486):665–75. [PMID: 16112304]

Pityriasis Rosea

 ## KEY FEATURES

ESSENTIALS OF DIAGNOSIS

- Oval, fawn-colored, scaly eruption following cleavage lines of trunk
- Herald patch precedes eruption by 1–2 weeks
- Occasional pruritus

GENERAL CONSIDERATIONS

- Common mild, acute inflammatory disease that is 50% more common in women
- The eruption usually lasts 4–8 weeks and heals without scarring

DEMOGRAPHICS

- Young adults are principally affected, mostly in the spring or fall

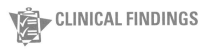 ## CLINICAL FINDINGS

SYMPTOMS AND SIGNS

- Diagnosis is made by finding one or more classic lesions
- The lesions consist of oval, fawn-colored plaques up to 2 cm in diameter
- The centers of the lesions have a crinkled or "cigarette paper" appearance and a collarette scale, ie, a thin bit of scale that is bound at the periphery and free in the center
- Only a few lesions in the eruption may have this characteristic appearance, however
- Lesions follow cleavage lines on the trunk (so-called Christmas tree pattern), and the proximal portions of the extremities are often involved
- Herald patch precedes eruption by 1–2 weeks
- Pruritus, if present, is usually mild

- Variants that affect the flexures (axillae and groin), so-called inverse pityriasis rosea, and papular variants, especially in black patients, also occur

DIFFERENTIAL DIAGNOSIS

- Secondary syphilis
- Tinea corporis (body ringworm)
- Seborrheic dermatitis
- Tinea versicolor (pityriasis versicolor)
- Lichen planus
- Psoriasis
- Nummular eczema
- Drug eruption
- Viral exanthem

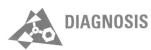 ## DIAGNOSIS

LABORATORY TESTS

- Clinical diagnosis

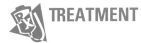 ## TREATMENT

MEDICATIONS

- See Table 150
- Often requires no treatment
- In Asians, Hispanics, or blacks, in whom lesions may remain hyperpigmented for some time, more aggressive management may be indicated
- The most effective management consists of daily UVB treatments for a week, or prednisone as used for contact dermatitis
- Topical corticosteroids of medium strength (triamcinolone 0.1% cream or ointment) may also be used if pruritus is bothersome
- Oral erythromycin 250 mg PO QID for 14 days was reported to clear 73% of patients within 2 weeks (compared with none of the patients taking placebo)

 ## OUTCOME

WHEN TO REFER

- If there is a question about the diagnosis, if recommended therapy is ineffective, or if specialized treatment is necessary

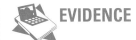 ## EVIDENCE

WEB SITE

- Dermatlas, Johns Hopkins University School of Medicine: Pityriasis Rosea Images

INFORMATION FOR PATIENTS

- American Academy of Dermatology: Pityriasis Rosea
- American Academy of Family Physicians: Pityriasis Rosea
- Mayo Clinic: Pityriasis Rosea
- MedlinePlus: Pityriasis Rosea

REFERENCE

- Cook B et al. Pityriasis rosea. Dermatol Nurs. 2006 Aug;18(4):370. [PMID: 16948385]

Plantar Fasciitis

 ## KEY FEATURES

- The most common cause of foot pain in outpatient medicine
- Results from constant strain on the plantar fascia at its insertion into the medial tubercle of the calcaneus
- The majority of cases occur in patients with no associated disease
- Most occur from excessive standing and improper footwear

 ## CLINICAL FINDINGS

- Severe pain on the bottoms of the feet in the morning—the first steps out of bed in particular—but the pain subsides after a few minutes of ambulation

 ## DIAGNOSIS

- Pain with palpation over the plantar fascia's insertion on the medial heel
- Radiographs have no role in the diagnosis of this condition; heel spurs frequently exist in patients without plantar fasciitis, and most symptomatic patients do not have heel spurs

- Differential diagnosis
  - Enthesopathy resulting from seronegative spondyloarthropathy
  - Achilles tendinitis
  - Metatarsal stress fracture
  - Genital herpes (referred pain from sacral ganglion)
  - Retrocalcaneal bursitis

 TREATMENT

- An interval of days without prolonged standing and the use of arch supports
- NSAIDs may provide some relief
- In severe cases, a corticosteroid with lidocaine injection (small volume—no more than a total of 1.5 mL) directly into the most tender area on the sole of the foot is helpful

Pleural Effusion

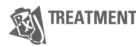 **KEY FEATURES**

ESSENTIALS OF DIAGNOSIS

- May be asymptomatic
- Chest pain seen in the setting of pleuritis, trauma, or infection
- Dyspnea is common with large effusions
- Dullness to percussion and decreased breath sounds over the effusion
- Radiographic evidence of pleural effusion
- Diagnostic findings on thoracentesis

GENERAL CONSIDERATIONS

- Pleural fluid is produced at 0.01 mL/kg/body weight/hour; a normal volume in the pleural space is 5–15 mL
- **Transudative** effusions (see Laboratory Tests) occur in the absence of pleural disease; 90% of cases result from congestive heart failure
- **Exudative** effusions are most commonly due to pneumonia (parapneumonic effusions) and malignancy (malignant effusions)
- Analysis of pleural fluid allows for identification of the pathophysiologic process leading to accumulation of pleural fluid
  - Increased production due to increased hydrostatic or decreased oncotic pressures (transudates)
  - Increased production due to abnormal capillary permeability (exudates)

- Decreased lymphatic clearance of fluid (exudates)
- Infection in the pleural space (empyema)
- Bleeding into the pleural space (hemothorax)
- A definitive diagnosis is made through cytology or identification of causative organism in 25% of cases
- In 50–60% of cases, classification of the effusion leads to a presumptive diagnosis

 CLINICAL FINDINGS

SYMPTOMS AND SIGNS

- Dyspnea, cough, or chest pain with respirations
- Symptoms are more common in patients with underlying cardiopulmonary disease
- Large effusions are more likely to be symptomatic
- Bronchial breath sounds and egophony above the effusion are caused by compressive atelectasis
- Massive effusions may cause contralateral shift of the trachea and bulging of intercostal spaces
- A pleural friction rub indicates infarction or pleuritis

DIFFERENTIAL DIAGNOSIS

- Atelectasis
- Chronic pleural thickening
- Lobar consolidation
- Subdiaphragmatic process
- Table 120

 DIAGNOSIS

LABORATORY TESTS

- See Table 121
- Pleural fluid should be sent for
  - Protein
  - Glucose
  - Lactate dehydrogenase (LDH)
  - Cell count
  - Gram stain
  - Culture
- Grossly purulent fluid signifies empyema; Gram stain and culture are confirmatory
- **Exudates** have one of the following
  - Pleural fluid protein/serum protein > 0.5
  - Pleural fluid LDH/serum LDH > 0.6

- Pleural fluid LDH more than two-thirds of the upper limit of normal serum LDH
- **Transudates** lack any of these features
- **Hemothorax** is defined as a pleural fluid hematocrit/peripheral hematocrit ratio > 0.5
- Elevated pleural fluid amylase suggests
  - Pancreatitis
  - Pancreatic pseudocyst
  - Adenocarcinoma of the lung
  - Esophageal rupture
- Pleural fluid triglyceride level > 100 mg/dL suggests disruption of the thoracic duct
- Pleural fluid cytology has a sensitivity of 50–65% for detecting malignancy
- Repeat cytologic examination, followed by thoracoscopy or video-assisted thoracoscopic surgery (VATS), is indicated if suspicion is high and cytology is negative

IMAGING STUDIES

- Chest radiographs can detect
  - 175–200 mL of pleural fluid on a frontal view
  - 75–100 mL of fluid on a lateral view
- Chest CT can identify 10 mL of pleural fluid
- Lateral decubitus chest films can determine whether blind thoracentesis may be performed; a minimum 1 cm of fluid must be seen for the procedure to be done safely
- Ultrasonography should be used to safely guide thoracentesis of small effusions

DIAGNOSTIC PROCEDURES

- Diagnostic paracentesis should be performed for any new pleural effusion without apparent cause
- Pleural biopsy should be performed in cases of suspected tuberculous effusion
- Pleural fluid culture is only 44% sensitive for tuberculous effusion; culture and histologic examination of pleural tissue increases sensitivity to 70–90%

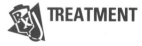 **TREATMENT**

MEDICATIONS

- Appropriate antibiotics for pleural infections (see Tables 62 and 63)

SURGERY

- Thoracotomy may be required in hemothorax to control hemorrhage, remove clot, and treat complications

- Chest tube insertion (tube thoracostomy)
  - Rarely indicated for transudates
  - May be useful in malignant effusions
  - Indicated for some complicated parapneumonic effusions and empyema

THERAPEUTIC PROCEDURES

- Pleurodesis involves placing an irritant into the pleural space to obliterate it by producing adhesions; side effects are pain and fever; premedication is necessary
  - Doxycycline is 70–75% effective
  - Talc is 90% effective
  - Rarely indicated for transudates
  - Often used for recurrent malignant effusions
- Intrapleural fibrinolysis
  - Streptokinase, 250,000 units or urokinase 100,000 units in 100 mL of saline can improve drainage of empyema or complicated parapneumonic effusions with loculations

Transudative effusions

- Treatment is directed at the underlying cause
- Therapeutic thoracentesis may offer only transient relief from dyspnea
- Tube thoracostomy and pleurodesis are rarely indicated

Malignant effusions

- Systemic therapy may address the underlying malignancy
- Repeated thoracentesis or chest tube insertion (tube thoracostomy) may be needed as local therapy to relieve symptoms related to the effusion itself
- Pleurodesis can reduce reaccumulation of fluid
- Alternative strategy is indwelling pleural catheter (eg, Pleurex)
  - Facilitates home drainage for suitable ambulatory patients
  - Provides relief while avoiding hospitalization
  - Has about 40% rate of spontaneous pleurodesis

Parapneumonic effusions

- Simple effusions (free-flowing, sterile) will resolve with treatment of the pneumonia and do not require drainage
- Complicated effusions should be drained via chest tube if fluid analysis reveals pH < 7.2 *or* glucose < 60 mg/dL; drainage should be considered for pH 7.2–7.3 or LDH > 1000 mg/dL
- Empyema should be drained via chest tube

Hemothorax

- If small-volume and stable, observation is adequate

- All other cases should be treated with immediate drainage via a large-bore chest tube

OUTCOME

FOLLOW-UP

- Serial chest radiographs to ensure resolution

COMPLICATIONS

- Fibrothorax can occur if hemothorax is not evacuated

PROGNOSIS

- Depends on the cause of the effusion

WHEN TO REFER

- All large effusions, exudative effusions, and complicated transudative effusions should be evaluated with the assistance of a pulmonologist

WHEN TO ADMIT

- For large-volume thoracentesis, chest tube placement, or complicated closed pleural biopsy

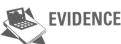
EVIDENCE

PRACTICE GUIDELINES

- Antunes G et al. BTS guidelines for the management of malignant pleural effusions. Thorax. 2003;58(Suppl 2):ii29. [PMID: 12728148]
- Maskell NA et al. BTS guidelines for the investigation of a unilateral pleural effusion in adults. Thorax. 2003;58(Suppl 2):ii8. [PMID: 12728146]

REFERENCES

- Colice GL et al. Medical and surgical treatment of parapneumonic effusions: an evidence-based guideline. Chest. 2000 Oct;118(4):1158–71. [PMID: 11035692]
- Shaw P et al. Pleurodesis for malignant pleural effusions. Cochrane Database Syst Rev. 2004;(1):CD002916. [PMID: 14973997]
- Yataco JC et al. Pleural effusions: evaluation and management. Cleve Clin J Med. 2005 Oct;72(10):854–6. [PMID: 16231684]

Pleuritis

KEY FEATURES

- Irritation of the parietal pleura causes the pain associated with pleuritis

CLINICAL FINDINGS

- Pain
  - Localized, sharp, and fleeting
  - Worsened by cough, sneeze, movement, or deep breathing
- Pain may be referred to the shoulder when there is irritation of the central portion of the ipsilateral diaphragmatic pleura

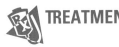
DIAGNOSIS

- The setting in which pain occurs can often narrow the broad list of potential causes
- In young, healthy individuals, pleuritis is usually due to a viral respiratory infection
- Pleural effusion, pleural thickening, or pneumothorax require additional diagnostic and therapeutic measures

TREATMENT

- Treatment is directed at the underlying disease
- NSAIDs (indomethacin, 25 mg PO BID–TID) may help pain relief
- Codeine (30–60 mg PO TID) may control cough
- Intercostal nerve blocks are occasionally helpful

Pneumocystis Pneumonia

KEY FEATURES

ESSENTIALS OF DIAGNOSIS

- *Pneumocystis* is a fungus found in lungs of many domesticated and wild mammals and *Pneumocystis jiroveci* in humans worldwide

- Infection causes pneumonia, with fever, dyspnea, nonproductive cough
- Bibasilar crackles on auscultation in many cases, others have no findings
- Bilateral diffuse interstitial disease without hilar adenopathy on chest radiograph
- Reduced partial pressure of oxygen
- *P jiroveci* in sputum, bronchoalveolar lavage fluid, or lung tissue

GENERAL CONSIDERATIONS

- Based on serology, asymptomatic infections occur at a young age in most persons
- Whether disease in adults represents reinfection or reactivation of existing infection is debated

DEMOGRAPHICS

- Most common in patients with AIDS, also occurs in patients with cancer, severe malnutrition, or in those undergoing immunosuppressive or radiation therapy (eg, for organ transplants, cancer)
- Mode of transmission unknown but likely airborne
- *Pneumocystis* pneumonia occurs in up to 80% of AIDS patients not receiving prophylaxis, usually at CD4 cell counts < 200/mcL
- Infection outside of the lungs is rare
- In non-AIDS patients taking immunosuppressives, symptoms often begin when corticosteroids are tapered or discontinued

 ## CLINICAL FINDINGS

SYMPTOMS AND SIGNS

- Fever; tachypnea; shortness of breath; and cough, usually nonproductive
- Normal lung examination or bibasilar crackles; findings may be slight compared with degree of illness and chest radiographic abnormality
- Spontaneous pneumothorax may occur if patient had previous episodes or received aerosolized pentamidine prophylaxis
- In AIDS: fever, fatigue, and weight loss may occur weeks or months before pulmonary symptoms

DIFFERENTIAL DIAGNOSIS

- Bacterial pneumonia
- Tuberculosis
- Coccidioidomycosis
- Histoplasmosis

- Cytomegalovirus
- Kaposi's sarcoma
- Lymphoma (including lymphocytic interstitial pneumonitis)
- Pulmonary embolism

 ## DIAGNOSIS

LABORATORY TESTS

- Lactate dehydrogenase elevation sensitive but not specific
- Lymphopenia with low CD4 count common
- Arterial blood gas shows hypoxemia and hypocapnia; peripheral oxygen saturation may be normal at rest but decreases rapidly with exercise
- Serologic tests not helpful
- Culture not possible
- Specimens of induced sputum can be stained to demonstrate cysts
- If induced sputum is negative and suspicion is high, diagnostic specimens may be obtained by bronchoalveolar lavage (sensitivity 86–97%) or, if necessary, by transbronchial lung biopsy (sensitivity 85–97%)
- Polymerase chain reaction test for *P jiroveci* appears sensitive but does not provide more rapid diagnosis

IMAGING STUDIES

- Chest radiograph
  - Usually shows diffuse interstitial infiltrates, but early in infection, these may be heterogeneous, miliary, or patchy
  - May also show diffuse or focal consolidation, cystic changes, nodules, or cavitation within nodules
  - Pleural effusions not seen
- Chest radiograph is normal in 5–10%; high-resolution chest CT better able to demonstrate mild disease
- Upper lobe infiltrates common if patient received aerosolized pentamidine prophylaxis
- Gallium lung scanning shows diffuse uptake. While sensitivity is high (> 95%), specificity is low (20–40%), so test usually obtained only if high suspicion and normal chest radiograph and PFTs

DIAGNOSTIC PROCEDURES

- Fine-needle aspiration and open lung biopsy are infrequently done but may need to be performed to diagnose a granulomatous form of *Pneumocystis* pneumonia

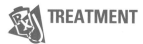 ## TREATMENT

MEDICATIONS

- If disease suspected clinically, initiate empiric therapy while work-up proceeds
- Trimethoprim-sulfamethoxazole (TMP-SMZ) is preferred therapy when tolerated and no sulfa allergy
- Oral TMP-SMZ generates same blood levels as IV and should be used when gastrointestinal tract is functioning
- Dose is based on TMP: 15–20 mg/kg once daily divided TID or QID for 14–21 days; usual adult dose is two double-strength tablets TID
- Hypersensitivity to sulfonamide is especially common in AIDS patients
- Symptoms often persist for 4–6 days after starting therapy and may worsen in first 3–5 days presumably due to immune response to dying organisms
- If $Pao_2 < 70$ mm Hg, add prednisone 40 mg BID for 5 days, then 40 mg once daily for 5 days, then 20 mg once daily until therapy complete
- For severe cases where TMP-SMZ is not tolerated, then pentamidine 3 mg/kg IV/IM once daily for 14–21 days
- For mild to moderate disease in patients intolerant of or not responding to TMP-SMZ
  - Clindamycin, 600 mg PO TID, plus primaquine, 15 mg PO once daily
  - Dapsone, 100 mg PO once daily, plus TMP, 15 mg/kg/day divided TID
  - Atovaquone, 750 mg PO BID
- If patient with known *P jiroveci* is not responding to therapy after 4–6 days, then
  - Need to assess for other concomitant infectious or noninfectious pulmonary processes (cytomegalovirus, tuberculosis, atypical pneumonia, congestive heart failure)
  - Add prednisone if not added at baseline
  - If taking TMP-SMZ, consider switch to alternative therapy
  - If not taking TMP-SMZ because of allergy, consider desensitization and use of TMP-SMZ

 ## OUTCOME

PROGNOSIS

- Without treatment, mortality of pneumocytosis approaches 100%
- With treatment, survival is most closely correlated with pretreatment arterial-alveolar gradient

- Early treatment reduces mortality to 10–20% in AIDS and to 30–50% in other immunodeficient patients
- Recurrence is common without prophylaxis
- In patients who have *P jiroveci* pneumonia associated with AIDS, initiation of highly active antiretroviral treatment may result in "paradoxical deterioration" presumably due to increased immune response against residual microbial antigens

PREVENTION

- Primary prophylaxis is indicated for all AIDS patients with CD4 cell count < 200/mcL
- Secondary prophylaxis indicated for AIDS patients until durable response to antiretroviral therapy has increased CD4 cell count to > 200/mcL on two occasions
- Primary prophylaxis also indicated in bone marrow transplant patients and in stem cell transplant patients who are receiving conditioning regimens; therapy usually continued for 6 months after transplant or longer for those with graft-versus-host disease
- First-line prophylaxis is TMP-SMZ one double-strength tablet three times weekly or once daily. Hypersensitivity is common but if mild may be able to continue therapy through to resolution
- Alternative to TMP-SMZ for prevention
  - Dapsone, 50–100 mg PO once daily; need to check glucose-6-phosphate dehydrogenase levels prior to initiation
  - Oral atovaquone, 1500 mg once daily, has some efficacy but also much more expensive than other regimens
  - Aerosolized pentamidine 300 mg monthly less effective compared with TMP-SMZ and predisposes to extrapulmonary pneumocystosis and pneumothorax

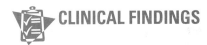

EVIDENCE

PRACTICE GUIDELINES

- Centers for Disease Control and Prevention—Guidelines for PCP prophylaxis
- Infectious Diseases Society of America—Summary of the guidelines for preventing opportunistic infections among hematopoietic stem cell transplant recipients
- 2002 USPHS/IDSA Guidelines for the Prevention of Opportunistic Infections in Persons Infected with Human Immunodeficiency Virus. US Department of

Health and Human Services, Public Health Service
- 2004 USPHS Guidelines for Treating Opportunistic Infections Among HIV-Infected Adults and Adolescents

WEB SITES

- AIDS Info by the USDHHS
- Project Inform

INFORMATION FOR PATIENTS

- Centers for Disease Control and Prevention
- JAMA patient page. HIV infection: the basics. JAMA. 2002;288:268. [PMID: 12123237]
- MedlinePlus

REFERENCES

- Briel M et al. Adjunctive corticosteroids for *Pneumocystis jiroveci* pneumonia in patients with HIV-infection. Cochrane Database Syst Rev. 2006 Jul 19; 3:CD006150. [PMID: 16856118]
- Festic E et al. Acute respiratory failure due to pneumocystis pneumonia in patients without human immunodeficiency virus infection: outcome and associated features. Chest. 2005 Aug; 128(2):573–9. [PMID: 16100140]

Pneumonia, Anaerobic, & Lung Abscess

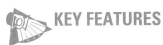

KEY FEATURES

ESSENTIALS OF DIAGNOSIS

- History of or predisposition to aspiration
- Indolent symptoms, including fever, weight loss, malaise
- Poor dentition
- Foul-smelling purulent sputum (in many patients)
- Opacity in dependent lung zone, with single or multiple areas of cavitation or pleural effusion

GENERAL CONSIDERATIONS

- Nocturnal aspiration of small amounts of oropharyngeal secretions is typically not pathologic

- Larger aspirations may cause
  - Nocturnal asthma
  - Chemical pneumonitis
  - Bronchiectasis
  - Mechanical obstruction
  - Pleuropulmonary infection
- Predisposing factors include
  - Drug or alcohol use
  - Seizures
  - Anesthesia
  - Central nervous system disease
  - Trachea or nasogastric tubes
- Periodontal disease and poor oral hygiene are associated with a greater likelihood of pleuropulmonary infection
- Disease usually occurs in dependent lung zones
- Most infections include multiple anaerobic bacteria
  - *Prevotella melaninogenica*
  - *Peptostreptococcus*
  - *Fusobacterium nucleatum*
  - *Bacteroides*

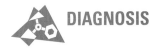

CLINICAL FINDINGS

SYMPTOMS AND SIGNS

- Onset is insidious; necrotizing pneumonia, abscess, or empyema may be apparent at presentation
- Constitutional symptoms of fever, malaise, and weight loss are common
- Cough with foul-smelling expectorant suggests anaerobic infection
- Poor dentition is typical; patients are rarely edentulous
- Occurrence in an edentulous patient suggests an obstructing bronchial lesion

DIFFERENTIAL DIAGNOSIS

- Other causes of cavitary lung disease
  - Tuberculosis
  - Fungal infection
  - Bronchogenic cancer
  - Pulmonary infarction
  - Wegener's granulomatosis
  - Cavitary bacterial pneumonia
- Fungal infection, eg, histoplasmosis
- Bronchiectasis

DIAGNOSIS

LABORATORY TESTS

- Culture of expectorated sputum is not useful due to contamination with oral flora

IMAGING STUDIES

- Chest radiograph in a lung abscess shows a thick-walled cavity surrounded by consolidation, occasionally with an air-fluid level
- Chest radiograph in necrotizing pneumonia demonstrates multiple areas of cavitation within an area of consolidation
- Empyema is characterized by purulent pleural fluid and may accompany the findings of abscess or necrotizing pneumonia
- Ultrasonography may identify loculations or help localize fluid for safe thoracentesis

DIAGNOSTIC PROCEDURES

- Thoracentesis with pleural fluid analysis should be performed on all effusions

TREATMENT

MEDICATIONS

- Clindamycin (600 mg IV q8h, then 300 mg PO q6h after initial improvement)
- Amoxicillin-clavulanate (875 mg PO q12h)
- Penicillin (amoxicillin 500 mg PO TID or penicillin G 1–2 million units IV q4–6h) plus metronidazole 500 mg PO or IV q8–12h
- Therapy should be continued until the chest radiograph improves, usually for a month or more

SURGERY

- Open pleural drainage is sometimes needed because of loculations associated with a parapneumonic effusion

THERAPEUTIC PROCEDURES

- Thoracentesis
- Thoracostomy tube drainage for empyema in anaerobic pleuropulmonary infection

OUTCOME

FOLLOW-UP

- Monitor with chest radiography; if radiograph does not improve, consider other causes

COMPLICATIONS

- Sepsis
- Parapneumonic effusion

- Empyema with loculations and/or pleural scarring may require surgical decortication via thoracotomy

PROGNOSIS

- Excellent with appropriate antimicrobial therapy

WHEN TO REFER

- Refer to infectious disease expert, pulmonary specialist, or thoracic surgeon if no response to antibiotic therapy or concern about the presence of another process (eg, cancer)

WHEN TO ADMIT

- Hypoxemia
- Severe malnutrition
- Marked systemic symptoms

PREVENTION

- Good dental hygiene

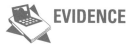

PRACTICE GUIDELINES

- Tablan OC et al; Healthcare Infection Control Practices Advisory Committee. Guidelines for preventing health-care–associated pneumonia, 2003: recommendations of CDC and the Healthcare Infection Control Practices Advisory Committee. MMWR Recomm Rep. 2004;53(RR-3):1. [PMID: 15048056]

REFERENCE

- Schiza S et al. Clinical presentation and management of empyema, lung abscess and pleural effusion. Curr Opin Pulm Med. 2006 May;12(3):205–11. [PMID: 16582676]

Pneumonia, *Chlamydophila*

 KEY FEATURES

- *Chlamydophila pneumoniae* (formerly known as *Chlamydia pneumoniae*) causes pneumonia and bronchitis
- *C pneumoniae* causes approximately 10% of community-acquired pneumonias

- *C pneumoniae* is second only to *Mycoplasma* as an agent of atypical pneumonia

 CLINICAL FINDINGS

- The clinical presentation is that of an atypical pneumonia

 DIAGNOSIS

- Microimmunofluorescence or complement fixation test of acute and convalescent sera

 TREATMENT

- Strains of *C pneumoniae* are resistant to sulfonamides
- Erythromycin or tetracycline, 500 mg PO QID for 10–14 days, appears to be effective
- Fluoroquinolones, such as levofloxacin, 500 mg or moxifloxacin 400 mg once daily for 7–14 days, are active in vitro against *C pneumoniae* and are probably effective; ciprofloxacin has inferior antichlamydial activity compared with the newer fluoroquinolones
- It is unclear if empiric coverage for atypical pathogens in hospitalized patients with community-acquired pneumonia provides a survival benefit or improves clinical outcome

Pneumonia, Community-Acquired

 KEY FEATURES

ESSENTIALS OF DIAGNOSIS

- Symptoms and signs of an acute lung infection
  - Fever or hypothermia
  - Cough with or without sputum
  - Dyspnea
  - Chest discomfort
  - Sweats or rigors
- Bronchial breath sounds or rales are common auscultatory findings

- Parenchymal opacity on chest radiograph
- Occurs outside of the hospital or less than 48 hours after admission

GENERAL CONSIDERATIONS

- Defined as beginning outside of the hospital or within 48 hours of admission in a patient who has not been hospitalized or residing in a long-term care facility for 14 days or more before the onset of symptoms
- The most deadly infectious disease in the United States and the sixth leading cause of death overall
- Mortality rate is 14% among hospitalized patients and 1% among outpatients
- Prospective studies fail to identify the cause in 40–60% of cases, although bacteria are more commonly identified than viruses
- The most common bacterial pathogens
  - *Streptococcus pneumoniae* (two-thirds of cases)
  - *Haemophilus influenzae*
  - *Mycoplasma pneumoniae*
  - *Chlamydia pneumoniae*
  - *Staphylococcus aureus*
  - *Neisseria meningitidis*
  - *Moraxella catarrhalis*
  - *Klebsiella pneumoniae*
- Common viral causes
  - Influenza
  - Respiratory syncytial virus
  - Adenovirus
  - Parainfluenza virus
- Assessment of epidemiologic risk factors may help in diagnosing pneumonia due to the following
  - *Chlamydia psittaci* (psittacosis)
  - *Coxiella burnetii* (Q fever)
  - *Francisella tularensis* (tularemia)
  - Endemic fungi (*Blastomyces, Coccidioides, Histoplasma*)
  - Sin Nombre virus (hantavirus pulmonary syndrome)

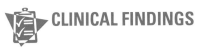 **CLINICAL FINDINGS**

SYMPTOMS AND SIGNS

- Acute or subacute onset of fever, cough with or without sputum, and dyspnea
- Rigors, sweats, chills, pleurisy, and chest discomfort are common
- Fatigue, anorexia, headache, myalgias, and abdominal pain can be present
- Physical findings include
  - Fever or hypothermia
  - Tachypnea
  - Tachycardia
  - Mild oxygen desaturation

- Altered breath sounds or rales are common
- Dullness to percussion may be present with a parapneumonic effusion

DIFFERENTIAL DIAGNOSIS

- Bacterial pneumonia
- Viral pneumonia
- Aspiration pneumonia
- *Pneumocystis jiroveci* pneumonia
- Bronchitis
- Lung abscess
- Tuberculosis
- Pulmonary embolism
- Myocardial infarction
- Sarcoidosis
- Lung neoplasm
- Hypersensitivity pneumonitis
- Bronchiolitis, cryptogenic (bronchiolitis obliterans) organizing pneumonia

 DIAGNOSIS

LABORATORY TESTS

- See Table 103
- Gram stain and culture of sputum are controversial but recommended in hospitalized patients
- Blood cultures obtained prior to antibiotics are generally recommended for hospitalized patients
- Recommended for all hospitalized patients
  - Arterial blood gases
  - Complete blood cell count
  - A comprehensive metabolic panel
- HIV serology should be considered in hospitalized patients

IMAGING STUDIES

- Chest radiograph can confirm the diagnosis and detect associated lung diseases
- Findings range from patchy airspace opacities to diffuse alveolar or interstitial opacities
- Clearing of opacities can take 6 weeks

DIAGNOSTIC PROCEDURES

- Sputum induction is reserved for patients who cannot provide expectorated samples or who may have *Pneumocystis jiroveci* or *Mycobacterium tuberculosis* pneumonia
- Thoracentesis with pleural fluid analysis should be performed in all patients with effusions

 TREATMENT

MEDICATIONS

- See Table 103
- Outpatient therapy
  - Macrolides: clarithromycin, 500 mg PO BID; azithromycyin, 500 mg PO initially, then 250 mg once daily for 4 days or 500 mg/day for 3 days
  - Doxycycline, 100 mg PO BID
  - Fluoroquinolones with enhanced *S pneumoniae* activity: levofloxacin, 500 mg PO once daily; or moxifloxacin 400 mg PO once daily
  - Alternatives are erythromycin, amoxicillin-clavulanate, and some second- or third-generation cephalosporins
- Hospitalized patients on a general medical ward
  - Extended-spectrum β-lactam (ceftriaxone or cefotaxime) with a macrolide (clarithromycin or azithromycin)
  - Fluoroquinolones with enhanced *S pneumoniae* activity (levofloxacin, moxifloxacin)
  - β-Lactam/β-lactamase inhibitor (ampicillin-sulbactam or piperacillin-tazobactam) with a macrolide
- Patients in intensive care unit
  - Macrolide or fluoroquinolone plus an extended-spectrum cephalosporin or β-lactam/β-lactamase inhibitor
  - Penicillin-allergic patients may receive a fluoroquinolone with or without clindamycin
  - Suspected aspiration pneumonia should be treated with fluoroquinolone with or without clindamycin, metronidazole, or β-lactam/β-lactamase inhibitor
- Patients with cystic fibrosis or bronchiectasis should receive empiric antipseudomonal therapy
- Duration of therapy
  - Influenced by the severity of illness, the etiologic agent, response to therapy, and other medical problems
  - For *S pneumoniae*, treat for 72 hours after the patient becomes afebrile
  - 2 weeks is minimum for pneumonia due to *S aureus, P aeruginosa, Klebsiella*, anaerobes, *M pneumoniae, C pneumoniae*, or *Legionella*

 OUTCOME

FOLLOW-UP

- Chest radiograph 6 weeks after therapy

COMPLICATIONS

- Parapneumonic effusion—simple or complicated
- Empyema
- Sepsis
- Respiratory failure or acute respiratory distress syndrome (ARDS), or both
- Pneumotocele
- Lung abscess
- Focal bronchiectasis

PROGNOSIS

- Excellent with appropriate antimicrobial and supportive care

WHEN TO REFER

- Extensive disease or seriously ill patient
- Progression of disease or failure to improve on antibiotics

WHEN TO ADMIT

- The PORT score stratifies patients by mortality and can assist in decisions regarding admission (Tables 104 and 105)

PREVENTION

- Polyvalent pneumococcal vaccine (Tables 67 and 68)
  - Can prevent or lessen the severity of pneumococcal infections
  - Indications are age > 65 or any chronic illness increasing the risk of community-acquired pneumonia
- Influenza vaccine
  - Effective at preventing primary influenza pneumonia and secondary bacterial pneumonia
  - Given annually to patients who are age > 65, are residents of long-term care facilities, have cardiopulmonary disease, or were recently hospitalized with chronic metabolic disorders
- Hospitalized patients who would benefit from vaccine should receive it in hospital
- Pneumococcal and influenza vaccines can be given simultaneously and are not contraindicated immediately after a pneumonia

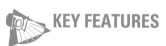

EVIDENCE

PRACTICE GUIDELINES

- American College of Emergency Physicians. Clinical policy for the management and risk stratification of community-acquired pneumonia in adults in the emergency department.

Ann Emerg Med. 2001;38:107. [PMID: 11859897]
- Mandell LA et al. Infectious Diseases Society of America. Update of practice guidelines for the management of community-acquired pneumonia in immunocompetent adults. Clin Infect Dis. 2003;37:1405. [PMID: 14614663]

REFERENCES

- Bodi M et al; Community-Acquired Pneumonia Intensive Care Units (CAPUCI) Study Investigators. Antibiotic prescription for community-acquired pneumonia in the intensive care unit: impact of adherence to IDSA guidelines on survival. Clin Infect Dis. 2005 Dec 15;41(12):1709–16. [PMID: 16288392]
- File TM Jr et al. Guidelines for empiric antimicrobial prescribing in community-acquired pneumonia. Chest. 2004 May;125(5):1888–901. [PMID: 15136404]
- Lutfiyya MN et al. Diagnosis and treatment of community-acquired pneumonia. Am Fam Physician. 2006 Feb 1; 73(3):442–50. [PMID: 16477891]
- Niederman MS et al. Guidelines for the management of adults with community-acquired pneumonia. Diagnosis, assessment of severity, antimicrobial therapy, and prevention. Am J Respir Crit Care Med. 2001 Jun;163(7):1730–54. [PMID: 11401897]
- Wunderink RG et al. Community-acquired pneumonia: pathophysiology and host factors with focus on possible new approaches to management of lower respiratory tract infections. Infect Dis Clin North Am. 2004 Dec; 18(4):743–59. [PMID: 15555822]

Pneumonia, Idiopathic Fibrosing Interstitial

KEY FEATURES

ESSENTIALS OF DIAGNOSIS

- Progressive dyspnea and cough
- Diffuse dry rales on auscultation of the chest

- Restrictive ventilatory defect and abnormal gas exchange
- Bibasilar, peripheral interstitial fibrosis on chest radiograph or CT
- Exclusion of known causes of interstitial lung disease

GENERAL CONSIDERATIONS

- Formerly known as idiopathic pulmonary fibrosis (IPF) and in Britain as cryptogenic fibrosing alveolitis
- Historically, diagnosis was based on clinical and radiographic criteria, with lung biopsy uncommon
- Several histologic patterns once grouped together as IPF are now recognized to be associated with different natural histories and responses to therapy
- Evaluation must first identify patients whose disease is truly idiopathic
- Most identifiable causes of interstitial lung diseases
  - Infectious
  - Drug-related
  - Exposures
  - Associated with other medical conditions
- A specific diagnosis allows providers to give accurate information on natural history and to distinguish patients most likely to benefit from treatment
- See Table 113

DEMOGRAPHICS

- Age range usually 40–70 years
- Slight male predominance
- More common in cigarette smokers than nonsmokers

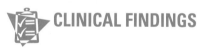

CLINICAL FINDINGS

SYMPTOMS AND SIGNS

- Insidious dry cough and exertional dyspnea lasting months
- Diffuse, fine late inspiratory crackles on auscultation of the lungs
- Clubbing is present at the time of diagnosis in 25–50%

DIFFERENTIAL DIAGNOSIS

- Bronchiolitis obliterans with organizing pneumonia (BOOP), now more commonly referred to as cryptogenic organizing pneumonia (COP)
- Interstitial lung disease due to infection (eg, fungal, viral, *Pneumocystis jiroveci*, tuberculosis)

- Drug-induced fibrosis (eg, amiodarone, bleomycin)
- Sarcoidosis
- Pneumoconiosis
- Hypersensitivity pneumonitis
- Asbestosis
- See Table 112

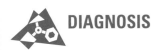

DIAGNOSIS

LABORATORY TESTS

- To exclude other causes
  - ANA, rheumatoid factor
  - Erythrocyte sedimentation rate
  - Aldolase, anti-Jo-1 antibody

IMAGING STUDIES

- Chest radiographs and high-resolution CT scans demonstrate
  - Low lung volumes
  - Diffuse, patchy fibrosis with pleural-based honeycombing

DIAGNOSTIC PROCEDURES

- Transbronchial biopsy cannot be used to definitively diagnose usual interstitial pneumonitis, though it may exclude it by confirming an alternative diagnosis
- Pulmonary function testing shows restrictive physiology with decreased diffusing capacity

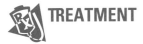

TREATMENT

MEDICATIONS

- Treatment is controversial: no randomized study has demonstrated that treatment improves survival

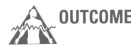

OUTCOME

FOLLOW-UP

- Serial pulmonary function tests and assessment of gas exchange

COMPLICATIONS

- Hypoxemia requiring oxygen therapy
- Respiratory failure

PROGNOSIS

- Median survival approximately 3 years, depending on stage at presentation

WHEN TO REFER

- All patients should be evaluated by a pulmonologist at the time of diagnosis to assist with diagnosis, consider treatment options, and evaluate for lung transplantation

WHEN TO ADMIT

- Progressive respiratory failure

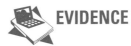

EVIDENCE

INFORMATION FOR PATIENTS

- Coalition for Pulmonary Fibrosis

REFERENCES

- King TE Jr. Clinical advances in the diagnosis and therapy of the interstitial lung diseases. Am J Respir Crit Care Med. 2005 Aug 1;172(3):268–79. [PMID: 15879420]
- Leslie KO. Pathology of interstitial lung disease. Clin Chest Med. 2004 Dec; 25(4):657–703. [PMID: 15564015]
- Lynch DA et al. Idiopathic interstitial pneumonias: CT features. Radiology. 2005 Jul;236(1):10–21. [PMID: 15987960]
- Swigris JJ et al. Idiopathic pulmonary fibrosis: challenges and opportunities for the clinician and investigator. Chest. 2005 Jan;127(1):275–83. [PMID: 15653995]

Pneumonia, Pneumococcal

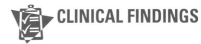

KEY FEATURES

ESSENTIALS OF DIAGNOSIS

- Productive cough, fever, rigors, dyspnea, early pleuritic chest pain
- Consolidating lobar pneumonia on chest radiograph
- Lancet-shaped gram-positive diplococci on Gram stain of sputum

GENERAL CONSIDERATIONS

- The most common cause of community-acquired pyogenic bacterial pneumonia
- Predisposing factors
  - Alcoholism

  - Asthma
  - HIV infection
  - Sickle cell disease
  - Splenectomy
  - Hematologic disorders
- Up to 40% of infections are caused by pneumococci resistant to at least one drug and 15% are due to a strain resistant to three or more drugs

DEMOGRAPHICS

- Until 2000, *Streptococcus pneumoniae* infections caused 100,000–135,000 hospitalizations for pneumonia, 6 million cases of otitis media, and 60,000 cases of invasive disease, including 3300 cases of meningitis
- Disease figures are now changing due to conjugate vaccine introduction

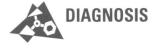

CLINICAL FINDINGS

SYMPTOMS AND SIGNS

- High fever, productive cough, occasionally hemoptysis, and pleuritic chest pain
- Rigors can occur within the first few hours of infection
- Bronchial breath sounds are an early sign
- Differentiating pneumococcal from other bacterial pneumonias is not possible clinically or radiographically because of significant overlap in presentations

DIFFERENTIAL DIAGNOSIS

- Pneumonia due to other causes, eg, *Haemophilus influenzae*, influenza
- Aspiration pneumonia or lung abscess
- Pulmonary embolism
- Myocardial infarction
- Acute exacerbation of chronic bronchitis
- Acute bronchitis
- Hypersensitivity pneumonitis

DIAGNOSIS

LABORATORY TESTS

- A good-quality sputum sample (less than 10 epithelial cells and more than 25 polymorphonuclear leukocytes per high-power field) shows gram-positive diplococci in 80–90% of cases
- Blood cultures are positive in up to 25% of selected cases and much more commonly so in HIV-positive patients

IMAGING STUDIES

- Chest radiograph shows findings of consolidation, often with a lobar distribution, infiltrates, pleural effusion

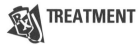

TREATMENT

MEDICATIONS

- Initial antimicrobial therapy of pneumonia is empiric pending isolation and identification of the causative agent (Table 103)

Outpatient

- Amoxicillin, 750 mg PO BID for 7–10 days
- Alternatives are azithromycin, one 500-mg dose PO on the first day and 250 mg PO for the next 4 days; clarithromycin, 500 mg PO BID for 10 days; or doxycycline, 100 mg PO BID for 10 days

Inpatient

- Aqueous penicillin G (susceptible strains), 2 million units IV q4h
- Ceftriaxone, 1 g IV q24h
- For a highly penicillin-resistant strain, vancomycin, 1 g IV q12h
- For community-acquired pneumonia, including that caused by penicillin-resistant strains of *S pneumonia* (with MIC ≥ 2 mcg/mL), amoxicillin-clavulanate extended-release 1000 mg-62.5 mg per tablet) 2 tablets PO q12h for 7–10 days
- Fluoroquinolones with enhanced gram-positive activity (eg, levofloxacin, 500 mg once daily; moxifloxacin, 400 mg once daily; or gatifloxacin, 400 mg once daily) are effective oral alternatives

THERAPEUTIC PROCEDURES

- Pleural effusions developing after initiation of antimicrobial therapy usually are sterile, and thoracentesis need not be performed if the patient is otherwise improving
- Thoracentesis is indicated for an effusion present prior to initiation of therapy and in the patient who has not responded to antibiotics after 3–4 days

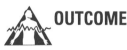

OUTCOME

FOLLOW-UP

- Repeat chest radiograph 6–8 weeks after treatment to ensure resolution of infiltrate

COMPLICATIONS

- Parapneumonic effusion is common cause of recurrent or persistent fever
- Empyema occurs in ≤ 5%
- Pneumococcal pericarditis (rare)
- Pneumococcal endocarditis usually involves aortic valve and often in association with meningitis

PROGNOSIS

- High mortality rate in the elderly, with multilobar disease, severe hypoxemia, extrapulmonary complications, or bacteremia

WHEN TO REFER

- Early referral to a pulmonologist for management of seriously ill patients

WHEN TO ADMIT

- The Pneumonia Patient Outcomes Research Team (PORT) model and clinical judgment guide whether to hospitalize a patient (Tables 104 and 105)
- Patients under 50 years old without comorbid conditions or physical examination abnormalities listed in Table 104 have the lowest risk

PREVENTION

Pneumococcal vaccine

- 23-valent purified polysaccharide from most common serotypes of *S pneumoniae*
- Current recommendations
  - Tables 67 and 68
  - Patients at increased risk for developing severe pneumococcal disease (eg, asplenic patients, those with sickle cell disease)
  - Chronic illnesses (eg, cardiopulmonary disease, alcoholism, renal disease, cancer)
  - Persons over 65 years of age
  - Elderly individuals with unknown immunization status should be immunized once
- Revaccination
  - Recommended regardless of age for those with the highest risk of fatal pneumococcal disease (eg, asplenic patients, nephrotic syndrome or renal failure, HIV, leukemia, lymphoma, myeloma, immunosuppressive medications, transplant patients)
  - 65 years of age if primary vaccine was at least 5 years before
  - High-risk individuals previously immunized with 14-valent vaccine

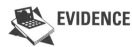

EVIDENCE

WEB SITE

- CDC—Division of Bacterial and Mycotic Diseases

INFORMATION FOR PATIENTS

- JAMA patient page. Pneumonia. JAMA. 2000;283:1922. [PMID: 10683063]
- NIH—National Institute of Allergy and Infectious Disease

REFERENCES

- Lexau CA et al; Active Bacterial Core Surveillance Team. Changing epidemiology of invasive pneumococcal disease among older adults in the era of pediatric pneumococcal conjugate vaccine. JAMA. 2005 Oct 26;294(16):2043–51. [PMID: 16249418]
- Siquier B et al; 620 Clinical Study Group. Efficacy and safety of twice-daily pharmacokinetically enhanced amoxicillin/clavulanate (2000/125 mg) in the treatment of adults with community-acquired pneumonia in a country with a high prevalence of penicillin-resistant *Streptococcus pneumoniae*. J Antimicrob Chemother. 2006 Mar;57(3):536–45. [PMID: 16446376]
- Talbot TR et al. Asthma as a risk factor for invasive pneumococcal disease. N Engl J Med. 2005 May 19; 352(20):2082–90. [PMID: 15901861]
- Tleyjeh IM et al. The impact of penicillin resistance on short-term mortality in hospitalized adults with pneumococcal pneumonia: a systematic review and meta-analysis. Clin Infect Dis. 2006 Mar 15;42(6):788–97. [PMID: 16477555]

Pneumothorax, Spontaneous

KEY FEATURES

ESSENTIALS OF DIAGNOSIS

- Acute onset of unilateral chest pain and dyspnea
- Minimal physical findings in mild cases
  - Unilateral chest expansion
  - Decreased tactile fremitus

– Hyperresonance
– Diminished breath sounds
• Tension pneumothorax
– Mediastinal shift
– Cyanosis
– Hypotension
• Pleural air on chest radiograph

GENERAL CONSIDERATIONS

• Spontaneous pneumothorax occurs without trauma and is classified as
– Secondary—complicating preexisting lung disease
– Primary—no prior lung disease
• Traumatic pneumothorax occurs as a result of penetrating or blunt trauma
• Iatrogenic pneumothorax may follow procedures such as central line placement and transbronchial biopsy
• Risk factors for secondary pneumothorax include
– Chronic obstructive pulmonary disease (COPD)
– Asthma
– Cystic fibrosis
– Tuberculosis
– Prior *Pneumocystis* pneumonia
– Menstruation (catemenial pneumothorax)
– Many interstitial lung diseases
• Tension pneumothorax usually occurs in the setting of
– Penetrating trauma
– Lung infection
– Cardiopulmonary resuscitation
– Positive pressure ventilation

DEMOGRAPHICS

• Primary pneumothorax affects mainly tall, thin males between 10 and 30 years of age
• Family history and smoking may be contributing factors in primary spontaneous pneumothorax

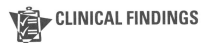 **CLINICAL FINDINGS**

SYMPTOMS AND SIGNS

• Chest pain ranges from minimal to severe
• Dyspnea is almost always present
• Symptoms usually begin at rest and resolve within 24 hours, even if the pneumothorax persists
• In the setting of COPD or asthma, patients may present with life-threatening respiratory failure
• Often seen with large pneumothoraces
– Unilateral chest expansion

– Hyperresonance
– Diminished breath sounds
– Decreased tactile fremitus
– Decreased movement of the chest
• Physical findings may be absent in small (< 15%) pneumothoraces
• Tension pneumothorax should be suspected if marked tachycardia, mediastinal or tracheal shift, or hypotension is present
• Crepitus may be found over the chest wall and adjacent structures

DIFFERENTIAL DIAGNOSIS

• Emphysematous bleb mimicking loculated pneumothorax
• Myocardial infarction
• Pneumonia
• Pulmonary embolism
• Pneumomediastinum caused by rupture of the esophagus or bronchus
• Upper respiratory tract infection
• Rib fracture
• Pericarditis
• Mesothelioma

 DIAGNOSIS

LABORATORY TESTS

• Arterial blood gas usually reveals hypoxemia and acute respiratory alkalosis
• Electrocardiogram: QRS axis and precordial T-wave changes may mimic acute myocardial infarction in left-sided pneumothorax

IMAGING STUDIES

• A visceral pleural line on chest radiograph is diagnostic; an expiratory film will increase sensitivity
• Secondary pleural effusion can occur
• Supine patients may demonstrate the "deep sulcus sign"—an abnormally radiolucent costophrenic angle
• Large amounts of subpleural air with contralateral mediastinal shift are present in tension pneumothorax

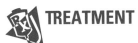 **TREATMENT**

MEDICATIONS

• Symptomatic treatment for cough and chest pain is appropriate
• Supplemental oxygen may increase the rate of reabsorption of pleural air

• Reliable patients with small (< 15%) primary pneumothoraces may be observed

SURGERY

• Simple aspiration of pleural air through a small-bore catheter can be performed for large or progressive pneumothoraces
• Placement of a small-bore chest tube (7F–14F) attached to a one-way Heimlich valve protects against development of a tension pneumothorax and may permit observation at home
• Chest tube placement (tube thoracostomy) may be indicated
– For secondary, large, or tension pneumothorax
– For severe symptoms or mechanically ventilated patients
• Thoracoscopy or open thoracotomy for removal of blebs or pleurodesis may be indicated in recurrent primary pneumothorax or with failed tube thoracostomy

THERAPEUTIC PROCEDURES

• Pleurodesis is indicated in recurrent or refractory cases

 OUTCOME

FOLLOW-UP

• Serial chest radiographs should be obtained at 24-hour intervals
• Chest tubes may be removed when the air leak subsides

COMPLICATIONS

• Tension pneumothorax, which may be life-threatening
• Pneumomediastinum and subcutaneous emphysema

PROGNOSIS

• 50% recurrence rate in smokers
• 30% risk of recurrence in spontaneous pneumothorax treated with observation or chest tube placement
• Recurrence after surgical therapy is less common

WHEN TO ADMIT

• Large, severely symptomatic, or progressive primary pneumothorax
• Secondary pneumothorax

PREVENTION

• Smokers should be counseled to quit

- Future exposure to high altitudes, unpressurized flight, and scuba diving should be avoided

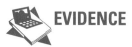 **EVIDENCE**

PRACTICE GUIDELINES

- Baumann MH et al. AACP Pneumothorax Consensus Group. Management of spontaneous pneumothorax: an American College of Chest Physicians Delphi consensus statement. Chest. 2001;119:590. [PMID: 11171742]
- Henry M et al. BTS guidelines for the management of spontaneous pneumothorax. Thorax. 2003;58(Suppl 2):ii39. [PMID: 12728149]

REFERENCES

- Baumann MH. Management of spontaneous pneumothorax. Clin Chest Med. 2006 Jun;27(2):369–81. [PMID: 16716824]
- Sahn SA et al. Spontaneous pneumothorax. N Engl J Med. 2000 Mar 23; 342(12):868–74. [PMID: 10727592]

Polyarteritis Nodosa & Microscopic Polyangiitis

 KEY FEATURES

ESSENTIALS OF DIAGNOSIS

- Classic polyarteritis nodosa affects only medium-sized arteries; smaller arterioles are sometimes involved
- Clinical findings depend on the arteries involved
- Common features include
  - Fever
  - Abdominal pain
  - Livedo reticularis
  - Mononeuritis multiplex
  - Anemia
  - Elevated acute phase reactants (erythrocyte sedimentation rate (ESR) or C-reactive protein or both)

- Classic polyarteritis nodosa spares the lung but often affects the kidney, causing renin-mediated hypertension
- Associated with hepatitis B (10% of cases)

GENERAL CONSIDERATIONS

- PAN is a medium-sized necrotizing arteritis with a predilection for involving peripheral nerves, mesenteric vessels (including renal arteries), heart, and brain but the capability of involving most organs
- Microscopic polyangiitis is a nongranulomatous vasculitis involving small blood vessels; it is often associated with antineutrophil cytoplasmic antibodies (ANCAs) that produce a perinuclear (p-ANCA) pattern on immunofluorescence testing and are directed against myeloperoxidase, a constituent of neutrophil granules
- Clinical findings depend on the arteries involved

 CLINICAL FINDINGS

SYMPTOMS AND SIGNS

- Common symptoms of both disorders
  - Insidious onset
  - Fever and other constitutional symptoms
  - Abdominal pain, particularly diffuse periumbilical pain precipitated by eating
  - Nausea and vomiting are frequently associated
  - Livedo reticularis
- Pain in the extremities is often a prominent early feature caused by arthralgia, myalgia (particularly affecting the calves), or neuropathy
- Mononeuritis multiplex (most common: foot-drop)
- Microscopic polyangiitis
  - Pulmonary hemorrhage and glomerulonephritis
- PAN
  - Skin: livedo reticularis, subcutaneous nodules, and skin ulcers
  - Involvement of the renal arteries leads to a renin-mediated hypertension
  - Seldom involves the lung
- Infarction compromises the function of major viscera and may lead to acalculous cholecystitis or appendicitis
- Some patients present dramatically with an acute abdomen caused by mesenteric vasculitis and gut perforation or with hypotension resulting from rupture of a microaneurysm in the liver, kidney, or bowel

DIFFERENTIAL DIAGNOSIS

- Wegener's granulomatosis
- Churg-Strauss syndrome
- Endocarditis
- Cryoglobulinemia
- Cholesterol atheroembolic disease
- Other systemic causes of peripheral neuropathy
  - Rheumatoid arthritis
  - Diabetes mellitus
  - Amyloidosis
  - Sarcoidosis
  - Multiple myeloma
- Other causes of mesenteric ischemia, eg, embolism, atherosclerosis

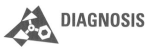 **DIAGNOSIS**

LABORATORY TESTS

- Anemia, and a sedimentation rate that is almost always elevated, often strikingly so
- Leukocytosis is common
- 75% of patients with microscopic polyangiitis are ANCA positive (usually with antibodies directed against myeloperoxidase, causing a p-ANCA pattern on immunofluorescence testing)
- Patients with classic PAN are ANCA negative
- Serologic tests for hepatitis B or C are positive in 10–30% of patients with PAN
- Microscopic polyangiitis: hematuria, proteinuria, and red blood cell casts in the urine

IMAGING STUDIES

- Mesenteric angiogram revealing microaneurysms is diagnostic

DIAGNOSTIC PROCEDURES

- Biopsies of symptomatic sites (eg, nerve, muscle, lung, or kidney) have high sensitivities and specificities
- The diagnosis of both of these disorders requires confirmation with either a tissue biopsy or, in the case of PAN, an angiogram
- The angiographic finding of aneurysmal dilations in the renal, mesenteric, or hepatic arteries may be diagnostic in patients in whom PAN is suspected— eg, on the basis of mesenteric ischemia or new-onset hypertension occurring in the setting of a systemic illness

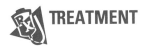

TREATMENT

MEDICATIONS

- For PAN, corticosteroids in high doses (up to 60 mg of prednisone daily) may control fever and constitutional symptoms and heal vascular lesions
- Pulse methylprednisolone (eg, 1 g intravenously daily for 3 days) may be necessary for patients who are critically ill at presentation
- Immunosuppressive agents, especially cyclophosphamide, appear to improve the survival of patients when given with corticosteroids
- In microscopic polyangiitis, patients are more likely to require cyclophosphamide because of the urgency in treating pulmonary hemorrhage and glomerulonephritis

OUTCOME

COMPLICATIONS

- Mesenteric vasculitis can cause bowel ischemia with bleeding or perforation

PROGNOSIS

- Without treatment, the 5-year survival rate in these disorders is poor—on the order of 10%
- With appropriate therapy, remissions are possible in many cases and the 5-year survival rate has improved to 60–90%
- Relapses may occur in both disorders—approximately 35% among patients with microscopic polyangiitis and perhaps less in those with PAN

WHEN TO REFER

- Refer to a rheumatologist to assist with establishing the diagnosis and planning therapy

WHEN TO ADMIT

- Admit for therapy whenever new visceral complications such as bowel ischemia, cardiomyopathy, or rapidly progressive neuropathy, develop

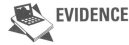

EVIDENCE

INFORMATION FOR PATIENTS

- Cleveland Clinic Foundation
- Johns Hopkins University

REFERENCES

- Bourgarit A et al; French Vasculitis Study Group. Deaths occurring during the first year after treatment onset for polyarteritis nodosa, microscopic polyangiitis, and Churg-Strauss syndrome: a retrospective analysis of causes and factors predictive of mortality based on 595 patients. Medicine (Baltimore). 2005 Sep;84(5):323–30. [PMID: 16148732]
- Guillevin L et al; French Vasculitis Study Group. Hepatitis B virus-associated polyarteritis nodosa: clinical characteristics, outcome, and impact of treatment in 115 patients. Medicine (Baltimore). 2005 Sep;84(5):313–22. [PMID: 16148731]
- Segelmark M et al. The challenge of managing patients with polyarteritis nodosa. Curr Opin Rheumatol. 2007 Jan;19(1):33–8. [PMID: 17143093]

Polycystic Kidney Disease

KEY FEATURES

- Common hereditary disease, affecting 1:1000 to 1:400 individuals in United States
- End-stage renal disease develops in 50% of patients by age 60
- Seen in 10% of dialysis patients
- Family history is positive in 75%
- Variable penetrance
- At least two genes in disorder
  - ADPKD1 on the short arm of chromosome 16 (85–90% of patients)
  - ADPKD2 on chromosome 4 (10–15% of patients)

CLINICAL FINDINGS

- Abdominal or flank pain caused by infection, bleeding into cysts, nephrolithiasis, rupture of cyst, urinary tract infection, renal cell carcinoma
- Fever caused by infection
- Nephrolithiasis, primarily calcium oxalate stones, in up to 20%
- Hypertension in 50%
- Abdominal mass
- Arterial aneurysms in the circle of Willis in 10–15%
- Mitral valve prolapse in up to 25%
- Aortic aneurysms
- Aortic valve abnormalities

DIAGNOSIS

- Renal ultrasonogram: diagnostic depending on age and number of cysts
- Urinalysis: may be normal because cysts do not communicate directly with the urinary tract, but blood cultures may be positive
- CT scan: infected cyst has increased wall thickness
- Cerebral arteriography screening: not recommended unless family history of aneurysms or patient undergoing elective surgery prone to cause hypertension

TREATMENT

- Cyst rupture
  - Bed rest
  - Analgesics, not nonsteroidal anti-inflammatory drugs
- Cyst pain: decompression
- Cyst infection:
  - Antibiotics: fluoroquinolones, trimethoprim-sulfamethoxazole, or chloramphenicol IV for 2 weeks followed by long-term PO therapy
- Hydration (2–3 L/day)
- Antihypertensive agents, but diuretics used cautiously because effect on renal cyst formation is unknown
- Caffeine may worsen cyst formation; patients may want to limit total intake

Polycystic Ovary Syndrome (Persistent Anovulation)

KEY FEATURES

ESSENTIALS OF DIAGNOSIS

- Clinical or biochemical evidence of hyperandrogenism
- Oligoovulation or anovulation
- Polycystic ovaries on ultrasonography

GENERAL CONSIDERATIONS

- The primary lesion is unknown
- There is a steady state of elevated estrogen (estrone), androgen, and luteinizing hormone (LH) levels rather than the fluctuating levels in ovulating women
- Increased estrone comes from conversion of androgens to estrone in body fat or from excessive levels of androgens seen in some women of normal weight
- High estrone levels may cause suppression of pituitary follicle-stimulating hormone (FSH) and a relative increase in LH
- Constant LH stimulation of the ovary results in anovulation, multiple cysts, and theca cell hyperplasia with excess androgen output
- The polycystic ovary has a thickened, pearly white capsule and may not be enlarged

DEMOGRAPHICS

- Affects 4–7% of women of reproductive age

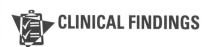

CLINICAL FINDINGS

SYMPTOMS AND SIGNS

- Hirsutism (50% of cases)
- Obesity (40%)
- Virilization (20%)
- Amenorrhea (50% of cases) and abnormal uterine bleeding (30%); 20% have normal menstruation
- Women are generally infertile, although they may ovulate occasionally

DIFFERENTIAL DIAGNOSIS

- Hypothalamic amenorrhea, eg, stress, weight change, exercise
- Obesity
- Hypothyroidism
- Hyperprolactinemia
- Premature ovarian failure
- Cushing's syndrome
- Congenital adrenal hyperplasia
- Androgen-secreting tumor (adrenal, ovarian)
- Pregnancy

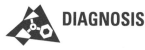

DIAGNOSIS

LABORATORY TESTS

- Check FSH, LH, prolactin, thyroid-stimulating hormone (TSH), and dehydroepiandrosterone sulfate (DHEAS) when amenorrhea has persisted for 6 months
- 2-h glucose tolerance test
- Lipoprotein profile

IMAGING STUDIES

- Pelvic ultrasound may document polycystic ovaries (not necessary for diagnosis)

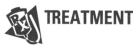

TREATMENT

MEDICATIONS

- **If the patient wishes to become pregnant**
  - Clomiphene or other drugs can be used for ovulatory stimulation The addition of dexamethasone, 0.5 mg PO at bedtime, to a clomiphene regimen may increase the likelihood of ovulation
  - If unresponsive to clomiphene, 3- to 6-month courses of metformin, 500 mg PO TID, rosiglitazone 4 mg daily, or pioglitazone 30–45 mg daily may bring resumption of regular cycles and ovulation
- **If the patient does not desire pregnancy**
  - Medroxyprogesterone acetate, 10 mg PO orally daily for the first 10 days of each month
  - If contraception is desired, a low-dose combination oral contraceptive can be used; this is also useful in controlling hirsutism, for which treatment must be continued for 6–12 months before results are seen
- Hirsutism
  - Dexamethasone, 0.5 mg PO each night, is helpful in women with excess adrenal androgen secretion
  - Spironolactone, an aldosterone antagonist, is also useful in doses of 25 mg PO TID or QID
  - Flutamide, 250 mg PO once daily, and finasteride, 5 mg PO once daily, are also effective
  - Because spironolactone, flutamide, and finasteride are potentially teratogenic, they should only be used with secure contraception

THERAPEUTIC PROCEDURES

- In obese patients with polycystic ovaries, weight reduction is often effective; a decrease in body fat will lower the conversion of androgens to estrone and thereby help restore ovulation
- Hirsutism may be managed with epilation and electrolysis

OUTCOME

FOLLOW-UP

- In long-term anovular patients over age 35, it is wise to search for an estrogen-stimulated cancer with mammography and endometrial aspiration

PROGNOSIS

- Women have insulin resistance and hyperinsulinemia when infused with glucose and are at increased risk for early-onset type 2 diabetes mellitus
- Women have an increased long-term risk of cancer of the breast and endometrium because of unopposed estrogen secretion

WHEN TO REFER

- If expertise in diagnosis is needed
- If the patient is having infertility problems

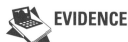

EVIDENCE

PRACTICE GUIDELINES

- American College of Obstetricians and Gynecologists. ACOG practice bulletin. Polycycstic ovary syndrome.
- American Association of Clinical Endocrinologists medical guidelines for clinical practice for the diagnosis and treatment of hyperandrogenic disorders.

INFORMATION FOR PATIENTS

- American Association of Family Physicians: Polycystic Ovary Syndrome
- American Society for Reproductive Medicine: Hirsutism and Polycystic Ovarian Syndrome
- International Council on Infertility Information Dissemination: PCOS FAQ
- MedlinePlus: Ovarian Cysts Interactive Tutorial
- National Women's Health Information Center: Polycystic Ovarian Syndrome

REFERENCES

- Ehrmann DA. Polycystic ovarian syndrome. N Engl J Med. 2005 Mar 24; 352(12):1223–36. [PMID: 15788499]
- Lakhani K et al. Polycystic ovaries. Br J Radiol. 2002;75:9. [PMID: 11806952]

- Lane DE. Polycystic ovary syndrome and its differential diagnosis. Obstet Gynecol Surv. 2006;61:125–35. [PMID: 16433936]

Polymyalgia Rheumatica & Giant Cell Arteritis

 KEY FEATURES

ESSENTIALS OF DIAGNOSIS

- Giant cell arteritis is characterized by headache, jaw claudication, polymyalgia rheumatica, visual abnormalities, and a markedly elevated erythrocyte sedimentation rate (ESR)
- The hallmark of polymyalgia rheumatica is pain and stiffness in shoulders and hips

GENERAL CONSIDERATIONS

- Polymyalgia rheumatica and giant cell arteritis probably represent a spectrum of one disease and frequently coexist
- The important difference between the two conditions is that polymyalgia rheumatica alone does not cause blindness and responds to low-dose (10–20 mg/day) prednisone therapy, whereas giant cell arteritis can cause blindness and large artery complications and requires high-dose therapy (40–60 mg/day)

DEMOGRAPHICS

- Both affect patients over age 50
- Giant cell arteritis is more common in northern Europeans and their descendants

 CLINICAL FINDINGS

SYMPTOMS AND SIGNS

Polymyalgia rheumatica

- Pain and stiffness of the shoulder and pelvic girdle areas
- Fever, malaise, and weight loss
- Anemia and a markedly elevated sedimentation rate are almost always present
- Muscle pain much greater than muscle weakness

Giant cell arteritis

- Headache, scalp tenderness, visual symptoms, jaw claudication, or throat pain
- The temporal artery is usually normal on physical examination but may be nodular, enlarged, tender, or pulseless
- Blindness
  - Results from occlusive arteritis of the posterior ciliary branch of the ophthalmic artery
  - Ischemic optic neuropathy may produce no funduscopic findings for the first 24–48 h after the onset of blindness
- Asymmetry of pulses in the arms, a murmur of aortic regurgitation, or bruits heard near the clavicle resulting from subclavian artery stenoses identify an affected aorta or its major branches
- Forty percent of patients with giant cell arteritis have nonclassic symptoms at presentation, primarily respiratory tract problems (most frequently dry cough), mononeuritis multiplex (most frequently with painful paralysis of a shoulder), or fever of unknown origin
- The fever can be as high as 40°C and is frequently associated with rigors and sweats
- Unexplained head or neck pain in an older patient may signal the presence of giant cell arteritis

DIFFERENTIAL DIAGNOSIS

Polymyalgia rheumatica

- Rheumatoid arthritis
- Polymyositis
- Chronic infection, eg, endocarditis
- Multiple myeloma
- Malignancy
- Fibromyalgia
- Polyarteritis nodosa

Giant cell (temporal) arteritis

- Migraine
- Glaucoma
- Takayasu's arteritis
- Uveitis
- Carotid plaque with embolic amaurosis fugax
- Trigeminal neuralgia

 DIAGNOSIS

LABORATORY TESTS

- An elevated ESR, with a median result of about 65 mm/h, occurs in more than 90% of patients with polymyalgia rheumatica or giant cell arteritis

- Most patients also have a mild normochromic, normocytic anemia and thrombocytosis

IMAGING STUDIES

- Role of ultrasonography of temporal arteries is controversial
- Angiography is helpful in the subset of patients that has large-artery disease (especially the subclavian artery)

DIAGNOSTIC PROCEDURES

- Temporal artery biopsy
- Diagnostic findings of giant cell arteritis may still be present 2 weeks (or even considerably longer) after starting corticosteroids
- An adequate biopsy specimen (2 cm in length) is essential, because the disease may be segmental

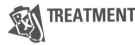 **TREATMENT**

MEDICATIONS

Polymyalgia rheumatica

- Prednisone, 10–20 mg/day PO; if no dramatic improvement within 72 h, the diagnosis should be revisited
- Weekly methotrexate may increase the chance of successfully tapering prednisone in some patients

Giant cell arteritis

- The urgency of early diagnosis and treatment in giant cell arteritis relates to the prevention of blindness
- When a patient has symptoms and findings suggestive of temporal arteritis, therapy with prednisone, 60 mg PO daily, is initiated immediately
- Prednisone should be continued in a dosage of 60 mg/day for 1–2 months before tapering
- IV pulse methylprednisolone (eg, 1 g/day for 3 days) may help patients with visual loss and may increase chance of remission; however, data supporting this recommendation are preliminary
- Low-dose aspirin (~81 mg/day PO) may reduce the risk of visual loss or stroke and should be added to prednisone

 OUTCOME

FOLLOW-UP

- Course is monitored by a composite of the patient's symptoms and laboratory markers of inflammation (ie, hematocrit, ESR, and C-reactive protein)

- In adjusting the dosage of corticosteroid, the ESR is a useful but not absolute guide to disease activity. A common error is treating the ESR rather than the patient
- Within 1–2 months after beginning treatment, the patient's symptoms and laboratory abnormalities will resolve
- Disease flares are common (50% or more) as prednisone is tapered
- The total duration of treatment varies considerably but ranges from 6 months to more than 2 years

COMPLICATIONS

- Blindness; once blindness develops, it is usually permanent
- Thoracic aortic aneurysms occur 17 times more frequently in patients with giant cell arteritis than in normal individuals

PROGNOSIS

- Impact on survival appears small

WHEN TO REFER

- Refer to a rheumatologist to establish the diagnosis, plan therapy, and monitor treatment
- Consult an ophthalmologist for visual changes

WHEN TO ADMIT

- Admit for evaluation and high-dose intravenous methylprednisolone if the patient acutely develops visual loss

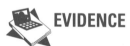 **EVIDENCE**

REFERENCES

- Blockmans D et al. Repetitive 18F-fluorodeoxyglucose positron emission tomography in giant cell arteritis: a prospective study of 35 patients. Arthritis Rheum. 2006 Feb 15;55(1):131–7. [PMID: 16463425]
- Gonzalez-Gay MA et al. Giant cell arteritis: disease patterns of clinical presentation in a series of 240 patients. Medicine (Baltimore). 2005 Sep; 84(5):269–76. [PMID: 16148727]
- Lee MS et al. Antiplatelet and anticoagulant therapy in patients with giant cell arteritis. Arthritis Rheum. 2006 Oct; 54(10):3306–9. [PMID: 17009265]
- Mazlumzadeh M et al. Treatment of giant cell arteritis using induction therapy with high-dose glucocorticoids: a double-blind, placebo-controlled, randomized prospective clinical trial. Arthritis Rheum. 2006 Oct; 54(10):3310–8. [PMID: 17009270]
- Nesher G et al. Low-dose aspirin and prevention of cranial ischemic complications in giant cell arteritis. Arthritis Rheum. 2004 Apr;50(4):1332–7. [PMID: 15077317]
- Parikh M et al. Prevalence of a normal C-reactive protein with an elevated erythrocyte sedimentation rate in biopsy-proven giant cell arteritis. Ophthalmology. 2006 Oct;113(10):1842–5. [PMID: 16884778]

Polyps, Colonic & Small Intestinal

 KEY FEATURES

ESSENTIALS OF DIAGNOSIS

- Discrete mass lesions that are flat or protrude into the intestinal lumen
- Most commonly sporadic, may be inherited as part of familial polyposis syndrome
- Three major pathological groups
  - Mucosal neoplastic (adenomatous) polyps
  - Mucosal nonneoplastic (hyperplastic, juvenile polyps, hamartomas, inflammatory) polyps
  - Submucosal lesions (lipomas, lymphoid aggregates, carcinoids, pneumatosis cystoides intestinalis)
- Nonneoplastic mucosal polyps have no malignant potential; adenomatous polyps do
- Of polyps removed at colonoscopy, over 70% are adenomatous; most of the remainder are hyperplastic; distinguished by histology

GENERAL CONSIDERATIONS

- Adenomatous polyps are tubular, villous, tubulovillous, or serrated adenomas; sessile or pedunculated
- > 95% of adenocarcinoma arise from adenomas
- Small adenomas (< 1 cm) have a low risk of being malignant; larger adenomas (> 1 cm) have a much higher risk (> 10%) of harboring malignancy or high-grade dysplasia

DEMOGRAPHICS

- Adenomatous polyps are present in 35% of adults aged > 50 years

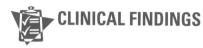 **CLINICAL FINDINGS**

SYMPTOMS AND SIGNS

- Usually asymptomatic
- Chronic occult blood loss may lead to iron deficiency anemia
- Large polyps may ulcerate, resulting in intermittent hematochezia

DIFFERENTIAL DIAGNOSIS

- Colorectal cancer
- Nonneoplastic polyp, eg, hyperplastic, inflammatory
- Submucosal polyp, eg, lipoma, lymphoid aggregate
- Other causes of occult gastrointestinal bleeding, eg, arteriovenous malformation, inflammatory bowel disease

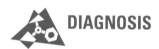 **DIAGNOSIS**

LABORATORY TESTS

- Fecal occult blood tests detect < 20% of adenomas > 1 cm in diameter

IMAGING STUDIES

- Barium enema, whether single- or double-contrast, has unacceptably low sensitivity (~50%) and specificity for the detection of colorectal polyps
- Spiral CT colonography ("virtual colonoscopy") detects over 80–90%

DIAGNOSTIC PROCEDURES

- Flexible sigmoidoscopy: about one-half to two-thirds of colonic adenomas are within the reach of the flexible sigmoidoscope
- Colonoscopy is best means of detecting and removing adenomatous polyps

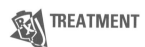 **TREATMENT**

SURGERY

- Primary surgical resection may be required for large (> 2–3 cm) sessile polyps
- Malignant polyps are adenomas that appear grossly benign at endoscopy but on histologic assessment are found to contain cancer

- Malignant polyps (termed "favorable") are adequately treated by polypectomy alone if the polyp is completely excised, well differentiated, the margin is not involved, and there is no vascular or lymphatic invasion
- Risk of residual cancer or nodal metastasis is 0.3% for pedunculated malignant polyps and 1.5% for sessile malignant polyps
- "Unfavorable" malignant polyps are treated by surgical resection

THERAPEUTIC PROCEDURES

- Colonoscopic polypectomy is possible for most polyps, particularly pedunculated polyps

 OUTCOME

FOLLOW-UP

- Periodic colonoscopic surveillance is recommended to detect "metachronous" adenomas
- Obtain colonoscopy
  - In 5–10 years for patients with 1–2 small (< 1 cm) tubular adenomas (without villous features or high-grade dysplasia)
  - In 3 years for patients with 3–10 adenomas, an adenoma > 1 cm, or an adenoma with villous features or high grade dysplasia
  - In 1–2 years for patients with > 10 adenomas; consider evaluating these patients for a familial polyposis syndrome

COMPLICATIONS

- Complications of colonoscopic polypectomy include perforation in 0.2%, bleeding in 1%

PREVENTION

- Nonsteroidal anti-inflammatory drugs (NSAIDs), aspirin, and cyclooxygenase (COX)-2 selective NSAIDs may decrease the incidence of colorectal adenomas and the progression to cancer; however, due to their other side effects, routine prophylaxis with these agents is not currently recommended

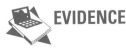 EVIDENCE

PRACTICE GUIDELINES

- Atkin WS et al. Surveillance guidelines after removal of colorectal adenoma-tous polyps. Gut 2002;51(Suppl 5):V6. [PMID: 12221031]
- Jenkins PJ et al. Screening guidelines for colorectal cancer and polyps in patients with acromegaly. Gut 2002;51(Suppl 5):V13.

INFORMATION FOR PATIENTS

- National Institute of Diabetes and Digestive and Kidney Diseases—What I need to know about colon polyps
- Torpy JM et al. JAMA patient page. Colon cancer screening. JAMA. 2003; 289:1334. [PMID: 12633198]

REFERENCES

- Butterly LF et al. Prevalence of clinically important histology on small adenomas. Clin Gastroenterol Hepatol. 2006 Mar; 4(3):343–8. [PMID: 16527698]
- Lauwers GY et al. The serrated polyp comes of age. Gastroenterology. 2006 Nov;131(5):1631–4. [PMID: 17067594]
- Levine JS et al. Adenomatous polyps of the colon. N Engl J Med. 2006 Dec 14; 355(24):2551–7. [PMID: 17167138]
- Rockey DC et al. Analysis of air contrast barium enema, computed tomographic colonography, and colonoscopy: prospective comparison. Lancet. 2005 Jan 22-28;365(9456):305–11. [PMID: 15664225]
- Schoen RE et al. Yield of advanced adenoma and cancer based on polyp size detected at screening flexible sigmoidoscopy. Gastroenterology. 2006 Dec; 131(6):1683–9. [PMID: 17188959]
- Winawer SJ et al. Guidelines for colonoscopy surveillance after polypectomy: a consensus update by the US Multi-Society Task Force on Colorectal Cancer and the American Cancer Society. Gastroenterology. 2006 May; 130(6):1872–85. [PMID: 16697750]

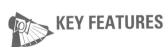

Porphyria, Acute Intermittent

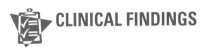 KEY FEATURES

ESSENTIALS OF DIAGNOSIS

- Unexplained abdominal crisis, generally in young women
- Acute central or peripheral nervous system dysfunction
- Recurrent psychiatric illnesses
- Hyponatremia
- Porphobilinogen in the urine during an attack

GENERAL CONSIDERATIONS

- Acute intermittent porphyria is caused by deficiency of porphobilinogen deaminase activity, leading to increased excretion of aminolevulinic acid and porphobilinogen in the urine
- Genetics: mutation in the porphobilinogen deaminase gene
- Autosomal dominant inheritance
- It remains clinically silent in the majority of patients who carry the trait
- Characteristic abdominal pain may be due to abnormalities in autonomic innervation in the gut
- Cutaneous photosensitivity is absent
- Attacks precipitated by numerous factors, including drugs and intercurrent infections
- Hyponatremia resulting from inappropriate release of antidiuretic hormone and gastrointestinal loss of sodium

DEMOGRAPHICS

- Usually presents in adulthood and has serious consequences
- Clinical illness usually develops in women
- Symptoms beginning in the teens or 20s, but in rare cases after menopause

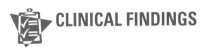 CLINICAL FINDINGS

SYMPTOMS AND SIGNS

- Intermittent abdominal pain of varying severity, sometimes simulating an acute abdomen
- Absence of fever and leukocytosis
- Complete recovery between attacks
- Autonomic neuropathy
- Peripheral neuropathy, symmetric or asymmetric, mild or profound
- CNS manifestations include
  - Seizures
  - Psychosis
  - Abnormalities of the basal ganglia

DIFFERENTIAL DIAGNOSIS

- Acute abdominal pain resulting from other cause, such as
  - Appendicitis
  - Peptic ulcer disease

– Cholecystitis
– Diverticulitis
– Ruptured ectopic pregnancy
– Familial Mediterranean fever
• Polyneuropathy resulting from other cause
• Guillain-Barré syndrome
• Lead or other heavy metal poisoning
• Psychosis resulting from other cause
• Syndrome of inappropriate antidiuretic hormone resulting from other cause
• Dark urine resulting from other cause (eg, alkaptonuria)

 DIAGNOSIS

LABORATORY TESTS

• Hyponatremia, often profound
• Freshly voided urine is of normal color but may turn dark upon standing in light and air
• Urine porphobilinogen increased during an acute attack
• Mutation detection in the gene for porphobilinogen deaminase

 TREATMENT

MEDICATIONS

• Analgesics
• IV glucose
• High-carbohydrate intake, a minimum of 300 g carbohydrate/day PO or IV
• Hematin up to 4 mg/kg IV QD or BID
• Adverse consequences of hematin therapy include phlebitis and coagulopathy

THERAPEUTIC PROCEDURES

• High-carbohydrate diet diminishes the number of attacks
• Withdrawal of the inciting agent
• Liver transplantation for extreme cases

 OUTCOME

FOLLOW-UP

• ECG
• Electrolytes
• Glucose
• Mental status

PROGNOSIS

• Acute attacks may be life-threatening and require prompt diagnosis

WHEN TO REFER

• Genetic counseling

WHEN TO ADMIT

• Abdominal crisis
• Marked hyponatremia
• Acute CNS dysfunction

PREVENTION

• Avoidance of factors known to precipitate attacks, especially drugs (Table 42)
• Starvation diets must be avoided

 EVIDENCE

WEB SITES

• American Porphyria Foundation
• National Center for Biotechnology Information: Online Mendelian Inheritance in Man

INFORMATION FOR PATIENTS

• American Porphyria Foundation: Acute Intermittent Porphyria (AIP)
• National Digestive Diseases Information Clearinghouse: Porphyria
• National Library of Medicine: Acute Intermittent Porphyria

REFERENCES

• Anderson KE et al. Recommendations for the diagnosis and treatment of the acute porphyrias. Ann Intern Med. 2005 Mar 15;142(6):439–50. [PMID: 15767622]
• Desnick RJ et al. Inherited porphyrias. In: *Emery and Rimoin's Principles and Practice of Medical Genetics*, 5th ed. Rimoin DL et al (editors). Churchill Livingstone, 2007.
• Herrick AL et al. Acute intermittent porphyria. Best Pract Res Clin Gastroenterol. 2005 Apr;19(2):235–49. [PMID: 15833690]
• Kauppinen R. Porphyrias. Lancet. 2005 Jan 15–21;365(9455):241–52. [PMID: 15652607]
• Norman RA. Past and future: porphyria and porphyrins. Skinmed. 2005 Sep–Oct;4(5):287–92. [PMID: 16282750]
• Soonawalla ZF et al. Liver transplantation as a cure for acute intermittent porphyria. Lancet. 2004 Feb 28; 363(9410):705–6. [PMID: 15001330]

Posttraumatic Stress Disorder

 KEY FEATURES

ESSENTIALS OF DIAGNOSIS

• A syndrome characterized by
  – "Reexperiencing" a traumatic event (eg, rape, severe burns, military combat)
  – Decreased responsiveness and avoidance of current events associated with the trauma
• Alcohol and other drugs are commonly used in self-treatment

GENERAL CONSIDERATIONS

• Included among the anxiety disorders in *DSM-IV*
• The symptoms may be precipitated or exacerbated by events that are a reminder of the original stress
• Symptoms frequently arise after a long latency period—eg, child abuse can result in later-onset posttraumatic stress disorder (PTSD)

 CLINICAL FINDINGS

SYMPTOMS AND SIGNS

• Physiologic hyperarousal
  – Startle reactions
  – Intrusive thoughts
  – Illusions
  – Overgeneralized associations
  – Sleep problems
  – Nightmares
  – Dreams about the precipitating event
  – Impulsivity
  – Difficulties in concentration
  – Hyperalertness

DIFFERENTIAL DIAGNOSIS

• Anxiety disorders
• Affective disorders
• Personality disorders exacerbated by stress
• Somatic disorders with psychic overlay

 DIAGNOSIS

LABORATORY TESTS

• Thyroid-stimulating hormone
• Complete blood cell count

- Toxicology screen (if suspected)
- Glucose

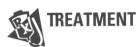 **TREATMENT**

MEDICATIONS

- Early treatment of anxious arousal with β-blockers (eg, propranolol, 80–160 mg PO daily), based on preliminary research, may
  - Lessen the peripheral symptoms of anxiety (eg, tremors, palpitations)
  - Help prevent the development of the disorder
- Antidepressant drugs—particularly selective serotonin reuptake inhibitors (SSRIs)—in full dosage
  - Helpful in ameliorating depression, panic attacks, sleep disruption, and startle responses in chronic PTSD
  - Sertraline and paroxetine are FDA approved for this purpose
- Antiseizure medications such as carbamazepine (400–800 mg PO daily) often mitigate impulsivity and difficulty with anger management
- Benzodiazepines (Table 145) such as clonazepam (1–4 mg PO daily)
  - Reduce anxiety and panic attacks when used in adequate dosage
  - Dependency problems are a concern, particularly when the patient has had such problems in the past

THERAPEUTIC PROCEDURES

- The therapeutic approach is to facilitate the normal recovery that was blocked at the time of the trauma
  - Therapy close to the event should be brief and simple (catharsis and working through of the traumatic experience), expecting quick recovery and promoting a sense of mastery and acceptance over the traumatic event
- Early cognitive-behavioral interventions can also speed recovery
- Treatment initiated later, when symptoms have crystallized, includes
  - Programs for cessation of alcohol and other drug abuse
  - Group and individual psychotherapy
  - Improved social support systems
- Psychological debriefing in a single session, once considered a mainstay in prevention of PTSD, is under scrutiny

 OUTCOME

PROGNOSIS

- The sooner the symptoms arise after the initial trauma and the sooner therapy is initiated, the better the prognosis
- Resolution may be delayed if others' responses to the patient's difficulties are thoughtlessly harmful or if the secondary gains outweigh the advantages of recovery
- The longer the symptoms persist, the worse the prognosis

WHEN TO REFER

- Marital problems are a major area of concern, and it is important that the clinician have available a dependable referral source when marriage counseling is indicated

 EVIDENCE

PRACTICE GUIDELINES

- American Academy of Family Physicians
- National Guideline Clearinghouse: VHA/DoD, 2004

WEB SITES

- American Psychiatric Association
- Internet Mental Health
- National Center for Posttraumatic Stress Disorder
- Posttraumatic stress disorder alliance

INFORMATION FOR PATIENTS

- American Psychiatric Association
- JAMA patient page. Posttraumatic stress disorder. JAMA. 2001;286:630. [PMID: 11508286]
- National Institute of Mental Health

REFERENCES

- Ehlers A et al. Early psychological interventions for survivors of trauma: a review. Biol Psychiatry. 2003 May 1; 53(9):817–26. [PMID: 12725974]
- Katon WJ et al. Dissemination of evidence-based mental health interventions: importance to the trauma field. J Trauma Stress. 2006 Oct;19(5):611–23. [PMID: 17075915]
- Vaiva G et al. Immediate treatment with propranolol decreases posttraumatic stress disorder two months after trauma. Biol Psychiatry. 2003 Nov 1;54(9):947–9. [PMID: 14573324]

Preeclampsia & Eclampsia

 KEY FEATURES

ESSENTIALS OF DIAGNOSIS

- Preeclampsia
  - Blood pressure of ≥ 140 mm Hg systolic or ≥ 90 mm Hg diastolic after 20 weeks gestation
  - Proteinuria of ≥ 0.3 g in 24 h
- Severe preeclampsia
  - Blood pressure of ≥ 160 mm Hg systolic or ≥ 110 mm Hg diastolic
  - Proteinuria ≥ 5 g in 24 h or 4+ on dipstick
  - Oliguria of < 500 mL in 24 h
  - Thrombocytopenia
  - Hemolysis elevated liver enzymes low platelets (HELLP)
  - Pulmonary edema
- Eclampsia
  - Same as severe preeclampsia, plus seizures
- Fetal growth restriction

GENERAL CONSIDERATIONS

- Cause is unknown, but an immunologic cause is suspected
- The only cure is delivery of the fetus and placenta
- Uncontrolled eclampsia is a significant cause of maternal death
- Use of diuretics, dietary changes, aspirin, and vitamin-mineral supplements such as calcium, or vitamin C or E have not been confirmed to be effective in clinical studies
- Early diagnosis is the key to treatment
- Many cases are asymptomatic early
- 5% of women with preeclampsia progress to eclampsia

DEMOGRAPHICS

- Occurs in 7% of pregnant women in the United States
- Higher incidence in primiparas
- Other risk factors
  - Multiple gestations
  - Chronic hypertension
  - Diabetes mellitus
  - Renal disease
  - Collagen-vascular and autoimmune disease
  - Gestational trophoblastic disease

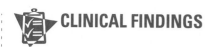 **CLINICAL FINDINGS**

SYMPTOMS AND SIGNS

- See Table 139
- Hypertension, proteinuria, and edema are classically required for the diagnosis, but presentation varies greatly
- Can occur any time after 20 weeks' gestation and up to 6 weeks postpartum
- Severity can be assessed with reference to the six sites where disease has its effects
  - CNS
  - Kidneys
  - Liver
  - Hematologic system
  - Vascular system
  - Fetal placental unit
- Few complaints are present in mild disease; antepartum fetal testing is reassuring
- Symptoms are dramatic and persist in severe disease; thrombocytopenia may progress to disseminated intravascular coagulation

DIFFERENTIAL DIAGNOSIS

- Essential hypertension or other cause of secondary hypertension
- Chronic renal failure or proteinuria due to other cause
- Primary seizure disorder
- Thrombotic thrombocytopenic purpura
- Other cause of abdominal pain, eg, cholecystitis, appendicitis, acute fatty liver of pregnancy
- Gallbladder and pancreatic disease
- Hemolytic-uremic syndrome

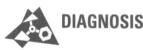 **DIAGNOSIS**

LABORATORY TESTS

- See Table 139
- Platelet count is over 100,000/mcL in mild to moderate disease
- Thrombocytopenia seen in severe disease
- Abnormal findings in the HELLP syndrome: hemolysis, elevated liver enzymes, and low platelets
- Hyperuricemia is helpful in diagnosis, as in pregnancy, it is seen only with gout, renal failure, or preeclampsia-eclampsia

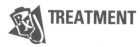 **TREATMENT**

MEDICATIONS

- Avoid sedatives and opiates, as they interfere with fetal assessment

---

- Administer two doses of corticosteroids IM (betamethasone, 12 mg or dexamethasone, 16 mg) 12–24 h apart if fetal lung immaturity is present
- Diazepam (5–10 mg IV over 4 minutes) or magnesium sulfate (4 g over 4 minutes, then 2–3 g/h unless abnormal renal function is present) is used to stop seizures
- Hydralazine, 5–10 mg IV Q 20 min, nifedipine, 10 mg SL or PO, or labetalol, 10–20 mg IV every 20 min can be used to control blood pressure
- Oxytocin may be used to induce or augment labor
- Magnesium sulfate infusion should be continued postpartum until preeclampsia-eclampsia begins to resolve (1–7 days), as indicated by the onset of diuresis (100–200 mL/h)
- Antihypertensive therapy is used if diastolic blood pressure > 110 mm Hg, with a target of 90–100 mm Hg

SURGERY

- Cesarean section is reserved for the usual fetal indications or when rapid delivery is needed
- Regional anesthesia or analgesia is acceptable

THERAPEUTIC PROCEDURES

- Nonstress and stress fetal testing or a biophysical profile should be obtained serially to confirm fetal well-being
- Daily fetal kick counts can be recorded by the mother
- Amniocentesis should be considered to evaluate lung maturity if hospitalization occurs at 30–37 weeks

Preeclampsia

- Disease of any severity at 36 weeks or later is managed by delivery
- Before 36 weeks, severe disease requires delivery except with extreme fetal prematurity
- Bed rest is the cornerstone of therapy for mild to moderate preeclampsia; it may be attempted at home or in the hospital depending on the degree of organ system involvement
- Epigastric pain, thrombocytopenia, and visual disturbances are strong indications for delivery

Eclampsia

- Patients having seizures are placed on their side to increase placental blood flow and avoid aspiration
- Maternal and fetal status determine the method of delivery

 OUTCOME

FOLLOW-UP

- Blood pressure, reflexes, proteinuria, and fetal monitoring must be checked regularly in hospitalized patients
- Blood cell count, electrolytes, proteinuria, and liver enzymes should be checked every 1–2 days in hospitalized patients
- 24-h urine protein and creatinine clearance on admission and as indicated
- Magnesium levels are checked q4–6h and infusions titrated to serum levels of 4–6 mEq/L
- Urinary output is checked hourly in severe disease or eclampsia
- Patients receiving magnesium infusions are monitored for signs of toxicity such as loss of deep tendon reflexes or respiratory depression; calcium gluconate can be used for reversal

WHEN TO ADMIT

- Moderate or severe preeclampsia or an unreliable home situation warrants hospitalization

 EVIDENCE

PRACTICE GUIDELINES

- ACOG Committee on Obstetrics Practice. ACOG practice bulletin. Diagnosis and management of preeclampsia and eclampsia. Number 33, January 2002. American College of Obstetricians and Gynecologists. Int J Gynaecol Obstet. 2002;77:67. [PMID: 12094777]
- Roberts JM et al; NHLBI. Report of the Working Group on Research on Hypertension During Pregnancy, 2001.

WEB SITE

- National Heart, Lung, and Blood Institute: Prevention of Preeclampsia

INFORMATION FOR PATIENTS

- American Academy of Family Physicians: Preeclampsia
- MedlinePlus: Preeclampsia
- MedlinePlus: Eclampsia
- National Heart, Lung, and Blood Institute: High Blood Pressure in Pregnancy

REFERENCES

- Levine R et al. Soluble endoglin and other circulating antiangiogenic factors in preeclampsia. N EngJ Med. 2006 Sep 7; 355(10):992–1005. [PMID: 16957146]

• Sibai BM. Diagnosis, prevention, and management of eclampsia. Obstet Gynecol. 2005 Feb;105(2):402–10. [PMID: 15684172]

Pregnancy

KEY FEATURES

ESSENTIALS OF DIAGNOSIS

• Amenorrhea, weight gain, nausea and vomiting, and breast changes
• Positive pregnancy test

GENERAL CONSIDERATIONS

• Prompt diagnosis of pregnancy allows early prenatal care and avoidance of harmful activities or exposures
• In the event of an unwanted pregnancy, early diagnosis allows for counseling regarding adoption or termination

CLINICAL FINDINGS

SYMPTOMS AND SIGNS

• No symptoms or signs are diagnostic
• Amenorrhea, weight gain
• Nausea and vomiting
• Breast tenderness and tingling
• Urinary frequency and urgency
• "Quickening" (perception of the first fetal movement) is noted at about 18 weeks' gestation
• Signs
  – Breast changes, abdominal enlargement, and cyanosis of the vagina and cervical portio (week 7)
  – Softening of the cervix (week 7)
  – Generalized enlargement and softening of the corpus (post-week 8)
  – Uterine fundus is palpable above the pubic symphysis by 12–15 weeks from last menstrual period
  – Fundus reaches the umbilicus by 20–22 weeks
  – Fetal heart tones heard by Doppler at 10–12 weeks

DIFFERENTIAL DIAGNOSIS

• Myomas can be confused with a gravid uterus

• A midline ovarian tumor may displace a nonpregnant uterus
• Ectopic pregnancies may show lower levels of human chorionic gonadotropin (hCG) that level off or fall
• Premature menopause

DIAGNOSIS

LABORATORY TESTS

Diagnostic tests

• All urine or blood pregnancy tests rely on detection of placental hCG and are accurate at the time of a missed period or shortly after it
• Laboratory and home assays use monoclonal antibodies specific for hCG
• hCG levels increase shortly after implantation, double every 48 h, peak at 50–75 days, and fall in second and third trimesters

Screening at the time of diagnosis

• The following are recommended
  – Urinalysis; culture of a mid-stream urine sample
  – Complete blood count (CBC)
  – Serologic test for syphilis
  – Rubella antibody titer
  – History of varicella
  – Blood group and Rh type
  – Atypical antibody screening
  – Hepatitis B surface antigen testing
• HIV testing should be encouraged
• Cervical cultures for *Neisseria gonorrhoea* and *Chlamydia* as well as Papanicolaou smear are indicated
• Testing for abnormal hemoglobins should be done in patients at risk for sickle cell or thalassemia traits
• Tuberculosis skin testing is recommended for high-risk groups
• Screening for Tay-Sachs and Canavan disease should be offered to
  – Jewish women with Jewish partners (especially those of Ashkenazi descent)
  – Couples of French-Canadian or Cajun ancestry
• Hepatitis C screening should be offered to mothers at high risk

Screening during pregnancy

• Maternal serum α-fetoprotein (AFP) is offered to all women to screen for neural tube defects and is mandatory in some states (16–20 weeks)
• hCG, estriol levels and inhibin A are combined with AFP (quad screen) for detection of fetal Down syndrome
• First trimester aneuploidy screening with nuchal translucency, serum levels

of PAPP-A, and free β-subunit of HCG can be offered at 11–13 weeks
• Screening for gestational diabetes by checking glucose 1 h post a 50-g glucose load (26–28 weeks)
• 3-h glucose tolerance test follows up an abnormal 1-h glucose load test
• Repeat Rh testing for negative patients (28 weeks, though result is not required before Rho(D) Ig is given)
• CBC to evaluate for anemia of pregnancy (28–32 weeks)
• Repeat tests for syphilis, HIV, and cervical cultures in at-risk patients (36 weeks to delivery)
• Screening for group B streptococcal (GBS) colonization can be done by rectovaginal culture at 35–37 weeks
  – If negative, no prophylaxis is given
  – Intrapartum prophylaxis with penicillin or clindamycin is given if screening cultures are positive and organism is sensitive
  – Patients with risk factors for GBS or who deliver at < 37 weeks receive intrapartum prophylaxis
  – Patients without a culture at 35–37 weeks receive prophylaxis only for a history of GBS bacteriuria or prior GBS disease in an infant, intrapartum fevers, or membrane rupture > 18 h

IMAGING STUDIES

• Radiographs should be avoided unless essential and approved by a physician and utilize shielding
• Fetal ultrasound for accurate dating and to evaluate fetal anatomy is usually done at 18–20 weeks' gestation
• In multiple pregnancies, ultrasound is repeated every 4 weeks to identify discordant growth

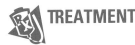

TREATMENT

MEDICATIONS

• Prenatal vitamins with iron and folic acid are indicated
• Medications should not be taken unless prescribed or authorized by the patient's provider (Tables 138 and 141)
• Penicillin (5 million units followed by 2.5 million units q4h until delivery), or clindamycin (900 mg IV q8h) are given for prophylaxis of group B streptococcal infection with susceptible isolates

THERAPEUTIC PROCEDURES

• Genetic counseling with the option of chorionic villous sampling or amniocentesis should be offered to women 35 or older at delivery, a family history of congenital abnormalities, or previous child with a metabolic disease, chromosomal abnormality, or neural tube defect

OUTCOME

FOLLOW-UP

- Prenatal visits should be scheduled
  - Every 4 weeks from 0–28 weeks
  - Every 2 weeks from 28–36 weeks
  - Weekly from 36 weeks to delivery

COMPLICATIONS

- Fetal alcohol syndrome: no safe level of alcohol intake has been established for pregnancy
- Cigarette smoking increases risk of abruptio placentae, placenta previa, and premature rupture of the membranes
- Premature delivery and lower birth weights are more common in children born to smokers
- Maternal cocaine, amphetamine, and opioid use in pregnancy is associated with numerous complications

WHEN TO REFER

- If the practitioner has no training or experience in prenatal care

WHEN TO ADMIT

- For any major medical or pregnancy-related complication

PREVENTION

- Hepatitis B vaccination for women with potential occupational exposure or household contacts
- Live virus immunizations (measles, rubella, varicella, yellow fever) are contraindicated during pregnancy
- Influenza vaccine is indicated in all women who will be in their second or third trimester during "flu season"
- Decrease caffeine intake
- Avoid ingestion of raw meat, all tobacco, alcohol, and recreational drugs, exposure to environmental tobacco smoke, excessive heat, hot tubs, and saunas, and handling of cat feces or litter
- Exercise should be mild to moderate, with heart rate kept below 140 beats/min

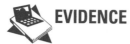

EVIDENCE

PRACTICE GUIDELINES

- American College of Obstetricians and Gynecologists. Immunization during pregnancy. Int J Gynaecol Obstet. 2003;81:123. [PMID: 12737148]
- National Collaborating Centre for Women's and Children's Health. Antenatal care: routine care for the healthy pregnant woman. 2003.

INFORMATION FOR PATIENTS

- National Women's Health Information Center
- Nemours Foundation: Medical Care During Pregnancy
- Nemours Foundation: Staying Healthy During Pregnancy
- New York Online Access to Health: Pregnancy

REFERENCES

- American College of Obstetricians and Gynecologists Committee on Health Care for Underserved Women. ACOG Committee Opinion No. 343: Psychosocial risk factors: perinatal screening and intervention. Obstet Gynecol. 2006 Aug; 108(2):469–77. [PMID: 16880322]
- Kirkham C et al. Evidence-based prenatal care: Part I. General prenatal care and counseling issues. Am Fam Physician. 2005 Apr 1;71(7):1307–16. [PMID: 15832534]

Prostate Cancer

KEY FEATURES

ESSENTIALS OF DIAGNOSIS

- Prostatic induration on digital rectal examination (DRE) or elevated level of serum prostate-specific antigen (PSA)
- Most often asymptomatic
- Rarely, systemic symptoms (weight loss, bone pain)

GENERAL CONSIDERATIONS

- Most common cancer detected in American men
- Second leading cause of cancer-related death in men

- In 2006, about 234,500 new cases of prostate cancer, about 27,350 deaths
- At autopsy, > 40% of men aged > 50 years have prostate carcinoma, most often occult
- Incidence increases with age: autopsy incidence ~30% of men aged 60–69 versus 67% in men aged 80–89 years
- Risk factors
  - Black race
  - Family history of prostate cancer
  - History of high dietary fat intake
- A 50-year-old American man has a lifetime risk of 40% for latent cancer, of 16% for clinically apparent cancer, and of 2.9% for death from prostate cancer
- Majority of prostate cancers are adenocarcinomas

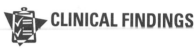

CLINICAL FINDINGS

SYMPTOMS AND SIGNS

- Focal nodules or areas of induration within the prostate on DRE
- Obstructive voiding symptoms
- Lymph node metastases
- Lower extremity lymphedema
- Back pain or pathologic fractures
- Rarely, signs of urinary retention (palpable bladder) or neurologic symptoms as a result of epidural metastases and cord compression

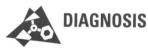

DIAGNOSIS

LABORATORY TESTS

- Elevations in serum PSA (normal < 4 ng/mL)
- PSA correlates with the volume of both benign and malignant prostate tissue
- 18–30% of men with PSA 4.1–10.0 ng/mL have prostate cancer
- Age-specific PSA reference ranges exist
- Most organ-confined cancers have PSA levels < 10 ng/mL
- Advanced disease (seminal vesicle invasion, lymph node involvement, or occult distant metastases) have PSA levels > 40 ng/mL
- Elevations in serum urea nitrogen or creatinine in patients with urinary retention or those with ureteral obstruction due to locally or regionally advanced prostate cancers
- Elevations in alkaline phosphatase or hypercalcemia in patients with bony metastases

- Disseminated intravascular coagulation (DIC) in patients with advanced prostate cancers

IMAGING STUDIES

- Transrectal ultrasound (TRUS): most prostate cancers are hypoechoic
- MRI of the prostate
- Positive predictive value for detection of both capsular penetration and seminal vesicle invasion is similar for both TRUS and MRI
- CT imaging can be useful in detecting regional lymphatic and intra-abdominal metastases
- Radionuclide bone scan for PSA level > 20 ng/mL

DIAGNOSTIC PROCEDURES

- TRUS-guided biopsy from the apex, mid portion, and base of the prostate
  - Done in men who have an abnormal DRE or an elevated PSA
  - Systematic rather than only lesion-directed biopsies are recommended
  - Extended pattern biopsies, including a total of at least 10 biopsies, are associated with improved cancer detection and risk stratification of newly diagnosed patients
- Fine-needle aspiration biopsies should be considered in patients at increased risk for bleeding

TREATMENT

MEDICATIONS

- Adrenal
  - Ketoconazole, 400 mg PO TID (adrenal insufficiency, nausea, rash, ataxia)
  - Aminoglutethimide, 250 mg PO QID (adrenal insufficiency, nausea, rash, ataxia)
  - Corticosteroids: prednisone, 20–40 mg PO once daily (gastrointestinal bleeding, fluid retention)
- Pituitary, hypothalamus
  - Estrogens, 1–3 mg PO once daily (gynecomastia, hot flushes, thromboembolic disease, erectile dysfunction)
  - Luteinizing hormone-releasing hormone (LHRH) agonists, monthly or 3-monthly depot injection (erectile dysfunction, hot flushes, gynecomastia, rarely anemia)
- Prostate cell
  - Antiandrogens: flutamide, 250 mg PO TID, or bicalutamide, 50 mg PO

once daily (no erectile dysfunction when used alone; nausea, diarrhea)
- Testis
  - Orchiectomy (gynecomastia, hot flushes, impotence)
  - Ketoconazole for patients who have advanced prostate cancer with spinal cord compression, bilateral ureteral obstruction, or DIC
  - Complete androgen blockade by combining an antiandrogen with use of an LHRH agonist or orchiectomy
- Chemotherapy: Docetaxel improves survival in men with hormone-refractory prostate cancer

THERAPEUTIC PROCEDURES

- Patients need to be advised of all treatment options, including surveillance (watchful waiting), benefits, risks, and limitations
- For lower stage and grade cancers and those with lower serum PSA at diagnosis, consider surveillance
- For minimal capsular penetration, standard irradiation or surgery
- For locally extensive cancers, including seminal vesicle and bladder neck invasion, combination therapy (androgen deprivation combined with surgery or irradiation)
- For metastatic disease, androgen deprivation
- For localized disease
  - Optimal form of treatment controversial
  - Selected patients may be candidates for surveillance
  - Patients with an anticipated survival of > 10 years should be considered for radical prostatectomy, radiation therapy
- Radical prostatectomy
  - For stages T1 and T2 prostatic cancers, local recurrence is uncommon after radical prostatectomy
    □ Organ-confined cancers rarely recur
    □ Locally extensive cancers (capsular penetration, seminal vesicle invasion) have higher local (10–25%) and distant (20–50%) relapse rates
  - Adjuvant therapy (radiation for patients with positive surgical margins or androgen deprivation for lymph node metastases)
- Radiation therapy
  - External beam radiotherapy
  - Transperineal implantation of radioisotopes
- Morbidity is limited; survival with localized cancers is 65% at 10 years
- Newer techniques of radiation (implantation, conformal therapy using three-

dimensional reconstruction of CT-based tumor volumes, heavy particle, charged particle, and heavy charged particle) improve local control rates
- Brachytherapy is implantation of permanent or temporary radioactive sources (palladium, iodine, or iridium)

 OUTCOME

FOLLOW-UP

- Surveillance alone may be appropriate for patients who are older and have very small and well-differentiated cancers

PROGNOSIS

- Risk assessment tools can help predict the likelihood of success of surveillance or treatment by combining stage, grade, PSA level, and number and extent of positive prostate biopsies
  - Kattan nomogram
    □ Predicts the likelihood that a patient will be disease-free by serum PSA at 5 years after radical prostatectomy or radiation therapy, depending on the tumor stage, grade, and PSA

PREVENTION

Screening for prostate cancer

- Screening tests currently available include DRE, serum PSA, TRUS
- Detection rates with DRE are low, varying from 1.5% to 7.0%
- TRUS has low specificity (and therefore high biopsy rate)
- TRUS increases the detection rate very little when compared with the combined use of DRE and PSA testing
- With PSA testing, 2.0–2.5% of men older than age 50 have prostate cancer; with DRE alone, rate is 1.5%
- However, elevation of PSA is not specific for cancer, occurs in BPH
- Age-specific reference ranges for PSA have been established and increase specificity
  - For men aged 40–49 years, range is < 2.5 ng/mL
  - For men 50–59, < 3.5 ng/mL
  - For men 60–69, < 4.5 ng/mL
  - For men 70–79, < 6.5 ng/mL
- PSA velocity (serial measurement of PSA), PSA density (serum PSA/volume of the prostate as measured by ultrasound), and PSA transition zone density (the zone of the prostate that undergoes enlargement with BPH)

- Free and protein-bound PSA levels: cancer patients have a lower percentage of free serum PSA
- PSA testing should be performed yearly in men with a normal DRE and a PSA > 2.5 ng/mL and biennially in those with a normal DRE and serum PSA < 2.5 ng/mL

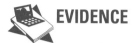

EVIDENCE

PRACTICE GUIDELINES

- Loblaw DA et al; American Society of Clinical Oncology. American Society of Clinical Oncology recommendations for the initial hormonal management of androgen-sensitive metastatic, recurrent, or progressive prostate cancer. J Clin Oncol. 2004;22:2927. [PMID: 15184404]

INFORMATION FOR PATIENTS

- Cleveland Clinic—Prostate cancer

REFERENCES

- Bill-Axelson A et al; Scandinavian Prostate Cancer Study Group No. 4. Radical prostatectomy versus watchful waiting in early prostate cancer. N Engl J Med. 2005 May 12;352(19):1977–84. [PMID: 15888698]
- Cooperberg MR et al. The University of California, San Francisco Cancer of the Prostate Risk Assessment Score: a straightforward and reliable preoperative predictor of disease recurrence after radical prostatectomy. J Urol. 2005 Jun; 173(6):1938–42. [PMID: 15879786]
- Han M et al. Prostate-specific antigen and screening for prostate cancer. Med Clin North Am. 2004 Mar;88(2):245–65. [PMID: 15049577]
- Meng MV et al. Treatment of patients with high risk localized prostate cancer: results from cancer of the prostate strategic urological research endeavor (CaPSURE). J Urol. 2005 May; 173(5):1557–61. [PMID: 15821485]
- Parnes HL et al. Prostate cancer chemoprevention agent development: the National Cancer Institute, Division of Cancer Prevention portfolio. J Urol. 2004 Feb;171(2 Pt 2):S68–74. [PMID: 14713758]
- Petrylak DP et al. Docetaxel and estramustine compared with mitoxantrone and prednisone for advanced refractory prostate cancer. N Engl J Med. 2004 Oct 7;351(15):1513–20. [PMID: 15470214]

Prostatitis, Acute Bacterial

KEY FEATURES

ESSENTIALS OF DIAGNOSIS

- Fever
- Irritative voiding symptoms
- Perineal or suprapubic pain
- Exquisite tenderness on rectal examination
- Positive urine culture

GENERAL CONSIDERATIONS

- Usual causative organisms: *Escherichia coli* and *Pseudomonas*
- Less common: *Enterococcus*

CLINICAL FINDINGS

SYMPTOMS AND SIGNS

- Perineal, sacral, or suprapubic pain
- Fever
- Irritative voiding complaints
- Obstructive symptoms
- Urinary retention
- Exquisitely tender prostate

DIFFERENTIAL DIAGNOSIS

- Epididymitis
- Diverticulitis
- Urinary retention from benign or malignant prostatic enlargement
- Chronic bacterial prostatitis
- Nonbacterial prostatitis
- Prostatodynia

DIAGNOSIS

LABORATORY TESTS

- Complete blood cell count: leukocytosis and a left shift
- Urinalysis: pyuria, bacteriuria, hematuria
- Urine culture: positive

TREATMENT

MEDICATIONS

- IV ampicillin and an aminoglycoside until afebrile for 24–48 h, then PO quinolone for 4–6 weeks
- Ampicillin, IV 1 g q6h, and gentamicin, IV 1 mg/kg q8h for 21 days
- Ciprofloxacin, PO 750 mg q12h for 21 days
- Ofloxacin, PO 200–300 mg q12h for 21 days
- Trimethoprim-sulfamethoxazole, PO 160/800 mg q12h for 21 days (increasing resistance noted [up to 20%])

THERAPEUTIC PROCEDURES

- Suprapubic drainage if urinary retention
- Urethral catheterization, instrumentation, and prostatic massage is contraindicated

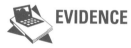

OUTCOME

FOLLOW-UP

- Posttreatment urine culture
- Posttreatment examination of expressed prostatic secretions after completion of therapy

PROGNOSIS

- With effective treatment, chronic bacterial prostatitis is rare

EVIDENCE

PRACTICE GUIDELINES

- Naber KG et al. EAU guidelines for the management of urinary and male genital tract infections. Urinary Tract Infection (UTI) Working Group of the Health Care Office (HCO) of the European Association of Urology (EAU). Eur Urol. 2001;40:576. [PMID: 11752870]

INFORMATION FOR PATIENTS

- Cleveland Clinic—Prostatitis
- Mayo Clinic—Prostatitis

REFERENCE

- Hua VN et al. Acute and chronic prostatitis. Med Clin North Am. 2004 Mar; 88(2):483–94. [PMID: 15049589]

Prostatitis, Chronic Bacterial

KEY FEATURES

- Irritative voiding symptoms
- Perineal or suprapubic discomfort, often dull and poorly localized
- Positive expressed prostatic secretions and culture
- Although chronic bacterial prostatitis may evolve from acute bacterial prostatitis, many men have no history of acute infection
- Most common: gram-negative rods
- Less common: *Enterococcus*

CLINICAL FINDINGS

- Variable; some patients are asymptomatic; most have irritative voiding symptoms, low back and perineal pain
- Many report a history of urinary tract infections
- Physical examination often unremarkable; prostate may feel normal, boggy, or indurated

DIAGNOSIS

- Culture secretions or postprostatic massage urine specimen
- Urinalysis: normal unless a secondary cystitis is present
- Expressed prostatic secretions: > 10 leukocytes/hpf, especially lipid-laden macrophages
- Differential diagnosis
  - Chronic urethritis
  - Cystitis
  - Perianal disease

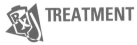

TREATMENT

- Anti-inflammatory agents (indomethacin, ibuprofen)
- Quinolones, trimethoprim-sulfamethoxazole, carbenicillin, erythromycin, or cephalexin, for 6–12 weeks
- Regimens
  - Ciprofloxacin, 250–500 mg PO q12h for 1–3 months
  - Ofloxacin, 200–400 mg PO q12h for 1–3 months
  - Trimethoprim-sulfamethoxazole, 160/800 mg PO q12h for 1–3 months (increasing resistance noted [up to 20%])
- Hot sitz baths
- Relax pelvic floor with micturition
- Difficult to cure
- Symptoms and recurrent urinary tract infections can be controlled by suppressive antibiotic therapy

Pruritus

KEY FEATURES

- Causes of generalized pruritus
  - Dry skin
  - Scabies
  - Dermatitis herpetiformis
  - Atopic dermatitis
  - Pruritus vulvae et ani
  - Miliaria
  - Insect bites, pediculosis
  - Contact dermatitis, fiberglass dermatitis
  - Drug reactions
  - Urticaria, urticarial eruptions of pregnancy
  - Psoriasis
  - Lichen planus, lichen simplex chronicus
  - Folliculitis
  - Bullous pemphigoid
- Persistent pruritus not explained by cutaneous disease should prompt a staged workup for systemic causes
- Other causes
  - Endocrine disorders, such as hypothyroidism or hyperthyroidism
  - Psychiatric disturbances
  - Lymphoma
  - Leukemia
  - Iron deficiency anemia
  - Certain neurologic disorders

CLINICAL FINDINGS

- Bilirubin may be normal in patients with hepatic pruritus, and the severity of the liver disease may not correlate with the degree of itching
- Burning or itching involving the face, scalp, and genitalia may be manifestations of primary depression and is treatable with antidepressant drugs such as
  - Tricyclics (amitriptyline, imipramine, doxepin)
  - Selective serotonin reuptake inhibitors (SSRIs)
  - Others

TREATMENT

- Naltrexone and nalmefene relieve the pruritus of liver disease
- Uremia in conjunction with hemodialysis and the pruritus of obstructive biliary disease may be helped by phototherapy with ultraviolet B or PUVA, or with gabapentin 300–400 mg PO after each dialysis
- Idiopathic pruritus and pruritus accompanying serious internal disease may not respond to any type of therapy
- Pruritus accompanying specific skin disease will subside when the disease is controlled

Pruritus, Anogenital

KEY FEATURES

ESSENTIALS OF DIAGNOSIS

- Itching, chiefly nocturnal, of the anogenital area
- Examination is highly variable, ranging from no skin findings to excoriations and inflammation of any degree, including lichenification

GENERAL CONSIDERATIONS

- May be due to
  - Intertrigo
  - Psoriasis
  - Lichen simplex chronicus
  - Seborrheic or contact dermatitis (from soaps, colognes, douches, contraceptives, and perhaps scented toilet tissue)
  - Irritating secretions (eg, diarrhea, leukorrhea, or trichomoniasis)
  - Local disease (candidiasis, dermatophytosis, erythrasma)
- Uncleanliness may be the cause

- In pruritus ani, hemorrhoids are often found, and leakage of mucus and bacteria from the distal rectum onto the perianal skin may be important in cases in which no other skin abnormality is found
- **In women**, pruritus ani by itself is rare, and pruritus vulvae does not usually involve the anal area, though anal itching usually spreads to the vulva
- **In men**, pruritus of the scrotum is most commonly seen in the absence of pruritus ani
- When all possible known causes have been ruled out, the condition is diagnosed as idiopathic or essential pruritus—by no means rare; some of these cases are due to lumbosacral radiculopathy

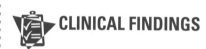 CLINICAL FINDINGS

SYMPTOMS AND SIGNS

- The only symptom is itching, which is primarily nocturnal
- Physical findings are usually not present, but there may be
  - Erythema
  - Fissuring
  - Maceration
  - Lichenification
  - Excoriations
  - Changes suggestive of candidiasis or tinea

DIFFERENTIAL DIAGNOSIS

- Idiopathic
- Intertrigo
- Psoriasis
- Hemorrhoids
- Lichen simplex chronicus
- Seborrheic dermatitis
- Contact dermatitis
- Candidiasis
- Tinea
- Erythrasma
- Irritants: diarrhea, vaginal discharge
- Lichen sclerosis et atrophicus
- Pinworm infestation

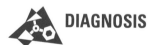 DIAGNOSIS

LABORATORY TESTS

- Urinalysis and blood glucose testing may lead to a diagnosis of diabetes mellitus
- Microscopic examination or culture of tissue scrapings may reveal yeasts or fungi

- Stool examination may show pinworms
- CT or MRI of the lumbosacral spine may show nerve root impingements

 TREATMENT

MEDICATIONS

General measures

- Treating constipation, preferably with high-fiber management (psyllium), may help

Local measures

- Pramoxine 1% cream or hydrocortisone/pramoxine (Pramosone), 1%/1% or 2.5%/1% cream, lotion, or ointment, is helpful in managing pruritus in the anogenital area; the ointment or cream should be applied after a bowel movement
- The use of strong corticosteroids on the scrotum may lead to persistent severe burning on withdrawal of the drug
- Soaks with aluminum subacetate solution, 1:20, are of value if the area is acutely inflamed and oozing
- Affected areas may be painted with Castellani's solution
- Balneol Perianal Cleansing Lotion, or Tucks premoistened pads, ointment, or cream may be very useful for pruritus ani
- In men with anogenital pruritus, capsaicin 0.006% cream BID may be beneficial

THERAPEUTIC PROCEDURES

- Instruct the patient to use very soft or moistened tissue or cotton after bowel movements and to clean the perianal area thoroughly with cool water if possible
- Women should use similar precautions after urinating
- Underclothing should be changed daily

 OUTCOME

PROGNOSIS

- Although benign, anogenital pruritus may be persistent and recurrent

WHEN TO REFER

- If there is a question about the diagnosis, if recommended therapy is ineffective, or if specialized treatment is necessary

PREVENTION

- Instruct the patient in proper anogenital hygiene after treating systemic or local conditions

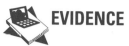 EVIDENCE

INFORMATION FOR PATIENTS

- American Academy of Family Physicians: Fiber: How to Increase the Amount in Your Diet
- American Society of Colon and Rectal Surgeons: Pruritus Ani
- Mayo Clinic: Anal Itch
- MedlinePlus: Vaginal Itching

REFERENCES

- Boardman LA et al. Recurrent vulvar itching. Obstet Gynecol. 2005 Jun; 105(6):1451–5. [PMID: 15932843]
- Cohen AD et al. Neuropathic scrotal pruritus: anogenital pruritus is a symptom of lumbosacral radiculopathy. J Am Acad Dermatol. 2005 Jan;52(1):61–6. [PMID: 15627082]

Pseudogout & Chondrocalcinosis

 KEY FEATURES

- Also known as calcium pyrophosphate dihydrate deposition disease (CPPD)
- Chondrocalcinosis is the presence of calcium-containing salts in articular cartilage
- May be familial and is associated with hemochromatosis, hyperparathyroidism, ochronosis, diabetes mellitus, true gout, hypothyroidism, Wilson's disease
- Usually seen in individuals 60 yr and older
- Pseudogout attacks of the knee especially common 1–2 days after general surgery

 CLINICAL FINDINGS

- CPPD can be asymptomatic, cause recurrent, acute attacks of monoarthritis (pseudogout), or result in chronic arthritis resembling either osteoarthritis or rheumatoid arthritis
- Pseudogout, like gout, frequently develops 24–48 h after major surgery
- CPPD with osteoarthritic changes of second and third metacarpophalangeals suggests hemochromatosis

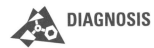
DIAGNOSIS

- Identification of calcium pyrophosphate crystals in joint aspirates is diagnostic
- Rhomboid-shaped pseudogout crystals are blue when parallel and yellow when perpendicular to the axis of the compensator with polarized light microscopy. Needle-shaped gout crystals give the opposite color pattern
- Radiographic examination shows not only calcification (usually symmetric) of cartilaginous structures but also signs of osteoarthritis
- Normal serum urate levels

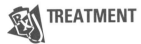
TREATMENT

- Treatment is directed at the primary disease, if present
- NSAIDs are used for acute episodes
- Colchicine, 0.6 mg PO BID, is more effective for prophylaxis than for acute episodes
- Intra-articular injection of triamcinolone, 10–40 mg

Pseudotumor Cerebri

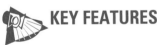
KEY FEATURES

ESSENTIALS OF DIAGNOSIS

- Headache, worse on straining
- Visual obscurations or diplopia may occur
- Level of consciousness may be impaired
- Other deficits depend on cause of intracranial hypertension or on herniation
- Examination reveals papilledema

GENERAL CONSIDERATIONS

- Pseudotumor cerebri is a diagnosis of exclusion in the setting of elevated intracranial pressure and normal cerebrospinal fluid
- Thrombosis of the transverse venous sinus as a noninfectious complication of otitis media or chronic mastoiditis is one cause, and sagittal sinus thrombosis may lead to a clinically similar picture

- Other causes
  - Chronic pulmonary disease
  - Endocrine disturbances such as hypoparathyroidism or Addison's disease
  - Vitamin A toxicity
  - Use of tetracycline or oral contraceptives
- Cases have also followed withdrawal of corticosteroids after long-term use

DEMOGRAPHICS

- Most patients are young, frequently obese, women

CLINICAL FINDINGS

SYMPTOMS AND SIGNS

- Symptoms
  - Headache
  - Diplopia
  - Other visual disturbances due to papilledema and abducens nerve dysfunction
- Examination reveals
  - Papilledema
  - Some enlargement of the blind spots
  - Abducens palsy is common
  - Patients otherwise look well

DIFFERENTIAL DIAGNOSIS

- Venous sinus thrombosis
- Dural arteriovenous malformation
- Space-occupying lesion, eg, brain tumor
- Meningitis
- Systemic hypertension
- Migraine
- Glaucoma
- Associated conditions
  - Hypoparathyroidism
  - Addison's disease
  - Chronic pulmonary disease
- Associated drugs
  - Vitamin A
  - Tetracycline
  - Minocycline
  - Oral contraceptives
  - Corticosteroid withdrawal
  - Isotretinoin
  - Danazol

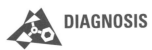
DIAGNOSIS

LABORATORY TESTS

- Lumbar puncture confirms intracranial hypertension, but the cerebrospinal fluid is normal

IMAGING STUDIES

- CT scan shows small or normal ventricles and no evidence of a space-occupying lesion
- MR venography can help detect thrombosis of the transverse venous sinus and sagittal sinus thrombosis

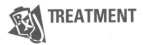
TREATMENT

MEDICATIONS

- Acetazolamide (250 mg PO TID) reduces formation of cerebrospinal fluid and can be initial therapy
- Corticosteroids (eg, prednisone, 60–80 mg PO once daily) may also be necessary
- Any specific cause of pseudotumor cerebri requires appropriate treatment
  - Hormone therapy should be initiated if there is an underlying endocrine disturbance
  - Discontinue the use of tetracycline, oral contraceptives, or vitamin A
  - If corticosteroid withdrawal is responsible, the medication should be reintroduced and then tapered more gradually

SURGERY

- If medical treatment fails to control the intracranial pressure, surgical placement of a lumboperitoneal or other shunt—or subtemporal decompression or optic nerve sheath fenestration—should be undertaken to preserve vision

THERAPEUTIC PROCEDURES

- Obese patients should be advised to lose weight
- Repeated lumbar puncture to lower the intracranial pressure by removal of cerebrospinal fluid is effective on a short-term basis
- However, pharmacologic treatment is also necessary

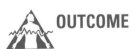
OUTCOME

FOLLOW-UP

- Treatment is monitored by checking visual acuity and visual fields, funduscopic appearance, and pressure of the cerebrospinal fluid

COMPLICATIONS

- Untreated pseudotumor cerebri can lead to secondary optic atrophy and permanent visual loss

PROGNOSIS

- Discontinuing the use of tetracycline, oral contraceptives, or vitamin A allows for resolution of pseudotumor cerebri due to these agents
- In many instances no specific cause is found, and the disorder remits spontaneously after several months

WHEN TO REFER

- All patients benefit from specialist referral to exclude specific causes and from specialized care to monitor treatment response with visual acuity and field checks, and from funduscopic examination

WHEN TO ADMIT

- Need for surgical placement of a device to reduce intracranial hypertension

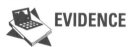 EVIDENCE

INFORMATION FOR PATIENTS

- National Institute of Neurological Diseases and Stroke

REFERENCE

- Skau M et al. What is new about idiopathic intracranial hypertension? An updated review of mechanism and treatment. Cephalalgia. 2006 Apr; 26(4):384–99. [PMID: 16556239]

Psoriasis

 KEY FEATURES

ESSENTIALS OF DIAGNOSIS

- Silvery scales on bright red, well-demarcated plaques, usually on the knees, elbows, and scalp
- Nail findings include pitting and onycholysis (separation of the nail plate from the bed)
- Mild itching (usually)
- May be associated with psoriatic arthritis
- Histopathology is not often useful and can be confusing

GENERAL CONSIDERATIONS

- A common benign, acute or chronic inflammatory skin disease based on a genetic predisposition
- Injury or irritation of normal skin tends to induce lesions of psoriasis at the site (Koebner phenomenon)
- Psoriasis has several variants—the most common is the plaque type

 CLINICAL FINDINGS

- There are often no symptoms, but itching may occur
- Although psoriasis may occur anywhere, examine the scalp, elbows, knees, palms and soles, umbilicus, and nails
- The lesions are red, sharply defined plaques covered with silvery scales; the glans penis and vulva may be affected; occasionally, only the flexures (axillae, inguinal areas) are involved
- Fine stippling ("pitting") in the nails is highly suggestive
- Psoriatics often have a pink or red intergluteal fold
- There may be associated seronegative arthritis, often involving the distal interphalangeal joints
- Eruptive (guttate) psoriasis consisting of myriad lesions 3–10 mm in diameter occurs occasionally after streptococcal pharyngitis
- Plaque type or extensive erythrodermic psoriasis with abrupt onset may accompany HIV infection

DIFFERENTIAL DIAGNOSIS

- Atopic dermatitis (eczema)
- Contact dermatitis
- Nummular eczema (discoid eczema, nummular dermatitis)
- Tinea
- Candidiasis
- Intertrigo
- Seborrheic dermatitis
- Pityriasis rosea
- Secondary syphilis
- Pityriasis rubra pilaris
- Onychomycosis (nail findings)
- Cutaneous features of reactive arthritis
- Cutaneous T cell lymphoma (mycosis fungoides)

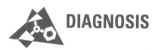 DIAGNOSIS

DIAGNOSTIC PROCEDURES

- The combination of red plaques with silvery scales on elbows and knees, with scaliness in the scalp or nail findings, is diagnostic
- Psoriasis lesions are well demarcated and affect extensor surfaces—in contrast to atopic dermatitis, with poorly demarcated plaques in flexural distribution
- In body folds, scraping and culture for *Candida* and examination of scalp and nails will distinguish psoriasis from intertrigo and candidiasis

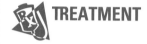 TREATMENT

MEDICATIONS

- See Table 150

Limited disease (mild to moderate)

- Topical corticosteroid cream or ointment
  - Restrict the highest-potency corticosteroids to 2–3 weeks of BID use; then three or four times on weekends or switch to a midpotency corticosteroid
  - Rarely induces a lasting remission
- Calcipotriene ointment 0.005%, a vitamin D analog, is used BID
  - It is the second most commonly used topical treatment (after topical corticosteroids)
  - Substitute calcipotriene once the topical corticosteroids have controlled the lesions
  - Once- or twice-daily calcipotriene is then continued long-term
  - It usually cannot be applied to the groin or the face because of irritation
  - Incompatible with many topical corticosteroids; it must be applied at a different time
- Occlusion alone clears isolated plaques in 30–40% of patients
  - Duoderm is placed on the lesions and left undisturbed for 5–7 days and then replaced
  - Responses may be seen within several weeks
- For the scalp
  - Start with a tar shampoo once daily
  - Thick scales: 6% salicylic acid gel (eg, Keralyt), P & S solution (phenol, mineral oil, and glycerin), or oil-based fluocinolone acetonide 0.01% (Derma-Smoothe/FS) under a shower cap at night, followed by a shampoo in the morning

– In order of increasing potency, triamcinolone 0.1%, or fluocinolone, betamethasone dipropionate, fluocinonide or amcinonide, and clobetasol are available in solution form for use on the scalp BID

• Psoriasis in the body folds

– Potent corticosteroids cannot be used

– Tacrolimus (Protopic 0.1% or 0.03%) ointment or pimecrolimus (Elidel 1%) cream applied BID can be effective in intertriginous psoriasis (but not plaques type); burning can occur and may be avoided by applying a mild corticosteroid (hydrocortisone 1.0–2.5%) BID for the week of treatment

Moderate to severe disease (more than 30% of the body surface)

• Parenteral corticosteroids should not be used because of possible induction of pustular lesions

• Methotrexate is very effective in doses up to 25 mg PO once weekly

• Acitretin, a synthetic retinoid, is most effective for pustular psoriasis at 0.5–1.0 mg/kg/day PO

– It also improves erythrodermic and plaque types and psoriatic arthritis

– Liver enzymes and serum lipids must be checked periodically

– Because acitretin is a teratogen, women must wait at least 3 years after completing treatment before considering pregnancy

• Cyclosporine dramatically improves severe cases of psoriasis

• Systemic immunomodulators (etanercept, 50 mg SQ twice weekly × 12, then once weekly; infliximab, 5 mg/kg IV weekly at weeks 0, 2, and 6, then every 8 weeks, and adalimumab, 40 mg SQ every 2 weeks) can be effective; all three can also induce psoriasis

• Alefacept 7.5 mg IV or 15 mg IM weekly × 12 weeks and efalizumab 0.7–1.0 mg/kg SQ weekly have moderate efficacy

THERAPEUTIC PROCEDURES

• Moderate to severe disease

– The treatment of choice is narrowband UVB light exposure three times weekly; clearing usually occurs in ~7 weeks; maintenance may be needed since relapses are frequent

– Severe disease unresponsive to ultraviolet light may be treated in a psoriasis day care center with the Goeckerman regimen, using crude coal tar for many hours and exposure to UVB light; this offers the best chance for prolonged remissions

– PUVA (psoralen plus ultraviolet A) may be effective even if standard UVB treatment has failed; may be used with other therapy, eg, acitretin

 OUTCOME

COMPLICATIONS

• Treatment with calcipotriene may result in hypercalcemia

• Long-term use of PUVA is associated with an increased risk of skin cancer (especially squamous cell carcinoma and perhaps melanoma)

PROGNOSIS

• The course tends to be chronic and unpredictable, and the disease may be refractory to treatment

WHEN TO REFER

• If there is a question about the diagnosis, if recommended therapy is ineffective, or if specialized treatment is necessary

 EVIDENCE

INFORMATION FOR PATIENTS

• American Academy of Dermatology: What is Psoriasis?

• MedlinePlus: Psoriasis Interactive Tutorial

• National Institute of Arthritis and Musculoskeletal and Skin Diseases: Psoriasis

REFERENCES

• Lee HH et al. Cutaneous side-effects in patients with rheumatic diseases during application of tumour necrosis factor-alpha antagonists. Br J Dermatol. 2007 Mar;156(3):486–91. [PMID: 17300238]

• Luba KM et al. Chronic plaque psoriasis. Am Fam Physician. 2006 Feb 15; 73(4):636–44. [PMID: 16506705]

• Pitarch G et al. Treatment of psoriasis with adalimumab. Clin Exp Dermatol. 2007 Jan;32(1):18–22. [PMID: 17305904]

• Schon MP et al. Psoriasis. N Engl J Med. 2005 May 5;352(18):1899–912. [PMID: 15872205]

• Smith CH et al. Psoriasis and its management. BMJ. 2006 Aug 19;333(7564): 380–4. [PMID: 16916825]

Psoriatic Arthritis

 KEY FEATURES

ESSENTIALS OF DIAGNOSIS

• Psoriasis precedes onset of arthritis in 80% of cases

• Arthritis usually asymmetric, with "sausage" appearance of fingers and toes

• Resembles rheumatoid arthritis; rheumatoid factor is negative

• Sacroiliac joint involvement common; ankylosis of the sacroiliac joints may occur

GENERAL CONSIDERATIONS

Patterns or subsets of arthritis accompanying psoriasis

• Joint disease that resembles rheumatoid arthritis with symmetric polyarthritis

• An oligoarticular form that may lead to considerable destruction of the affected joints

• Predominant involvement of the distal interphalangeal joints; pitting of the nails and onycholysis are frequently associated

• A severe deforming arthritis (arthritis mutilans) with marked osteolysis

• A spondylitic form in which sacroiliitis and spinal involvement predominate; 50% of these patients are HLA-B27 positive

DEMOGRAPHICS

• Arthritis is at least five times more common in patients with severe skin disease than in those with only mild skin findings

 CLINICAL FINDINGS

SYMPTOMS AND SIGNS

• Although psoriasis usually precedes the onset of arthritis, arthritis precedes or occurs simultaneously with the skin disease in approximately 20% of cases

• May be a single patch of psoriasis (typically hidden in the scalp, gluteal cleft, or umbilicus)

• Nail pitting, a residue of previous psoriasis, is sometimes the only clue

• "Sausage" swelling of one or more digits is a common manifestation of enthesopathy in psoriatic arthritis

DIFFERENTIAL DIAGNOSIS

- Rheumatoid arthritis
- Gout
- Osteoarthritis
- Other causes of sacroiliitis
  - Reactive arthritis (Reiter's syndrome)
  - Ankylosing spondylitis
  - Inflammatory bowel disease

 DIAGNOSIS

LABORATORY TESTS

- Elevation of the sedimentation rate
- Rheumatoid factor is not present

IMAGING STUDIES

- Radiographic findings are most helpful in distinguishing the disease from other forms of arthritis
- There are marginal erosions of bone and irregular destruction of joint and bone, which, in the phalanx, may give the appearance of a sharpened pencil ("pencil-in-cup")
- Fluffy periosteal new bone may be marked, especially at the insertion of muscles and ligaments into bone. Such changes will also be seen along the shafts of metacarpals, metatarsals, and phalanges
- Asymmetric sacroiliitis

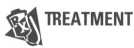 **TREATMENT**

MEDICATIONS

- Nonsteroidal anti-inflammatory drugs (NSAIDs) are usually sufficient for mild cases
- Corticosteroids are less effective in psoriatic arthritis than in other forms of inflammatory arthritis
- Methotrexate (7.5–15 mg per week PO) is considered the drug of choice for patients who have not responded to NSAIDs
- For cases with disease that is refractory to methotrexate, etanercept or infliximab is usually effective for both arthritis and psoriatic skin disease
- Successful treatment of the skin lesions (eg, by PUVA therapy) commonly—though not invariably—is accompanied by an improvement in peripheral articular symptoms

THERAPEUTIC PROCEDURES

- Treatment regimens are symptomatic

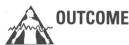 **OUTCOME**

COMPLICATIONS

- Fusion of peripheral or spinal joints

PROGNOSIS

- Generally better than rheumatoid arthritis, but severe cases occur

WHEN TO REFER

- Refer when joint disease does not respond to NSAIDs or when skin disease is severe

 EVIDENCE

WEB SITES

- American College of Rheumatology
- Arthritis Foundation

INFORMATION FOR PATIENTS

- Arthritis Foundation
- National Psoriasis Foundation

REFERENCES

- Antoni CE et al. Sustained benefits of infliximab therapy for dermatologic and articular manifestations of psoriatic arthritis: results from the infliximab multinational psoriatic arthritis controlled trial (IMPACT). Arthritis Rheum. 2005 Apr;52(4):1227–36. [PMID: 15818699]
- Gottlieb AB. Alefacept for psoriasis and psoriatic arthritis. Ann Rheum Dis. 2005 Nov;64 Suppl 4:iv58–60. [PMID: 16239390]

Pulmonary Edema, Acute

 KEY FINDINGS

- Acute onset or worsening of dyspnea at rest
- Tachycardia, diaphoresis, cyanosis
- Pulmonary rales, rhonchi, expiratory wheezes
- Chest radiograph shows interstitial and alveolar edema with or without cardiomegaly

- Arterial hypoxemia
- Cardiac causes include
  - Acute myocardial infarction (MI) or ischemia
  - Congestive heart failure (CHF)
  - Valvular regurgitation
  - Mitral stenosis
- Noncardiac causes include
  - Injection drug (opioid) use
  - Increased intracerebral pressure
  - High altitude
  - Sepsis
  - Medications
  - Inhaled toxins
  - Transfusion reactions
  - Shock
  - Disseminated intravascular coagulation

 CLINICAL FINDINGS

- Severe dyspnea
- Pink, frothy sputum
- Diaphoresis
- Cyanosis
- Rales, wheezing, or rhonchi in all lung fields
- Sudden onset in acute exacerbations of CHF or acute MI

 DIAGNOSIS

- Characteristic clinical findings
- Chest radiograph
  - Pulmonary vascular congestion
  - Increased interstitial markings
  - Butterfly pattern of alveolar edema
  - Heart enlarged or normal in size
- Echocardiography: assesses ejection fraction, atrial pressure
- Pulmonary capillary wedge pressure
  - Always elevated (usually > 25 mm Hg) in cardiogenic pulmonary edema
  - Normal or even low in noncardiogenic pulmonary edema

 TREATMENT

- Place patient in a sitting position with legs dangling over the side of the bed
- Give oxygen by mask for Pao_2 < 60 mm Hg
- Noninvasive pressure support ventilation or endotracheal intubation and mechanical ventilation for respiratory distress
- Morphine, 4–8 mg IV or SQ, repeated PRN after 2–4 h (avoid in patients with

opioid-induced and neurogenic pulmonary edema)
- Diuretic IV (Table 16)
- Nitroglycerin SL, PO, or IV
- Inhaled β-adrenergic agonists or IV aminophylline for bronchospasm
- Parenteral vasodilator (eg, nitroprusside IV) for elevated arterial pressure
- Positive inotropic agents in low-output states, hypotension

Pulmonary Embolism

KEY FEATURES

ESSENTIALS OF DIAGNOSIS

- Predisposition to venous thrombosis, usually of the lower extremities
- Usually dyspnea, chest pain, hemoptysis, or syncope
- Tachypnea and a widened alveolar–arterial P_{O_2} difference
- Characteristic defects on ventilation-perfusion lung scan, spiral CT scan of the chest, or pulmonary angiogram

GENERAL CONSIDERATIONS

- Cause of an estimated 50,000 deaths annually in the United States and the third most common cause of death in hospitalized patients
- Most cases are not recognized antemortem: < 10% with fatal emboli receive specific treatment
- Pulmonary thromboembolism (PE) and deep venous thrombosis (DVT) are manifestations of the same disease, with the same risk factors
  - Immobility (bed rest, stroke, obesity)
  - Hyperviscosity (polycythemia)
  - Increased central venous pressures (low cardiac output, pregnancy)
  - Vessel damage (prior DVT, orthopedic surgery, trauma)
  - Hypercoagulable states, either acquired or inherited
- Pulmonary thromboemboli most often originate in deep veins of the lower extremities
- PE develops in 50–60% of patients with proximal lower extremity DVT; 50% of these events are asymptomatic

- Hypoxemia results from vascular obstruction leading to dead space ventilation, right-to-left shunting, and decreased cardiac output
- Other types of pulmonary emboli
  - Fat embolism
  - Air embolism
  - Amniotic fluid embolism
  - Septic embolism (eg, endocarditis)
  - Tumor embolism (eg, renal cell carcinoma)
  - Foreign body embolism (eg, talc in injection drug use)
  - Parasite egg embolism (schistosomiasis)

CLINICAL FINDINGS

SYMPTOMS AND SIGNS

- See Table 114
- Clinical findings depend on the size of the embolus and the patient's preexisting cardiopulmonary status
- Dyspnea occurs in 75–85% and chest pain in 65–75% of patients
- Tachypnea is the only sign reliably found in more than 50% of patients
- 97% of patients in the PIOPED study had **at least one** of the following
  - Dyspnea
  - Tachypnea
  - Chest pain with breathing

DIFFERENTIAL DIAGNOSIS

- Myocardial infarction (heart attack)
- Pneumonia
- Pericarditis
- Congestive heart failure
- Pleuritis (pleurisy)
- Pneumothorax
- Pericardial tamponade

DIAGNOSIS

LABORATORY TESTS

- ECG is abnormal in 70% of patients
  - Sinus tachycardia and nonspecific ST-T changes are the most common findings
- Acute respiratory alkalosis, hypoxemia, and widened arterial–alveolar O_2 gradient (A–a D_{O_2}), but these findings are not diagnostic (Table 114)
- A normal D-dimer level by the ELISA assay virtually rules out DVT (sensitivity is 97%); however, many hospitals use a less-sensitive latex-agglutination assay

IMAGING STUDIES

- Chest radiograph—most common findings
  - Atelectasis
  - Infiltrates
  - Pleural effusions
  - Westermark's sign is focal oligemia with a prominent central pulmonary artery
  - Hampton's hump is a pleural-based area of increased intensity from intraparenchymal hemorrhage
- Lung scanning (V/Q scan)
  - A normal scan can exclude PE
  - A high-probability scan is sufficient to make the diagnosis in most cases
  - Indeterminate scans are common and do not further refine clinical pretest probabilities
- Helical CT arteriography is supplanting V/Q scanning as the initial diagnostic study
  - It requires administration of intravenous radiocontrast dye but is otherwise noninvasive
  - It is very sensitive for the detection of thrombus in the proximal pulmonary arteries but less so in the segmental and subsegmental arteries
- Venous thrombosis studies
  - Venous ultrasonography is the test of choice in most centers
  - Diagnosing DVT establishes the need for treatment and may preclude invasive testing in patients in whom there is a high suspicion for PE
- In the setting of a nondiagnostic V/Q scan, negative serial DVT studies over 2 weeks predict a low risk (< 2%) of subsequent DVT over the next 6 weeks
- Pulmonary angiography is the reference standard for the diagnosis of PE
  - Invasive, but safe—minor complications in < 5%
  - Role in the diagnosis of PE controversial, but generally used when there is a high clinical probability and negative noninvasive studies
- MRI is a research tool for the diagnosis of PE
- Integrated approach is used (Figure 2)

TREATMENT

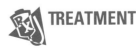

MEDICATIONS

- See Tables 117 and 118
- Classic anticoagulation regimen: unfractionated heparin (UFH) followed by warfarin to maintain the INR 2.0–3.0

- Compared with UFH, low-molecular-weight heparins (LMWH)
  - Are easier to dose and require no test monitoring
  - Have similar hemorrhage rates
  - Are at least as effective
  - Enable home-based therapy in selected patients
- Warfarin is contraindicated in pregnancy; LMWHs are safe alternatives
- Guidelines for the duration of full anticoagulation
  - 6 months for an initial episode with a reversible risk factor
  - 12 months after an initial, idiopathic episode
  - 6–12 months to indefinitely in patients with irreversible risk factors or recurrent disease
- Recent data support the use of long-term low-intensity warfarin (INR 1.5–2.0) after full anticoagulation is completed
- **Thrombolytic therapy** accelerates resolution of thrombi when compared with heparin, but does not improve mortality
  - Carries 10-fold greater risk of intracranial hemorrhage compared with heparin (0.2–2.1%)
  - Indicated in patients who are hemodynamically unstable while on heparin
- **Venal caval interruption** (IVC filters) may be indicated when a significant contraindication to anticoagulation exists or when recurrence occurs despite adequate anticoagulation
- IVC filters decrease the short-term incidence of PE, but increase the rate of recurrent DVT

SURGERY

- Pulmonary embolectomy is an emergency procedure with a high mortality rate performed at few centers

THERAPEUTIC PROCEDURES

- Catheter devices that fragment and extract thrombus have been used on small numbers of patients
- Platelet counts should be monitored for the first 14 days of UFH due to the risk of immune-mediated thrombocytopenia
- Warfarin has interactions with many drugs

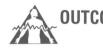

OUTCOME

COMPLICATIONS

- Immune-mediated thrombocytopenia occurs in 3% of patients taking UFH

- Hemorrhage is the major complication of anticoagulation with heparin: risk of any hemorrhage is 0–7%; risk of fatal hemorrhage is 0–2%
- Risk of hemorrhage with warfarin therapy is 3–4% per patient year, but correlates with INR
- Chronic thromboembolic pulmonary hypertension occurs in about 1% of patients; selected patients may benefit from pulmonary endarterectomy

PROGNOSIS

- Overall prognosis depends on the underlying disease rather than the thromboembolic event
- Death from recurrent PE occurs in only 3% of cases; 6 months of anticoagulation therapy reduces the risk of recurrent thrombosis and death by 80–90%
- Perfusion defects resolve in most survivors

WHEN TO REFER

- All patients evaluated for or diagnosed with a PE should be evaluated by an expert (typically a pulmonologist, hematologist, or internist)

WHEN TO ADMIT

- Patients with an acute PE should be admitted for stabilization, initiation of therapy, evaluation of cause of PE, and education

PREVENTION

- See Tables 115 and 116

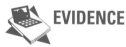

EVIDENCE

PRACTICE GUIDELINES

- American College of Emergency Physicians Clinical Policies Committee; Clinical Policies Committee Subcommittee on Suspected Pulmonary Embolism. Clinical policy: critical issues in the evaluation and management of adult patients presenting with suspected pulmonary embolism. Ann Emerg Med. 2003;41:257. [PMID: 12548278]
- British Thoracic Society Standards of Care Committee Pulmonary Embolism Guideline Development Group. British Thoracic Society guidelines for the management of suspected acute pulmonary embolism. Thorax. 2003;58:470. [PMID: 12775856]
- Buller HR et al. Antithrombotic therapy for venous thromboembolic disease: the

Seventh ACCP Conference on Antithrombotic and Thrombolytic Therapy. Chest. 2004;126:401S. [PMID: 15383479]

INFORMATION FOR PATIENTS

- JAMA patient page. Pulmonary embolism. JAMA. 2003;290:2828. [PMID: 14657080]

REFERENCES

- Buller HR et al. Antithrombotic therapy for venous thromboembolic disease: the Seventh ACCP Conference on Antithrombotic and Thrombolytic Therapy. Chest. 2004 Sep;126(3 Suppl):401S–428S. [PMID: 15383479]
- Geerts WH et al. Prevention of venous thromboembolism: the Seventh ACCP Conference on Antithrombotic and Thrombolytic Therapy. Chest. 2004 Sep;126(3 Suppl):338S–400S. [PMID: 15383478]
- Hirsh J et al. New anticoagulants. Blood. 2005 Jan 15;105(2):453–63. [PMID: 15191946]
- Hull RD. Revisiting the past strengthens the present: an evidence-based medicine approach for the diagnosis of deep venous thrombosis. Ann Intern Med. 2005 Apr 5;142(7):583–5. [PMID: 15809468]
- Perrier A et al. Multidetector-row computed tomography in suspected pulmonary embolism. N Engl J Med. 2005 Apr 28;352(17):1760–8. [PMID: 15858185]
- Quiroz R et al. Clinical validity of a negative computed tomography scan in patients with suspected pulmonary embolism: a systematic review. JAMA. 2005 Apr 27;293(16):2012–7. [PMID: 15855435]
- Roy PM et al. Systematic review and meta-analysis of strategies for the diagnosis of suspected pulmonary embolism. BMJ. 2005 Jul 30;331(7511):259. [PMID: 16052017]
- Segal JB et al. Management of venous thromboembolism: a systematic review for a practice guideline. Ann Intern Med. 2007 Feb 6;146(3):211–22. [PMID: 17261856]
- Snow V et al. Management of venous thromboembolism: a clinical practice guideline from the American College of Physicians and the American Academy of Family Physicians. Ann Intern Med. 2007 Feb 6;146(3):204–10. [PMID: 17261857]
- van Belle A et al; Christopher Study Investigators. Effectiveness of managing

suspected pulmonary embolism using an algorithm combining clinical probability, D-dimer testing, and computed tomography. JAMA. 2006 Jan 11; 295(2):172–9. [PMID: 16403929]

- Wells PS et al. Does this patient have deep vein thrombosis? JAMA. 2006 Jan 11;295(2):199–207. [PMID: 16403932]

Pulmonary Hypertension, Idiopathic

 ## KEY FEATURES

- Elevated pulmonary vascular resistance and hypertension in the absence of other cardiac or pulmonary disease
- Some evidence for genetic associations
- Pathologic findings: diffuse narrowing of pulmonary arterioles
- The diet pills fenfluramine, dexfenfluramine, and phentermine may cause a picture indistinguishable from primary pulmonary hypertension

 ## CLINICAL FINDINGS

- Clinical findings are similar to pulmonary hypertension from other causes (eg, cor pulmonale)
- Characteristically occurs in young women
- Weakness and fatigue from right-sided heart failure, low cardiac output
- Edema, ascites, peripheral cyanosis, and effort-related syncope as right-sided heart failure advances

 ## DIAGNOSIS

- ECG: RV and RA hypertrophy
- Obtain tests for collagen vascular diseases
- Check for sleep apnea
- Chest radiograph
  - Enlarged RV
  - Enlarged main pulmonary arteries (PAs) with reduced peripheral branches

- If patchy, pulmonary edema is present; suspect pulmonary veno-occlusive disease or pulmonary vein stenosis
- Echocardiography
  - Often diagnostic
  - Provides evidence of RV function and estimate of PA pressures
  - Excludes left heart disease, shunts, valvular disease
- Cardiac catheterization
  - Measures PA pressures
  - Can calculate pulmonary vascular resistance
- Nitric oxide inhalation can provide data regarding the degree of vasoactivity still present in the lungs; positive response is reflected by
  - > 20% fall in the PA pressure
  - > 20% drop in pulmonary vascular resistance
  - Final mean PA pressure of < 45 mm Hg

 ## TREATMENT

- Death usually occurs in 2–8 yr
- Long-term anticoagulation is recommended by most experts because of in-situ thrombosis
- Oxygen recommended (at least at night)
- Epoprostenol (a prostacyclin) by continuous IV infusion may slow (but not halt) symptom progression in advanced disease
- Bosentan (an oral endothelin antagonist) now available and in wide use
- Iloprost (an inhaled prostacyclin) is also available
- Sildenafil should be considered in patients who respond to therapy
- Lung transplantation and, occasionaly, heart-lung transplantation is required in some patients

Pulmonary Nodule, Solitary

 ## KEY FEATURES

ESSENTIALS OF DIAGNOSIS

- An isolated, < 3-cm rounded opacity on chest radiograph that is outlined by normal lung and not associated with infiltrate, atelectasis, or adenopathy

GENERAL CONSIDERATIONS

- Most are asymptomatic and represent an unexpected radiographic finding
- Associated with a 10–68% risk of malignancy
- Most benign nodules are infectious granulomas; benign neoplasms such as hamartomas account for 5% of solitary nodules
- Symptoms alone rarely establish etiology, but can be used with radiographic data to assess the probability of malignancy
- The goal of evaluation is to determine the probability of malignancy in any nodule in order to justify resection or biopsy versus observation

DEMOGRAPHICS

- Malignant nodules are rare in persons under age 30
- Over age 30, risk for malignancy increases with age
- Smokers are at increased risk, with the likelihood of cancer increasing with the number of daily cigarettes smoked
- A history of malignancy increases the likelihood that a nodule represents cancer

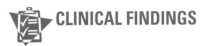 ## CLINICAL FINDINGS

SYMPTOMS AND SIGNS

- Solitary nodules are discovered incidentally on radiographic studies

DIFFERENTIAL DIAGNOSIS

- Granulomatous disease
- Benign neoplasm
- Bronchogenic carcinoma
- Granuloma (tuberculous, fungal)
- Lung abscess
- Hamartoma
- Metastatic cancer
- Arteriovenous malformation
- Resolving pneumonia
- Rheumatoid nodule
- Pulmonary infarction
- Carcinoid
- Pseudotumor (loculated fluid in a fissure)

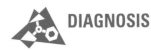 ## DIAGNOSIS

LABORATORY TESTS

- Sputum cytology is highly specific, but insensitive for detecting malignant nodules

IMAGING STUDIES

- Comparison with prior radiographic studies allows estimation of doubling time: rapid doubling time (< 30 days) suggests infection; slow doubling time (< 465 days) suggests benignity
- High-resolution CT (HRCT) scanning for any nodule
- Increasing size on CT scan correlates with risk of malignancy
  - 1% malignancy rate for 2–5 mm
  - 33% for 11–20 mm
  - 80% for 21–45 mm
- CT features suggesting malignancy
  - Spiculations or a peripheral halo
  - Sparse stippled or eccentric calcifications
  - Thick-walled (> 16 mm) cavitary lesions
- CT features associated with benign processes
  - Smooth, well-defined margins
  - Dense central or laminar calcifications
- Positron emission tomography (PET) is highly sensitive (85–95%) and specific (70–85%) for detecting malignant nodules and is incorporated in many diagnostic algorithms with HRCT

DIAGNOSTIC PROCEDURES

- In patients with a high probability of malignancy, biopsies rarely yield a specific benign diagnosis
- Bronchoscopy yields a diagnosis in 10–80%, depending on the size and location of the nodule; complications are rare
- Transthoracic needle aspiration (TTNA) has a diagnostic yield of 50–97%, with a 30% risk of pneumothorax
- Video-assisted thoracoscopic surgery (VATS) is used for initial evaluation of intermediate risk nodules; frozen sections can direct treatment in the operating room

 TREATMENT

SURGERY

- Surgical resection via open thoracotomy or VATS is indicated for
  - Proven malignancies
  - Nodules likely to be malignant
  - Certain intermediate risk nodules

THERAPEUTIC PROCEDURES

- A probability of malignancy should be assigned to each nodule based on clinical and radiographic features
- Watchful waiting is appropriate for patients with low probability (< 8%) of malignancy (2 years, benign calcification pattern)
- Resection is indicated for patients with a high probability (> 70%) of malignancy and no contraindications to surgery
- Optimal management of patients with an intermediate probability (8–70%) of malignancy is controversial; bronchoscopy, transthoracic needle biopsy, VATS, PET scan, and contrast-enhanced HRCT are used

 OUTCOME

FOLLOW-UP

- For a nodule with a low probability of malignancy, patients should have chest radiograph every 3 months for 1 year, then every 6 months for 1 year

WHEN TO REFER

- For specialized diagnostic procedures such as bronchoscopy, transthoracic needle aspiration, or thoracoscopic surgery

 EVIDENCE

PRACTICE GUIDELINES

- MacMahon H et al. Guidelines for management of small pulmonary nodules detected on CT scans: a statement from the Fleischner Society. Radiology. 2005;237:395. [PMID: 16244247]

REFERENCES

- Gurney JW. Determining the likelihood of malignancy in solitary pulmonary nodules with Bayesian analysis. Part I. Theory. Radiology. 1993 Feb; 186(2):405–13. [PMID: 8421743]
- MacMahon H et al. Guidelines for management of small pulmonary nodules detected on CT scans: a statement from the Fleischner Society. Radiology. 2005 Nov;237(2):395–400. [PMID: 16244247]
- Winer-Muram HT. The solitary pulmonary nodule. Radiology. 2006 Apr; 239(1):34–49. [PMID: 16567482]

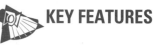
Pyelonephritis, Acute

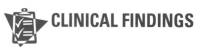 **KEY FEATURES**

ESSENTIALS OF DIAGNOSIS

- Fever
- Flank pain
- Irritative voiding symptoms
- Positive urine culture

GENERAL CONSIDERATIONS

- Acute pyelonephritis is an infectious inflammatory disease involving the kidney parenchyma and renal pelvis
- Most common causative organisms
  - *Escherichia coli*
  - *Proteus*
  - *Klebsiella*
  - *Enterobacter*
  - *Pseudomonas*
- Less common causative organisms
  - *Enterococcus faecalis*
  - *Staphylococcus aureus*

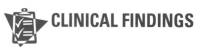 **CLINICAL FINDINGS**

SYMPTOMS AND SIGNS

- Fever
- Flank pain
- Shaking chills
- Urgency, frequency, dysuria
- Nausea, vomiting, diarrhea
- Tachycardia
- Costovertebral angle tenderness

DIFFERENTIAL DIAGNOSIS

- Appendicitis
- Cholecystitis
- Pancreatitis
- Diverticulitis
- Lower lobe pneumonia

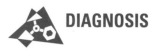 **DIAGNOSIS**

LABORATORY TESTS

- Complete blood cell count: leukocytosis and a left shift
- Urinalysis: pyuria, bacteriuria, hematuria, white blood cell casts
- Urine (and sometimes blood) culture positive

IMAGING STUDIES

- Renal ultrasound or abdominal CT (in complicated cases) to evaluate for hydronephrosis from stone or other obstruction

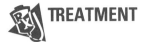 **TREATMENT**

MEDICATIONS

- Inpatients: IV ampicillin and an aminoglycoside until afebrile for 24 h, then PO antibiotics for 3 weeks
- Outpatients: quinolones or nitrofurantoin

Regimens

- Ampicillin, 1 g q6h, and gentamicin, 1 mg/kg q8h IV for 21 days
- Ciprofloxacin, 750 mg q12h PO for 21 days
- Ofloxacin, 200–300 mg q12h PO for 21 days
- Trimethoprim-sulfamethoxasole, 160/800 mg q12h PO for 21 days (increasing resistance noted [up to 20%])

SURGERY

- Nephrostomy drainage or double-J ureteral stent if ureteral obstruction

THERAPEUTIC PROCEDURES

- Failure to respond warrants abdominal imaging to exclude obstruction
- Catheter drainage

 OUTCOME

FOLLOW-UP

- Follow-up urine culture after completion of treatment

PROGNOSIS

- With prompt diagnosis and treatment, good prognosis
- With complicating factors, underlying renal disease, and increasing patient age, less favorable prognosis

WHEN TO ADMIT

- Admit if severe infections or complicating factors; obtain urine and blood cultures

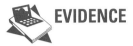 **EVIDENCE**

PRACTICE GUIDELINES

- Bass PF 3rd et al. Urinary tract infections. Prim Care. 2003;30:41. [PMID: 12838910]

INFORMATION FOR PATIENTS

- Mayo Clinic—Urinary tract infection
- National Kidney and Urologic Diseases Information Clearinghouse

REFERENCE

- Meng MV et al. Infections of the upper urinary tract. In: *Urologic Emergencies,* Humana Press, 2005.

Raynaud Phenomenon

 KEY FEATURES

ESSENTIALS OF DIAGNOSIS

- Paroxysmal bilateral symmetric pallor and cyanosis followed by rubor of the skin of the digits
- Precipitated by cold or emotional stress; relieved by warmth
- Primarily affects young women
- Primary form benign
- Secondary form can cause digital ulceration or gangrene

GENERAL CONSIDERATIONS

- Raynaud phenomenon (RP) is a syndrome of paroxysmal digital ischemia
- Most commonly caused by an exaggerated response of digital arterioles to cold or emotional stress
- Toes and other acral areas (eg, nose and ears) can be affected as well as fingers
- Classified as primary (idiopathic or Raynaud disease) or secondary
- Primary form
  - Appears between ages 15 and 30, almost always in women
  - Tends to be mildly progressive

DEMOGRAPHICS

- Primary RP occurs in 2–6% of adults

 CLINICAL FINDINGS

SYMPTOMS AND SIGNS

- Only one or two fingertips may be affected in early attacks
- All fingers down to the distal palm may be involved as condition progresses
- Thumbs are rarely affected
- Well-demarcated digital pallor or cyanosis in initial phase
- Intense rubor, throbbing, paresthesia, pain, and slight swelling during recovery phase
- Patient usually asymptomatic between attacks
- Sensory changes that often accompany vasomotor manifestations
  - Numbness
  - Stiffness
  - Diminished sensation
  - Aching pain

- Primary RP
  - Symmetric involvement of the fingers of both hands
  - Spasm becomes more frequent and prolonged
  - Does not cause digital pitting, ulceration, or gangrene
- Secondary RP
  - May be unilateral and may involve only one or two fingers
  - Nailfold capillary abnormalities
  - Digital pitting or ulceration
  - Skin tightening
  - Loss of extremity pulse
  - Rash
  - Swollen joints

DIFFERENTIAL DIAGNOSIS

- RP occasionally the first manifestation of such rheumatic conditions as
  - Systemic sclerosis (including its CREST variant)
  - Systemic lupus erythematosus
  - Mixed connective tissue disease
- Thromboangiitis obliterans (Buerger's disease)
- Thoracic outlet syndromes
- Acrocyanosis
- Frostbite
- Ergot poisoning (unusual)
- Bleomycin and vincristine chemotherapy
- Cryoglobulinemia

 DIAGNOSIS

LABORATORY TESTS

- Serologic tests for rheumatic diseases (Table 123)

DIAGNOSTIC PROCEDURES

- Evaluate nailfold capillary pattern
  - Place a drop of grade B immersion oil at cuticle
  - View area with an ophthalmoscope set to 20–40 diopters
- Dilation or dropout of the capillary loops indicates presence of secondary form of RP, most commonly scleroderma
- While highly specific for secondary RP, nailfold capillary changes have a low sensitivity

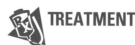 **TREATMENT**

MEDICATIONS

- Calcium channel blockers
  - First-line therapy

- Produce a modest benefit
- More effective in primary RP than secondary RP
- Slow release nifedipine (30–180 mg/day) or amlodipine (5–20 mg/day), felodipine, or nisoldipine are popular and more effective than verapamil and diltiazem
- Other medications that are sometimes effective
  - Angiotensin-converting enzyme inhibitors
  - Sympatholytic agents (eg, prazosin)
  - Topical nitrates
  - Phosphodiesterase inhibitors (eg, sildenafil, tadalafil, and vardenafil)
  - Selective serotonin reuptake inhibitors (fluoxetine)
  - Endothelin-receptor inhibitors (ie, bosentan)

SURGERY

- Sympathectomy indications
  - Frequent and severe attacks
  - Interference with work and well being
  - Development of trophic changes and failure of medical measures
- Cervical sympathectomy is modestly effective for primary but not secondary RP
- Digital sympathectomy may improve secondary RP

THERAPEUTIC PROCEDURES

- Keep the body warm
- Protect hands from injury at all times
- Softening and lubricating lotion
- Smoking cessation

 OUTCOME

PROGNOSIS

- Primary PR is benign and largely a nuisance for affected individuals
- Prognosis of secondary RP depends on severity of the underlying disease

PREVENTION

- Avoidance of cold exposure
- Reduction of emotional stress

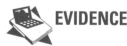 **EVIDENCE**

INFORMATION FOR PATIENTS

- Cleveland Clinic: Raynaud's Phenomenon
- Mayo Clinic: Raynaud's Disease
- MedlinePlus: Raynaud's Phenomenon

REFERENCES

- Sule SD, Wigley FM. Raynaud Phenomenon. In: *Current Diagnosis & Treatment Rheumatology*, 2nd edition. Imboden J et al (editors). McGraw-Hill, New York; 2007.
- Wigley FM. Clinical practice. Raynaud's phenomenon. N Engl J Med. 2002 Sep 26;347(13):1001–8. [PMID: 12324557]

Renal Artery Stenosis

 KEY FEATURES

ESSENTIALS OF DIAGNOSIS

- Produced by atherosclerotic occlusive disease (most patients) or fibromuscular dysplasia
- Hypertension
- Renal failure with initiation of angiotensin-converting enzyme (ACE) inhibitor therapy

GENERAL CONSIDERATIONS

- Atherosclerotic ischemic renal disease
  - Accounts for nearly all cases of renal artery stenosis
  - Occurs most commonly in persons over age 45 who have a history of atherosclerotic disease
- Other risk factors include
  - Renal insufficiency
  - Diabetes mellitus
  - Tobacco use
  - Hypertension
- Fibromuscular dysplasia primarily affects young women

DEMOGRAPHICS

- Approximately 5% of Americans with hypertension suffer from renal artery stenosis

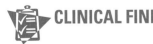 CLINICAL FINDINGS

SYMPTOMS AND SIGNS

- Refractory hypertension
- New-onset hypertension in older patient
- Pulmonary edema with poorly controlled blood pressure
- Acute renal failure upon starting an ACE inhibitor
- Abdominal bruit on affected side

DIFFERENTIAL DIAGNOSIS

 DIAGNOSIS

LABORATORY TESTS

- Elevated blood urea nitrogen and serum creatinine

IMAGING STUDIES

- Abdominal ultrasound shows asymmetric kidney size
- Initial screening tests: Doppler ultrasonography, captopril renography, and magnetic resonance angiography (MRA)
- **Doppler ultrasonography**
  - Measure blood flow at aorta and along each third of renal artery
  - Highly sensitive and specific (> 90%) and relatively inexpensive
  - Poor choice for patients who are obese, unable to lie supine, or have interfering bowel gas patterns
- **Captopril renography**
  - Capitalizes on difference in renal perfusion with and without ACE inhibitors
  - Sensitivity ranges from 75% to 100% and specificity from 60% to 90%
  - Not as accurate in moderate to severe kidney disease
- **MRA**
  - Excellent but expensive
  - Sensitivity is 99–100% and specificity ranges from 71% to 96%
  - Turbulent blood flow can cause false-positive results
- **Renal angiography**
  - Gold standard for diagnosis
  - CO_2 subtraction angiography used when risk of dye nephropathy exists (eg, diabetic patients with renal insufficiency)
  - Risk of atheroembolic phenomena after angiography ranges from 5% to 10%
  - Fibromuscular dysplasia has characteristic "beads-on-a-string" appearance

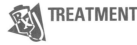 TREATMENT

MEDICATIONS

- Antihypertensive pharmacologic agents that avoid ACE inhibitors and ACE receptor blockers

SURGERY

- Surgical bypass an option for atherosclerotic ischemic renal disease

THERAPEUTIC PROCEDURES

- Angioplasty for atherosclerotic ischemic renal disease
  - Might reduce number of antihypertensive medications
  - Equally as effective as, and safer than, surgical revision
- Stenting
  - Produces significantly better angioplastic results
  - However, blood pressure is equally improved, and serum creatinines are similar at 6 months of observation
- Percutaneous transluminal angioplasty curative for fibromuscular dysplasia

 OUTCOME

FOLLOW-UP

- Monitor blood pressure, renal function, serum lipids

COMPLICATIONS

- Resistent hypertension
- Chronic kidney disease

WHEN TO REFER

- Inability to control hypertension
- Renal insufficiency

WHEN TO ADMIT

- Malignant hypertension

PREVENTION

- Risk factor modification (eg, treatment of hyperlipidemia) to reduce atherosclerosis

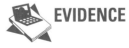 EVIDENCE

PRACTICE GUIDELINES

- Martin LG et al. Quality improvement guidelines for angiography, angioplasty, and stent placement in the diagnosis and treatment of renal artery stenosis in adults. J Vasc Interv Radiol. 2002 Nov; 13(11):1069–83. [PMID: 12427805]

INFORMATION FOR PATIENTS

- American College of Physicians: Summaries for Patients: Diagnosis of Renal Artery Stenosis
- MedlinePlus: Renal Artery Stenosis

REFERENCES

- Bloch MJ et al. Clinical insights into the diagnosis and management of renovascular disease. An evidence-based review. Minerva Med. 2004 Oct;95(5):357–73. [PMID: 15467512]
- Kalra PA et al. Atherosclerotic renovascular disease in United States patients aged 67 years or older: risk factors, revascularization, and prognosis. Kidney Int. 2005 Jul;68(1):293–301. [PMID: 15954920]
- Korsakas S et al. Delay of dialysis in end-stage renal failure: prospective study on percutaneous renal artery interventions. Kidney Int. 2004 Jan; 65(1):251–8. [PMID: 14675057]
- Nordmann AJ et al. Balloon angioplasty versus medical therapy for hypertensive patients with renal artery obstruction. Cochrane Database Syst Rev 2003; (3):CD002944. [PMID: 12917937]
- Safian RD et al. Renal artery stenosis. N Engl J Med. 2001 Feb 8;344(6):431–42. [PMID: 11172181]

Renal Cell Carcinoma

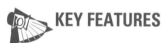 **KEY FEATURES**

ESSENTIALS OF DIAGNOSIS

- Gross or microscopic hematuria
- Flank pain or mass in some patients
- Systemic symptoms such as fever, weight loss may be prominent
- Solid renal mass on imaging

GENERAL CONSIDERATIONS

- ~2.6% of all adult cancers
- In 2005, ~36,160 cases of renal cell carcinoma and ~12,660 deaths in the United States

DEMOGRAPHICS

- Peak incidence in sixth decade of life
- Male-to-female ratio = 2:1
- Cause is unknown
- Risk factor: cigarette smoking
- Familial: von Hippel-Lindau syndrome
- Association with dialysis-related acquired cystic disease

 CLINICAL FINDINGS

SYMPTOMS AND SIGNS

- Hematuria (gross or microscopic) in 60% of cases
- Flank pain or an abdominal mass in ~30%
- Triad of flank pain, hematuria, and mass in ~10–15%, often a sign of advanced disease
- Symptoms of metastatic disease (cough, bone pain) in ~20–30% at presentation
- Often detected incidentally

DIFFERENTIAL DIAGNOSIS

- Angiomyolipomas (fat density usually visible by CT)
- Urothelial cell cancers of the renal pelvis (more centrally located, involvement of the collecting system, positive urinary cytology reports)
- Adrenal tumors (superoanterior to the kidney)
- Oncocytomas
- Renal abscesses

 DIAGNOSIS

LABORATORY TESTS

- Hematuria in 60%
- Paraneoplastic syndromes
- Erythrocytosis from increased erythropoietin production in ~5% (anemia far more common)
- Hypercalcemia in 10%
- Stauffer's syndrome, a reversible syndrome of hepatic dysfunction

IMAGING STUDIES

- Renal mass on abdominal ultrasonography, CT or MRI scan

DIAGNOSTIC PROCEDURES

- CT scanning is the most valuable imaging test; it confirms character of the mass, stages the lesion
- Chest radiographs for pulmonary metastases
- Bone scans for large tumors, bone pain, elevated alkaline phosphatase levels
- MRI and duplex Doppler ultrasonography can assess for the presence and extent of tumor thrombus within the renal vein or vena cava in selected patients

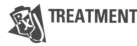 **TREATMENT**

MEDICATIONS

- For metastatic renal cell carcinoma, no effective chemotherapy is available
- Vinblastine yields short-term partial response rates of 15%
- Biologic response modifiers: α-interferon yields partial response rate of 15–20% and interleukin-2, partial response rate of 15–35%
- Vascular endothelial growth factor (VEGF) and Raf-kinase inhibitors: oral agents, well-tolerated, with demonstrated effectiveness in patients with advanced kidney cancer, especially clear cell carcinoma (~40% response rate)

SURGERY

- Laparoscopic or open radical nephrectomy for localized renal cell carcinoma
- Partial nephrectomy for patients with a small cancer, single kidney, bilateral lesions, or significant medical renal disease
- Cytoreductive nephrectomy for patients with metastatic kidney cancer and good performance status who have resectable primary tumors

THERAPEUTIC PROCEDURES

- Cell type and histologic pattern do not affect treatment
- Patients with metastatic disease usually should be considered for palliative surgery followed by systemic therapy with biologic response modifiers

 OUTCOME

PROGNOSIS

- For patients with solitary resectable metastases, radical nephrectomy with resection of the metastasis has resulted in 5-year disease-free survival rates of 15–30%

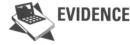 **EVIDENCE**

PRACTICE GUIDELINES

- Motzer RJ et al. NCCN Kidney Cancer Practice Guidelines Panel. National Comprehensive Cancer Network: Kidney Cancer v.1.2005.

WEB SITE

- National Cancer Institute: Kidney Cancer Information for Patients and Health Professionals

INFORMATION FOR PATIENTS

- American Cancer Society: Kidney Cancer
- Mayo Clinic: Kidney Cancer
- National Cancer Institute: Kidney Cancer
- Torpy JM et al. JAMA patient page. Kidney cancer. JAMA. 2004;292:134. [PMID: 15238600]

REFERENCES

- Dhote R et al. Risk factors for adult renal cell carcinoma. Urol Clin North Am. 2004 May;31(2):237–47. [PMID: 15123404]
- Flanigan RC et al. Nephrectomy followed by interferon alfa-2b compared with interferon alfa-2b alone for metastatic renal-cell cancer. N Engl J Med. 2001 Dec 6;345(23):1655–9. [PMID: 11759643]
- Mickisch GH et al; European Organisation for Research and Treatment of Cancer (EORTC) Genitourinary Group. Radical nephrectomy plus interferon-alfa-based immunotherapy compared with interferon alfa alone in metastatic renal-cell carcinoma: a randomised trial. Lancet. 2001 Sep 22;358(9286):966–70. [PMID: 11583750]
- Motzer RJ et al. Activity of SU11248, a multitargeted inhibitor of vascular endothelial growth factor receptor and platelet-derived growth factor receptor, in patients with metastatic renal cell carcinoma. J Clin Oncol. 2006 Jan 1;24(1):16–24. [PMID: 16330672]
- Motzer RJ et al. Prognostic factors for survival in previously treated patients with metastatic renal cell carcinoma. J Clin Oncol. 2004 Feb 1;22(3):454–63. [PMID: 14752067]
- Rini BI. New approaches in advanced renal cell carcinoma. Urol Oncol. 2005 Jan-Feb;23(1):65–6. [PMID: 15885585]
- Saika T et al. Long-term outcome of laparoscopic radical nephrectomy for pathologic T1 renal cell carcinoma. Urology. 2003 Dec;62(6):1018–23. [PMID: 14665347]

Renal Failure, Acute

 KEY FEATURES

ESSENTIALS OF DIAGNOSIS

- Defined as a sudden decrease in renal function, resulting in an inability to maintain fluid and electrolyte balance and to excrete nitrogenous wastes
- Sudden increase in blood urea nitrogen (BUN) or serum creatinine
- Oliguria often associated
- Symptoms and signs depend on cause

GENERAL CONSIDERATIONS

- 5% of hospital admissions and 30% of ICU admissions have acute renal failure
- 25% of hospitalized patients develop acute renal failure
- Serum creatinine concentration can typically increase 1.0–1.5 mg/dL daily
- Three categories of acute kidney injury
  - Prerenal azotemia
  - Intrinsic renal failure
  - Postrenal azotemia

CLINICAL FINDINGS

SYMPTOMS AND SIGNS

- Nausea, vomiting
- Malaise
- Hypertension
- Pericardial friction rub, effusions, and cardiac tamponade
- Arrhythmias
- Rales
- Abdominal pain and ileus
- Bleeding secondary to platelet dysfunction
- Encephalopathy, altered sensorium, asterixis, seizures
- Oliguria, defined as urinary output < 500 mL/day or < 20 mL/hour

DIFFERENTIAL DIAGNOSIS

Prerenal azotemia
- Dehydration
- Hemorrhage (eg, gastrointestinal bleeding)
- Congestive heart failure
- Renal artery stenosis, including fibromuscular dysplasia

- Nonsteroidal anti-inflammatory drugs (NSAIDs), angiotensin-converting enzyme inhibitors

Postrenal azotemia
- Obstruction (eg, benign prostatic hyperplasia, bladder tumor)

Intrinsic renal disease
- Acute tubular necrosis
  - Toxins
    - NSAIDs
    - Antibiotics
    - Contrast
    - Multiple myeloma
    - Rhabdomyolysis
    - Hemolysis
    - Chemotherapy
    - Hyperuricemia
    - Cyclosporine
  - Ischemia (eg, prolonged prerenal azotemia)
- Acute glomerulonephritis
  - Immune complex
    - IgA nephropathy
    - Endocarditis
    - Systemic lupus erythematosus (SLE)
    - Cryoglobulinemia
    - Postinfectious
    - Membranoproliferative
  - Pauci-immune (ANCA+)
    - Wegener's granulomatosis
    - Churg-Strauss syndrome
    - Microscopic polyarteritis
  - Antiglomerular basement membrane (anti-GBM)
    - Goodpasture's disease
    - Anti-GBM glomerulonephritis
- Vascular
  - Malignant hypertension
  - Thrombotic thrombocytopenia purpura
  - Atheroembolism
- Acute interstitial nephritis
  - Drugs
    - β-Lactams
    - Sulfa
    - Diuretics
    - NSAIDs
    - Rifampin
    - Phenytoin
    - Allopurinol
  - Infections
    - *Streptococcus*
    - Leptospirosis
    - Cytomegalovirus
    - Histoplasmosis
    - Rocky Mountain spotted fever
  - Immune
    - SLE
    - Sjögren's syndrome
    - Sarcoidosis
    - Cryoglobulinemia

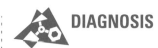

DIAGNOSIS

LABORATORY TESTS

- Serum creatinine and BUN elevated
- BUN–creatinine ratio > 20:1 in prerenal and postrenal azotemia, and acute glomerulonephritis; < 20:1 in acute tubular necrosis and acute interstitial nephritis
- Hyperkalemia
- Anion gap metabolic acidosis
- Hyperphosphatemia
- Hypocalcemia
- Anemia
- Fractional excretion of sodium (FE_{Na}) can be useful in oliguric states:
  FE_{Na} = clearance of Na^+/GFR = clearance of Na^+/creatinine clearance
  FE_{Na} = (urine Na^+/plasma Na^+)/(urine Cr/plasma Cr) $\times$ 100
- FE_{Na} low (< 1%) in prerenal azotemia; high (> 1%) in acute tubular necrosis; variable in postrenal azotemia, acute interstitial nephritis, acute glomerulonephritis

IMAGING STUDIES

- Renal ultrasonography to exclude obstruction or other anatomic abnormalities; check renal size and echotexture
- CT or MRI if retroperitoneal fibrosis from tumor or radiation suspected

DIAGNOSTIC PROCEDURES

- ECG: peaked T waves, PR prolongation, and QRS widening in hyperkalemia, long QT interval with hypocalcemia

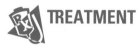

TREATMENT

THERAPEUTIC PROCEDURES

- Prerenal azotemia
  - Treatment depends on cause
  - Maintain euvolemia
  - Monitor serum potassium
  - Avoid nephrotoxic drugs
- Postrenal azotemia: relief of obstruction if present
  - Place catheters or stents to treat obstruction
  - Catheterize the bladder if hydroureter and hydronephrosis are present with an enlarged bladder on ultrasonography
- Intrinsic renal failure: treatment depends on cause (see Tubular Necrosis, Acute); hold offending agents

- Hemodialysis, peritoneal dialysis: indications include
  - Uremic symptoms such as pericarditis, encephalopathy, or coagulopathy
  - Fluid overload unresponsive to diuresis
  - Refractory hyperkalemia
  - Severe metabolic acidosis (pH < 7.20)
  - Neurologic symptoms such as seizures or neuropathy

OUTCOME

WHEN TO REFER

- Persistence of acute renal failure for 2–4 weeks or sooner if uremic symptoms or dialysis needs are present

WHEN TO ADMIT

- Significant acid–base, fluid, or electrolyte abnormalities or uremia

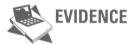

EVIDENCE

WEB SITE

- National Kidney and Urologic Diseases Information Clearinghouse

INFORMATION FOR PATIENTS

- Mayo Clinic: Kidney Failure
- MedlinePlus: Kidney Failure
- Parmet S et al. JAMA patient page: Acute renal failure. JAMA. 2002; 288:2634. [PMID: 12444873]

REFERENCES

- Cantarovich F et al. High-dose furosemide for established ARF: a prospective, randomized, double-blind, placebo-controlled, multicenter trial. Am J Kidney Dis. 2004 Sep;44(3):402–9. [PMID: 15332212]
- Mehta R et al. Diuretics, mortality, and nonrecovery of renal function in acute renal failure. JAMA. 2002 Nov 27; 288(20):2547–53. [PMID: 12444861]
- Perazella MA. Drug-induced renal failure: update on new medications and unique mechanisms of nephrotoxicity. Am J Med Sci. 2003 Jun;325(6):349–62. [PMID: 12811231]
- Warnock DG. Towards a definition and classification of acute kidney injury. J Am Soc Nephrol. 2005 Nov; 16(11):3149–50. [PMID: 16207828]
- Weisbord S et al. Radiocontrast-induced acute renal failure. J Intensive Care Med. 2005 Mar–Apr;20(2):63–75. [PMID: 15855219]

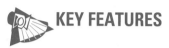

Renal Failure, Chronic

KEY FEATURES

ESSENTIALS OF DIAGNOSIS

- Progressive azotemia over months to years
- Symptoms and signs of uremia when nearing end-stage disease
- Hypertension in the majority
- Isosthenuria and broad casts in urinary sediment are common
- Bilateral small kidneys on ultrasonogram are diagnostic

GENERAL CONSIDERATIONS

- Major causes (> 50% of cases) are diabetes mellitus and hypertension
- Glomerulonephritis, cystic diseases, other urologic diseases account for another 20–25%, and unknown causes ~15% (Table 85)
- Rarely reversible
- Progressive decline in renal function

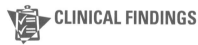

CLINICAL FINDINGS

SYMPTOMS AND SIGNS

- Symptoms develop slowly and are nonspecific
- Can be asymptomatic until renal failure is far advanced (glomerular filtration rate [GFR] < 10–15 mL/min)
- Fatigue, weakness, and malaise
- Gastrointestinal complaints such as anorexia, nausea, vomiting, a metallic taste in the mouth, and hiccups
- Neurologic irritability, difficulty concentrating, insomnia, restless legs, and twitching
- Pruritus
- Decreased libido, menstrual irregularities
- Chest pain from pericarditis
- Renal osteodystrophy (osteitis fibrosa cystica), osteomalacia, and adynamic bone disease

DIFFERENTIAL DIAGNOSIS

- See Table 86

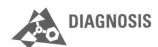

DIAGNOSIS

LABORATORY TESTS

- Serum creatinine and blood urea nitrogen (BUN) elevated; evidence of previously elevated creatinine and BUN, abnormal prior urinalyses help differentiate between acute and chronic renal failure
- Plot of the inverse of serum creatinine ($1/S_{Cr}$) versus time if three or more prior measurements are available helps estimate time to end-stage renal disease
- Anemia
- Platelet dysfunction, bleeding time prolongation
- Metabolic acidosis
- Hyperphosphatemia, hypocalcemia
- Hyperkalemia
- Isosthenuria
- Urinary sediment: broad waxy casts

IMAGING STUDIES

- Renal ultrasonogram for anatomic abnormalities, kidney size, and echogenicity

DIAGNOSTIC PROCEDURES

- Possible renal biopsy

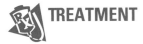

TREATMENT

MEDICATIONS

- Acute hyperkalemia: calcium chloride or gluconate IV, insulin administration with glucose IV, bicarbonate IV, and ion exchange resin (sodium polystyrene sulfonate) PO or PR, cardiac monitoring
- Chronic hyperkalemia: dietary potassium restriction, sodium polystyrene sulfonate, 15–30 g PO once daily in juice or sorbitol
- Acid–base disorders: sodium bicarbonate, calcium bicarbonate, or sodium citrate 20–30 mmol/day divided into two doses, titrated to maintain serum bicarbonate at > 20 mEq/L
- Hypertension
  – Salt and water restriction, weight loss, decreased salt diet (4–6 to 2 g/day)
  – Angiotensin-converting enzyme (ACE) inhibitors or angiotensin II receptor blockers (if serum potassium and GFR permit)
  – Calcium channel-blocking agents, diuretics, and β-blocking agents
  – Clonidine, hydralazine, minoxidil as adjunctive drugs
- Congestive heart failure
  – Salt and water restriction, loop diuretics
  – Avoid ACE inhibitors if serum creatinine > 3 mg/dL
- Anemia
  – Recombinant erythropoietin, 50 U/kg (3000–4000 U/dose) 1× or 2× week IV or SQ
  – Ferrous sulfate, 325 mg one to three times daily if serum ferritin < 100 ng/mL or if iron saturation < 20–25%
- Coagulopathy: dialysis
  – Desmopressin, 25 mcg IV q8–12h for two doses for surgery
  – Conjugated estrogens, 0.6 mg/kg diluted in 50 mL of 0.9% sodium chloride infused over 30–40 min once daily, or 2.5–5.0 mg PO once daily for 5–7 days; effect lasts several weeks
- Renal osteodystrophy, osteomalacia
  – Dietary phosphorus restriction
  – Oral phosphorus-binding agents such as calcium carbonate or calcium acetate given in divided doses 3–4× daily with meals titrated to a serum calcium of 10 mg/dL and serum phosphorus < 4.5 mg/dL
  – Vitamin D or vitamin D analogs (if iPTH > 2–3× normal), serum phosphate and calcium adequately low
  – Calcitriol 0.25–0.5 mcg once daily or every other day

NONPHARMACOLOGIC APPROACH

Diet

- Protein restriction to < 1 g/kg/day; if beneficial, < 0.6 g/kg/day
- Salt restriction to < 2 g/day sodium for nondialysis patient approaching end-stage renal disease
- Water restriction to < 1–2 L /day
- Potassium restriction to < 50–60 mEq/day
- Phosphorus restriction to < 5–10 mg/kg/day
- Magnesium-containing laxatives and antacids contraindicated

THERAPEUTIC PROCEDURES

- Renal transplantation
- Hemodialysis, peritoneal dialysis
  – Uremic symptoms (eg, pericarditis, encephalopathy, coagulopathy)
  – Fluid overload unresponsive to diuresis
  – Refractory hyperkalemia
  – Severe metabolic acidosis (pH < 7.20)
  – Neurologic symptoms (eg, seizures, neuropathy)
- Dialysis Outcomes Quality Initiative guidelines: Begin dialysis in nondiabetics at GFR of 10 mL/min or serum creatinine of 8 mg/dL, in diabetics at GFR of 15 mL/min or serum creatinine of 6 mg/dL

OUTCOME

FOLLOW-UP

- Check serum creatinine and potassium within 9–10 days if ACE inhibitors used

PROGNOSIS

- Mortality is higher for patients receiving dialysis than for age-matched controls; annual mortality rate is 22.4 deaths per 100 patient-years
- Common causes of death
  – Cardiac dysfunction (48%)
  – Infection (15%)
  – Cerebrovascular disease (6%)
  – Malignancy (4%)

WHEN TO REFER

- Refer to nephrologist when GFR < 60 mL/min for comanagement

WHEN TO ADMIT

- Congestive heart failure, pericarditis
- Severe acid–base or electrolyte disturbances or uremia

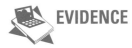

EVIDENCE

PRACTICE GUIDELINES

- Knoll G et al; Kidney Transplant Working Group of the Canadian Society of Transplantation. Canadian Society of Transplantation: consensus guidelines on eligibility for kidney transplantation. CMAJ. 2005;173:S1. [PMID: 16275956]
- Locatelli F et al. Revised European best practice guidelines for the management of anaemia in patients with chronic renal failure. Nephrol Dial Transplant. 2004;19(Suppl 2):ii1. [PMID: 15206425]
- National Kidney Foundation: Kidney Disease Outcomes Quality Initiative (K/DOQI) Practice Guidelines
- Parker TF III et al. The chronic kidney disease initiative. J Am Soc Nephrol. 2004;15:708. [PMID: 14978173]

WEB SITE

- National Kidney Foundation

INFORMATION FOR PATIENTS

- Mayo Clinic: Kidney Failure
- MedlinePlus: Kidney Failure
- National Kidney Foundation: Dialysis

REFERENCES

- Barry JM. Current status of renal transplantation. Patient evaluations and outcomes. Urol Clin North Am. 2001 Nov; 28(4):677–86. [PMID: 11791486]
- Block GA et al. Cinacalcet for secondary hyperparathyroidism in patients receiving hemodialysis. N Engl J Med. 2004 Apr 8;350(15):1516–25. [PMID: 15071126]
- Bolton WK et al. Preparing the patient for renal replacement therapy. Teamwork optimizes outcomes. Postgrad Med. 2002 Jun;111(6):97–8, 101–4, 107–8. [PMID: 12082923]
- Collins AJ et al. Cardiovascular disease in end-stage renal disease patients. Am J Kidney Dis. 2001 Oct;38(4 Suppl 1):S26–9. [PMID: 11576917]
- Fan SL et al. Bisphosphonates in renal osteodystrophy. Curr Opin Nephrol Hypertens. 2001 Sep;10(5):581–8. [PMID: 11496050]
- Go AS et al. Chronic kidney disease and the risks of death, cardiovascular events, and hospitalization. N Engl J Med. 2004 Sep 23;351(13):1296–305. [PMID: 15385656]
- JAMA patient page. Kidney failure. JAMA. 2001 Dec 12;286(22):2898. [PMID: 11767735]
- Levey AS et al; National Kidney Foundation. National Kidney Foundation practice guidelines for chronic kidney disease: evaluation, classification, and stratification. Ann Intern Med. 2003 Jul 15;139(2):137–47. [PMID: 12859163]
- Mathur RV et al. Calciphylaxis. Postgrad Med J. 2001 Sep;77(911):557–61. [PMID: 11524512]
- Ramanathan V et al. Renal transplantation. Semin Nephrol. 2001 Mar; 21(2):213–9. [PMID: 11245782]
- Ruggenenti P et al. Progression, remission, regression of chronic renal diseases. Lancet. 2001 May 19; 357(9268):1601–8. [PMID: 11377666]
- Smogorzewski MJ. Central nervous dysfunction in uremia. Am J Kidney Dis. 2001 Oct;38(4 Suppl 1):S122–8. [PMID: 11576937]

Rhabdomyolysis

 KEY FEATURES

ESSENTIALS OF DIAGNOSIS

- Necrosis of skeletal muscle
- Can be encountered in a wide variety of clinical settings, alone or in concert with other disorders of muscle

GENERAL CONSIDERATIONS

- Rhabdomyolysis is generally seen with concomitant myopathy, though the term "rhabdomyolysis" refers only to a test abnormality
- Commonly due to a syndrome of crush injury to muscle, associated with
  - Myoglobinuria
  - Renal insufficiency
  - Markedly elevated creatine kinase (CK) levels
  - Frequently, multiorgan failure as a consequence of other complications of the trauma

Causes
- Crush injury
- Prolonged immobility, eg, drug overdose, exposure, hypothermia
- Statin use
- Myositis, eg, polymyositis, dermatomyositis
- Seizure
- Strenuous exercise or heat stroke
- Hypokalemia or hypophosphatemia
- Severe volume contraction
- Acute alcoholic intoxication (rare)

 CLINICAL FINDINGS

SYMPTOMS AND SIGNS

- Often there is little evidence for muscle injury on external examination of these patients—and specifically, neither myalgia nor myopathy is present
- Can be associated with myopathy (objective weakness of muscle) or myalgias (pain in the muscle)

DIFFERENTIAL DIAGNOSIS

- Myopathy without muscle necrosis or elevated creatine phosphokinase, eg, endocrine causes of hyperthyroidism, Cushing's syndrome
- Other cause of myalgia, eg, influenza
- Polymyalgia rheumatica

- A simple intramuscular injection may cause some elevation of CK

 DIAGNOSIS

LABORATORY TESTS

- Elevated serum CK is the biochemical indicator of skeletal muscle necrosis
- A urinary dipstick testing positive for blood (due to myoglobinuria) in the absence of red blood cells in the sediment
- Elevations of alanine aminotransferase and lactate dehydrogenase may be present, and may have been obtained for other reasons, such as suspected liver disease or hemolysis
- When these tests are disproportionately elevated, confirm that they are not of muscle origin with a CK determination

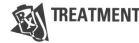 **TREATMENT**

MEDICATIONS

- Vigorous fluid resuscitation
- Mannitol, 100 mg IV once daily for 3 days
- Alkalinization of the urine with 2 ampules of sodium bicarbonate in 1 L D_5 $^1/_2$ normal saline

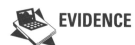 **OUTCOME**

COMPLICATIONS

- Renal insufficiency due to myoglobinuria is caused by tubular damage resulting from filtered myoglobin and is nearly always associated with hypovolemia

PROGNOSIS

- Renal insufficiency is usually reversible with hydration. The role of urine alkalinization is unproven

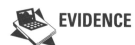 **EVIDENCE**

REFERENCES

- Kashani A et al. Risks associated with statin therapy: a systematic overview of randomized clinical trials. Circulation. 2006 Dec 19;114(25):2788–97. [PMID: 17159064]
- Thompson PD et al. Statin-associated myopathy. JAMA. 2003 Apr 2; 289(13):1681–90. [PMID: 12672737]

Rheumatoid Arthritis

 KEY FEATURES

ESSENTIALS OF DIAGNOSIS

- Usually insidious onset with morning stiffness and pain in affected joints
- Symmetric polyarthritis with predilection for small joints of the hands and feet; deformities common with progressive disease
- Radiographic findings
  - Juxta-articular osteoporosis
  - Joint erosions
  - Joint space narrowing
- Rheumatoid factor and antibodies to cyclic citrullinated peptides (anti-CCP) are present in 70–80%
- Extra-articular manifestations
  - Subcutaneous nodules
  - Pleural effusion
  - Pericarditis
  - Lymphadenopathy
  - Splenomegaly with leukopenia
  - Vasculitis

GENERAL CONSIDERATIONS

- A chronic systemic inflammatory disease of unknown cause; major manifestation is synovitis of multiple joints
- The pathological findings in the joint include chronic synovitis with pannus formation
- The pannus erodes cartilage, bone, ligaments, and tendons

DEMOGRAPHICS

- Female patients outnumber males almost 3:1
- Can begin at any age but peak onset is in fourth or fifth decade for women and sixth to eighth decades for men

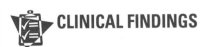 **CLINICAL FINDINGS**

SYMPTOMS AND SIGNS

- Joint symptoms
  - Onset of articular signs of inflammation is usually insidious, with prodromal symptoms of vague periarticular pain or stiffness
  - Symmetric swelling of multiple joints with tenderness and pain is characteristic

- Monarticular disease is occasionally seen initially
- Stiffness persisting for more than 30 minutes (and usually many hours) is prominent in the morning; the duration of morning stiffness is a useful indicator of disease activity
- Stiffness may recur after daytime inactivity and be much more severe after strenuous activity
- PIP joints of the fingers, MCP joints, wrists, knees, ankles, and MTP joints are most often involved
- Synovial cysts and rupture of tendons may occur
- Entrapment syndromes are not unusual—particularly of the median nerve at the carpal tunnel of the wrist
- Neck can be affected but the other components of the spine are usually spared and sacroiliac joints are not involved
- Rheumatoid nodules
  - Present in about 20% of patients
  - Most commonly situated over bony prominences but also observed in the bursae and tendon sheaths
  - Occasionally seen in the lungs, the sclerae, and other tissues
  - Correlate with the presence of rheumatoid factor in serum ("seropositivity"), as do most other extra-articular manifestations
- Ocular symptoms
  - Dryness of the eyes, mouth, and other mucous membranes is found especially in advanced disease (see Sjögren's Syndrome)
  - Other manifestations include episcleritis, scleritis, and scleromalacia due to scleral nodules
- Other symptoms
  - Palmar erythema is common
  - Occasionally, a small vessel vasculitis develops and manifests as as tiny hemorrhagic infarcts in the nail folds or finger pulps
  - Necrotizing arteritis is well reported but rare
  - Pericarditis and pleural disease, when present, are usually silent clinically
  - Additional extra-articular manifestations of rheumatoid arthritis include pulmonary fibrosis, mononuclear cell infiltration of skeletal muscle and perineurium, and hyperplasia of lymph nodes

DIFFERENTIAL DIAGNOSIS

- Gout with tophi (mistaken for nodules)
- Systemic lupus erythematosus
- Parvovirus B19 infection

- Osteoarthritis or inflammatory osteoarthritis
- Polymyalgia rheumatica
- Hemochromatosis (MCP and wrist joints)
- Lyme disease
- Rheumatic fever
- Rubella arthritis
- Hepatitis B or C
- Palindromic rheumatism
- Hypertrophic pulmonary osteoarthropathy (paraneoplastic)
- Systemic vasculitis, especially
  - Polyarteritis nodosa
  - Mixed cryoglobulinemia
  - Antineutrophil cytoplasmic antibody-associated vasculitides

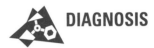 **DIAGNOSIS**

LABORATORY TESTS

- Anti-CCP antibodies and rheumatoid factor are present in 70–80% of patients with established rheumatoid arthritis but have sensitivities of only 50% in early disease
- Anti-CCP antibodies are the most specific blood test (specificity ~95%)
- Approximately 20% of patients have antinuclear antibodies
- Erythrocyte sedimentation rate and levels of C-reactive protein are typically elevated in proportion to disease activity
- A moderate hypochromic normocytic anemia is common
- The white blood cell count is normal or slightly elevated, but leukopenia may occur, often in the presence of splenomegaly (eg, Felty's syndrome)
- The platelet count is often elevated, roughly in proportion to the severity of overall joint inflammation
- Joint fluid examination is valuable, reflecting abnormalities that are associated with varying degrees of inflammation (see Table 124)

IMAGING STUDIES

- Radiographic changes are the most specific for rheumatoid arthritis (RA)
- However, radiographs are not sensitive in that most of those taken during the first 6 months are read as normal
- The earliest changes occur in the wrists or feet and consist of soft tissue swelling and juxta-articular demineralization
- Later, diagnostic changes of uniform joint space narrowing and erosions develop

DIAGNOSTIC PROCEDURES

- Arthrocentesis is needed to diagnose superimposed septic arthritis, which is a common complication of rheumatoid arthritis and should be considered whenever one joint is inflamed out of proportion to the rest

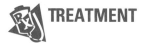 TREATMENT

MEDICATIONS

- **Nonsteroidal anti-inflammatory drugs (NSAIDs)**
  - Provide some symptomatic relief but do not prevent erosions or alter disease progression
  - Not appropriate for monotherapy and should only be used in conjunction with disease modifying drugs
- **Cyclooxygenase (COX)-2 inhibitors**
  - Just as effective as NSAIDs
  - However, they are less likely to cause clinically significant upper gastrointestinal hemorrhage or ulceration
  - Long-term use, particularly without concomitant aspirin use, increases the risk of cardiovascular events
- **Disease-modifying antirheumatic drugs (DMARDs)** should be started as soon as the diagnosis is certain
- **Methotrexate**
  - Initial synthetic DMARD of choice
  - Is generally well tolerated and often produces a beneficial effect in 2–6 weeks
- **Tumor necrosis factor inhibitors** work faster than methotrexate and may replace that drug as the remitting agent of first choice
- **Hydroxychloroquine** is useful for patients with mild disease
- **Corticosteroids**
  - Low doses (eg, oral prednisone 5–10 mg/day) produce a prompt anti-inflammatory effect and slow the rate of bony destruction
  - However, multiple side effects limit their long-term use
- **Sulfasalazine**
  - Second-line agent
  - Dosing: start at 0.5 g orally twice daily and then increased each week by 0.5 g until the patient improves or the daily dose reaches 3 g
- **Leflunomide**, a pyrimidine synthesis inhibitor, is also FDA approved for treatment of RA
- **Abatacept**, a recombinant protein made by fusing a fragment of the Fc domain of human IgG with the extracellular domain of a T cell inhibitory molecule (CTLA4), is FDA approved for use in RA
- **Rituximab** can be effective for disease refractory to the combination of methotrexate and a TNF inhibitor

SURGERY

- Long-standing, severe, erosive disease may benefit from joint replacements
- Hips, knees, shoulders, and MCP joints may benefit from replacement in cases of advanced destruction

THERAPEUTIC PROCEDURES

- Nonpharmacologic
  - Physical therapy
  - Occupational therapy
  - Joint rest
  - Exercise
  - Splinting
  - Heat and cold
  - Assist devices
  - Splints
- Intra-articular corticosteroids (triamcinolone, 10–40 mg) may be helpful if one or two joints are the primary source of difficulty

 OUTCOME

FOLLOW-UP

- Frequent follow-up early after diagnosis to ensure appropriate patient education and response to treatment
- Patients taking DMARDs require monitoring of blood cell counts and hepatic and renal function every 6–8 weeks

COMPLICATIONS

- Joint destruction
- Septic arthritis
- Rheumatoid vasculitis (eg, skin ulcers, vasculitic neuropathy, pericarditis)
- Osteoporosis
- Cushing's syndrome from corticosteroids

PROGNOSIS

- Most common deformities
  - Ulnar deviation of the fingers
  - Boutonnière deformity (hyperextension of the DIP joint with flexion of the PIP joint)
  - "Swan-neck" deformity (flexion of the DIP joint with extension of the PIP joint)
  - Valgus deformity of the knee
  - Volar subluxation of the MTP joints
- The excess mortality is largely due to cardiovascular disease

WHEN TO REFER

- Early referral to a rheumatologist is essential for appropriate diagnosis and the timely introduction of effective therapy

WHEN TO ADMIT

- Admission is sometimes required at diagnosis to exclude other entities
- Superimposed septic arthritis
- Rheumatoid vasculitis
- Severe ocular inflammatory disease (eg, impending corneal melt)

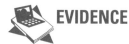 EVIDENCE

PRACTICE GUIDELINES

- American College of Rheumatology

WEB SITES

- American College of Rheumatology
- Arthritis Foundation

INFORMATION FOR PATIENTS

- Arthritis Foundation
- National Institute of Arthritis and Musculoskeletal and Skin Diseases

REFERENCES

- Cohen SB et al; REFLEX Trial Group. Rituximab for rheumatoid arthritis refractory to anti-tumor necrosis factor therapy: Results of a multicenter, randomized, double-blind, placebo-controlled, phase III trial evaluating primary efficacy and safety at twenty-four weeks. Arthritis Rheum. 2006 Sep; 54(9):2793–806. [PMID: 16947627]
- Genovese MC et al. Abatacept for rheumatoid arthritis refractory to tumor necrosis factor alpha inhibition. N Engl J Med. 2005 Sep 15;353(11):1114–23. [PMID: 16162882]
- Goekoop-Ruiterman YP et al. Clinical and radiographic outcomes of four different treatment strategies in patients with early rheumatoid arthritis (the BeSt study): a randomized, controlled trial. Arthritis Rheum. 2005 Nov; 52(11):3381–90. [PMID: 16258899]
- O'Dell JR. Therapeutic strategies for rheumatoid arthritis. N Engl J Med. 2004 Jun 17;350(25):2591–602. [PMID: 15201416]
- Raza K et al. Predictive value of antibodies to cyclic citrullinated peptide in

patients with very early inflammatory arthritis. J Rheumatol. 2005 Feb; 32(2):231–8. [PMID: 15693082]

- Wassenberg S et al. Very low-dose prednisolone in early rheumatoid arthritis retards radiographic progression over two years: a multicenter, double-blind, placebo-controlled trial. Arthritis Rheum. 2005 Nov;52(11):3371–80. [PMID: 16255011]

Rocky Mountain Spotted Fever

 ## KEY FEATURES

- Caused by *Rickettsia rickettsii*, a parasite of ticks, transmitted by tick bites
- Most cases occur in the middle and southern Atlantic seaboard and the central Mississippi River valley
- Most cases occur in late spring and summer
- Typical incubation period is 2–14 days (median, 7 days)

 ## CLINICAL FINDINGS

- Initial symptoms include fevers, chills, headache, nausea and vomiting
- Cough and pneumonitis often occur early in the disease
- Rash (not always found) begins as a faint macule that progresses to large maculopapules and often petechiae
- Rash begins on the wrists and ankles, characteristically involves palms and soles, and spreads to arms, legs, and trunk
- About 3–5% of recognized cases in the United States are fatal

 ## DIAGNOSIS

- Thrombocytopenia
- Hyponatremia
- Hepatitis
- CSF low glucose
- Immunohistologic staining for *R rickettsii* in skin biopsy specimens and serologic testing are the keys to a definitive diagnosis

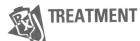 TREATMENT

- Doxycycline or chloramphenicol (where available) are usually highly effective
- Prevention: protective clothing and avoiding tick bites

Rosacea

 ## KEY FEATURES

ESSENTIALS OF DIAGNOSIS

- A chronic facial disorder of middle-aged and older people
- A vascular component (erythema and telangiectasis) and a tendency to flush easily
- An acneiform component (papules and pustules) may also be present
- A glandular component accompanied by hyperplasia of the soft tissue of the nose (rhinophyma)

GENERAL CONSIDERATIONS

- Rosacea is usually a lifelong affliction, so maintenance therapy is required

 ## CLINICAL FINDINGS

SYMPTOMS AND SIGNS

- The cheeks, nose, and chin—at times the entire face—may have a rosy hue
- No comedones
- Inflammatory papules are prominent, and there may be pustules
- Associated seborrhea may be found
- The patient often complains of burning or stinging with episodes of flushing
- It is not uncommon for patients to have associated ophthalmic disease, including blepharitis and keratitis

DIFFERENTIAL DIAGNOSIS

- Acne vulgaris
- Seborrheic dermatitis
- Perioral dermatitis
- Systemic lupus erythematosus
- Carcinoid
- Dermatomyositis

- Rosacea
  - Distinguished from acne by age, the presence of the vascular component, and the absence of comedones
  - The rosy hue is due to inflammation and telangiectases and generally will pinpoint the diagnosis
- Topical corticosteroids can change trivial dermatoses of the face into perioral dermatitis and steroid rosacea

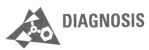 DIAGNOSIS

LABORATORY TESTS

- Clinical diagnosis

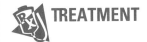 TREATMENT

MEDICATIONS

- See Table 150
- Medications are directed only at the inflammatory papules and pustules and the erythema that surrounds them

Local therapy

- Metronidazole, 0.75% gel applied twice daily or 1% cream once daily, is the topical treatment of choice
- If metronidazole is not tolerated, topical clindamycin (solution, gel, or lotion) used twice daily is effective
- Erythromycin as described above may be helpful (see Acne vulgaris)
- For significant response, may need 5–8 weeks of treatment

Systemic therapy

- Tetracycline or erythromycin, 250 or 500 mg PO BID on an empty stomach, should be used when topical therapy is inadequate
- Minocycline or doxycycline, 50–100 mg PO once or twice daily, may work in refractory cases
- Isotretinoin may succeed where other measures fail; a dosage of 0.5–1.0 mg/kg/day PO for 12–28 weeks is recommended
- Metronidazole, 250 mg PO BID for 3 weeks
  - May be worth trying but is seldom required
  - Side effects are few, though may produce a disulfiram-like effect when the patient ingests alcohol and it may cause neuropathy with long-term use

SURGERY

- The only satisfactory treatment for the telangiectasias is laser surgery

- Rhinophyma (soft tissue and sebaceous hyperplasia of the nose) responds to surgical debulking

OUTCOME

PROGNOSIS

- Rosacea tends to be a stubborn and persistent process
- With the regimens described above, it can usually be controlled adequately

WHEN TO REFER

- If there is a question about the diagnosis, if recommended therapy is ineffective, or if specialized treatment is necessary

EVIDENCE

PRACTICE GUIDELINES

- Wilkin J et al. Standard classification of rosacea: Report of the National Rosacea Society Expert Committee on the Classification and Staging of Rosacea. J Am Acad Dermatol. 2002;46:584. [PMID: 11907512]

WEB SITE

- National Rosacea Society: Physician Information

INFORMATION FOR PATIENTS

- American Academy of Dermatology: What is Rosacea?

- American Academy of Family Physicians: Rosacea and Its Treatment
- National Institute for Arthritis and Musculoskeletal and Skin Diseases: Questions and Answers About Rosacea
- National Rosacea Society: Frequently Asked Questions

REFERENCES

- Powell FC. Rosacea. N Engl J Med. 2005 Feb 24;352(8):793–803. [PMID: 15728812]
- van Zuuren EJ et al. Interventions for rosacea. Cochrane Database Syst Rev. 2005 Jul 20;(3):CD003262. [PMID: 16034895]

Rubella

KEY FEATURES

- Spread by respiratory droplets
- Rare disease in United States
- Nonspecific features makes it difficult to distinguish from other viral infections

CLINICAL FINDINGS

- Mild fever, malaise, and arthralgias, which are more common in women

- Cervical, postauricular lymphadenopathy common
- Fine, pink rash lasts 3 days in each area
- Rash typically starts on the face and spreads to trunk and extremities
- Exposure during pregnancy can lead to fetal infection and death
- Postinfectious encephalopathy is rare; few long-term sequelae
- Congenital rubella associated with CNS, cutaneous, ophthalmic (cataracts), otic (deafness), and cardiac disease

DIAGNOSIS

- Exposure 14–21 days before symptom onset
- Leukopenia common
- Definitive diagnosis is based on
  - Elevated IgM antibody
  - Fourfold or greater rise in IgG antibody titers
  - Isolation of the virus

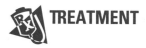
TREATMENT

- Symptomatic treatment and supportive measures
- Prevention: live attenuated virus is safe and highly effective (Tables 67 and 68)
- Women should be immunized when not pregnant

Sarcoidosis

 ## KEY FEATURES

ESSENTIALS OF DIAGNOSIS

- Symptoms related to
  - Lung
  - Skin
  - Eyes
  - Peripheral nerves
  - Liver
  - Kidney
  - Heart
  - Other tissues
- Demonstration of noncaseating granulomas in biopsy specimen
- Exclusion of other granulomatous disorders

GENERAL CONSIDERATIONS

- A systemic disease of unknown etiology
- Granulomatous inflammation of the lungs is present in 90% of cases

DEMOGRAPHICS

- Highest incidence in North American blacks and northern European whites
- Among blacks, women are more frequently affected than men
- Disease onset is usually in the third or fourth decade

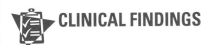 ## CLINICAL FINDINGS

SYMPTOMS AND SIGNS

- Malaise, fever, and insidious dyspnea
- Symptoms referable to the skin, eyes, peripheral nerves, liver, kidney, or heart may also prompt initial evaluation
- Some patients are asymptomatic, and diagnosis is made after abnormal findings are noted on chest radiograph
- Crackles are uncommon on chest examination
- Erythema nodosum, parotid gland enlargement, hepatosplenomegaly, and lymphadenopathy may be noted
- Myocardial sarcoidosis is found in 5% of patients and can lead to
  - Restrictive cardiomyopathy
  - Arrhythmias
  - Conduction disturbances

DIFFERENTIAL DIAGNOSIS

- Other granulomatous diseases must be excluded
- Tuberculosis
- Lymphoma (including lymphocytic interstitial pneumonitis)
- Histoplasmosis
- Coccidioidomycosis
- Idiopathic pulmonary fibrosis
- Pneumoconiosis (especially berylliosis)
- Syphilis

 ## DIAGNOSIS

LABORATORY TESTS

- Leukopenia
- Elevation of erythrocyte sedimentation rate
- Hypercalcemia in 5%, hypercalciuria in 20%
- Angiotensin-converting enzyme (ACE) levels
  - Commonly elevated in active disease
  - Neither sensitive nor specific enough to be of diagnostic value
- Pulmonary function tests may show obstruction or restriction, with diminished diffusion capacity

IMAGING STUDIES

- Radiographic findings are variable
  - Stage I: hilar adenopathy alone
  - Stage II: hilar adenopathy with parenchymal involvement
  - Stage III: parenchymal involvement alone
- Parenchymal involvement usually manifests as diffuse reticular infiltrates, but focal infiltrates, acinar shadows, nodules, and rare cavitation are seen
- Pleural effusion occurs in < 10% of patients

DIAGNOSTIC PROCEDURES

- Biopsy demonstrating noncaseating granulomas is required for diagnosis
- Easily accessible biopsy sites include lymph nodes, skin lesions, and salivary glands
- Transbronchial biopsy has a yield of 75–90%
- Bronchoalveolar lavage is usually characterized by an increase in lymphocytes with a high CD4/CD8 ratio; this may be used to follow disease activity, but not for diagnosis

- Some experts believe biopsy is unnecessary in stage I disease with a presentation highly suggestive of sarcoidosis

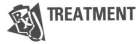 ## TREATMENT

MEDICATIONS

- Corticosteroids (oral prednisone, 0.5–1.0 mg/kg/day) are indicated for
  - Constitutional symptoms
  - Hypercalcemia
  - Iritis
  - Arthritis
  - Central nervous system involvement
  - Cardiac involvement
  - Hepatitis
  - Cutaneous lesions other than erythema nodosum
  - Symptomatic pulmonary lesions
- Long-term therapy is usually required over months to years
- Immunosuppressive drugs and cyclosporine have been tried when benefits of corticosteroid therapy have been exhausted
- Anti-TNF therapy with infliximab has shown some promise in extrapulmonary sarcoidosis

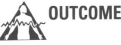 ## OUTCOME

FOLLOW-UP

- At a minimum, yearly physical examination, pulmonary function studies, chemistry panel, ophthalmologic evaluation, chest radiograph, and ECG

COMPLICATIONS

- Hemoptysis
- Pneumothorax
- Mycetoma formation in lung cavities
- Respiratory failure in advanced disease

PROGNOSIS

- 20% of patients with lung involvement suffer irreversible lung impairment, with progressive fibrosis, bronchiectasis, and cavitation
- Outlook is best for patients with stage I disease, worse with radiographic parenchymal involvement
- Erythema nodosum is associated with a good outcome
- Death from pulmonary insufficiency occurs in about 5% of patients

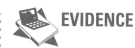

EVIDENCE

INFORMATION FOR PATIENTS

- American Lung Association
- National Heart, Lung, and Blood Institute

REFERENCES

- Baughman RP. Pulmonary sarcoidosis. Clin Chest Med. 2004 Sep;25(3):521–30. [PMID: 15331189]
- Cox CE et al. Sarcoidosis. Med Clin North Am. 2005 Jul;89(4):817–28. [PMID: 15925652]
- Paramothayan NS et al. Corticosteroids for pulmonary sarcoidosis. Cochrane Database Syst Rev. 2005 Apr 18; (2):CD001114. [PMID: 15846612]

Scabies

KEY FEATURES

ESSENTIALS OF DIAGNOSIS

- Generalized very severe itching
- Pruritic burrows, vesicles, and pustules, especially on finger webs and in wrist creases
- Mites, ova, and brown dots of feces visible microscopically
- Red papules or nodules on the scrotum and on the penile glans and shaft are pathognomonic

GENERAL CONSIDERATIONS

- Caused by *Sarcoptes scabiei*
- Usually spares the head and neck (though these areas may be involved in the elderly, and in patients with AIDS)
- Usually acquired through the bedding of an infested individual or by other close contact

CLINICAL FINDINGS

SYMPTOMS AND SIGNS

- Itching is almost always present and can be quite severe
- Lesions are more or less generalized excoriations with small pruritic vesicles, pustules, and "burrows" in the web spaces and on the heels of the palms, wrists, elbows, and around the axillae
- Often, burrows are found only on the feet, as they have been scratched off in other locations
- The burrow appears as a short irregular mark, 2–3 mm long and the width of a hair
- Characteristic lesions may occur on the nipples in females and as pruritic papules on the scrotum or penis in males
- Pruritic papules may be seen over the buttocks

DIFFERENTIAL DIAGNOSIS

- Pediculosis (lice)
- Atopic dermatitis (eczema)
- Contact dermatitis
- Arthropod bites (insect bites)
- Urticaria
- Dermatitis herpetiformis

DIAGNOSIS

LABORATORY TESTS

- The diagnosis should be confirmed by microscopic demonstration of the organism, ova, or feces in a mounted specimen, best done on unexcoriated lesions from interdigital webs, wrists, elbows, or feet
- A No. 15 blade is used to perform a very superficial shave biopsy by sawing off the burrow

TREATMENT

MEDICATIONS

- Treat mites and control the dermatitis, which can last months after eradication of the mites, with mid-potency topical corticosteroids (0.1% triamcinolone cream) (Table 150)
- Treatment consists of disinfestation; add systemic antibiotics for secondary pyoderma
- Permethrin 5% cream; treat with a single application for 8–12 h; may repeat in 1 week
- Crotamiton cream or lotion
  - An alternative, applied in the same way as permethrin but is used nightly for 4 nights
  - It is far less effective if used for only 48 h
- Benzyl benzoate
  - A lotion or emulsion in strengths from 20% to 35% and used as generalized applications (from collarbones down) overnight for two treatments 1 week apart
  - It is cosmetically acceptable, clean, and not overly irritating
- **Pregnant patients**
  - Treat only if they have documented scabies
  - Use permethrin 5% cream once for 12 h—or 5% or 6% sulfur in petrolatum applied nightly for 3 nights from the collarbones down
- **Treatment failures**
  - In immunocompetent persons, most are due to incorrect use or incomplete treatment of the housing unit
    □ Repeat treatment with permethrin once weekly for 2 weeks, with reeducation regarding the method and extent of application
    □ Alternatively, ivermectin 200 mcg/kg, single dose, is effective in about 75% of cases and in 95% of cases with two doses 2 weeks apart
  - In immunosuppressed persons and those with crusted (hyperkeratotic) scabies
    □ Multiple doses of ivermectin (every 2 weeks for two or three doses) plus topical therapy with permethrin once or twice weekly may be effective when topical treatment and oral therapy alone fail
- Persistent pruritic **postscabietic papules**: mid- to high-potency corticosteroids or intralesional triamcinolone acetonide (2.5–5.0 mg/mL)

THERAPEUTIC PROCEDURES

- Bedding and clothing should be laundered or cleaned or set aside for 14 days in plastic bags
- Must treat all persons in a family or institutionalized group

OUTCOME

WHEN TO REFER

- If there is a question about the diagnosis, if recommended therapy is ineffective, or if specialized treatment is necessary

EVIDENCE

PRACTICE GUIDELINES

- Association for Genitourinary Medicine, Medical Society for the Study of Venereal Disease (London). 2002 national guideline on the management of scabies

WEB SITE

- Centers for Disease Control and Prevention: Scabies Professional Information

INFORMATION FOR PATIENTS

- American Academy of Dermatology: Scabies
- American Social Health Association: Scabies
  - MedlinePlus: Scabies

REFERENCES

- Chosidow O. Clinical practices. Scabies. N Engl J Med. 2006 Apr 20; 354(16):1718–27. [PMID: 16625010]
- Heukelbach J et al. Scabies. Lancet. 2006 May 27;367(9524):1767–74. [PMID: 16731272]

Schistosomiasis

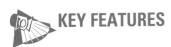 **KEY FEATURES**

ESSENTIALS OF DIAGNOSIS

- History of fresh water exposure in an endemic area
- Diagnosis based on characteristic eggs in feces or urine; biopsy of rectal or bladder mucosa; positive serology

Acute schistosomiasis

- Fever, headache, cough, malaise
- Myalgias
- Urticaria
- Diarrhea
- Eosinophilia

Intestinal schistosomiasis

- Abdominal pain, diarrhea
- Fatigue
- Hepatomegaly, progressing to anorexia, weight loss, and features of portal hypertension

Urinary schistosomiasis

- Hematuria and dysuria, progressing to hydroureter, hydronephrosis, urinary infections, and renal failure

GENERAL CONSIDERATIONS

- Disease is caused by five species of trematode blood flukes
- Intestinal schistosomiasis caused by
  - *Schistosoma mansoni,* which is present in Africa, the Arabian peninsula, South America, and the Caribbean
  - *Schistosoma japonicum,* which is endemic in China and Southeast Asia
  - *Schistosoma mekongi,* which is endemic near the Mekong River in Southeast Asia
  - *Schistosoma intercalatum,* which occurs in parts of Africa
- Urinary schistosomiasis caused by *Schistosoma haematobium* , which is endemic in Africa and the Middle East
- Humans are infected after contact with fresh water containing cercariae released by infected snails
- Disease in endemic areas primarily due to host response to eggs, with granuloma formation and inflammation, leading to fibrosis
- Chronic infection can result in scarring of mesenteric or vesicular blood vessels, leading to portal hypertension and alterations in urinary tract

DEMOGRAPHICS

- Affects more than 200 million persons worldwide
- Leads to severe consequences in 20 million persons and about 100,000 deaths annually
- Transmission is focal, with greatest prevalence in poor rural areas
- Control efforts have diminished transmission significantly in many areas, but high level transmission remains common in sub-Saharan Africa and some other areas
- Prevalence of infection and illness typically peaks at about 15–20 years of age

CLINICAL FINDINGS

SYMPTOMS AND SIGNS

- Cercarial dermatitis
  - Localized erythema develops
  - Can progress to pruritic maculopapular rash persisting for days
  - Can be caused by human schistosomes and, in nontropical areas, by bird schistosomes that cannot complete their life cycle in humans (swimmer's itch)

Acute schistosomiasis (Katayama syndrome)

- Febrile illness may develop 2–8 weeks after exposure in persons without prior infection, most commonly after heavy infection with *S mansoni* or *S japonicum*
- Presenting symptoms and signs
  - Acute onset of fever
  - Headache, cough, malaise
  - Myalgias
  - Urticaria
  - Diarrhea, which may be bloody
- Laboratory findings
  - Hepatosplenomegaly
  - Lymphadenopathy
  - Pulmonary infiltrates
  - Leukocytosis
  - Marked eosinophilia
- Stool may be negative for eggs, especially early in disease
- Localized lesions may occasionally cause severe manifestations, including CNS abnormalities and death
- Usually resolves in 2–8 weeks

Chronic schistosomiasis

- Infections may be light and asymptomatic
- However, about 50–60% of patients have symptoms and 5–10% have advanced organ damage
- Asymptomatic infected children may suffer from anemia and growth retardation
- **Intestinal schistosomiasis**
  - Abdominal pain, diarrhea
  - Fatigue
  - Hepatomegaly
  - Over years, anorexia, weight loss, weakness, colonic polyps, and features of portal hypertension develop
  - Late manifestations include hematemesis from esophageal varices, hepatic failure, and pulmonary hypertension
- **Urinary schistosomiasis**
  - May present within months of infection with hematuria and dysuria, most commonly in children and young adults
  - Fibrotic changes in the urinary tract can lead to hydroureter, hydronephrosis, bacterial urinary infections and, ultimately, renal failure or bladder cancer

DIFFERENTIAL DIAGNOSIS

- Acute
  - Amebiasis
  - Bacterial dysentery, eg, *Shigella, Salmonella*
  - Viral hepatitis
  - Typhoid fever
  - Malaria
- Chronic
  - Typhoid fever
  - Visceral leishmaniasis
  - Lymphoma
  - Amebiasis
  - Portal hypertension due to other causes, eg, cirrhosis, portal vein thrombosis
  - Hematuria due to other causes, eg, urinary tract infections, renal cell carcinoma

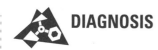

DIAGNOSIS

LABORATORY TESTS

- Complete blood count
- Smears of stool or urine
  - Can identify characteristic eggs
  - Filtration or concentration techniques can improve yields
- Quantitative tests that yield > 400 eggs per gram of feces or 10 mL of urine indicate heavy infections
- Serologic tests include an ELISA available from the CDC that is 99% specific for all species but sensitivity varies
  - 99% sensitive for *S mansoni*
  - 95% sensitive for *S haematobium*
  - < 50% sensitive for *S japonicum*
- Species-specific immunoblots can increase sensitivity
- In acute schistosomiasis, serologic tests may become positive before eggs are seen in stool or urine
- After therapy, eggs may be shed in stool or urine for months, and so the identification of eggs in fluids or tissue or positive serologic tests cannot distinguish past or active disease
- Tests for egg viability are available

IMAGING STUDIES

- Ultrasonography or other imaging modality helpful in evaluating extent of disease
- Chest radiography

DIAGNOSTIC PROCEDURES

- Liver function studies can establish extent of disease
- Biopsy of rectum, colon, liver, or bladder can confirm diagnosis

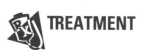

TREATMENT

MEDICATIONS

- Treatment is indicated for all schistosome infections
- In areas where recurrent infection is common, treatment is valuable in reducing worm burdens and limiting clinical complications
- Praziquantel
  - Drug of choice
  - 40 mg/kg/day (in one or two doses) for *S mansoni*, *S haematobium,* and *S intercalatum* infections
  - 60 mg/kg/day (in two or three doses) for *S japonicum* and *S mekongi*

- May not prevent illness when given after exposure
- Repeat course after a few weeks may be needed for recent infections
- Combining with corticosteroids for severe disease may decrease complications
- May be used during pregnancy
- Resistance has been reported
- Side effects include abdominal pain, diarrhea, urticaria, headache, nausea, vomiting, and fever
- Oxamniquine
  - Alternative therapy for *S mansoni* infection
  - Not available in the United States
  - Resistance may be a problem
- Metrifonate
  - Alternative therapy for *S haemotobium* infection
  - Not available in the United States
  - Resistance may be a problem
- No second-line drug is available for *S japonicum* infections
- Artemether
  - Active against schistosomulae and adult worms
  - May be effective in chemoprophylaxis
  - However, it is expensive, and long-term use in malarious areas might select for resistant malaria parasites

OUTCOME

FOLLOW-UP

- Examine for eggs about every 3 months for 1 year after therapy, with re-treatment if eggs are seen

COMPLICATIONS

- Portal hypertension (contracted liver, splenomegaly, pancytopenia, esophageal varices)
- Pulmonary hypertension with cor pulmonale
- Large bowel stricture, granulomatous masses, colonic polyposis, and persistent *Salmonella* infection may occur
- Transverse myelitis, epilepsy, or optic neuritis may result from collateral circulation of eggs or ectopic worms
- Sequelae of *S haematobium* infection include
  - Bladder polyp formation
  - Cystitis
  - Chronic *Salmonella* infection
  - Pyelitis
  - Pyelonephritis
  - Urolithiasis

  - Hydronephrosis due to ureteral obstruction
  - Renal failure
  - Death
  - Severe liver, lung, genital, or neurologic disease is rare
- Bladder cancer has been associated with vesicular schistosomiasis

PROGNOSIS

- Cure rates with praziquantel are generally > 80% after a single treatment
- Intensity of infection markedly reduced in those not cured

WHEN TO REFER

- All patients with chronic schistosomiasis

WHEN TO ADMIT

- In areas where cysticercosis may coexist with a schistosomal infection being treated with praziquantel, treatment is best conducted in a hospital to monitor for death of cysticerci, which may be followed by neurologic complications

PREVENTION

- Travelers to endemic areas should avoid fresh water exposure
- Vigorous toweling after exposure may limit cercarial penetration
- Chemoprophylaxis with artemether has shown efficacy but is not standard practice
- Community control includes improved sanitation and water supplies, elimination of snail habitats, and intermittent administration of treatment to limit worm burdens

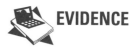

EVIDENCE

WEB SITES

- CDC—Division of Parasitic Diseases
- Travelers' Health

REFERENCES

- Da Silva LC et al. Schistosomiasis mansoni—clinical features. Gastroenterol Hepatol. 2005 Jan;28(1):30–9. [PMID: 15691467]
- Fenwick A et al. Implementation of human schistosomiasis control: challenges and prospects. Adv Parasitol. 2006;61:567–622. [PMID: 16735173]
- Fenwick A et al. Schistosomiasis: challenges for control, treatment and drug resistance. Curr Opin Infect Dis. 2006 Dec;19(6):577–82. [PMID: 17075334]

- Gryseels B et al. Human schistosomiasis. Lancet. 2006 Sep 23; 368(9541):1106–18. [PMID: 16997665]
- Meltzer E et al. Schistosomiasis among travelers: new aspects of an old disease. Emerg Infect Dis. 2006 Nov; 12(11):1696–700. [PMID: 17283619]
- Ross AG et al. Katayama syndrome. Lancet Infect Dis. 2007 Mar;7(3):218–24. [PMID: 17317603]

Schizophrenia

KEY FEATURES

ESSENTIALS OF DIAGNOSIS

- Massive disruption of thinking, mood, and overall behavior, as well as poor filtering of stimuli
- Schizophrenic disorders subdivided into types by prominent phenomena
  - **Disorganized (hebephrenic)**: incoherence and incongruous or silly affect
  - **Catatonic**: psychomotor disturbance or either excitement or rigidity
  - **Paranoid**: persecutory or grandiose delusions, and hallucinations
  - **Undifferentiated**: lack of symptoms specific enough to fit other types
  - **Residual**: for persons with a history of clear schizophrenia, but who presently exhibit only milder signs without overt psychosis

GENERAL CONSIDERATIONS

- Origin believed to have genetic, environmental, and neurotransmitter pathophysiologic components

CLINICAL FINDINGS

SYMPTOMS AND SIGNS

- A history of a major disruption in the individual's life may precede gross psychotic deterioration
- Gradual decompensation usually predates the acute episode
- Symptoms of at least 6 months' duration
- **Positive** symptoms
  - Delusions are often paranoid, involving perceived threat from others

- Hallucinations are typically auditory
- Hypersensitivity to environmental stimuli, with feelings of enhanced sensory awareness
- **Negative** symptoms
  - Diminished sociability
  - Restricted affect
  - Impoverished speech
- **Appearance**: may be bizarre, though usually patients are just mildly unkempt
- **Motor activity**: generally reduced, although a broad spectrum is seen
- **Social function**: marked withdrawal, often with deterioration in personal care, disturbed interpersonal relationships
- **Speech**
  - Neologisms (made-up words or phrases)
  - Echolalia (repetition of others' words)
  - Verbigeration (repetition of senseless words or phrases)
- **Affect**: flat, occasionally inappropriate
- **Mood**: depression in most patients, less apparent during acute psychosis, may have rapidly alternating mood shifts irrespective of circumstances
- **Thought content**
  - Varies from paucity of ideas to rich delusions
  - Concrete thinking with inability to abstract
  - Inappropriate symbolism

DIFFERENTIAL DIAGNOSIS

- Schizophrenia should be distinguished from other psychoses
  - **Delusional disorders** are characterized by nonbizarre delusions with minimal impairment on daily life
  - **Schizoaffective disorders** fail to fit within the definitions of either schizophrenia or affective disorders
  - **Schizophreniform disorders** have a duration of less than 6 months, but more than 1 week
  - **Brief psychotic disorders** result from psychological stress, last less than 1 week, and have a much better prognosis
  - Late-life psychosis occurs after age 60 and is accompanied by cognitive impairment
  - **Atypical psychoses** are psychotic symptoms arising from a cause that may be apparent only later
  - Clues are precipitous onset and a good premorbid history
- Manic episodes
- Obsessive-compulsive disorder
- Psychotic depression
- Drug intoxication and abuse

- Thyroid, adrenal, and pituitary disorders
- Complex partial seizures and temporal lobe dysfunction may produce psychotic symptoms
- Drug toxicities, particularly overdoses of typical antipsychotics, can produce catatonia

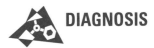

DIAGNOSIS

LABORATORY TESTS

- Tests to rule out metabolic and endocrine disorders, such as
  - Electrolytes, blood urea nitrogen (BUN), creatinine
  - Glucose, thyroid-stimulating hormone (TSH); tests for endocrine disorders may be appropriate
- Toxicology screen

IMAGING STUDIES

- Ventricular enlargement and cortical atrophy on CT have been correlated with chronicity, cognitive impairment, and poor response to neuroleptics
- Decreased frontal lobe activity on positron emission tomography scan has been associated with negative symptoms
- MRI can exclude temporal lobe disorders

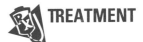

TREATMENT

MEDICATIONS

- See Tables 146 and 147
- Typical neuroleptic agents
  - Phenothiazines
  - Thioxanthenes
  - Butyrophenones
  - Dihydroindolones
  - Dibenzoxazepines
  - Benzisoxazoles
- Newer, atypical neuroleptics (clozapine, risperidone, olanzapine, quetiapine, ziprasidone, and aripiprazole)
  - Cause less tardive dyskinesia and extrapyramidal symptoms
  - Are more effective than typical agents on negative symptoms
- Antidepressant drugs may be used with antipsychotics if significant depression is present
- Resistant cases may require addition of lithium, carbamazepine, or valproate
- Addition of benzodiazepine can resolve catatonic symptoms and allow a lower neuroleptic dose

THERAPEUTIC PROCEDURES

- Social
  - Board and care homes with experienced staff can improve functioning and limit hospitalizations
  - Nonresidential self-help groups (Recovery, Inc.) should be used
  - Vocational rehabilitation and work agencies (Goodwill Industries, Inc.) can provide structured work situations
- Psychological
  - Need for psychotherapy varies markedly with patient status and history
  - Insight-oriented psychotherapy is often counterproductive
  - Cognitive-behavioral therapy with medication management may be efficacious
  - Family therapy may alleviate the patient's stress and assist relatives in coping
- Behavioral
  - Music from portable players with headphones can divert attention from auditory hallucinations

 OUTCOME

FOLLOW-UP

- Clozapine
  - 1% risk of agranulocytosis
  - Weekly white blood cell counts (WBCs) for 6 months, then every other week thereafter
  - Weekly WBCs for 1 month after discontinuation of clozapine
- Ziprasidone
  - Can cause QT prolongation
  - Pretreatment ECG and cardiac risk factor screen are necessary
- Quetiapine
  - Associated with cataracts
  - Ophthalmologic examination at initiation and biannually

COMPLICATIONS

- Neuroleptic malignant syndrome is uncommon but serious side effect of neuroleptics
- Tardive dyskinesia may occur after long-term use of neuroleptics
- Anticholinergic and adrenergic side effects are more frequent with low-potency neuroleptics
- Extrapyramidal symptoms are seen with high-potency neuroleptics
- Olanzapine has been associated with significant weight gain with case reports of type 2 diabetes

PROGNOSIS

- After removal of positive symptoms, prognosis is excellent in most patients
- Negative symptoms are more difficult to treat
- Prognosis is guarded when psychosis is associated with a history of serious drug abuse, owing to likely CNS damage
- Life expectancy is 20% shorter in schizophrenics, mostly because of higher mortality rates among young patients

WHEN TO ADMIT

- Gross disorganization
- Risk of self-harm or harm to others

 EVIDENCE

PRACTICE GUIDELINES

- American Psychiatric Association: adult schizophrenia, 2004

WEB SITES

- American Psychiatric Association
- Internet Mental Health
- National Institutes of Health—National Institute of Mental Health

INFORMATION FOR PATIENTS

- JAMA patient page. Schizophrenia. JAMA. 2001;286:494. [PMID: 11484732]

REFERENCES

- Freedman R. Schizophrenia. N Engl J Med. 2003 Oct 30;349(18):1738–49. [PMID: 14585943]
- Koro CE et al. Assessment of independent effect of olanzapine and risperidone on risk of diabetes among patients with schizophrenia: population-based nested case-control study. BMJ. 2002 Aug 3;325(7358):243. [PMID: 12153919]
- Lieberman JA et al; Clinical Antipsychotic Trials of Intervention Effectiveness (CATIE) Investigators. Effectiveness of antipsychotic drugs in patients with chronic schizophrenia. N Engl J Med. 2005 Sep 22;353(12):1209–23. [PMID: 16172203]
- Newcomer JW. Second-generation (atypical) antipsychotics and metabolic effects: a comprehensive literature review. CNS Drugs. 2005;19(Suppl 1):1-93. [PMID: 15998156]
- Wang PS et al. Risk of death in elderly users of conventional vs. atypical anti- psychotic medications. N Engl J Med. 2005 Dec 1;353(22):2335–41. [PMID: 16319382]

Scleroderma (Systemic Sclerosis)

 KEY FEATURES

ESSENTIALS OF DIAGNOSIS

- Limited disease (80% of patients): thickening of skin confined to the face and neck, distal arms, feet and hands
- Diffuse disease (20%): widespread thickening of skin, including truncal involvement, with areas of increased pigmentation and depigmentation
- Raynaud's phenomenon in 90% of patients
- Dysphagia
- Hypomotility of gastrointestinal tract
- Pulmonary fibrosis
- Cardiac and renal involvement
- Positive test for antinuclear antibodies nearly universal

GENERAL CONSIDERATIONS

- A chronic disorder characterized by diffuse fibrosis of the skin and internal organs
- Microchimerism (long-term persisting cells from pregnancy) could be involved in the pathogenesis
- Patients presenting with systemic sclerosis or an eosinophilic fasciitis-like syndrome should be asked about tryptophan use, which is banned by the Food and Drug Administration

Eosinophilic fasciitis

- A rare disorder presenting with skin changes that resemble diffuse systemic sclerosis
- The inflammatory abnormalities, however, are limited to the fascia rather than the dermis and epidermis
- Unlike patients with systemic sclerosis, patients have peripheral blood eosinophilia, absence of Raynaud's phenomenon, a good response to prednisone, and an increased risk of developing aplastic anemia

DEMOGRAPHICS

- Symptoms usually appear in the third to sixth decades
- Women are affected about four times as frequently as men

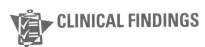 **CLINICAL FINDINGS**

SYMPTOMS AND SIGNS

- Skin
  - Most frequently, skin involvement precedes visceral involvement
  - With time the skin becomes thickened and hidebound, with loss of normal folds
  - Telangiectasia, pigmentation, and depigmentation are characteristic
  - Ulceration about the fingertips and subcutaneous calcification are seen
- Joints
  - Polyarthralgia and Raynaud's phenomenon (present in 90% of patients) are early manifestations
- Gastrointestinal tract
  - Dysphagia from esophageal dysfunction (abnormalities in motility and later from fibrosis) is common
  - Fibrosis and atrophy of the gastrointestinal tract cause hypomotility, and malabsorption results from bacterial overgrowth
- Pulmonary
  - Diffuse pulmonary fibrosis and pulmonary vascular disease are reflected in low diffusing capacity and decreased lung compliance
- Cardiac abnormalities
  - Pericarditis, heart block, myocardial fibrosis
  - Right heart failure secondary to pulmonary hypertension
- Renal crisis
  - Results from obstruction of smaller renal blood vessels
  - Indicates a grave prognosis

DIFFERENTIAL DIAGNOSIS

- Several conditions classified as "localized" sclerosis may mimic systemic morphea and limited systemic sclerosis. These disorders are generally limited to the skin (typically in a localized fashion) and are associated with excellent prognoses
- Eosinophilic fasciitis
- Eosinophilic-myalgia syndrome (due to tryptophan use)
- Overlap syndrome ("mixed connective tissue disease")
- Raynaud's disease
- Morphea
- Amyloidosis
- Graft-versus-host disease
- Cryoglobulinemia

 DIAGNOSIS

LABORATORY TESTS

- Antinuclear antibody tests are nearly always positive (Table 123)
- The scleroderma antibody (SCL-70) directed against topoisomerase III is found in one-third of patients with diffuse systemic sclerosis and in 20% of those with CREST syndrome
- Anticentromere antibody is seen in 50% of those with CREST syndrome and in 1% of individuals with diffuse systemic sclerosis
- Elevation of the sedimentation rate is unusual
- Mild anemia is often present
- Proteinuria and cylindruria appear in association with renal involvement

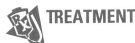 **TREATMENT**

MEDICATIONS

- Severe Raynaud's syndrome may respond to calcium channel blockers, eg, long-acting nifedipine, 30–120 mg PO once daily, or to losartan, 50 mg PO once daily
- IV epoprostenol, a prostacyclin analog that causes vasodilation and platelet inhibition, is moderately effective in healing digital ulcers
- IV iloprost also effective but not available in the United States
- IV prostaglandins (epoprostenol or PGE_2) or a SQ prostacyclin analog (treprostinil) may be effective in pulmonary hypertension. An endothelin-1 antagonist, bosentan, improves symptoms and exercise tolerance in pulmonary hypertension
- Esophageal reflux can be reduced using antacids, H_2-blockers, and proton pump inhibitors (eg, omeprazole, 20–40 mg PO once daily)
- Malabsorption due to bacterial overgrowth also responds to antibiotics, eg, tetracycline, 500 mg PO QID
- The hypertensive crises associated with systemic sclerosis renal crisis must be treated early and aggressively (in the hospital) with angiotensin-converting enzyme inhibitors, eg, captopril, initi-

ated at 25 mg q6h and titrated as needed to a maximum of 100 mg q6h
- Prednisone has little or no role in the treatment of scleroderma
- Cyclophosphamide, a drug with many important side effects, may improve dyspnea and pulmonary function tests modestly in patients with severe interstitial lung disease

SURGERY

- Digital sympathectomy may provide at least temporary relief in severe digital ischemia

THERAPEUTIC PROCEDURES

- Treatment is symptomatic and supportive

 OUTCOME

COMPLICATIONS

- End-stage renal disease and often death from the malignant hypertension associated with scleroderma renal crisis
- Pulmonary hypertension
- Pulmonary fibrosis
- Profound gastrointestinal hypomotility and bacterial overgrowth
- Digital loss

PROGNOSIS

- Patients with CREST syndrome have a much better prognosis than those with diffuse disease, in large part because patients with limited disease do not develop renal failure or interstitial lung disease
- The 9-year survival rate in scleroderma averages approximately 40%
- The prognosis tends to be worse in those with diffuse scleroderma, in blacks, in males, and in older patients

WHEN TO REFER

- Patients should be managed in consultation with a rheumatologist

WHEN TO ADMIT

- Scleroderma renal crisis
- Advanced pulmonary hypertension

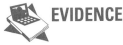 **EVIDENCE**

WEB SITES

- American College of Rheumatology
- Scleroderma Foundation

INFORMATION FOR PATIENTS

- American College of Rheumatology
- National Institute of Arthritis and Musculoskeletal and Skin Diseases

REFERENCES

- Baroni SS et al. Stimulatory autoantibodies to the PDGF receptor in systemic sclerosis. N Engl J Med. 2006 Jun 22;354(25):2667–76. [PMID: 16790699]
- Denton CP et al. Bosentan treatment for pulmonary arterial hypertension related to connective tissue disease: a subgroup analysis of the pivotal clinical trials and their open-label extensions. Ann Rheum Dis. 2006 Oct;65(10):1336–40. [PMID: 16793845]
- Ioannidis JP et al. Mortality in systemic sclerosis: an international meta-analysis of individual patient data. Am J Med. 2005 Jan;118(1):2–10. [PMID: 15639201]
- Korn JH et al. Digital ulcers in systemic sclerosis: prevention by treatment with bosentan, an oral endothelin receptor antagonist. Arthritis Rheum. 2004 Dec; 50(12):3985–93. [PMID: 15593188]
- Tashkin DP et al; Scleroderma Lung Study Research Group. Cyclophosphamide versus placebo in scleroderma lung disease. N Engl J Med. 2006 Jun 22; 354(25):2655–66. [PMID: 16790698]

Sclerosing Cholangitis, Primary

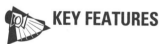 ## KEY FEATURES

ESSENTIALS OF DIAGNOSIS

- Males, aged 20–50 years old
- Often associated with ulcerative colitis
- Progressive jaundice, itching, and other features of cholestasis
- Diagnosis based on characteristic cholangiographic findings
- 10% risk of cholangiocarcinoma

GENERAL CONSIDERATIONS

- Characterized by a diffuse inflammation of the biliary tract leading to fibrosis and strictures of the biliary system

- Associated with the histocompatibility antigens HLA-B8 and -DR3 or -DR4
- In patients with AIDS, sclerosing cholangitis may result from infections caused by cytomegalovirus (CMV), *Cryptosporidium*, or microsporum
- Occasional patients have clinical and histologic features of both sclerosing cholangitis and autoimmune hepatitis
- Even more rarely, an association with chronic pancreatitis (sclerosing pancreaticocholangitis) is seen, and this entity is often responsive to corticosteroids
- The diagnosis is difficult to make after biliary surgery or intrahepatic artery chemotherapy, which may result in bile duct injury
- Primary sclerosing cholangitis must be distinguished from idiopathic adulthood ductopenia, a rare disorder affecting young to middle-aged adults who manifest cholestasis resulting from loss of interlobular and septal bile ducts yet who have a normal cholangiogram

DEMOGRAPHICS

- Most common in men aged 20–50
- Closely associated with ulcerative colitis (and occasionally Crohn's colitis), which is present in approximately two-thirds of patients
- However, clinically significant sclerosing cholangitis develops in only 1–4% of patients with ulcerative colitis
- As in ulcerative colitis, smoking is associated with a decreased risk of primary sclerosing cholangitis

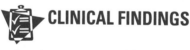 ## CLINICAL FINDINGS

SYMPTOMS AND SIGNS

- Progressive obstructive jaundice, frequently associated with fatigue, pruritus, anorexia, and indigestion
- Occasional patients have clinical and histologic features of both sclerosing cholangitis and autoimmune hepatitis

DIFFERENTIAL DIAGNOSIS

- Primary biliary cirrhosis
- Choledocholithiasis
- Cancer of pancreas or biliary tree
- Biliary stricture
- Drug-induced cholestasis, eg, chlorpromazine
- Inflammatory bowel disease complicated by cholestatic liver disease
- Idiopathic adulthood ductopenia
- *Clonorchis sinensis* (Chinese liver fluke)

- *Fasciola hepatica* (sheep liver fluke)
- Sclerosing cholangitis due to
  - CMV
  - Cryptosporidiosis
  - Microsporidiosis (in AIDS)

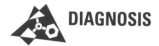 ## DIAGNOSIS

LABORATORY TESTS

- Condition may be diagnosed in the presymptomatic phase because of an elevated alkaline phosphatase level
- Progressive disease is associated with rising alkaline phosphatase and bilirubin levels; eventually hepatic failure ensues
- Perinuclear ANCA as well as antinuclear, anticardiolipin, antithyroperoxidase, and anti-*Saccharomyces cerevisiae* antibodies and rheumatoid factor are frequently detected in serum

IMAGING STUDIES

- The diagnosis is generally made by magnetic resonance cholangiography (MRC), which shows characteristic segmental fibrosis of the bile ducts with saccular dilatations between strictures
- MRC is nearly as sensitive as ERCP for visualizing the intrahepatic ducts. Biliary obstruction by a stone or tumor should be excluded

DIAGNOSTIC PROCEDURES

- The disease may be confined to small intrahepatic bile ducts, in which case ERCP is normal and the diagnosis is suggested by liver biopsy
- Liver biopsy is needed for staging, which is based on the degree of inflammation and fibrosis

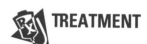 ## TREATMENT

MEDICATIONS

- Episodes of acute bacterial cholangitis may be treated with ciprofloxacin (750 mg twice daily PO or IV)
- Ursodeoxycholic acid in standard doses (10–15 mg/kg/day) may improve liver biochemical test results but does not appear to alter the natural history
- Whether high-dose ursodeoxycholic acid (25–30 mg/kg orally daily) reduces cholangiographic progression and liver fibrosis is controversial, but it does not appear to improve survival or prevent cholangiocarcinoma

SURGERY

- In patients without cirrhosis, surgical resection of a dominant bile duct stricture may lead to longer survival than endoscopic therapy by decreasing the subsequent risk of cholangiocarcinoma
- For patients with cirrhosis and clinical decompensation, liver transplantation is the procedure of choice

THERAPEUTIC PROCEDURES

- Careful endoscopic evaluation of the biliary tree may permit balloon dilation of localized strictures
- If there is a major stricture, short-term placement of a stent may relieve symptoms and improve biochemical abnormalities with sustained improvement after the stent is removed
- Repeated balloon dilation of a recurrent dominant bile duct stricture may improve survival
- However, long-term stenting may increase the rate of complications such as cholangitis

 OUTCOME

COMPLICATIONS

- Complications of chronic cholestasis, such as osteoporosis and malabsorption of fat-soluble vitamins, may occur
- Cholangiocarcinoma
  - Occurs in up to 20% of cases
  - May be difficult to diagnose by cytologic examination or biopsy because of false-negative results
  - A serum CA 19-9 level > 100 units/mL is suggestive but not diagnostic of cholangiocarcinoma
  - Positron emission tomography and choledochoscopy may have roles in early detection

PROGNOSIS

- Survival averages 12–17 years
- Adverse prognostic markers
  - Older age
  - Hepatosplenomegaly
  - Higher serum bilirubin and aspartate aminotransferase levels
  - Lower albumin levels
  - History of variceal bleeding; variceal bleeding is also a risk factor for cholangiocarcinoma
  - Dominant bile duct stricture
  - Extrahepatic duct changes
- Actuarial survival rates with liver transplantation are as high as 85% at 3 years,

but rates are much lower once cholangiocarcinoma has developed

- Following transplantation, patients have an increased risk of nonanastomotic biliary strictures and—in those with ulcerative colitis—colon cancer
- Patients who are unable to undergo liver transplantation will ultimately require high-quality palliative care
- When the disease is confined to small intrahepatic bile ducts, the survival is longer and there is a lower rate of cholangiocarcinoma than with involvement of the large ducts

WHEN TO REFER

- All patients

PREVENTION

- In patients with ulcerative colitis, primary sclerosing cholangitis is an independent risk factor for the development of colorectal dysplasia and cancer, and strict adherence to a colonoscopic surveillance program is recommended

 EVIDENCE

PRACTICE GUIDELINES

- Lee Y-M et al. Management of primary sclerosing cholangitis. Am J Gastroenterol. 2002;97:528. [PMID: 11922543]

INFORMATION FOR PATIENTS

- National Digestive Diseases Information Clearinghouse

REFERENCES

- Abdalian R et al. Sclerosing cholangitis: a focus on secondary causes. Hepatology. 2006 Nov;44(5):1063–74. [PMID: 17058222]
- Berstad AE et al. Diagnostic accuracy of magnetic resonance and endoscopic retrograde cholangiography in primary sclerosing cholangitis. Clin Gastroenterol Hepatol. 2006 Apr;4(4):514–20. [PMID: 16616358]
- LaRusso NF et al. Primary sclerosing cholangitis: summary of a workshop. Hepatology. 2006 Sep;44(3):746–64. [PMID: 16941705]
- Prytz H et al; Swedish Internal Medicine Liver Club. Dynamic FDG-PET is useful for detection of cholangiocarcinoma in patients with PSC listed for liver transplantation. Hepatology. 2006 Dec;44(6):1572–80. [PMID: 17133469]
- Tischendorf JJ et al. Characterization, outcome, and prognosis in 273 patients with primary sclerosing cholangitis: a single center study. Am J Gastroenterol. 2007 Jan;102(1):107–14. [PMID: 17037993]

Seafood Poisoning

 KEY FEATURES

- In most cases, the seafood has a normal appearance and taste
- Scombroid may have a peppery taste

 CLINICAL FINDINGS

- A variety of intoxications may occur, including scombroid, ciguatera, paralytic shellfish, and puffer fish poisoning (Table 143)
- Abrupt respiratory arrest may occur with acute paralytic shellfish and puffer fish poisoning

 DIAGNOSIS

- Table 143

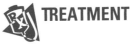 **TREATMENT**

- Observe patients for at least 4–6 h
- Replace fluid and electrolyte losses from gastroenteritis with IV saline or other crystalloid solution
- Administer activated charcoal for recent ingestions
  - 60–100 g PO or via gastric tube, mixed in aqueous slurry
  - Do not use for comatose or convulsing patients unless it can be given by gastric tube and the airway is first protected by a cuffed endotracheal tube
- There is no specific antidote for paralytic shellfish or puffer fish poisoning
- **Ciguatera**
  - Acute neurologic symptoms may respond to mannitol, 1 g/kg IV (anecdotal)
- **Scombroid**
  - Antihistamines such as diphenhydramine, 25–50 mg IV, and the H_2-

blocker cimetidine, 300 mg IV, are usually effective
– For severe reactions, also give epinephrine, 0.3–0.5 mL of a 1:1000 solution SQ

Serum Sickness (Immune Complex Disease)

 ## KEY FEATURES

ESSENTIALS OF DIAGNOSIS

- Fever, pruritus, and arthropathy
- Reaction is delayed in onset, usually 7–10 days after allergen exposure, when specific IgG antibodies are generated against the allergen
- Immune complexes found circulating in serum or deposited in affected tissues

GENERAL CONSIDERATIONS

- Serum sickness reactions occur when immune complexes are formed by the binding of drugs or heterologous serum to antibodies
- These complexes deposit in the vascular endothelium, activate the complement cascade and produce immune-mediated tissue injury
- The commonly affected organs include skin (urticaria, vasculitis), joints (arthritis), and kidney (nephritis)

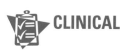 ## CLINICAL FINDINGS

SYMPTOMS AND SIGNS

- Usually a self-limited illness, but can be a severe vasculitis
- Constitutional symptoms are common
- Fever
- Urticaria
- Arthritis
- Nephritis

DIFFERENTIAL DIAGNOSIS

- Infection
- Autoimmune hypersensitivity
- Vasculitis
- Systemic lupus erythematosus (SLE)
- Rheumatoid arthritis (RA)

 ## DIAGNOSIS

LABORATORY TESTS

- The specific IgG antibody may be present in sufficient quantity in serum to be detected by the precipitin-in-gel method; ELISA will detect antibodies present in lesser amounts
- Decreased C3, C4, or CH50 is nonspecific evidence of immune complex disease
- Immune complexes can be detected circulating in serum or deposited in affected tissues
- Increased erythrocyte sedimentation rate
- Red blood cell casts if nephritis is present

 ## TREATMENT

MEDICATIONS

- Aspirin or nonsteroidal anti-inflammatory drugs for fever and arthritis
- Antihistamines and topical corticosteroids for dermatitis
- Systemic corticosteroids are used for systemic vasculitis manifesting as glomerulonephritis or neuropathy

 ## OUTCOME

PROGNOSIS

- Good to excellent if inciting antigen is identified and withdrawn (eg, drug, serum, etc)

WHEN TO REFER

- To an allergist for assistance in identifying inciting agent(s)
- To a rheumatologist if autoimmune disorder is suspected (eg, SLE, RA, or vasculitis)

PREVENTION

- Avoid known inciting agents

 ## EVIDENCE

INFORMATION FOR PATIENTS

- MedlinePlus: Serum Sickness

REFERENCES

- Katta R et al. Serum sickness-like reaction to cefuroxime: a case report and review of the literature. J Drugs Dermatol. 2007 Jul;6(7):747–8. [PMID: 17763603]
- Knowles SR et al. Recognition and management of severe cutaneous drug reactions. Dermatol Clin. 2007 Apr; 25(2):245–53, viii. [PMID: 17430761]

Sexual Dysfunction

 ## KEY FEATURES

ESSENTIALS OF DIAGNOSIS

- Large category of vasocongestive and orgasmic disorders
- Often involve problems of sexual adaptation, education, and technique

GENERAL CONSIDERATIONS

- Two most common conditions in men
  - Erectile dysfunction
  - Ejaculation disturbances
- Two most common conditions in women
  - Vaginismus
  - Frigidity

Erectile dysfunction
- The inability to achieve an erection adequate for satisfactory intercourse
- Causes can be psychological, physiologic, or both
- A history of occasional erections—especially nocturnal tumescence—can demonstrate a psychological origin

Ejaculation disturbances
- Ejaculation control is an acquired behavior that is minimal in adolescence and increases with experience
- Sexual ignorance, anxiety, guilt, depression, and relationship problems may interfere with learning control
- Interference with the sympathetic nerve distribution through surgery or trauma can be responsible

Vaginismus
- Conditioned response in which a spasm of the perineal muscles occurs when there is any stimulation of the area
- The desire is to avoid penetration

Frigidity
- Characterized by a general lack of sexual responsiveness
- Sexual activity varies from avoidance to an occasional orgasm

- Possible causes
  - Poor sexual techniques
  - Early traumatic sexual experiences
  - Marital problems
- Organic causes include
  - Conditions causing dyspareunia
  - Pelvic pathology
  - Mechanical obstruction
  - Neurologic deficits

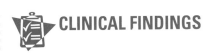 CLINICAL FINDINGS

SYMPTOMS AND SIGNS

Erectile dysfunction

- Often mentioned only after direct questioning
- Patients sometimes use the term "impotence" to describe premature ejaculation

Ejaculation disturbances

- Patients may not relate symptoms without direct questions regarding their sex lives

Frigidity

- Difficulty in experiencing erotic sensation and lack of vasocongestive response
- Should be differentiated from orgasmic dysfunction, in which varying degrees of difficulty are experienced in achieving orgasm

DIFFERENTIAL DIAGNOSIS

- Depression or anxiety
- Underlying medical condition, eg, diabetes, peripheral vascular disease, hyperprolactinemia, hypogonadism
- Dyspareunia or chronic pelvic pain
- Drugs or substance use, eg, selective serotonin reuptake inhibitors (SSRIs), tricyclic antidepressants, alcohol

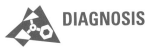 DIAGNOSIS

DIAGNOSTIC PROCEDURES

- Erectile dysfunction
  - Depression must be ruled out
  - Workup must differentiate between anatomic, endocrine, neurologic, and psychological causes
  - Even if an irreversible cause is identified, this knowledge may help the patient to accept the condition
- Other conditions
  - Clinical diagnosis

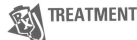 TREATMENT

MEDICATIONS

Erectile dysfunction

- Sildenafil (25–100 mg), vardenafil (2.5–20 mg), or tadalafil (5–20 mg) 1 hour before intercourse is useful
- Sildenafil, vardenafil, and tadalafil must not be used concurrently with nitrates owing to a risk of hypotension leading to sudden death

Ejaculation disturbances

- SSRIs have been effective because of their common effect in delaying ejaculation

THERAPEUTIC PROCEDURES

- Anxiety and guilt about parental injunctions against sex may contribute to sexual dysfunction

Erectile dysfunction

- The effect of this problem on relationships must be considered and addressed

Ejaculation disturbances

- Psychotherapy is best suited to cases in which interpersonal or intrapsychic problems predominate
- A combined behavioral-psychological approach is most effective

Vaginismus

- Responds well to desensitization with graduated Hegar dilators along with relaxation techniques
- Masters and Johnson have used behavioral approaches in all of the sexual dysfunctions, with concomitant supportive psychotherapy and with improvement of the communication patterns of the couple

Frigidity

- Organic causes (conditions causing dyspareunia, pelvic pathology, mechanical obstruction, and neurologic deficits) and contributing intrapersonal issues must be uncovered and addressed
- As with other psychosexual disorders, behavioral approaches with supportive psychotherapy and improved communication within couples can be effective

 OUTCOME

PREVENTION

- The proximity of other people (eg, mother-in-law) in a household is frequently an inhibiting factor in sexual relationships; some social engineering may alleviate the problem

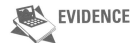 EVIDENCE

PRACTICE GUIDELINES

- American Academy of Family Physicians: Female Sexual Dysfunction: evaluation and treatment
- National Guideline Clearinghouse: American Association of Clinical Endocrinologists: Male sexual dysfunction, 2003

WEB SITE

- American Psychiatric Association

INFORMATION FOR PATIENTS

- American Academy of Family Physicians
- The Cleveland Clinic
- JAMA patient page. Male sexual dysfunction. JAMA. 2004;291:3076. [PMID: 15213218]
- JAMA patient page. Sexual dysfunction. JAMA. 1999;281:584. [PMID: 10022117]

REFERENCES

- Kostis JB et al. Sexual dysfunction and cardiac risk (The Second Princeton Consensus Conference). Am J Cardiol. 2005 Jul 15;96(2):313–21. [PMID: 16018863]
- Sivalingam S et al. An overview of the diagnosis and treatment of erectile dysfunction. Drugs. 2006;66(18):2339–55. [PMID: 17181376]
- Taylor MJ. Strategies for managing antidepressant induced sexual dysfunction: a review. Curr Psychiatry Rep. 2006 Dec;8(6):431–6. [PMID: 17094922]

Sexually Transmitted Diseases

 KEY FEATURES

GENERAL CONSIDERATIONS

- The most common sexually transmitted diseases (STDs) are
  - Gonorrhea
  - Syphilis
  - Condyloma acuminatum
  - Chlamydial genital infections
  - Herpesvirus genital infections

- *Trichomonas* vaginitis
- Chancroid
- Granuloma inguinale
- Scabies
- Louse infestation
- Bacterial vaginosis (among women who have sex with women)

- Shigellosis, hepatitis A, B, and C, amebiasis, giardiasis, cryptosporidiosis, salmonellosis, and campylobacteriosis may also be transmitted by sexual (oral–anal) contact, especially in men who have sex with men

- Homosexual contact and increasing, bidirectional heterosexual transmission are the typical methods of transmission of HIV

- In most infections caused by sexually transmitted bacteria, spirochetes, chlamydiae, viruses, or protozoal agents, early lesions occur on genitalia or other sexually exposed mucous membranes

- However, wide dissemination may occur, and involvement of nongenital tissues and organs may mimic many noninfectious disorders

- All STDs have subclinical phases that play an important role in long-term persistence or in the infection's transmission from infected (but largely asymptomatic) persons to other contacts

Sexual assault

- Victims of assault have a high baseline rate of infection
  - *Neisseria gonorrhoeae,* 6%
  - *Chlamydia trachomatis,* 10%
  - *Trichomonas vaginalis,* 15%
  - Bacterial vaginosis, 34%

- The risk of acquiring infection as a result of the assault is significant but is often lower than the preexisting rate
  - *N gonorrhoeae,* 6–12%
  - *C trachomatis,* 4–17%
  - *T vaginalis,* 12%
  - Syphilis, 0.5–3%
  - Bacterial vaginosis, 19%

- The likelihood of HIV transmission from vaginal or anal receptive intercourse when the source is known to be HIV positive is 1–5 per 1000, respectively

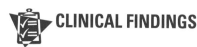 **CLINICAL FINDINGS**

SYMPTOMS AND SIGNS

- See individual diseases

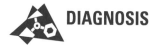 **DIAGNOSIS**

LABORATORY TESTS

- Simultaneous infection by several different agents is common

- Any person with an STD should be tested for syphilis; a repeat study should be done in 3 months if negative, since seroconversion is delayed after primary infection

- Laboratory examinations are of particular importance in the diagnosis of asymptomatic patients during the subclinical or latent phases of STDs

- All patients who seek STD testing should also undergo routine testing for HIV

Sexual assault

- Victims should be evaluated within 24 h after the assault and cultures or nucleic acid amplification tests for *N gonorrhoeae* and *C trachomatis* should be obtained

- Vaginal secretions are cultured and examined for *Trichomonas*

- If a discharge is present, if there is itching, or if secretions are malodorous, a wet mount should be examined for *Candida* and bacterial vaginosis

- A blood sample should be obtained for immediate serologic testing for syphilis, hepatitis B, and HIV

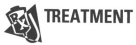 **TREATMENT**

MEDICATIONS

- The usefulness of presumptive therapy for victims of sexual assault is controversial

- If therapy is given, a reasonable regimen would be hepatitis B vaccination (without hepatitis B immune globulin, the first dose given at the initial evaluation and follow-up doses at 1–2 months and 4–6 months) and one dose of ceftriaxone, 125 mg IM, plus metronidazole, 2 g PO as a single dose, plus doxycycline, 100 mg PO BID for 7 days, or azithromycin, 1 g PO as a single dose instead of doxycycline

  - In premenopausal women, azithromycin should be used instead of doxycycline until the pregnancy status is determined

  - If the pregnancy test is positive, metronidazole should be given only after the first trimester

- Prophylactic postexposure treatment for HIV is recommended with HAART for 28 days if

  - The individual seeks care within 72 hours of the assault
  - The source is known to be HIV infected
  - The exposure is associated with a substantial risk of transmission

- If the status of the source is not known, and the victim presents within 72 hours

of the assault, no firm recommendations can be made and the decision to treat is case-by-case

- If the patient seeks care > 72 hours after the assault, prophylaxis is not recommended

THERAPEUTIC PROCEDURES

- As a rule, sexual partners should be treated simultaneously to avoid prompt reinfection

- Prompt treatment of contacts is facilitated by giving antibiotics to the index case to distribute to contacts and has been shown to prevent further transmission

 OUTCOME

FOLLOW-UP

- Follow-up examination for STD after an assault should be repeated within 1–2 weeks, since concentrations of infecting organisms may not have been sufficient to produce a positive test result at the time of initial examination

- If prophylactic treatment was given, tests should be repeated only if the victim has symptoms

- If prophylaxis was not administered, the victim should be seen in 1 week so that any positive tests can be treated

- Follow-up serologic testing for syphilis and HIV infection should be performed in 6, 12, and 24 weeks if the initial tests are negative

 EVIDENCE

PRACTICE GUIDELINES

- Centers for Disease Control and Prevention. Sexually transmitted diseases treatment guidelines 2006. MMWR Recomm Rep. 2006;51(RR-11):1. [PMID: 16888612]

WEB SITE

- Centers for Disease Control and Prevention—National Center for STD, HIV, and TB Prevention, Division of Sexually Transmitted Diseases

INFORMATION FOR PATIENTS

- American Academy of Family Physicians

- CDC National Prevention Information Network

- National Institute of Allergy and Infectious Diseases

REFERENCES

- Aragon TJ et al. Case-control study of shigellosis in San Francisco: The role of sexual transmission and HIV infection. Clin Infect Dis. 2007 Feb 1;44(3):327–34. [PMID: 17205436]
- Golden MR et al. Effect of expedited treatment of sex partners on recurrent or persistent gonorrhea or chlamydial infection. N Engl J Med. 2005 Feb 17; 352(7):676–85. [PMID: 15716561]
- Peterman TA et al. High incidence of new sexually transmitted infections in the year following a sexually transmitted infection: a case for rescreening. Ann Intern Med. 2006 Oct 17;145(8):564–72. [PMID: 17043338]
- Sexually transmitted diseases treatment guidelines 2006. Centers for Disease Control and Prevention. MMWR Recomm Rep. 2006 Aug 4;55(RR-11):1–94. [PMID: 16888612]
- Smith DK et al. Antiretroviral postexposure prophylaxis after sexual, injection-drug use, or other nonoccupational exposure to HIV in the United States: recommendations from the U.S. Department of Health and Human Services. MMWR Recomm Rep. 2005 Jan 21;54(RR-2):1–20. [PMID: 15660015]

Shock

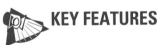 **KEY FEATURES**

ESSENTIALS OF DIAGNOSIS

- Hypotension
- Hypoperfusion and impaired oxygen delivery

GENERAL CONSIDERATIONS

- Can be classified as
  - Hypovolemic
  - Cardiogenic
  - Obstructive
  - Distributive, including septic and neurogenic
- **Hypovolemic**
  - Results from decreased intravascular volume secondary to loss of blood or fluids
  - > 15% loss of intravascular volume can result in hypotension and progressive tissue hypoxia
- **Cardiogenic**
  - Results from pump failure (eg, complication of myocardial infarction, congestive heart failure)
- **Obstructive**
  - Results from acute decrease in cardiac output due to cardiac tamponade, tension pneumothorax, or massive pulmonary embolism
- **Distributive**
  - Causes include sepsis (most common), anaphylaxis, systemic inflammatory response syndrome produced by severe pancreatitis or burns, or acute adrenal insufficiency
  - Reduction in systemic vascular resistance (SVR) results in inadequate cardiac output and tissue hypoperfusion despite normal circulatory volume
- **Septic**
  - Typically secondary to gram-negative bacteremia
  - May also occur from gram-positive cocci and gram-negative anaerobes
- **Neurogenic**
  - Caused by spinal cord injury or epidural or spinal anesthetic agents
  - Pain, gastric dilation, or fright may enduce reflex vagal parasympathetic stimulation which results in hypotension, bradycardia, and syncope

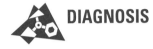 **CLINICAL FINDINGS**

SYMPTOMS AND SIGNS

- Hypotension
- Weak or thready peripheral pulses
- "Clamped down" extremities (cold, mottled)
- Splanchnic vasoconstriction may lead to oliguria, bowel ischemia, and hepatic dysfunction
- Mentation may be normal or altered (eg, restlessness, agitation, confusion, lethargy, or coma)
- **Hypovolemic**
  - Jugular venous pressure is low
  - Narrow pulse pressure indicative of reduced stroke volume
- **Cardiogenic**
  - Jugular venous pressure is elevated
  - May be evidence of pulmonary edema in the setting of left sided heart failure and evidence of ECG changes
- **Obstructive**
  - Central venous pressure may be elevated
- **Distributive**
  - Hyperdynamic heart sounds
  - Warm extremities
  - Wide pulse pressure indicative of large stroke volume
- **Septic**
  - Evidence of infection in the setting of persistent hypotension
  - Evidence of organ hypoperfusion, such as in lactic acidosis, decreased urinary output, or altered mental status despite volume resuscitation
- **Neurogenic**
  - Loss of sympathetic tone with a reduction in SVR
  - Hypotension without a compensatory tachycardia

DIAGNOSIS

LABORATORY TESTS

- Complete blood count
- Serum electrolytes
- Serum glucose
- Arterial blood gas determinations
- Coagulation parameters
- Typing and cross-matching
- Blood cultures

IMAGING STUDIES

- Transesophageal echocardiography shows
  - Reduced left ventricular filling in hypovolemic and obstructive shock
  - Enlarged left ventricle in cardiogenic shock

DIAGNOSTIC PROCEDURES

- An arterial line should be placed for blood pressure and arterial oxygen monitoring
- Foley catheter should be inserted to monitor urinary output
- Pulmonary artery catheter
  - Can distinguish cardiogenic from septic shock
  - Can monitor effects of volume resuscitation or pressor medications
- Central venous pressure (CVP) or pulmonary capillary wedge pressure (PCWP)
  - < 5 mm Hg suggests hypovolemia
  - > 18 mm Hg suggests volume overload, cardiac failure, tamponade, or pulmonary hypertension
- Cardiac index
  - < 2 L/min/m^2 indicates need for inotropic support
  - > 4 L/min/m^2 in a hypotensive patient is consistent with early septic shock
- SVR
  - Low (< 800 dyne × s/cm^{-5}) in septic and neurogenic shock

– High (> 1500 dyne × s/cm^{-5}) in hypovolemic and cardiogenic shock

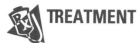

TREATMENT

MEDICATIONS

- Dobutamine
  - First-line drug for cardiogenic shock
  - Initial dosage: 0.5–1 mcg/kg/min as continuous IV infusion, then titrated every few minutes
  - Usual dosage: 2–20 mcg/kg/min IV
- Amrinone or milrinone can be substituted for dobutamine
- Norepinephrine
  - Generally used for vasodilatory shock
  - Initial dosage: 0.5–1 mcg/min as an IV infusion, titrated to maintain the systolic blood pressure to at least 80 mm Hg
  - Usual maintenance dosage: 2–4 mcg/min (maximum dose is 30 mcg/min)
  - Patients with refractory shock may require dosages of 8–30 mcg/min
- Epinephrine
  - May be used in severe shock and during acute resuscitation
  - Initial dosage: 1 mcg/min as a continuous IV infusion
  - Usual dosage: 2–10 mcg/min IV
- Dopamine
  - Low doses (2–3 mcg/kg/min) stimulate dopaminergic and β-agonist receptors, producing increased glomerular filtration, heart rate, and contractility
  - With higher doses (> 5 mcg/kg/min), α-adrenergic effects predominate, resulting in peripheral vasoconstriction
- Vasopressin for distributive or vasodilatory shock
- Nitric oxide plays an important role in the vasodilatation associated with septic shock
- Low-dose corticosteroids in septic shock with acute adrenal insufficiency
  - Hydrocortisone 50 mg q6h and 50 mcg of 9-alpha-fludrocortisone once daily, both for 7 days
  - Hydrocortisone 50 mg by IV bolus, followed by a continuous infusion of 0.18 mg/kg of body weight/hour until cessation of vasopressor support
- Activated protein C (drotrecogin alpha) has antithrombotic, profibrinolytic, and anti-inflammatory properties
- Broad-spectrum antibiotics for septic shock
- Sodium bicarbonate for patients with sepsis of any etiology and lactic acidosis

VOLUME REPLACEMENT

- Critical in initial management of shock
- Hemorrhagic shock
  - Rapid infusions of type-specific or type O negative packed red blood cells (PRBC) or whole blood, which also provides extra volume and clotting factors
  - Each unit of PRBC or whole blood is expected to raise the hematocrit by 3%
- Hypovolemic shock secondary to dehydration: rapid boluses of isotonic crystalloid, usually in 1 L increments
- Cardiogenic shock in absence of fluid overload: requires smaller fluid challenges usually in increments of 250 mL
- Septic shock: usually requires large volumes of fluid for resuscitation

SURGERY

- Transcutaneous or transvenous pacing or placement of an intra-arterial balloon pump for cardiac failure
- Emergent revascularization by percutaneous angioplasty or coronary artery bypass surgery appears to improve long-term outcome

THERAPEUTIC PROCEDURES

- IV access and fluid resuscitation should be instituted along with cardiac monitoring and assessment of hemodynamic parameters such as blood pressure and heart rate
- Treatment is directed at maintaining a
  - CVP of 8–12 mm Hg
  - Mean arterial pressure of 65–90 mm Hg
  - Cardiac index of 2–4 L/min/m^2
  - Central venous oxygen saturation > 70%
- Pulmonary artery catheters most useful in managing cardiogenic shock
- Central venous line may be adequate in other types of shock
- In obstructive shock, pericardiocentesis or pericardial window, chest tube placement, or catheter-directed thrombolytic therapy can be lifesaving
- Urgent hemodialysis or continuous venovenous hemofiltration may be indicated for maintenance of fluid and electrolyte balance during acute renal insufficiency resulting in shock

OUTCOME

PROGNOSIS

- Septic shock mortality is 30–87%

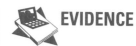

EVIDENCE

PRACTICE GUIDELINES

- Dellinger RP et al. Surviving Sepsis Campaign guidelines for management of severe sepsis and septic shock. Crit Care Med. 2004 Mar;32(3):858–73. [PMID: 15090974]
- Guidelines for the management of severe sepsis and septic shock. The International Sepsis Forum. Intensive Care Med. 2001;27(Suppl 1):S1–134. [PMID: 11519475]
- Martel MJ et al. Hemorrhagic shock. J Obstet Gynaecol Can. 2002 Jun; 24(6):504–20. [PMID: 12196857]

INFORMATION FOR PATIENTS

- Mayo Clinic: Shock

REFERENCES

- Alam HB et al. New developments in fluid resuscitation. Surg Clin North Am. 2007 Feb;87(1):55–72. [PMID: 17127123]
- Annane D et al; Ger-Inf-05 Study Group. Effect of low doses of corticosteroids in septic shock patients with or without early acute respiratory distress syndrome. Crit Care Med. 2006 Jan; 34(1):22–30. [PMID: 16374152]
- Fourrier F. Recombinant human activated protein C in the treatment of severe sepsis: an evidence-based review. Crit Care Med. 2004 Nov;32(11 Suppl):S534–41. [PMID: 15542961]
- Nguyen HB et al; Emergency Department Sepsis Education Program and Strategies to Improve Survival (ED-SEPSIS) Working Group. Severe sepsis and septic shock: review of the literature and emergency department management guidelines. Ann Emerg Med. 2006 Jul;48(1):28–54. [PMID: 16781920]
- Oppert M et al. Low-dose hydrocortisone improves shock reversal and reduces cytokine levels in early hyperdynamic septic shock. Crit Care Med. 2005 Nov;33(11):2457–64. [PMID: 16276166]
- Siraux V et al. Relative adrenal insufficiency in patients with septic shock: comparison of low-dose and conventional corticotropin tests. Crit Care Med. 2005 Nov;33(11):2479–86. [PMID: 16276169]

Sickle Cell Anemia

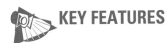

KEY FEATURES

ESSENTIALS OF DIAGNOSIS

- Irreversibly sickled cells on peripheral blood smear
- Positive family history and lifelong personal history of hemolytic anemia
- Recurrent painful episodes
- Hemoglobin S is the major hemoglobin seen on electrophoresis

GENERAL CONSIDERATIONS

- Autosomal recessive disorder in which abnormal hemoglobin leads to chronic hemolytic anemia with numerous clinical consequences
- Single DNA base change leads to amino acid substitution of valine for glutamine in the sixth position on β-globin chain
- Sickling is increased by increased red blood cell (RBC) hemoglobin S concentration, RBC dehydration, acidosis, and hypoxemia
- Sickling is retarded markedly by hemoglobin F; high hemoglobin F levels are associated with more benign course
- Patients with heterozygous genotype (hemoglobin AS) have sickle cell trait
- Acute painful episodes as a result of vasoocclusion by sickled RBCs occur spontaneously or they are provoked by infection, dehydration, or hypoxia

DEMOGRAPHICS

- Hemoglobin S gene is carried in 8% of African Americans
- Sickle cell anemia occurs in 1 birth in 400 in African Americans
- Onset during first year of life, when hemoglobin F levels fall

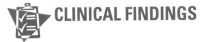

CLINICAL FINDINGS

SYMPTOMS AND SIGNS

- Chronic hemolytic anemia produces
  - Jaundice
  - Pigment (calcium bilirubinate) gallstones
  - Splenomegaly
  - Poorly healing ulcers over the lower tibia
- Anemia may be life-threatening during hemolytic or aplastic crises

- Hemolytic crises result from splenic sequestration of sickled cells (primarily in childhood, before spleen has infarcted) or with coexistent disorders such as glucose-6-phosphate dehydrogenase deficiency
- Aplastic crises occur when bone marrow compensation is reduced by infection or folate deficiency
- Acute painful episodes, commonly in bones and chest, last hours to days and produce low-grade fever
- Acute vasoocclusion may cause priapism and strokes
- Repeated vasoocclusion affects
  - Heart (cardiomegaly, hyperdynamic precordium, systolic murmurs)
  - Lungs
  - Liver
  - Bone (ischemic necrosis, staphylococcal or salmonella osteomyelitis)
  - Spleen (infarction, asplenia)
  - Kidney (infarction of renal medullary papillae, renal tubular concentrating defects, and gross hematuria)
- Pulmonary hypertension is associated with decreased survival
- Increased susceptibility to infection occurs as a result of hyposplenism and complement defects
- **Sickle cell trait**
  - Asymptomatic most often
  - Acute vasoocclusion occurs only under extreme conditions
  - Gross hematuria or renal tubular defect causing inability to concentrate urine may occur

DIFFERENTIAL DIAGNOSIS

- Other sickle cell syndromes
  - Sickle cell trait
  - Sickle thalassemia
  - Hemoglobin SC disease
- Osteomyelitis
- Hematuria from other cause
- Acute rheumatic fever

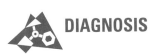

DIAGNOSIS

LABORATORY TESTS

- Elevated serum indirect bilirubin and lactase dehydrogenase; serum haptoglobin low
- Hematocrit usually 20–30%
- Reticulocyte count elevated
- Peripheral blood smear: irreversibly sickled cells comprise 5–50% of RBCs; reticulocytosis (10–25%); nucleated RBCs; Howell-Jolly bodies and target cells

- White blood cell count characteristically elevated to 12,000–15,000/mcL; thrombocytosis may occur
- Screening test for sickle hemoglobin positive
- Hemoglobin electrophoresis confirms diagnosis
- Sickle cell anemia (homozygous S)
  - Hemoglobin S usually comprises 85–98% of hemoglobin and no hemoglobin A is present
  - Hemoglobin F levels variably increased
- Sickle cell trait
  - Complete blood cell count and peripheral blood smear normal
  - Hemoglobin electrophoresis shows that hemoglobin S comprises ~40% of hemoglobin

IMAGING STUDIES

- Chest radiograph in acute chest syndrome
- Bone radiographs show characteristic abnormalities
- CT shows hepatomegaly and absence of spleen

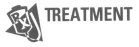

TREATMENT

MEDICATIONS

- Folic acid, 1 mg PO once daily
- Hydroxyurea, 500–750 mg PO once daily
  - Increases hemoglobin F levels
  - Reduces frequency of painful crises in patients whose quality of life is disrupted by frequent pain crises
  - Long-term safety uncertain
  - Concern exists about potential for secondary malignancies

THERAPEUTIC PROCEDURES

- Prenatal diagnosis and genetic counseling should be made available to those with personal or family history
- No specific treatment is available for sickle cell anemia
- Pneumococcal vaccination reduces incidence of infections
- Acute painful episodes
  - Identify precipitating factors
  - Treat infections if present
  - Maintain good hydration
  - Administer oxygen if hypoxic
- Sickle cell trait
  - No treatment necessary
  - Genetic counseling appropriate

- Exchange transfusion primarily indicated for treatment of intractable pain crises, priapism, and stroke
- Long-term transfusion therapy shown to reduce risk of recurrent stroke in children
- Allogeneic bone marrow transplantation under investigation as possible curative option for severely affected young patients

OUTCOME

COMPLICATIONS

- Sickle cell anemia becomes a chronic multisystem disease, with death from organ failure
- Acute chest syndrome

PROGNOSIS

- With improved supportive care, average life expectancy is between ages 40 and 50

EVIDENCE

PRACTICE GUIDELINES

- Rees DC et al. Guidelines for the management of the acute painful crisis in sickle cell disease. Br J Haematol. 2003; 120:744. [PMID: 12614204]

WEB SITES

- Georgia Comprehensive Sickle Cell Center at Grady Health System
- National Library of Medicine Genetics Home Reference: Sickle Cell Anemia

INFORMATION FOR PATIENTS

- JAMA patient page. Sickle cell anemia. JAMA. 1999;281:1768. [PMID: 10328078]
- National Heart, Lung, and Blood Institute: What Is Sickle Cell Anemia?
- Dolan DNA Learning Center: Sickle Cell Disease
- Sickle Cell Disease Association of America

REFERENCES

- Adams RJ et al; The Optimizing Primary Stroke Prevention in Sickle Cell Anemia (STOP 2) Trial Investigators. Discontinuing prophylactic transfusions used to prevent stroke in sickle cell disease. N Engl J Med. 2005 Dec 29; 353(26):2769–78. [PMID: 16382063]
- Alexander N et al. Are there clinical phenotypes of homozygous sickle cell disease? Br J Haematol. 2004 Aug; 126(4):606–11. [PMID: 15287956]
- Hankins JS et al. Long-term hydroxyurea therapy for infants with sickle cell anemia: the HUSOFT extension study. Blood. 2005 Oct 1;106(7):2269–75. [PMID: 16172253]
- Stuart MJ et al. Sickle-cell disease. Lancet. 2004 Oct 9-15;364(9442):1343–60. [PMID: 15474138]

Sinusitis, Acute

KEY FEATURES

ESSENTIALS OF DIAGNOSIS

- Pain is usually unilateral over the maxillary sinus or toothache-like
- Symptoms usually last for more than 1 week but less than 4 weeks
- Change of secretions from mucoid to purulent green or yellow or bloody
- Occasional visible swelling or erythema over a sinus
- Postnasal drainage, headache, and cough may also be present

GENERAL CONSIDERATIONS

- Diseases that swell the nasal mucous membrane, such as viral or allergic rhinitis, are usually the underlying cause
- Usually is a result of impaired mucociliary clearance and obstruction of the osteomeatal complex, resulting in the accumulation of mucous secretion in the sinus cavity that becomes secondarily infected by bacteria
- The terms "rhinosinusitis" or "acute bacterial rhinosinusitis" are used by otolaryngologists to emphasize the importance of intranasal obstruction in the pathogenesis of sinusitis
- The typical pathogens are the same as those that cause acute otitis media
  - *Streptococcus pneumoniae*
  - Other streptococci
  - *Haemophilus influenzae*
  - Less commonly, *Staphylococcus aureus* and *Moraxella catarrhalis*
- About 25% of healthy asymptomatic individuals may, if sinus aspirates are cultured, harbor these bacteria
- Discolored nasal discharge and poor response to decongestants suggest sinusitis

DEMOGRAPHICS

- Uncommon compared with viral rhinitis, but still affects nearly 20 million Americans annually
- The prevalence of nosocomial sinusitis is as high as 40% in critically ill intubated patients

CLINICAL FINDINGS

SYMPTOMS AND SIGNS

- **Maxillary sinusitis**
  - Unilateral facial fullness, pressure, and tenderness over the cheek
  - Pain may refer to the upper incisor and canine teeth
  - May result from dental infection, and tender teeth should be carefully examined for abscess
  - Purulent nasal drainage helps differentiate sinusitis from acute rhinitis
  - Nonspecific symptoms include fever, malaise, halitosis, headache, nasal congestion, hyposmia, cough
- **Ethmoid sinusitis**
  - Usually accompanied by maxillary sinusitis; the symptoms of maxillary sinusitis generally predominate
  - Pain and pressure over the high lateral wall of the nose between the eyes that may radiate to the orbit
  - Periorbital cellulitis may be present
- **Sphenoid sinusitis**
  - Usually seen in the setting of pansinusitis, or infection of all the paranasal sinuses on at least one side
  - The patient may complain of a headache "in the middle of the head" and often points to the vertex
- **Frontal sinusitis**
  - Usually pain and tenderness of the forehead
  - This is most easily elicited by palpation of the orbital roof just below the medial end of the eyebrow
- **Hospital-acquired sinusitis**
  - May present without any symptoms in head and neck
  - Common source of fever in critically ill patients
  - Often associated with prolonged presence of nasogastric tube
  - Pansinusitis on side of tube commonly seen on imaging studies

DIFFERENTIAL DIAGNOSIS

- Upper respiratory tract infection
- Viral rhinitis
- Allergic rhinitis
- Nasal polyposis

- Dental abscess
- Rhinocerebral mucormycosis
- Otitis media
- Pharyngitis
- Dacryocystitis
- Paranasal sinus cancer

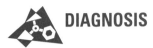 **DIAGNOSIS**

LABORATORY TESTS

- Diagnosis usually made on clinical grounds alone

IMAGING STUDIES

- Routine radiographs
  - Not cost-effective
  - May be helpful when clinically based criteria are difficult to evaluate or when symptoms of more serious infection are noted
- Noncontrast coronal CT scans
  - More cost-effective and provide more information than conventional sinus films
  - Provide a rapid and effective means to assess all of the paranasal sinuses, to identify areas of greater concern (such as bony dehiscence, periosteal elevation or maxillary tooth root exposure within the sinus), and to direct therapy
- Sinusitis is a clinical diagnosis for which CT may be helpful in confirming, excluding, or monitoring

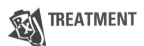 **TREATMENT**

MEDICATIONS

Criteria for antibiotic therapy

- Symptoms lasting more than 10–14 days
- Severe symptoms, including fever, facial pain, and periorbital swelling

First-line antibiotic therapy

- Amoxicillin, 1000 mg PO TID for 7–10 days
- Trimethoprim-sulfamethoxazole (TMP-SMZ)
  - 160/800 mg PO BID for 7–10 days
  - Suitable in penicillin allergy
- Doxycycline
  - 200 mg PO once daily × 1 day, then 100 mg PO BID thereafter for 7–10 days
  - Suitable in penicillin allergy
- Broad-spectrum antibiotics given for hospital-acquired infections

First-line therapy after recent antibiotic use

- Levofloxacin, 500 mg PO once daily for 10 days
- Amoxicillin-clavulanate, 875/125 mg PO BID for 10 days

Second-line antibiotic therapy

- Amoxicillin-clavulanate
  - 1000/62.5 mg two extended-release tablets PO BID for 10 days
  - Consider if no improvement after 3 days of first-line therapy
- Moxifloxacin
  - 400 mg PO once daily for 10 days
  - Consider if no improvement after 3 days of first-line therapy
- Telithromycin
  - 800 mg PO once daily for 10 days
  - Consider if no improvement after 3 days of first-line therapy
  - Contraindicated in myasthenia gravis; recent reports of hepatic failure

Decongestants

- For symptom improvement, use oral or nasal decongestants or both
  - Oral pseudoephedrine, 30–120 mg/dose, up to 240 mg/day
  - Nasal oxymetazoline, 0.05%, or xylometazoline, 0.05–0.1%, one or two sprays in each nostril q6–8h for up to 3 days

THERAPEUTIC PROCEDURES

- For hospital-acquired sinusitis
  - Remove nasogastric tube
  - Improve nasal hygiene (saline sprays, humidification of supplemental nasal oxygen, nasal decongestants)
  - Endoscopic or transantral cultures may help direct antibiotic therapy in complicated cases

 OUTCOME

COMPLICATIONS

- Orbital cellulitis and abscess
- Osteomyelitis
- Intracranial extension
- Cavernous sinus thrombosis

PROGNOSIS

- Two-thirds of untreated patients will improve symptomatically within 2 weeks

WHEN TO REFER

- Recurrent sinusitis or sinusitis that does not appear to respond clinically warrants evaluation by a specialist
- Any complication of sinusitis

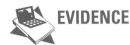 **EVIDENCE**

PRACTICE GUIDELINES

- Institute for Clinical Systems Improvement: Acute Sinusitis in Adults, 2004.

WEB SITE

- Baylor College of Medicine Otolaryngology Resources on the Internet

INFORMATION FOR PATIENTS

- American Academy of Allergy, Asthma & Immunology: Sinusitis
- American Academy of Family Physicians: Sinusitis
- American Academy of Otolaryngology—Head and Neck Surgery: Doctor, What Is Sinusitis?
- National Institute of Allergy and Infectious Diseases: Sinusitis

REFERENCES

- Mafee MF et al. Imaging of rhinosinusitis and its complications: plain film, CT and MRI. Clin Rev Allergy Immunol. 2006 Jun;30(3):165–86. [PMID: 16785588]
- Marple BF et al. Acute bacterial rhinosinusitis: a review of US treatment guidelines. Otolaryngol Head Neck Surg. 2006 Sep;135(3):341–8. [PMID: 16949962]
- Merenstein D et al. Are antibiotics beneficial for patients with sinusitis complaints? A randomized double-blind clinical trial. J Fam Pract. 2005 Feb; 54(2):144–51. [PMID: 15689289]
- Piccirillo JF. Clinical practice. Acute bacterial sinusitis. N Engl J Med. 2004 Aug 26;351(9):902–10. [PMID: 15329428]

Sjögren's Syndrome

 KEY FEATURES

ESSENTIALS FOR DIAGNOSIS

- Dryness of eyes and dry mouth (sicca components); they occur alone or in association with rheumatoid arthritis or other connective tissue disease

- Rheumatoid factor and other autoanti-bodies common
- Increased incidence of lymphoma

GENERAL CONSIDERATIONS

- Chronic autoimmune dysfunction of exocrine glands in many areas of the body
- Dryness of the eyes, mouth, and other areas covered by mucous membranes
- Keratoconjunctivitis sicca results from inadequate tear production caused by lymphocyte and plasma cell infiltration of the lacrimal glands
- Frequently associated with a rheumatic disease, most often rheumatoid arthritis

Associated conditions
- Rheumatoid arthritis
- Systemic lupus erythematosus (SLE)
- Primary biliary cirrhosis
- Scleroderma
- Polymyositis
- Hashimoto's thyroiditis
- Polyarteritis nodosa
- Idiopathic pulmonary fibrosis

DEMOGRAPHICS

- The disorder is predominantly a disease of women, in a ratio of 9:1
- Greatest incidence between ages 40 and 60 years

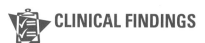

CLINICAL FINDINGS

SYMPTOMS AND SIGNS

- Eyes
  - Ocular burning, itching, ropy secre-tions
  - "Grain of sand in the eye" sensation
- Parotid glands
  - Enlargement may be chronic or re-lapsing
  - Develops in one-third of patients
- Dryness of the mouth (xerostomia) leads to difficulty in swallowing dry foods (like crackers), to constant thirst for fluids, and to severe dental caries
- There may be loss of taste and smell
- Systemic manifestations
  - Dysphagia, pancreatitis
  - Pleuritis, obstructive lung disease (in the absence of smoking)
  - Neuropsychiatric dysfunction
  - Vasculitis
- Kidney
  - Renal tubular acidosis (type I, distal) occurs in 20% of patients

- Chronic interstitial nephritis, which may result in impaired renal func-tion, may be seen

DIFFERENTIAL DIAGNOSIS

- Sicca complex associated with other autoimmune disease, eg, sarcoidosis, rheumatoid arthritis, SLE, scleroderma
- Other causes of dry mouth or eyes, eg, anticholinergics, mumps, irradiation, sea-sonal allergies, irritation from smoking

DIAGNOSIS

LABORATORY TESTS

- Rheumatoid factor is found in 70% of patients
- Antibodies against the cytoplasmic anti-gens SS-A and SS-B (also called Ro and La, respectively) are often present (Table 123)
- When SS-A antibodies are present, extraglandular manifestations are far more common

DIAGNOSTIC PROCEDURES

- Lip biopsy is the only specific diagnostic technique and has minimal risk; if lym-phoid foci are seen in accessory salivary glands, the diagnosis is confirmed
- Biopsy of the parotid gland should be reserved for patients with atypical pre-sentations such as unilateral gland enlargement
- The Schirmer test measures the quantity of tears secreted

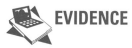

TREATMENT

MEDICATIONS

- Pilocarpine (5 mg QID) and the acetyl-choline derivative cevimeline (30 mg TID) are helpful for severe xerostomia
- Atropinic drugs and decongestants decrease salivary secretions and should be avoided

THERAPEUTIC PROCEDURES

- Treatment is symptomatic and supportive
- Artificial tears applied frequently will relieve ocular symptoms and avert fur-ther desiccation
- Sipping water frequently or using sugar-free gums and hard candies usually relieves dry mouth symptoms
- A program of oral hygiene is essential to preserve dentition

OUTCOME

COMPLICATIONS

- A spectrum of lymphoproliferation ranging from benign to malignant may be found
- Malignant lymphomas and Walden-ström's macroglobulinemia occur nearly 50 times more frequently than can be explained by chance alone in primary Sjögren's syndrome

PROGNOSIS

- Usually benign and consistent with a normal life span
- Prognosis is mainly influenced by the nature of the associated disease
- The patients (3–10% of the total Sjögren's population) at greatest risk for developing lymphoma have
  - Severe dryness
  - Marked parotid gland enlargement
  - Splenomegaly
  - Vasculitis
  - Peripheral neuropathy
  - Anemia
  - Mixed monoclonal cryoglobulinemia

EVIDENCE

PRACTICE GUIDELINES

- Johns Hopkins University

WEB SITE

- Sjögren's Syndrome Foundation

INFORMATION FOR PATIENTS

- National Institute of Arthritis and Mus-culoskeletal and Skin Diseases
- National Institute of Neurological Dis-orders and Stroke

REFERENCES

- Brito-Zeron P et al. Circulating mono-clonal immunoglobulins in Sjögren syn-drome: prevalence and clinical significance in 237 patients. Medicine (Baltimore). 2005 Mar;84(2):90–7. [PMID: 15758838]
- Goransson LG et al. Peripheral neuropa-thy in primary Sjögren syndrome: a population-based study. Arch Neurol. 2006 Nov;63(11):1612–5. [PMID: 17101831]
- Ono M et al. Therapeutic effect of cevimeline on dry eye in patients with Sjögren's syndrome: a randomized, dou-ble-blind clinical study. Am J Ophthal-

mol. 2004 Jul;138(1):6–17. [PMID: 15234277]

- Ramos-Casals M et al. Cutaneous vasculitis in primary Sjögren syndrome: classification and clinical significance of 52 patients. Medicine (Baltimore). 2004 Mar;83(2):96–106. [PMID: 15028963]

Sleep Apnea, Obstructive

 ## KEY FEATURES

ESSENTIALS OF DIAGNOSIS

- Daytime somnolence or fatigue
- A history of loud snoring with witnessed apneic events
- Overnight polysomnography demonstrates apneic episodes with hypoxemia

GENERAL CONSIDERATIONS

- Upper airway obstruction results from a loss of pharyngeal muscle tone during sleep
- Patients with narrowed upper airways are predisposed to the condition
- Ingestion of alcohol or sedatives before sleep and nasal obstruction from any cause may precipitate or worsen the condition
- Cigarette smoking and hypothyroidism are risk factors

DEMOGRAPHICS

- Most patients are obese, middle-aged men

 ## CLINICAL FINDINGS

SYMPTOMS AND SIGNS

- Patients complain of daytime somnolence or fatigue, morning sluggishness, or cognitive impairment
- Recent weight gain, headaches, and impotence may be present
- Bed partners usually report loud cyclical snoring and witnessed apneas with restlessness and thrashing movements during sleep
- Systemic hypertension is usually present
- Physical examination may show evidence of pulmonary hypertension with cor pulmonale

- Oropharyngeal narrowing due to excessive soft tissue may be seen
- A short, thick neck is common
- Bradydysrhythmias may occur during sleep
- Tachydysrhythmias may be seen once airflow is reestablished following an apneic episode

DIFFERENTIAL DIAGNOSIS

- Central sleep apnea
- Mixed sleep apnea
- Obesity-hypoventilation syndrome (Pickwickian syndrome)
- Narcolepsy
- Alcohol or sedative abuse
- Depression
- Hypothyroidism
- Seizure disorder

 ## DIAGNOSIS

LABORATORY TESTS

- Erythrocytosis is common
- Serum thyroid-stimulating hormone (TSH) should be checked

DIAGNOSTIC PROCEDURES

- Overnight polysomnography is essential to make the diagnosis
- Apneic episodes are defined as breath cessation for 10 seconds or more
- Hypopnea is defined as a decrement in airflow with a drop in oxyhemoglobin saturation of 4% or more
- An otolaryngologic examination should be performed
- Screening with home nocturnal pulse oximetry has a high negative predictive value if no desaturations are seen

 ## TREATMENT

MEDICATIONS

- Pharmacologic therapy is not successful

SURGERY

- Uvulopalatopharyngoplasty, the resection of pharyngeal tissue and removal of a portion of the soft palate and uvula, is helpful in approximately half of selected patients
- Nasal septoplasty is performed if gross nasal septal deformity is present
- Tracheostomy is the definitive therapy, but is reserved for life-threatening, refractory cases

THERAPEUTIC PROCEDURES

- Weight loss and avoidance of alcohol and hypnotic medications are initial steps
- 10–20% weight loss may be curative
- Nasal continuous positive airway pressure (CPAP) is curative in many patients
- Polysomnography is often necessary to determine the level of CPAP (usually 5–15 mm Hg) required
- Prosthetic devices inserted into the mouth to prevent pharyngeal occlusion can be modestly effective, but compliance is limiting

 ## OUTCOME

COMPLICATIONS

- Cor pulmonale
- Life-threatening cardiac dysrhythmias
- Systemic hypertension

PROGNOSIS

- Only 75% of patients continue to use CPAP after 1 year

WHEN TO REFER

- For a sleep study

EVIDENCE

PRACTICE GUIDELINES

- Littner M et al. Practice parameters for the use of laser-assisted uvulopalatoplasty: an update for 2000. Sleep. 2001; 24:603. [PMID: 11480657]

INFORMATION FOR PATIENTS

- National Institute of Neurological Disorders and Stroke

REFERENCES

- Bao G et al. Upper airway resistance syndrome—one decade later. Curr Opin Pulm Med. 2004 Nov;10(6):461–7. [PMID: 15510051]
- Caples SM et al. Obstructive sleep apnea. Ann Intern Med. 2005 Feb 1; 142(3):187–97. [PMID: 15684207]
- Pack AI. Advances in sleep-disordered breathing. Am J Respir Crit Care Med. 2006 Jan 1;173(1):7–15. [PMID: 16284108]
- White DP. Pathogenesis of obstructive and central sleep apnea. Am J Respir Crit Care Med. 2005 Dec 1; 172(11):1363–70. [PMID: 16100008]

Status Epilepticus

 ## KEY FEATURES

ESSENTIALS OF DIAGNOSIS

- Occurrence of two or more convulsions without recovery of consciousness between attacks
- A fixed and enduring epileptic condition (for 30 minutes or more)

GENERAL CONSIDERATIONS

- Status epilepticus is a medical emergency
- Causes
  - Poor compliance with the anticonvulsant drug (most common)
  - Alcohol withdrawal
  - Intracranial infection or neoplasms
  - Stroke
  - Metabolic disorders
  - Drug overdose
- Mortality rate of convulsive status may be as high as 20%, with a high incidence of neurologic and mental sequelae
- Prognosis relates to the length of time between onset of status epilepticus and start of effective treatment

 ## CLINICAL FINDINGS

SYMPTOMS AND SIGNS

- Two clinical subtypes
  - Tonic-clonic convulsive status epilepticus
  - Nonconvulsive status epilepticus
- Nonconvulsive status epilepticus is characterized by
  - Fluctuating abnormal mental status
  - Confusion
  - Impaired responsiveness
  - Automatism
  - Two subtypes: absence (petit mal) and complex partial status epilepticus

DIFFERENTIAL DIAGNOSIS

- Seizure due to
  - Hypoglycemia
  - Electrolyte abnormality
  - Alcohol withdrawal
  - Cocaine
  - Bacterial meningitis
  - Herpes encephalitis
  - Brain tumor
  - CNS vasculitis
- Syncope
- Cardiac arrhythmia
- Stroke or transient ischemic attack
- Pseudoseizure
- Panic attack
- Migraine
- Narcolepsy

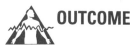 ## DIAGNOSIS

LABORATORY TESTS

- Electroencephalography (EEG) is essential in establishing the diagnosis of nonconvulsive status epilepticus and its two subtypes

TREATMENT

MEDICATIONS

- See Table 133
- Initial treatment with IV lorazepam or diazepam is usually helpful regardless of the type of status epilepticus
- Phenytoin, phenobarbital, carbamazepine, and other drugs are also needed

Initial management

- Maintenance of the airway and 50% dextrose (25–50 mL) IV in case of hypoglycemia
- Lorazepam
  - Give 4 mg IV bolus, repeat once after 10 minutes if necessary
  - Effective in halting seizures for a brief period
  - However, occasionally causes respiratory depression
- Diazepam
  - An alternative to lorazepam
  - Give 10 mg IV over 2 minutes and repeat after 10 minutes if necessary
  - Hypotension and respiratory depression may occur
- Also give phenytoin (18–20 mg/kg) IV at 50 mg/min for initiation of longer seizure control
  - Best injected directly but can also be given in saline; it precipitates if injected into glucose-containing solutions
  - Arrhythmias may develop during rapid administration; ECG monitoring is prudent
  - May cause hypotension, especially if diazepam has also been given
  - Has been widely replaced by injectable fosphenytoin, which is rapidly and completely converted to phenytoin following IV administration
  - No dosing adjustments are necessary because fosphenytoin is expressed in terms of phenytoin equivalents (PE)
- Fosphenytoin
  - Less likely to cause reactions at the infusion site than phenytoin
  - Can be given with all common IV solutions
  - May be administered at a faster rate (150 mg PE/min)
  - More expensive than phenytoin

If seizures continue

- Phenobarbital
  - Give in a loading dose of 10–20 mg/kg IV by slow or intermittent injection (50 mg/min)
  - Respiratory depression and hypotension are common complications and should be anticipated
- If these measures fail, general anesthesia with ventilatory assistance and neuromuscular junction blockade may be required
- Midazolam
  - An alternative to phenobarbital
  - IV midazolam may control refractory status epilepticus
  - Suggested loading dose is 0.2 mg/kg, followed by 0.05–0.2 mg/kg/h

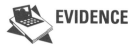 ## OUTCOME

FOLLOW-UP

- After status epilepticus is controlled, an oral drug program for the long-term management of seizures is started, and investigations into the cause of the disorder are pursued

WHEN TO REFER

- Many patients can benefit from the expertise of a neurologist

WHEN TO ADMIT

- All patients until seizure control is obtained

EVIDENCE

INFORMATION FOR PATIENTS

- Epilepsy Foundation
- National Institute of Neurological Disorders and Stroke

REFERENCES

- Brathen G et al. EFNS guidelines on the diagnosis and management of alcohol-related seizures: report of a EFNS task force. Eur J Neurol. 2005 Aug; 12(8):575–81. [PMID: 16053464]

- Chen JW et al. Status epilepticus: pathophysiology and management in adults. Lancet Neurol. 2006 Mar; 5(3):246–56. [PMID: 16488380]
- Duncan JS et al. Adult epilepsy. Lancet. 2006 Apr 1;367(9516):1087–100. [PMID: 16581409]
- Hitiris N et al. Modern antiepileptic drugs: guidelines and beyond. Curr Opin Neurol. 2006 Apr;19(2):175–80. [PMID: 16538093]
- Kelso AR et al. Advances in epilepsy. Br Med Bull. 2005 Apr 21;72:135–48. [PMID: 15845748]
- Vazquez B. Monotherapy in epilepsy: role of the newer antiepileptic drugs. Arch Neurol. 2004 Sep;61(9):1361–5. [PMID: 15364680]

Still's Disease, Adult

 KEY FEATURES

- A form of juvenile chronic arthritis
- High spiking fevers are much more prominent, especially at the outset, than in rheumatoid arthritis

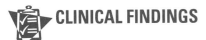 **CLINICAL FINDINGS**

- The fever is dramatic, often spiking to 40°C, associated with sweats and chills, and then plunging to several degrees below normal
- An evanescent salmon-colored nonpruritic rash, chiefly on the chest and abdomen, is a characteristic feature but is easily missed because it often appears only with the fever spike
- Sore throat
- Lymphadenopathy
- Joint symptoms are mild or absent in the beginning, but a destructive arthritis, especially of the wrists, may develop months later
- Anemia and leukocytosis, with white blood cell counts sometimes exceeding 40,000/mcL, are the rule
- About one-third of patients have recurrent episodes
- Ferritin levels are exceptionally high (> 3000 mg/mL) in more than 70% of adult Still's disease

 DIAGNOSIS

- A diagnosis of exclusion (of other causes of fever and arthritis)
- Strongly suggested by the fever pattern, sore throat, and classic rash

 TREATMENT

- About half of the patients respond to high-dose aspirin (eg, 1 g TID) or other nonsteroidal anti-inflammatory drugs
- About half require prednisone, sometimes in doses > 60 mg/day
- Dramatic responses have been achieved with the IL-1 receptor antagonist anakinra

Stress & Adjustment Disorders

 KEY FEATURES

ESSENTIALS OF DIAGNOSIS

- Anxiety or depression clearly secondary to an identifiable stress
- Subsequent symptoms of anxiety or depression commonly elicited by similar stress of lesser magnitude
- Alcohol and other drugs are commonly used in self-treatment

GENERAL CONSIDERATIONS

- Stress exists when the adaptive capacity of the individual is overwhelmed by events
- The event may be an insignificant one objectively considered
- Even favorable changes (eg, promotion and transfer) requiring adaptive behavior can produce stress
- For each individual, stress is subjectively defined, and the response to stress is a function of each person's personality and physiologic endowment
- The causes or sources of stress are different at different ages
  - Young adulthood
    - Marriage or parent-child relationship
    - Employment relationship
    - Struggle to achieve financial stability
  - Middle years
    - Changing spousal relationships
    - Problems with aging parents
    - Problems associated with having young adult offspring who themselves are encountering stressful situations
  - Old age
    - Retirement
    - Loss of physical capacity
    - Major personal losses
    - Thoughts of death
- Maladaptive behavior in response to stress is called adjustment disorder, with the major symptom specified (eg, "adjustment disorder with depressed mood")

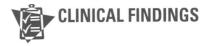 **CLINICAL FINDINGS**

SYMPTOMS AND SIGNS

- Common subjective responses
  - Fear (of repetition of the stress-inducing event)
  - Rage (at frustration)
  - Guilt (over aggressive impulses)
  - Shame (over helplessness)
- Acute and reactivated stress manifestations
  - Restlessness
  - Irritability
  - Fatigue
  - Increased startle reaction
  - A feeling of tension
- Inability to concentrate, sleep disturbances (insomnia, bad dreams), and somatic preoccupations often lead to self-medication, most commonly with alcohol or other central nervous system depressants

DIFFERENTIAL DIAGNOSIS

- Anxiety disorders
- Affective disorders
- Personality disorders exacerbated by stress
- Somatic disorders with psychic overlay

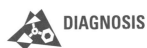 **DIAGNOSIS**

DIAGNOSTIC PROCEDURES

- Obtain history
- Identify precipitating sources of stress

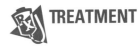 **TREATMENT**

MEDICATIONS

- Judicious use of sedatives (Table 145) (eg, lorazepam, 1–2 mg PO daily) for a limited time and as part of an overall treatment plan can provide relief

THERAPEUTIC PROCEDURES

- Behavioral
  - Stress reduction techniques include immediate symptom reduction (eg, rebreathing in a bag for hyperventilation) or early recognition and removal from a stress source before full-blown symptoms appear
  - It is often helpful for the patient to keep a daily log of stress precipitators, responses, and alleviators
  - Relaxation and exercise techniques are also helpful in reducing the reaction to stressful events
- Social
  - While it is not easy for the patient to make necessary changes (or they would have been made long ago), it is important for the clinician to establish the framework of the problem, since the patient's denial system may obscure the issues
  - Clarifying the problem allows the patient to begin viewing it within the proper context and facilitates the sometimes difficult decisions the patient eventually must make (eg, change of job or relocation of adult dependent offspring)
- Psychological
  - Prolonged in-depth psychotherapy is seldom necessary in cases of isolated stress response or adjustment disorder
  - Supportive psychotherapy with an emphasis on the here and now and strengthening of existing coping mechanisms is a helpful approach

 OUTCOME

PROGNOSIS

- A return to satisfactory function after a short period is part of the clinical picture of this syndrome
- Resolution may be delayed if others' responses to the patient's difficulties are thoughtlessly harmful or if the secondary gains outweigh the advantages of recovery
- The longer the symptoms persist, the worse the prognosis

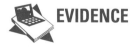 **EVIDENCE**

WEB SITES

- American Psychiatric Association
- Internet Mental Health

INFORMATION FOR PATIENTS

- American Academy of Family Physicians: Stress: Who Has Time for It? (for teens)
- American Academy of Family Physicians: When You Are the Caregiver
- National Cancer Institute
- National Institutes of Health: Adjustment Disorders

REFERENCES

- Ehlers A et al. Early psychological interventions for survivors of trauma: a review. Biol Psychiatry. 2003 May 1; 53(9):817–26. [PMID: 12725974]
- Katon WJ et al. Dissemination of evidence-based mental health interventions: importance to the trauma field. J Trauma Stress. 2006 Oct;19(5):611–23. [PMID: 17075915]
- Vaiva G et al. Immediate treatment with propranolol decreases posttraumatic stress disorder two months after trauma. Biol Psychiatry. 2003 Nov 1;54(9):947–9. [PMID: 14573324]

Stroke, Intracerebral Hemorrhage

 KEY FEATURES

ESSENTIALS OF DIAGNOSIS

- Hypertension is the usual cause
- Usually occurs suddenly and without warning, often during activity

GENERAL CONSIDERATIONS

Hypertensive intracerebral hemorrhage

- Spontaneous intracerebral hemorrhage in patients with no angiographic evidence of an associated vascular anomaly (eg, aneurysm or angioma) is usually due to hypertension
- Likely pathologic basis is microaneurysms that develop on perforating vessels 100–300 mcm in diameter in hypertensive patients
- Occurs most frequently in the basal ganglia and less commonly in the pons, thalamus, cerebellum, and cerebral white matter

- Extension into the ventricular system or subarachnoid space may cause signs of meningeal irritation

Other causes

- May occur with
  - Hematologic and bleeding disorders (eg, leukemia, thrombocytopenia, hemophilia, or disseminated intravascular coagulation)
  - Anticoagulant therapy
  - Liver disease
  - Cerebral amyloid angiopathy
  - Primary or secondary brain tumors
- There is also an association with advancing age, male sex, and high alcohol intake
- Bleeding from an intracranial aneurysm or arteriovenous malformation is primarily into the subarachnoid space, but it may also be partly intraparenchymal
- In some cases, no specific cause for cerebral hemorrhage can be identified

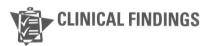 **CLINICAL FINDINGS**

SYMPTOMS AND SIGNS

Hemorrhage into the cerebral hemisphere

- Consciousness is initially lost or impaired in about 50% of patients
- Vomiting is frequent at the onset, and headache is sometimes present
- Focal symptoms and signs follow, depending on the site of the bleed
- With hypertensive hemorrhage, there is generally a rapidly evolving neurologic deficit with hemiplegia or hemiparesis
- A hemisensory disturbance occurs with more deeply placed lesions
- With lesions of the putamen, loss of conjugate lateral gaze may be present
- With thalamic hemorrhage, there may be a loss of upward gaze, downward or skew deviation of the eyes, lateral gaze palsies, and pupillary inequalities

Cerebellar hemorrhage

- Sudden onset of nausea and vomiting, disequilibrium, headache, and loss of consciousness that may be fatal within 48 hours
- Less commonly, the onset is gradual and episodic or slowly progressive, suggesting an expanding cerebellar lesion
- Onset and course can be intermediate
  - Lateral conjugate gaze palsies to the side of the lesion
  - Small reactive pupils
  - Contralateral hemiplegia; peripheral facial weakness

– Ataxia of gait, limbs, or trunk
– Periodic respiration
– Some combination of these findings

DIFFERENTIAL DIAGNOSIS

- Ischemic stroke
- Subarachnoid hemorrhage
- Space-occupying lesion, eg, brain tumor
- Subdural or epidural hemorrhage

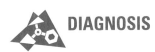 DIAGNOSIS

LABORATORY TESTS

- A predisposing cause may be revealed by
  – Complete blood cell count
  – Platelet count
  – Bleeding time
  – Prothrombin and partial thrombo-plastin times
  – Liver and renal function tests
- Lumbar puncture is contraindicated because it may cause herniation in patients with a large hematoma

IMAGING STUDIES

- CT scanning (without contrast) is important in confirming hemorrhage and for determining the size and site of the hematoma
- CT is superior to MRI for detecting intracranial hemorrhage of less than 48 hours' duration
- If the patient's condition permits further intervention, cerebral angiography may reveal an aneurysm or arteriovenous malformation

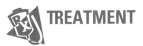 TREATMENT

SURGERY

- In cerebellar hemorrhage, prompt surgical evacuation of the hematoma is appropriate
- Decompression is helpful when a superficial hematoma in cerebral white matter is causing mass effect and herniation
- Ventricular drainage may be required in patients with intraventricular hemorrhage and acute hydrocephalus

THERAPEUTIC PROCEDURES

- In noncerebellar hemorrhage, neurologic management is generally conservative and supportive, either in cases of profound deficit with associated brainstem compression or more localized deficits

- The treatment of underlying structural lesions or bleeding disorders depends on their nature
- Randomized trials of recombinant activated factor Vll given within a few hours of onset are in progress

 OUTCOME

PROGNOSIS

- Surgery for cerebellar hemorrhage may lead to complete resolution of the clinical deficit
- Untreated cerebellar hemorrhage can spontaneously deteriorate with a fatal outcome from brainstem herniation

WHEN TO ADMIT

- All patients

 EVIDENCE

PRACTICE GUIDELINES

- American Academy of Neurology

INFORMATION FOR PATIENTS

- Parmet S et al. JAMA patient page: Hemorrhagic stroke. JAMA. 2004; 292:1916. [PMID: 15494591]
- National Institute of Neurological Disorders and Stroke

REFERENCE

- Mayer SA et al. Treatment of intracerebral haemorrhage. Lancet Neurol. 2005 Oct;4(10):662–72. [PMID: 16168935]

Stroke, Ischemic

 KEY FEATURES

ESSENTIALS OF DIAGNOSIS

- Thrombotic or embolic occlusion of a major vessel leads to cerebral infarction
- The resulting deficit depends on the particular vessel involved and the extent of any collateral circulation

GENERAL CONSIDERATIONS

- Strokes are traditionally subdivided into infarcts (thrombotic or embolic) and

hemorrhages, but clinical distinction may not be possible
- A previous stroke is a risk factor for a subsequent stroke

DEMOGRAPHICS

- The third leading cause of death in the United States, despite a general decline in the incidence of stroke in the last 30 years

 CLINICAL FINDINGS

SYMPTOMS AND SIGNS

- See Table 131
- Onset is usually abrupt, and there may then be very little progression except that due to brain swelling
- Examine the heart for murmur or arrhythmia and the carotid and subclavian arteries for bruits
- In hemiplegia of pontine origin, the eyes often deviate toward the paralyzed side
- In a hemispheric lesion, the eyes commonly deviate away from the hemiplegic side

Carotid circulation

- Ophthalmic artery occlusion
  – Symptomless in most
  – May produce amaurosis fugax—sudden and brief loss of vision in one eye
- Anterior cerebral artery occlusion distal to junction with anterior communicating artery
  – Weakness and cortical sensory loss in the contralateral leg and sometimes mild proximal arm weakness
  – May see contralateral grasp reflex, paratonic rigidity, and abulia (lack of initiative) or frank confusion
  – Urinary incontinence is common
- Middle cerebral artery occlusion
  – Contralateral hemiplegia, hemisensory loss, and homonymous hemianopia (ie, bilaterally symmetric loss of vision in half of the visual fields), with the eyes deviated to the side of the lesion
  – If the dominant hemisphere is involved, global aphasia is present
  – May be impossible to distinguish from occlusion of the internal carotid artery
  – May see considerable swelling of the hemisphere, leading to drowsiness, stupor, and coma
- Anterior main division occlusion of the middle cerebral artery
  – Expressive dysphasia

– Contralateral paralysis and loss of sensations in the arm, the face, and, to a lesser extent, the leg
- Posterior branch occlusion of the middle cerebral artery
  – Receptive (Wernicke's) aphasia
  – Homonymous visual field defect

Vertebrobasilar circulation

- Posterior cerebral artery occlusion may lead to
  – Thalamic syndrome of sensory loss
  – Ipsilateral facial, ninth and tenth cranial nerve lesions
  – Limb ataxia and numbness
  – Horner's syndrome, combined with contralateral sensory loss of the limb
- Occlusion of both vertebral arteries or the basilar artery
  – Coma with pinpoint pupils
  – Flaccid quadriplegia
  – Sensory loss
  – Variable cranial nerve abnormalities
- Partial basilar artery occlusion
  – Diplopia
  – Visual loss
  – Vertigo
  – Dysarthria
  – Ataxia
  – Weakness or sensory disturbances in some or all of the limbs
  – Discrete cranial nerve palsies
- Occlusion of any major cerebellar artery
  – Vertigo
  – Nausea
  – Vomiting
  – Nystagmus
  – Ipsilateral limb ataxia
  – Contralateral spinothalamic sensory loss in the limbs
  – Massive cerebellar infarction may lead to coma, tonsillar herniation, and death

DIFFERENTIAL DIAGNOSIS

- Hypoglycemia
- Transient ischemic attack
- Intracerebral hemorrhage or other mass lesion (eg, tumor)
- Focal seizure (Todd's paralysis)
- Migraine
- Peripheral causes of vertigo (Ménière's disease)

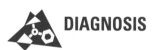 **DIAGNOSIS**

LABORATORY TESTS

- Complete blood cell count, sedimentation rate, blood glucose, and serologic tests for syphilis
- Antiphospholipid antibodies, serum lipids, and homocysteine
- ECG to help exclude a cardiac arrhythmia or recent myocardial infarction that might be a source of embolization
- Blood cultures if endocarditis is suspected

IMAGING STUDIES

- A CT scan of the head (without contrast) excludes cerebral hemorrhage but may not distinguish between a cerebral infarct and a tumor
- CT scanning is preferable to MRI in the acute stage because it is quicker and hemorrhage is not easily detected by MRI in the first 48 hours
- In selected patients, carotid duplex studies, MRI and MR angiography, and conventional angiography may also be necessary
- Diffusion-weighted MRI is more sensitive than standard MRI in detecting cerebral ischemia
- Echocardiography if heart disease is suspected

DIAGNOSTIC PROCEDURES

- Holter monitoring if paroxysmal cardiac arrhythmia suspected

 TREATMENT

MEDICATIONS

- If the CT shows no hemorrhage and there is a cardiac source of embolization, start intravenous heparin while warfarin is introduced, with a target INR of 2–3 for the prothrombin time
- Some physicians prefer to wait for 2 or 3 days before initiating anticoagulant treatment after repeat CT scan shows no evidence of hemorrhagic transformation
- Intravenous thrombolytic therapy with recombinant tissue plasminogen activator
  – 0.9 mg/kg to a maximum of 90 mg, with 10% given as a bolus over 1 minute and the remainder over 1 hour
  – Effective in reducing the neurologic deficit in selected patients who have no CT evidence of intracranial hemorrhage when given within 3 hours of symptom onset
  – Later administration has not been proved effective or safe
- Contraindications to thrombolytic therapy
  – Recent hemorrhage
  – Increased risk of hemorrhage (eg, treatment with anticoagulants), arterial puncture at a noncompressible site
  – Systolic pressure above 185 mm Hg or diastolic pressure above 110 mm Hg

THERAPEUTIC PROCEDURES

- Early management consists of general supportive measures
- Avoid lowering the blood pressure of hypertensive patients within 2 weeks of stroke because ischemic areas may be further compromised—unless the systolic pressure exceeds 200 mm Hg, in which case it can be lowered gradually to 170–200 mm Hg and then, after 2 weeks, reduced further
- Physical therapy with early mobilization and active rehabilitation are important
- Occupational therapy may improve morale and motor skills
- Speech therapy may be beneficial in patients with expressive dysphasia or dysarthria

 OUTCOME

PROGNOSIS

- The prognosis for survival after cerebral infarction is better than after cerebral or subarachnoid hemorrhage
- Loss of consciousness after a cerebral infarct implies a poorer prognosis than otherwise
- The extent of the infarct governs the potential for rehabilitation

PREVENTION

- Patients who have had a cerebral infarct are at risk for further strokes and for myocardial infarcts
- Statin therapy to lower serum lipid levels may reduce this risk
- Antiplatelet therapy with aspirin (325 mg PO once daily)
  – Reduces the recurrence rate by 30% among patients who have no cardiac cause for the stroke and who are not candidates for carotid endarterectomy
  – Nevertheless, the cumulative risk of recurrence of noncardioembolic stroke is still 3–7% annually
- A 2-year comparison did not show benefit of warfarin (INR 1.4–2.8) over aspirin (325 mg PO once daily)
- Higher doses of warfarin should be avoided because they lead to an increased incidence of major bleeding

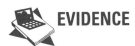

EVIDENCE

PRACTICE GUIDELINES

- Adams H et al. Guidelines for the early management of patients with ischemic stroke: 2005 guidelines update. A scientific statement from the Stroke Council of the American Heart Association/American Stroke Association. Stroke. 2005;36:916. [PMID: 15800252]
- Albers GW et al. Antithrombotic and thrombolytic therapy for ischemic stroke: the Seventh ACCP Conference on Antithrombotic and Thrombolytic Therapy. Chest. 2004;126(3 Suppl): 483S. [PMID: 15383482]
- American Stroke Association/American Academy of Neurology Joint Report: Anticoagulants and antiplatelet agents in acute ischemic stroke. Stroke. 2002; 33:1934. [PMID: 12105379]

INFORMATION FOR PATIENTS

- UCSF Neurocritical Care and Stroke

REFERENCES

- Amarenco P et al; Stroke Prevention by Aggressive Reduction in Cholesterol Levels (SPARCL) Investigators. High-dose atorvastatin after stroke or transient ischemic attack. N Engl J Med. 2006 Aug 10;355(6):549–59. [PMID: 16899775]
- Di Carlo A et al; European BIOMED Study of Stroke Care Group. Risk factors and outcome of subtypes of ischemic stroke. Data from a multicenter multinational hospital-based registry. The European Community Stroke Project. J Neurol Sci. 2006 May 15; 244(1–2):143–50. [PMID: 16530226]
- Edgell R et al. Acute endovascular stroke therapy. Curr Neurol Neurosci Rep. 2006 Nov;6(6):531–8. [PMID: 17074290]
- Hart RG et al. Lessons from the Stroke Prevention in Atrial Fibrillation trials. Ann Intern Med. 2003 May 20; 138(10):831–8. [PMID: 12755555]
- Subramaniam S et al. Massive cerebral infarction. Neurologist. 2005 May; 11(3):150–60. [PMID: 15860137]

Stroke, Lacunar

 KEY FEATURES

- Small lesions (usually < 5 mm in diameter) occur in the distribution of
  - Short, penetrating arteries in the basal ganglia
  - Pons
  - Cerebellum
  - Anterior limb of the internal capsule
  - Deep cerebral white matter (less common)
- Risk factors include poorly controlled hypertension and diabetes mellitus
- Generally has a good prognosis, with partial or complete resolution often occurring over 4–6 weeks

 CLINICAL FINDINGS

- There are several clinical syndromes
  - Contralateral pure motor or pure sensory deficit
  - Ipsilateral ataxia with crural paresis
  - Dysarthria with clumsiness of the hand
- Deficits may progress over 24–36 h before stabilizing

 DIAGNOSIS

- Sometimes visible on CT scans as small, punched-out, hypodense areas, but in other patients no abnormality is seen
- In some instances, patients with a clinical syndrome suggestive of lacunar infarction are found to have a severe hemispheric infarct on CT scanning

 TREATMENT

- Control hypertension or diabetes mellitus
- Avoid tobacco use
- Anticoagulation is not indicated
- Aspirin, 325 mg PO once daily, is of uncertain benefit

Stupor and Coma

 KEY FEATURES

ESSENTIALS OF DIAGNOSIS

- The stuporous patient is unresponsive except when subjected to repeated vigorous stimuli
- The comatose patient is unarousable and unable to respond to external events or inner needs, although reflex movements and posturing may be present

GENERAL CONSIDERATIONS

- Coma is a major complication of serious CNS disorders
- Abrupt onset of coma suggests
  - Subarachnoid hemorrhage
  - Brainstem stroke
  - Intracerebral hemorrhage
  - Acute herniation
- A slower onset and progression of coma occur with other structural or mass lesions
- A metabolic cause is likely with a preceding intoxicated state or agitated delirium
- **Intracranial causes**
  - Anoxic brain injury or head trauma
  - Ischemic stroke or intracerebral hemorrhage
  - Subarachnoid hemorrhage
  - Meningitis or encephalitis
  - Brainstem hemorrhage, infarct, or mass
  - Cerebral mass lesion causing brainstem compression
  - Subdural hematoma
  - Seizure
- **Metabolic causes**
  - Hypoglycemia
  - Diabetic ketoacidosis
  - Hyperglycemic hyperosmolar state
  - Drugs, eg, alcohol, opioids, sedatives, antidepressants, salicylates
  - Uremic or hepatic encephalopathy
  - Hypernatremia or hyponatremia
  - Hypercalcemia
  - Hypothermia
  - Heat stroke
  - Myxedema
  - Carbon monoxide poisoning

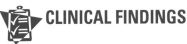 **CLINICAL FINDINGS**

SYMPTOMS AND SIGNS

- In stupor, response to painful stimuli
  - Purposive limb withdrawal from painful stimuli implies that sensory

pathways from and motor pathways to the stimulated limb are functionally intact

– Unilateral absence of responses to stimuli to both sides of the body implies a corticospinal lesion, bilateral absence of responses suggests brainstem involvement, bilateral pyramidal tract lesions, or psychogenic unresponsiveness

– Decorticate posturing occurs with lesions of the internal capsule and rostral cerebral peduncle, decerebrate posturing with dysfunction or destruction of the midbrain and rostral pons

• Pupils

– Hypothalamic disease processes may lead to unilateral Horner's syndrome

– Bilateral diencephalic involvement or destructive pontine lesions leads to small but reactive pupils

– Ipsilateral pupillary dilation with no response to light occurs with compression of the third cranial nerve, eg, with uncal herniation

– Pupils are slightly smaller than normal but responsive to light in many metabolic encephalopathies

– Pupils may be fixed and dilated following overdosage with atropine, scopolamine, or glutethimide

– Pupils may be pinpoint (but responsive) with opiates

– Pupillary dilation for several hours after cardiopulmonary arrest implies a poor prognosis

• Eye movements

– Conjugate deviation to the side suggests the presence of an ipsilateral hemispheric lesion or a contralateral pontine lesion

– A mesencephalic lesion leads to downward conjugate deviation

– Dysconjugate ocular deviation in coma implies a structural brainstem lesion (or preexisting strabismus)

• Oculomotor responses to passive head turning

– In response to brisk rotation, flexion, and extension of the head, conscious patients with open eyes do not exhibit contraversive conjugate eye deviation (doll's-head eye response) unless there is voluntary visual fixation or bilateral frontal pathology

– With cortical depression in lightly comatose patients, a brisk doll's-head eye response is seen

– With brainstem lesions, this oculocephalic reflex becomes impaired or lost, depending on the lesion site

• Oculovestibular reflex

– Tested by caloric stimulation using irrigation with ice water

– In normal persons, jerk nystagmus is elicited for about 2 or 3 minutes, with the slow component toward the irrigated ear

– In unconscious patients with an intact brainstem, the fast component of the nystagmus disappears, so that the eyes tonically deviate toward the irrigated side for 2–3 minutes before returning to their original position

– With impairment of brainstem function, the response is perverted and disappears

– In metabolic coma, oculocephalic and oculovestibular reflex responses are preserved, at least initially

• Respiratory patterns

– Cheyne-Stokes respiration may occur with bihemispheric or diencephalic disease or in metabolic disorders

– Hyperventilation occurs with lesions of the brainstem tegmentum

– Apneustic breathing (prominent end-inspiratory pauses) suggests damage at the pontine level

– Atactic breathing (completely irregular pattern, with deep and shallow breaths occurring randomly) associated with lesions of the lower pons and medulla

DIFFERENTIAL DIAGNOSIS

• Brain death
• Persistent vegetative state
• Locked-in syndrome

 DIAGNOSIS

LABORATORY TESTS

• Serum glucose, electrolyte, and calcium levels
• Arterial blood gases
• Liver and renal function tests
• Toxicologic studies

IMAGING STUDIES

• CT scan to identify a structural lesion

DIAGNOSTIC PROCEDURES

• The diagnostic workup of the comatose patient must proceed concomitantly with management
• Lumbar puncture (if CT scan reveals no structural lesion) to exclude subarachnoid hemorrhage or meningitis

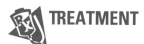 **TREATMENT**

MEDICATIONS

• Dextrose 50% (25 g), naloxone (0.4–1.2 mg), and thiamine (50 mg) are given intravenously

THERAPEUTIC PROCEDURES

• Treatment of coma depends on underlying cause
• Emergency measures
  – Supportive therapy for respiration or blood pressure is initiated
  – In hypothermia, all vital signs may be absent; all such patients should be rewarmed before the prognosis is assessed
  – The patient is positioned on one side with the neck partly extended, dentures removed, and secretions cleared by suction
  – If necessary, the patency of the airways is maintained with an oropharyngeal airway

 OUTCOME

WHEN TO ADMIT

• All patients to an ICU

PROGNOSIS

• In coma because of cerebral ischemia and hypoxia, the absence of pupillary light reflexes at the time of initial examination implies little chance of regaining independence
• By contrast, preserved pupillary light responses, the development of spontaneous eye movements (roving, conjugate, or better), and extensor, flexor, or withdrawal responses to pain at this early stage imply a relatively good prognosis

 EVIDENCE

INFORMATION FOR PATIENTS

• National Institute of Neurological Disorders and Stroke

REFERENCES

• Stevens RD et al. Approach to the comatose patient. Crit Care Med. 2006 Jan;34(1):31–41. [PMID: 16374153]
• Wijdicks EF et al. Practice parameter: prediction of outcome in comatose survivors after cardiopulmonary resuscita-

tion (an evidence-based review): report of the Quality Standards Subcommittee of the American Academy of Neurology. Neurology. 2006 Jul 25;67(2):203–10. [PMID: 16864809]

Subarachnoid Hemorrhage

 KEY FEATURES

ESSENTIALS OF DIAGNOSIS

- Sudden severe headache
- Signs of meningeal irritation usually present
- Obtundation or coma common
- Focal deficits frequently absent

GENERAL CONSIDERATIONS

- 5–10% of strokes are due to subarachnoid hemorrhage
- Hemorrhage is usually from rupture of an aneurysm or arteriovenous malformation
- No specific cause found in 20% of cases
- See Table 131

 CLINICAL FINDINGS

SYMPTOMS AND SIGNS

- Sudden onset of headache with severity never experienced previously by the patient
- May be followed by nausea and vomiting and loss or impairment of consciousness (transient, or progressing to coma and death)
- Patient is often confused and irritable and may show other symptoms of an altered mental status
- Nuchal rigidity and other signs of meningeal irritation are seen, except in deeply comatose patients
- Focal neurologic deficits may be present and may suggest the site of the underlying lesion

DIFFERENTIAL DIAGNOSIS

- Meningitis
- Migraine
- Intracerebral hemorrhage
- Ischemic stroke

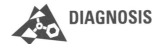 **DIAGNOSIS**

IMAGING STUDIES

- CT scan should be performed immediately to confirm that hemorrhage has occurred and to search for its source
- CT is faster and more sensitive in detecting hemorrhage in the first 24 hours than MRI
- Rarely, CT is normal in patients with suspected hemorrhage
- If CT is normal in such patients, examine cerebrospinal fluid for blood or xanthochromia before the possibility of subarachnoid hemorrhage is discounted

DIAGNOSTIC PROCEDURES

- Cerebral arteriography
  - Helps determine the source of bleeding
  - Performed when the patient's condition has stabilized and surgery is feasible
- Bilateral carotid and vertebral arteriography are necessary because aneurysms are often multiple, while arteriovenous malformations may be supplied from several sources
- MR angiography
  - May also permit visualization of vascular anomalies
  - Less sensitive than conventional arteriography

 TREATMENT

MEDICATIONS

- Phenytoin to prevent seizures

SURGERY

- Causal lesion is treated surgically or by interventional radiology

THERAPEUTIC PROCEDURES

- Major aim is to prevent further hemorrhage
- Conscious patients
  - Confine to bed
  - Advise against exertion or straining
  - Treat symptomatically for headache and anxiety
  - Give laxatives or stool softeners
- Lower blood pressure gradually for severe hypertension, but not below a diastolic level of 90 mm Hg

 OUTCOME

PROGNOSIS

- Approximately 20% of patients with aneurysms have further bleeding within 2 weeks and 40% within 6 months
- The greatest risk of further aneurysmal hemorrhage is within a few days of the initial bleed, thus early obliteration (within 2 days) is preferred
- When an arteriovenous malformation is responsible, treatment may be delayed until the patient's state is optimal

WHEN TO ADMIT

- All patients

PREVENTION

- See Aneurysm, Intracranial

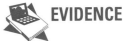 **EVIDENCE**

PRACTICE GUIDELINES

- American Society of Interventional and Therapeutic Neuroradiology. Mechanical and pharmacologic treatment of vasospasm. AJNR Am J Neuroradiol. 2001;22(8 Suppl):S26. [PMID: 11686071]

WEB SITE

- The Brain Aneurysm Foundation

INFORMATION FOR PATIENTS

- The Brain Aneurysm Foundation

REFERENCES

- Doerfler A et al. Endovascular treatment of cerebrovascular disease. Curr Opin Neurol. 2004 Aug;17(4):481–7. [PMID: 15247546]
- Molyneux AJ et al. International Subarachnoid Aneurysm Trial (ISAT) of neurosurgical clipping versus endovascular coiling in 2143 patients with ruptured intracranial aneurysms: a randomised comparison of effects on survival, dependency, seizures, rebleeding, subgroups, and aneurysm occlusion. Lancet. 2005 Sep 3–9; 366(9488):809–17. [PMID: 16139655]
- Nieuwkamp DJ et al. Subarachnoid haemorrhage in patients ≥ 75 years: clinical course, treatment and outcome. J Neurol Neurosurg Psychiatry. 2006 Aug;77(8):933-7. [PMID: 16638789]

- Pouratian N et al. Endovascular management of unruptured intracranial aneurysms. J Neurol Neurosurg Psychiatry. 2006 May;77(5):572–8. [PMID: 16614015]

Syncope

 KEY FEATURES

- Transient loss of consciousness and postural tone for few seconds to few minutes
- Caused by inadequate cerebral blood flow
- Prompt recovery without resuscitative measures
- Causes include cardiac, vascular, and neurologic processes
- More likely in those with heart disease, older men, and young women prone to vasovagal episodes
- 30% of adults will experience ≥ 1 syncopal episode
- Accounts for ~3% of ED visits

 CLINICAL FINDINGS

Vasomotor
- Caused by excessive vagal tone or impaired reflex control of the peripheral circulation
- "Common faint" most common
  - Often initiated by stressful situations
  - Common premonitory symptoms
    □ Nausea
    □ Diaphoresis
    □ Tachycardia
    □ Pallor
- Other varieties: carotid sinus hypersensitivity, postmicturition, or cough syncope

Orthostatic
- Caused by impaired vasoconstrictive response to assuming upright posture, leading to abrupt decrease in venous return
- Occurs in
  - Advanced age
  - Diabetes or other cause of autonomic neuropathy
  - Blood loss or hypovolemia
  - Vasodilator, diuretic, or adrenergic-blocker therapy

Cardiogenic
- Caused by
  - Rhythm disturbances (sick sinus syndrome, AV block, tachyarrhythmias)
  - Mechanical causes (aortic or pulmonary stenosis, hypertrophic obstructive cardiomyopathy, pulmonary hypertension, atrial myxoma)
- Episodes are often exertional

 DIAGNOSIS

- Examine for orthostatic changes in BP and pulse, cardiac abnormalities, and response to carotid sinus massage
- Specific cause found on initial examination in only 50%
- Resting ECG
  - Arrhythmias
  - Accessory pathways
  - Infarction
  - Hypertrophy
- Do tilt-table testing before invasive studies unless clinical and ambulatory ECG evaluation suggests a cardiac cause

Vasomotor
- Characteristic history
- Carotid sinus massage under carefully monitored conditions or tilt-table testing may be diagnostic

Orthostatic
- > 20 mm Hg decline in BP immediately on standing
- Tilt-table testing and Valsalva's maneuver are diagnostic

Cardiogenic
- Echocardiography to rule out mechanical causes
- If rhythm disturbance suspected, ambulatory ECG monitoring indicated; may need to repeat several times, up to 3 days
- Event recorder and transtelephone ECG monitoring indicated for more intermittent presyncopal episodes
- Electrophysiologic studies indicated for
  - Recurrent episodes
  - Nondiagnostic ambulatory ECGs
  - Ischemic cardiomyopathy

 TREATMENT

Vasomotor
- Avoid the inciting stimuli
- Lie down
- β-Blockers may be helpful
- Permanent pacing rarely indicated

Orthostatic
- Discontinue offending drugs
- Stand up slowly
- Fludrocortisone rarely effective

Cardiogenic
- Treat the underlying disorder
- Bradyarrhythmias: permanent pacemaker placement may be indicated
- Ventricular tachyarrhythmias: implantable cardioverter-defibrillator may be indicated

Syndrome of Inappropriate Antidiuretic Hormone (SIADH)

KEY FEATURES

ESSENTIALS OF DIAGNOSIS

- Serum Na^+ concentration < 130 mEq/L
- Hypotonic, euvolemic hyponatremia

GENERAL CONSIDERATIONS

- Hyponatremia occurs from abnormal water balance rather than abnormal sodium balance
- Inappropriate antidiuretic hormone (ADH) excess and consequent retention of water due to impaired excretion results in hyponatremia and low serum osmolality
- Hospitalized patients treated with hypotonic fluid are at increased risk for hyponatremia
- Patterns of abnormal ADH secretion
  - Random secretion (eg, carcinomas)
  - Reset osmostat (eg, elderly, pulmonary diseases)
  - Leak of ADH (eg, basilar skull fractures)

Etiology
- CNS disorders
  - Head trauma
  - Stroke
  - Subarachnoid hemorrhage
  - Hydrocephalus
  - Brain tumor
  - Encephalitis
  - Guillain-Barré syndrome
  - Meningitis

– Acute psychosis
– Acute intermittent porphyria
• **Pulmonary lesions**
– Tuberculosis
– Bacterial pneumonia
– Aspergillosis
– Bronchiectasis
– Neoplasms
– Positive pressure ventilation
• **Malignancies**
– Bronchogenic carcinoma
– Pancreatic carcinoma
– Prostatic carcinoma
– Renal cell carcinoma
– Adenocarcinoma of colon
– Thymoma
– Osteosarcoma
– Malignant lymphoma
– Leukemia
• **Drugs: Increased ADH production**
– Amiodarone
– Antidepressants: tricyclics, monoamine oxidase inhibitors, selective serotonin reuptake inhibitors
– Antineoplastics: cyclophosphamide, vincristine
– Carbamazepine
– Methylenedioxymethamphetamine (MDMA; Ecstasy)
– Clofibrate
– Neuroleptics: thiothixene, thioridazine, fluphenazine, haloperidol, trifluoperazine
• **Drugs: Potentiated ADH action**
– Carbamazepine
– Chlorpropamide, tolbutamide
– Cyclophosphamide
– Nonsteroidal anti-inflammatory drugs
– Somatostatin and analogs
• **Others**
– Postoperative
– Pain
– Stress
– AIDS
– Pregnancy (physiological)
– Hypokalemia

DEMOGRAPHICS

• Most common cause of hyponatremia in hospitalized patients

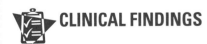 **CLINICAL FINDINGS**

SYMPTOMS AND SIGNS

• Frequently asymptomatic
• Symptoms usually seen with serum sodium levels < 120 mEq/L
• If symptomatic, primarily CNS symptoms of lethargy, weakness, confusion, delirium, and seizures

• Symptoms are often mistaken for primary neurologic or metabolic disorders

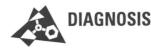 **DIAGNOSIS**

LABORATORY TESTS

• Serum Na^+ concentration < 130 mEq/L
• Decreased osmolality (< 280 mosm/kg) with inappropriately increased urine osmolality (> 150 mosm/kg)
• Low blood urea nitrogen (BUN) (< 10 mg/dL) and hypouricemia (< 4 mg/dL), which are not only dilutional but result from increased urea and uric acid clearances in response to the volume-expanded state
• A high BUN suggests a volume-contracted state, which excludes a diagnosis of SIADH

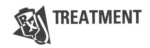 **TREATMENT**

MEDICATIONS

Symptomatic hyponatremia

• Initial goal: Achieve serum sodium concentration of 125–130 mEq/L, guarding against overly rapid correction
• Increase serum sodium concentration by ≤ 1–2 mEq/L/h and not > 25–30 mEq/L in first 2 days to prevent central pontine myelinolysis
• Rate should be reduced to 0.5–1.0 mEq/L/h as neurologic symptoms improve
• If CNS symptoms, hyponatremia should be immediately treated at any level of serum sodium concentration
• Hypertonic (eg, 3%) saline plus furosemide (0.5–1.0 mg/kg IV) indicated for symptomatic hyponatremia
– To determine how much 3% saline (513 mEq/L) to administer, obtain a spot urinary Na^+ after a furosemide diuresis has begun
– Excreted Na^+ is replaced with 3% saline, empirically begun at 1–2 mL/kg/h, and then adjusted based on urinary output and urinary sodium
– For example, after furosemide, urine volume may be 400 mL/h and sodium plus potassium excretion 100 mEq/L; excreted Na^+ is 40 mEq/h, which is replaced with 78 mL/h of 3% saline (40 mEq/h divided by 513 mEq/L)

Asymptomatic hyponatremia

• Increase serum sodium concentration by ≤ 0.5 mEq/L/h

– Restrict water intake to 0.5–1.0 L/day
– 0.9% saline with furosemide may be used when serum sodium < 120 mEq/L. Urinary sodium and potassium losses are replaced as above
– Demeclocycline, 300–600 mg PO BID
  ◻ Inhibits effect of ADH on distal tubule
  ◻ Useful for patients who cannot adhere to water restriction or need additional therapy
  ◻ Onset of action may be 1 week; concentrating may be permanently impaired
  ◻ Therapy with demeclocycline in cirrhosis appears to increase risk of renal failure
– For hospitalized patients with euvolemic SIADH, the selective V2 antagonist, conivaptan may be administered as a loading dose of 20 mg IV delivered continuously over 30 min, then as 20 mg IV continuously over 24 h. Subsequent infusions of 20–40 mg/d may be administered every 1–3 days
– Other selective V2 antagonists
  ◻ Mozavaptan is available in Japan, but not yet in the United States, for the treatment of paraneoplastic SIADH
  ◻ Tolvaptan is another promising agent, currently in clinical trials

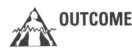 **OUTCOME**

FOLLOW-UP

• If symptomatic, measure plasma sodium ~q4h and observe the patient closely

COMPLICATIONS

• Central pontine myelinolysis may occur from osmotically induced demyelination as a result of overly rapid correction of serum sodium (an increase of more than 1 mEq/L/h, or 25 mEq/L within the first day of therapy)
• Hypoxic-anoxic episodes during hyponatremia may contribute to the demyelination

PROGNOSIS

• Associated with underlying cause of SIADH
• Premenopausal women in whom hyponatremic encephalopathy develops from rapidly acquired hyponatremia (eg, postoperative hyponatremia) are about 25 times more likely than postmenopausal women to die or to suffer permanent brain damage

WHEN TO ADMIT

- Symptomatic hyponatremia
- Serum sodium < 120 mEq/L

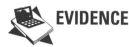

EVIDENCE

WEB SITE

- Fall PJ. Hyponatremia and hypernatremia: A systematic approach to causes and their correction. Postgraduate Medicine Online, 2000

INFORMATION FOR PATIENTS

- American Association for Clinical Chemistry: Lab Tests Online: Sodium
- Mayo Clinic: Low Blood Sodium in Older Adults
- MedlinePlus: ADH
- MedlinePlus: Dilutional Hyponatremia (SIADH)

REFERENCES

- Castello L et al. Hyponatremia in liver cirrhosis: pathophysiological principles of management. Dig Liver Dis. 2005 Feb;37(2):73–81. [PMID: 15733516]
- Ellison DH et al. Clinical practice. The syndrome of inappropriate antidiuresis. N Engl J Med. 2007 May 17; 356(20):2064–72. [PMID: 17507705]
- Goldsmith SR. Current treatments and novel pharmacologic treatments for hyponatremia in congestive heart failure. Am J Cardiol. 2005 May 2; 95(9A):14B–23B. [PMID: 15847853]
- Hoorn EJ et al. Diagnostic approach to a patient with hyponatremia: traditional versus physiology-based options. QJM. 2005 Jul;98(7):529–40. [PMID: 15955797]
- McDade G. Disorders of sodium balance: hyponatraemia and drug use (and abuse). BMJ. 2006 Apr 8; 332(7545):853. [PMID: 16601056]
- Reynolds RM et al. Disorders of sodium balance. BMJ. 2006 Mar 25; 332(7543):702–5. [PMID: 16565125]
- Riggs JE. Neurologic manifestations of electrolyte disturbances. Neurol Clin. 2002 Feb;20(1):227–39. [PMID: 11754308]
- Schrier RW et al; SALT Investigators. Tolvaptan, a selective oral vasopressin V2-receptor antagonist, for hyponatremia. N Engl J Med. 2006 Nov 16; 355(20):2099–112. [PMID: 17105757]

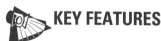

Syphilis

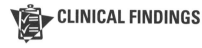

KEY FEATURES

ESSENTIALS OF DIAGNOSIS

- The spirochete can infect almost any organ or tissue in the body and cause protean clinical manifestations
- Transmission occurs most frequently during sexual contact
- Sites of inoculation are usually genital but may be extragenital

GENERAL CONSIDERATIONS

- The risk of syphilis after unprotected sex with an individual with infectious syphilis is ~30–50%
- Congenital syphilis: transmission from mother to fetus after the tenth week of pregnancy
- Two major clinical stages
  - Early (infectious) syphilis
  - Late syphilis
- Stages are separated by a symptom-free latent period
- During early latency (within the first year after infection) the infectious stage may recur
- **Early (infectious) syphilis**
  - Primary lesions (chancre and regional lymphadenopathy)
  - Secondary lesions (commonly involving skin and mucous membranes, occasionally bone, CNS, or liver)
  - Congenital lesions
- **Late syphilis** consists of
  - So-called benign (gummatous) lesions involving skin, bones, and viscera
  - Cardiovascular disease (principally aortitis)
  - CNS and ocular syndromes

DEMOGRAPHICS

- A dramatic increase in syphilis occurred from 1985 to 1990
- In 1998, a syphilis elimination program that emphasized screening, early treatment, contact tracing, and condom use began targeting high-risk populations
  - Women of childbearing age, sexually active teens
  - Drug users
  - Inmates of penal institutions
  - Persons with multiple sexual partners or those who have sex with sex workers

- Initially, there was a decrease in primary and secondary cases
  - However, in 2005 the number of cases increased to 8724; most likely due to lack of condom use and disinhibition in men having sex with men with availability of HAART

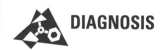

CLINICAL FINDINGS

SYMPTOMS AND SIGNS

Primary
- Painless ulcer (chancre) on genitalia, perianal area, rectum, pharynx, tongue, lip, or elsewhere 2–6 weeks after exposure
- Nontender enlargement of regional lymph nodes

Secondary
- Generalized maculopapular skin rash
- Mucous membrane lesions, including patches and ulcers
- Weeping papules (condylomas) in moist skin areas
- Generalized nontender lymphadenopathy
- Low-grade fever
- Meningitis, hepatitis, osteitis, arthritis, iritis

Relapsing, early latent
- No physical signs

Late latent ("hidden")
- No physical signs

Late (tertiary)
- Infiltrative tumors of skin, bones, liver (gummas)
- Aortitis, aneurysms, aortic regurgitation
- CNS disorders, including
  - Meningovascular and degenerative changes
  - Paresthesias
  - Sharp pains
  - Abnormal reflexes
  - Dementia
  - Psychosis

DIFFERENTIAL DIAGNOSIS

- Chancroid (usually painful)
- Lymphogranuloma venereum (uncommon in United States)
- Genital herpes
- Neoplasm
- Any lesion on genitalia should be considered possible primary syphilitic lesion

DIAGNOSIS

LABORATORY TESTS

- HIV test

Nontreponemal antigen tests

- VDRL and rapid plasma reagin (RPR)
  - Generally become positive 4–6 weeks after infection, or 1–3 weeks after a primary lesion
  - Not highly specific
- False-positive reactions are frequent in
  - Connective tissue or febrile diseases
  - Infectious mononucleosis
  - Malaria, leprosy
  - HIV
  - Injection drug use
  - Infective endocarditis
  - Old age
  - Hepatitis C
  - Pregnancy
- False-negative results when very high antibody titers are present (prozone phenomenon)
- RPR titers are often higher than VDRL titers and thus are not comparable
- Titers are used to assess adequacy of therapy
- The time required for titers to decrease is variable. In general, patients with recurrent infection, high initial titers and later stages of disease, or those who are HIV positive have slower seroconversion and some may remain serofast

Treponemal antibody tests

- The *T pallidum* hemagglutination (TPHA) test and the *T pallidum* particle agglutination (TPPA) test are comparable in specificity and sensitivity to the fluorescent treponemal antibody absorption test (FTA-ABS)
- The TPPA test is preferred method for confirming diagnosis because of its ease of performance
- These tests help determine whether a positive nontreponemal antigen test is false-positive or is indicative of syphilis
- Results are positive in most patients with primary syphilis and in almost all patients with secondary syphilis
- False-positive tests occur rarely in systemic lupus erythematosus and in other disorders associated with increased levels of γ-globulins
- Lyme disease may cause a false-positive treponemal test but rarely causes a false-positive reaginic test

DIAGNOSTIC PROCEDURES

- Dark-field microscopic examination
  - May show *T pallidum* in fresh exudate from lesions or aspirated material from regional lymph nodes in primary or secondary syphilis
  - Not recommended for oral lesions due to presence of non-pathogenic treponemes in the mouth

- Immunofluorescent staining for *T pallidum* of dried smears of fluid taken from early lesions may be helpful
- Cerebrospinal fluid (CSF) findings in neurosyphilis include
  - Elevated total protein
  - Lymphocytosis
  - Positive CSF VDRL; however may be negative in 30–70% of cases
- CSF may, however, be normal
- CSF FTA-ABS is not recommended

TREATMENT

MEDICATIONS

- For primary and secondary syphilis: benzathine penicillin G, 2.4 million units IM once
- For late latent syphilis or latent syphilis of unknown duration: benzathine penicillin G, 2.4 million units IM × 3 at 7-day intervals
- For neurosyphilis: aqueous penicillin G, 18–24 million units IV once daily (3–4 million units q4h or as a continuous infusion) for 10–14 days
- For patients allergic to penicillin
  - Doxycycline, 100 mg PO BID for 14 days, or tetracycline, 500 mg PO QID for 14 days, for infectious syphilis
  - In syphilis of more than 1-year duration or of unknown duration, treat for 28 days
- Ceftriaxone
  - Limited data available
  - Optimum dose and duration not well defined
- Azithromycin
  - Previously recommended as possible alternative treatment
  - Increasing resistance may limit its effectiveness
- Patients with gonorrhea and exposure to syphilis should be treated with separate regimens effective against both diseases

OUTCOME

FOLLOW-UP

- Patients must abstain from sexual activity until rendered noninfectious by antibiotic therapy
- Primary, secondary, early latent syphilis
  - Reexamine clinically and serologically at 3–6 month intervals
  - If VDRL or RPR titers fail to decrease fourfold by 6 months, repeat the HIV test
  - Consider lumbar puncture

- If careful follow-up cannot be ensured, repeat treatment with benzathine penicillin 2.4 million units IM weekly for 3 weeks
- Latent syphilis
  - Repeat serologies at 6, 12, and 24 months
  - If titers increase fourfold or if initially high titers (> 1:32) fail to decrease fourfold by 12–24 months, perform an HIV test and lumbar puncture and retreat
- Neurosyphilis
  - Repeat lumbar puncture every 6 months
  - If CSF cell count has not decreased by 6 months or is not normal at 2 years, give second course of treatment

COMPLICATIONS

- Jarisch-Herxheimer reaction
  - Manifests as fever and aggravation of the clinical picture
  - Usually begins within first 24 h of treatment and subsides within next 24 h
  - Treatment should not be discontinued unless symptoms become severe or threaten to be fatal or syphilitic laryngitis, auditory neuritis, or labyrinthitis is present
  - May be prevented or modified by simultaneous administration of antipyretics or corticosteroids

PROGNOSIS

- Late syphilis may be highly destructive, permanently disabling, and may lead to death
- If left untreated
  - Spontaneous cure will occur in ~one-third of patients
  - The latent phase will remain in ~one-third throughout their life
  - Serious late lesions will develop in ~one-third

WHEN TO REFER

- If uncertain about interpretation of serologic tests, need for lumbar puncture, or optimal therapy, or if patient has severe penicillin allergy

WHEN TO ADMIT

- Admit for complications (eg, stroke, meningoencephalitis, dementia) or for observation for Jarisch-Herxheimer reaction

PREVENTION

- Avoidance of sexual contact

- Latex condoms are effective but protects covered areas only

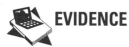

EVIDENCE

PRACTICE GUIDELINES

- National Guideline Clearinghouse: Screening for syphilis infection. United States Preventive Services Task Force, 2004.
- Sexually transmitted diseases treatment guidelines 2006. MMWR Recomm Rep. 2006 Aug 4;55(RR-11):1–94. [PMID: 16888612]

WEB SITE

- Centers for Disease Control and Prevention—National Center for HIV, STD and TB Prevention—Division of Sexually Transmitted Diseases

INFORMATION FOR PATIENTS

- American Social Health Organization
- Centers for Disease Control and Prevention—Division of Sexually Transmitted Diseases
- JAMA patient page. Syphilis. JAMA. 2000;284:520. [PMID: 10939892]

REFERENCES

- Goh BT. Syphilis in adults. Sex Transm Infect. 2005 Dec;81(6):448–52. [PMID: 16326843]
- Hall CS et al. Managing syphilis in the HIV-infected patient. Curr Infect Dis Rep. 2004 Feb;6(1):72–81. [PMID: 14733852]
- Marra CM et al. Normalization of cerebrospinal fluid abnormalities after neurosyphilis treatment: does HIV status matter? Clin Infect Dis. 2004 Feb 1; 189(3):369–76. [PMID: 14745693]
- O'Donnell JA et al. Neurosyphilis: A current review. Curr Infect Dis Rep. 2005 Jul;7(4):277–284. [PMID: 15963329]

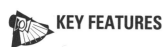

Systemic Lupus Erythematosus

KEY FEATURES

ESSENTIALS OF DIAGNOSIS

- Occurs mainly in young women
- Rash over areas exposed to sunlight
- Joint symptoms in 90% of patients
- Multiple system involvement
- Anemia, leukopenia, thrombocytopenia
- Antinuclear antibody with high titer to native DNA

GENERAL CONSIDERATIONS

- Systemic lupus erythematosus (SLE) is an inflammatory autoimmune disorder that affects multiple organ systems
- The clinical course is marked by spontaneous remission and relapses
- Four features of drug-induced lupus separate it from SLE
  - The sex ratio is nearly equal
  - Nephritis and central nervous system features are not ordinarily present
  - Hypocomplementemia and antibodies to native DNA are absent
  - The clinical features and most laboratory abnormalities usually revert toward normal when the offending drug is withdrawn

DEMOGRAPHICS

- 85% of patients are women
- Occurs in 1:1000 white women but in 1:250 black women

CLINICAL FINDINGS

SYMPTOMS AND SIGNS

- Fever, anorexia, malaise, and weight loss
- **Skin** lesions
  - Occur in most patients at some time
  - The characteristic "butterfly" rash affects less than 50%
  - Alopecia is common
- **Raynaud's** phenomenon (20% of patients) often antedates other symptoms
- **Joint** symptoms, with or without active synovitis
  - Occur in over 90% and are often the earliest manifestation
  - The arthritis is seldom deforming
- **Ocular**
  - Conjunctivitis
  - Photophobia
  - Blurring of vision
  - Transient or permanent monocular blindness
- **Pulmonary**
  - Pleurisy
  - Pleural effusion
  - Bronchopneumonia
  - Pneumonitis
  - Restrictive lung disease

- **Cardiac**
  - Pericarditis
  - Myocarditis
  - Arrhythmias
  - The typical verrucous endocarditis of Libman-Sacks is usually clinically silent but can produce acute or chronic valvular incompetence—most commonly mitral regurgitation—and can serve as a source of emboli
- **Mesenteric vasculitis**
  - Occasionally occurs and may resemble polyarteritis nodosa, including the presence of aneurysms in medium-sized blood vessels
  - Abdominal pain (particularly postprandial), ileus, peritonitis, and perforation may result
- **Neurologic**
  - Psychosis
  - Cognitive impairment
  - Seizures
  - Peripheral and cranial neuropathies
  - Transverse myelitis
  - Strokes
  - Severe depression and psychosis may be exacerbated by the administration of large doses of corticosteroids
- **Glomerulonephritis:** several forms may occur, including mesangial, focal and diffuse proliferative, and membranous

DIFFERENTIAL DIAGNOSIS

- Drug-induced lupus (Table 127) (especially procainamide, hydralazine, and isoniazid)
- Scleroderma
- Rheumatoid arthritis
- Inflammatory myopathy, especially dermatomyositis
- Rosacea
- Vasculitis, eg, polyarteritis nodosa
- Endocarditis
- Lyme disease

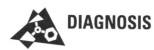

DIAGNOSIS

LABORATORY TESTS

- Production of many different autoantibodies (Table 123)
- Antinuclear antibody tests are sensitive but not specific for systemic lupus—ie, they are positive in most patients with lupus but are also positive in many patients with non-lupus conditions such as rheumatoid arthritis, hepatitis, and interstitial lung disease
- Antibodies to double-stranded DNA and to Sm are specific for SLE but not

sensitive, since they are present in only 60% and 30% of patients, respectively
- Depressed serum complement—a finding suggestive of disease activity—often returns toward normal in remission
- Three types of antiphospholipid antibodies occur
  - The first causes the biologic false-positive tests for syphilis
  - The second is lupus anticoagulant, a risk factor for venous and arterial thrombosis and miscarriage
  - The third is anticardiolipin antibody
- Abnormality of urinary sediment is almost always found in association with renal lesions. Red blood cells, with or without casts, and mild proteinuria are frequent

DIAGNOSTIC PROCEDURES

- The diagnosis can be made with reasonable probability if 4 of the 11 criteria set forth in Table 128 are met. These criteria should be viewed as rough guidelines that do not supplant clinical judgment in the diagnosis of SLE
- Renal biopsy is useful in deciding whether to treat with cyclophosphamide, and to rule out end-stage renal disease that may no longer benefit from treatment

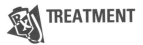 **TREATMENT**

MEDICATIONS

- Skin lesions often respond to the local administration of corticosteroids
- Minor joint symptoms can usually be alleviated by rest and nonsteroidal anti-inflammatory drugs (NSAIDs)
- Antimalarials (hydroxychloroquine) may be helpful in treating lupus rashes or joint symptoms that do not respond to NSAIDs
- Corticosteroids are required for the control of certain serious complications, such as
  - Thrombocytopenic purpura
  - Hemolytic anemia
  - Myocarditis
  - Pericarditis
  - Convulsions
  - Nephritis

- Immunosuppressive agents such as cyclophosphamide, chlorambucil, and azathioprine are used in cases resistant to corticosteroids
  - Cyclophosphamide improves renal survival
  - Overall patient survival, however, is no better than in the prednisone-treated group
- Systemic corticosteroids are not usually given for minor arthritis, skin rash, leukopenia, or the anemia associated with chronic disease

THERAPEUTIC PROCEDURES

- Avoid sun exposure and use sunscreen

 OUTCOME

COMPLICATIONS

- Thrombocytopenic purpura
- Hemolytic anemia
- Myocarditis
- Pericarditis
- Convulsions
- Nephritis

PROGNOSIS

- 10-year survival rate exceeds 85%
- In most patients, the illness pursues a relapsing and remitting course
- In some patients, the disease pursues a virulent course, leading to serious impairment of vital structures such as lung, heart, brain, or kidneys, and the disease may lead to death
- Accelerated atherosclerosis attributed, in part, to corticosteroid use, has been responsible for a rise in late deaths due to myocardial infarction

WHEN TO REFER

- Most patients should be monitored in consultation with a rheumatologist
- Severity of organ involvement dictates referral to other subspecialties, such as a nephrologist and pulmonologist

WHEN TO ADMIT

- Severe renal disease
- Pulmonary insufficiency

- Cardiac involvement
- Central nervous system disease
- Acute abdominal pain

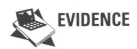 **EVIDENCE**

WEB SITES

- Arthritis Foundation
- Lupus Foundation of America

INFORMATION FOR PATIENTS

- National Institute of Arthritis and Musculoskeletal and Skin Diseases

REFERENCES

- Arbuckle MR et al. Development of autoantibodies before the clinical onset of systemic lupus erythematosus. N Engl J Med. 2003 Oct 16;349(16): 1526–33. [PMID: 14561795]
- Asanuma Y et al. Premature coronary-artery atherosclerosis in systemic lupus erythematosus. N Engl J Med. 2003 Dec 18;349(25):2407–15. [PMID: 14681506]
- Ginzler EM. Mycophenolate mofetil or intravenous cyclophosphamide for lupus nephritis. N Engl J Med. 2005 Nov 24;353(21):2219–28. [PMID: 16306519]
- Petri M et al; OC-SELENA Trial. Combined oral contraceptives in women with systemic lupus erythematosus. N Engl J Med. 2005 Dec 15;353(24): 2550–8. [PMID: 16354891]
- Somers EC et al. Use of a gonadotropin-releasing hormone analog for protection against premature ovarian failure during cyclophosphamide therapy in women with severe lupus. Arthritis Rheum. 2005 Sep;52(9):2761–7. [PMID: 16142702]
- Tseng CE et al. The effect of moderate-dose corticosteroids in preventing severe flares in patients with serologically active, but clinically stable, systemic lupus erythematosus: findings of a prospective, randomized, double-blind, placebo-controlled trial. Arthritis Rheum. 2006 Nov;54(11):3623–32. [PMID: 17075807]

Tardive Dyskinesia

 KEY FEATURES

- A syndrome of involuntary stereotyped movements of the face, mouth, tongue, trunk, limbs
- Occurs after months or (typically) years of neuroleptic treatment in 20–35% of patients
- Predisposing factors
  - Older age
  - Cigarette smoking
  - Diabetes mellitus
- Atypical antipsychotics appear to be lower risk
- Symptoms do not necessarily worsen and may improve even when neuroleptics are continued

 CLINICAL FINDINGS

- Early signs
  - Fine worm-like tongue movements
  - Difficulty sticking out the tongue
  - Facial tics
  - Increased blink frequency
  - Jaw movements
- Late signs
  - Lip smacking
  - Chewing motions
  - Disturbed gag reflex
  - Puffing of the cheeks
  - Respiratory distress
  - Disturbed speech
  - Choreoathetoid movements

 DIAGNOSIS

- Differentiate early signs of tardive dyskinesia from reversible side effects of medicines, such as tricyclic antidepressants and antiparkinsonism agents

 TREATMENT

- Emphasis should be on prevention by using lowest effective dose
- Stop anticholinergic drugs and gradually discontinue neuroleptic dose
- Benzodiazepines, buspirone, phosphatidylcholine, clonidine, calcium channel blockers, vitamin E, and propranolol are of limited usefulness in treating symptoms

Testicular Cancer

 KEY FEATURES

ESSENTIALS OF DIAGNOSIS

- Most common neoplasm in men aged 20–35
- Typical presentation as a patient-identified painless nodule
- Orchiectomy necessary for diagnosis

GENERAL CONSIDERATIONS

- Rare, 2–3 new cases per 100,000 males in the United States each year
- 90–95% of all primary testicular tumors are germ cell tumors (seminoma and nonseminoma); 5–10% are nongerminal neoplasms (Leydig cell, Sertoli cell, gonadoblastoma)
- Lifetime probability of developing testicular cancer is 0.2% for an American white male
- Slightly more common on the right than on the left, bilateral in 1–2%
- Cause unknown, though there may be a history of unilateral or bilateral cryptorchism
- Risk of development of malignancy is highest for an intra-abdominal testis (1:20) and lower for an inguinal testis (1:80)
- Orchiopexy does not alter the malignant potential of the cryptorchid testis; it does facilitate examination and tumor detection
- 5–10% of testicular tumors occur in the contralateral, normally descended testis

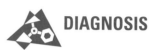 **CLINICAL FINDINGS**

SYMPTOMS AND SIGNS

- Most common symptom: painless enlargement of the testis
- Sensation of heaviness
- Acute testicular pain from intratesticular hemorrhage in ~10%
- Symptoms relating to metastatic disease, such as back pain (retroperitoneal metastases), cough (pulmonary metastases), or lower extremity edema (vena cava obstruction), in 10%
- Asymptomatic at presentation in 10%
- Physical examination: testicular mass or diffuse enlargement of the testis in most cases
- Secondary hydroceles in 5–10%
- Supraclavicular adenopathy
- Retroperitoneal mass
- Gynecomastia in 5% of germ cell tumors

DIFFERENTIAL DIAGNOSIS

- Epidermoid cyst

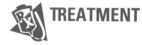 **DIAGNOSIS**

LABORATORY TESTS

- Serum human chorionic gonadotropin, α-fetoprotein, and lactate dehydrogenase
- Liver function tests

IMAGING STUDIES

- Scrotal ultrasound
- CT scan of abdomen and pelvis

TREATMENT

SURGERY

- Radical orchiectomy by inguinal exploration with early vascular control of the spermatic cord structures
- Scrotal approaches and open testicular biopsies should be avoided

Seminomas

- Stage I and IIa (retroperitoneal disease < 10 cm in diameter) seminomas treated by radical orchiectomy and retroperitoneal irradiation have 5-year disease-free survival rates of 98% and 92–94%, respectively
- Stage IIb (> 10 cm retroperitoneal involvement) and stage III seminomas are treated with primary chemotherapy (etoposide and cisplatin or cisplatin, etoposide, and bleomycin)
- Among stage III patients, 95% will attain a complete response following orchiectomy and chemotherapy

Nonseminomas

- Up to 75% of stage A nonseminomas are cured by orchiectomy alone
- Modified retroperitoneal lymph node dissections have been designed to preserve the sympathetic innervation required for ejaculation
- Selected patients who are reliable may be offered surveillance (watchful waiting) if
  - Tumor is confined within the tunica albuginea
  - Tumor does not demonstrate vascular invasion

– Tumor markers normalize after orchiectomy

– Radiographic imaging (chest radiograph and CT scan) shows no evidence of disease

• Surveillance is done monthly for the first 2 years and bimonthly in year 3

– Tumor markers at each visit

– Chest radiograph and CT scan every 3–4 months

– Majority of relapses occur within the first 8–10 months

– With rare exceptions, patients who relapse can be cured by chemotherapy or surgery

– The 5-year disease-free survival rate for stage A is 96% to 100%; for low-volume stage B disease, it is 90%

• Patients with bulky retroperitoneal disease (> 3 cm nodes) or metastases are treated with primary cisplatin-based combination chemotherapy following orchiectomy (cisplatin and etoposide or cisplatin, etoposide and bleomycin)

• For a residual mass > 3 cm, retroperitoneal lymph node resection is mandatory

• If tumor markers fail to normalize following primary chemotherapy, salvage chemotherapy is required (cisplatin, etoposide, bleomycin, ifosfamide)

 OUTCOME

PROGNOSIS

• Patients with bulky retroperitoneal or disseminated disease treated with primary chemotherapy followed by surgery have a 5-year disease-free survival rate of 55–80%

 EVIDENCE

PRACTICE GUIDELINES

• Laguna MP et al. EAU guidelines on testicular cancer. Eur Urol. 2001; 40:102. [PMID: 11528185]

• Segal R et al. Surveillance programs for early stage non-seminomatous testicular cancer: a practice guideline. Can J Urol. 2001;8:1184. [PMID: 11268306]

WEB SITES

• American Cancer Society—What is testicular cancer?

• National Cancer Institute—questions and answers about testicular cancer

• Testicular Cancer Resource Center

INFORMATION FOR PATIENTS

• Mayo Clinic—Testicular cancer

• MedlinePlus—Testicular cancer

• National Cancer Institute

REFERENCES

• Heidenreich A et al. Organ-sparing surgery for malignant germ cell tumor of the testis. J Urol. 2001 Dec;166(6): 2161–5. [PMID: 11696727]

• Huyghe E et al. Increasing incidence of testicular cancer worldwide: a review. J Urol. 2003 Jul;170(1):5–11. [PMID: 12796635]

• Jewett MA et al. Management of recurrence and follow-up strategies for patients with nonseminoma testis cancer. Urol Clin North Am. 2003 Nov; 30(4):819–30. [PMID: 14680317]

• Patel MI et al. Management of recurrence and follow-up strategies for patients with seminoma and selected high-risk groups. Urol Clin North Am. 2003 Nov;30(4):803–17. [PMID: 14680316]

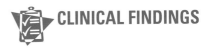

Tetanus

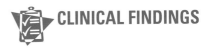 **KEY FEATURES**

ESSENTIALS OF DIAGNOSIS

• History of wound with possible contamination

• Jaw stiffness followed by spasms of jaw muscles (trismus)

• Stiffness of the neck and other muscles

• Dysphagia

• Irritability

• Hyperreflexia

• Finally, painful convulsions precipitated by minimal stimuli

GENERAL CONSIDERATIONS

• Caused by the neurotoxin tetanospasmin elaborated by *Clostridium tetani*

• Spores of this organism are ubiquitous in soil. When introduced into a wound, spores may germinate

• Tetanospasmin interferes with neurotransmission at spinal synapses of inhibitory neurons

• Minor stimuli result in uncontrolled spasms, and reflexes are exaggerated

• Most cases occur in unvaccinated individuals

• Persons at risk

– Elderly

– Migrant workers

– Newborns

– Injection drug users, who may acquire the disease through subcutaneous injections

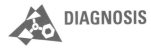 **CLINICAL FINDINGS**

SYMPTOMS AND SIGNS

• The first symptom may be pain and tingling at the site of inoculation, followed by spasticity of the muscles nearby

• Other early signs

– Stiffness of the jaw

– Neck stiffness

– Dysphagia

– Irritability

• Hyperreflexia develops later, with spasms of the jaw muscles (trismus) or facial muscles and rigidity and spasm of the muscles of the abdomen, neck, and back

• Painful tonic convulsions precipitated by minor stimuli are common

• Spasms of the glottis and respiratory muscles may cause acute asphyxia

• The patient is awake and alert throughout the illness. The sensory examination is normal. The temperature is normal or only slightly elevated

• Urinary retention and constipation may result from spasm of the sphincters

• Respiratory arrest and cardiac failure are late, life-threatening events

DIFFERENTIAL DIAGNOSIS

• Meningitis

• Rabies

• Tetany due to hypocalcemia

• Strychnine poisoning

• Neuroleptic malignant syndrome

• Trismus due to peritonsillar abscess

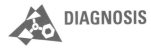 **DIAGNOSIS**

LABORATORY TESTS

• The diagnosis is made clinically

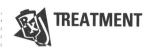

TREATMENT

MEDICATIONS

- Whenever a wound is contaminated or likely to have devitalized tissue
  - Passive tetanus immunization should be given
  - Administer 250 units of human tetanus immune globulin to nonimmunized individuals and those whose immunization status is uncertain
- Human tetanus immune globulin, 500 units, is given intramuscularly to those with clinical signs and symptoms of tetanus. Active immunization with tetanus toxoid should be started concurrently
- Table 69 provides a guide to prophylactic management
- Penicillin, 20 million units daily, is given to all patients with tetanus—even those with mild illness—to eradicate toxin-producing organisms

THERAPEUTIC PROCEDURES

- Minimal stimuli can provoke spasms, so the patient should be placed at bed rest and monitored under the quietest conditions possible
- Sedation, paralysis with curare-like agents, and mechanical ventilation are often necessary to control tetanic spasms

OUTCOME

COMPLICATIONS

- Respiratory arrest
- Pneumonia

PROGNOSIS

- High mortality rates are associated with
  - A short incubation period
  - Early onset of convulsions
  - Delay in treatment
- Contaminated lesions about the head and face are more dangerous than wounds on other parts of the body
- The overall mortality rate is about 40%, but this can be reduced with ventilator management

WHEN TO REFER

- For mechanical ventilation, refer to an intensivist or pulmonary specialist

WHEN TO ADMIT

- Any patient in whom there is clinical suspicion of the disease
- Intensive care unit may be needed

PREVENTION

- Tetanus is completely preventable by active immunization (Tables 67 and 68)
- For primary immunization of adults
  - Tetanus and diphtheria toxoids are administered as two doses 4–6 weeks apart, with a third dose 6–12 months later
  - Booster doses are given every 10 years or at the time of major injury if it occurs more than 5 years after a dose

EVIDENCE

PRACTICE GUIDELINES

- Kretsinger K et al; Centers for Disease Control and Prevention; Advisory Committee on Immunization Practices; Healthcare Infection Control Practices Advisory Committee. Preventing tetanus, diphtheria, and pertussis among adults: use of tetanus toxoid, reduced diphtheria toxoid and acellular pertussis vaccine recommendations of the Advisory Committee on Immunization Practices (ACIP) and recommendation of ACIP, supported by the Healthcare Infection Control Practices Advisory Committee (HICPAC), for use of Tdap among health-care personnel. MMWR Recomm Rep. 2006 Dec 15;55(RR-17):1–37. [PMID: 17167397]

WEB SITE

- CDC—National Immunization Program

INFORMATION FOR PATIENTS

- National Foundation for Infectious Diseases

REFERENCE

- Thwaites CL et al. Magnesium sulphate for treatment of severe tetanus: a randomised controlled trial. Lancet. 2006 Oct 21;368(9545):1436–43. [PMID: 17055945]

Thalassemia

KEY FEATURES

ESSENTIALS OF DIAGNOSIS

- Microcytosis out of proportion to degree of anemia
- Positive family history or lifelong personal history of microcytic anemia
- Abnormal red blood cell (RBC) morphology with microcytes, acanthocytes, and target cells
- In β-thalassemia, elevated levels of hemoglobin A_2 or F

GENERAL CONSIDERATIONS

- Hereditary disorders characterized by reduction in synthesis of globin chains (α or β), causing reduced hemoglobin synthesis and eventually hypochromic microcytic anemia
- Normal adult hemoglobin primarily hemoglobin A, a tetramer of two α-chains and two β-chains ($\alpha_2\beta_2$)
- Thalassemias are described as
  - **Trait,** when there are laboratory features without clinical impact
  - **Intermedia,** when there is a RBC transfusion requirement or other moderate clinical impact
  - **Major,** when the disorder is life-threatening
- α-Thalassemia syndromes determined by number of functional α-globin genes
  - Normal (four α-globin genes)
  - Silent carrier (three α-globin genes, normal hematocrit)
  - α-Thalassemia minor or trait (two α-globin genes, hematocrit 32–40%, mean cell volume [MCV] 60–75)
  - Hemoglobin H disease (one α-globin gene, hematocrit 22–32%, MCV 60-70)
  - Hydrops fetalis (0 α-globin genes)
- β-Thalassemia: Reduced β-globin chain synthesis results in relative increase in percentages of hemoglobins A_2 and F compared with hemoglobin A, because β-like globins (γ and δ) substitute for missing β-chains
- With reduced β-chains
  - Excess α-chains precipitate, causing hemolysis
  - Bone marrow becomes hyperplastic, resulting in bony deformities, osteopenia, and pathologic fractures

DEMOGRAPHICS

- α-Thalassemia occurs primarily in persons from southeast Asia and China and, less commonly, in blacks
- β-Thalassemia affects persons of Mediterranean origin (Italian, Greek) and to lesser extent Chinese, other Asians, and blacks

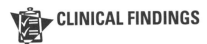 **CLINICAL FINDINGS**

SYMPTOMS AND SIGNS

- α-Thalassemia silent carriers: asymptomatic
- α-Thalassemia trait: clinically normal with mild microcytic anemia
- Hemoglobin H disease
  - Chronic hemolytic anemia of variable severity
  - Pallor
  - Splenomegaly
- Hydrops fetalis: fetal death
- Heterozygous for β-thalassemia (thalassemia minor): mild microcytic anemia
- Homozygous for mild β-thalassemia (thalassemia intermedia): chronic hemolytic anemia
- Homozygous for major β-thalassemia (thalassemia major)
  - Severe anemia requiring transfusion
  - Growth failure
  - Bony deformities (abnormal facial structure, pathologic fractures)
  - Hepatosplenomegaly and jaundice

DIFFERENTIAL DIAGNOSIS

- Iron deficiency anemia (thalassemia has lower MCV, normal iron studies, more normal RBC count, more abnormal peripheral blood smear at modest levels of anemia)
- Other hemoglobinopathy (eg, sickle thalassemia, hemoglobin C disorders)
- Sideroblastic anemia
- Anemia of chronic disease

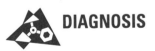 **DIAGNOSIS**

LABORATORY TESTS

α-Thalassemia trait

- Mild anemia (hematocrit 28–40%) with strikingly low MCV (60–75 fL)
- RBC count normal or increased
- Peripheral blood smear mildly abnormal
  - Microcytes
  - Hypochromia
  - Occasional target cells
  - Acanthocytes

- Reticulocyte count and iron studies normal
- Hemoglobin electrophoresis: no increase in percentage of hemoglobins A_2 or F and no hemoglobin H (thus usually a diagnosis of exclusion)
- See Table 3
- Hemoglobin H disease
- Variably severe hemolytic anemia (hematocrit 22–32%) with remarkably low MCV (60–70 fL)
- Peripheral blood smear markedly abnormal: hypochromia, microcytosis, target cells, poikilocytosis
- Reticulocyte count elevated
- Hemoglobin electrophoresis: shows hemoglobin H comprises 10–40% of the hemoglobin

β-Thalassemia minor

- Mild anemia (hematocrit 28–40%) with MCV 55–75 fL
- RBC count normal or increased
- Peripheral blood smear mildly abnormal
  - Hypochromia
  - Microcytosis
  - Target cells
  - Basophilic stippling
- Reticulocyte count normal or slightly elevated
- Hemoglobin electrophoresis: elevated hemoglobin A_2 to 4–8% and occasionally elevated hemoglobin F to 1–5%

β-Thalassemia major

- Severe anemia (hematocrit sometimes < 10% without transfusion)
- Peripheral blood smear bizarre
  - Severe poikilocytosis
  - Hypochromia
  - Microcytosis
  - Target cells
  - Basophilic stippling
  - Nucleated RBCs
- Hemoglobin electrophoresis
  - Little or no hemoglobin A
  - Variable amounts of hemoglobin A_2
  - Major hemoglobin present is hemoglobin F
  - See Table 4

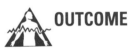 **TREATMENT**

MEDICATIONS

- Mild thalassemias (α-thalassemia trait or β-thalassemia minor)
  - Usually require no treatment
  - Should be identified to avoid repeated evaluations for iron deficiency and inappropriate administration of supplemental iron

- α-Thalassemia trait and thalassemia intermedia may require transfusion during infection or other stress
- Hemoglobin H disease
  - Folate supplementation
  - Avoid medicinal iron and oxidative drugs, such as sulfonamides
- Severe thalassemia
  - Regular transfusions
  - Folate supplementation
- Deferoxamine is routinely given as an iron-chelating agent to avoid or postpone hemosiderosis
- Deferasirox is a new oral iron chelator that has been approved for clinical use

SURGERY

- Splenectomy indicated if hypersplenism causes marked increase in transfusion requirement

THERAPEUTIC PROCEDURES

- Prenatal diagnosis and genetic counseling should be offered
- Blood transfusions as above
- Allogeneic bone marrow transplantation for β-thalassemia major in children who have not yet experienced iron overload and chronic organ toxicity

OUTCOME

COMPLICATIONS

- Bony deformities, osteopenia, and pathologic fractures in β-thalassemia
- Complications of blood transfusions as below
- Splenomegaly may result from chronic hemolysis

PROGNOSIS

- Mild thalassemia (α-thalassemia trait or β-thalassemia minor): normal life expectancy
- Thalassemia intermedia
  - Transfusional iron overload may develop
  - Patients survive into adulthood but with hepatosplenomegaly and bony deformities
- β-Thalassemia major
  - Clinical course modified significantly by transfusion therapy, but transfusional iron overload causes heart failure, cirrhosis, and endocrinopathies, usually after > 100 units of transfusion
  - Death from cardiac failure usually occurs between ages 20 and 30

– Long-term survival is > 80% in cases undergoing allogeneic bone marrow transplantation

PREVENTION

- Deferoxamine is routinely given as iron-chelating agent to avoid or postpone hemosiderosis in transfusion-dependent patients
- Low-iron diet may also help

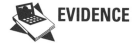 **EVIDENCE**

WEB SITES

- Children's Hospital Oakland: Thalassemia
- Cooley's Anemia Foundation
- Thalassemia Foundation of Canada

INFORMATION FOR PATIENTS

- MedlinePlus: Thalassemia
- National Heart, Lung, and Blood Institute: Thalassemia
- National Human Genome Research Institute: Learning About Thalassemia

REFERENCES

- Chaidos A et al. Treatment of beta-thalassemia patients with recombinant human erythropoietin: effect on transfusion requirements and soluble adhesion molecules. Acta Haematol. 2004; 111(4):189–95. [PMID: 15153710]
- Chui D et al. Hemoglobin H disease: not necessarily a benign disorder. Blood. 2003 Feb 1;101(3):791–800. [PMID: 12393486]
- Cohen AR. New advances in iron chelation therapy. Hematology Am Soc Hematol Educ Program. 2006:42–7. [PMID: 17124038]
- Cunningham MJ et al. Thalassemia Clinical Research Network. Complications of beta-thalassemia major in North America. Blood. 2004 Jul 1; 104(1):34–9. [PMID: 14988152]
- Rund D et al. β-Thalassemia. N Engl J Med 2005 Sep 15;353(11):1135–46. [PMID: 16162884]

Thoracic Aortic Aneurysm

 KEY FEATURES

ESSENTIALS OF DIAGNOSIS

- Widened mediastinum on chest radiograph
- With rupture, sudden onset chest pain radiating to the back

GENERAL CONSIDERATIONS

- Aneurysms of the thoracic aorta account for < 10% of aortic aneurysms
- Causes
  – Atherosclerosis
  – Trauma
  – Syphilis (rare)
  – Ehlers-Danlos and Marfan syndromes (also rare)

 CLINICAL FINDINGS

SYMPTOMS AND SIGNS

- Most are asymptomatic
- Substernal back or neck pain
- Pressure on the trachea, esophagus, or superior vena cava can result in
  – Dyspnea, stridor, or brassy cough
  – Dysphagia
  – Edema in the neck and arms
  – Distended neck veins
- Hoarseness due to stretching of the left recurrent laryngeal nerve
- Aortic regurgitation with aneurysms of the ascending aorta

DIFFERENTIAL DIAGNOSIS

 DIAGNOSIS

IMAGING STUDIES

- Chest radiograph shows calcified outline of the dilated aorta
- CT scanning is modality of choice
  – Demonstrates the anatomy and size of the aneurysm
  – Excludes lesions that can mimic aneurysms, such as neoplasms or substernal goiter
- MRI can also be useful

DIAGNOSTIC PROCEDURES

- Cardiac catheterization and echocardiography may be required to describe the relationship of the coronary vessels to an aneurysm of the ascending aorta

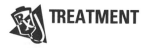 **TREATMENT**

SURGERY

- Indications for repair depend on
  – Location of dilation
  – Rate of growth
  – Associated symptoms
  – Overall condition of patient
- Aneurysms measuring ≥ 6 cm may be considered for repair

THERAPEUTIC PROCEDURES

- Endovascular grafting for aneurysms of the descending thoracic aorta
- Experimental branched endovascular reconstructions (custom made grafts with branches to the vessels that would be occluded by the grafts) for arch aneurysms

 OUTCOME

FOLLOW-UP

- CT scanning for stable aneurysms

COMPLICATIONS

- With the exception of endovascular repair for discrete saccular aneurysms of the descending thoracic aorta, the morbidity and mortality of thoracic repair is considerably higher than that for infrarenal abdominal aortic aneurysm repair
- Paraplegia (rare)
- Risk of stroke increased when aortic arch is involved, even when the aneurysm does not directly affect the carotid artery

PROGNOSIS

- Generally, degenerative aneurysms of the thoracic aorta will enlarge and require repair
- Good with endovascular repair of saccular aneurysms, particularly those distal to the left subclavian artery and the descending thoracic aorta
- Resection of large complex aneurysms of the aortic arch should only be attempted in low-risk patients
- Experimental branched technology for endovascular grafting holds promise for reduced morbidity and mortality

viduals with varicose veins or thromboangiitis obliterans

- May be associated with
  - Trauma
  - Occult deep vein thrombosis (DVT) (in about 20% of cases)
  - Short-term venous catheterization of superficial arm veins
  - Longer term peripherally inserted central catheter lines
- May also be a manifestation of systemic hypercoagulability secondary to abdominal cancer
- Pulmonary emboli are exceedingly rare and always from an associated DVT
- Observe IV catheter sites daily for signs of local inflammation

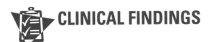 **CLINICAL FINDINGS**

SYMPTOMS AND SIGNS

- Dull pain in the region of the involved vein
- Induration, redness, and tenderness along the course of a vein
- Process may be localized, or it may involve most of the long saphenous vein and its tributaries
- Inflammatory reaction generally subsides in 1–2 weeks; a firm cord may remain for much longer
- Edema of the extremity is uncommon
- Chills and high fever suggest septic phlebitis

DIFFERENTIAL DIAGNOSIS

- Cellulitis
- Erythema nodosum
- Erythema induratum
- Panniculitis
- Fibrositis
- Lymphangitis
- Deep thrombophlebitis

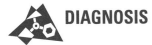 **DIAGNOSIS**

LABORATORY TESTS

- Blood culture: in septic thrombophlebitis, the causative organism is often *Staphylococcus*

IMAGING STUDIES

- Ultrasonography to assess extent of thrombosis

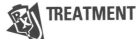 **TREATMENT**

MEDICATIONS

- Nonsteroidal anti-inflammatory drugs
- For septic thrombophlebitis
  - Broad-spectrum antibiotics (vancomycin +/- gentamicin) (Table 62); if cultures are positive, continue for 7–10 days or for 4–6 weeks if complicating endocarditis cannot be excluded
  - Systemic anticoagulation with heparin
- Anticoagulation for rapidly progressing disease or extension into the deep system

SURGERY

- Ligation and division of vein at junction of deep and superficial veins indicated when process is extensive or progressing toward the saphenofemoral or cephaloaxillary junction

THERAPEUTIC PROCEDURES

- Local heat
- Bed rest with leg elevation

 OUTCOME

COMPLICATIONS

- Serious thrombotic or septic complications can occur if IV catheters are not removed once local reaction develops in the vein

PROGNOSIS

- Course is generally benign and brief
- Prognosis depends on the underlying pathologic process
- In patients with phlebitis secondary to varicose veins, recurrent episodes are likely unless correction of the underlying venous reflux and excision of varicosities is done
- Mortality from septic thrombophlebitis
  - Low and prognosis is excellent with early treatment
  - ≥ 20% without aggressive treatment

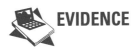 **EVIDENCE**

PRACTICE GUIDELINES

- Institute for Clinical Systems Improvement: Venous Thromboembolism, 2002

- Kalodiki E et al. Superficial thrombophlebitis and low-molecular-weight heparins. Angiology. 2002;53:659. [PMID: 12463618]

INFORMATION FOR PATIENTS

- Mayo Clinic: Thrombophlebitis
- MedlinePlus: Superficial Thrombophlebitis
- Merck Manual of Medical Information: Superficial Thrombophlebitis

REFERENCE

- van Weert H et al. Spontaneous superficial venous thrombophlebitis: does it increase risk for thromboembolism? A historic follow-up study in primary care. J Fam Pract. 2006 Jan;55(1):52–7. [PMID: 16388768]

Thrombotic Thrombocytopenic Purpura

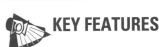 **KEY FEATURES**

ESSENTIALS OF DIAGNOSIS

- Thrombocytopenia
- Microangiopathic hemolytic anemia
- Normal coagulation tests
- Elevated serum lactate dehydrogenase (LDH)

GENERAL CONSIDERATIONS

- Uncommon syndrome characterized by
  - Microangiopathic hemolytic anemia
  - Thrombocytopenia
  - Noninfectious fever
  - Neurologic disorders
  - Renal insufficiency
- Markedly elevated serum LDH
- Pathogenesis appears to be deficiency of a von Willebrand factor–cleaving protease ADAMTS13, in some cases resulting from antibody against the protease
- Occasionally precipitated by estrogen use, pregnancy, drugs, or infections

DEMOGRAPHICS

- Occurs primarily in young adults between ages 20 and 50
- Slight female predominance

CLINICAL FINDINGS

SYMPTOMS AND SIGNS

- Fever may be present
- Pallor and symptoms of anemia
- Purpura, petechiae, and bleeding
- Neurologic symptoms and signs, including
  - Headache
  - Confusion
  - Aphasia
  - Alterations in consciousness from lethargy to coma, may wax and wane over minutes
  - Hemiparesis and seizures with more advanced disease
- Abdominal pain and tenderness resulting from pancreatitis

DIFFERENTIAL DIAGNOSIS

- Disseminated intravascular coagulation
- Hemolytic-uremic syndrome
- Preeclampsia–eclampsia
- Meningitis
- Evans's syndrome (idiopathic thrombocytopenic purpura with autoimmune hemolytic anemia)

DIAGNOSIS

LABORATORY TESTS

- Peripheral smear shows microangiopathic changes with fragmented red blood cells (RBCs) (schistocytes, helmet cells)
- Anemia is universal and may be marked
- Usually marked reticulocytosis and occasional circulating nucleated RBCs
- Thrombocytopenia is invariably present and may be severe
- Increased indirect bilirubin and occasionally hemoglobinemia and hemoglobinuria from hemolysis; methemalbuminemia may impart brown color to plasma
- LDH markedly elevated in proportion to severity of hemolysis; Coombs test negative
- Coagulation tests (prothrombin time, partial thromboplastin time, fibrinogen) normal unless ischemic tissue damage causes secondary disseminated intravascular coagulation
- Elevated fibrin degradation products may be seen, as in other acutely ill patients
- Renal insufficiency, with abnormal urinalysis

DIAGNOSTIC PROCEDURES

- Pathologically, may see thrombi in capillaries and small arteries, with no evidence of inflammation

TREATMENT

MEDICATIONS

- Prednisone and antiplatelet agents (aspirin, 325 mg PO TID, and dipyridamole, 75 mg PO TID) have been used in addition to plasmapheresis, but their role is unclear
- Management of refractory patients who do not respond to plasmapheresis or have rapid recurrences is controversial
- Combination of splenectomy, corticosteroids, and dextran used with success
- Immunosuppression (eg, cyclophosphamide, rituximab) also effective

SURGERY

- Splenectomy may be indicated for refractory disease
- Splenectomy during remission may prevent subsequent relapses

THERAPEUTIC PROCEDURES

- Emergent large-volume plasmapheresis is the treatment of choice for thrombotic thrombocytopenic purpura
  - 60–80 mL/kg of plasma removed and replaced with fresh-frozen plasma, continued daily until complete remission
  - Optimal duration of plasmapheresis after remission unknown

OUTCOME

PROGNOSIS

- With plasmapheresis, formerly dismal prognosis has dramatically changed; 80–90% now recover completely
- Neurologic abnormalities are usually reversed
- Most complete responses are durable, but 20% of cases are chronic and relapsing

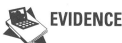

EVIDENCE

PRACTICE GUIDELINES

- Allford SL et al. Guidelines on the diagnosis and management of the thrombotic microangiopathic haemolytic anaemias. Br J Haematol. 2003; 120:556. [PMID: 12588343]

INFORMATION FOR PATIENTS

- MedlinePlus: Thrombotic Thrombocytopenic Purpura

REFERENCES

- Ahmad A et al. Rituximab for treatment of refractory/relapsing thrombotic thrombocytopenic purpura (TTP). Am J Hematol. 2004 Oct;77(2):171–6. [PMID: 15389904]
- Fakhouri F et al. Efficiency of curative and prophylactic treatment with rituximab in ADAMTS 13-deficient thrombotic thrombocytopenic purpura: a study of 11 cases. Blood. 2005 Sep 15; 106(6):1932–7. [PMID: 15933059]
- Sadler JE. Thrombotic thrombocytopenic purpura: a moving target. Hematology Am Soc Hematol Educ Program. 2006:415–20. [PMID: 17124092]

Thyroid Cancer

KEY FEATURES

ESSENTIALS OF DIAGNOSIS

- Painless swelling in region of thyroid
- Serum thyroid-stimulating hormone (TSH), free tetraiodothyronine (T$_4$) generally normal
- Positive thyroid fine-needle aspiration biopsy

GENERAL CONSIDERATIONS

- Most thyroid cancers are microscopic and indolent. Larger ones require treatment

Papillary carcinoma

- Pure papillary or mixed papillary-follicular most common thyroid cancer (80%)
- Childhood head–neck radiation or nuclear fallout exposure imparts increased lifelong risk
- May be familial or associated with adenomatous polyposis coli
- Least aggressive thyroid malignancy, but spreads via thyroid lymphatics; distant metastases may occur

Follicular carcinoma

- Second most common thyroid malignancy
- Generally more aggressive than papillary carcinoma
- Metastases commonly found in neck lymph nodes, bone, and lungs

Medullary thyroid carcinoma

- 3% of thyroid cancers
- One-third sporadic, one-third familial, one-third associated with MEN 2
- Early local metastases usually present, and late metastases may be in bones, lungs, adrenals, or liver
- Peptides (eg, serotonin) can cause symptoms and serve as tumor markers

Anaplastic thyroid carcinoma

- 2% of thyroid cancers
- Older patient with rapidly enlarging mass in multinodular goiter
- Most aggressive thyroid carcinoma
- Metastasizes early to surrounding lymph nodes and distant sites

Other thyroid malignancies

- 3% of thyroid cancers
- Lymphoma; metastatic bronchogenic, breast, and renal carcinomas, melanoma

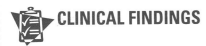 **CLINICAL FINDINGS**

SYMPTOMS AND SIGNS

- Usually presents as palpable, firm, nontender nodule
- Larger cancers can cause neck discomfort, dysphagia, or hoarseness
- ~3% present with metastasis to local lymph nodes and sometimes to distant sites such as bone or lung
- Metastatic differentiated carcinoma may secrete enough thyroxine to produce thyrotoxicosis
- Medullary carcinoma causes flushing, diarrhea, fatigue; ~5% develop Cushing's syndrome
- Anaplastic or long-standing tumors can produce hoarseness

DIFFERENTIAL DIAGNOSIS

- Benign thyroid nodule
- Subacute thyroiditis
- Benign multinodular goiter
- Lymphadenopathy due to other cause
- Metastasis from head and neck cancer
- Lymphoma

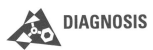 **DIAGNOSIS**

LABORATORY TESTS

- TSH and T_4 normal unless concomitant thyroiditis; metastatic follicular carcinoma may secrete enough thyroxine to suppress TSH

- Markers for recurrent or metastatic disease
  - Obtain levels preoperatively and follow postoperatively
  - Serum thyroglobulin high in most metastatic papillary and follicular tumors
    - Useful marker except if antithyroglobulin Ab present
  - Serum calcitonin frequently elevated in medullary thyroid carcinoma, but nonspecific test
  - Serum carcinoembryonic antigen (CEA) usually elevated with medullary carcinoma
- Genetic testing of siblings and children of patients with medullary carcinoma for *RET* protooncogene mutations, which occur in MEN 2 and familial medullary thyroid carcinoma

IMAGING STUDIES

- Preoperative neck ultrasound
  - Especially useful if known metastases, persistent elevation in serum thyroglobulin, or detectable levels of antithyroglobulin antibodies
  - Useful for postoperative surveillance
- Radioiodine scanning only useful postoperatively
- Chest radiograph or CT scan
  - May demonstrate metastases, but iodinated contrast reduces effectiveness of radioiodine scanning and therapy
  - Medullary carcinoma metastases in thyroid, nodes, and liver may calcify, but rarely in lung
- Positive emission tomography (PET) scanning sensitive for detecting metastases
  - Useful if serum thyroglobulin rising after thyroidectomy, especially > 10 mcg/mL, normal whole-body RAI scan and unrevealing neck ultrasound
  - Can be combined with a CT scan
  - The resultant PET/CT fusion scan is 60% sensitive for detecting metastases not visible by other methods
  - Pretreatment with recombinant human thyrotropin (rhTSH) can further increase sensitivity of PET

DIAGNOSTIC PROCEDURES

- Fine-needle aspiration biopsy for clinically suspicious nodules

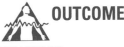 **TREATMENT**

MEDICATIONS

- Levothyroxine, 0.75–0.1 mg PO once daily begun immediately after thyroidectomy

  - Adjust dose using an ultrasensitive assay for serum TSH: suppress TSH below 0.1 mU/L for stage II disease and below 0.05 mU/L for stage III–IV disease

SURGERY

- Total or near-total thyroidectomy is treatment of choice for most patients
- Subtotal thyroidectomy acceptable for adults aged < 45 with single tumor < 1 cm
- Surgical resection of metastases to brain (radiation or radioactive iodide therapy ineffective), and of bulky recurrent tumor in neck region
- Total thyroidectomy for medullary thyroid carcinoma; repeated neck dissections often required over time
- Prophylactic total thyroidectomy, ideally at age 6, in persons with *RET* protooncogene mutations
- Local resection, combined with radiation therapy, for anaplastic carcinoma

THERAPEUTIC PROCEDURES

- After thyroidectomy, patients with differentiated thyroid carcinomas receive radioiodine (RAI) neck and whole-body scan after rhTSH administration or while hypothyroid
- Decision to treat with ^{131}I in patient with suspicious RAI uptake
  - Stage I differentiated thyroid cancer
  - ^{131}I therapy does not improve survival but does reduce local recurrence
  - Some advocate ^{131}I for those with a primary tumor > 1 cm diameter, tumor at the surgical margin, or lymph node involvement
  - Stage II–IV cancer
- ^{131}I therapy cautions
  - Pregnant women may not receive RAI therapy
  - Women are advised to avoid pregnancy for at least 4 months after therapy
  - Men have abnormal spermatozoa up to 6 months after therapy and must use contraceptive methods during that time
- External-beam radiation therapy for bone metastases
- Zoledronic acid (4 mg IV over 20 minutes) every 4–6 months for patients with bone metastases

OUTCOME

FOLLOW-UP

- Monitor serum TSH, and adjust thyroxine dose (as above)

- Whole-body ^{131}I or ^{123}I scans at 2–4 months postoperatively (detects ~65% of metastases) and then 6–12 months later
- Two successive whole-body scans without metastases are required for diagnosis of remission
- Monitor serum calcitonin and CEA periodically after surgery for medullary carcinoma
- Monitor bone densitometry periodically if patient receiving thyroxine suppression therapy
- Surveillance of family of patients with medullary thyroid carcinoma

COMPLICATIONS

- Medullary carcinomas may secrete serotonin and prostaglandins (flushing and diarrhea); or ACTH or corticotropin-releasing hormone (Cushing's syndrome). Coincident pheochromocytoma and hyperparathyroidism may occur in MEN-related cases
- Permanent hypothyroidism and vocal cord palsy after radical neck surgery
- Immediate autotransplantation of incidentally resected parathyroids reduces postoperative hypoparathyroidism

PROGNOSIS

- For papillary (and follicular) carcinoma, generally excellent
- Palpable lymph node metastases in papillary thyroid cancer do not increase mortality, but do increase risk of local recurrence
- Prognosis worsened with follicular instead of papillary carcinoma, older age, males, bone or brain metastases, large pulmonary metastases, and lack of ^{131}I uptake into metastases
- [^{18}F]fluorodeoxyglucose positron emission tomography ([18]FDG-PET) scan: Metastases with low standardized uptake value (SUV) are generally indolent
- Brain metastases (in 1%) reduce median survival to 12 months; prognosis improved by surgical resection
- Mortality increased twofold by 10 years and threefold by 25 years in patients not receiving ^{131}I ablation
- For medullary thyroid carcinoma, variable:
  - Overall 10-year survival rate 90% when confined to thyroid, 70% with metastases to cervical lymph nodes, and 20% with distant metastases

- In MEN 2A, less aggressive tumors and in MEN 2B, more aggressive
- Those staining heavily for calcitonin, usually less aggressive; prolonged survival despite extensive metastases
- For anaplastic thyroid carcinoma, poor

WHEN TO ADMIT

- Admit for thyroidectomy and keep for at least 1 day postoperatively to monitor for late bleeding, airway problems, and tetany
- Admit for high-dose ^{131}I therapy

 EVIDENCE

PRACTICE GUIDELINES

- AACE/AAES Medical/Surgical Guidelines for Clinical Practice: Management of Thyroid Carcinoma

WEB SITE

- American Thyroid Association

INFORMATION FOR PATIENTS

- American Thyroid Association—Thyroid cancer
- NIH Medline Plus Encyclopedia

REFERENCES

- Fernandes JK et al. Overview of the management of differentiated thyroid cancer. Curr Treat Options Oncol. 2005 Jan;6(1):47–57. [PMID: 15610714]
- Hamady ZZ et al. Surgical pathological second opinion in thyroid malignancy: impact on patients' management and prognosis. Eur J Surg Oncol. 2005 Feb; 31(1):74–7. [PMID: 15642429]
- Kim TY et al. Metastasis to the thyroid diagnosed by fine-needle aspiration biopsy. Clin Endocrinol (Oxf). 2005 Feb;62(2):236–41. [PMID: 15670202]
- Robbins RJ et al. Real-time prognosis for metastatic thyroid carcinoma based on 2-[18F]fluoro-2-deoxy-D-glucose-positron emission tomography scanning. J Clin Endocrinol Metab. 2006 Feb;91(2):498–505. [PMID: 16303836]

Thyroid Nodules & Multinodular Goiter

 KEY FEATURES

ESSENTIALS OF DIAGNOSIS

- Commonly found during careful thyroid examinations
- Thyroid function tests mandatory
- Thyroid biopsy for single or dominant nodules or if history of head–neck radiation
- Clinical follow-up required

GENERAL CONSIDERATIONS

- Most small thyroid nodules are asymptomatic and discovered incidentally on physical or radiologic examination
- Most patients with goiter are euthyroid, but many have hypothyroidism or hyperthyroidism
- Causes of diffuse and multinodular goiters include
  - Benign multinodular goiter
  - Iodine deficiency
  - Pregnancy (in areas of iodine deficiency)
  - Graves' disease
  - Hashimoto's thyroiditis
  - Subacute thyroiditis
  - Infections
- Causes of solitary thyroid nodule include
  - Benign adenoma
  - Colloid nodule
  - Cyst
  - Primary thyroid malignancy or (less frequently) metastatic neoplasm
- Higher risk of malignancy if
  - History of head-neck radiation in childhood
  - Family history of thyroid cancer
  - Personal history of another malignancy

DEMOGRAPHICS

- Each year in the United States, about 275,000 thyroid nodules are detected by palpation
- Incidence of goiter higher in iodine-deficient geographic areas (see Goiter, Endemic)

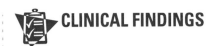 **CLINICAL FINDINGS**

SYMPTOMS AND SIGNS

- Small thyroid nodules usually asymptomatic
- Toxic multinodular goiter and hyperfunctioning nodules can cause hyperthyroidism
  - Sweating
  - Weight loss
  - Anxiety
  - Loose stools
  - Heat intolerance
  - Tachycardia
  - Tremor
- Hashimoto's thyroiditis may cause goiter and hypothyroidism
  - Fatigue
  - Cold intolerance
  - Constipation
  - Weight gain
  - Depression
  - Dry skin
  - Delayed return of deep tendon reflexes
- Thyroid nodules or multinodular goiter can grow and cause cosmetic embarrassment, discomfort, hoarseness, or dysphagia
- Large retrosternal multinodular goiters can cause dyspnea due to tracheal compression
- Malignancy is suggested by
  - Hoarseness or vocal cord paralysis
  - Nodules in men or young women
  - Nodule that is solitary, firm, large, or adherent to trachea or strap muscles
  - Enlarged lymph nodes
  - Distant metastases

DIFFERENTIAL DIAGNOSIS

- Iodine-deficient goiter
- Pregnancy (in areas of iodine deficiency)
- Graves' disease
- Hashimoto's thyroiditis
- Subacute (de Quervain's) thyroiditis
- Drugs causing hypothyroidism
  - Lithium
  - Amiodarone
  - Propylthiouracil
  - Methimazole
  - Phenylbutazone
  - Sulfonamides
  - Interferon-α
  - Iodide
- Infiltrating disease, eg, malignancy, sarcoidosis
- Suppurative thyroiditis
- Riedel's thyroiditis
- Nonthyroid neck mass, eg, lymphadenopathy, lymphoma, branchial cleft cyst

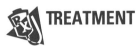 **DIAGNOSIS**

LABORATORY TESTS

- Thyroid-stimulating hormone (TSH) (sensitive assay) and free thyroxine (FT$_4$) can exclude hypothyroidism or hyperthyroidism
- Hashimoto's thyroiditis
  - Antithyroperoxidase or antithyroglobulin antibodies usually very high

IMAGING STUDIES

- Neck ultrasound indicated for most palpable nodules
  - To determine nodule size, consistency, whether it is part of a multinodular goiter
  - Solid nodules often malignant; cystic nodules usually benign
  - Monitor nodules
  - Preferred over CT and MRI because of accuracy

DIAGNOSTIC PROCEDURES

- Fine-needle aspiration (FNA) biopsy of suspicious nodules (thyroiditis frequently coexists with malignancy)
- FNA biopsy success is increased by ultrasound guidance
- Of thyroid FNA biopsies
  - ~70% are benign
  - 10% follicular neoplasm (suspicious cytology)
  - 5% malignant
  - 15% nondiagnostic
- Among patients with suspicious cytology, ~30% harbor malignancy; risk is higher in young patients and if nodule is fixed or > 3 cm
- Cytology should be done on cystic fluid obtained at FNA
  - Cystic nodules yielding serous fluid are usually benign
  - Nodules yielding bloody fluid have higher chance of malignancy
  - Repeat FNA biopsy if cytology nondiagnostic and nodule remains palpable
- Thyroid incidentalomas: nonpalpable small thyroid nodules incidentally found by 25–50% of scans of the neck (MRI, CT, ultrasound) done for other reasons
  - Require ultrasound-guided FNA biopsy (USGFNAB) only if > 1.5 cm or history of head-neck radiation in childhood
  - Consider USGFNAB for nodules < 1.5 cm diameter if history of head–neck irradiation or a family history of thyroid cancer or a suspicious appearance on ultrasound (calcified, solitary, or irregular)
  - Follow-up thyroid ultrasound in 3–4 months for nodules of borderline concern; growing lesions may be biopsied or resected

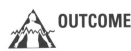 **TREATMENT**

MEDICATIONS

- Levothyroxine, 0.05–0.2 mg PO once daily, if elevated TSH
- Consider "suppression" of nodules > 2 cm with levothyroxine, 0.05–0.1 mg once daily, if TSH elevated or normal
  - Avoid if baseline TSH is low, suggesting autonomous thyroid hormone secretion, because levothyroxine will be ineffective and may cause thyrotoxicosis
  - Long-term suppression of TSH tends to keep nodules from enlarging and new nodules from developing, but few existing nodules actually shrink
  - Works best for younger patients
  - May increase risk for angina and arrhythmia in patients with cardiovascular disease
  - Causes small loss of bone density in many postmenopausal women not taking estrogen or bisphosphonate

SURGERY

- Surgical resection indicated for solitary nodule with history of head–neck radiation due to risk of malignancy
- Surgical resection of toxic adenoma cures hyperthyroidism
- Excision of multinodular goiters causing compressive symptoms

PROCEDURES

- Aspiration of cystic nodule with fluid sent for cytology. Multiple aspirations may be required because cysts tend to recur

OUTCOME

FOLLOW-UP

- Regular clinical evaluation and thyroid palpation or ultrasound examinations in all patients; even patients with a "negative" FNAB require follow-up because the false-negative rate for FNAB is 4%
- Monitor patients receiving levothyroxine suppression for atrial arrhythmias and osteoporosis

- Periodic bone densitometry in patients who are receiving levothyroxine suppression and at risk for osteoporosis

PROGNOSIS

- Benign nodules usually persist or grow slowly and may involute
- Malignant transformation is rare
- Prognosis of malignant nodules depends on histology (see Thyroid Cancer)
- Multinodular goiters tend to persist or grow slowly, even in iodine-deficient areas where iodine repletion usually does not shrink established goiters
- In Hashimoto's thyroiditis, a palpable solitary thyroid nodule of ≥ 1 cm diameter has ~8% chance of being malignant
- Patients with small incidentally discovered nonpalpable thyroid nodules are at very low risk for malignancy
  - Nonpalpable thyroid nodules < 1 cm diameter are benign in 98.4% of cases
  - Even those with malignancy have little morbidity and mortality

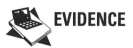

EVIDENCE

PRACTICE GUIDELINES

- AACE Medical Guidelines for Clinical Practice for the Diagnosis and Management of Thyroid Nodules

WEB SITE

- The American Thyroid Association

INFORMATION FOR PATIENTS

- American Thyroid Association—Thyroid nodule
- Mayo Clinic—Thyroid nodule

REFERENCES

- Bui A et al. New paradigms in the diagnosis and management of thyroid nodules. Endocrinologist. 2007;17:35.
- Hegedüs L. Clinical practice. The thyroid nodule. N Engl J Med. 2004 Oct 21;351(17):1764–71. [PMID: 15496625]
- Kang HW et al. Prevalence, clinical and ultrasonographic characteristics of thyroid incidentalomas. Thyroid. 2004 Jan; 14(1):29–33. [PMID: 15009911]
- Kessler A et al. Accuracy and consistency of fine-needle aspiration biopsy in the diagnosis and management of solitary thyroid nodules. Isr Med Assoc J. 2005 Jun;7(6):371–3. [PMID: 15984379]
- Liebeskind A et al. Rates of malignancy in incidentally discovered thyroid nodules evaluated with sonography and fine-needle aspiration. J Ultrasound Med. 2005 May;24(5):629–34. [PMID: 15840794]
- Nam-Goong IS et al. Ultrasonography-guided fine-needle aspiration of thyroid incidentaloma: correlation with pathological findings. Clin Endocrinol (Oxf). 2004 Jan;60(1):21–8. [PMID: 14678283]

Thyroiditis

 KEY FEATURES

ESSENTIALS OF DIAGNOSIS

- **Acute thyroiditis**: swelling of thyroid, sometimes causing pressure symptoms
- **Chronic thyroiditis**: painless enlargement of thyroid or rubbery firmness
- Thyroid function tests variable
- Serum antithyroperoxidase, antimicrosomal, antithyroglobulin antibody tests often positive

GENERAL CONSIDERATIONS

- Classification
  - **Hashimoto's** (chronic lymphocytic) thyroiditis
    - Most common thyroid disorder in the United States
    - Due to autoimmunity
    - Frequency increased by dietary iodine supplementation; certain drugs (eg, amiodarone, interferon-α)
    - Associated with other autoimmune diseases, eg, diabetes mellitus, pernicious anemia, adrenal insufficiency (Schmidt's syndrome), other endocrine deficiencies, inflammatory bowel disease, celiac disease; usually, concurrent with Graves' disease
  - **Subacute thyroiditis** (de Quervain's thyroiditis, granulomatous thyroiditis, and giant cell thyroiditis)
  - **Suppurative thyroiditis**: rare, caused by pyogenic organisms, usually during systemic infection
  - **Postpartum thyroiditis** (autoimmune): causes transient hyperthyroidism followed by hypothyroidism
  - **Riedel's thyroiditis**: rarest form
- Thyroiditis commonly occurs in patients with hepatitis C

DEMOGRAPHICS

- Hashimoto's thyroiditis
  - Often familial, varies by kindred and by race
  - Six times more common in women
- Antithyroid antibodies in US adolescents and adults found in
  - 3% of men and 13% of women
  - 25% of women over age 60 years
  - 14% of whites
  - 11% of Mexican Americans
  - 5% of African Americans
- Subacute thyroiditis usually affects young and middle-aged women
- Riedel's thyroiditis usually affects middle-aged or elderly women
- 40% of women and 20% of men exhibit focal thyroiditis at autopsy

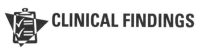 **CLINICAL FINDINGS**

SYMPTOMS AND SIGNS

Hashimoto's thyroiditis

- Thyroid gland usually diffusely enlarged, firm, and finely nodular
- One lobe may be asymmetrically enlarged, raising concern for neoplasm
- Neck tightness; pain and tenderness not usually present
- Thyroiditis often progresses to hypothyroidism, which is usually permanent
- Uncommonly, thyroiditis causes transient thyrotoxicosis
- Rarely, a hypofunctioning gland may become hyperfunctioning with onset of coexistent Graves' disease
- Mild dry mouth (xerostomia) or dry eyes (keratoconjunctivitis sicca) related to Sjögren's syndrome in ~33%
- Diplopia due to coexistent myasthenia gravis
- Manifestations of other autoimmune diseases listed above

Subacute thyroiditis

- Acute, usually painful, thyroid enlargement, with dysphagia. May have malaise or signs of thyrotoxicosis
- If no pain, called "silent thyroiditis"
- May persist for weeks or months

Suppurative thyroiditis

- Severe pain, tenderness, redness, and fluctuance around thyroid gland

Riedel's thyroiditis

- Usually causes hypothyroidism
- Enlargement often asymmetric

- Gland is stony hard and adherent to neck structures, causing dysphagia, dyspnea, pain, and hoarseness

DIFFERENTIAL DIAGNOSIS

- Benign multinodular goiter
- Iodine-deficient (endemic) goiter
- Graves' disease
- Thyroid cancer
- Other malignancies (eg, lymphoma)

 DIAGNOSIS

LABORATORY TESTS

- Thyroid-stimulating hormone (TSH) level is elevated if thyroiditis causes hypothyroidism, suppressed if it causes hyperthyroidism
- Serum-free tetraiodotyronine (T_4) usually elevated in acute and subacute thyroiditis with hyperthyroidism; normal or low in the chronic forms
- **Hashimoto's thyroiditis**
  – Antithyroperoxidase levels increased in 95%
  – Antithyroglobulin antibodies increased in 60% (very nonspecific)
- Thyroid autoantibodies also found in other types of thyroiditis
  – Mildly elevated titers found in 13% of asymptomatic women and 3% of asymptomatic men
  – Only 1% of the population has antibody titers > 1:6400
- **Subacute thyroiditis**
  – Erythrocyte sedimentation rate markedly elevated
  – Antithyroid antibody titers low

IMAGING STUDIES

- Radioiodine uptake and scan
  – Usually not required
  – Characteristically very low in initial, hyperthyroid phase of subacute thyroiditis, distinguishing thyroiditis from Graves' disease
- Radioiodine uptake may be high with an uneven scan in chronic thyroiditis, with enlargement of the gland, and low in Riedel's thyroiditis
- Ultrasound of thyroid helps distinguish thyroiditis from multinodular goiter or thyroid nodules that are suspicious for malignancy

DIAGNOSTIC PROCEDURES

- Biopsy may be required to distinguish asymmetric thyroiditis from carcinoma

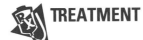 TREATMENT

MEDICATIONS

Hashimoto's thyroiditis

- Levothyroxine, 50–200 mcg PO once daily, if hypothyroidism or large goiter present
- If euthyroid (normal TSH) and minimal goiter, do not administer levothyroxine but follow patient until hypothyroidism develops

Subacute thyroiditis

- Aspirin is drug of choice, continue for several weeks
- Propranolol, 10–40 mg PO q6h, for thyrotoxic symptoms
- Iodinated contrast agents promptly normalize triiodothyronine (T_3) levels and dramatically improve thyrotoxic symptoms. Sodium ipodate (Oragrafin, Bilivist) or iopanoic acid (Telepaque), 500 mg PO once daily, until free T_4 normalizes
- Levothyroxine, 50–100 mcg PO once daily, if transient hypothyroidism is symptomatic

Suppurative thyroiditis

- Antibiotics

Riedel's thyroiditis

- Tamoxifen, 10 mg PO BID, usually induces partial to complete remissions within 3–6 months and must be continued for years
- Short-term corticosteroid treatment for relief of pain and compression symptoms

SURGERY

- Suppurative thyroiditis requires surgical drainage when fluctuance is marked
- For Riedel's thyroiditis, surgery usually fails to permanently alleviate compression and is difficult due to dense fibrous adhesions

 OUTCOME

FOLLOW-UP

- Euthyroid patients with Hashimoto's thyroiditis must be followed up long-term because hypothyroidism may develop years later

COMPLICATIONS

- Hashimoto's thyroiditis
  – Hypothyroidism or transient thyrotoxicosis
  – Associated with other autoimmune disorders

- Subacute and chronic thyroiditis can be complicated by dyspnea
- Riedel's thyroiditis
  – Vocal cord palsy from pressure on neck structures
  – Multifocal systemic fibrosis syndrome, eg, retroperitoneal fibrosis, fibrosing mediastinitis
- Perimenopausal women with high antithyroperoxidase titers are at risk for depression independent of thyroid hormone levels
- Graves' disease may develop in patients with Hashimoto's thyroiditis
- Carcinoma or lymphoma may be associated with chronic thyroiditis and must be considered if uneven painless enlargements continue despite treatment

PROGNOSIS

- Hashimoto's thyroiditis has an excellent prognosis, because it either remains stable for years or progresses slowly to hypothyroidism, which is easily treated
- Subacute thyroiditis may smolder for months; spontaneous remissions and exacerbations are common
- Postpartum thyroiditis usually resolves with return to normal thyroid function

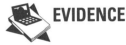 EVIDENCE

PRACTICE GUIDELINES

- Pearce EN et al. Thyroiditis. N Engl J Med. 2003;348:2646. [PMID: 12826640]
- Slatosky J et al. Thyroiditis: differential diagnosis and management. Am Fam Physician. 2000;61:1047. Erratum in Am Fam Physician. 2000;62:318. [PMID: 10706157]

WEB SITES

- American Association of Clinical Endocrinologists
- American Thyroid Association

INFORMATION FOR PATIENTS

- American Thyroid Association
- Mayo Clinic—Subacute thyroiditis
- MedlinePlus—Chronic thyroiditis
- MedlinePlus—Painless thyroiditis
- MedlinePlus—Subacute thyroiditis

REFERENCES

- Gullu S et al. In vivo and in vitro effects of statins on lymphocytes in patients with Hashimoto's thyroiditis. Eur J

Endocrinol. 2005 Jul;153(1):41–8. [PMID: 15994744]

- Jung YJ et al. A case of Riedel's thyroiditis treated with tamoxifen: another successful outcome. Endocr Pract. 2004 Nov–Dec;10(6):483–6. [PMID: 16033720]
- Pearce EN et al. Thyroiditis. N Engl J Med. 2003 Jun 26;348(26):2646–55. [PMID: 12826640]
- Smyth PP et al. Sequential studies on thyroid antibodies during pregnancy. Thyroid. 2005 May;15(5):474–7. [PMID: 15929669]
- Stagnaro-Green A. Postpartum thyroiditis. Best Pract Res Clin Endocrinol Metab. 2004 Jun;18(2):303–16. [PMID: 15157842]

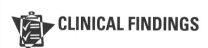

Tinea Corporis or Tinea Circinata

 KEY FEATURES

ESSENTIALS OF DIAGNOSIS

- Ring-shaped lesions with an advancing scaly border and central clearing or scaly patches with a distinct border
- On exposed skin surfaces or the trunk
- Microscopic examination of scrapings or culture confirms the diagnosis

GENERAL CONSIDERATIONS

- The lesions are often on exposed areas of the body such as the face and arms
- *Trichophyton rubrum* is the most common pathogen, usually representing extension onto the trunk or extremities of tinea cruris, pedis, or manuum
- Body ringworm usually responds promptly to conservative topical therapy or to griseofulvin by mouth within 4 weeks

 CLINICAL FINDINGS

SYMPTOMS AND SIGNS

- Ring-shaped lesions with an advancing scaly border and central clearing or scaly patches with a distinct border
- Location: on exposed skin surfaces or the trunk
- Itching may be present

- A history of exposure to an infected cat may occasionally be obtained, usually indicating *Microsporum* infection

DIFFERENTIAL DIAGNOSIS

- Psoriasis
- Impetigo
- Seborrheic dermatitis
- Secondary syphilis
- Pityriasis rosea
- Nummular eczema (discoid eczema, nummular dermatitis)
- Bacterial folliculitis

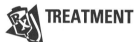 **DIAGNOSIS**

DIAGNOSTIC PROCEDURES

- The diagnosis may be confirmed by KOH preparation and culture

 TREATMENT

MEDICATIONS

- See Table 150

Local measures

- Most topical antifungals (eg, miconazole, clotrimazole, butenafine, and terbinafine, which are available OTC) are effective
- Terbinafine and butenafine require shorter courses and lead to the most rapid response
- In general, use of betamethasone-clotrimazole (Lotrisone) does not justify the expense

Systemic measures

- Griseofulvin (ultramicrosize), 250–500 mg PO twice daily, is used; typically, only 2–4 weeks of therapy are required
- Itraconazole as a single week-long pulse of 200 mg PO once daily is also effective in tinea corporis
- Terbinafine, 250 mg PO once daily for 1 month, is an alternative

THERAPEUTIC PROCEDURES

- Treatment should be continued for 1–2 weeks after clinical clearing

 OUTCOME

COMPLICATIONS

- Extension of disease down the hair follicles
- Pyoderma

PROGNOSIS

- Body ringworm usually responds promptly to conservative topical therapy or to griseofulvin by mouth within 4 weeks

WHEN TO REFER

- If there is a question about the diagnosis, if recommended therapy is ineffective, or if specialized treatment is necessary

PREVENTION

- Treat infected household pets (*Microsporum* infections)

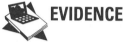 **EVIDENCE**

INFORMATION FOR PATIENTS

- American Academy of Family Physicians: Tinea Infections: Athlete's Foot, Jock Itch and Ringworm
- American Medical Association: Fungal Skin Infection
- Mayo Clinic: Ringworm of the Body
- MedlinePlus: Tinea Corporis

REFERENCE

- Gupta AK et al. Dermatophytosis: the management of fungal infections. Skinmed. 2005 Sep–Oct;4(5):305–10. [PMID: 16282753]

Tinea Manuum & Pedis

KEY FEATURES

ESSENTIALS OF DIAGNOSIS

- Most often presenting with asymptomatic scaling
- May progress to fissuring or maceration in toe web spaces
- Itching, burning, and stinging of interdigital webs, palms, and soles seen occasionally; deep vesicles in inflammatory cases
- The fungus is shown in skin scrapings examined microscopically or by culture of scrapings

GENERAL CONSIDERATIONS

- An extremely common acute or chronic dermatosis

- Certain individuals appear to be more susceptible than others
- Most infections are caused by *Trichophyton* species
- Interdigital tinea pedis is the most common cause of leg cellulitis in healthy individuals

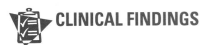

CLINICAL FINDINGS

SYMPTOMS AND SIGNS

- Most often presents with asymptomatic scaling that may progress to fissuring or maceration in toe web spaces
- Itching, burning, and stinging of interdigital webs, palms, and soles seen occasionally; deep vesicles in inflammatory cases
- Tinea pedis has several presentations that vary with the location
- On the sole and heel, may appear as chronic noninflammatory scaling, occasionally with thickening and cracking of the epidermis; this may extend over the sides of the feet in a "moccasin" distribution
- Often appears as a scaling or fissuring of the toe webs, perhaps with sodden maceration
- There may be grouped vesicles distributed anywhere on the soles or palms, generalized exfoliation of the skin of the soles, or nail involvement in the form of discoloration and thickening and crumbling of the nail plate

DIFFERENTIAL DIAGNOSIS

- Erythrasma
- Psoriasis
- Contact dermatitis
- Dyshidrosis (pomphylox)
- Scabies
- Pitted keratolysis
- Tinea pedis must be differentiated from other skin conditions involving the same areas, such as
  - Interdigital erythrasma (use Wood's light)
  - Psoriasis: repeated fungal cultures should be negative
- Contact dermatitis (from shoes) will often involve the dorsal surfaces and will respond to topical or systemic corticosteroids

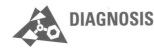

DIAGNOSIS

LABORATORY TESTS

- The KOH preparation is usually positive
- As the web spaces become more macerated, the KOH preparation and fungal culture are less often positive because bacterial species begin to dominate

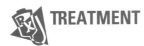

TREATMENT

MEDICATIONS

Local measures

- See Table 150
- Macerated stage—treat with aluminum subacetate solution soaks for 20 min BID
- Broad-spectrum antifungal creams and solutions (containing imidazoles or ciclopirox instead of tolnaftate and haloprogin) will help combat diphtheroids and other gram-positive organisms present at this stage and alone may be adequate therapy
- If topical imidazoles fail, try 1 week of once-daily allylamine treatment (terbinafine or butenafine)
- Dry and scaly stage—use any of the agents listed in Table 150
- The addition of urea 10% lotion or cream (Carmol) under an occlusive dressing may increase the efficacy of topical treatments in thick ("moccasin") tinea of the soles

Systemic measures

- Griseofulvin should be used only for severe cases or those recalcitrant to topical therapy
- Itraconazole, 200 mg PO once daily for 2 weeks or 400 mg once daily for 1 week, or terbinafine, 250 mg PO once daily for 2–4 weeks, may be used in refractory cases

THERAPEUTIC PROCEDURES

- Socks should be changed frequently, and absorbent nonsynthetic socks are preferred

OUTCOME

FOLLOW-UP

- The use of powders containing antifungal agents (eg, Zeasorb-AF) or long-term use of antifungal creams may prevent recurrences, which occur commonly

WHEN TO REFER

- If there is a question about the diagnosis, if recommended therapy is ineffective, or if specialized treatment is necessary

PREVENTION

- The essential factor in prevention is personal hygiene
- Wear open-toed sandals if possible; use of rubber or wooden sandals in community showers and bathing places is often recommended
- Careful drying between the toes after showering is essential; a hair dryer used on low setting may be used

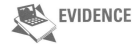

EVIDENCE

WEB SITES

- MedlinePlus: Tinea Manuum Image

INFORMATION FOR PATIENTS

- American Academy of Family Physicians: Tinea Infections: Athlete's Foot, Jock Itch and Ringworm
- Mayo Clinic: Athlete's Foot
- MedlinePlus: Athlete's Foot

REFERENCES

- Crawford F. Athlete's foot. Clin Evid. 2005 Dec;(14):2000–5. [PMID: 16620478]
- Gupta AK et al: Dermatophytosis: the management of fungal infections. Skinmed. 2005 Sep–Oct;4(5):305–10. [PMID: 16282753]

Tinea Versicolor

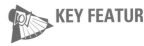

KEY FEATURES

ESSENTIALS OF DIAGNOSIS

- Pale macules with fine scales that will not tan, or hyperpigmented macules
- Velvety, tan, pink, whitish, or brown macules that scale with scraping
- Central upper trunk the most frequent site
- Yeast and short hyphae observed on microscopic examination of scales

GENERAL CONSIDERATIONS

- Mild, superficial *Malassezia furfur* infection of the skin (usually of the upper trunk)
- Patients often first notice that involved areas will not tan, causing hypopigmentation
- High recurrence rate after treatment

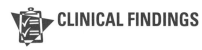

CLINICAL FINDINGS

SYMPTOMS AND SIGNS

- Lesions are asymptomatic, with occasional itching
- The lesions are velvety, tan, pink, white, or brown macules that vary from 4–5 mm in diameter to large confluent areas
- The lesions initially do not look scaly, but scales may be readily obtained by scraping the area
- Lesions may appear on the trunk, upper arms, neck, and groin

DIFFERENTIAL DIAGNOSIS

- Seborrheic dermatitis
- Pityriasis rosea
- Postinflammatory pigmentary change (eg, acne, atopic dermatitis)
- Secondary syphilis
- Hansen's disease (leprosy)
- Vitiligo
  - Usually presents with periorificial lesions or lesions on the tips of the fingers
  - Characterized by total depigmentation, not just a lessening of pigmentation as with tinea versicolor

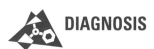

DIAGNOSIS

LABORATORY TESTS

- Large, blunt hyphae and thick-walled budding spores ("spaghetti and meatballs") are seen on KOH
- Fungal culture is not useful

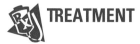

TREATMENT

MEDICATIONS

- See Table 150

Topical treatments

- Selenium sulfide lotion 2.5%
  - May be applied from neck to waist daily and left on for 5–15 min for 7 days
  - Repeat weekly for a month and then monthly for maintenance

- Ketoconazole shampoo lathered on the chest and back and left on for 5 min may also be used weekly for treatment and to prevent recurrence

Systemic therapy

- Ketoconazole
  - 200 mg orally daily for 1 week or 400 mg as a single oral dose, results in short-term cure of 90% of cases
  - Patients should be instructed not to shower for 8 to 12 h after taking ketoconazole because it is delivered in sweat to the skin
  - The single dose may not work in more hot and humid areas

THERAPEUTIC PROCEDURES

- Stress to the patient that the raised and scaly aspects of the rash are being treated; the alterations in pigmentation may take months to fade or fill in
- Irritation and odor from these agents are common complaints from patients

OUTCOME

COMPLICATIONS

- More protracted therapy with ketoconazole carries a small but finite risk of drug-induced hepatitis

PROGNOSIS

- Relapses are common
- Without maintenance therapy, recurrences will occur in over 80% of "cured" cases over the subsequent 2 years

WHEN TO REFER

- If there is a question about the diagnosis, if recommended therapy is ineffective, or if specialized treatment is necessary

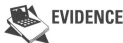

EVIDENCE

INFORMATION FOR PATIENTS

- American Academy of Dermatology: Tinea Versicolor
- American Medical Association: Fungal Skin Infection
- Mayo Clinic: Tinea Versicolor
- MedlinePlus: Tinea Versicolor

REFERENCE

- Khachemoune A. Tinea versicolor. Dermatol Nurs. 2006 Apr;18(2):167. [PMID: 16708681]

Tinnitus

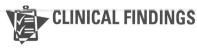

KEY FEATURES

- Tinnitus is the perception of abnormal ear or head noises
- Intermittent periods of mild, high-pitched tinnitus lasting for seconds to minutes are common in normal-hearing persons
- Persistent tinnitus often, but not always, indicates the presence of sensory hearing loss
- When severe and persistent, tinnitus may interfere with sleep and the ability to concentrate, resulting in considerable psychological distress

CLINICAL FINDINGS

- Pulsatile tinnitus
  - Often described as listening to one's own heartbeat
  - Should be distinguished from tonal tinnitus
  - Often caused by conductive hearing loss
  - May indicate a vascular abnormality, such as glomus tumor, carotid vaso-occlusive disease, venous sinus stenosis, arteriovenous malformation, or aneurysm
- A staccato "clicking" tinnitus
  - May result from middle-ear muscle spasm, sometimes associated with palatal myoclonus
  - Patient typically perceives a rapid series of popping noises, lasting seconds to a few minutes, accompanied by a fluttering feeling in the ear

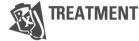

DIAGNOSIS

- Consider MR angiography and venography when vascular abnormality is suspected

TREATMENT

- Avoid exposure to excessive noise, ototoxic agents, and other factors that may cause cochlear damage
- Masking the tinnitus with music or through amplification of normal sounds with a hearing aid may bring relief
- Oral antidepressants (eg, nortriptyline at an initial dosage of 50 mg at bedtime)

often impact tinnitus-induced sleep disorder and depression

Tourette's Syndrome

KEY FEATURES

ESSENTIALS OF DIAGNOSIS

- Multiple motor and phonic tics
- Symptoms begin before age 21 years
- Tics occur frequently for at least 1 year
- Tics vary in number, frequency, and nature over time

GENERAL CONSIDERATIONS

- The diagnosis of the disorder is often delayed for years, the tics being interpreted as psychiatric illness or some other form of abnormal movement
- Patients are thus often subjected to unnecessary treatment before the disorder is recognized

DEMOGRAPHICS

- Tics are noted first in childhood, generally between the ages of 2 and 15
- A family history is sometimes obtained
  - Inheritance has been attributed to an autosomal dominant gene with variable penetrance
  - In some instances, mutations in the *SLITRK1* gene on chromosome 13q have been incriminated

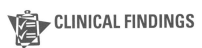

CLINICAL FINDINGS

SYMPTOMS AND SIGNS

- Motor tics
  - Initial manifestation in 80% of cases
  - Most commonly involve the face, head, shoulders, such as sniffing, blinking, frowning, shoulder shrugging, and head thrusting
- Phonic tics
  - Initial symptoms in 20% of cases
  - Commonly consist of grunts, barks, hisses, throat clearing, coughs, verbal utterances including coprolalia (obscene speech)
- A combination of different motor and phonic tics ultimately develop in all patients

- Echolalia (repetition of the speech of others)
- Echopraxia (imitation of others' movements)
- Palilalia (repetition of words or phrases)
- Some tics may be self-mutilating in nature
  - Nail-biting
  - Hair-pulling
  - Biting of the lips or tongue
- Obsessive-compulsive behaviors are commonly associated and may be more disabling than the tics themselves
- In addition to obsessive-compulsive behavior disorders, psychiatric disturbances may occur because of the associated cosmetic and social embarrassment

DIFFERENTIAL DIAGNOSIS

- Wilson's disease

DIAGNOSIS

DIAGNOSTIC PROCEDURES

- Examination usually reveals no abnormalities other than the tics

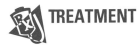

TREATMENT

MEDICATIONS

- Oral clonazepam (in a dose that depends on response and tolerance) or oral clonidine (2–5 mcg/kg/day) may be helpful and prevents some of the long-term extrapyramidal side effects of haloperidol
- Haloperidol
  - Started in a low daily dose (0.25 mg PO)
  - Gradually increase dose by 0.25 mg every 4 or 5 days until there is maximum benefit with a minimum of side effects or until side effects limit further increments
  - A total daily dose of between 2 and 8 mg is usually optimal, but higher doses are sometimes necessary
- Phenothiazines, such as fluphenazine (2–15 mg PO daily), have been used
  - Patients unresponsive to haloperidol are usually unresponsive to phenothiazines as well
- Pimozide is a dopamine blocker related to haloperidol
  - May be helpful in patients who cannot tolerate or have not responded to haloperidol
  - Starting dose is 1 mg PO daily

  - Daily dose is increased by 1–2 mg every 10 days
  - Average dose is between 7 and 16 mg PO daily
- Treatment with risperidone, calcium channel blockers, tetrabenazine, clomipramine, or metoclopramide has yielded mixed results
- Injection of botulinum toxin type A at the site of the most distressing tics is sometimes worthwhile
- Bilateral high-frequency thalamic stimulation may help in otherwise intractable cases and is being studied

THERAPEUTIC PROCEDURES

- Treatment is symptomatic and may need to be continued indefinitely

OUTCOME

PROGNOSIS

- The disorder is chronic, but the course may be punctuated by relapses and remissions

WHEN TO REFER

- When the diagnosis is uncertain
- For expertise in management, particularly when patients do not respond to conventional therapy

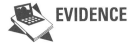

EVIDENCE

PRACTICE GUIDELINES

- Tourette Syndrome Association

INFORMATION FOR PATIENTS

- National Institute of Neurological Disorders and Stroke
- Tourette Syndrome Association

REFERENCE

- Albin RL et al. Recent advances in Tourette syndrome research. Trends Neurosci. 2006 Mar;29(3):175–82. [PMID: 16430974]

Toxic Shock Syndrome, *Staphylococcus aureus*

 KEY FEATURES

- Strains of staphylococci may produce toxins that can cause four important entities
  - Scalded skin syndrome, typically in children, or bullous impetigo in adults
  - Necrotizing pneumonitis in children
  - Toxic shock syndrome (TSS)
  - Enterotoxin food poisoning
- Most cases (≥ 90%) of TSS were initially reported in women of childbearing age, especially common within 5 days of the onset of a menstrual period in women who have used tampons
- Nonmenstrual cases of TSS are now about as common as menstrual cases
- Organisms from various sites, including the nasopharynx, bones, vagina, and rectum, or wounds have all been associated with the illness

 CLINICAL FINDINGS

- Toxic shock is characterized by abrupt onset of fever, vomiting, and watery diarrhea
- A diffuse macular erythematous rash and nonpurulent conjunctivitis are common, and desquamation, especially of the palms and soles, is typical during recovery

 DIAGNOSIS

- Blood cultures classically are negative because symptoms are due to the effects of the toxin and not to the invasive properties of the organism

 TREATMENT

- Rapid rehydration, antistaphylococcal antibiotics (eg, parenteral nafcillin or oxacillin or, in the penicillin allergic patient, clindamycin), management of renal or cardiac failure, and most impor-

tantly removal of sources of toxin (eg, removal of tampon, drainage of abscess)

Toxoplasmosis in the Immuno-competent Patient

 KEY FEATURES

ESSENTIALS OF DIAGNOSIS

Primary infection
- Fever, malaise, headache, sore throat
- Lymphadenopathy
- Positive IgG and IgM serologic tests

Congenital infection
- Follows acute infection of seronegative women and leads to CNS abnormalities and retinochoroiditis

GENERAL CONSIDERATIONS

- *Toxoplasma gondii,* an obligate intracellular protozoan, is found worldwide in humans and in many species of animals and birds
- Cats are the definitive hosts
- Humans are infected after
  - Ingestion of cysts in raw or undercooked meat
  - Ingestion of oocysts in food or water contaminated by cats
  - Transplacental transmission of trophozoites
  - Direct inoculation of trophozoites via blood transfusion or organ transplantation (rare)
- Congenital transmission occurs as a result of infection, which may be symptomatic or asymptomatic, in a nonimmune woman during pregnancy

DEMOGRAPHICS

- Seroprevalence varies widely
  - In the United States, has decreased to about 20–30%
  - In other countries, may exceed 80%
- Congenital infections
  - 400 to 4000 new cases each year in the United States
  - Fetal infection follows maternal infection in 30–50% of cases
  - Risk of transmission varies by trimester: 10–25%, 30–50%, and 60% or

higher during first, second, and third trimesters, respectively

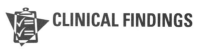 **CLINICAL FINDINGS**

SYMPTOMS AND SIGNS

- Most acute infections are asymptomatic
- About 10–20% are symptomatic after an incubation period of 1–2 weeks

Primary infection
- Nontender cervical or diffuse lymphadenopathy may persist for weeks to months
- Systemic findings
  - Fever, malaise
  - Headache, sore throat
  - Rash
  - Myalgias
  - Hepatosplenomegaly
  - Atypical lymphocytosis
- Rare severe manifestations
  - Pneumonitis
  - Meningoencephalitis
  - Hepatitis
  - Myocarditis
  - Polymyositis
  - Retinochoroiditis

Congenital infection occurring early in pregnancy
- Commonly leads to
  - Spontaneous abortion
  - Stillbirths
  - Severe neonatal disease, including neurologic manifestations
- Neurologic findings can include
  - Seizures
  - Psychomotor retardation
  - Deafness
  - Hydrocephalus
- Retinochoroiditis and other sight-threatening eye lesions may develop
- Systemic findings
  - Fever or hypothermia
  - Jaundice
  - Vomiting, diarrhea
  - Hepatosplenomegaly
  - Pneumonitis, myocarditis
  - Rash

Congenital infection occurring later in pregnancy
- Less commonly leads to major fetal problems
- Most infants appear normal at birth, but subtle abnormalities may be present
- Hepatosplenomegaly and lymphadenopathy may develop in the first few months of life
- CNS and eye disease often present later

Retinochoroiditis

- Late presentation of congenital toxoplasmosis
- Uveitis
- Pain
- Photophobia
- Visual changes, usually without systemic symptoms
- Signs and symptoms eventually improve, but visual defects may persist
- Progression may result in glaucoma and blindness (rarely)

DIAGNOSIS

LABORATORY TESTS

- Isolation of *T gondii* or identification of tachyzoites in tissue or body fluids confirms diagnosis
  - Demonstration of tachyzoites indicates acute infection
  - Cysts may represent either acute or chronic infection
- Histologic evaluation of lymph nodes can show characteristic morphology, with or without organisms

Polymerase chain reaction

- Can be used for sensitive identification of organisms in
  - Amniotic fluid
  - Blood
  - Cerebrospinal fluid
  - Aqueous humor
  - Bronchoalveolar lavage fluid
- Offers a sensitive assessment for congenital disease when acute infection during pregnancy is suspected; should be performed at 18 weeks of gestation

Serologic tests

- Multiple methods are used, including
  - Sabin-Feldman dye test
  - Enzyme-linked immunosorbent assay (ELISA)
  - Indirect fluorescent antibody test
  - Agglutination tests
- Seroconversion, a 16-fold rise in antibody titer, or an IgM titer > 1:64 suggest acute infection, although false-positive results may occur
- IgG antibodies
  - Seen within 1–2 weeks of infection
  - Usually persist for life
- IgM antibodies
  - Peak earlier than IgG and decline more rapidly
  - May persist for years
- During pregnancy
  - Tests not routinely performed

- When tests are done, negative IgG and IgM assays exclude active infection
- Positive IgG with negative IgM is highly suggestive of chronic infection, with no risk of congenital disease unless the mother is severely immunocompromised
- Positive IgM test is concerning for new infection because of the risk of congenital disease
- Confirmatory testing should be performed before consideration of treatment or possible termination of pregnancy due to the limitations of available tests
- Tests of the avidity of anti-IgG antibodies can be helpful, but a battery of tests is needed for confirmation of acute infection during pregnancy
- In newborns
  - Positive IgM or IgA antibody tests are indicative of congenital infection, although the diagnosis is not ruled out by a negative test
  - Positive IgG assays may represent transfer of maternal antibodies without infection of the infant

TREATMENT

MEDICATIONS

- Treatment indications
  - Not necessary for otherwise healthy persons, since primary infection is self-limited
  - Severe, persistent, or visceral disease should be treated for 2–4 weeks
  - Decreases in visual acuity, multiple or large lesions, macular lesions, significant inflammation, or persistence for > 1 month in retinochoroiditis
- Drugs for toxoplasmosis are active only against tachyzoites, so they do not eradicate infection
- Pyrimethamine plus sulfadiazine
  - Pyrimethamine: 200 mg loading dose then 50–75 mg (1 mg/kg) PO once daily
  - Sulfadiazine: 1–1.5 g PO QID
  - Coadminister folinic acid (10–20 mg PO once daily) to prevent bone marrow suppression
- Pyrimethamine
  - Side effects include headache and gastrointestinal symptoms
  - Avoid during first trimester of pregnancy due to its teratogenicity
- Alternatives to sulfadiazine
  - Clindamycin: 600 mg PO QID (first-line)
  - Trimethoprim-sulfamethoxazole

- Combining pyrimethamine with atovaquone, clarithromycin, azithromycin, or dapsone
- Spiramycin: 1 g PO TID until delivery
  - Used only to decrease the risk of fetal infection
  - Reduces frequency of transmission to the fetus by about 60%
  - Does not cross the placenta
  - When fetal infection is documented or for acute infections late in pregnancy, treatment with combination regimens as described above is indicated

OUTCOME

FOLLOW-UP

- Platelet and white blood cell counts should be monitored at least weekly while taking pyrimethamine plus sulfadiazine and folinic acid therapy

COMPLICATIONS

- Patients should be screened for a history of sulfonamide sensitivity
  - Skin rashes
  - Gastrointestinal symptoms
  - Hepatotoxicity
- To prevent crystal-induced nephrotoxicity
  - Good urinary output should be maintained
  - Alkalinization with sodium bicarbonate may also be useful

PROGNOSIS

- Symptoms of primary infection may fluctuate, but most patients recover spontaneously within a few months

PREVENTION

- Avoid undercooked meat or contact with material contaminated by cat feces
- For meat, irradiation, cooking to 66 °C, or freezing to –20 °C kills tissue cysts
- Avoid ingestion of dried meat
- Thorough cleaning of hands and surfaces is needed after contact with raw meat or areas contaminated by cats
- Litter boxes should be changed daily and soaked in boiling water for 5 minutes since fresh oocysts are not infective for 48 hours
- Wear gloves when gardening
- Fruits and vegetables should be washed thoroughly

EVIDENCE

INFORMATION FOR PATIENTS

- National Toxicology Program

REFERENCES

- Miro JM. Discontinuation of primary and secondary *Toxoplasma gondii* prophylaxis is safe in HIV-infected patients after immunological restoration with highly active antiretroviral therapy: results of an open, randomized, multi-center clinical trial. Clin Infect Dis. 2006 Jul 1;43(1):79–89. [PMID: 16758422].
- Montoya JG et al. Diagnosis and management of toxoplasmosis. Clin Perinatol. 2005 Sep;32(3):705–26. [PMID: 16085028]
- Montoya JG et al. Toxoplasmosis. Lancet. 2004 Jun 12;363(9425):1965–76. [PMID: 15194258]
- Remington JS et al. Recent developments for diagnosis of toxoplasmosis. J Clin Microbiol. 2004 Mar;42(3):941–5. [PMID: 15004036]

Toxoplasmosis in the Immunocompromised Patient

 KEY FEATURES

ESSENTIALS OF DIAGNOSIS

- Reactivation leads to encephalitis, retinochoroiditis, pneumonitis, myocarditis
- Positive IgG but negative IgM serologic tests

GENERAL CONSIDERATIONS

- *Toxoplasma gondii* is an obligate intracellular protozoan
  - Found worldwide in humans and many species of animals and birds
  - The cat is the definitive host
- Humans are infected after
  - Ingestion of cysts in raw or undercooked meat
  - Ingestion of oocysts in food or water contaminated by cats
  - Transplacental transmission of trophozoites
  - Direct inoculation of trophozoites via blood transfusion or organ transplantation (rare)

DEMOGRAPHICS

- Seroprevalence varies widely
  - In the United States, has decreased to about 20–30%
  - In other countries, may exceed 80%

 CLINICAL FINDINGS

SYMPTOMS AND SIGNS

- Reactivated toxoplasmosis occurs in patients with AIDS or hematologic malignancies, or those given immunosuppressive drugs
- AIDS
  - Encephalitis, with multiple necrotizing brain lesions
    - Fever
    - Headache
    - Altered mental status
    - Focal neurologic findings
    - Other evidence of brain lesions
  - Chorioretinitis
    - Ocular pain
    - Alterations in vision
  - Pneumonitis
    - Fever
    - Cough
    - Dyspnea
- Toxoplasmosis can develop in seronegative recipients of solid organ or bone marrow transplants due to reactivation or transmission of infection
- Immunodeficiency due to malignancy or immunosuppressive drugs
  - Symptoms similar to those seen in persons with AIDS
  - However, pneumonitis and myocarditis are more common
- Other organ systems are less commonly involved in generalized toxoplasmosis

DIFFERENTIAL DIAGNOSIS

- CNS lymphoma
- Tuberculoma
- Bacterial brain abscess
- Fungal abscess
- Carcinoma

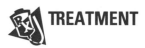 DIAGNOSIS

LABORATORY TESTS

- Serologic tests can be done on blood, cerebrospinal fluid, aqueous humor, and other body fluids
- IgM and IgG antibodies (see Toxoplasmosis in the Immunocompetent Patient)

IMAGING STUDIES

- CT and MRI scans
  - Typically show multiple ring-enhancing cerebral lesions, most commonly involving the corticomedullary junction and basal ganglia
  - MRI is the more sensitive imaging modality

DIAGNOSTIC PROCEDURES

- Diagnosis of CNS toxoplasmosis is most typically made after a therapeutic trial, with clinical and radiologic improvement expected within 2–3 weeks
- Brain biopsy and search for organisms and typical histology provides definitive diagnosis
- In retinochoroiditis, fundoscopic examination shows
  - Vitreous inflammatory reaction
  - White retinal lesions
  - Pigmented scars
- Diagnosis of other clinical entities in immunocompromised individuals is generally based on histology

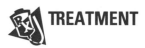 TREATMENT

MEDICATIONS

- Active infection must be treated
- For persons with transient immunodeficiency, therapy can be continued for 4–6 weeks after cessation of symptoms
- For persons with persistent immunodeficiency, such as AIDS patients, full therapy for 4–6 weeks is followed by maintenance therapy with lower doses of drugs
- Immunodeficient patients who are asymptomatic but have a positive IgG serologic test should receive long-term chemoprophylaxis
- Chemoprophylaxis
  - Pyrimethamine, 25 mg/d orally for 6 weeks
  - Trimethoprim-sulfamethoxazole (TMP-SMZ), one double-strength tablet daily or two tablets three times weekly)
  - Alternatives to TMP-SMZ are pyrimethamine plus either sulfadoxine or dapsone (various regimens)

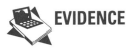

OUTCOME

PREVENTION

- Avoidance of undercooked meat or contact with material contaminated by cat feces, particularly for seronegative pregnant women and immunocompromised persons
- For meat, irradiation, cooking to 66 °C, or freezing to –20 °C kills tissue cysts
- Avoid eating dried meats
- Thorough cleaning of hands and surfaces is needed after contact with raw meat or areas contaminated by cats
- Litter boxes should be changed daily and soaked in boiling water for 5 minutes, since fresh oocysts are not infective for 48 hours
- Wear gloves when gardening
- Fruits and vegetables should be thoroughly washed

EVIDENCE

WEB SITE

- CDC—Division of Parasitic Diseases

INFORMATION FOR PATIENTS

- American Academy of Family Physicians

REFERENCES

- Miro JM. Discontinuation of primary and secondary *Toxoplasma gondii* prophylaxis is safe in HIV-infected patients after immunological restoration with highly active antiretroviral therapy: results of an open, randomized, multicenter clinical trial. Clin Infect Dis. 2006 Jul 1;43(1):79–89. [PMID: 16758422]
- Montoya JG et al. Diagnosis and management of toxoplasmosis. Clin Perinatol. 2005 Sep;32(3):705–26. [PMID: 16085028]
- Montoya JG et al. Toxoplasmosis. Lancet. 2004 Jun 12;363(9425):1965–76. [PMID: 15194258]
- Remington JS et al. Recent developments for diagnosis of toxoplasmosis. J Clin Microbiol. 2004 Mar;42(3):941–5. [PMID: 15004036]

Transient Ischemic Attack

KEY FEATURES

ESSENTIALS OF DIAGNOSIS

- Acute, focal neurologic deficit
- Clinical deficit resolves completely within 24 hours

GENERAL CONSIDERATIONS

- Focal, ischemic, cerebral neurologic deficits that last for < 24 h (usually < 1–2 h)
- Embolization is an important etiology and may explain why separate attacks may affect different parts of the territory supplied by the same vessel
- Cardiac embolic sources
  - Rheumatic heart disease
  - Mitral valve disease
  - Cardiac arrhythmia
  - Infective endocarditis
  - Atrial myxoma
  - Mural thrombi after myocardial infarction (MI)
  - Atrial septal defects and patent foramen ovale may permit emboli from the veins to reach the brain ("paradoxical emboli")
- Cerebrovascular sources
  - An ulcerated plaque on a major artery to the brain may be a source of emboli
  - In the anterior circulation, atherosclerotic changes occur most commonly near the carotid bifurcation extracranially and may cause a bruit
  - Other (less common) abnormalities of blood vessels that may cause transient ischemic attacks (TIAs): fibromuscular dysplasia (particularly affects the cervical internal carotid artery); atherosclerosis of the aortic arch; inflammatory arterial disorders such as giant cell arteritis, systemic lupus erythematosus, polyarteritis, and granulomatous angiitis; and meningovascular syphilis
- Hypotension may reduce cerebral blood flow and rarely cause a TIA if a major extracranial artery to the brain is markedly stenosed
- The subclavian steal syndrome may lead to transient vertebrobasilar ischemia from stenosis or occlusion of one subclavian artery proximal to the source of the vertebral artery

- Hematologic causes
  - Polycythemia
  - Sickle cell disease
  - Hyperviscosity

DEMOGRAPHICS

- Proper treatment of TIAs can help prevent strokes
- About 30% of patients with stroke have a history of TIAs
- Risk of stroke is highest within 1 month after a TIA and then progressively declines
- Incidence of stroke is not related to the number or duration of individual TIAs but is increased in patients with hypertension or diabetes mellitus

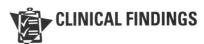

CLINICAL FINDINGS

SYMPTOMS AND SIGNS

- Symptoms vary markedly among patients, but tend to be consistent in a given individual
- Onset abrupt, and recovery often occurs within a few minutes
- TIA in the carotid territory may manifest with
  - Weakness and heaviness of the contralateral arm, leg, or face, singly or in combination
  - Numbness or paresthesias may occur either as sole manifestation or with motor deficits
  - Dysphagia
  - Visual loss in the eye contralateral to affected limbs may occur
  - During an attack, examination may reveal flaccid weakness with pyramidal distribution, sensory changes, hyperreflexia or an extensor plantar response on the affected side, dysphasia, or any combination of these
  - A carotid bruit or cardiac abnormality may be present
- Vertebrobasilar TIA may manifest with
  - Vertigo
  - Ataxia
  - Diplopia
  - Dysarthria
  - Dimness or blurring of vision
  - Perioral numbness and paresthesias
  - Weakness or sensory complaints on one, both, or alternating sides of the body
  - Drop attacks due to bilateral leg weakness, without headache or loss of consciousness, may occur, in relation to head movements
  - Attacks may occur intermittently and stop spontaneously

- Findings in the subclavian steal syndrome may include
  - A bruit in the supraclavicular fossa
  - Unequal radial pulses
  - A difference of 20 mm Hg or more between the systolic blood pressures in the arms

DIFFERENTIAL DIAGNOSIS

- Stroke
- Hypoglycemia
- Focal seizure (Todd's paralysis)
- Syncope
- Migraine
- Peripheral causes of vertigo (eg, Ménière's disease)

 DIAGNOSIS

LABORATORY TESTS

- Complete blood cell count
- Fasting blood glucose and serum cholesterol and homocysteine
- Serologic test for syphilis
- Blood cultures if endocarditis is suspected

IMAGING STUDIES

- Chest radiograph
- CT or MRI scan of the head to exclude a cerebral hemorrhage or a rare tumor masquerading as a TIA
- Carotid duplex ultrasonography can detect significant stenosis of the internal carotid artery
- MR or CT angiography
  - May reveal stenotic lesions of large vessels
  - Less sensitive than conventional arteriography
- Patients with vertebrobasilar TIA are treated medically and are not subjected to arteriography unless there is clinical evidence of stenosis in carotid or subclavian arteries
- Echocardiography with bubble contrast is performed if a cardiac source is likely

DIAGNOSTIC PROCEDURES

- ECG
- Holter monitoring if a paroxysmal cardiac arrhythmia is suspected
- Assessment for
  - Hypertension
  - Heart disease
  - Hematologic disorders
  - Diabetes mellitus
  - Hyperlipidemia
  - Peripheral vascular disease

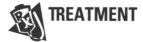 **TREATMENT**

MEDICATIONS

Embolization from the heart

- Anticoagulants should be started immediately unless contraindicated
- The fear of causing hemorrhage into an infarcted area is misplaced, since there is a far greater risk of further embolism to the cerebral circulation if treatment is withheld
- Use IV heparin while warfarin in introduced
  - Loading dose of 5000–10,000 units of standard molecular weight heparin
  - Maintenance infusion of 1000–2000 units/h, depending on the partial thromboplastin time
- Warfarin is more effective than aspirin in reducing the incidence of cardioembolic events, but when contraindicated, aspirin (325 mg PO once daily) may be used in nonrheumatic atrial fibrillation

Noncardioembolic attacks

- In presumed or angiographically verified atherosclerotic changes in the extracranial or intracranial cerebrovascular circulation, antithrombotic medication is prescribed
- Treatment with aspirin, 325 mg PO once daily, significantly reduces the frequency of TIA and stroke
- Sustained-release dipyridamole (200 mg BID) can be added to aspirin for optimal stroke prevention
- In patients intolerant of aspirin, clopidogrel, 75 mg PO once daily, may be used
- Anticoagulant drugs are not recommended; there is no benefit over antiplatelet therapy and risk of serious hemorrhagic adverse effects is greater

SURGERY

- Carotid endarterectomy
  - Reduces the risk of ipsilateral carotid stroke, especially when TIAs are of recent onset (< 2 months)
  - Indicated when there is a surgically accessible high-grade stenosis (70–99% in luminal diameter) on the side appropriate to carotid ischemic attacks and there is relatively little atherosclerosis elsewhere in the cerebrovascular system
- Surgery is not indicated for mild stenosis (< 30%); its benefits are unclear with severe stenosis plus diffuse intracranial atherosclerotic disease
- Surgical extracranial-intracranial arterial anastomosis is generally not helpful

in TIAs associated with stenotic lesions of the distal internal carotid or the proximal middle cerebral arteries

THERAPEUTIC PROCEDURES

- Cigarette smoking should be stopped
- Treat cardiac sources of embolization, hypertension, diabetes mellitus, hyperlipidemia, arteritis, or hematologic disorders appropriately
- Weight reduction and regular physical activity should be encouraged when appropriate

 OUTCOME

PROGNOSIS

- In general, carotid TIAs are more likely than vertebrobasilar TIAs to be followed by stroke
- The stroke risk is greater
  - In patients older than 60 years
  - In diabetic persons
  - After TIAs that last longer than 10 minutes
  - With symptoms or signs of weakness, speech impairment, or gait disturbance

WHEN TO REFER

- If CT scan is normal, there is no cardiac source of embolization, and patient is a good operative risk, refer for possible endarterectomy

WHEN TO ADMIT

- Consider hospitalization for patients seen within 48 hours of first attack; or with crescendo attacks, symptoms lasting for more than 1 h; symptomatic carotid stenosis; or a known cardiac source of emboli or hypercoagulable state

PREVENTION

- Anticoagulation of atrial fibrillation (except lone atrial fibrillation)
- Control of hypertension
- Control of lipids

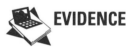 **EVIDENCE**

PRACTICE GUIDELINES

- Adams RJ et al. Coronary risk evaluation in patients with transient ischemic attack and ischemic stroke: a scientific statement for healthcare professionals from the Stroke Council and the Council on Clinical Cardiology of the American Heart Association/American Stroke Association. Stroke. 2003;34:2310. [PMID: 12958318]

- Albers GW et al. Antithrombotic and thrombolytic therapy for ischemic stroke: the Seventh ACCP Conference on Antithrombotic and Thrombolytic Therapy. Chest. 2004;126(3 Suppl):483S. [PMID: 15383482]
- Johnston SC et al. National Stroke Association guidelines for the management of transient ischemic attacks. Ann Neurol. 2006 Sep;60(3):301–13. [PMID: 16912978]

INFORMATION FOR PATIENTS

- American Heart Association
- National Institute of Neurological Disorders and Stroke

REFERENCES

- Chimowitz MI et al; Warfarin-Aspirin Symptomatic Intracranial Disease Trial Investigators. Comparison of warfarin and aspirin for symptomatic intracranial arterial stenosis. N Engl J Med. 2005 Mar 31;352(13):1305–16. [PMID: 15800226]
- Nguyen-Huynh MN et al. Transient ischemic attack: a neurologic emergency. Curr Neurol Neurosci Rep. 2005 Feb;5(1):13–20. [PMID: 15676103]
- Rothwell PM et al. Recent advances in management of transient ischaemic attacks and minor ischaemic strokes. Lancet Neurol. 2006 Apr;5(4):323–31. [PMID: 16545749]

Trigeminal Neuralgia

 KEY FEATURES

ESSENTIALS OF DIAGNOSIS

- Brief episodes of stabbing facial pain
- Pain is in the territory of the second and third division of the trigeminal nerve
- Pain exacerbated by touch

GENERAL CONSIDERATIONS

- Trigeminal neuralgia (tic douloureux) is most common in middle and later life
- It affects women more frequently than men

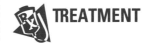 **CLINICAL FINDINGS**

SYMPTOMS AND SIGNS

- Momentary episodes of sudden lancinating facial pain
- Commonly arises near one side of the mouth and shoots toward the ear, eye, or nostril on that side
- The pain may be triggered by touch, movement, drafts, and eating
- To prevent further attacks, many patients try to hold the face still
- Symptoms remain confined to the distribution of the trigeminal nerve (usually the second or third division) on one side only
- Neurologic examination shows no abnormality unless trigeminal neuralgia is symptomatic of some underlying lesion, such as multiple sclerosis or a brainstem neoplasm

DIFFERENTIAL DIAGNOSIS

- Atypical facial pain
  - Especially common in middle-aged women
  - Generally a constant burning pain that may have a restricted distribution at onset but soon spreads to the rest of the face on the affected side and sometimes involves the other side of the face, the neck, and the back of the head as well
- Temporomandibular joint dysfunction
  - Occurs with malocclusion, abnormal bite, or faulty dentures
  - May cause tenderness of the masticatory muscles
  - An association between pain onset and jaw movement
  - Diagnosis requires dental examination and x-rays
- Giant cell arteritis—may have pain on mastication
- Sinusitis and ear infections
- Glaucoma
- Multiple sclerosis
- Brainstem tumor
- Dental caries or abscess
- Otitis media
- Glossopharyngeal neuralgia
- Postherpetic neuralgia

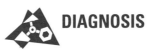 **DIAGNOSIS**

IMAGING STUDIES

- Cerebral CT scans and MRIs are normal in patients with classic trigeminal

neuralgia but should nevertheless be performed to exclude structural causes

DIAGNOSTIC PROCEDURES

- The characteristic features of the pain in trigeminal neuralgia usually distinguish it from other causes of facial pain
- In a young patient presenting with trigeminal neuralgia, multiple sclerosis must be suspected even if there are no other neurologic signs
  - In such a patient, findings on evoked potential testing, head MRI, and examination of cerebrospinal fluid may be corroborative

 TREATMENT

MEDICATIONS

- Oxcarbazepine (300–600 mg PO BID) or carbamazepine (200–400 mg PO BID) is most helpful (monitor blood cell counts and liver function tests)
- Phenytoin is second choice (Table 133)
- Baclofen (10–20 mg PO TID or QID) may be helpful, alone or in combination with carbamazepine or phenytoin
- Gabapentin
  - Up to 2400 mg PO daily is given in divided doses
  - May relieve pain in patients refractory to conventional therapy and those with multiple sclerosis

SURGERY

- Surgical exploration, radiofrequency rhizotomy, and gamma radiosurgery should be reserved for specialized centers

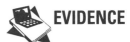 **OUTCOME**

PROGNOSIS

- Spontaneous remissions may occur for several months or longer
- Progression of the disorder
  - Episodes of pain become more frequent
  - Remissions become shorter and less common
  - A dull ache may persist between the episodes of stabbing pain

 EVIDENCE

INFORMATION FOR PATIENTS

- National Institute of Neurological Disorders and Stroke

REFERENCES

- Liu JK et al. Treatment of trigeminal neuralgia. Neurosurg Clin North Am. 2004 Jul;15(3):319–34. [PMID: 15246340]
- Rozen TD. Trigeminal neuralgia and glossopharyngeal neuralgia. Neurol Clin. 2004 Feb;22(1):185–206. [PMID: 15062534]

Tuberculosis, Latent Infection

KEY FEATURES

ESSENTIALS OF DIAGNOSIS

- Positive tuberculin skin test
- No evidence of active infection with tuberculosis
- History (knowingly or not) of exposure to *Mycobacterium tuberculosis* (MTB)

GENERAL CONSIDERATIONS

- Targeted skin testing used to identify
  - Persons at high risk for tuberculosis (TB)
  - Persons who would benefit from treatment of latent tuberculosis infection (LTBI)
- LTBI describes patients who have been infected with *M tuberculosis* but do not have active disease
- Individuals with LTBI have contained but not eradicated infection
- The importance of identifying and treating LTBI is to prevent reactivation disease
- LTBI is nontransmissible but may become active disease if a person's immune function becomes impaired
- Without preventive therapy, 10% of patients with LTBI will have reactivation during their lifetime, with 50% of cases occurring within 2 years of primary infection
- Reactivation occurs within 2 years in up to 50% of HIV-positive patients with LTBI
- Patients with primary infection require 2–10 weeks to manifest an immune response to skin testing
- Persons who have received bacillus Calmette-Guérin (BCG) vaccination may have a positive purified protein derivative (PPD) tuberculin test for the rest of their lives

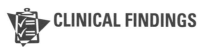

CLINICAL FINDINGS

SYMPTOMS AND SIGNS

- Patients are asymptomatic
- LTBI is uncovered by screening with the tuberculin skin test
- Any pulmonary or constitutional symptoms should prompt an evaluation for active disease prior to prophylactic treatment

DIFFERENTIAL DIAGNOSIS

- BCG vaccination

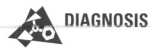

DIAGNOSIS

LABORATORY TESTS

- All patients with risk factors should be tested for HIV

IMAGING STUDIES

- Chest radiograph is required to rule out active pulmonary tuberculosis

DIAGNOSTIC PROCEDURES

- The Mantoux test is the preferred skin test (Table 106)
  - 0.1 mL of PPD containing 5 tuberculin units is injected intradermally on the volar forearm
  - Transverse width in millimeters of induration is measured at 48–72 hours
- False-positive tuberculin skin test reactions occur in patients previously vaccinated against MTB with BCG
- Prior vaccination with BCG does not alter the interpretation of the tuberculin skin test
- False-negative tests may result from
  - Improper technique
  - Concurrent infections
  - Malnutrition
  - Advanced age
  - Immunosuppression of any kind
  - Fulminant MTB infection
- Because of waning immunity, some patients with LTBI may have a negative skin test many years after exposure
- Two-step testing or "boosting"
  - Performed to reduce the likelihood that a boosted reaction will later be misinterpreted as a recent infection in individuals who will be tested repeatedly (health care workers)
  - A second test is performed 1–3 weeks after a negative test
  - If negative, the patient is uninfected or anergic; if positive, a "boosted reaction" is likely
- Anergy testing is not recommended to distinguish a true-negative test from anergy

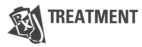

TREATMENT

MEDICATIONS

- Treatment substantially reduces the risk that infection will reactivate and progress to clinical disease
- Patients in whom active disease is suspected should be treated with multidrug regimens until the diagnosis is confirmed or excluded
- Exposed persons who are skin-test–negative and HIV-negative may be observed without treatment or treated with 6 months of oral therapy
- Isoniazid (INH)
  - 9 months oral regimen (= 270 doses within 12 months)
  - 300 mg once daily or 15 mg/kg twice weekly
  - Coadministration of pyridoxine, 10–50 mg PO once daily, for patients at risk for INH-related neuropathy (diabetes mellitus, uremia, malnutrition, alcoholism, HIV infection, pregnancy, seizure disorder) and pregnant or lactating women
- Rifampin/pyrazinamide (RIF/PZA)
  - 2 months oral regimen (= 60 doses within 3 months)
  - RIF 10 mg/kg PO once daily to maximum of 600 mg/day and PZA 15–20 mg/day to maximum of 2 g/day
- Rifampin (RIF)
  - 4-month oral regimen (= 120 doses over 4 months)
  - RIF 10 mg/kg PO once daily to maximum of 600 mg/day
  - Used for patients who cannot receive INH or PZA
- Contacts of persons with INH-resistant, RIF-sensitive MTB should receive RIF/PZA or RIF regimens
- Contacts of persons with multidrug-resistant TB (MDRTB) should receive two drugs to which the organism is sensitive
- HIV-positive contacts should be treated for 12 months

THERAPEUTIC PROCEDURES

- It is not necessary to routinely monitor liver function tests unless there are abnormalities at baseline or clinical reasons to obtain the measurements

OUTCOME

FOLLOW-UP

- All contacts of persons with MDRTB should be monitored for 2 years regardless of treatment
- Patients being treated for LTBI should be seen monthly to evaluate for evidence of active TB, side effects (eg, INH hepatitis), and adherence to treatment

COMPLICATIONS

- Development of active TB
- Drug toxicity

PROGNOSIS

- Almost all properly treated patients with TB can be cured
- Relapse rates are < 5% with current regimens
- Treatment failure is most commonly due to medication nonadherence

WHEN TO REFER

- HIV-positive patients receiving antiretroviral therapy should be referred to TB and HIV experts if they are to receive rifampin therapy

PREVENTION

- Close contacts of patients with active TB should be retested 10–12 weeks after a negative tuberculin skin test
- Despite a negative skin test, close contacts of patients with TB should consider treatment if they are immunosuppressed

EVIDENCE

PRACTICE GUIDELINES

- Centers for Disease Control and Prevention; American Thoracic Society. Update: adverse event data and revised American Thoracic Society/CDC recommendations against the use of rifampin and pyrazinamide for treatment of latent tuberculosis infection—United States, 2003. MMWR Morb Mortal Wkly Rep. 2003;52(31):735. [PMID: 12904741]
- Neff M et al. ATS, CDC, and IDSA update recommendations on the treatment of tuberculosis. Am Fam Physi-

cian. 2003;68:1854,1857,1861. [PMID: 14620606]

INFORMATION FOR PATIENTS

- National Institute of Allergy and Infectious Disease

REFERENCES

- American Thoracic Society; Centers for Disease Control and Prevention; Infectious Diseases Society of America. American Thoracic Society; Centers for Disease Control and Prevention; Infectious Diseases Society of America. Controlling tuberculosis in the United States. Am J Respir Crit Care Med. 2005 Nov 1;172(9):1169–227. [PMID: 16249321]
- Blumberg HM et al. American Thoracic Society/Centers for Disease Control and Prevention/Infectious Diseases Society of America. Treatment of tuberculosis. Am J Respir Crit Care Med. 2003 Feb 15;167(4):603–62. [PMID: 12588714]
- Blumberg HM et al. Update on the treatment of tuberculosis and latent tuberculosis infection. JAMA. 2005 Jun 8;293(22):2776–84. [PMID: 15941808]
- Brodie D et al. The diagnosis of tuberculosis. Clin Chest Med. 2005 Jun; 26(2):247–71. [PMID: 15837109]
- Diagnostic Standards and Classification of Tuberculosis in Adults and Children. American Thoracic Society and Centers for Disease Control and Prevention. Am J Respir Crit Care Med 2000 Apr;161(4 Part 1):1376–95. [PMID: 10764337]

Tuberculosis, Pulmonary

KEY FEATURES

ESSENTIALS OF DIAGNOSIS

- Cough and constitutional symptoms
- Pulmonary infiltrates on chest radiograph, most often apical
- Positive tuberculin skin test reaction (most cases)
- Sputum smear showing acid-fast bacilli or sputum culture positive for *Mycobacterium tuberculosis* (MTB)

GENERAL CONSIDERATIONS

- **Primary infection**
  - Occurs with inhalation of airborne droplets containing viable tubercle bacilli and subsequent lymphangitic and hematogenous spread before immunity develops
  - Up to one-third of new urban cases are from primary infection acquired by person-to-person transmission
- **Progressive primary tuberculosis**
  - Occurs in 5% of cases, with pulmonary and constitutional symptoms
- **Latent tuberculosis infection** (LTBI)
  - Occurs when bacilli are contained within granulomata
  - Nontransmissible, but may become active disease if a person's immune function becomes impaired
- Resistance to one or more drugs is seen in 15% of tuberculosis patients in the United States and is increasing
- Nonadherence is a major cause of treatment failure, disease transmission, and development of drug resistance

DEMOGRAPHICS

- Infects 20–40% of the world population annually (3 million deaths)
- Occurs disproportionately among malnourished, homeless, and marginally housed individuals
- Risk factors for reactivation
  - Gastrectomy
  - Silicosis
  - Diabetes mellitus
  - HIV
  - Immunosuppressive drugs
- Risk factors for drug resistance
  - Immigration from regions with drug-resistant tuberculosis
  - Close contact with patients infected with drug-resistant tuberculosis
  - Unsuccessful prior therapy
  - Patient noncompliance with treatment

CLINICAL FINDINGS

SYMPTOMS AND SIGNS

- Cough is the most common symptom
- Blood-streaked sputum is common, frank hemoptysis is rare
- Slowly progressive constitutional symptoms include malaise, anorexia, weight loss, fever, and night sweats
- Patients appear chronically ill
- Chest examination is nonspecific; posttussive apical rales are classic

- Atypical presentations are becoming more common, usually among the elderly and HIV-positive patients

DIFFERENTIAL DIAGNOSIS

- Pneumonia or lung abscess
- Lung cancer or lymphoma
- *Mycobacterium avium* complex (or other nontuberculous mycobacteria)
- Sarcoidosis
- Fungal infection, eg, histoplasmosis
- Endocarditis
- Silicosis or asbestosis
- Nocardiosis

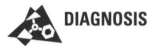

DIAGNOSIS

LABORATORY TESTS

- Tuberculin skin test (Table 106)
- Definitive diagnosis is *M tuberculosis* on culture or identification with DNA or RNA amplification techniques
- Three consecutive first morning sputum samples are advised
- Cultures on solid media may require 12 weeks; liquid medium culture systems can identify growth in several days
- Pleural fluid cultures are positive in only 25% of tuberculous effusions

IMAGING STUDIES

Chest radiograph

- Primary disease
  - There may be homogeneous infiltrates, hilar and paratracheal lymph node enlargement, and/or segmental atelectasis
  - Cavitation may be seen with progressive disease
- Reactivation disease
  - There may be fibrocavitary apical disease, nodules, and infiltrates, usually in apical or posterior segments of upper lobes, but in other locations in 30% of cases
  - More commonly in elderly patients
- Miliary pattern (diffuse small nodular densities) reflects hematologic or lymphangitic spread
- Ghon (calcified primary focus) and Ranke (calcified primary focus with calcified hilar lymph node) complexes represent healed primary infection

DIAGNOSTIC PROCEDURES

- Sputum induction is required for patients unable to voluntarily produce a sample

- Bronchoscopy may be considered in smear-negative patients in whom there is a high suspicion of disease
- Needle biopsy of the pleura reveals granulomatous inflammation in 60% of tuberculous pleural effusions
- Culture of three pleural biopsy specimens combined with microscopic examination increases the diagnostic yield to 90%

TREATMENT

MEDICATIONS

- Medications: see dosages in Table 108
- Multiple drugs to which the organism is susceptible are used
  - At least two new drugs are added when treatment failure is suspected
  - When a twice- or thrice-weekly regimen is used, dosages are increased (Tables 107 and 108)
- Coadminister pyridoxine, 10–50 mg/day, for patients at risk for INH-related neuropathy (diabetes mellitus, uremia, malnutrition, alcoholism, HIV infection, seizure disorder) or pregnancy and lactation

HIV-infected patients

- 6-month rather than 9-month regimen
- Daily isoniazid (INH), rifampin (RIF), and pyrazinamide (PZA) for 2 months
- Ethambutol (EMB) or streptomycin added where prevalence of INH resistance is 4% or higher
- If isolate is RIF- and INH-sensitive, continue these two drugs for 4 months
- Therapy is continued for at least 3 months beyond documentation of sputum cultures negative for MTB
- Directly observed therapy (DOT) regimens
  - INH/RIF/PZA plus EMB or streptomycin daily for 2 months, then INH/RIF 2–3 times/week for 4 months if susceptibility is demonstrated
  - INH/RIF/PZA plus EMB or streptomycin daily for 2 weeks, then 2 times/week for 6 weeks, then INH/RIF 2 times/week for 4 months if susceptibility is demonstrated
  - INH/RIF/PZA plus EMB or streptomycin 3 times/week for 6 months

Drug-resistant TB

- MTB resistant only to INH can be treated with 6 months of RIF/PZA plus EMB or streptomycin or 12 months of RIF/EMB
- Treatment requires individualized daily treatment with DOT under an experienced clinician

- Most resistant MTB strains have at least INH or RIF resistance and require three drugs to which susceptibility is proven
- The three-drug regimen is continued until negative cultures are documented; a two-drug regimen is continued for another 12–24 months

Pregnant or lactating women

- INH, RIF, and EMB, with EMB excluded if INH resistance is unlikely
- Teratogenicity of PZA is unknown; streptomycin is contraindicated owing to a risk of congenital deafness
- Pyridoxine should be given with INH
- Breast-feeding is not contraindicated

Extrapulmonary disease

- In most cases, regimens effective for pulmonary disease are adequate
- Miliary, meningeal, bone, or joint involvement require 9 months of therapy
- Corticosteroids reduce complications of tuberculous pericarditis and meningitis

SURGERY

- Early débridement and drainage are recommended for skeletal involvement

OUTCOME

FOLLOW-UP

- Complete blood cell counts, pulmonary function tests, and renal function should be checked at baseline
- Visual acuity and red-green color vision testing prior to EMB use and audiometry prior to streptomycin use
- Routine monitoring for evidence of drug toxicity is not recommended unless baseline results are abnormal or liver disease is suspected
- Monthly visits with monthly sputum smears and cultures until documented negative
- If sputum is negative after 2 months of therapy, repeat smear and culture at the end of therapy
- Patients with multidrug-resistant tuberculosis (MDRTB) should have sputum smear and culture monthly throughout therapy
- Chest radiograph is recommended at conclusion of successful therapy
- Patients whose cultures do not turn negative or have persistent symptoms after 3 months of therapy should be evaluated for MDRTB

COMPLICATIONS

- Development of drug resistance

PROGNOSIS

- Almost all properly treated patients with tuberculosis can be cured; relapse rates are less than 5% with current regimens
- The main cause of treatment failure is medication nonadherence

WHEN TO REFER

- All cases of drug-resistant TB
- DOT is recommended with MDRTB and those receiving twice- or thrice-weekly therapy

WHEN TO ADMIT

- Hospitalization is not necessary for initial therapy in most patients
- Admit patients who are incapable of self-care or likely to expose susceptible individuals to tuberculosis
- Hospitalized patients require isolation in an appropriately ventilated room until three sputums from different days are negative for MTB organisms

PREVENTION

- Bacillus Calmette-Guérin (BCG) vaccination
- BCG vaccination is not recommended in the United States because of its variable effectiveness, the low prevalence of TB infection, and the interference of the vaccine with determination of LTBI
- All suspected and confirmed cases of MTB should be reported to local and state public health authorities

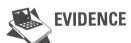 **EVIDENCE**

PRACTICE GUIDELINES

- American Thoracic Society; Centers for Disease Control and Prevention; Infectious Diseases Society of America. American Thoracic Society; Centers for Disease Control and Prevention; Infectious Diseases Society of America. Controlling tuberculosis in the United States. Am J Respir Crit Care Med. 2005 Nov 1;172(9):1169–227. [PMID: 16249321]
- Blumberg HM et al; American Thoracic Society/Centers for Disease Control and Prevention/Infectious Diseases Society of America. Treatment of tuberculosis. Am J Respir Crit Care Med. 2003 Feb 15;167(4):603–62. [PMID: 12588714]

- Diagnostic Standards and Classification of Tuberculosis in Adults and Children. American Thoracic Society and Centers for Disease Control and Prevention. Am J Respir Crit Care Med 2000 Apr;161(4 Part 1):1376–95. [PMID: 10764337]

WEB SITE

- CDC's Division of Tuberculosis Elimination

INFORMATION FOR PATIENTS

- National Institute of Allergy and Infectious Disease

REFERENCES

- Blumberg HM et al. Update on the treatment of tuberculosis and latent tuberculosis infection. JAMA. 2005 Jun 8;293(22):2776–84. [PMID: 15941808]
- Brodie D et al. The diagnosis of tuberculosis. Clin Chest Med. 2005 Jun; 26(2):247–71. [PMID: 15837109]
- Burman WJ. Issues in the management of HIV-related tuberculosis. Clin Chest Med. 2005 Jun;26(2):283–94. [PMID: 15837111]

Tubular Necrosis, Acute

 KEY FEATURES

ESSENTIALS OF DIAGNOSIS

- Acute kidney injury
- Fractional excretion of sodium (FE_{Na}) > 1% if oliguric
- Pigmented granular casts and renal tubular epithelial cells in urine sediment are pathognomonic but not always present

GENERAL CONSIDERATIONS

- Acute renal failure as a result of tubular damage
- Accounts for 85% of intrinsic acute renal failure
- Two major causes are ischemia and nephrotoxin exposure
- Ischemic acute renal failure occurs in prolonged hypotension or hypoxemia such as with dehydration, shock, and sepsis and after major surgical procedures

- Nephrotoxin exposure includes both exogenous and endogenous toxins

Exogenous nephrotoxins

- Aminoglycosides
- Vancomycin, IV acyclovir, several cephalosporins
- Radiographic contrast media
- Antineoplastics, such as cisplatin and organic solvents, and heavy metals (mercury, cadmium, and arsenic)

Endogenous nephrotoxins

- Myoglobinuria as a consequence of rhabdomyolysis
- Hemoglobinuria, massive intravascular hemolysis
- Hyperuricemia
- Bence Jones protein, paraproteins

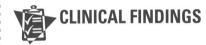 **CLINICAL FINDINGS**

SYMPTOMS AND SIGNS

- See Renal Failure, Acute

DIFFERENTIAL DIAGNOSIS

- Prerenal azotemia (eg, dehydration)
- Postrenal azotemia (benign prostatic hyperplasia)
- Other renal causes of acute renal failure
  - Acute glomerulonephritis: immune complex (eg, IgA nephropathy), pauci-immune (eg, Wegener's granulomatosis), antiglomerular basement membrane disease
  - Acute interstitial nephritis: drugs (eg, β-lactams), infections (eg, *Streptococcus*), immune (eg, systemic lupus erythematosus)

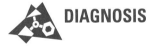 **DIAGNOSIS**

LABORATORY TESTS

- Serum creatinine (Cr) and blood urea nitrogen (BUN) elevated
- BUN–creatinine ratio < 20:1 in acute tubular necrosis
- Hyperkalemia
- Anion gap metabolic acidosis
- Hyperphosphatemia
- Urinalysis: Urine may be brown with pigmented granular casts or "muddy brown" casts; renal tubular epithelial cells and epithelial cell casts
- FE_{Na} = clearance of Na^+/GFR = clearance of Na^+/creatinine clearance = (urine Na^+/plasma Na^+)/(urine Cr/plasma Cr) × 100

- FE_{Na} high (>1%) in acute tubular necrosis

IMAGING STUDIES

- Renal ultrasonography

DIAGNOSTIC PROCEDURES

- Renal biopsy is rarely indicated

 TREATMENT

MEDICATIONS

- Stop offending agent and correct ischemia
- Loop diuretics in moderation, with or without thiazide, for volume maintenance
- Phosphate-binding agents
  - Aluminum hydroxide, 500 mg PO TID with meals
  - Calcium carbonate, 500–1500 mg PO TID with meals
  - Calcium acetate, 667 mg 2–4 tabs PO TID with meals
  - Sevelamer, 800–1600 mg PO TID with meals
  - Lanthanum carbonate (1000 mg orally with meals) is a new but less well-studied option

THERAPEUTIC PROCEDURES

- Dietary protein restriction of 0.6 g/kg/ day in certain settings
- Nutritional support
- Avoid volume overload
- Avoid potassium-containing foods, salt substitutes, and medications known to cause hyperkalemia (ACE inhibitors, ARBs, spironolactone, eplerenone, triamterene)
- Avoid magnesium-containing antacids and laxatives
- Hemodialysis, peritoneal dialysis: indications include
  - Uremic symptoms such as pericarditis, encephalopathy, or coagulopathy
  - Fluid overload unresponsive to diuresis
  - Refractory hyperkalemia
  - Severe metabolic acidosis (pH < 7.20)
  - Neurologic symptoms such as seizures or neuropathy

 OUTCOME

COMPLICATIONS

- Loop diuretics in large doses may cause deafness

PROGNOSIS

- Nonoliguric acute tubular necrosis has a better outcome
- Mortality from acute renal failure is 20–50% in medical illness and up to 70% in a surgical setting
- Increased mortality with advanced age, severe underlying disease, and multisystem organ failure
- Leading causes of death are
  - Infections
  - Fluid and electrolyte disturbances
  - Worsening of underlying disease

WHEN TO REFER

- Refer to a nephrologist when the etiology is unclear or renal function continues to worsen despite intervention
- Referral is also appropriate if fluid, electrolyte, and acid-base abnormalities are recalcitrant

WHEN TO ADMIT

- When a patient has signs or symptoms of acute renal failure that require immediate intervention, such as intravenous fluids, dialytic therapy

PREVENTION

- Monitor patients closely with rising serum creatinine after radiographic contrast media

 EVIDENCE

WEB SITE

- National Kidney and Urologic Diseases Information Clearinghouse

INFORMATION FOR PATIENTS

- Mayo Clinic: Kidney Failure
- MedlinePlus: Acute Tubular Necrosis
- MedlinePlus: Kidney Failure Interactive Tutorial

REFERENCES

- Esson ML et al. Diagnosis and treatment of acute tubular necrosis. Ann Intern Med. 2002 Nov 5;137(9):744–52. [PMID: 12416948]
- Gill N et al. Renal failure secondary to acute tubular necrosis: epidemiology, diagnosis, and management. Chest. 2005 Oct;128(4):2847–63. [PMID: 16236963]
- Musso CG et al. Acute renal failure in the elderly: particular characteristics. Int Urol Nephrol. 2006;38(3–4):787–93. [PMID: 17160631]

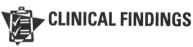

Turner Syndrome (Gonadal Dysgenesis)

 KEY FEATURES

- Patients with classic syndrome lack one X chromosome (45,XO karyotype)
- Common cause of primary amenorrhea and early ovarian failure
- Associated with primary hypogonadism, short stature, other phenotypic anomalies
- Incidence: 40 cases per million live-born girls
- Diagnosis suspected: at birth, small newborns, often with lymphedema; in childhood, short stature

CLINICAL FINDINGS

- Features variable and may be subtle if mosaicism
- Short stature
- Hypogonadism
- Webbed neck
- High-arched palate
- Short fourth metacarpals
- Wide-spaced nipples
- Recurrent otitis media
- Hypertension
- Renal abnormalities
- Coarctation of aorta
- Hypogonadism presents as delayed adolescence (80%) or early ovarian failure (20%)
- Prone to:
  - Keloid formation after ear piercing or surgery
  - Hypothyroidism
  - Diabetes mellitus
  - Dyslipidemia
  - Hypertension
  - Osteoporosis

DIAGNOSIS

- Serum FSH and LH levels elevated
- Karyotype shows 45,XO (or X chromosome abnormalities, or mosaicism)
- Serum growth hormone and IGF-I levels normal
- Yearly physical examinations and periodic thyroid, lipid, and glucose testing recommended

TREATMENT

- Growth hormone, 0.1 unit/kg/day SQ for ≥ 4 years before epiphyseal fusion increases final height by ~10 cm over mean predicted height of 144.2 cm
- Estrogen therapy after age 12 (eg, conjugated estrogens, 0.3 mg PO on days 1–21/month)
- Estrogen plus progestin hormone replacement therapy after growth stops
- Life expectancy reduced

Typhoid Fever

KEY FEATURES

ESSENTIALS OF DIAGNOSIS

- Gradual onset of malaise, headache, sore throat, cough, and either diarrhea or constipation
- Rose spots, relative bradycardia, splenomegaly, and abdominal distention and tenderness
- Leukopenia; blood, stool, and urine culture positive for *Salmonella*

GENERAL CONSIDERATIONS

- The term "typhoid fever" applies when *Salmonella enterica* subspecies *enterica* serotype typhi is the cause of enteric fever accompanied by bacteremia
- Enteric fever generally refers to a typhoidal type illness caused by serotypes other than typhi
- Infection is transmitted by consumption of contaminated food, water, or drink
- Infection begins when organisms cross the intestinal mucosa
  - Bacteremia occurs, and the infection then localizes principally in the lymphoid tissue of the small intestine

(particularly within 60 cm of the ileocecal valve)
  - Peyer's patches become inflamed and may ulcerate, with involvement greatest during the third week of disease
- The incubation period is 5–14 days

DEMOGRAPHICS

- 400 cases per year in the United States, mostly among travelers
- An estimated 21 million cases of typhoid fever and 200,000 deaths occur worldwide

CLINICAL FINDINGS

SYMPTOMS AND SIGNS

Prodromal stage
- Increasing malaise, headache, cough, and sore throat
- Abdominal pain and constipation are often present while the fever ascends in a stepwise fashion
- During the early prodrome, physical findings are few
- There may be marked constipation

Later stage
- After about 7–10 days, the fever reaches a plateau and the patient is much more ill, appearing exhausted and often prostrated
- Marked constipation may develop into "pea soup" diarrhea
- Splenomegaly, abdominal distention and tenderness, relative bradycardia, dicrotic pulse, and occasionally meningismus appear
- The rash (rose spots) commonly appears during the second week of disease
  - The individual spot, found principally on the trunk, is a pink papule 2–3 mm in diameter that fades on pressure
  - It disappears in 3–4 days

DIFFERENTIAL DIAGNOSIS

- Brucellosis
- Tuberculosis
- Infective endocarditis
- Q fever and other rickettsial infections
- Other causes of acute diarrhea
- Viral hepatitis
- Lymphoma
- Adult Still's disease
- Malaria

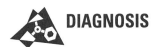
DIAGNOSIS

LABORATORY TESTS

- Best diagnosed by isolation of the organism from blood culture, which is positive in the first week of illness in 80% of patients who have not taken antibiotics
- Cultures of bone marrow occasionally are positive when blood cultures are not
- Stool culture is not reliable because it may be positive in gastroenteritis without typhoid fever

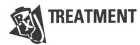
TREATMENT

MEDICATIONS

- Ciprofloxacin, 500 mg PO BID or 400 mg IV BID for 5–7 days (10–14 days for severe typhoid)
- Azithromycin, 1 g PO once daily for 7 days (not recommended for severe disease)
- Ceftriaxone, 2 g IV once daily for 10–14 days for severe typhoid
- Dexamethasone
  - 3 mg/kg over 30 min IV, then 1 mg/kg q6h for eight doses
  - Reduces mortality in patients with severe typhoid fever (eg, those with delirium, coma, shock)
- Many strains are resistant to ampicillin and chloramphenicol
- Resistance to trimethoprim-sulfamethoxazole is increasing

OUTCOME

FOLLOW-UP

- Follow-up examination, with blood cultures for fever, since relapse can occur

COMPLICATIONS

- Complications occur in about 30% of untreated cases and account for 75% of all deaths
- Intestinal hemorrhage, manifested by a sudden drop in temperature and signs of shock followed by dark or fresh blood in the stool, or intestinal perforation, accompanied by abdominal pain and tenderness, is most likely to occur during the third week

PROGNOSIS

- Mortality rate is about 2% in treated cases

- With complications, the prognosis is poor
- Relapses occur in 5–10% of cases; these are treated the same as primary infection
- A residual carrier state frequently persists in spite of chemotherapy

WHEN TO REFER

- Report to the public health department to trace contacts or carriers
- Refer early to an infectious disease specialist

WHEN TO ADMIT

- For intravenous antibiotics or supportive care

PREVENTION

- Immunization is not always effective but should be provided for household contacts of a typhoid carrier, for travelers to endemic areas, and during epidemic outbreaks
- A multiple-dose oral vaccine and a single-dose parenteral vaccine are available
- Adequate waste disposal and protection of food and water supplies from contamination are important public health measures to prevent salmonellosis
- Carriers must not be permitted to work as food handlers

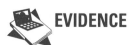 **EVIDENCE**

PRACTICE GUIDELINES

- Advisory Committee on Immunization Practices Recommendations

WEB SITE

- CDC—Division of Bacterial and Mycotic Diseases

REFERENCES

- Bhan MK et al. Typhoid and paratyphoid fever. Lancet. 2005 Aug 27–Sep 2;366(9487):749–62. [PMID: 16125594]
- Parry CM et al. A randomised controlled comparison of ofloxacin, azithromycin and an ofloxacin-azithromycin combination for treatment of multi-drug-resistant and nalidixic acid resistant typhoid fever. Antimicrob Agents Chemother. 2007 Mar;51(3):819–25. [PMID: 17145784]
- Roumagnac P et al. Evolutionary history of *Salmonella* typhi. Science. 2006 Nov 24;314(5803):1301 4. [PMID: 17124322]

Typhus, Scrub

 KEY FEATURES

- Caused by *Orientia tsutsugamushi*, a parasite of rodents, and transmitted by mites
- Mites live on vegetation, but bite humans who contact infested vegetation
- Occurs most commonly in Southeast Asia, western Pacific, and Australia
- Typical incubation period is 7–21 days

 CLINICAL FINDINGS

- Malaise, chills, severe headache, backache
- Site of the bite turns from a papule to a flat black eschar with enlarged regional lymph nodes
- Gradual onset of fever with an accompanying macular rash
- Late complications
  - Pneumonitis
  - Myocarditis
  - Encephalitis
  - Granulomatous hepatitis
  - GI hemorrhage

 DIAGNOSIS

- Serologic testing with immunofluorescence and immunoperoxidase assays or enzyme-linked immunoassays (ELISA) are available to make the diagnosis
- Polymerase chain reaction (PCR) test is an increasingly used and very sensitive way to confirm the diagnosis

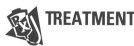 **TREATMENT**

- Doxycycline or chloramphenicol for 3–7 days
- Mortality rate for untreated patients may be as high as 30%
- Prevention: long-acting miticides and insecticides

Ulcerative Colitis

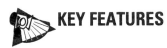 **KEY FEATURES**

ESSENTIALS OF DIAGNOSIS

- Bloody diarrhea
- Lower abdominal cramps and fecal urgency
- Anemia, low serum albumin
- Negative stool cultures
- Sigmoidoscopy is key to diagnosis

GENERAL CONSIDERATIONS

- Idiopathic inflammatory condition that involves the mucosal surface of the colon, resulting in diffuse friability and erosions with bleeding
- In 50% of cases, disease is confined to the rectosigmoid region (proctosigmoiditis); 30% extend to the splenic flexure (left-sided colitis); < 20% extend more proximally (extensive colitis)
- Most affected patients experience periods of symptomatic flare-ups and remissions

DEMOGRAPHICS

- More common in nonsmokers and former smokers, severity may worsen in patients who stop smoking
- Appendectomy at age < 20 reduces risk

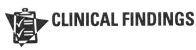 **CLINICAL FINDINGS**

SYMPTOMS AND SIGNS

- Bloody diarrhea
- Cramps, abdominal pain
- Fecal urgency and tenesmus
- Abdominal pain and tenderness
- Bright red blood on digital rectal examination

Mild disease
- Diarrhea infrequent
- Rectal bleeding and mucus intermittent
- Left lower quadrant cramps, relieved by defecation
- No significant abdominal tenderness

Moderate disease
- Diarrhea more severe with frequent bleeding
- Abdominal pain and tenderness
- Mild fever

Severe disease
- > 6–10 bloody bowel movements per day

- Signs of hypovolemia and impaired nutrition
- Abdominal pain and tenderness

Fulminant disease
- Rapid progression of symptoms and signs of severe toxicity (hypovolemia, hemorrhage requiring transfusion, and abdominal distention with tenderness) over 1–2 weeks

Toxic megacolon
- Colonic dilation of > 6 cm on radiographs with signs of toxicity, occurring in < 2%, heightens risk of perforation

Extracolonic manifestations
- Occur in 25% of cases
- Erythema nodosum, pyoderma gangrenosum
- Episcleritis
- Thromboembolic events
- Oligoarticular, nondeforming arthritis
- Sclerosing cholangitis, with risk of cholangiocarcinoma

DIFFERENTIAL DIAGNOSIS

- Infectious colitis
  - Salmonella
  - Shigella
  - Campylobacter
  - Amebiasis
  - Clostridium difficile
  - Enteroinvasive Escherichia coli
- Ischemic colitis
- Crohn's disease
- Diverticular disease
- Colon cancer
- Antibiotic-associated diarrhea or pseudomembranous colitis
- Infectious proctitis: gonorrhea, chlamydia, herpes, syphilis
- Radiation colitis or proctitis
- Cytomegalovirus colitis in AIDS

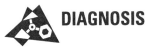 **DIAGNOSIS**

LABORATORY TESTS

- Hematocrit, erythrocyte sedimentation rate, and serum albumin
  - Anemia in moderate to severe disease
  - Hypoalbuminemia in moderate to severe disease
- Antineutrophil cytoplasmic antibodies with perinuclear staining (p-ANCA) in 50–70%; sometimes useful to distinguish from Crohn's disease in patients with indeterminate colitis
- Stools for bacterial (including C difficile) culture, ova and parasites

IMAGING STUDIES

- Abdominal radiographs
- Barium enema is of little usefulness and may precipitate toxic megacolon

DIAGNOSTIC PROCEDURES

- Sigmoidoscopy establishes diagnosis
- Colonoscopy should not be performed in patients with severe disease because of the risk of perforation
- However, after improvement, colonoscopy is recommended to determine extent of disease and for cancer surveillance

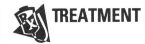 **TREATMENT**

MEDICATIONS

Mild to moderate colitis
- Mesalamine delayed release tables (Lialda) 2.4–4.8 g PO once daily or mesalamine delayed release tablets (Pentasa), 2.0–4.0 g once daily; balsalazide, 2.25 g PO TID; or sulfasalazine, 500 mg PO BID and increased gradually over 1–2 weeks to 2 g PO BID; 50–70% improve
- Folic acid, 1 mg PO once daily, should be given to all patients taking sulfasalazine
- Corticosteroid therapy to patients who do not improve after 2–3 weeks
- Hydrocortisone foam or enemas (80–100 mg BID), or prednisone, 20–30 mg BID, tapering after 2 weeks by no more than 5 mg/week, slower tapering after 15 mg/day
- Antidiarrheal agents (eg, loperamide, 2 mg, diphenoxylate with atropine, 1 tablet, or tincture of opium, 8–15 drops up to four times daily), but should not be given in the acute phase of illness

Distal colitis
- Mesalamine rectal suppositories (Canasa) 1000 mg PR once daily for proctitis or mesalamine rectal suspension (Rowasa), 4 g/60 mL suspension PR QHS for proctosigmoiditis, for 3–12 weeks; 75% of patients improve
- Hydrocortisone suppository or foam for proctitis and hydrocortisone enema (80–100 mg) for proctosigmoiditis; less effective

Moderate to severe colitis
- Corticosteroid therapy improves 50–75%
  - Prednisone 20–30 mg PO BID for 1–2 weeks; then taper by 5–10 mg per week

– Severe disease: methylprednisolone, 48–64 mg IV, or hydrocortisone 300 mg IV, in three divided doses or by continuous infusion

– Hydrocortisone enema, 100 mg IV BID as a drip over 30 min

• Infliximab 5 mg/kg IV

– Moderate to severe disease: given at 0, 2, and 6 weeks for patients with inadequate response to corticosteroids or mesalamine; clinical response in 65% and remission in 35%

– Severe to fulminant disease: 5 mg/kg IV given to patients with inadequate response to 4–7 days of IV corticosteroids

• Cyclosporine, 4 mg/kg/day IV, improves 60–75% of patients with severe colitis who did not improve after 7–10 days of IV corticosteroids

Fulminant colitis and toxic megacolon

• Broad-spectrum antibiotics targeting anaerobes and gram-negative bacteria

• IV corticosteroids, infliximab or cyclosporine, as discussed above

Maintenance therapy

• Sulfasalazine, 1.0–1.5 g PO BID; olsalazine, 500 mg PO BID; and mesalamine, 800 mg PO BID–TID (Asacol) or 500 mg PO QID (Pentasa) reduce relapse rate from 75% to < 35%

• For distal colitis: oral mesalamine, balsalazide, or sulfasalazine reduce the relapse rate from 80–90% to < 20% within 1 year

• Immunomodulators: 6-mercaptopurine 1.0–1.5 mg/kg or azathioprine 2.0–2.5 mg/kg of benefit in 60% of patients with severe or refractory disease, allowing tapering of corticosteroids and maintenance of remission

• Infliximab 5 mg/kg IV every 8 weeks for moderate to severe disease; up to half of patients maintain clinical response at 1 year

Refractory disease

• Mercaptopurine or azathioprine

SURGERY

• Total proctocolectomy with ileostomy (standard ileostomy, continent ileostomy, or ileoanal anastomosis) required in 25% of patients

• Indications for surgery include

– Patients with severe disease (eg, severe hemorrhage) who do not improve at 7–10 days

– Patients with fulminant disease who do not improve after 48–72 hours of corticosteroid, infliximab, or cyclosporine therapy

– Perforation

– Refractory disease requiring long-term corticosteroids to control symptoms

– Dysplasia or carcinoma on surveillance colonoscopic biopsies

THERAPEUTIC PROCEDURES

Mild to moderate colitis

• Regular diet

• Limit intake of caffeine and gas-producing vegetables

• Fiber supplements (eg, psyllium, 3.4 g PO BID; methylcellulose, 2 g PO BID; bran powder, 1 tbsp PO BID)

Severe colitis

• Discontinue all oral intake

• Avoid opioid and anticholinergic agents

• Restore circulating volume with fluids and blood

• Correct electrolyte abnormalities

Fulminant colitis and toxic megacolon

• Nasogastric suction, roll patients from side to side and onto the abdomen

• Serial examinations and abdominal radiographs to look for worsening dilation

OUTCOME

COMPLICATIONS

• Toxic megacolon

• Colon cancer

• Sclerosing cholangitis with risk of cholangiocarcinoma

PROGNOSIS

• Lifelong disease characterized by exacerbations and remissions

• In most patients, disease is readily controlled by medical therapy without need for surgery

• Majority never require hospitalization

• Surgery results in complete cure of the disease

WHEN TO REFER

• Patients with severe or refractory disease requiring immunomodulatory therapy

WHEN TO ADMIT

• Severe colitis

PREVENTION

• Colon cancer occurs in ~0.5–1.0% per year of patients who have had colitis for > 10 years

• Colonoscopy with multiple random mucosal biopsies recommended every

1–2 years in patients with extensive colitis, beginning 8–10 years after diagnosis

• Folic acid, 1 mg PO QD, decreases risk of colon cancer

EVIDENCE

PRACTICE GUIDELINES

• Bebb JR et al. Systematic review: how effective are the usual treatments for ulcerative colitis? Aliment Pharmacol Ther. 2004;20:143. [PMID: 15362049]

• Itzkowitz SH et al; Crohn's and Colitis Foundation of America Colon Cancer in IBD Study Group. Consensus Conference: Colorectal cancer screening and surveillance in inflammatory bowel disease. Inflam Bowel Dis. 2005 Mar; 11(3):314–21. [PMID: 15735438]

• Kornbluth A et al. Ulcerative colitis practice guidelines in adults (update): American College of Gastroenterology, Practice Parameters Committee. Am J Gastroenterol. 2004;99:1371. [PMID: 15233681]

WEB SITES

• Crohn's & Colitis Foundation of America

• National Digestive Diseases Information Clearinghouse—Ulcerative Colitis

• WebPath Gastrointestinal Pathology Index

REFERENCES

• Cohen RD. Azathioprine versus mesalamine in steroid-dependent ulcerative colitis: long awaited results? Gastroenterology. 2006 Feb;130(2):607–8. [PMID: 16472614]

• Bergman R et al. Systematic review: the use of mesalazine in inflammatory bowel disease. Aliment Pharmacol Ther. 2006 Apr 1;23(7):841–55. [PMID: 16573787]

• Gisbert JP et al. Systematic review: infliximab therapy in ulcerative colitis. Aliment Pharmacol Ther. 2007 Jan 1; 25(1):19–37. [PMID: 17229218]

• Hanauer SB et al. Delayed-release oral mesalamine at 4.8 g/day (800 mg tablet) for the treatment of moderately active ulcerative colitis: the ASCEND II Trial. Am J Gastroenterol. 2005 Nov; 100(11):2478–85. [PMID: 16279903]

• Leighton JA et al. ASGE guideline: endoscopy in the diagnosis and treatment of inflammatory bowel disease. Gastrointest Endosc. 2006 Apr; 63(4):558–65. [PMID: 16564852]

- Moskovitz DN et al. Incidence of colectomy during long-term follow-up after cyclosporine-induced remission of severe ulcerative colitis. Clin Gastroenterol Hepatol. 2006 Jun;4(6):760–5. [PMID: 16716758]
- Pardi DS et al. Systematic review: the management of pouchitis. Aliment Pharmacol Ther. 2006 Apr 15; 23(8):1087–96. [PMID: 16611268]
- Regueiro M et al. Clinical guidelines for the medical management of left-sided ulcerative colitis and ulcerative proctitis: summary statement. Inflamm Bowel Dis. 2006 Oct;12(10):972–8. [PMID: 17012968]
- Rutter MD et al. Thirty-year analysis of a colonoscopic surveillance program for neoplasia in ulcerative colitis. Gastroenterology. 2006 Apr;130(4):1030–8. [PMID: 16618396]
- Velayos FS et al. Effect of 5-aminosalicylate use on colorectal cancer and dysplasia risk: a systematic review and meta-analysis of observational studies. Am J Gastroenterol. 2005 Jun; 100(6):1345–53. [PMID: 15929768]

Urinary Incontinence in Elderly

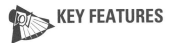

KEY FEATURES

ESSENTIALS OF DIAGNOSIS

- Ruling out transient causes is the first step in incontinence evaluation
- Detrusor overactivity (urge incontinence) is the most common cause of established incontinence

GENERAL CONSIDERATIONS

Transient causes (the mnemonic "DIAPPERS")

- Delirium (a common cause in hospitalized patients)
- Infection (symptomatic urinary tract infection)
- Atrophic urethritis and vaginitis
- Pharmaceuticals
  - Potent diuretics
  - Anticholinergics
  - Psychotropics
  - Opioid analgesics
  - α-Blockers (in women)
  - α-Agonists (in men)
  - Calcium channel blockers
- Psychological factors (severe depression with psychomotor retardation)
- Excess urinary output caused by
  - Diuretics
  - Excess fluid intake
  - Hyperglycemia
  - Peripheral edema and its associated nocturia
- Restricted mobility (see Immobility in Elderly)
- Stool impaction

Established causes

- Detrusor overactivity (urge incontinence)
  - Uninhibited bladder contractions that cause leakage
  - Most common cause of established geriatric incontinence, accounting for two-thirds of cases; usually idiopathic
  - Detrusor hyperactivity with incomplete contractions (DHIC) is a subtype of urge incontinence that can present with urgency with incomplete bladder emptying
- Stress incontinence
- Overflow incontinence
  - Urethral obstruction (most common cause is benign prostatic hyperplasia [BPH])
  - Impaired detrusor contractility
- Mixed incontinence (most commonly combined stress and urge in older women)

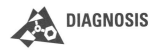

CLINICAL FINDINGS

SYMPTOMS AND SIGNS

- Atrophic urethritis and vaginitis
  - Vaginal mucosal friability
  - Erosions
  - Telangiectasia
  - Petechiae
  - Erythema
- **Detrusor overactivity (urge incontinence)**
  - Complaint of urinary leakage after the onset of an intense urge to urinate that cannot be forestalled
  - Examination often normal with a low (< 100 mL) postvoid residual urine volume
  - A standing full bladder stress test (asking the patient to cough while standing) may result in a few second delay in release of urine
- **Urethral incompetence (stress incontinence)**
  - Urinary loss occurs with laughing, coughing, or lifting heavy objects
  - Most commonly seen in women but can be seen following prostatectomy in men
  - Postvoid residual urine volume usually < 100 mL
  - A standing full bladder stress test (asking the patient to cough while standing) should result in immediate release of urine
- **Urethral obstruction**
  - Commonly due to BPH in men, can be seen in women with cystoceles or other anatomic problems
  - Common symptoms include dribbling, frequency, and slow urinary stream
  - The AUA (American Urologic Association) Score is helpful in evaluation of BPH
  - Detrusor overactivity (which coexists in two-thirds of cases) may cause symptoms of urgency
  - Overflow incontinence due to urinary retention
  - Postvoid residual urine volume almost always > 100 mL
- **Detrusor underactivity (overflow incontinence)**
  - Urinary frequency, nocturia, and frequent leakage of small amounts
  - Postvoid residual urine volume high (> 200 mL)

DIAGNOSIS

LABORATORY TESTS

- Review medications
- Check urinalysis, urine culture for infection
- Consider tests for hyperglycemia, hypercalcemia, diabetes insipidus

IMAGING STUDIES

- Ultrasonography can determine postvoid residual
- Renal ultrasound to exclude hydronephrosis in men whose postvoid residual exceeds 150 mL, particularly if the incontinence developed suddenly
- In older men for whom surgery is planned, urodynamic confirmation of obstruction is strongly advised

DIAGNOSTIC PROCEDURES

- To test for **stress incontinence**, have the patient relax her perineum and cough vigorously (a single cough) while standing with a full bladder
  - Instantaneous leakage indicates stress incontinence if urinary retention has

been excluded by postvoid residual determination using ultrasound

– A delay of several seconds or persistent leakage suggests the problem is caused by an uninhibited bladder contraction induced by coughing

• Because **detrusor overactivity** may be due to bladder stones or tumor, the abrupt onset of otherwise unexplained urge incontinence—especially if accompanied by perineal or suprapubic discomfort or sterile hematuria—should be investigated by cystoscopy and cytologic examination of the urine

• An elevated postvoid residual (generally over 450 mL) distinguishes detrusor underactivity from detrusor overactivity and stress incontinence, but only urodynamic testing differentiates it from urethral obstruction in men

 TREATMENT

NONPHARMACOLOGIC APPROACHES

• **Detrusor overactivity**

– The cornerstone of treatment is behavioral therapy

– Patients are instructed to void every 1–2 h while awake (increased by 30 min until the interval is 4–5 h)

– Pelvic floor exercises, behavioral approaches, and biofeedback can be extremely helpful

– In refractory cases, where intermittent catheterization is feasible, the physician may choose to induce urinary retention with a bladder relaxant and have the patient empty the bladder three or four times daily

• **Urethral incompetence (stress incontinence)**

– Lifestyle modifications, including limiting caffeine intake and timed voiding, may be helpful for some women, particularly women with mixed stress/urge incontinence

– Pelvic muscle and pelvic floor exercises are effective for mild to moderate stress incontinence; they can be combined with biofeedback, electrical stimulation, or vaginal cones

– A pessary or a tampon (for women with exercise-associated stress incontinence); patients are instructed to void every 1–2 h while awake (increased by 30 min until the interval is 4–5 h)

– In refractory cases, where intermittent catheterization is feasible, the physician may choose to induce urinary retention with a bladder relaxant and have the patient empty the bladder three or four times daily

• **Urethral obstruction** and **detrusor underactivity**

– For the nonoperative candidate, use an intermittent or indwelling catheter

– Augmented voiding techniques (eg, double voiding, suprapubic pressure)

– Intermittent or indwelling catheterization

MEDICATIONS

Transient causes

• Discontinue all anticholinergic agents or substitute with less anticholinergic effects (eg, sertraline instead of desipramine)

• Other aggravating medications might include

– Loop diuretics

– Sedative-hypnotics

– Calcium channel blockers

– α-Blockers (which may exacerbate stress)

– α-Agonists (which may precipitate retention with BPH)

• Alcohol and caffeine may exacerbate urge incontinence

Established causes

• **Detrusor overactivity**

– Oxybutynin (2.5–5.0 mg PO TID or QID), long-acting oxybutynin (5–15 mg PO once daily), or tolterodine (1–2 mg PO BID), trospium (20 mg BID or once daily), darifenicin (7.5–15.0 mg once daily), or solifenicin (5–10 mg once daily) may reduce episodes of incontinence

– Watch for delirium, dry mouth, or urinary retention

• **Urethral incompetence (stress incontinence)**

– Topical estrogens may be helpful if atrophic vaginitis with urethral irritation is present

– Duloxetine may reduce episodes in women

• **Urethral obstruction**

– For prostatic obstruction without retention, treatment with α-blocking agents (eg, terazosin, 1–10 mg PO once daily; prazosin, 1–5 mg PO BID; doxazosin, 1–8 mg PO once daily; tamsulosin, 0.4–0.8 mg PO once daily) with or without 5-α-reductase inhibitor finasteride (5 mg PO once daily) may improve symptoms

• **Detrusor underactivity**

– Antibiotics (only for symptomatic upper urinary tract infection or as prophylaxis against recurrent symptomatic infections with intermittent catheterization)

SURGERY

• Although a last resort, surgery is the most effective treatment for stress incontinence, resulting in a cure rate of 75–85% even in older women

• Surgical decompression is the most effective treatment for urethral obstruction, especially in the setting of urinary retention

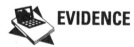 **OUTCOME**

COMPLICATIONS

• The most important complication is restriction of social activity

• In immobile patients, incontinence increases the risk for pressure ulcers

PROGNOSIS

• Some incontinence resolves spontaneously

• In most patients, treatment of exacerbating factors, and pharmacologic and nonpharmacologic treatments can substantially reduce the severity

WHEN TO REFER

• Refer to a multidisciplinary incontinence clinic or geriatrician if there is no response to first-line measures

• Most patients with high postvoid residual volumes (> 200 mL) should be referred to a specialist unless the cause is immediately reversible

PREVENTION

• Weight loss may be beneficial especially for stress incontinence

EVIDENCE

PRACTICE GUIDELINES

• Urinary incontinence in adults: acute and chronic management. Clinical Practice Guideline, No. 2, 1996 update. United States Department of Health and Human Services. Public Health Service, AHCPR. Publication No. 96-0682.

• National Guidelines Clearinghouse

– Urinary Incontinence. The John A. Hartford Foundation Institute for Geriatric Nursing, 2003.

WEB SITES

• MedlinePlus: Urinary Incontinence

• The ACOVE Project Tools for Physicians and Information for Patients

REFERENCES

- Norton P et al. Urinary incontinence in women. Lancet. 2006 Jan 7;367(9504): 57–67. [PMID: 16399154]
- Ouslander JG. Management of overactive bladder. N Engl J Med. 2004 Feb 19;350(8):786–99. [PMID: 14973214]

Urinary Stone Disease

 KEY FEATURES

ESSENTIALS OF DIAGNOSIS

- Flank pain
- Nausea and vomiting
- Identification on noncontrast CT scan

GENERAL CONSIDERATIONS

- Affects 240,000–720,000 Americans per year
- Males > females (3:1)
- Initial presentation predominates in the third and fourth decades
- Incidence is greatest during hot summer months
- Contributing factors to urinary stone formation
  - Geographic factors
    - High humidity
    - Elevated temperatures
  - Genetic factors
    - Cystinuria
    - Distal renal tubular acidosis
  - Diet
    - Sodium and protein intake
    - Excess intake of oxalate and purines
  - Fluid intake
- Five major types of urinary stones
  - Calcium oxalate
  - Calcium phosphate
  - Struvite
  - Uric acid
  - Cystine
- Most urinary stones contain calcium (85%) and are radiopaque; uric acid stones are radiolucent
- **Hypercalciuric calcium nephrolithiasis** (> 250 mg/24 h) can be caused by absorptive, resorptive, and renal disorders (Table 35)
  - **Absorptive hypercalciuria**
    - Secondary to increased absorption of calcium at the level of the small bowel, predominantly in the jejunum
    - Can be further subdivided into types I, II, and III
    - *Type I*: Independent of calcium intake. There is increased urinary calcium on a regular or even a calcium-restricted diet
    - *Type II*: Diet dependent
    - *Type III*: Secondary to a renal phosphate leak, which results in increased vitamin D synthesis and secondarily increased small bowel absorption of calcium
  - **Resorptive hypercalciuria**
    - Secondary to hyperparathyroidism
    - Hypercalcemia, hypophosphatemia, hypercalciuria, and an elevated serum parathyroid hormone level are found
  - **Renal hypercalciuria**
    - Occurs when the renal tubules are unable to efficiently reabsorb filtered calcium
    - Hypercalciuria and secondary hyperparathyroidism result
- **Hyperuricosuric calcium nephrolithiasis** is secondary to dietary excesses or uric acid metabolic defects
- **Hyperoxaluric calcium nephrolithiasis** is usually due to primary intestinal disorders, including chronic diarrhea, inflammatory bowel disease, or steatorrhea
- **Hypocitraturic calcium nephrolithiasis** is secondary to disorders associated with metabolic acidosis including chronic diarrhea, type I (distal) renal tubular acidosis, and long-term hydrochlorothiazide treatment
- **Uric acid calculi**: Contributing factors include
  - Low urinary pH
  - Myeloproliferative disorders
  - Malignancy with increased uric acid production
  - Abrupt and dramatic weight loss
  - Uricosuric medications
- **Struvite calculi** (magnesium-ammonium-phosphate, "staghorn" calculi)
  - Occur with recurrent urinary tract infections with urease-producing organisms, including *Proteus*, *Pseudomonas*, *Providencia* and, less commonly, *Klebsiella*, staphylococci, and *Mycoplasma*
  - Urine pH ≥ 7.2
- **Cystine calculi**: Inherited disorder with recurrent stone disease

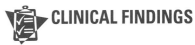 **CLINICAL FINDINGS**

SYMPTOMS AND SIGNS

- Colicky pain in the flank, usually severe
- Nausea and vomiting
- Patients constantly moving—in sharp contrast to those with an acute abdomen
- Pain episodic and radiates anteriorly over the abdomen
- With stone in the ureter, pain may be referred into the ipsilateral testis or labium
- With stone at the ureterovesical junction, marked urinary urgency and frequency
- Stone size does not correlate with severity of symptoms

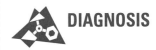 **DIAGNOSIS**

LABORATORY TESTS

- Urinalysis
  - Microscopic or gross (~10%) hematuria
  - Absence of microhematuria does not exclude urinary stones
- Urinary pH
  - Persistent urinary pH < 5.0 is suggestive of uric acid or cystine stones
  - Persistent pH ≥ 7.2 is suggestive of a struvite stone

Metabolic evaluation

- Stone analysis on recovered stones
- Uncomplicated first-time stone formers: serum calcium, phosphate, electrolytes, and uric acid
- Recurrent stone formers or patients with a family history of stone disease: 24-h urine collection on a random diet for volume, urinary pH, and calcium, uric acid, oxalate, phosphate, and citrate excretion
- To subcategorize patients, if necessary: a second 24-h urine collection on a restricted calcium (400 mg/day) and sodium (100 mEq/day) diet
- Serum parathyroid hormone

IMAGING STUDIES

- Spiral CT sensitivity exceeds that of ultrasound or intravenous urography
- Plain film of the abdomen and renal ultrasound will diagnose most stones
- Plain film of the abdomen: radiopaque stones
- Abdominal ultrasonography: stones at the ureterovesical junction can be imaged if patient has a full bladder

TREATMENT

MEDICATIONS

- **Type I absorptive hypercalciuria**
  - Cellulose phosphate, 10–15 g in 3 divided doses given with meals to decrease bowel absorption of calcium
  - Follow-up metabolic surveillance every 6–8 months to exclude hypomagnesemia, secondary hyperoxaluria, and recurrent calculi
  - Thiazide therapy can decrease renal calcium excretion
- **Type II absorptive hypercalciuria**
  - Decrease calcium intake by 50% (to approximately 400 mg once daily)
  - There is no specific medical therapy
- **Type III absorptive hypercalciuria**: orthophosphates (250 mg TID) to inhibit vitamin D synthesis
- **Renal hypercalciuria**: thiazides (effective long-term)
- **Hyperuricosuric calcium nephrolithiasis**: dietary purine restrictions or allopurinol, 300 mg PO once daily, (or both)
- **Hyperoxaluric calcium nephrolithiasis**
  - Measures to curtail the diarrhea or steatorrhea
  - Oral calcium supplements with meals
  - Encourage increased fluid intake
- **Hypocitraturic calcium nephrolithiasis**: potassium citrate, 20 mEq PO TID
- **Uric acid calculi**
  - Potassium citrate, 20 mEq PO TID, to increase urinary pH above 6.2
  - Patients should monitor their urinary alkalinization with Nitrazine pH paper
  - If hyperuricemia is present, allopurinol, 300 mg PO once daily
- **Struvite calculi**
  - After stone extraction, consider suppressive antibiotics
  - Acetohydroxamic acid, an effective urease inhibitor, is poorly tolerated
- **Cystine calculi**
  - Difficult to manage medically
  - Prevention by increased fluid intake, alkalinization of the urine above pH 7.5 (monitored with Nitrazine pH paper), penicillamine and tiopronin

SURGERY

- **Resorptive hypercalciuria**: surgical resection of the parathyroid adenoma
- **Infection with ureteral obstruction**: a medical emergency requiring both antibiotics and prompt drainage by a ureteral catheter or a percutaneous nephrostomy tube
- **Ureteral stones**
  - Stones < 6 mm in diameter will usually pass spontaneously
  - Conservative observation with appropriate pain medications for up to 6 weeks
  - Therapeutic intervention required if spontaneous passage does not occur
  - Indications for earlier intervention include
    - Severe pain unresponsive to medications
    - Fever
    - Persistent nausea and vomiting requiring IV hydration
  - Oral corticosteroids, α-blockers, and calcium channel blockers may enhance stone passage of observed ureteral stones
  - α-Blockers are safe and well tolerated
    - Tamsulosin, 0.4 mg PO once daily
    - Terazosin, 5 mg PO once daily
    - Doxazosin, 4 mg PO once daily
  - Distal ureteral stones: either ureteroscopic stone extraction or in situ extracorporeal shock wave lithotripsy (ESWL)
  - Proximal and midureteral stones can be treated with ESWL or ureteroscopic extraction, and a double-J ureteral stent to ensure adequate drainage
- **Renal stones**
  - Conservative observation for patients presenting without pain, urinary tract infections, or obstruction
  - Intervention if calculi become symptomatic or grow in size
  - For renal stones < 2.5 cm, treat by ESWL
  - For stones in the inferior calix or those > 3 cm, treat by percutaneous nephrolithotomy
  - Perioperative antibiotics as indicated by preoperative urine cultures

THERAPEUTIC PROCEDURES

- Forced IV fluid diuresis is not productive and exacerbates pain

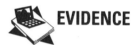

OUTCOME

PREVENTION

- Increased fluid intake to void 1.5–2.0 L/day to reduce stone recurrence
- Patients are encouraged to ingest fluids during meals, 2 h after each meal, prior to going to sleep in the evening, and during the night
- Reduce sodium intake
- Reduce animal protein intake during individual meals

EVIDENCE

PRACTICE GUIDELINES

- Sandhu C et al. Urinary tract stones–Part II. current status of treatment. Clin Radiol. 2003;58:422. [PMID: 12788311]

INFORMATION FOR PATIENTS

- Cleveland Clinic—Kidney Stones
- Mayo Clinic—Kidney Stones
- NIH MedlinePlus—Kidney Stone Tutorial

REFERENCES

- Dellabella M et al. Randomized trial of the efficacy of tamsulosin, nifedipine and phloroglucinol in medical expulsive therapy for distal ureteral calculi. J Urol. 2005 Jul;174(1):167–72. [PMID: 15947613]
- Pak CY. Medical management of urinary stone disease. Nephron Clin Pract. 2004;98(2):c49–53. [PMID: 15499203]
- Pak CY et al. Predictive value of kidney stone composition in the detection of metabolic abnormalities. Am J Med. 2003 Jul;115(1):26–32. [PMID: 12867231]
- Parmar MS. Kidney stones. BMJ. 2004 Jun 12;328(7453):1420–4. [PMID: 15191979]
- Stoller ML et al. The primary stone event: a new hypothesis involving a vascular etiology. J Urol. 2004 May; 171(5):1920–4. [PMID: 15076312]
- Tiselius HG. Epidemiology and medical management of stone disease. BJU Int. 2003 May;91(8):758–67. [PMID: 12709088]

Urticaria & Angioedema

KEY FEATURES

ESSENTIALS OF DIAGNOSIS

- Eruptions of evanescent wheals or hives
- Itching is usually intense but may on rare occasions be absent
- Special forms of urticaria have special features (dermographism; cholinergic, solar, or cold urticaria)
- Most incidents are acute and self-limited over a period of 1–2 weeks
- Chronic urticaria (episodes lasting > 6 weeks) may have an autoimmune basis

GENERAL CONSIDERATIONS

- The most common causes of acute urticaria are foods, viral infections, and medications
- **Nonallergic** causes of urticaria
  - Drugs, eg, atropine, pilocarpine, morphine, and codeine
  - Arthropod bites, eg, insect bites and bee stings
  - Physical factors such as heat, cold, sunlight, and pressure
  - Neurogenic factors such as in cholinergic urticaria induced by exercise, excitement, hot showers
- **Allergic** causes of urticaria
  - Penicillins, aspirin, and other medications
  - Inhalants, eg, feathers and animal danders
  - Ingestion of shellfish, tomatoes, or strawberries
  - Injections of sera and vaccines; external contactants, eg, various chemicals and cosmetics
  - Infections such as hepatitis
- Chronic urticaria (episodes lasting > 6 weeks) may have an autoimmune basis; the cause is often not found
- Autoimmune thyroid disease may coexist, but treatment of the thyroid disease does not improve the urticaria
- Physical forms of urticaria have special features (dermographism; cholinergic, solar, or cold urticaria)

DEMOGRAPHICS

- Chronic urticaria is most common in young adult women

CLINICAL FINDINGS

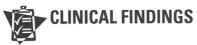

SYMPTOMS AND SIGNS

- Lesions are itchy red swellings of a few millimeters to many centimeters
- The morphology of the lesions may vary over a period of minutes to hours
- Individual lesions in true urticaria last less than 24 h, and often only 2–4 h
- Angioedema is involvement of deeper vessels, with swelling of the lips, eyelids, palms, soles, and genitalia in association with more typical lesions
- Angioedema is no more likely than urticaria to be associated with systemic complications such as laryngeal edema or hypotension
- In cholinergic urticaria, triggered by a rise in core body temperature (hot showers, exercise), wheals are 2–3 mm in diameter with a large surrounding red flare

DIFFERENTIAL DIAGNOSIS

- Vasculitis
- Erythema multiforme
- Contact dermatitis (eg, poison oak or ivy)
- Cellulitis

DIAGNOSIS

LABORATORY TESTS

- Laboratory studies are not likely to be helpful in the evaluation of acute or chronic urticaria unless there are suggestive findings in the history and physical examination
- Quantitative immunoglobulins, cryoglobulins, cryofibrinogens, and antinuclear antibodies are often sought in urticaria but are rarely found
- Liver tests may be elevated, since a serum sickness-like prodrome, with urticaria, may be associated with acute hepatitis B infection

DIAGNOSTIC PROCEDURES

- In patients with individual slightly purpuric lesions that persist past 24 h, a skin biopsy may help exclude urticarial vasculitis

TREATMENT

MEDICATIONS

- H_1-antihistamines
  - Hydroxyzine, 10 mg PO BID to 25 mg TID or one dose of 50–75 mg at night to reduce sedation, is initial therapy
  - Cyproheptadine, 4 mg PO QID, may be useful for cold urticaria
- Add "nonsedating" or less sedating antihistamines if the generic sedating antihistamines are not effective
  - Fexofenadine is given in a dosage of 60–180 mg PO BID
  - Loratadine in a dosage of 10 mg PO once daily is similar to the other H_1-antihistamines in effectiveness
  - Cetirizine, a metabolite of hydroxyzine, may be sedating (13% of patients) and is given in a dosage of 10 mg PO once daily
- Doxepin (a tricyclic antidepressant), 25 mg PO TID or, more commonly, 25–75 mg at bedtime
  - Can be very effective in chronic urticaria
  - Has anticholinergic side effects
- H_2-antihistamines in combination with H_1-blockers may be helpful in patients with symptomatic dermatographism
- Adjuvants
  - Calcium channel blockers (used for at least 4 weeks)
  - Systemic corticosteroids, eg, prednisone ~40 mg PO once daily usually suppresses acute and chronic urticaria
  - However, the use of corticosteroids is rarely indicated
  - In the most refractory and life-altering cases, other immunosuppressives may be required
  - Topical treatment is rarely rewarding

THERAPEUTIC PROCEDURES

- UVB phototherapy can suppress some cases of chronic urticaria

OUTCOME

PROGNOSIS

- Acute urticaria usually lasts only a few days to 6 weeks
- 50% of patients whose urticaria persists for more than 6 weeks will have it for years

WHEN TO REFER

- If there is a question about the diagnosis, if recommended therapy is ineffective, or if specialized treatment is necessary

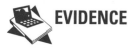 **EVIDENCE**

PRACTICE GUIDELINES

- Grattan C et al. British Association of Dermatologists. Management and diagnostic guidelines for urticaria and angiooedema. Br J Dermatol. 2001;144:708. [PMID: 11298527]

INFORMATION FOR PATIENTS

- American Academy of Allergy, Asthma & Immunology: Allergic Skin Conditions
- American Academy of Dermatology: Urticaria—Hives
- Mayo Clinic: Hives and Angioedema

REFERENCES

- Caproni M et al. Chronic idiopathic and chronic autoimmune urticaria: clinical and immunopathological features of 68 subjects. Acta Derm Venereol. 2004; 84(4):288–90. [PMID: 15339073]
- Dibbern DA Jr. Urticaria: selected highlights and recent advances. Med Clin North Am. 2006 Jan;90(1):187–209. [PMID: 16310530]
- Hennino A et al. Pathophysiology of urticaria. Clin Rev Allergy Immunol. 2006 Feb;30(1):3–11. [PMID: 16461989]
- Kaplan AP et al. Angioedema. J Am Acad Dermatol. 2005 Sep;53(3):373–88. [PMID: 16112343]
- Kostis JB et al. Incidence and characteristics of angioedema associated with enalapril. Arch Intern Med. 2005 Jul 25;165(14):1637–42. [PMID: 16043683]

Vaginal Bleeding, Abnormal Premenopausal

KEY FEATURES

ESSENTIALS OF DIAGNOSIS

- Blood loss of over 80 mL per cycle
- Excessive bleeding, often with the passage of clots, may occur at regular menstrual intervals (**menorrhagia**) or irregular intervals (**dysfunctional uterine bleeding**)
- Etiology most commonly involves dysfunctional uterine bleeding on a hormonal basis

GENERAL CONSIDERATIONS

- Average normal menstrual bleeding lasts 4 days (range, 2–7 days), with a mean blood loss of 40 mL
- Bleeding cycles less than 21 days apart are likely anovular
- Blood loss of over 80 mL per cycle is abnormal and frequently produces anemia
- **Ovulation bleeding**, a single episode of spotting between regular menses, is quite common. Heavier or irregular intermenstrual bleeding warrants investigation
- **Anovulatory bleeding** (dysfunctional uterine bleeding) is usually caused by overgrowth of endometrium due to estrogen stimulation without adequate progesterone to stabilize growth

DEMOGRAPHICS

- Anovulation associated with high estrogen levels commonly occurs in teenagers, in women aged late 30s to late 40s, and in extremely obese women or those with polycystic ovary syndrome

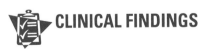

CLINICAL FINDINGS

SYMPTOMS AND SIGNS

- Obtain
  - A careful description of the duration and amount of flow, related pain, and relationship to the last menstrual period (LMP). The presence of blood clots or the degree of inconvenience caused by the bleeding may be more useful indicators
  - A history of pertinent illnesses or weight change
  - A history of all medications taken in the past month
  - A history of coagulation disorders in the patient or family members
- Perform a careful pelvic examination to look for
  - Vaginal or cervical lesions
  - Pregnancy
  - Uterine myomas
  - Adnexal masses
  - Infection

DIFFERENTIAL DIAGNOSIS

- Ovulation bleeding (spotting episode between menses)
- Anovulatory cycle (dysfunctional uterine bleeding)
- Polycystic ovary syndrome (type of anovulatory cycle)
- Pregnancy
- Ectopic pregnancy
- Spontaneous abortion
- Uterine leiomyomas (fibroids)
- Endometrial polyp
- Cervicitis or pelvic inflammatory disease
- Adenomyosis (uterine endometriosis)
- Cervical cancer
- Cervical polyp
- Endometrial hyperplasia
- Endometrial cancer
- Hypothyroidism
- Hyperprolactinemia
- Diabetes mellitus
- Bleeding disorder, eg, von Willebrand's disease

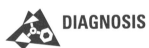

DIAGNOSIS

LABORATORY TESTS

- Cervical smears as needed for cytologic and culture studies
- Complete blood cell count, sedimentation rate, and glucose levels
- Pregnancy test
- Thyroid function and blood clotting should be considered
- Tests for ovulation in cyclic menorrhagia include
  - Basal body temperature records
  - Serum progesterone measured 1 week before the expected onset of menses
  - Analysis of an endometrial biopsy specimen for secretory activity shortly before the onset of menstruation

IMAGING STUDIES

- Ultrasound can evaluate endometrial thickness or diagnose intrauterine or ectopic pregnancy or adnexal masses
- Endovaginal ultrasound with saline infusion sonohysterography can diagnose endometrial polyps or subserous myomas
- MRI can definitively diagnose submucous myomas and adenomyosis

DIAGNOSTIC PROCEDURES

- In women over age 35, perform endometrial sampling to rule out endometrial hyperplasia or carcinoma prior to initiation of hormonal therapy for dysfunctional uterine bleeding
- If cancer of the cervix is suspected, colposcopically directed biopsies and endocervical curettage are indicated as first steps
- Hysteroscopy can visualize endometrial polyps, submucous myomas, and exophytic endometrial cancers. It is useful immediately before D&C

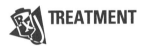

TREATMENT

MEDICATIONS

Dysfunctional uterine bleeding

- Give medroxyprogesterone acetate, 10 mg PO once daily, or norethindrone acetate, 5 mg once daily, for 10–14 days starting on day 15 of the cycle, following which withdrawal bleeding (medical curettage) occurs
- Repeat treatment for several cycles and reinstitute if amenorrhea or dysfunctional bleeding recurs
- In women who are bleeding actively
  - Any combination oral contraceptive can be given QID for 1 or 2 days followed by two pills daily through day 5 and then one pill daily through day 20
  - After withdrawal bleeding occurs, pills are taken in the usual dosage for three cycles

Heavy bleeding

- For intractable heavy bleeding, danazol, 200 mg PO QID, is sometimes used to create an atrophic endometrium
- Alternatively, a gonadotropin-releasing hormone agonist can be used for up to 6 months to create a temporary cessation of menstruation by ovarian suppression; for example
  - Depot leuprolide, 3.75 mg IM monthly

– Nafarelin, 0.2–0.4 mg intranasally BID

- IV conjugated estrogens, 25 mg q4h for three or four doses, can be used followed by oral conjugated estrogens, 2.5 mg PO once daily, or ethinyl estradiol, 20 mcg PO once daily, for 3 weeks, with the addition of medroxyprogesterone acetate, 10 mg PO once daily for the last 10 days of treatment, or a combination oral contraceptive daily for 3 weeks
  – This will thicken the endometrium and control the bleeding

Menorrhagia

- Nonsteroidal anti-inflammatory drugs in the usual anti-inflammatory doses will often reduce blood loss in menorrhagia—even that associated with a copper intrauterine device
- Prolonged use of a progestin, as in a minipill, in injectable contraceptives, or in the therapy of endometriosis, can also lead to intermittent bleeding, sometimes severe
  – In this instance, the endometrium is atrophic and fragile
  – If bleeding occurs, it should be treated with estrogen as follows: ethinyl estradiol, 20 mcg PO once daily for 7 days, or conjugated estrogens, 1.25 mg PO once daily for 7 days

THERAPEUTIC PROCEDURES

- Discuss stressful situations that may contribute to anovulation, such as prolonged emotional turmoil or excessive use of drugs or alcohol
- If the abnormal bleeding is not controlled by hormonal treatment, a D&C is necessary to check for
  – Incomplete abortion
  – Polyps
  – Submucous myomas
  – Endometrial cancer
- D&C usually not necessary in women under age 40
- In the absence of specific pathology, bleeding unresponsive to medical therapy may be treated with endometrial ablation, levonorgestrel-releasing IUD, or hysterectomy
- Endometrial ablation through the hysteroscope with laser photocoagulation or electrocautery
- Newer non-hysteroscopic techniques include
  – Balloon thermal ablation
  – Cryoablation
  – Free-fluid thermal ablation
  – Impedence bipolar radiofrequency ablation
  – Microwave ablation

OUTCOME

FOLLOW-UP

- Monitor for the development of iron deficiency anemia

PROGNOSIS

- While short-term results with endometrial ablation and levonorgestrel-releasing IUD are satisfactory, up to 40% of women will have had either repeat ablation procedures or a hysterectomy at 5 years

WHEN TO REFER

- Refer if bleeding does not stop with first-line therapy or if expertise is needed with a procedure

WHEN TO ADMIT

- If bleeding is uncontrollable with first-line therapy and patient is not hemodynamically stable

EVIDENCE

PRACTICE GUIDELINES

- American College of Obstetricians and Gynecologists (ACOG). Management of anovulatory bleeding, 2000
- Brigham and Women's Hospital. Common gynecologic problems: a guide to diagnosis and treatment, 2002

INFORMATION FOR PATIENTS

- American Academy of Family Physicians: Abnormal Uterine Bleeding
- Mayo Clinic: Vaginal Bleeding
- MedlinePlus: Vaginal Bleeding Between Periods
- MedlinePlus: Dysfunctional Uterine Bleeding

REFERENCES

- Lethaby AE et al. Progesterone or progestogen-releasing intrauterine systems for heavy menstrual bleeding. Cochrane Database Syst Rev. 2005; (4):CD002126. [PMID: 16235297]
- Marjoribanks J et al. Surgery versus medical therapy for heavy menstrual bleeding. Cochrane Database Syst Rev. 2006;(2):CD003855. [PMID: 16625593]
- Munro M. Endometrial ablation:Where have we been? Where are we going? Clin Obstet Gynecol. 2006 Dec;49(4):736–66. [PMID: 17082671]

Vaginal Bleeding, Postmenopausal

 KEY FEATURES

ESSENTIALS OF DIAGNOSIS

- Vaginal bleeding that occurs 6 months or more following cessation of menstrual function
- Bleeding is usually painless
- Bleeding may be a single episode of spotting or profuse bleeding for days or months

GENERAL CONSIDERATIONS

- Most common causes
  – Atrophic endometrium
  – Endometrial proliferation or hyperplasia
  – Endometrial or cervical cancer
  – Administration of estrogens without added progestin
- Risk factors
  – Obesity
  – Nulliparity
  – Diabetes
  – History of anovulation
  – Tamoxifen therapy

 CLINICAL FINDINGS

SYMPTOMS AND SIGNS

- Uterine bleeding is usually painless, but pain will be present if
  – Cervix is stenotic
  – Bleeding is severe and rapid
  – Infection or torsion or extrusion of a tumor is present
- The vulva and vagina should be inspected for areas of bleeding, ulcers, or neoplasms

DIFFERENTIAL DIAGNOSIS

- Atrophic endometrium
- Endometrial hyperplasia or proliferation
- Endometrial cancer
- Atrophic vaginitis
- Perimenopausal bleeding
- Endometrial polyp

- Unopposed exogenous estrogen
- Cervical cancer
- Uterine leiomyomas (fibroids)
- Trauma
- Bleeding disorder
- Cervical polyp
- Cervical ulcer
- Vaginal cancer
- Vulvar cancer

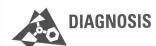

DIAGNOSIS

LABORATORY TESTS

- A cytologic smear of the cervix and vaginal pool should be taken

IMAGING STUDIES

- Transvaginal sonography should be used to measure endometrial thickness
- A measurement of 5 mm or less indicates a low likelihood of hyperplasia or endometrial cancer, although up to 4% of endometrial cancers may be missed with sonography

DIAGNOSTIC PROCEDURES

- If the endometrial thickness by transvaginal sonography is > 5 mm, endocervical curettage and endometrial aspiration should be performed, preferably in conjunction with hysteroscopy

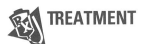

TREATMENT

MEDICATIONS

- Treat simple endometrial hyperplasia with cyclic progestin therapy for 21 days of each month for 3 months
  - Medroxyprogesterone acetate, 10 mg PO once daily
  - Norethindrone acetate, 5 mg PO once daily
- A repeat D&C or endometrial biopsy should be performed, and if tissues are normal and estrogen replacement therapy is reinstituted, a progestin should be prescribed in a cyclic or continuous regimen

SURGERY

- Aspiration curettage (with polypectomy if indicated) will frequently be curative
- If endometrial hyperplasia with atypical cells or carcinoma of the endometrium is found, hysterectomy is necessary

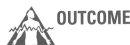

OUTCOME

FOLLOW-UP

- Annual visit for pelvic examination and transvaginal sonography

COMPLICATIONS

- Endometrial cancer
- Complex hyperplasia with atypia has a high risk of becoming adenocarcinoma of the endometrium and requires hysterectomy

WHEN TO REFER

- Complex endometrial hyperplasia with atypia
- Hysteroscopy is indicated

PREVENTION

- Avoidance of unopposed estrogen therapy
- Weight reduction
- Simple endometrial hyperplasia responds well to medical therapy

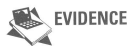

EVIDENCE

PRACTICE GUIDELINES

- Scottish Intercollegiate Guidelines Network. Investigation of post-menopausal bleeding. A national clinical guideline. 2002.
- American Cancer Society guidelines on testing for early endometrial cancer detection-update 2001.

INFORMATION FOR PATIENTS

- American Academy of Family Physicians: Abnormal Uterine Bleeding
- American College of Obstetricians and Gynecologists: Endometrial Hyperplasia
- American College of Surgeons: About D&C for Uterine Bleeding Problems
- American College of Surgeons: Hysteroscopy
- Mayo Clinic: Vaginal Bleeding

REFERENCE

- Clark TJ et al. Investigating postmenopausal bleeding for endometrial cancer: cost-effectiveness of initial diagnostic strategies. BJOG. 2006 May;113(5): 502–10. [PMID: 16637894]

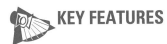

Vaginitis

KEY FEATURES

ESSENTIALS OF DIAGNOSIS

- Vaginal irritation, pruritus, pain, or unusual discharge

GENERAL CONSIDERATIONS

- Inflammation and infection of the vagina are common
- Results from a variety of pathogens, allergic reactions to vaginal contraceptives or other products, or the friction of coitus
- The normal vaginal pH is 4.5 or less, and *Lactobacillus* is the predominant organism
- At the time of the midcycle estrogen surge, clear, elastic, mucoid secretions from the cervical os are often profuse
- In the luteal phase and during pregnancy, vaginal secretions are thicker, white, and sometimes adherent to the vaginal walls
- These normal secretions can be confused with vaginitis by concerned women

Candida albicans

- Pregnancy, diabetes, and use of broad-spectrum antibiotics or corticosteroids predispose to *Candida* infections
- Heat, moisture, and occlusive clothing also contribute to the risk

Trichomonas vaginalis

- This protozoal flagellate infects the vagina, Skene's ducts, and lower urinary tract in women and the lower genitourinary tract in men
- It is sexually transmitted

Bacterial vaginosis

- This condition is considered to be a polymicrobial (overgrowth of *Gardnerella vaginalis* and other anaerobes) and is not sexually transmitted

Condylomata acuminata *(genital warts)*

- Caused by various types of the human papillomavirus
- Sexually transmitted
- Pregnancy and immunosuppression favor growth

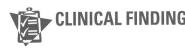

CLINICAL FINDINGS

SYMPTOMS AND SIGNS

- Careful history regarding
  - Onset of the last menstrual period

– Recent sexual activity
– Use of contraceptives, tampons, or douches
– Vaginal burning, pain, pruritus
– Profuse or malodorous discharge
• Physical examination: careful inspection of the vulva and speculum examination of the vagina and cervix

Candida albicans

• Pruritus
• Vulvovaginal erythema
• White curd-like discharge that is not malodorous

Trichomonas vaginalis

• Pruritus and a malodorous frothy, yellow-green discharge
• Diffuse vaginal erythema and red macular lesions on the cervix in severe cases

Bacterial vaginosis

• Increased malodorous discharge without obvious vulvitis or vaginitis
• Discharge is grayish, frothy

Condylomata acuminata

• Warty growths on the vulva, perianal area, vaginal walls, or cervix
• Vulvar lesions: obviously wart-like
• Fissures may be at the fourchette
• Vaginal lesions may show diffuse hypertrophy or a cobblestone appearance
• These lesions may be related to dysplasia and cervical cancer

DIFFERENTIAL DIAGNOSIS

• Normal vaginal discharge
• Bacterial vaginosis
• Trichomonas vaginitis
• Candida vulvovaginitis
• Atrophic vaginitis
• Genital warts (condyloma acuminata)
• Friction from intercourse
• Reaction to douches, tampons, condoms, soap

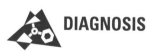 DIAGNOSIS

LABORATORY TESTS

• The cervix is sampled for *Gonococcus* or *Chlamydia* if applicable
• The vaginal pH is frequently > 4.5 in infections due to trichomonads (pH of 5.0–5.5) and bacterial vaginosis
• Examine a specimen of vaginal discharge microscopically
  – In a drop of 0.9% saline solution (wet mount) to search for motile organisms with flagella (trichomonads) and epithelial cells covered with bacteria

to such an extent that cell borders are obscured (clue cells)
  – In a drop of 10% potassium hydroxide to search for the filaments and spores of *Candida* and an amine-like "fishy" odor of *Trichomonas*
• Cultures with Nickerson's medium may be used if *Candida* is suspected but not demonstrated
• Vaginal cultures are generally not useful in diagnosis

DIAGNOSTIC PROCEDURES

• Vulvar or cervical lesions of condylomata acuminata may be visible by colposcopy only after pretreatment with 4% acetic acid, when they appear whitish, with prominent papillae

 TREATMENT

MEDICATIONS

Candida albicans

• Women with uncomplicated vulvovaginal candidiasis will usually respond to a 1- to 3-day regimen of a topical azole
• Women should receive 7–14 days of a topical regimen or two doses of fluconazole 3 days apart for complicated infection, which includes
  – Four or more episodes in 1 year
  – Severe signs and symptoms
  – Nonalbicans species
  – Uncontrolled diabetes
  – HIV infection
  – Corticosteroid treatment
  – Pregnancy (pregnant women should use only topical azoles)
• Single-dose regimens
  – Miconazole (200-mg vaginal suppository)
  – Tioconazole ointment (6.5%, 5 g)
  – Butoconazole sustained-release (2% cream, 5 g)
• Three-day regimens
  – Butoconazole (2% cream, 5 g) once daily
  – Clotrimazole (two 100-mg vaginal tablets) once daily
  – Terconazole (0.8% cream, 5 g, or 80 mg suppository) once daily
  – Miconazole (200-mg vaginal suppository) once daily
• Seven-day regimens
  – Clotrimazole (1% cream or 100-mg vaginal tablet) once daily
  – Miconazole (2% cream, 5 g, or 100-mg vaginal suppository) once daily
  – Terconazole (0.4% cream, 5 g) once daily

• Fourteen-day regimen
  – Nystatin (100,000-unit vaginal tablet once daily)
• Recurrent candidal vulvovaginitis (maintenance therapy for up to 6 months)
  – Clotrimazole (500-mg vaginal suppository) once weekly or clotrimazole (200 mg cream) twice weekly
  – Fluconazole (100, 150 or 200 mg PO) once weekly

Trichomonas vaginalis

• Recommend treatment of both partners
  – Metronidazole, 2 g PO, single dose
  – For treatment failure in the absence of reexposure, retreat with metronidazole, 500 mg BID for 7 days
  – If this is not effective, metronidazole susceptibility testing can be arranged with the Centers for Disease Control and Prevention

Bacterial vaginosis

• Metronidazole, 500 mg PO BID for 7 days
• Clindamycin vaginal cream (2%, 5 g), QD for 7 days
• Metronidazole gel (0.75%, 5 g), BID for 5 days
• Metronidazole, 2 g PO as a single dose
• Clindamycin, 300 mg PO BID for 7 days

Condylomata acuminata

• For vulvar warts
  – Podophyllum resin 25% in tincture of benzoin (do not use during pregnancy or on bleeding lesions). Wash off after 2–4 h
  – 80–90% trichloroacetic or bichloroacetic acid. Apply carefully to avoid the surrounding skin
• Freezing with liquid nitrogen
• Patient-applied regimens include podofilox 0.5% solution or gel and imiquimod 5% cream
• Vaginal warts may be treated with cryotherapy with liquid nitrogen, trichloroacetic acid, or podophyllum resin
• Interferon is not recommended for routine use

THERAPEUTIC PROCEDURES

• Routine examination of sex partners is not necessary for the management of genital warts
• However, partners may wish to be examined for detection and treatment of genital warts and other sexually transmitted diseases

Condylomata acuminata

• Vulvar warts: freezing with cryoprobe and electrocautery

- Vaginal warts: extensive warts may require treatment with CO_2 laser under anesthesia

OUTCOME

FOLLOW-UP

- Examination for pelvic infection

EVIDENCE

PRACTICE GUIDELINES

- ACOG Committee on Practice Bulletins—Gynecology. ACOG Practice Bulletin. Clinical management guidelines for obstetrician-gynecologists, Number 72, May 2006: Vaginitis. Obstet Gynecol. 2006 May;107(5):1195–1206. [PMID: 16648432]
- Centers for Disease Control and Prevention. Sexually Transmitted Diseases Treatment Guidelines—2006

INFORMATION FOR PATIENTS

- American Social Health Association: Vaginitis
- MedlinePlus: Sexually Transmitted Diseases Interactive Tutorial
- National Institute of Allergy and Infectious Diseases: Vaginitis Due to Vaginal Infections
- National Institute of Child Health & Human Development: Vaginitis

REFERENCE

- Sexually transmitted disease treatment guidelines 2006. Centers for Disease Control and Prevention. MMWR Recomm Rep. 2006 Aug 4;55(RR-11):1–94. [PMID: 16888612]

Varicella & Herpes Zoster

KEY FEATURES

ESSENTIALS OF DIAGNOSIS

- Fever and malaise before visible skin lesions (varicella)
- Pain before onset of skin lesions in a dermatome (herpes zoster)

- Typical incubation period of 2–3 weeks between exposure and clinical onset

GENERAL CONSIDERATIONS

- Chickenpox is spread by inhalation of infective droplets or by contact with skin lesions

DEMOGRAPHICS

- Disease manifestations include
  - Chickenpox (varicella), which occurs typically in children
  - Shingles (zoster), which occurs more commonly in elderly or immunocompromised persons

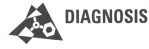

CLINICAL FINDINGS

SYMPTOMS AND SIGNS

Varicella (chickenpox)

- Fever and malaise mild in children, marked in adults
- Vesicular eruptions often first involve oropharynx
- Rash involves face, scalp, and trunk and then moves out to the extremities
- Lesions erupt over 1–5 days so all stages of eruption present simultaneously
- Vesicles and pustules are superficial, elliptical, with slightly serrated borders
- Multinucleated giant cells on Tzanck smear of materials from vesicle bases

Herpes zoster (shingles)

- Pain is often severe and precedes the lesions
- Lesions follow any nerve route distribution (thoracic and lumbar most common)
- Vesicular skin lesions resemble varicella
- Lesions on tip of nose, inner corner of eye, and root and side of nose (Hutchinson's sign) indicate potential ophthalmic involvement
- Facial palsy, vertigo, tinnitus, deafness, or external ear lesions suggest geniculate ganglion involvement

DIFFERENTIAL DIAGNOSIS

Varicella (chickenpox)

- Herpes simplex (cold or fever sore; genital herpes)
- Herpes zoster (shingles)
- Contact dermatitis
- Scabies
- Atopic dermatitis (eczema) (acute)
- Miliaria (heat rash)
- Photodermatitis
- Smallpox

- Rickettsialpox
- Hand, foot, and mouth disease

Herpes zoster (shingles)

- Contact dermatitis (eg, poison oak or ivy)
- Herpes simplex
- Varicella (chickenpox)
- Erysipelas
- Prodromal pain mimics angina, peptic ulcer, appendicitis, biliary or renal colic

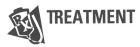

DIAGNOSIS

LABORATORY TESTS

- Leukopenia often present in varicella
- Zoster symptoms and signs often highly characteristic, not requiring further diagnostic testing
- When diagnosis remains in doubt, direct fluorescent antibody (DFA) testing, viral culture, and polymerase chain reaction (PCR) testing can be helpful

DIAGNOSTIC FINDINGS

- Most patients with a history of exposure and clinical symptoms and signs of varicella do not need further diagnostic testing

TREATMENT

MEDICATIONS

- Acyclovir or related drugs (valacyclovir, famciclovir)
  - Can reduce the duration and severity of chickenpox or zoster infection, especially when started early
  - However, seldom needed in immunocompetent patients
- Acyclovir may reduce the likelihood and severity of postherpetic neuralgia
- Acyclovir is usually indicated in immunocompromised patients with systemic varicella infection
- Foscarnet may be useful in acyclovir-resistant varicella, especially in patients receiving long-term acyclovir therapy
- Prevention: varicella immunoglobulin is effective in preventing chickenpox in exposed individuals
- Vaccination with live, attenuated virus
  - 85% effective at preventing disease
  - 95% effective at preventing serious complications
- Adults should receive a second vaccine dose 1–2 months after the first dose
- Postherpetic neuralgia: initial treatment with acyclovir or related drugs and cor-

ticosteroids may reduce the incidence and severity

- Once established, pain may be treated with
  - Tricyclic antidepressants
  - Lidocaine patches
  - Antiepileptics, such as gabapentin or carbamazepine

THERAPEUTIC PROCEDURES

- Isolate patients with active vesicles or pneumonia from susceptible (seronegative) patients

PREVENTION

- Varicella-zoster vaccine reduces the incidence of zoster as well as the development of postherpetic neuralgia (Tables 67 and 68)

 OUTCOME

COMPLICATIONS

Varicella (chickenpox)

- Interstitial pneumonia more common in adults than children
- Ischemic strokes, though uncommon, may be due to an associated vasculitis
- Hepatitis occurs in 0.1%
- Encephalitis, characterized by ataxia, nystagmus, and even death, is rare (0.025%)
- Reye's syndrome may occur in conjunction with aspirin use, usually in children
- Congenital malformations occur with first-trimester infections

Herpes zoster (shingles)

- Skin lesions beyond the dermatome, visceral lesions, and encephalitis occur in immunocompromised individuals
- Postherpetic neuralgia
  - Occurs in 60–70% of elderly patients
  - Early treatment with acyclovir (or related drugs) and corticosteroids (tapered over 21 days) may have some benefit in preventing postherpetic neuralgia

PROGNOSIS

- Total duration of varicella from onset of symptoms to disappearance of crusts usually < 2 weeks
- Zoster symptoms and lesions usually resolve within 6 weeks

WHEN TO REFER

- Refer patients with synchronous progression of the lesions, which raises the concern for smallpox, to local health

department and infectious disease experts for confirmation

WHEN TO ADMIT

- Consider hospitalization for signs of visceral involvement, especially pulmonary involvement. Varicella pneumonia can be lethal, especially in adults and in immunocompromised patients

 EVIDENCE

PRACTICE GUIDELINES

- General recommendations on immunization: recommendations of the Advisory Committee on Immunization Practices (ACIP) and the American Academy of Family Physicians (AAFP). American Academy of Family Physicians; Centers for Disease Control and Prevention, 2002

WEB SITE

- National Institute of Allergy and Infectious Diseases, National Institutes of Health

INFORMATION FOR PATIENTS

- NIAID Facts About Shingles (Varicella-Zoster Virus)
- Web MD Varicella

REFERENCES

- Boeckh M et al. Long-term acyclovir for prevention of varicella zoster virus disease after allogeneic hematopoietic cell transplantation—a randomized double-blind placebo-controlled study. Blood. 2006 Mar 1;107(5):1800–5. [PMID: 16282339]
- Gilden DH et al. VZV vasculopathy and postherpetic neuralgia: progress and perspective on antiviral therapy. Neurology. 2005 Jan 11;64(1):21–5. [PMID: 15642898]
- Heininger U et al. Varicella. Lancet. 2006 Oct 14;368(9544):1365–76. [PMID: 17046469]
- Opstelten W et al. Managing ophthalmic herpes zoster in primary care. BMJ. 2005 Jul 16;331(7509):147–51. [PMID: 16020856]
- Oxman MN et al; Shingles Prevention Study Group. A vaccine to prevent herpes zoster and postherpetic neuralgia in older adults. N Engl J Med. 2005 Jun 2; 352(22):2271–84. [PMID: 15930418]
- van Wijck AJ et al. The PINE study of epidural steroids and local anaesthetics to prevent postherpetic neuralgia: a randomised controlled trial. Lancet. 2006 Jan 21;367(9506):219–24. [PMID: 16427490]

Varicose Veins

 KEY FEATURES

ESSENTIALS OF DIAGNOSIS

- Dilated, tortuous superficial veins in the lower extremities
- May be asymptomatic or associated with fatigue, aching discomfort, or pain
- Edema, pigmentation, and stasis ulcers of the skin may develop
- Usually hereditary, with most patients reporting a family member with similar lesions
- Increased frequency after pregnancy

GENERAL CONSIDERATIONS

- Varicose veins consist of abnormally dilated, elongated, and tortuous alterations usually in the saphenous veins and their tributaries
- Secondary varicosities can develop as a result of
  - Obstructive changes and valve damage in the deep venous system following thrombophlebitis
  - Proximal venous occlusion due to neoplasm (rarely)
- Congenital or acquired arteriovenous fistulas or venous malformations are also associated with varicosities

DEMOGRAPHICS

- Highest incidence in women after pregnancy
- Develop in 15% of all adults

 CLINICAL FINDINGS

SYMPTOMS AND SIGNS

- Extensive varicose veins may produce no subjective symptoms, whereas minimal varicosities may produce many symptoms
- Dull, aching heaviness or a feeling of fatigue
- Itching from a venous stasis dermatitis
- Dilated, tortuous, elongated veins beneath the skin in the thigh and leg are

- generally visible in the standing individual
- However, palpation may be necessary in very obese patients
- Secondary tissue changes may be absent even in extensive varicosities
- However, brownish pigmentation and thinning of the skin above the ankle are often present if varicosities are of long duration
- Swelling may occur, but signs of severe chronic venous stasis are unusual

DIFFERENTIAL DIAGNOSIS

- Primary varicose veins should be differentiated from those secondary to
  - Chronic venous insufficiency of the deep system of veins
  - Retroperitoneal vein obstruction from extrinsic pressure or fibrosis
  - Arteriovenous fistula (congenital or acquired)
  - Congenital venous malformation
- Pain or discomfort secondary to arthritis, radiculopathy, or arterial insufficiency
- Arteriosclerotic peripheral vascular disease

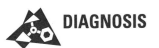 **DIAGNOSIS**

IMAGING STUDIES

- Duplex ultrasonography is modality of choice
- Imaging is important in adolescent patients with varicose veins to exclude a congenital malformation or atresia of the deep veins

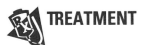 **TREATMENT**

SURGERY

- Endovenous ablation (with either radiofrequency or laser)
- Greater saphenous vein stripping less common
- Excision of the symptomatic varicose veins; correction of reflux done at same time
- Phlebectomy without correction of reflux results in a high rate of recurrent varicosities
- Concurrent reflux detected by ultrasonography in the deep system is not a contraindication to treatment of superficial reflux

- Occlusive arterial disease is usually a contraindication to the operative treatment of varicosities distal to the knee
- Surgical treatment of varicose veins in adolescent patients is usually contraindicated because the varicosities may play a significant role in venous drainage of the limb

THERAPEUTIC PROCEDURES

- Elastic graduated compression stockings (medium or heavy weight)
- Limb elevation when possible
- Sclerotherapy
  - Obliterates and produces permanent fibrosis of the involved veins
  - Generally reserved for varicose veins < 4 mm in diameter
  - Use of foam sclerotherapy can allow treatment of larger veins, although systemic embolization of the foam sclerosant is a concern

 OUTCOME

COMPLICATIONS

- Phlebitis within a varicose vein from sluggish blood flow, which predisposes to localized thrombosis
- Predisposing conditions for phlebitis
  - Pregnancy
  - Local trauma
  - Prolonged period of sitting
- Tissue necrosis or infection may occur with sclerotherapy

PROGNOSIS

- Excellent with correction of the venous insufficiency and excision of varicose veins
- 5-year success rate is 85–90%
- Simple excision (phlebectomy) or injection sclerotherapy without correction of reflux is associated with higher rates of recurrence
- Even after adequate treatment, secondary tissue changes, such as lipodermosclerosis, may persist

 EVIDENCE

INFORMATION FOR PATIENTS

- Cleveland Clinic: Varicose and Spider Veins
- MedlinePlus: Varicose Veins
- MedlinePlus: Varicose Veins interactive tutorial

REFERENCES

- Bergan JJ et al. Chronic venous disease. N Engl J Med. 2006 Aug 3;355(5): 488–98. [PMID: 16885552]
- Campbell B. Varicose veins and their management. BMJ. 2006 Aug 5; 333(7562):287–92. [PMID: 16888305]

Venous Stasis Ulcers

 KEY FEATURES

ESSENTIALS OF DIAGNOSIS

- History of varicosities, thrombophlebitis, or postphlebitic syndrome
- Irregular ulceration, often on the medial aspect of the lower legs above the malleolus
- Edema of the legs, hyperpigmentation, and red and scaly areas (stasis dermatitis) support the diagnosis

GENERAL CONSIDERATIONS

- Patients at risk may have a history of venous insufficiency, either with obvious varicosities or with a past history of thrombophlebitis, or with immobility of the calf muscle group (paraplegics, etc)
- Red, pruritic patches of stasis dermatitis often precede ulceration
- Because venous insufficiency is the most common cause of lower leg ulceration, testing of venous competence is a required part of the evaluation even when no changes of venous insufficiency are present

 CLINICAL FINDINGS

SYMPTOMS AND SIGNS

- Classically, chronic edema is followed by a dermatitis, which is often pruritic; these changes are followed by hyperpigmentation, skin breakdown, and eventually sclerosis of the skin of the lower leg
- The ulcer base may be clean, but it may have a yellow fibrin eschar that often requires surgical treatment
- Ulceration is often on the *medial* aspect of the lower legs above the malleolus

- Edema of the legs, varicosities, hyperpigmentation, and red and scaly areas (stasis dermatitis) and scars from old ulcers support the diagnosis
- Ulcers that appear on the feet, toes, or above the knees are atypical for venous stasis—consider other diagnoses

DIFFERENTIAL DIAGNOSIS

- Arterial insufficiency (arterial ulcer)
- Bacterial pyoderma (eg, infected wound or bite)
- Trauma
- Diabetic ulcer
- Pressure ulcer
- Vasculitis
- Pyoderma gangrenosum
- Skin cancer
- Infection (eg, mycobacterial, fungal, tertiary syphilis, leishmaniasis, amebiasis)
- Sickle cell anemia
- Embolic disease (including cholesterol emboli)
- Cryoglobulinemia
- Calciphylaxis

 DIAGNOSIS

LABORATORY TESTS

- Thorough evaluation of the patient's vascular system (including measurement of the ankle-brachial index) is essential

IMAGING STUDIES

- Doppler ultrasound is usually sufficient (except in the diabetic) to elucidate the cause of most vascular cases of lower leg ulceration

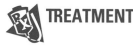 **TREATMENT**

MEDICATIONS

Cleaning of the ulcer

- The patient is instructed to clean the base with saline or cleansers such as Safclens or Cara-klenz daily
- Once the base is clean
  - The ulcer is treated with metronidazole 1% gel to reduce bacterial growth and odor
  - Any red dermatitic skin is treated with a medium- to high-potency corticosteroid ointment
  - The ulcer is then covered with an occlusive hydroactive dressing (Duoderm or Cutinova) or a polyurethane

foam (Allevyn) followed by an Unna zinc paste boot, changed weekly

Systemic therapy

- Pentoxifylline, 400 mg PO TID, administered with compression accelerates healing
- Zinc supplementation is occasionally beneficial in patients with low serum zinc levels
- If cellulitis accompanies the ulcer, systemic antibiotics are recommended

SURGERY

- A curette or small scissors can be used to remove the yellow fibrin eschar, under local anesthesia if the areas are very tender
- Grafting for severe or nonhealing ulcers
  - Full- or split-thickness grafts often do not take, and pinch grafts (small shaves of skin laid onto the bed) may be more effective
  - Cultured epidermal cell grafts may accelerate wound healing, but they are very expensive

 OUTCOME

PROGNOSIS

- The ulcer should begin to heal within weeks, and healing should be complete within 3–4 months

WHEN TO REFER

- If there is a question about the diagnosis, if recommended therapy is ineffective, or if specialized treatment is necessary

PREVENTION

- Elevation of an edematous leg above the heart for more than 2 h BID
- Compression stockings to reduce edema
  - Compression should achieve a pressure of 30 mm Hg below the knee and 40 mm Hg at the ankle
  - The stockings should not be used in patients with arterial insufficiency with an ankle-brachial pressure index less than 0.7
  - Pneumatic sequential compression devices may be of great benefit

 EVIDENCE

PRACTICE GUIDELINES

- Registered Nurses Association of Ontario. Assessment and management of venous leg ulcers, 2004

- Smith & Nephew Ltd. Grace P, editor. Guidelines for the management of leg ulcers in Ireland, 2002

INFORMATION FOR PATIENTS

- MedlinePlus: Stasis Dermatitis
- MedlinePlus: Varicose Veins
- Radiological Society of North America: Venous Ultrasound

REFERENCES

- Grey JE et al. Venous and arterial leg ulcers. BMJ. 2006 Feb 11;332(7537):347–50. [PMID: 16470058]
- Jones JE et al. Skin grafting for venous leg ulcers. Cochrane Database Syst Rev. 2005 Jan 25;(1):CD001737. [PMID: 15674883]
- LayFlurrie K. Assessment and good technique are key to effective compression therapy. Prof Nurse. 2005 Mar; 20(7):31–4. [PMID: 15754720]

Ventricular Septal Defect

 KEY FEATURES

- Location of ventricular septal defect (VSD) varies
  - Inlet or membranous VSD common
  - VSD may be high and committed to both ventricles or may be in the muscular septum
- Presentation in adults depends on size of left-to-right shunt and presence or absence of associated pulmonic or subpulmonic stenosis
- Small defects may be asymptomatic
- Moderate to large shunts may lead to pulmonary hypertension (Eisenmenger's physiology) and right heart failure or left heart failure
- Cyanosis prominent when shunt becomes right-to-left

 CLINICAL FINDINGS

- The smaller the size of the VSD, the smaller the shunt and the louder the murmur
- Small shunts: loud, harsh holosystolic murmur in third and fourth left inter-

spaces along the sternum and, occasionally, mid-diastolic flow murmur
- Systolic thrill common
- Large shunts: RV volume and pressure overload may cause pulmonary hypertension and cyanosis

DIAGNOSIS

- ECG: LV and RV hypertrophy
- Chest radiograph
  - Increased pulmonary vascularity
  - Enlarged pulmonary artery and left atrium
- Doppler echocardiography
  - Diagnostic
  - Can assess magnitude and location of shunt and estimate gradient across the VSD
  - Can also estimate pulmonary artery pressure and address associated lesions
- Cardiac CT and MRI can visualize defect and other anatomic abnormalities
- Cardiac catheterization
  - Usually reserved for those with at least moderate shunting
  - Can measure pulmonary vascular resistance and degree of pulmonary hypertension

TREATMENT

- Endocarditis occurs more often with smaller shunts; antibiotic prophylaxis is important
- Small shunts do not require closure in asymptomatic patients
- Large shunts should be surgically or percutaneously repaired
- Surgical mortality is 2–3%, but ≥ 50% if pulmonary hypertension is present
- Surgery is contraindicated in Eisenmenger's syndrome
- Percutaneous closure devices are available and effective in some situations

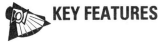

KEY FEATURES

ESSENTIALS OF DIAGNOSIS

- Either a sensation of motion when there is no motion or an exaggerated sense of motion in response to a given bodily movement
- Duration of discrete vertiginous events
- Must differentiate peripheral from central causes of vestibular dysfunction

GENERAL CONSIDERATIONS

- Causes can be determined based on the duration of symptoms (seconds, hours, days, months) and whether auditory symptoms are present (Table 22)
- Vertigo can occur as a side effect of
  - Anticonvulsants (eg, phenytoin)
  - Antibiotics (eg, aminoglycosides, doxycycline, metronidazole)
  - Hypnotics (eg, diazepam)
  - Analgesics (eg, aspirin)
  - Tranquilizing drugs and alcohol

Positioning vertigo
- Commonly known as benign paroxysmal positioning vertigo (BPPV) or benign positioning vertigo (BPV)
- Associated with changes in head position, often rolling over in bed

Endolymphatic hydrops (Ménière's disease)
- Cause is unknown
- Presumably, results from distention of the endolymphatic compartment of the inner ear
- Two known causes are syphilis and head trauma

CLINICAL FINDINGS

SYMPTOMS AND SIGNS

- See Table 22
- A thorough history often narrows, if not confirms, the diagnosis
- Triggers should also be sought
  - Diet (eg, high salt in Ménière's disease)
  - Stress
  - Fatigue
  - Bright lights
- Perform Romberg test; evaluate gait; observe for nystagmus

Peripheral vestibulopathy
- Vertigo usually sudden; may be so severe that patient is unable to walk or stand; frequently accompanied by nausea and vomiting
- Tinnitus and hearing loss may accompany; support otologic origin
- **Nystagmus** usually horizontal with rotary component; fast phase usually beats away from diseased side

- Visual fixation tends to inhibit nystagmus except in very acute peripheral lesions or with CNS disease
- **Dix-Hallpike test**
  - Patient is quickly lowered into supine position with head extending over the edge and placed 30° lower than the body, turned either to left or right
  - Elicits delayed onset (about 15 s) of fatiguable nystagmus in cases of benign positioning vertigo
  - Nonfatiguable nystagmus indicates central etiology for dizziness
- Subtle forms of nystagmus may be observed by using Fresnel goggles, which prevent visual fixation
- **Fukuda test**
  - Patient walks in place with eyes closed
  - Can also demonstrate vestibular asymmetry
- **Positional vertigo**
  - Typical symptoms occur in clusters that persist for several days
  - A brief latency period (10–15 s) follows head movement before symptoms develop
  - Acute vertigo subsides within 10–60 s, but patient may remain imbalanced for several hours
  - Constant repetition of positional change leads to habituation
  - In central lesions, there is no latent period, fatigability, or habituation
- **Ménière's syndrome**
  - Classic syndrome consists of episodic vertigo, with discrete vertigo spells lasting 20 min to several hours in association with
    □ Fluctuating low-frequency sensorineural hearing loss
    □ Tinnitus (usually low-tone and "blowing" in quality)
    □ Sensation of aural pressure
  - Symptoms wax and wane as endolymphatic pressure rises and falls
  - Caloric testing commonly reveals loss or impairment of thermally induced nystagmus on the involved side
- **Labyrinthitis**
  - Acute onset of continuous, usually severe vertigo lasting several days to a week, hearing loss, tinnitus
  - During recovery (several weeks), vertigo gradually improves
  - Hearing may return to normal or be permanently impaired in involved ear

Central vestibulopathy
- Vertigo tends to develop gradually, often progressively more severe and debilitating
- Nystagmus
  - Not always present but can occur in any direction and may be dissociated in both eyes

– Often nonfatigable, vertical rather than horizontal, without latency, unsuppressed by visual fixation

DIFFERENTIAL DIAGNOSIS

- Imbalance
- Light-headedness
- Syncope

 DIAGNOSIS

IMAGING STUDIES

- MRI to evaluate central audiovestibular dysfunction

DIAGNOSTIC PROCEDURES

- Electronystagmography or videonystagmography useful in differentiating central from peripheral causes of vertigo

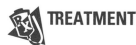 **TREATMENT**

MEDICATIONS

- Diazepam or meclizine
  – For acute phases of vertigo only
  – Discontinue as soon as feasible to avoid long-term dysequilibrium
- **Ménière's disease:** low-salt diet and diuretics (eg, acetazolamide)
- **Labyrinthitis**
  – Antibiotics if patient is febrile or has symptoms of bacterial infection
  – Vestibular suppressants (eg, diazepam or meclizine)

THERAPEUTIC PROCEDURES

- **Positioning vertigo:** involves physical therapy protocols (eg, the Epley maneuver or Brandt-Daroff exercises)
- For refractory cases of **Ménière's disease**
  – Endolymphatic sac decompression
  – Vestibular ablation either through transtympanic gentamicin, vestibular nerve section, or surgical labyrinthectomy

 OUTCOME

WHEN TO REFER

- Audiologic evaluation, caloric stimulation, electronystagmography, videonystagmography, and MRI are indicated in patients with persistent vertigo or when CNS disease is suspected

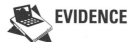 **EVIDENCE**

PRACTICE GUIDELINES

- Cesarani A et al. The treatment of acute vertigo. Neurol Sci. 2004;25(Suppl 1):S26. [PMID: 15045617]

WEB SITE

- Baylor College of Medicine Otolaryngology Resources on the Internet

INFORMATION FOR PATIENTS

- American Hearing Research Foundation: Benign Paroxysmal Positional Vertigo (BPPV)
- MedlinePlus: Vertigo-Associated Disorders
- National Institute on Deafness and Other Communication Disorders: Balance Disorders
- National Institute on Deafness and Other Communication Disorders: Ménière's Disease
- Vestibular Disorders Association

REFERENCES

- Brandt T et al. General vestibular testing. Clin Neurophysiol. 2005 Feb; 116(2):406–26. [PMID: 15661119]
- Guilemany JM et al. Clinical and epidemiological study of vertigo at an outpatient clinic. Acta Otolaryngol. 2004 Jan;124(1):49–52. [PMID: 14977078]
- Lempert T et al. Episodic vertigo. Curr Opin Neurol. 2005 Feb;18(1):5–9. [PMID: 15655395]
- Kim HH et al. Trends in the diagnosis and the management of Meniere's disease: results of a survey. Otolaryngol Head Neck Surg. 2005 May; 132(5):722–6. [PMID: 15886625]
- Kovar M et al. Diagnosing and treating benign paroxysmal positional vertigo. J Gerontol Nurs. 2006 Dec;32(12):22–9. [PMID: 17190403]
- Seemungal BM. Neuro-otological emergencies. Curr Opin Neurol. 2007 Feb; 20(1):32–9. [PMID: 17215686]

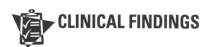

Vitamin B$_{12}$ Deficiency

 KEY FEATURES

ESSENTIALS OF DIAGNOSIS

- Macrocytic anemia
- Macroovalocytes and hypersegmented neutrophils on peripheral blood smear
- Serum vitamin B$_{12}$ level < 100 pg/mL

GENERAL CONSIDERATIONS

- All vitamin B$_{12}$ is absorbed from the diet (foods of animal origin)
- After ingestion, vitamin B$_{12}$ binds to intrinsic factor, a protein secreted by gastric parietal cells
- Vitamin B$_{12}$-intrinsic factor complex is absorbed in the terminal ileum by cells with specific receptors for the complex; it is then transported through the plasma and stored in the liver
- Liver stores are of such magnitude that it takes at least 3 years for vitamin B$_{12}$ deficiency to develop after vitamin B$_{12}$ absorption ceases
- Causes of vitamin B$_{12}$ deficiency
  – Decreased intrinsic factor production: pernicious anemia (most common cause), gastrectomy
  – Dietary deficiency (only in vegans)
  – Competition for B$_{12}$ in gut: blind loop syndrome, fish tapeworm (rare)
  – Decreased ileal B$_{12}$ absorption: surgical resection, Crohn's disease, metformin
  – Pancreatic insufficiency
  – *Helicobacter pylori* infection
  – Transcobalamin II deficiency (rare)
- Pernicious anemia is associated with atrophic gastritis and other autoimmune diseases, eg, immunoglobulin A (IgA) deficiency, polyglandular endocrine failure syndromes

DEMOGRAPHICS

- Pernicious anemia is hereditary, though rare clinically before age 35

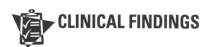 **CLINICAL FINDINGS**

SYMPTOMS AND SIGNS

- Megaloblastic anemia, which may be severe
- Pallor and mild icterus

- Glossitis and vague gastrointestinal disturbances (eg, anorexia, diarrhea)
- Neurologic manifestations
  - Peripheral neuropathy usually occurs first
  - Then, subacute combined degeneration of the spinal cord affecting posterior columns may develop, causing difficulty with position and vibration sensation and balance
  - In advanced cases, dementia and other neuropsychiatric changes may occur
  - Neurologic manifestations occasionally precede hematologic changes; patients with suspicious neurologic symptoms and signs should be evaluated for vitamin B_{12} deficiency despite normal mean cell volume (MCV) and absence of anemia

DIFFERENTIAL DIAGNOSIS

- Folic acid deficiency (other cause of megaloblastic anemia)
- Myelodysplastic syndrome (other cause of macrocytic anemia with abnormal morphology)
- Other cause of peripheral neuropathy, ataxia, or dementia

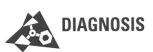 **DIAGNOSIS**

LABORATORY TESTS

- Anemia of variable severity; hematocrit may be as low as 10–15%
- MCV
  - Strikingly elevated: 110–140 fL
  - May be normal if coexistent thalassemia or iron deficiency is present
- Low serum vitamin B_{12} level, often < 100 pg/mL (normal 150–350 pg/mL), establishes diagnosis
- Serum methylmalonic acid or homocysteine level elevations can confirm diagnosis
- Peripheral blood smear
  - Macroovalocytes are characteristic
  - Hypersegmented neutrophils with mean lobe count > 4, or ≥ 1 six-lobed neutrophils
  - Anisocytosis and poikilocytosis
- Reticulocyte count reduced
- Pancytopenia present in severe cases
- Serum lactate dehydrogenase (LDH) is elevated and indirect bilirubin modestly increased

DIAGNOSTIC PROCEDURES

- Schilling test is now rarely used
- Bone marrow morphology is characteristic
  - Marked erythroid hyperplasia

- Megaloblastic changes in erythroid series
- Giant metamyelocytes in myeloid series

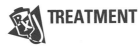 **TREATMENT**

MEDICATIONS

- For pernicious anemia
  - Vitamin B_{12}, 100 mcg IM once daily for 1 week, then every week for 1 month, then every month for life
  - Oral cobalamin, 1000 mcg PO once daily, may be tried instead of parenteral therapy but must be continued indefinitely
- Antibiotics if vitamin B_{12} deficiency is caused by bacterial overgrowth in a blind loop
- Pancreatic enzymes if deficiency is due to pancreatic insufficiency
- Anthelmintic agent if deficiency is due to fish tapeworm
- **Note**: Large doses of folic acid may produce hematologic responses in cases of vitamin B_{12} deficiency but allow neurologic damage to progress

 OUTCOME

FOLLOW-UP

- Pernicous anemia is a lifelong disorder; if patients discontinue monthly therapy, the vitamin deficiency will recur
- Brisk reticulocytosis occurs 5–7 days after therapy, and the hematologic picture normalizes in 2 months
- Follow serum vitamin B_{12} level

COMPLICATIONS

- Nervous system complications include subacute combined degeneration of the spinal cord, psychosis, and dementia
- Atrophic gastritis in pernicious anemia is associated with increased risk of gastric carcinoma
- Hypokalemia may complicate the first several days of parenteral vitamin B_{12} therapy in pernicious anemia, particularly if anemia is severe

PROGNOSIS

- Patients with pernicious anemia respond to parenteral vitamin B_{12} therapy with immediate improvement in sense of well-being
- Nervous system manifestations are reversible if they are of relatively short duration (< 6 months) but may be permanent if treatment is not initiated promptly

 EVIDENCE

WEB SITE

- National Institutes of Health, Office of Dietary Supplements: Vitamin B_{12}

INFORMATION FOR PATIENTS

- American Academy of Family Physicians: Vitamin B_{12}
- Mayo Clinic: Vitamin Deficiency Anemia
- MedlinePlus: Pernicious Anemia
- MedlinePlus: Vitamin B_{12} (Systemic)

REFERENCES

- Andres E et al. Vitamin B_{12} (cobalamin) deficiency in elderly patients. CMAJ. 2004 Aug 3;171(3):251–9. [PMID: 15289425]
- Bolaman Z et al. Oral versus intramuscular cobalamin treatment in megaloblastic anemia: a single-center, prospective, randomized, open-label study. Clin Ther. 2003 Dec; 25(12):3124–34. [PMID: 14749150]
- Carmel R. Current concepts in cobalamin deficiency. Annu Rev Med. 2000; 51:357–75. [PMID: 10774470]

von Willebrand's Disease

 KEY FEATURES

ESSENTIALS OF DIAGNOSIS

- Family history with autosomal dominant pattern of inheritance
- Prolonged bleeding time, either at baseline or after challenge with aspirin
- Factor VIII antigen or ristocetin cofactor levels are reduced
- Factor VIII coagulant activity levels are reduced in some patients

GENERAL CONSIDERATIONS

- Most common congenital disorder of hemostasis
- Autosomal dominant transmission
- Characterized by deficient or defective von Willebrand factor (vWF), a protein that mediates platelet adhesion
- Platelets adhere to subendothelium via vWF, which binds to platelet receptor

composed of glycoprotein Ib (missing in Bernard-Soulier syndrome)

- Platelet aggregation is normal in von Willebrand's disease
- vWF has a separate function of binding the factor VIII coagulant protein (factor VIII:C), and protecting it from degradation (factor VIII:C is deficient in classic hemophilia A); may thus secondarily cause coagulation disturbance because of deficient factor VIII:C levels, but coagulopathy is rarely severe
- Subtypes of von Willebrand's disease (Table 5)
  - Type I (80% of cases): quantitative decrease in vWF
  - Type IIa: qualitative abnormality prevents multimer formation; only small multimers present that cannot mediate platelet adhesion
  - Type IIb: qualitative abnormality causes rapid clearance of functional large multimeric forms
  - Type III: rare autosomal recessive disorder in which vWF nearly absent
  - Pseudo-von Willebrand disease: rare disorder in which platelets bind large vWF multimers with excessive avidity, causing their clearance from plasma

DEMOGRAPHICS

- Common disorder affecting both men and women

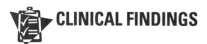

CLINICAL FINDINGS

SYMPTOMS AND SIGNS

- Mild bleeding occurs in most cases but rarely is it as severe as that which occurs in patients with hemophilia; spontaneous hemarthroses do not occur
- Mucosa is the usual site of bleeding (epistaxis, gingival bleeding, menorrhagia), but gastrointestinal bleeding may occur
- Incisional bleeding usually occurs after surgery or dental extractions
- Bleeding tendency is exacerbated by aspirin
- Bleeding tendency decreases during pregnancy or estrogen use

DIFFERENTIAL DIAGNOSIS

- Other qualitative platelet disorders, eg, uremia, aspirin use, Glanzmann's thrombasthenia
- Thrombocytopenia
- Hemophilia
- Waldenström's macroglobulinemia

DIAGNOSIS

LABORATORY TESTS

- See Table 5
- Platelet number and morphology are normal
- Bleeding time usually (not always) is prolonged; measure whenever the diagnosis is considered because it correlates most closely with clinical bleeding
- When the bleeding time is normal in von Willebrand's disease, it will be prolonged markedly by aspirin; normal persons prolong their bleeding time to a minor extent with aspirin but rarely out of the normal range
- In the most common form of von Willebrand's disease (type I), vWF plasma levels are reduced, as measured by factor VIII antigen or by ristocetin cofactor activity
- When factor VIII antigen is reduced, there may also be a decrease in factor VIII coagulant (factor VIII:C) levels; when factor VIII:C levels < 25%, partial thromboplastin time is prolonged
- Platelet aggregation studies with standard agonists (ADP, collagen, thrombin) are normal, but platelet aggregation in response to ristocetin may be subnormal
- In difficult cases, it may be helpful to perform a direct assay of the multimeric composition of vWF

TREATMENT

MEDICATIONS

- Desmopressin, 0.3 mcg/kg IV × 1, is useful for mild type I von Willebrand's disease
  - vWF levels usually rise twofold to threefold in 30–90 min, apparently via release of stored vWF from endothelial cells
  - Can be given only every 24 h as stores of vWF become depleted
- Desmopressin is not effective in type IIa von Willebrand's disease, in which no endothelial stores are present
- Desmopressin may be harmful in type IIb, leading to thrombocytopenia and increased bleeding
- Factor VIII concentrate, eg, Humate-P (Armour), 20–50 U/kg depending on disease severity, is treatment of choice if factor replacement is required; some (not all) of these products contain functional vWF and they do not transmit HIV or hepatitis

- ε-Aminocaproic acid (EACA; Amicar) is useful as adjunctive therapy during dental procedures; after either cryoprecipitate or desmopressin, 4 g PO q4h to reduce the likelihood of bleeding

THERAPEUTIC PROCEDURES

- In mild bleeding disorder, no treatment is routinely given other than aspirin avoidance
- In preparation for surgical or dental procedures, measure bleeding time as the best indicator of bleeding likelihood; prophylactic therapy may be reasonably withheld if the procedure is minor and bleeding time is normal

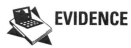

OUTCOME

PROGNOSIS

- Prognosis is excellent
- In most cases, bleeding disorder is mild
- In more serious cases, replacement therapy is effective

EVIDENCE

PRACTICE GUIDELINES

- Laffan M et al. The diagnosis of von Willebrand disease: a guideline from the UK Haemophilia Centre Doctors' Organization. Haemophilia. 2004 May; 10(3):199–217. [PMID: 15086318]
- Pasi KJ et al. Management of von Willebrand disease: a guideline from the UK Haemophilia Centre Doctors' Organization. Haemophilia. 2004;10:218. [PMID: 15086319]

WEB SITE

- National Hemophilia Foundation

INFORMATION FOR PATIENTS

- MedlinePlus: von Willebrand's Disease
- National Heart, Lung, and Blood Institute: von Willebrand Disease
- National Hemophilia Foundation: von Willebrand Disease

REFERENCE

- Federici AB et al. Biologic response to desmopressin in patients with severe type 1 and type 2 von Willebrand disease: results of a multicenter European study. Blood. 2004 Mar 15;103(6): 2032–8. [PMID: 14630825]

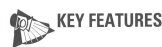

Waldenström's Macroglobulinemia

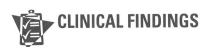

KEY FEATURES

ESSENTIALS OF DIAGNOSIS

- Monoclonal immunoglobulin M (IgM) paraprotein
- Infiltration of bone marrow by plasmacytic lymphocytes
- Absence of lytic bone disease

GENERAL CONSIDERATIONS

- Malignant disease of B cells that appears to be a hybrid of lymphocytes and plasma cells
- Cells characteristically secrete IgM paraprotein, and this macroglobulin causes many clinical manifestations

DEMOGRAPHICS

- Occurs mainly in patients aged 60–79

CLINICAL FINDINGS

SYMPTOMS AND SIGNS

- Insidious fatigue related to anemia
- Mucosal or gastrointestinal bleeding is related to engorged blood vessels and platelet dysfunction with hyperviscosity syndrome (usually when viscosity > 4 times that of water)
- Nausea, vertigo, or visual disturbances
- Alterations in consciousness from mild lethargy to stupor and coma with hyperviscosity syndrome
- Symptoms of cold agglutinin disease or peripheral neuropathy from IgM paraprotein
- Hepatosplenomegaly or lymphadenopathy may be present
- Retinal vein engorgement
- Purpura may be present
- Bone tenderness absent

DIFFERENTIAL DIAGNOSIS

- Monoclonal gammopathy of uncertain significance
- Multiple myeloma
- Chronic lymphocytic leukemia
- Lymphoma

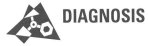

DIAGNOSIS

LABORATORY TESTS

- Anemia is nearly universal, and rouleau formation common
- White blood cell and platelet count are usually normal
- Peripheral blood smear: abnormal plasmacytic lymphocytes may be present in small numbers
- Serum protein electrophoresis (SPEP) demonstrates monoclonal IgM spike in β- or γ-globulin region
- Serum viscosity is usually increased above normal (> 1.4–1.8 times viscosity of water)
- No direct correlation between paraprotein concentration and serum viscosity
- Coombs, cold agglutinin, or cryoglobulin tests may be positive because of IgM paraprotein
- If macroglobulinemia is suspected but the SPEP shows only hypogammaglobulinemia, repeat the SPEP while maintaining blood at 37°C, because the paraprotein may precipitate at room temperature
- No evidence of renal failure

IMAGING STUDIES

- Bone radiographs are normal

DIAGNOSTIC PROCEDURES

- Bone marrow aspiration and biopsy: characteristic infiltration by the plasmacytic lymphocytes

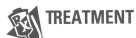

TREATMENT

MEDICATIONS

- Chemotherapy with fludarabine
- Rituximab and fludarabine
- See Table 7

THERAPEUTIC PROCEDURES

- Emergent plasmapheresis for marked hyperviscosity syndrome (stupor or coma)
- Plasmapheresis alone periodically for some patients
- Autologous stem cell transplantation in younger patients with more aggressive disease

OUTCOME

PROGNOSIS

- Median survival rate is 3–5 years; some patients may survive 10 years or longer

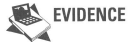

EVIDENCE

PRACTICE GUIDELINES

- Gertz MA et al. Treatment recommendations in Waldenström's macroglobulinemia: consensus panel recommendations from the Second International Workshop on Waldenström's Macroglobulinemia. Semin Oncol. 2003;30:121. [PMID: 12720120]
- Kyle RA et al. Prognostic markers and criteria to initiate therapy in Waldenström's macroglobulinemia: consensus panel recommendations from the Second International Workshop on Waldenström's Macroglobulinemia. Semin Oncol. 2003;30:116. [PMID: 12720119]

WEB SITE

- International Waldenström's Macroglobulinemia Foundation

INFORMATION FOR PATIENTS

- American Cancer Society: Detailed Guide: Waldenström's Macroglobulinemia
- MedlinePlus: Macroglobulinemia of Waldenström
- National Cancer Institute: Waldenström's Macroglobulinemia Facts
- Research Fund for Waldenström's: What Is Waldenström's Macroglobulinemia?

REFERENCES

- Dimopoulos MA et al. Diagnosis and management of Waldenstrom's macroglobulinemia. J Clin Oncol. 2005 Mar 1;23(7):1564–77. [PMID: 15735132]
- Munshi NC et al. Role for high-dose therapy with autologous hematopoietic stem cell support in Waldenstrom's macroglobulinemia. Semin Oncol. 2003 Apr;30(2):282–5. [PMID: 12720153]

Warts

 KEY FEATURES

ESSENTIALS OF DIAGNOSIS

- Verrucous papules anywhere on the skin or mucous membranes, usually no larger than 1 cm in diameter
- Prolonged incubation period (average 2–18 months); spontaneous "cures" are frequent (50%)
- "Recurrences" (new lesions) are frequent

GENERAL CONSIDERATIONS

- Caused by human papillomaviruses (HPVs)
- Especially in genital warts, simultaneous infection with numerous wart types is common
- Genital HPVs are divided into low-risk and high-risk types depending on the likelihood of their association with cervical and anal cancer

 CLINICAL FINDINGS

SYMPTOMS AND SIGNS

- There are usually no symptoms
- Tenderness on pressure occurs with plantar warts; itching occurs with anogenital warts
- Flat warts are most evident under oblique illumination
- Subungual warts may be dry, fissured, and hyperkeratotic and may resemble hangnails or other nonspecific changes
- Plantar warts resemble plantar corns or calluses

DIFFERENTIAL DIAGNOSIS

- Nongenital warts
  - Actinic keratosis
  - Squamous cell carcinoma
  - Molluscum contagiosum
  - Skin tag (acrochordon)
  - Nevus
  - Verrucous zoster (in AIDS)
- Genital warts (condyloma acuminata)
  - Secondary syphilis (condyloma lata)
  - Psoriasis
  - Seborrheic keratosis
  - Molluscum contagiosum
  - Bowenoid papulosis and squamous cell carcinoma
  - Lichen planus
  - Pearly penile papules
  - Skin tag (acrochordon)

 DIAGNOSIS

LABORATORY TESTS

- Clinical diagnosis

DIAGNOSTIC PROCEDURES

- Biopsy may be necessary for definitive diagnosis

TREATMENT

MEDICATIONS

Liquid nitrogen

- Apply to achieve a thaw time of 20–45 s; two freeze-thaw cycles are used every 2–4 weeks for several visits
- Scarring will occur if used incorrectly
- May cause permanent depigmentation in darkly pigmented individuals
- It is useful on dry penile warts and on filiform warts on the face and body

Keratolytic agents and occlusion

- Any of the following salicylic acid products may be used against common warts or plantar warts: Occlusal, Trans-Ver-Sal, and Duofilm
- Plantar warts may be treated by applying a 40% salicylic acid plaster (Mediplast) after paring; the plaster may be left on for 5–6 days, then removed, the lesion pared down, and another plaster applied; it may take months to eradicate
- Chronic occlusion alone with water-impermeable tape (duct tape, adhesive tape) for months may be effective

Podophyllum resin

- Paint each anogenital wart carefully (protecting normal skin) every 2–3 weeks with 25% podophyllum resin (podophyllin) in compound tincture of benzoin
- Avoid use in pregnancy
- The purified active component of the resin, podofilox, is available for use at home twice daily three consecutive days a week for cycles of 4–6 weeks; it is less irritating and more effective than podophyllum resin
- May need multiple cycles of treatment

Imiquimod

- A 5% cream of this local interferon inducer can clear external genital warts, particularly in women
- Treatment is once daily on 3 alternate days per week; response may take up to 12 weeks; recurrences may occur
- There is less risk in pregnancy than with podophyllum resin and it appears to be the "patient-administered" treatment of choice in women
- In men, the more rapid response, lower cost, and similar efficacy make podophyllotoxin the initial treatment of choice, with imiquimod used for recurrences or refractory cases
- May be used to treat superficial flat warts

Other agents

- Bleomycin diluted to 1 unit/mL injected into plantar and common warts; do not use on digital warts because of the potential complications of Raynaud's phenomenon, nail loss, and terminal digital necrosis
- Cimetidine, 35–50 mg/kg daily, for younger patients with common warts as an adjunct to immunotherapies listed below
- Apply aquaric acid dibutylester 0.2–2.0% directly to the warts from once weekly to five times weekly to induce a mild contact dermatitis; most warts clear over 10–20 weeks
- Injection of candida antigen may be used in the same way

Retinoids

- Tretinoin (Retin-A) cream or gel applied topically twice daily may be effective for facial or beard flat warts
- Extensive warts may remit after 4–8 weeks of oral retinoids

THERAPEUTIC PROCEDURES

- Soaking warts in hot (42.2°C) water for 10–30 min daily for 6 weeks can result in involution

Operative removal

- For genital warts, snip biopsy (scissors) removal followed by light electrocautery is more effective than cryotherapy

Laser therapy

- The CO_2 laser
  - Can be used for recurrent warts, periungual warts, plantar warts, and condylomata acuminata
  - Should be reserved for refractory cases that have failed the more standard treatments listed above
  - Leaves open wounds that must fill in with granulation tissue over 4–6 weeks and is best reserved for warts resistant to other modalities

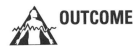

OUTCOME

PROGNOSIS

- Development of new lesions is common
- Warts may disappear spontaneously or may be unresponsive to treatment

WHEN TO REFER

- If there is a question about the diagnosis, if recommended therapy is ineffective, or if specialized treatment is necessary

PREVENTION

- The use of condoms may reduce transmission of genital warts

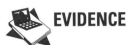

EVIDENCE

PRACTICE GUIDELINES

- American College of Obstetricians and Gynecologists. ACOG Practice Bulletin. Clinical Management Guidelines for Obstetrician-Gynecologists. Number 61, April 2005. Human papillomavirus. Obstet Gynecol. 2005 Apr;105(4):905–18. [PMID: 15802436]

INFORMATION FOR PATIENTS

- American Academy of Dermatology: Warts
- American Academy of Family Physicians: Warts
- MedlinePlus: Warts

REFERENCES

- Abernethy H et al. Clinical inquiries. What nonpharmacological treatments are effective against common nongenital warts? J Fam Pract. 2006 Sep;55(9):801–2. [PMID: 16948965]
- Bacelieri R et al. Cutaneous warts: an evidence-based approach to therapy. Am Fam Physician. 2005 Aug 15;72(4):647–52. [PMID: 16127954]
- Warren T et al. Counseling the patient who has genital herpes or genital human papillomavirus infection. Infect Dis Clin North Am. 2005 Jun;19(2):459–76. [PMID: 15963883]

Wegener's Granulomatosis

KEY FEATURES

ESSENTIALS OF DIAGNOSIS

- Triad of
  - Upper respiratory tract disease
  - Lower respiratory disease
  - Glomerulonephritis
- Suspect this diagnosis whenever mundane respiratory systems (eg, nasal congestion, sinusitis) are refractory to usual treatment
- Pathology defined by the triad of
  - Small vessel vasculitis
  - Granulomatous inflammation
  - Necrosis
- ANCAs, usually directed against proteinase-3 (less commonly against myeloperoxidase present in severe, active disease) (90% of patients)
- Renal disease often rapidly progressive

GENERAL CONSIDERATIONS

- The disease presents as vasculitis of small arteries, arterioles, and capillaries, necrotizing granulomatous lesions of both upper and lower respiratory tract, and glomerulonephritis

DEMOGRAPHICS

- Annual incidence of 10 per million
- Occurs most commonly in the fourth and fifth decades of life
- Affects men and women with equal frequency

CLINICAL FINDINGS

SYMPTOMS AND SIGNS

- Usually develops over 4–12 months
- Fever, malaise, and weight loss
- 90% of patients present with upper or lower respiratory tract symptoms or both
- Upper respiratory tract symptoms can include
  - Nasal congestion, sinusitis
  - Otitis media, mastoiditis
  - Inflammation of the gums
  - Stridor due to subglottic stenosis
- Physical examination can be remarkable for congestion, crusting, ulceration, bleeding, and even perforation of the nasal mucosa

- The lung is affected initially in 40% and eventually in 80%, with symptoms including cough, dyspnea, and hemoptysis
- Renal involvement (75%) may be subclinical until renal insufficiency is advanced
- Other early symptoms can include
  - Unilateral proptosis (from pseudotumor)
  - Red eye from scleritis
  - Arthritis
  - Purpura
  - Dysesthesia due to neuropathy
  - Destruction of the nasal cartilage with "saddle nose" deformity occurs late
- Patients are at high risk for venous thrombotic events (deep venous thrombosis, pulmonary embolism)

DIFFERENTIAL DIAGNOSIS

- Polyarteritis nodosa
- Microscopic polyangiitis
- Churg-Strauss syndrome
- Chronic sinusitis
- Goodpasture's disease
- Systemic lupus erythematosus
- Sarcoidosis

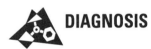

DIAGNOSIS

LABORATORY TESTS

- c-ANCA
  - Caused by antibodies to proteinase-3, a constituent of neutrophil granules
  - Has a high specificity (> 90%)
  - In the setting of active disease, the sensitivity of c-ANCA is also reasonably high (= 70%)
- p-ANCA
  - Caused by antibodies to myeloperoxidase and is much less specific than c-ANCA
  - Approximately 10–25% of patients with classic Wegener's granulomatosis have p-ANCA
- The urinary sediment in the renal disease invariably contains red cells, with or without white cells, and red cell casts

IMAGING STUDIES

- Chest CT is more sensitive than chest radiograph for infiltrates, nodules, masses, and cavities

PROCEDURES

- ANCA testing does not eliminate the need in most cases for confirmation of the diagnosis by tissue biopsy

- The full range of pathologic changes is usually evident only on thoracoscopic lung biopsy
- Histologic features include
  – Vasculitis
  – Granulomatous inflammation
  – Geographic necrosis
  – Acute and chronic inflammation
- Renal biopsy discloses a segmental necrotizing glomerulonephritis with multiple crescents (characteristic but not diagnostic)

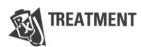 TREATMENT

MEDICATIONS

- Prednisone and oral cyclophosphamide for induction treatment
- Methotrexate, 20–25 mg/week, is a reasonable substitute for oral cyclophosphamide in patients who do not have immediately life-threatening disease
- Azathioprine (up to 2 mg/kg/day PO) can be substituted for cyclophosphamide once remission has been achieved
- Before the institution of azathioprine, patients should be tested for deficiencies in the level of thiopurine methyltransferase, an enzyme essential to the metabolism of azathioprine
- Rituximab, which depletes B cells and thereby reduces ANCA levels, appears promising and may help reveal whether ANCA plays a critical role in the pathogenesis of Wegener's granulomatosis

THERAPEUTIC PROCEDURES

- Early treatment is crucial in preventing renal failure and may be lifesaving

 OUTCOME

FOLLOW-UP

- Complete blood cell count every 2 weeks for patients on daily cyclophosphamide

COMPLICATIONS

Permanent disease-related complications

- Suffered by 85% of patients
- End-stage renal disease
- Decreased hearing
- Visual impairment
- Subglottic stenosis
- Saddle-nose deformity

- Deep venous thrombophlebitis or pulmonary embolism

Permanent treatment-related complications

- Suffered by 40% of patients
- Multitudinous effects of corticosteroids
- Cyclophosphamide
  – Bone marrow hypoplasia
  – Secondary malignancy (bladder, leukemia)
  – Hemorrhagic cystitis
  – Infertility

PROGNOSIS

- Without treatment it is invariably fatal, most patients surviving < 1 year after diagnosis
- Remissions have been induced in up to 75% of patients treated with cyclophosphamide and prednisone, though half of these patients eventually suffer disease recurrences

WHEN TO REFER

- All patients should be monitored by a rheumatologist. Other subspecialty consultations may be appropriate

WHEN TO ADMIT

- Alveolar hemorrhage
- Rapidly progressive glomerulonephritis

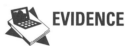 EVIDENCE

WEB SITE

- The Johns Hopkins Vasculitis Center

REFERENCES

- Bosch X et al. Antineutrophil cytoplasmic antibodies. Lancet. 2006 Jul 29; 368(9533):404–18. [PMID: 16876669]
- Merkel PA et al. High incidence of venous thrombotic events among patients with Wegener granulomatosis: the Wegener's Clinical Occurrence of Thrombosis (WeCLOT) Study. Ann Intern Med. 2005 Apr 19;142(8):620–6. [PMID: 15838068]
- Seo P et al. Damage caused by Wegener's granulomatosis and its treatment: prospective data from the Wegener's Granulomatosis Etanercept Trial (WGET). Arthritis Rheum. 2005 Jul; 52(7):2168–78. [PMID: 15986348]
- Wegener's Granulomatosis Etanercept Trial (WGET) Research Group: Etanercept plus standard therapy for Wegener's granulomatosis. N Engl J Med. 2005 Jan 27;352(4):351–61. [PMID: 15673801]

Weight Loss & Malnutrition in Elderly

 KEY FEATURES

ESSENTIALS OF DIAGNOSIS

- The definition of unintended weight loss varies according to setting
  – For elders in long term care: it is defined as weight loss exceeding 5% in 1 month or 10% in 6 months (OBRA 1987)
  – For community dwelling elders it is weight loss exceeding 5% in 6 months or 10% in 1 year
- Failure to thrive

GENERAL CONSIDERATIONS

- Undernutrition affects substantial numbers of elderly persons and often precedes hospitalization for "failure to thrive"
- "Failure to thrive"
  – A syndrome lacking a consensus definition but generally represents a constellation of weight loss, weakness, and progressive functional decline
  – The label is typically applied when some triggering event—loss of social support, a bout of depression or pneumonia, the addition of a new medication—pulls a struggling elderly person below the threshold of successful independent living
- Poor fitting dentures or oral health problems may contribute to nutritional problems, particularly in those with dementia
- Medications may alter taste or appetite
- Total caloric needs are reduced by about 30% in the elderly, but protein needs may be increased
- Risk factors for malnutrition include
  – Chronic disease
  – Functional and cognitive impairment
  – Depression

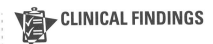 **CLINICAL FINDINGS**

SYMPTOMS AND SIGNS

- A 10% loss of weight suggests severe malnutrition
- A loss of 5% suggests moderate malnutrition
- Subcutaneous tissue loss can be best evaluated in the subscapular, suprailiac, and triceps skinfolds
- A body mass index under 22 should raise concern about significant malnutrition

DIFFERENTIAL DIAGNOSIS

Medical
- Chronic heart, lung disease
- Dementia
- Oral problems (eg, poor denture fit)
- Dysphagia
- Dysgeusia
- Mesenteric ischemia
- Cancer
- Diabetes
- Hyperthyroidism
- Malabsorption

Psychosocial
- Alcoholism/substance use
- Depression/dementia
- Social isolation
- Limited funds
- Problems with shopping or food preparation
- Inadequate assistance with feeding

Drug-related
- Nonsteroidal anti-inflammatory drugs
- Antiepileptics
- Digoxin
- Selective serotonin reuptake inhibitors
- Anticholinergics

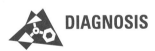 **DIAGNOSIS**

LABORATORY TESTS

- Laboratory studies are intended to uncover an occult metabolic or neoplastic cause
- Useful laboratory studies include
  - Complete blood cell count
  - Serum chemistries (eg, glucose, TSH, creatinine, calcium)
  - Urinalysis

IMAGING STUDIES

- Chest radiograph

- Further imaging (eg, mammography, colonoscopy) as dictated by the clinical presentation

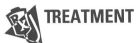 **TREATMENT**

THERAPEUTIC PROCEDURES

- Aim for a caloric intake of about 25 kcal/kg, based on ideal body weight
- Nutritional supplements may lead to weight gain; use of instant breakfast powder in whole milk (for those who can tolerate dairy products) is a less costly alternative
- For those who have lost the ability to feed themselves, assiduous hand feeding may allow maintenance of weight
- Artificial nutrition and hydration ("tube feeding") is an alternative, but it deprives the patient of the taste and texture of food as well as the social milieu typically associated with mealtime
- If the patient makes repeated attempts to pull out the tube during a trial of artificial nutrition, the treatment burden becomes substantial, and the utility of tube feeding should be reconsidered
- Megestrol acetate has not been shown to increase body mass in the elderly
- Treatment of depression with mirtazapine has been associated with modest weight gain

 OUTCOME

FOLLOW-UP

- Patients with malnutrition are at higher risk for death, functional decline, and nursing home placement

COMPLICATIONS

- Hospitalized patients with malnutrition are more likely to experience multiple life-threatening complications

PROGNOSIS

- Though commonly used, there is no evidence that tube feeding prolongs life in patients with end-stage dementia
- Nutritional supplements may increase weight, but a recent meta-analysis suggested a mortality benefit only for malnourished hospitalized elders

WHEN TO REFER

- Early involvement of a nutritionist may be helpful
- Consider dental or denture evaluation

WHEN TO ADMIT

- Malnutrition is rarely an indication for admission in and of itself
- The threshold for admission should be lower when a malnourished patient presents with an acute illness such as pneumonia

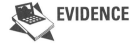 **EVIDENCE**

PRACTICE GUIDELINES

- American Academy of Family Physicians
- National Guidelines Clearinghouse: American Medical Directors Association, 2001

WEB SITES

- Administration on Aging
- American Geriatrics Society
- Merck Manual of Geriatrics

INFORMATION FOR PATIENTS

- Federal nutrition.gov
- JAMA patient page. Healthy diet. JAMA. 2000;283:2198. [PMID: 10791513]
- National Institute on Aging

REFERENCE

- Milne AC et al. Meta-analysis: Protein and energy supplementation in older people. Ann Intern Med. 2006 Jan 3; 144(1):37–48. [PMID: 16389253]

Weight Loss, Involuntary

 KEY FEATURES

ESSENTIALS OF DIAGNOSIS

- Decreased caloric intake
- Fever
- Change in bowel habits
- Secondary confirmation (eg, changes in clothing size)
- Substance abuse
- History of age-appropriate cancer screening

GENERAL CONSIDERATIONS

- Body weight is determined by
  - Person's caloric intake

– Absorptive capacity
– Metabolic rate
– Energy losses

• Involuntary weight loss is clinically significant when it exceeds 5% or more of usual body weight over a 6- to 12-month period

• Often indicates serious physical or psychological illness

• Most common causes
– Cancer (~30% of cases)
– Gastrointestinal disorders (~15%)
– Dementia or depression (~15%)

• In approximately 15–25% of cases, no cause for the weight loss can be found

 CLINICAL FINDINGS

SYMPTOMS AND SIGNS

• History should include medication profile and 24-h diet recall
• Cancer
– Night sweats
– Cough
– Breast mass
– Constipation
– Hematochezia
– Bone pain
• Gastrointestinal disease
– Nausea
– Vomiting
– Diarrhea
– Abdominal pain
• Depression
– Anhedonia
– Sleep disorder
– Suicidal ideation
– Recent psychosocial stressors
• Dementia
– Memory loss
– Wandering
– Isolation
• Physical examination for evidence of cancer

DIFFERENTIAL DIAGNOSIS

Medical

• Malignancy
• Gastrointestinal disorders, eg, malabsorption, pancreatic insufficiency, peptic ulcer
• Hyperthyroidism
• Chronic heart, lung, or renal disease
• Uncontrolled diabetes mellitus
• Mesenteric ischemia (ischemic bowel)
• Dysphagia
• Anorexia due to azotemia
• Hypercalcemia
• Tuberculosis
• Subacute bacterial endocarditis

Psychosocial

• Depression
• Dementia
• Alcoholism
• Anorexia nervosa
• Loss of teeth, poor denture fit
• Social isolation
• Poverty
• Inability to shop or prepare food

Drug-related

• Nonsteroidal anti-inflammatory drugs
• Antiepileptics
• Digoxin
• Selective serotonin reuptake inhibitors

 DIAGNOSIS

LABORATORY TESTS

• Complete blood cell count
• Serologic tests
• Serum thyroid-stimulating hormone
• Urinalysis
• Fecal occult blood tests

IMAGING STUDIES

• Chest radiograph
• Abdominal CT scan or upper gastrointestinal series, or both
• When these tests are normal, more definitive gastrointestinal investigation (eg, tests for malabsorption; endoscopy) and cancer screening (eg, Pap smear, mammography, prostate-specific antigen)

DIAGNOSTIC PROCEDURES

• If initial diagnostic workup is unrevealing, follow-up is preferable to further diagnostic testing

 TREATMENT

MEDICATIONS

• Appetite stimulants (mild to moderate effectiveness)
– Corticosteroids
– Progestational agents
– Dronabinol
– Serotonin antagonists
• Anabolic agents
– Growth hormone
– Testosterone derivatives
• Anticatabolic agents
– Omega-3 fatty acids
– Pentoxifylline

– Hydrazine sulfate
– Thalidomide

THERAPEUTIC PROCEDURES

• Treatment of the underlying disorder
• Consultation with dietician
• Caloric supplementation to achieve intake of 30–40 kcal/kg/day
• Oral feeding is preferred, but temporary nasojejunal tube, or permanent cutaneous gastric or jejunal tube may be necessary

 OUTCOME

PROGNOSIS

• Rapid unintentional weight loss is predictive of morbidity and mortality
• Mortality rates at 2-year follow-up
– 8% for unexplained involuntary weight loss
– 19% for weight loss due to nonmalignant disease
– 79% for weight loss due to malignant disease

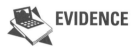 **EVIDENCE**

PRACTICE GUIDELINES

• American Academy of Family Physicians, American Dietetic Association, Nutrition Screening Initiative: Nutrition Management for Older Adults (Specific Guidelines for Cancer, COPD, CHF, CHD, Dementia, Diabetes Mellitus, Hypertension, Osteoporosis), 2002.
• American Medical Directors Association: Altered Nutritional Status, 2001.

INFORMATION FOR PATIENTS

• Mayo Clinic: When you have no appetite: Tips to get the nutrition you need
• Mayo Clinic: Illness and appetite: What to do when nothing tastes right
• MedlinePlus: Unintentional Weight Loss
• National Institutes of Health: The Widespread Effects of Depression

REFERENCES

• Alibhai SM et al. An approach to the management of unintentional weight loss in elderly people. CMAJ. 2005 Mar 15;172(6):773–80. [PMID: 15767612]
• Collins N. Protein-energy malnutrition and involuntary weight loss: nutritional and pharmacological strategies to enhance wound healing. Expert Opin

Pharmacother. 2003 Jul;4(7):1121–40. [PMID. 12831338]

- Hernandez JL et al. Clinical evaluation for cancer in patients with involuntary weight loss without specific symptoms. Am J Med. 2003 Jun 1;114(8):631–7. [PMID: 12798450]
- Lankisch P et al. Unintentional weight loss: diagnosis and prognosis. The first prospective follow-up study from a secondary referral centre. J Intern Med. 2001 Jan;249(1):41–6. [PMID: 11168783]
- Sahyoun NR et al. The epidemiology of recent involuntary weight loss in the United States population. J Nutr Health Aging. 2004;8(6):510–7. [PMID: 15543425]

Wernicke's Encephalopathy

 ## KEY FEATURES

- Caused by thiamine deficiency
- In United States, occurs most commonly in alcoholic patients
- It may also occur in patients with AIDS, in patients with hyperemesis gravidarum, or after surgery for morbid obesity

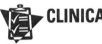 ## CLINICAL FINDINGS

- Triad of confusion, ataxia, and nystagmus leading to ophthalmoplegia (lateral rectus muscle weakness, conjugate gaze palsies)
- Peripheral neuropathy may be present

 ## DIAGNOSIS

- Confirmed by the response to treatment within 1 or 2 days, which must not be delayed while laboratory confirmation is obtained

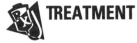 ## TREATMENT

- In suspected cases, thiamine 50 mg, is given IV immediately and then IM on a daily basis until a satisfactory diet can be ensured

- IV glucose given before thiamine may precipitate the syndrome or worsen the symptoms

Whipple's Disease

 ## KEY FEATURES

ESSENTIALS OF DIAGNOSIS

- Multisystem disease
- Fever, lymphadenopathy, arthralgias
- Malabsorption
- Duodenal biopsy with PAS-positive macrophages with characteristic bacillus

GENERAL CONSIDERATIONS

- Rare multisystem illness caused by infection with the bacillus *Tropheryma whippelii*
- Source of infection is unknown; no cases of human-to-human spread have been documented

DEMOGRAPHICS

- May occur at any age but most commonly affects white men in the fourth to sixth decades

 ## CLINICAL FINDINGS

SYMPTOMS AND SIGNS

- Clinical manifestations are protean
- Arthralgias or a migratory, nondeforming arthritis in 80%
- Gastrointestinal symptoms in 75% include
  - Abdominal pain
  - Diarrhea
  - Variable malabsorption with distention, flatulence, and steatorrhea
- Weight loss in almost all patients
- Protein-losing enteropathy with hypoalbuminemia and edema
- Intermittent low-grade fever in > 50%
- Chronic cough
- Generalized lymphadenopathy
- Myocardial involvement: congestive heart failure or valvular regurgitation
- Ocular
  - Uveitis
  - Vitreitis
  - Keratitis
  - Retinitis
  - Retinal hemorrhages
- CNS involvement
  - Dementia
  - Lethargy
  - Coma
  - Seizures
  - Myoclonus
  - Hypothalamic signs
- Cranial nerve findings: ophthalmoplegia or nystagmus
- Physical examination
  - Low-grade fever
  - Hypotension (late)
  - Lymphadenopathy in 50%
  - Heart murmurs
  - Peripheral joint inflammation, swelling
  - Neurologic findings
  - Hyperpigmentation on sun-exposed areas in up to 40%

DIFFERENTIAL DIAGNOSIS

- Malabsorption due to other cause, eg, celiac or tropical sprue
- Inflammatory bowel disease
- Sarcoidosis
- Reactive arthritis (Reiter's syndrome)
- Systemic vasculitis
- Infective endocarditis
- Intestinal lymphoma
- Familial Mediterranean fever
- Behçet's syndrome
- Intestinal *Mycobacterium avium-intracellulare* (in AIDS)

 ## DIAGNOSIS

LABORATORY TESTS

- Polymerase chain reaction (PCR)
  - Confirms diagnosis by demonstrating the presence of 16S ribosomal RNA of *T whippelii* in blood, cerebrospinal fluid, vitreous fluid, synovial fluid, or cardiac valves
  - Sensitivity of 97%
  - Specificity of 100%

DIAGNOSTIC PROCEDURES

- Endoscopic biopsy of the duodenum demonstrates infiltration of the lamina propria with PAS-positive macrophages that contain gram-positive, non–acid-fast bacilli, and dilatation of the lacteals
- Biopsy of other involved organs or lymph nodes for histologic evaluation of the involved tissues may be necessary

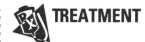

TREATMENT

MEDICATIONS

- Trimethoprim-sulfamethoxazole (1 double-strength tablet PO BID) is recommended as first-line therapy
- In severely ill patients, administer 2 g/day of IV ceftriaxone for 2 weeks
- For patients allergic to sulfonamides or resistant to therapy, consider long-term treatment with doxycycline or hydroxychloroquine
- Prolonged treatment for at least 1 year is required

THERAPEUTIC PROCEDURES

- After antibiotic treatment, repeat biopsies for PCR; negative results predict a low likelihood of clinical relapse

OUTCOME

FOLLOW-UP

- Patients must be monitored closely after treatment for recurrence

COMPLICATIONS

- Some neurologic signs may be permanent

PROGNOSIS

- Antibiotic therapy results in a dramatic clinical improvement within several weeks
- Complete response within 1–3 months
- Relapse may occur in up to one-third of patients after discontinuation of treatment
- If untreated, the disease is fatal

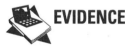

EVIDENCE

INFORMATION FOR PATIENTS

- Cleveland Clinic—Whipple's disease
- Medical College of Wisconsin—Whipple's disease
- National Digestive Diseases Information Clearinghouse
- National Institute of Neurological Disorders and Stroke

REFERENCE

- Fenollar F et al. Whipple's disease. N Engl J Med. 2007 Jan 4;356(1):55–66. [PMID: 17202456]

Wilson's Disease

KEY FEATURES

ESSENTIALS OF DIAGNOSIS

- Excessive deposition of copper in the liver and brain
- Rare autosomal recessive disorder that usually occurs in persons under age 40
- Serum ceruloplasmin, the plasma copper-carrying protein, is low
- Urinary excretion of copper is high

GENERAL CONSIDERATIONS

- The genetic defect, localized to chromosome 13, affects a copper-transporting adenosine triphosphatase (ATP7B) in the liver and leads to oxidative damage of hepatic mitochondria
- Over 200 different mutations in the Wilson disease gene have been identified
  - Genetic diagnosis is therefore impractical except within families in which the mutation has been identified in the index case
  - Most patients are compound heterozygotes (ie, carry two different mutations)
- The major physiologic aberration is excessive absorption of copper from the small intestine and decreased excretion of copper by the liver, resulting in increased tissue deposition, especially in the liver, brain, cornea, and kidney

DEMOGRAPHICS

- Adolescents and young adults but can manifest in persons over age 40

CLINICAL FINDINGS

SYMPTOMS AND SIGNS

- Consider the diagnosis in any child or young adult with the following
  - Hepatitis, splenomegaly with hypersplenism, portal hypertension
  - Hemolytic anemia
  - Neurologic or psychiatric abnormalities
  - Chronic or fulminant hepatitis
- Hepatic involvement may range from elevated liver tests (although the alkaline phosphatase may be low) to cirrhosis and portal hypertension
- Neurologic manifestations
  - Related to basal ganglia dysfunction
  - Resting, postural, or kinetic tremor
  - Dystonia of the bulbar musculature with resulting dysarthria and dysphagia
- Psychiatric features include behavioral and personality changes and emotional lability
- **Kayser-Fleischer ring**
  - Pathognomonic sign
  - Brownish or gray-green pigmented granular deposits in Descemet's membrane in the cornea close to the endothelial surface
  - Usually most marked at the superior and inferior poles of the cornea
  - It is sometimes seen with the naked eye and is readily detected by slit-lamp examination
  - It may be absent in patients with hepatic manifestations only but is usually present in those with neuropsychiatric disease

DIFFERENTIAL DIAGNOSIS

- Acute hepatitis
- Cholestasis
- Acute hepatic failure
- Chronic hepatitis
- Cirrhosis
- Hepatomegaly
- Other cause of hepatitis, fulminant hepatic failure, or cirrhosis, eg, viral, toxins, hemochromatosis
- Tremor due to other causes, eg, Parkinson's disease, essential tremor
- Dementia due to other causes, eg, Huntington's disease
- Behavior change due to other medical illness, eg, neurosyphilis, brain tumor

DIAGNOSIS

LABORATORY TESTS

- Increased urinary copper excretion (> 100 mcg/24 h) or low serum ceruloplasmin levels (< 20 mcg/dL), and elevated hepatic copper concentration (> 250 mcg/g of dry liver)
- However, increased urinary copper and low serum ceruloplasmin levels are not specific for Wilson's disease
- In equivocal cases (when the serum ceruloplasmin level is normal), the diagnosis may require demonstration of low radiolabeled copper incorporation into ceruloplasmin or urinary copper determination after a penicillamine challenge

DIAGNOSTIC PROCEDURES

- Liver biopsy may show acute or chronic hepatitis or cirrhosis and is used to quantify hepatic copper

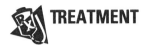 TREATMENT

MEDICATIONS

- Oral penicillamine (0.75–2.0 g/day in divided doses) is the drug of choice, enhancing urinary excretion of chelated copper. Add pyridoxine, 25–50 mg/week, since penicillamine is an antimetabolite of this vitamin
- If penicillamine treatment cannot be tolerated because of gastrointestinal, hypersensitivity, or autoimmune reactions, consider the use of trientine, 250–500 mg three times a day
- Oral zinc acetate, 50 mg three times a day
  - Interferes with intestinal absorption of copper
  - Promotes fecal copper excretion
  - May be used as maintenance therapy after decoppering with a chelating agent or as first-line therapy in presymptomatic or pregnant patients
- Ammonium tetrathiomolybdate complexes copper in the intestinal tract and has shown promise as initial therapy for neurologic Wilson's disease
- Treatment should continue indefinitely
- Once the serum nonceruloplasmin copper level is within the normal range, the dose of chelating agent can be reduced to the minimum necessary for maintaining that level

SURGERY

- Indications for liver transplantation
  - Fulminant hepatitis (often after plasma exchange as a stabilizing measure)
  - End-stage cirrhosis
  - Intractable neurologic disease (in selected cases)
- Survival is lower when transplantation is undertaken for neurologic disease than for liver disease

THERAPEUTIC PROCEDURES

- Early treatment to remove excess copper is essential before it can produce hepatic or neurologic damage
- Early in the treatment phase, restrict dietary copper (shellfish, organ foods, and legumes)

 OUTCOME

FOLLOW-UP

- Serum nonceruloplasmin copper
- Urine copper

COMPLICATIONS

- Fulminant hepatitis and cirrhosis
- Renal calculi, the Fanconi defect, renal tubular acidosis, hypoparathyroidism, and hemolytic anemia may occur

PROGNOSIS

- The prognosis is good if effective treatment occurs before liver or brain damage
- The disease may stabilize with treatment in cirrhosis

PREVENTION

- Family members, especially siblings, require screening with serum ceruloplasmin, liver biochemical tests, and slit-lamp examination

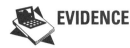 EVIDENCE

PRACTICE GUIDELINES

- National Guideline Clearinghouse
- Roberts EA et al. A practice guideline on Wilson disease. Hepatology. 2003; 37:1475. [PMID: 12774027]

INFORMATION FOR PATIENTS

- Mayo Clinic
- National Digestive Diseases Information Clearinghouse
- National Institute of Neurological Disorders and Stroke

REFERENCES

- Ferenci P. Wilson's disease. Clin Gastroenterol Hepatol. 2005 Aug;3(8):726–33. [PMID: 16233999]
- Medici V et al. Diagnosis and management of Wilson's disease: results of a single center experience. J Clin Gastroenterol. 2006 Nov–Dec; 40(10):936–41. [PMID: 17063115]
- Merle U et al. Clinical presentation, diagnosis and long-term outcome of Wilson's disease: a cohort study. Gut. 2007 Jan;56(1):115–20. [PMID: 16709660]

Zollinger-Ellison Syndrome

KEY FEATURES

ESSENTIALS OF DIAGNOSIS

- Peptic ulcer disease, may be severe and atypical
- Gastric acid hypersecretion
- Diarrhea common, relieved by nasogastric suction
- Most cases are sporadic; 25% with multiple endocrine neoplasia (MEN) type 1

GENERAL CONSIDERATIONS

- Caused by gastrin-secreting gut neuroendocrine tumors (gastrinomas), which result in hypergastrinemia and acid hypersecretion
- Gastrinomas cause < 1% of peptic ulcers
- Primary gastrinomas may arise in the pancreas (25%), duodenal wall (45%), lymph nodes (5–15%), or other locations (20%)
- Most gastrinomas are solitary or multifocal nodules that are potentially resectable; 25% are small multicentric gastrinomas associated with MEN 1 that are more difficult to resect
- Gastrinomas are malignant in less than two-thirds; one-third have already metastasized to the liver at initial presentation
- Screening for Zollinger-Ellison syndrome with fasting gastrin levels indicated for patients with
  – Ulcers refractory to standard therapies
  – Giant ulcers (> 2 cm)
  – Ulcers located distal to the duodenal bulb
  – Multiple duodenal ulcers
  – Frequent ulcer recurrences
  – Ulcers associated with diarrhea
  – Ulcers occurring after ulcer surgery
  – Ulcers with complications
  – Ulcers with hypercalcemia
  – Family history of ulcers
  – Ulcers not related to *Helicobacter pylori* or nonsteroidal anti-inflammatory drugs (NSAIDs)

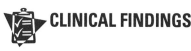

CLINICAL FINDINGS

SYMPTOMS AND SIGNS

- Peptic ulcers in > 90%, usually solitary and in proximal duodenal bulb, but may be multiple or in distal duodenum
- Isolated gastric ulcers do not occur
- Gastroesophageal reflux symptoms
- Diarrhea, steatorrhea, and weight loss (in ~33%) secondary to pancreatic enzyme inactivation

DIFFERENTIAL DIAGNOSIS

- Peptic ulcer disease due to other cause, eg, NSAIDs, *H pylori*
- Gastroesophageal reflux disease, esophagitis, gastritis, pancreatitis, or cholecystitis
- Diarrhea due to other cause
- Other gut neuroendocrine tumor
  – Carcinoid
  – Insulinoma
  – VIPoma
  – Glucagonoma
  – Somatostatinoma
- Hypergastrinemia due to other cause
  – Atrophic gastritis
  – Gastric outlet obstruction
  – Pernicious anemia
  – Chronic renal failure

DIAGNOSIS

LABORATORY TESTS

- Fasting serum gastrin concentration increased (> 150 pg/mL) in patients not taking H_2-receptor antagonists for 24 h or proton pump inhibitor for 6 days
- Serum calcium, parathyroid hormone, prolactin, leutinizing hormone, follicle-stimulating hormone, and growth hormone level in all patients with Zollinger-Ellison syndrome to exclude MEN 1
- Gastric pH of > 3.0 implies hypochlorhydria and excludes gastrinoma

IMAGING STUDIES

- CT, MRI, and transabdominal ultrasound have sensitivity of < 50–70% for hepatic metastases and 35% for primary tumors
- Somatostatin receptor scintigraphy (SRS) with SPECT has high sensitivity (> 80%) for detecting hepatic metastases, as well as primary tumors
- Endoscopic ultrasonography (EUS)
  – Indicated in patients with negative SRS
  – Has sensitivity of > 90% for tumors of the pancreatic head and ~50% for tumors in the duodenal wall or adjacent lymph nodes
- Combination of SRS and EUS can localize > 90% of primary gastrinomas preoperatively

DIAGNOSTIC PROCEDURES

- Secretin stimulation test distinguishes Zollinger-Ellison syndrome from other causes of hypergastrinemia
- Secretin, 2 units/kg IV, produces a rise in serum gastrin of > 200 pg/mL within 2–30 min in 85% of patients with gastrinoma

TREATMENT

MEDICATIONS

- Proton pump inhibitors (omeprazole, rabeprazole, pantoprazole, esomeprazole, or lansoprazole), 40–120 mg/day, titrated to achieve a basal acid output of < 10 mEq/h for metastatic disease

SURGERY

- Primary resection of gastrinoma at laparotomy for localized disease
- Preoperative studies and intraoperative palpation and sonography allow successful localization and resection in the majority of cases
- Surgical resection of isolated hepatic metastases

OUTCOME

COMPLICATIONS

- In patients with unresectable disease, complications of gastric acid hypersecretion can be prevented in almost all cases by sufficient doses of proton pump inhibitors
- Treatment options for metastatic disease include interferon, octreotide, combination therapy, and chemoembolization

PROGNOSIS

- 15-year survival of patients without liver metastases at initial presentation is > 80%
- 10-year survival of patients with hepatic metastases is 30%

WHEN TO REFER

- All patients with Zollinger-Ellison syndrome should be referred to a gastrointestinal surgeon with expertise in evaluation and management

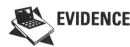

EVIDENCE

PRACTICE GUIDELINES

- Gibril F et al. Zollinger-Ellison syndrome revisited: diagnosis, biologic markers, associated inherited disorders, and acid hypersecretion. Curr Gastroenterol Rep. 2004;6:454. [PMID: 15527675]

• Quan C et al. Management of peptic ulcer disease not related to *Helicobacter pylori* or NSAIDs. Am J Gastroenterol. 2002;97:2950. [PMID: 12492176]

WEB SITES

• MedlinePlus—Zollinger-Ellison syndrome
• National Digestive Diseases Information Clearinghouse—Zollinger-Ellison syndrome

INFORMATION FOR PATIENTS

• Cleveland Clinic—Zollinger-Ellison syndrome

• Florida State University College of Medicine—Zollinger-Ellison Syndrome
• Mayo Clinic—Zollinger-Ellison syndrome

REFERENCE

• Libutti SK et al. Gastrinoma: sporadic and familial disease. Surg Oncol Clin N Am. 2006 Jul;15(3):479–96. [PMID: 16882493]

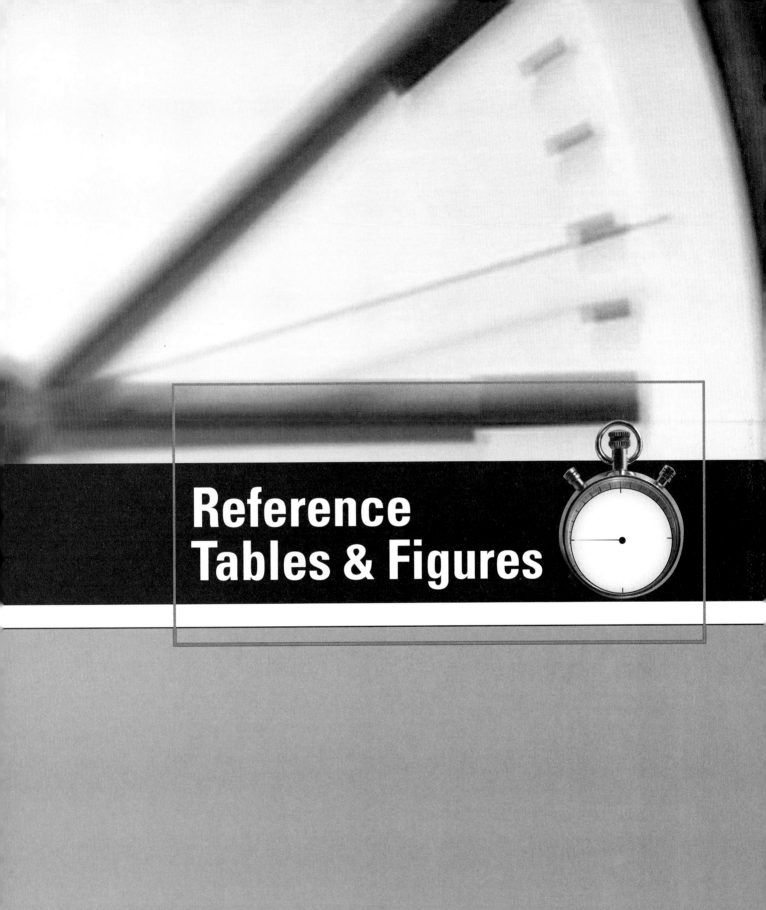

Reference
Tables & Figures

CONTENTS: Reference Tables & Figures

Figures

Table 1. Acetaminophen, COX-2 inhibitors, and useful nonsteroidal anti-inflammatory drugs.

Drug	Usual Dose for Adults ≥ 50 kg	Usual Dose for Adults < 50 kg[1]	Cost per Unit	Cost for 30 Days[2]	Comments[3]
Acetaminophen[4] (Tylenol, Datril, etc)	650 mg q4h or 975 mg q6h	10–15 mg/kg q4h (oral); 15–20 mg/kg q4h (rectal)	$0.02/325 mg (oral) OTC; $0.52/650 mg (rectal) OTC	$7.20 (oral); $93.60 (rectal)	Not an NSAID because it lacks peripheral anti-inflammatory effects. Equivalent to aspirin as analgesic and antipyretic agent.
Aspirin[5]	650 mg q4h or 975 mg q6h	10–15 mg/kg q4h (oral); 15–20 mg/kg q4h (rectal)	$0.02/325 mg OTC; $0.31/600 mg (rectal) OTC	$7.20 (oral); $55.80 (rectal)	Available also in enteric-coated form that is more slowly absorbed but better tolerated.
Celecoxib[4] (Celebrex)	200 mg once daily (osteoarthritis); 100–200 mg twice daily (rheumatoid arthritis)	100 mg once or twice daily	$2.29/100 mg; $3.76/200 mg	$112.80 OA; $225.60 RA	Cyclooxygenase-2 inhibitor. No antiplatelet effects. Lower doses for elderly who weigh < 50 kg. Lower incidence of endoscopic gastrointestinal ulceration. Not known if true lower incidence of gastrointestinal bleeding. Possible link to cardiovascular toxicity. Celecoxib is contraindicated in sulfonamide allergy.
Choline magnesium salicylate[6] (Trilasate, others)	1000–1500 mg three times daily	25 mg/kg three times daily	$0.57/500 mg	$153.90	Salicylates cause less gastrointestinal distress and renal impairment than NSAIDs but are probably less effective in pain management than NSAIDs.
Diclofenac (Voltaren, Cataflam, others)	50–75 mg two or three times daily		$0.86/50 mg; $1.04/75 mg	$77.40; $93.60	May impose higher risk of hepatotoxicity. Low incidence of gastrointestinal side effects. Enteric-coated product; slow onset.
Diclofenac sustained release (Voltaren-XR, others)	100–200 mg once daily		$2.81/100 mg	$168.60	
Diflunisal[7] (Dolobid, others)	500 mg q12h		$1.29/500 mg	$77.40	Fluorinated acetylsalicylic acid derivative.
Etodolac (Lodine, others)	200–400 mg q6–8h		$1.47/400 mg	$176.40	Perhaps less gastrointestinal toxicity.
Fenoprofen calcium (Nalfon, others)	300–600 mg q6h		$0.51/600 mg	$61.20	Perhaps more side effects than others, including tubulointerstitial nephritis.
Flurbiprofen (Ansaid)	50–100 mg three or four times daily		$0.79/50 mg; $1.19/100 mg	$94.80; $142.80	Adverse gastrointestinal effects may be more common among elderly.
Ibuprofen (Motrin, Advil, Rufen, others)	400–800 mg q6h	10 mg/kg q6–8h	$0.28/600 mg Rx; $0.05/200 mg OTC	$33.60; $9.00	Relatively well tolerated. Less gastrointestinal toxicity.
Indomethacin (Indocin, Indometh, others)	25–50 mg two to four times daily		$0.38/25 mg; $0.64/50 mg	$45.60; $76.80	Higher incidence of dose-related toxic effects, especially gastrointestinal and bone marrow effects.
Ketoprofen (Orudis, Oruvail, others)	25–75 mg q6–8h (max 300 mg/d)		$0.96/50 mg Rx; $1.07/75 mg Rx; $0.09/12.5 mg OTC	$172.80; $128.40; $16.20	Lower doses for elderly.
Ketorolac tromethamine (Toradol)	10 mg q4–6h to a maximum of 40 mg/d orally		$1.02/10 mg	Not recommended	Short-term use (< 5 days) only; otherwise, increased risk of gastrointestinal side effects.
Ketorolac tromethamine[8] (Toradol)	60 mg IM or 30 mg IV initially, then 30 mg q6h IM or IV		$1.80/30 mg	Not recommended	Intramuscular or intravenous NSAID as alternative to opioid. Lower doses for elderly. Short-term use (< 5 days) only.
Magnesium salicylate (various)	467 mg q4h		$0.08/467 mg OTC	$9.60	
Meclofenamate sodium[9] (Meclomen)	50–100 mg q6h		$3.40/100 mg	$408.00	Diarrhea more common.
Mefenamic acid (Ponstel)	250 mg q6h		$5.85/250 mg	$702.00	

(continued)

Table 1. Acetaminophen, COX-2 inhibitors, and useful nonsteroidal anti-inflammatory drugs. (continued)

Drug	Usual Dose for Adults ≥ 50 kg	Usual Dose for Adults < 50 kg[1]	Cost per Unit	Cost for 30 Days[2]	Comments[3]
Nabumetone (Relafen)	500–1000 mg once daily (max dose 2000 mg/d)		$1.30/500 mg; $1.53/750 mg	$91.80	May be less ulcerogenic than ibuprofen, but overall side effects may not be less.
Naproxen (Naprosyn, Anaprox, Aleve [OTC], others)	250–500 mg q6–8h	5 mg/kg q8h	$1.30/500 mg Rx; $0.08/220 mg OTC	$156.00; $7.20 OTC	Generally well tolerated. Lower doses for elderly.
Oxaprozin (Daypro, others)	600–1200 mg once daily		$1.51/600 mg	$90.60	Similar to ibuprofen. May cause rash, pruritus, photosensitivity.
Piroxicam (Feldene, others)	20 mg daily		$2.64/20 mg	$79.20	Not recommended in the elderly due to high adverse drug reaction rate. Single daily dose convenient. Long half-life. May cause higher rate of gastrointestinal bleeding and dermatologic side effects.
Sodium salicylate	325–650 mg q3–4h		$0.08/650 mg OTC	$19.20	
Sulindac (Clinoril, others)	150–200 mg twice daily		$0.98/150 mg; $1.21/200 mg	$58.80; $72.60	May cause higher rate of gastrointestinal bleeding. May have less nephrotoxic potential.
Tolmetin (Tolectin)	200–600 mg four times daily		$0.75/200 mg; $1.80/600 mg	$90.00; $216.00	Perhaps more side effects than others, including anaphylactic reactions.

[1]Acetaminophen and NSAID dosages for adults weighing less than 50 kg should be adjusted for weight.

[2]Average wholesale price (AWP, for AB-rated generic when available) for quantity listed. Source: *Red Book* Update, Vol. 27, No. 2, February 2008. AWP may not accurately represent the actual pharmacy cost because wide contractual variations exist among institutions.

[3]The adverse effects of headache, tinnitus, dizziness, confusion, rashes, anorexia, nausea, vomiting, gastrointestinal bleeding, diarrhea, nephrotoxicity, visual disturbances, etc, can occur with any of these drugs. Tolerance and efficacy are subject to great individual variations among patients. Note: All NSAIDs can increase serum lithium levels.

[4]Acetaminophen and celecoxib lack antiplatelet effects.

[5]May inhibit platelet aggregation for 1 week or more and may cause bleeding.

[6]May have minimal antiplatelet activity.

[7]Administration with antacids may decrease absorption.

[8]Has the same gastrointestinal toxicities as oral NSAIDs.

[9]Coombs-positive autoimmune hemolytic anemia has been associated with prolonged use.

OTC, over-the-counter; Rx, prescription; OA, osteoarthritis; RA, rheumatoid arthritis.

Adapted from Jacox AK et al: *Management of Cancer Pain: Quick Reference Guide for Clinicians No. 9.* AHCPR Publication No. 94–0593. Rockville, MD: Agency for Health Care Policy and Research, Public Health Service, U.S. Department of Health and Human Services. March 1994.

Table 2. Useful opioid agonist analgesics.

Drug	Approximate Equianalgesic Dose[1]		Usual Starting Dose				Potential Advantages	Potential Disadvantages
			Adults ≥ 50 kg Body Weight		Adults < 50 kg Body Weight[1]			
	Oral	Parenteral	Oral	Parenteral	Oral	Parenteral		
Opioid agonists[2]								
Fentanyl	Not available	0.1 (100 mcg) q1h	Not available	50–100 mcg IV/IM q1h or 0.5–1.5 mcg/kg/h IV infusion $0.86/100 mcg	Not available	0.5–1 mcg/kg IV q1–4h or 1–2 mcg/kg IV × 1, then 0.5–1 mcg/kg/h infusion	Possibly less neuroexcitatory effects, including in renal failure.	
Fentanyl oral transmucosal (Actiq); buccal (Fentora)		Not available	200 mcg transmucosal; 100 mcg buccal; $25.12/200 mcg transmucosal; $15.90/200 mcg buccal	Not available		Not available	For pain breaking through long-acting opioid medication.	Transmucosal and buccal formulations are not bioequivalent; there is higher bioavailability of buccal formulation.
Fentanyl transdermal	Not available orally, but clinician can use "2:1 Rule"[2] for transdermal formulation	Not available	Not available orally 12.5–25 mcg/h patch q72h; $14.42/25 mcg/h	Not available	12.5–25 mcg/h patch q72h	Not available	Stable medication blood levels.	Not for use in opioid-naive patients.
Hydromorphone[3] (Dilaudid)	7.5 mg q3–4h	1.5 mg q3–4h	1–4 mg q3–4h; $0.37/2 mg	1.5 mg q3–4h; $1.02/2 mg	0.06 mg/q3–4h	0.015 mg/kg q3–4h	Similar to morphine. Available in injectable high-potency preparation, rectal suppository.	Short duration.
Levorphanol (Levo-Dromoran)	4 mg q6–8h	2 mg q6–8h	4 mg q6–8h; $1.07/2 mg	2 mg q6–8h; $3.96/2 mg	0.04 mg/kg q6–8h	0.02 mg q6–8h	Longer-acting than morphine sulfate.	
Meperidine[4] (Demerol)	300 mg q2–3h; normal dose 50–150 mg q3–4h	100 mg q3h; $0.69/50 mg	Not recommended; $0.69/50 mg	100 mg q3h; $0.56/100 mg	Not recommended	0.75 mg/kg q2–3h	Use only when single dose, short duration analgesia is needed as for outpatient procedures like colonoscopy. Not recommended for chronic pain or for repeated dosing.	Short duration. Normeperidine metabolite accumulates in renal failure and other situations, and in high concentrations may cause irritability and seizures.
Methadone (Dolophine, others)	10–20 mg q6–8h (when converting from < 100 mg long-term daily oral morphine)	5–10 mg q6–8h	5–20 mg q6–8h; $0.15/10 mg	2.5–10 mg q6–8h; $4.10/10 mg	0.2 mg/kg q6–8h	0.1 mg/kg q6–8h	Somewhat longer-acting than morphine. Useful in cases of intolerance to morphine. May be particularly useful for neuropathic pain. Available in liquid formulation.	Analgesic duration shorter than plasma duration. May accumulate, requiring close monitoring during first weeks of treatment. Equianalgesic ratios vary with opioid dose.
Morphine[3] immediate release (Morphine sulfate tablets, Roxanol liquid)	30 mg q3–4h (repeat around-the-clock dosing); 60 mg q3–4h (single or intermittent dosing)	10 mg q3–4h	4–12 mg q3–4h; $0.18/15 mg	10 mg q3–4h; $1.20/10 mg	0.3 mg/kg q3–4h	0.1 mg/kg q3–4h	Standard of comparison; multiple dosage forms available.	No unique problems when compared with other opioids.

Drug	Approximate equianalgesic oral dose	Approximate equianalgesic parenteral dose	Recommended starting dose (adults): Oral	Recommended starting dose (adults): Parenteral	Recommended starting dose (children): Oral	Recommended starting dose (children): Parenteral	Comments
Morphine controlled-release[3] (MS Contin, Oramorph)	90–120 mg q12h	Not available	15–60 mg q12h; $1.69/30 mg	Not available	Not available	Not available	
Morphine extended release (Kadian, Avinza)	180–240 mg q24h	Not available	20–30 mg q24h; $3.24/30 mg	Not available	Not available	Not available	Once-daily dosing.
Oxycodone (Roxicodone, OxyIR)	20–30 mg q3–4h	Not available	5–10 mg q3–4h; $0.36/5 mg	Not available	0.2 mg/kg q3–4h	Not available	Similar to morphine.
Oxycodone controlled release (Oxycontin)	40 mg q12h	Not available	20–40 mg q12h; $3.31/20 mg				
Oxymorphone[5] injectable (Numorphan)	Not available	1 mg q3–4h	Not available	1 mg q3–4h; $3.13/1 mg			Active metabolite of oxycodone.
Oxymorphone[5] oral, immediate release (Opana)	10 mg q3–4h	Not available	5–10 mg q3–4h; $2.28/5 mg	Not available			New formulation with less known about equianalgesic dosing.
Oxymorphone[5] extended release (Opana ER)	30–40 mg q12h	Not available	15–30 mg q12h; $3.18/10 mg	Not available			New formulation with less known about equianalgesic dosing.
Combination Opioid-NSAID Preparations							
Codeine[6,7] (with aspirin or acetaminophen)[8]	180–200 mg q3–4h; normal dose, 15–60 mg q4–6h	130 mg q3–4h	60 mg q4–6h; $0.64/60 mg	60 mg q2h (IM/SC); $2.34/60 mg	0.5–1 mg/kg q3–4h	Not recommended	Similar to morphine. Closely monitor for efficacy as patients vary in their ability to convert the pro-drug codeine to morphine.
Hydrocodone[5] (in Loret, Lortab, Vicodin, others)[8]	30 mg q3–4h	Not available	10 mg q3–4h; $0.32/5 mg	Not available	0.2 mg/kg q3–4h	Not available	Combination with acetaminophen limits dosage titration.
Oxycodone[6] (in Percocet, Percodan, Tylox, others)[8]	30 mg q3–4h	Not available	10 mg q3–4h; $0.31/5 mg	Not available	0.2 mg/kg q3–4h	Not available	Similar to morphine. Combination with acetaminophen and aspirin limits dosage titration.

[1] Published tables vary in the suggested doses that are equianalgesic to morphine. Clinical response is the criterion that must be applied for each patient; titration to clinical efficacy is necessary. Because there is not complete cross-tolerance among these drugs, it is usually necessary to use a lower than equianalgesic dose initially when changing drugs and to retitrate to response.

[2] Dosing of transdermal fentanyl can be based on the "2:1 Rule"—the approximate equianalgesic dose of transdermal fentanyl in mcg/h is half the 24-hour mg dose of oral morphine.

[3] *Caution:* For morphine, hydromorphone, and oxymorphone, rectal administration is an alternative route for patients unable to take oral medications. Equianalgesic doses may differ from oral and parenteral doses. A short-acting opioid should normally be used for initial therapy.

[4] Not recommended for chronic pain. Doses listed are for brief therapy of acute pain only. Switch to another opioid for long-term therapy.

[5] *Caution:* Recommended doses do not apply for adult patients with renal or hepatic insufficiency or other conditions affecting drug metabolism.

[6] *Caution:* Doses of aspirin and acetaminophen in combination products must also be adjusted to the patient's body weight.

[7] *Caution:* Doses of codeine above 60 mg often are not appropriate because of diminishing incremental analgesia with increasing doses but continually increasing nausea, constipation, and other side effects.

[8] *Caution:* Monitor total acetaminophen dose carefully, including any OTC use. Total acetaminophen dose maximum 4 g/d. If liver impairment or heavy alcohol use, maximum is 2 g/d.

Note: Average wholesale price (AWP, generic when available) for quantity listed. Source: *Red Book Update*, Vol. 27, No. 2, February 2008. AWP may not accurately represent the actual pharmacy cost because wide contractual variations exist among institutions.

Adapted from Jacox AK et al. *Management of Cancer Pain: Quick Reference Guide for Clinicians No. 9.* AHCPR Publication No. 94-0593. Rockville, MD. Agency for Health Care Policy and Research, Public Health Service, U.S. Department of Health and Human Services. March 1994. (Erstad BL. A rational approach to the management of acute pain states.) Advanstar Communications, Inc. Reproduced in part, with permission, from Hosp Formul 1994;29(8 Part 2):586.

Table 3. α-Thalassemia syndromes.

α-Globin Genes	Syndrome	Hematocrit	MCV
4	Normal	Normal	
3	Silent carrier	Normal	
2	Thalassemia minor	28–40%	60–75 fL
1	Hemoglobin H disease	22–32%	60–70 fL
0	Hydrops fetalis		

MCV, mean cell volume.

Table 4. β-Thalassemia syndromes.

	β-Globin Genes	Hb A	Hb A$_2$	Hb F
Normal	Homozygous β	97–99%	1–3%	< 1%
Thalassemia major	Homozygous β^0	0%	4 10%	90–96%
Thalassemia major	Homozygous β$^+$	0–10%	4–10%	90–96%
Thalassemia intermedia	Homozygous β$^+$ (mild)	0–30%	0–10%	6–100%
Thalassemia minor	Heterozygous β^0	80–95%	4–8%	1–5%
	Heterozygous β$^+$	80–95%	4–8%	1–5%

Hb, hemoglobin.

Table 5. Laboratory diagnosis of von Willebrand disease.

Type		vWF Activity	vWF Antigen	FVIII	RIPA	Multimer Analysis
1		↓	↓	Nl or ↓	↓	Uniform ↓ in intensity
	A	↓↓	↓	↓	↓	Large and intermediate multimers decreased or absent
2	B	↓↓	↓	↓	↑	Large multimers decreased or absent
	M	↓	↓	↓	↓	Nl
	N	Nl	Nl	↓↓	Nl	Nl
3		↓↓↓	↓↓↓	↓↓↓	↓↓↓	Absent

RIPA, ristocetin-induced platelet aggregation, Nl, normal.

Table 6. Cancer screening recommendations for average-risk adults.

Test	ACS[1]	CTF[2]	USPSTF[3]
Breast self-examination (BSE)	An option for women over age 20.	Fair evidence that BSE *should not* be used.	Insufficient evidence to recommend for or against.
Clinical breast examination	Every 3 years age 20–40 and annually thereafter.	Good evidence for annual screening women aged 50–69 by clinical examination and mammography.	Insufficient evidence to recommend for or against.
Mammography	Annually age 40 and older.	Current evidence does not support the recommendation that screening mammography be included in or excluded from the periodic health examination of women aged 40–49.	Recommended every 1–2 years for women aged 40 and over (B).
Papanicolaou test	Annually beginning within 3 years after first vaginal intercourse or no later than age 21. Screening may be done every 2 years with the liquid-based Pap test. After age 30, women with three normal tests may be screened every 2–3 years or every 3 years by Pap test plus the HPV DNA test. Women may choose to stop screening after age 70 if they have had three normal (and no abnormal) results within the last 10 years.	Annually at age of first intercourse or by age 18; can move to every-2-year screening after two normal results to age 69.	Every 3 years beginning at onset of sexual activity or age 21 (A). Recommends against routinely screening women older than age 65 if they have had adequate recent screening with normal Pap tests and are not otherwise at high risk for cervical cancer (D).
Annual stool test for occult blood[4] or fecal immunochemical test (FIT) Sigmoidoscopy (every 5 years) Double-contrast barium enema (every 5 years) Colonoscopy (every 10 years)	Screening recommended, with the combination of fecal occult blood test or fecal immunochemical test (FIT) and sigmoidoscopy preferred over stool test or sigmoidoscopy alone. Double-contrast barium enema and colonoscopy also considered reasonable alternatives.	Good evidence for screening every 1–2 years over age 50. Fair evidence for screening over age 50 (insufficient evidence about combining stool test and sigmoidoscopy). Not addressed. Insufficient evidence for or against use in screening.	Screening strongly recommended (A), but insufficient evidence to determine best test.
Prostate-specific antigen (PSA) blood test Digital rectal examination (DRE)	PSA and DRE should be offered annually to men age 50 and older who have at least a 10-year life expectancy. Men at high risk (African-American men and men with a strong family history) should begin at age 45. Information should be provided to men about the benefits and risks, and they should be allowed to participate in the decision. Men without a clear preference should be screened.	Fair evidence *against* including in routine care. Insufficient evidence for or against including in routine care.	Insufficient evidence to recommend for or against. Insufficient evidence to recommend for or against.
Cancer-related checkup	For people aged 20 or older having periodic health exams, a cancer-related checkup should include counseling and perhaps oral cavity, thyroid, lymph node, or testicular examinations.	Not assessed.	Not assessed.

[1]American Cancer Society recommendations, available at http://www.cancer.org.
[2]Canadian Task Force on Preventive Health Care recommendations available at http://www.ctfphc.org.
[3]United States Preventive Services Task Force recommendations available at http://www.ahrq.gov.
Recommendation A: The USPSTF strongly recommends that clinicians routinely provide the service to eligible patients. (The USPSTF found good evidence that the service improves important health outcomes and concludes that benefits substantially outweigh harms.)
Recommendation B: The USPSTF recommends that clinicians routinely provide the service to eligible patients. (The USPSTF found at least fair evidence that the service improves important health outcomes and concludes that benefits substantially outweigh harms.)
Recommendation D: The USPSTF recommends against routinely providing the service to asymptomatic patients. (The USPSTF found at least fair evidence that the service is ineffective or that harms outweigh benefits.)
[4]Home test with three samples.

Table 7. Treatment choices for cancers responsive to systemic agents.

Diagnosis	Current Treatment of Choice	Other Valuable Agents and Procedures
Acute lymphocytic leukemia	**Induction:** combination chemotherapy. *Adults:* Vincristine, prednisone, daunorubicin, and asparaginase (DVPasp). **Consolidation:** multiagent alternating chemotherapy. Allogeneic bone marrow transplant for young adults or high-risk disease or second remission. Central nervous system prophylaxis with intrathecal methotrexate with or without whole brain radiation. **Remission maintenance:** methotrexate, thioguanine.	Doxorubicin, cytarabine, cyclophosphamide, etoposide, teniposide, clofarabine, allopurinol,[1] autologous bone marrow transplantation T cell disease: Nelarabine (relapsed or refractory)
Acute myelocytic and myelomonocytic leukemia	**Induction:** combination chemotherapy with cytarabine and an anthracycline (daunorubicin, idarubicin). Tretinoin with idarubicin for acute promyelocytic leukemia. **Consolidation:** high-dose cytarabine. Autologous (with or without purging) or allogeneic bone marrow transplantation for high-risk disease or second remission.	Gemtuzumab ozogamicin (Mylotarg), mitoxantrone, idarubicin, etoposide, mercaptopurine, thioguanine, azacitidine,[2] amsacrine,[2] methotrexate, doxorubicin, tretinoin, allopurinol,[1] leukapheresis, prednisone, arsenic trioxide for acute promyelocytic leukemia
Chronic myelocytic leukemia	Imatinib mesylate (Gleevec), dasatinib, nilotinib. Allogeneic bone marrow transplantation for imatinib-resistant or high-risk disease.	Hydroxyurea, busulfan, cytarabine, autologous bone marrow transplantation,[2] allopurinol[1]
Chronic lymphocytic leukemia	Fludarabine, chlorambucil, and prednisone (if treatment is indicated), rituximab with fludarabine or cyclophosphamide. Bendamustine. Second-line therapy: alemtuzumab (Campath-1H).	Rituximab, vincristine, cyclophosphamide, doxorubicin, chlorambucil, cladribine (2-chlorodeoxyadenosine; CdA), allogeneic bone marrow transplantation, androgens,[2] allopurinol[1]
Hairy cell leukemia	Cladribine (2-chlorodeoxyadenosine; CdA).	Pentostatin (deoxycoformycin), interferon-α
Hodgkin disease (stages III and IV)	**Combination chemotherapy:** doxorubicin (Adriamycin), bleomycin, vinblastine, dacarbazine (ABVD) or alternative combination therapy without mechlorethamine. Autologous bone marrow transplantation for high-risk patients or relapsed disease.	Mechlorethamine, vincristine, prednisone, procarbazine (MOPP); carmustine, lomustine, etoposide, thiotepa, autologous bone marrow transplantation
Non-Hodgkin lymphoma (intermediate to high grade)	**Combination therapy:** depending on histologic classification but usually including cyclophosphamide, vincristine, doxorubicin, and prednisone (CHOP) with or without rituximab in older patients. Autologous bone marrow transplantation in high-risk first remission or first relapse.	Bleomycin, methotrexate, etoposide, chlorambucil, fludarabine, lomustine, carmustine, cytarabine, thiotepa, amsacrine, mitoxantrone, allogeneic bone marrow transplantation
Non-Hodgkin lymphoma (low grade)	Fludarabine, rituximab, if CD20 positive; ibritumomab tiuxetan or ^{131}I tositumomab for relapsed or refractory disease.	**Combination chemotherapy:** cyclophosphamide, prednisone, doxorubicin, vincristine; chlorambucil, autologous or allogeneic transplantation
Cutaneous T cell lymphoma (mycosis fungoides)	Topical carmustine, electron beam radiotherapy, photochemotherapy, targretin, denileukin diftitox (ONTAK) or vorinostat for refractory disease.	Interferon, denileukin diftitox (ONTAK), vorinostat, combination chemotherapy, targretin
Multiple myeloma	**Combination chemotherapy:** vincristine, doxorubicin, dexamethasone; melphalan and prednisone; melphalan, cyclophosphamide, carmustine, vincristine, doxorubicin, prednisone, thalidomide. Autologous transplantation in first complete or partial remission, miniallogeneic transplant for poor-prognosis disease. Bortezomib or lenalidomide or thalidomide with dexamethasone for relapsed or refractory disease.	Thalidomide, lenalidomide, bortezomib, etoposide, cytarabine, dexamethasone, autologous bone marrow transplantation
Waldenström macroglobulinemia	Fludarabine or chlorambucil or cyclophosphamide, vincristine, prednisone. Allogeneic bone marrow transplantation for high-risk young patients.	Cladribine, etoposide, interferon-α, doxorubicin, dexamethasone, plasmapheresis, autologous bone marrow transplantation
Polycythemia vera, essential thrombocytosis	Hydroxyurea, phlebotomy for polycythemia. Hydroxyrea or anagrelide for thrombocytosis.	Busulfan, chlorambucil, cyclophosphamide, interferon-α, radiophosphorus [32]P
Carcinoma of the lung		
Small cell	**Combination chemotherapy:** cisplatin and etoposide. Palliative radiation therapy. Topotecan for relapsed disease.	Cyclophosphamide, doxorubicin, vincristine
Non–small cell[3]	**Localized disease:** cisplatin or carboplatin, docetaxel. **Advanced disease:** cisplatin or carboplatin, docetaxel, gemcitabine, erlotinib, etoposide, vinblastine, vinorelbine.	Doxorubicin, etoposide, pemetrexed, mitomycin, ifosfamide, paclitaxel, capecitabine, radiation therapy
Malignant pleural mesothelioma	Pemetrexed with cisplatin.	Doxorubicin, radiation, pleurectomy
Carcinoma of the head and neck[3]	**Combination chemotherapy:** cisplatin and fluorouracil, paclitaxel, cetuximab with radiation (locally advanced) or alone (second-line metastatic).	Methotrexate, bleomycin, hydroxyurea, doxorubicin, vinblastine
Carcinoma of the esophagus[3]	**Combination chemotherapy:** fluorouracil, cisplatin, mitomycin.	Methotrexate, bleomycin, doxorubicin, mitomycin
Carcinoma of the stomach and pancreas[3]	**Stomach:** etoposide, leucovorin,[1] fluorouracil (ELF). **Pancreas:** fluorouracil or ELF, gemcitabine with or without erlotinib.	Carmustine, mitomycin, lomustine, doxorubicin, gemcitabine, methotrexate, cisplatin, combinations for stomach

(continued)

Table 7. Treatment choices for cancers responsive to systemic agents. (continued)

Diagnosis	Current Treatment of Choice	Other Valuable Agents and Procedures
Carcinoma of the colon and rectum[3]	**Colon:** oxaliplatin with infusional 5-fluorouracil (5-FU)/leucovorin (FOLFOX4) (adjuvant); bevacizumab with irinotecan, 5-FU/leucovorin with irinotecan, cetuximab, panitumumab, capecitabine (advanced). **Rectum:** fluorouracil with radiation therapy (adjuvant), advanced similar to colon cancer.	Methotrexate, mitomycin, carmustine, cisplatin, floxuridine
Carcinoma of the kidney[3]	Sunitinib, sorafenib, temsirolimus; consider miniallogeneic transplantation.[2]	Floxuridine, vinblastine, interleukin-2 (IL-2), interferon-α, progestins, infusional fluorodeoxyuridine, fluorouracil
Carcinoma of the bladder[3]	Intravesical bacillus Calmette-Guérin (BCG) or thiotepa. **Combination chemotherapy:** methotrexate, vinblastine, doxorubicin (Adriamycin), cisplatin (M-VAC) or CMV alone.	Cyclophosphamide, fluorouracil, intravesical valrubicin, gemcitabine, cisplatin
Carcinoma of the testis[3]	**Combination chemotherapy:** etoposide and cisplatin. Autologous bone marrow transplantation for high-risk or relapsed disease.	Bleomycin, vinblastine, ifosfamide, mesna,[1] carmustine, carboplatin
Carcinoma of the prostate[3]	Estrogens or luteinizing hormone-releasing hormone analog (leuprolide, goserelin, or triptorelin) plus an antiandrogen (flutamide).	Ketoconazole, doxorubicin, aminoglutethimide, progestins, cyclophosphamide, cisplatin, vinblastine, etoposide, suramin[2]; PC-SPES; estramustine phosphate
Carcinoma of the uterus[3]	Progestins or tamoxifen.	Doxorubicin, cisplatin, fluorouracil, ifosfamide
Carcinoma of the ovary[3]	**Combination chemotherapy:** paclitaxel and cisplatin or carboplatin. Intraperitoneal chemotherapy with cisplatin and paclitaxel combined with intravenous paclitaxel.[1]	Docetaxel, doxorubicin, topotecan, cyclophosphamide, etoposide, liposomal doxorubicin
Carcinoma of the cervix[3]	**Combination chemotherapy:** methotrexate, doxorubicin, cisplatin, and vinblastine; or mitomycin, bleomycin, vincristine, and cisplatin with radiation therapy.	Carboplatin, ifosfamide, lomustine
Carcinoma of the breast[3]	**Combination chemotherapy:** a variety of regimens are used for adjuvant therapy. For node-positive disease—combinations including doxorubicin or epirubicin and at least one of the following additional drugs: 5-FU, cyclophosphamide, docetaxel, paclitaxel. For node-negative disease—a combination of the drugs listed above or cyclophosphamide, methotrexate, and 5-FU (CMF), or docetaxel and cyclophosphamide. For HER2/neu-positive disease, anthracycline-based chemotherapy followed by trastuzumab with paclitaxel or docetaxel or a combination of docetaxel, carboplatin and trastuzumab. For estrogen- or progesterone-positive disease, tamoxifen with or without ovarian suppression of estrogen production (premenopausal women) or anastrozole/letrozole/exemestane following or instead of tamoxifen (postmenopausal women) is given for 5 years regardless of the use of adjuvant chemotherapy.	Trastuzumab (Herceptin) with chemotherapy, lapatinib in combination with capecitabine (HER2+), bevacizumab in combination with paclitaxel or docetaxel, paclitaxel, docetaxel, nab-paclitaxel, epirubicin, mitoxantrone, pegylated doxorubicin, capecitabine, gemcitabine, ixabepilone alone or in combination with capecitabine, vinorelbine, thiotepa, vincristine, vinblastine, carboplatin or cisplatin, anastrozole, letrozole, exemestane, fulvestrant, toremifine, progestins, goserelin, leuprolide, triptorelin
Choriocarcinoma (trophoblastic neoplasms)[3]	Methotrexate or dactinomycin (or both) plus chlorambucil.	Vinblastine, cisplatin, mercaptopurine, doxorubicin, bleomycin, etoposide
Carcinoma of the thyroid gland[3]	Radioiodine (^{131}I).	Doxorubicin, cisplatin, bleomycin, melphalan
Carcinoma of the adrenal gland[3]	Mitotane.	Doxorubicin, suramin[2]
Carcinoid[3]	Fluorouracil plus streptozocin with or without interferon-α.	Doxorubicin, cyclophosphamide, octreotide, cyproheptadine,[1] methysergide[1]
Osteogenic sarcoma[3]	High-dose methotrexate, doxorubicin, vincristine.	Cyclophosphamide, ifosfamide, bleomycin, dacarbazine, cisplatin, dactinomycin
Soft tissue sarcoma[3]	Doxorubicin, dacarbazine.	Ifosfamide, cyclosphosphamide, etoposide, cisplatin, high-dose methotrexate, vincristine
Melanoma[3]	Dacarbazine, interferon-α, interleukin-2.	Carmustine, lomustine, melphalan, thiotepa, cisplatin, paclitaxel, tamoxifen, vincristine, vaccine therapy (Melacine)[2]
Kaposi sarcoma	Doxorubicin, vincristine alternating with vinblastine or vincristine alone. Palliative radiation therapy.	Interferon-α bleomycin, etoposide, doxorubicin
Neuroblastoma[3]	**Combination chemotherapy:** variations of cyclophosphamide, cisplatin, vincristine, doxorubicin, dacarbazine.	Melphalan, ifosfamide, autologous or allogeneic bone marrow transplantation
Hepatocellular carcinoma	Sunitinib, surgical resection.	

[1]Supportive agent; not oncolytic.

[2]Investigational agent or procedure. Treatment is available through qualified investigators and centers authorized by the National Cancer Institute and Cooperative Oncology Groups.

[3]These tumors are generally managed initially with surgery with or without radiation therapy and with or without adjuvant chemotherapy. For metastatic disease, the role of palliative radiation therapy is as important as that of chemotherapy.

Table 8. Single-agent dosage and toxicity of anticancer drugs.[1]

Drug	Dosage	Acute Toxicity	Delayed Toxicity
Alkylating agents			
Mechlorethamine	6–10 mg/m² intravenously every 3 weeks	Severe vesicant; severe nausea and vomiting	Moderate suppression of blood counts. Melphalan effect may be delayed 4–6 weeks. High doses produce severe bone marrow suppression with leukopenia, thrombocytopenia, and bleeding. Alopecia and hemorrhagic cystitis occur with cyclophosphamide, while busulfan can cause hyperpigmentation, pulmonary fibrosis, and weakness (see text). Ifosfamide is always given with mesna to prevent cystitis. Acute leukemia may develop in 5–10% of patients receiving prolonged therapy with melphalan, mechlorethamine, or chlorambucil; all alkylators probably increase the risk of secondary malignancies with prolonged use. Most cause either temporary or permanent aspermia or amenorrhea.
Chlorambucil	0.1–0.2 mg/kg/d orally (6–12 mg/d) or 0.4 mg/kg pulse every 4 weeks	None	
Cyclophosphamide	100 mg/m²/d orally for 14 days; 400 mg/m² orally for 5 days; 1–1.5 g/m² intravenously every 3–4 weeks	Nausea and vomiting with higher doses	
Melphalan	0.25 mg/kg/d orally for 4 days every 6 weeks	None	
Busulfan	2–8 mg/d orally; 150–250 mg/course	None	
Estramustine	14 mg/kg orally in three or four divided doses	Nausea, vomiting, diarrhea	Thrombosis, thrombocytopenia, hypertension, gynecomastia, glucose intolerance, edema.
Carmustine (BCNU)	200 mg/m² intravenously every 6 weeks	Local irritant	Prolonged leukopenia and thrombocytopenia. Rarely hepatitis. Acute leukemia has been observed to occur in some patients receiving nitrosoureas. Nitrosoureas can cause delayed pulmonary fibrosis with prolonged use.
Lomustine (CCNU)	100–130 mg orally every 6–8 weeks	Nausea and vomiting	
Procarbazine	100 mg/m²/d orally for 14 days every 4 weeks	Nausea and vomiting	Bone marrow suppression, mental suppression, MAO inhibition, disulfiram-like effect.
Dacarbazine	250 mg/m²/d intravenously for 5 days every 3 weeks; 1500 mg/m² intravenously as single dose	Severe nausea and vomiting; anorexia	Bone marrow suppression; flu-like syndrome.
Cisplatin	50–100 mg/m² intravenously every 3 weeks; 20 mg/m² intravenously for 5 days every 4 weeks	Severe nausea and vomiting	Nephrotoxicity, mild otic and bone marrow toxicity, neurotoxicity.
Carboplatin	360 mg/m² intravenously every 4 weeks	Severe nausea and vomiting	Bone marrow suppression, prolonged anemia; same as cisplatin but milder.
Oxaliplatin	85 mg/m² intravenously in 250–500 mL D₅W over 2 hours on day 1, with infusional 5-FU/leucovorin on days 1 and 2 every 2 weeks (FOLFOX4)	Nausea, vomiting, diarrhea, fatigue, rare anaphylactic reactions	Peripheral neuropathy, cytopenias, pulmonary toxicity (rare).
Bendamustine (Treanda)	100 mg/m² intravenously on days 1 and 2 every 28 days	Fever, nausea, vomiting, hypersensitivity reaction	Myelosuppression, infection.
Structural analogs or antimetabolites			
Methotrexate	2.5–5 mg/d orally; 20–25 mg intramuscularly twice weekly; high-dose: 500–1000 mg/m² every 2–3 weeks; 12–15 mg intrathecally every week for 4–6 doses	None	Bone marrow suppression, oral and gastrointestinal ulceration, acute renal failure; hepatotoxicity, rash, increased toxicity when effusions are present. Note: Citrovorum factor (leucovorin) rescue for doses over 100 mg/m².
Pemetrexed (Alimta)	500 mg/m² intravenously every 3 weeks; given with cisplatin or alone; requires folate and vitamin B₁₂ supplementation	Skin rash, cytopenias, decreased clearance of agent if given with NSAIDs, nausea, diarrhea, mucositis, hypersensitivity reactions	Cytopenias, rash, neuropathy.
Mercaptopurine	2.5 mg/kg/d orally; 100 mg/m²/d orally for 5 days for induction	None	Well tolerated. Larger doses cause bone marrow suppression.
Thioguanine	2 mg/kg/d orally; 100 mg/m²/d intravenously for 7 days for induction	Mild nausea, diarrhea	Well tolerated. Larger doses cause bone marrow suppression.
Fluorouracil	15 mg/kg/d intravenously for 3–5 days every 3 weeks; 15 mg/kg weekly as tolerated; 500–1000 mg/m² intravenously every 4 weeks	None	Nausea, diarrhea, oral and gastrointestinal ulceration, bone marrow suppression, dacrocystitis.
Capecitabine	2500 mg/m² orally twice daily on days 1–14 every 3 weeks	Nausea, diarrhea	Hand and foot syndrome, mucositis.

(continued)

Table 8. Single-agent dosage and toxicity of anticancer drugs.[1] (continued)

Drug	Dosage	Acute Toxicity	Delayed Toxicity
Cytarabine	100–200 mg/m^2/d for 5–10 days by continuous intravenous infusion; 2–3 g/m^2 intravenously every 12 hours for 3–7 days; 20 mg/m^2 subcutaneously daily in divided doses	High-dose: nausea, vomiting, diarrhea, anorexia	Nausea and vomiting; cystitis; severe bone marrow suppression; megaloblastosis; CNS toxicity with high-dose cytarabine.
Temozolomide	150 mg/m^2 orally for 5 days; repeat every 4 weeks	Headache, nausea, vomiting	Unknown.
Clofarabine	52 mg/m^2 intravenously daily for 5 days every 2–6 weeks	Nausea, vomiting	Bone marrow suppression, hepatobiliary and renal toxicity, capillary leak syndrome.
Androgens and androgen antagonists			
Testosterone propionate	100 mg intramuscularly three times weekly	None	Fluid retention, masculinization, leg cramps. Cholestatic jaundice in some patients receiving fluoxymesterone.
Fluoxymesterone	20–40 mg/d orally	None	
Flutamide	250 mg three times a day orally	None	Gynecomastia, hot flushes, decreased libido, mild gastrointestinal side effects, hepatotoxicity.
Bicalutamide	50 mg/d orally		
Nilutamide	300 mg/d orally for 30 days, then 150 mg/d		
Ethinyl estradiol	3 mg/d orally	None	Fluid retention, feminization, uterine bleeding, exacerbation of cardiovascular disease, painful gynecomastia, thromboembolic disease.
Selective estrogen receptor modulators			
Tamoxifen	20 mg/d orally	Hot flushes, joint aching, vaginal discharge or dryness, vaginal bleeding, reduced libido, acne, nausea, transient flare of bone pain (metastatic disease only)	Thromboembolic disease, anovulation, endometrial cancer, endometrial polyps, ovarian cysts, cataracts, weight gain.
Toremifene	60 mg/d orally		
Aromatase inhibitors			
Anastrozole	1 mg/d orally	Hot flushes, joint and muscle aching, joint stiffness, vaginal dryness, reduced libido	Accelerated bone mineral density loss, possible exacerbation of hyperlipidemia.
Letrozole	2.5 mg/d orally		
Exemestane	25 mg/d orally		
Pure estrogen receptor antagonist			
Fulvestrant	250 mg intramuscularly once a month	Transient injection site reactions, hot flushes	Nausea, vomiting, constipation, diarrhea, abdominal pain, headache, back pain.
Progestins			
Megestrol acetate	40 mg orally four times daily	Hot flushes	Fluid retention; rare thrombosis, weight gain.
Medroxyprogesterone	100–200 mg/d orally; 200–600 mg orally twice weekly	None	
GnRH analogs			
Leuprolide	7.5 mg intramuscularly (depot) once a month or 22.5 mg every 3 months as depot injection	Local irritation, transient flare of symptoms	Hot flushes, decreased libido, impotence, gynecomastia, mild gastrointestinal side effects, nausea, diarrhea, fatigue.
Goserelin acetate	3.6 mg subcutaneously monthly or 10.8 mg every 3 months as depot injection		
Triptorelin pamoate	3.75 mg intramuscularly once a month (a 3-month depot formulation also exists)		
Adrenocorticosteroids			
Prednisone	20–100 mg/d orally or 50–100 mg every other day orally with systemic chemotherapy	Alteration in mood	Fluid retention, hypertension, diabetes, increased susceptibility to infection, "moon facies," osteoporosis, electrolyte abnormalities, gastritis.
Dexamethasone	5–10 mg orally daily or twice daily		
Ketoconazole	400 mg orally three times daily	Acute nausea	Gynecomastia, hepatotoxicity.

(continued)

Table 8. Single-agent dosage and toxicity of anticancer drugs.[1] (continued)

Drug	Dosage	Acute Toxicity	Delayed Toxicity
Biologic response modifiers			
Interferon-α-2a Interferon-α-2b	3–5 million units subcutaneously three times weekly or daily	Fever, chills, fatigue, anorexia	General malaise, weight loss, confusion, hypothyroidism, retinopathy, autoimmune disease.
Aldesleukin (IL-2)	600,000 units/kg intravenously over 15 minutes every 8 hours for 14 doses, repeated after 9-day rest period. Some doses may be withheld or interrupted because of toxicity. **Caution:** High doses must be administered in an ICU setting by experienced personnel.	Hypotension, fever, chills, rigors, diarrhea, nausea, vomiting, pruritus; liver, kidney, and CNS toxicity; capillary leak (primarily at high doses), pruritic skin rash, infections (can be severe)	Hypoglycemia, anemia.
Peptide hormone inhibitor			
Octreotide acetate	100–600 mcg/d subcutaneously in two divided doses	Local irritant; nausea and vomiting	Diarrhea, abdominal pain, hypoglycemia.
Natural products and miscellaneous agents			
Vinblastine	0.1–0.2 mg/kg or 6 mg/m^2 intravenously weekly	Mild nausea and vomiting; severe vesicant	Alopecia, peripheral neuropathy, bone marrow suppression, constipation, SIADH, areflexia.
Vincristine	1.5 mg/m^2 (maximum: 2 mg weekly)	Severe vesicant	Areflexia, muscle weakness, peripheral neuropathy, paralytic ileus, alopecia (see text), SIADH.
Vinorelbine	25–30 mg/m^2 intravenously weekly	Mild nausea and vomiting, fatigue, severe vesicant	Granulocytopenia, constipation, peripheral neuropathy, alopecia.
Paclitaxel (Taxol)	175 mg/m^2 over 3 hours every 2 to 3 weeks or 80 mg/m^2 over 1 hour every week	Hypersensitivity reaction (premedicate with diphenhydramine and dexamethasone), mild nausea and vomiting	Peripheral neuropathy, bone marrow suppression, sensory neuropathy fluid retention, myalgia/arthralgias, asthenia, alopecia.
Nab-paclitaxel (Abraxane)	260 mg/m^2 intravenously every 3 weeks		
Docetaxel (Taxotere)	60–100 mg/m^2 intravenously every 3 weeks		
Ixabepilone	40 mg/m^2 intravenously every 3 weeks		
Dactinomycin	0.04 mg/kg intravenously weekly	Nausea and vomiting; severe vesicant	Alopecia, stomatitis, diarrhea, bone marrow suppression.
Daunorubicin	30–60 mg/m^2 daily intravenously for 3 days, or 30–60 mg/m^2 intravenously weekly		Alopecia, stomatitis, bone marrow suppression, late cardiotoxicity. Risk of cardiotoxicity increases with radiation, cyclophosphamide.
Idarubicin	12 mg/m^2 daily intravenously for 3 days		
Doxorubicin	60 mg/m^2 intravenously every 3 weeks to a maximum total dose of 550 mg/m^2		
Epirubicin	60–100 mg/m^2 intravenously every 3 weeks		
Liposomal doxorubicin (Doxil)	35–40 mg/m^2 intravenously every 4 weeks	Mild nausea	Hand and foot syndrome; alopecia, stomatitis, and bone marrow suppression uncommon.
Liposomal daunorubicin (DaunoXome)	40 mg/m^2 intravenously every 2 weeks		
Etoposide	100 mg/m^2/d intravenously for 5 days or 50–150 mg/d orally	Nausea and vomiting; occasionally hypotension	Alopecia, bone marrow suppression, secondary leukemia.
Mitomycin	10–20 mg/m^2 every 6–8 weeks	Severe vesicant; nausea	Prolonged bone marrow suppression, rare hemolytic-uremic syndrome.
Mitoxantrone	12–15 mg/m^2/d intravenously for 3 days with cytarabine; 8–12 mg/m^2 intravenously every 3 weeks	Mild nausea and vomiting	Alopecia, mild mucositis, bone marrow suppression.
Bleomycin	Up to 15 units/m^2 intramuscularly, intravenously, or subcutaneously twice weekly to a total dose of 200 units/m^2	Allergic reactions, fever, hypotension	Fever, dermatitis, pulmonary fibrosis.
Hydroxyurea	500–1500 mg/d orally	Mild nausea and vomiting	Hyperpigmentation, bone marrow suppression.
Mitotane	6–12 g/d orally	Nausea and vomiting	Dermatitis, diarrhea, mental suppression, muscle tremors.

(continued)

Table 8. Single-agent dosage and toxicity of anticancer drugs.[1] (continued)

Drug	Dosage	Acute Toxicity	Delayed Toxicity
Fludarabine	25 mg/m^2/d intravenously for 5 days every 4 weeks	Nausea and vomiting	Bone marrow suppression, diarrhea, mild hepatotoxicity, immune suppression.
Cladribine (CdA)	0.09 mg/kg/d by continuous intravenous infusion for 7 days	Mild nausea, rash, fatigue	Bone marrow suppression, fever, immune suppression.
Topotecan	1.5 mg/m^2 intravenously daily for 5 days every 3 weeks	Nausea, vomiting, diarrhea, headache, dyspnea	Alopecia, bone marrow suppression.
Gemcitabine	1000 mg/m^2 every week up to 7 weeks, then 1 week off, then weekly for 3 of 4 weeks	Nausea, vomiting, diarrhea, fever, dyspnea	Bone marrow suppression, rash, fluid retention, mouth sores, flu-like symptoms, paresthesias.
Irinotecan	125 mg/m^2 weekly for 4 weeks, then a 2-week rest, then repeat; given with bevacizumab, 5-FU, and leucovorin Dose reduced for homozygous polymorphism in the *UGT1A1* gene	Flushing, salivation, lacrimation, bradycardia, abdominal cramps, diarrhea	Bone marrow suppression, diarrhea.
Azacitidine	75 mg/m^2 subcutaneously daily for 7 days, repeat every 4 weeks. May increase to 100 mg/m^2 after two cycles if no response	Nausea, fever, injection site infection	Neutropenia, thrombocytopenia, fatigue, anorexia, liver and renal toxicity (rare).
Novel therapeutic agents			
Imatinib mesylate (Gleevec)	400–600 mg/d orally	Mild nausea	Myalgias, edema, bone marrow suppression, abnormal liver function tests.
Dasatinib (Sprycel)	100 mg/d orally or 70 mg twice a day	Fever, diarrhea, musculoskeletal pain, headache	Myelosuppression, bleeding, fluid retention, dyspnea.
Nilotinib (Tasigna)	400 mg twice a day orally	Rash, itching, nausea, headache, constipation, diarrhea, vomiting	Fatigue, thrombocytopenia, neutropenia, rash.
Erlotinib (Tarceva)	150 mg by mouth daily	Mild nausea	Rash, diarrhea, anorexia, fatigue, transaminitis, interstitial lung disease (rare).
Alemtuzumab (Campath-1H)	30 mg three times a week by subcutaneous injection for up to 12 weeks. (Use dose escalation to reduce infusion-related events.)	Severe infusion-related events, injection site irritation	Infections, short-term bone marrow suppression, autoimmune hemolytic anemia.
Gemtuzumab ozogamicin (Mylotarg)	9 mg/m^2 for two doses given 14 days apart	Infusion-related events	Profound bone marrow suppression.
Tretinoin	45 mg/m^2 by mouth daily until remission or for 90 days	Retinoic acid syndrome (fever, dyspnea, pleural or pericardial effusion) must be treated emergently with dexamethasone	Headache, dry skin, rash, flushing.
Arsenic trioxide	**Induction:** 0.15 mg/kg intravenously daily until remission; maximum 60 doses	Same as tretinoin	Nausea, vomiting, diarrhea, edema.
	Consolidation: 0.15 mg/kg intravenously daily for 25 doses	Retinoic acid syndrome (fever, dyspnea, pleural or pericardial effusion) must be treated emergently with dexamethasone	Headache, dry skin, rash, flushing.
Trastuzumab (Herceptin) Lapatinib	**Load:** 4 mg/kg intravenously followed by 2 mg/kg weekly	Low-grade fever, chills, fatigue, constitutional symptoms with first infusion	Cardiac toxicity, especially when given with anthracyclines.
	1250 mg by mouth daily in combination with capecitabine, 2000 mg/m^2 in two divided doses daily. Capecitabine is given on a 2 weeks on, 1 week off schedule	Rash, diarrhea, skin toxicity, mild bone marrow suppression	None known.
Denileukin diftitox (ONTAK)	9–10 mcg/kg/d intravenously for 5 days every 21 days	Hypersensitivity type reactions with first infusion	Vascular leak syndrome, low albumin, increased risk of infections, diarrhea, rash.
Rituximab	375 mg/m^2 intravenously weekly for 4–8 doses	Hypersensitivity type reactions with first infusion; fever, tumor lysis syndrome (can be life-threatening)	Mild cytopenias, rare red cell aplasia or aplastic anemia, severe mucocutaneous reactions.
Ibritumomab tiuxetan (Zevalin)	0.3–0.4 mCi/kg (not to exceed 32 mCi); dosing must follow rituximab	Rituximab infusion reaction symptom complex	Prolonged and severe myelosuppression, nausea, vomiting, abdominal pain, arthralgias.

(continued)

Table 8. Single-agent dosage and toxicity of anticancer drugs.[1] (continued)

Drug	Dosage	Acute Toxicity	Delayed Toxicity
Bortezomib (Velcade)	1.3 mg/m² by intravenous bolus twice a week for 2 weeks followed by a 10-day rest. Repeat every 3 weeks.	Low-grade nausea, diarrhea, low-grade fever, weakness	Peripheral neuropathy, thrombocytopenia, edema.
[131]I Tositumomab (Bexxar)	[131]I Tositumomab must be given with tositumomab (T). **Dosimetric step:** 450 mg T over 60 minutes followed by [131]I T containing 35 mg T with 5 mCi [131]I. **Therapeutic step:** Calculated to deliver 75 cGy total body irradiation with 35 mg T.	Hypersensitivity reactions	Prolonged and severe myelosuppression, nausea, vomiting, abdominal pains, arthralgias.
Targretin	300 mg/m²/d orally	Nausea	Hyperlipidemia, dry mouth, dry skin, constipation, leukopenia, edema.
Bevacizumab (Avastin)	5 mg/kg intravenously every 2 weeks; given with irinotecan, 5-FU, and leucovorin (IFL), 10 mg/kg every 2 weeks given with paclitaxel.	Asthenia, hypertension, diarrhea, hypersensitivity reactions	Proteinuria, hypertension, thromboembolism, gastrointestinal perforation, wound dehiscence, hemoptysis (lung cancer), reversible posterior leukoencephalopathy syndrome (RPLS), tracheoesophageal fistula.
Cetuximab (Erbitux)	400 mg/m² intravenous loading dose, then 250 mg/m² once a week; given alone or with irinotecan; requires special tubing	Rare severe infusion reactions, diarrhea, nausea, abdominal pain	Interstitial lung disease, acneiform rash, sun sensitivity, fatigue.
Panitumumab (Vectibix)	6 mg/kg every 14 days	Nausea, diarrhea, constipation, mucositis, abdominal pain	Sun sensitivity, acneiform rash and other dermatologic reactions including abscesses, mouth pain and mucositis, ocular toxicities, hypomagnesemia, fatigue.
Sunitinib (Sutent)	50 mg/d orally for 4 weeks, then 2 weeks off treatment. Adjust dose for patient tolerability	Fatigue, diarrhea, anorexia, nausea, mucositis, rash, skin discoloration	Bone marrow suppression, fall in left ventricular ejection fraction.
Sorafenib (Nexavar)	400 mg twice daily by mouth, dose reduce for toxicity to 400 mg/d	Diarrhea, rash, desquamation, fatigue, hand/foot syndrome, pruritus, skin erythema and blisters	Bone marrow suppression, bleeding, sensory neuropathy.
Temsirolimus (Torisel)	25 mg intravenously weekly	Rash, nausea, anorexia	Mucositis, weakness, fatigue, edema.
Vorinostat (Zolinza)	400 mg/d orally	Diarrhea, nausea, anorexia	Fatigue, pulmonary embolism, hypercholesterolemia, hypertriglyceridemia, hyperglycemia, increased creatinine, myelosuppression.
Thalidomide	200 mg/d orally	Diarrhea, rash	Teratogenic risk, venous thromboembolism, constipation, rash, somnolence, neuropathy.
Lenalidomide (Revlimid)	10 mg/d orally	Diarrhea, itching, rash, nausea, constipation, fever	Myelosuppression, teratogenic risk, fatigue, nasopharyngitis, arthralgia, back pain, peripheral edema.
Supportive agents (antiemetics are covered in detail in the text, under Chemotherapy-Induced Nausea and Vomiting)			
Allopurinol (Prevent hyperuricemia from tumor lysis syndrome)	300–900 mg/d orally for prevention or relief of hyperuricemia	None	Rash, Stevens-Johnson syndrome; enhances effects and toxicity of mercaptopurine when used in combination.
Mesna (Prevent ifosfamide bladder toxicity)	20% of ifosfamide dosage at the time of ifosfamide administration, then 4 and 8 hours after each dose of chemotherapy to prevent hemorrhagic cystitis	Nausea, vomiting, diarrhea	None.
Leucovorin (Protect against methotrexate toxicity to normal cells)	10 mg/m² every 6 hours intravenously or orally until serum methotrexate levels are below 5×10^{-8} mol/L with hydration and urinary alkalinization (about 72 hours)	None	Enhances toxic effects of fluorouracil.
Amifostine (Prevent radiation toxicity)	910 mg/m² intravenously daily, 30 minutes prior to chemotherapy with cyclophosphamide or ifosphamide	Hypotension, nausea, vomiting, flushing	Decrease in serum calcium.
Dexrazoxane (Protect against anthracycline cardiac toxicity)	10:1 ratio of anthracycline intravenously, before (within 30 minutes of) chemotherapy infusion	Pain on injection	Increased bone marrow suppression.

(continued)

Table 8. Single-agent dosage and toxicity of anticancer drugs.[1] (continued)

Drug	Dosage	Acute Toxicity	Delayed Toxicity
Palifermin (Prevent mucositis)	60 mcg/kg/d intravenous bolus daily for 3 days before and 3 days after myelotoxic chemotherapy (total of six doses separated from chemotherapy by at least 24 hours)	None	Skin rash, skin erythema, edema, pruritus, oral dysesthesias.
Pilocarpine hydro-chloride (Ameliorate dry mouth from radiation)	5–10 mg orally three times daily	Sweating, headache, flushing; nausea, chills, rhinitis, dizziness, and urinary frequency at high dosage	
Pamidronate (Treat hypercalcemia, reduce effects of bone metastases)	90 mg intravenously every month	Symptomatic hypoglycemia (rare), flare of bone pain, local irritation	Osteonecrosis, renal insufficiency.
Zoledronic acid (Treat hypercalcemia, reduce effects of bone metastases)	4 mg intravenously every month		
Epoetin alfa (erythropoietin) (Treat cancer or chemotherapy-related anemia)	100–300 units/kg intravenously or subcutaneously 3 times a week	Skin irritation or pain at injection site	Hypertension, headache, seizures in patients on dialysis (rare).
Darbepoetin alfa (Long-acting erythropoietin)	200 mcg subcutaneously every other week or 300 mcg subcutaneously every 3 weeks[2]	Injection site pain	Hypertension, thromboses, headache, diarrhea.
Filgrastim (G-CSF) (Reduce severity and duration of chemotherapy-induced neutropenia)	5 mcg/kg/d subcutaneously or intravenously daily until neutrophils recover	Mild to moderate bone pain, mild hypotension (rare), irritation at injection sites (rare)	Bone pain, hypoxia.
Pegfilgrastim (Long-acting neupogen)	6 mg subcutaneously on day 2 of each 2- to 3-week chemotherapy cycle[2]	Injection site reactions	Bone pain, hypoxia.
Sargramostim (GM-CSF)	250 mcg/kg/d as a 2-hour intravenous infusion (can be given subcutaneously)	Fluid retention, dyspnea, capillary leak (rare), supraventricular tachycardia (rare), mild to moderate bone pain, irritation at injection sites	
Neumega (IL-11) (Treat chemotherapy-induced thrombocytopenia)	50 mcg/kg/d subcutaneously	Fluid retention, arrhythmias, headache, arthralgias, myalgias	Unknown.
Gallium nitrate (Treat hypercalcemia, bone pain from cancer)	200 mg/m² intravenously daily by continuous infusion for 5 days	Hypocalcemia, transient hypophosphatemia	Renal insufficiency, hypocalcemia.
Samarium-153 lexidronam (Sm-153 EDTMP) (Treat bone metastases)	1 mCi/kg intravenously as single dose	None	Hematopoietic suppression.
Strontium-89 (Treat bone metastases)	4 mCi every 3 months intravenously	None	Hematopoietic suppression.

[1]5-FU, 5-fluorouracil; NSAIDs, nonsteroidal anti-inflammatory drugs; MAO, monoamine oxidase; GnRH, gonadotropin-releasing hormone; CNS, central nervous system; IL, interleukin; SIADH, syndrome of inappropriate antidiuretic hormone; G-CSF, granulocyte colony-stimulating factor; GM-CSF, granulocyte-macrophage colony-stimulating factor.
[2]Off label.

Table 9. A common scheme for dose modification of cancer chemotherapeutic agents.[1]

Granulocyte Count	Platelet Count	Suggested Dosage (% of Full Dose)
> 2000/mcL	> 100,000/mcL	100%
1000–2000/mcL	75,000–100,000/mcL	50%
< 1000/mcL	< 50,000/mcL	0%

[1]In general, dose modification should be avoided to maintain therapeutic efficacy. The use of myeloid growth factors or a delay in the start of the next cycle of chemotherapy is usually effective.

Table 10. Paraneoplastic syndromes associated with common cancers.[1]

Syndromes; Hormone Excess	Small Cell Lung Cancer	Non-Small Cell Lung Cancer	Breast Cancer	Multiple Myeloma	Gastro-intestinal Cancers	Hepato-cellular Cancer	Gestational Trophoblastic Disease	Lymphoma	Renal Cell Cancer	Carcinoid	Thymoma	Ovarian Cancer	Prostate Cancer	Myelopro-liferative Disease	Adreno-cortical Tumors	Cerebellar Hemangio-blastomas
Endocrine																
Cushing syndrome	XX	X														
SIADH	XX	X														
Hypercalcemia	XX	X	X	X				X				X				
Hypoglycemia					X	X										
Gonadotropin excess	XX	X			X		X		X	X						
Hyperthyroidism							X									
Neuromuscular																
Subacute cerebellar degeneration	XX	X			X			X				X				
Sensorimotor peripheral neuropathy	XX	X														
Lambert-Eaton syndrome	XX		X		X							X				
Stiff man syndrome			X									X				
Dermatomyositis/polymyositis	XX	X	X		XX							X		X		
Skin																
Dermatomyositis	XX	X	X		XX							X		X		
Acanthosis nigricans		X	X		X					X			X	X		
Sweet syndrome		X	X		X			XX	X			X	X	XX		
Hematologic																
Erythrocytosis						X			X			X			X	X
Pure red cell aplasia			X		X			X			XX					
Eosinophilia								XX								
Thrombocytosis	X	X	X		X	X		X	X	X		X	X	X	X	X
Coagulopathy			X					X	X				X	X		
Fever	X	X	X	X	X	X		X	X	X	X	X	X	X	X	X
Amyloidosis				X				X	X							

[1]XX, strong association; X, reported association.
SIADH, syndrome of inappropriate antidiuretic hormone.

Table 11. Thrombolytic therapy for acute myocardial infarction.

	Streptokinase	Alteplase; Tissue Plasminogen Activator (t-PA)	Reteplase	Tenecteplase (TNK-t-PA)
Source	Group C streptococcus	Recombinant DNA	Recombinant DNA	Recombinant DNA
Half-life	20 minutes	5 minutes	15 minutes	20 minutes
Usual dose	1.5 million units	100 mg	20 units	40 mg
Administration	750,000 units over 20 minutes followed by 750,000 units over 40 minutes	Initial bolus of 15 mg, followed by 50 mg infused over the next 30 minutes and 35 mg over the following 60 minutes	10 units as a bolus over 2 minutes, repeated after 30 minutes	Single weight-adjusted bolus, 0.5 mg/kg
Anticoagulation after infusion	Aspirin, 325 mg daily; there is no evidence that adjunctive heparin improves outcome following streptokinase	Aspirin, 325 mg daily; heparin, 5000 units as bolus, followed by 1000 units per hour infusion, subsequently adjusted to maintain PTT 1.5–2 times control	Aspirin, 325 mg; heparin as with t-PA	Aspirin, 325 mg daily
Clot selectivity	Low	High	High	High
Fibrinogenolysis	+++	+	+	+
Bleeding	+	+	+	+
Hypotension	+++	+	+	+
Allergic reactions	++	0	0	+
Reocclusion	5–20%	10–30%	—	5–20%
Approximate cost[1]	$563.00	$3940.00	$2895.00	$2917.00

[1]Average wholesale price (AWP, for AB-rated generic when available) for quantity listed. Source: *Red Book Update*, Vol. 27, No. 2, February 2008. AWP may not accurately represent the actual pharmacy cost because wide contractual variations exist among institutions.
PTT, partial thromboplastin time.

Table 12. Antiarrhythmic drugs.

Agent	Intravenous Dosage	Oral Dosage	Therapeutic Plasma Level	Route of Elimination	Side Effects
Class Ia: Action: Sodium channel blockers: Depress phase 0 depolarization; slow conduction; prolong repolarization.					
Indications: Supraventricular tachycardia, ventricular tachycardia, prevention of ventricular fibrillation, symptomatic ventricular premature beats.					
Quinidine	6–10 mg/kg (intramuscularly or intravenously) over 20 min (rarely used parenterally)	200–400 mg every 4–6 h or every 8 h (long-acting)	2–5 mg/mL	Hepatic	GI, ↓LVF, ↑Dig
Procainamide	100 mg/1–3 min to 500–1000 mg; maintain at 2–6 mg/min	50 mg/kg/d in divided doses every 3–4 h or every 6 h (long-acting)	4–10 mg/mL; NAPA (active metabolite), 10–20 mcg/mL	Renal	SLE, hypersensitivity, ↓LVF
Disopyramide		100–200 mg every 6–8 h	2–8 mg/mL	Renal	Urinary retention, dry mouth, markedly ↓LVF
Moricizine		200–300 mg every 8 h	**Note:** Active metabolites	Hepatic	Dizziness, nausea, headache, ↓theophylline level, ↓LVF
Class Ib: Action: Shorten repolarization.					
Indications: Ventricular tachycardia, prevention of ventricular fibrillation, symptomatic ventricular beats.					
Lidocaine	1–2 mg/kg at 50 mg/min; maintain at 1–4 mg/min		1–5 mg/mL	Hepatic	CNS, GI
Mexiletine		100–300 mg every 6–12 h; maximum: 1200 mg/d	0.5–2 mg/mL	Hepatic	CNS, GI, leukopenia
Class Ic: Action: Depress phase 0 repolarization; slow conduction. *Propafenone* is a weak calcium channel blocker and β-blocker and prolongs action potential and refractoriness.					
Indications: Life-threatening ventricular tachycardia or fibrillation, refractory supraventricular tachycardia.					
Flecainide		100–200 mg twice daily	0.2–1 mg/mL	Hepatic	CNS, GI, ↓↓LVF, incessant VT, sudden death
Propafenone		150–300 mg every 8–12 h	**Note:** Active metabolites	Hepatic	CNS, GI, ↓↓LVF, ↑Dig

(*continued*)

Table 12. Antiarrhythmic drugs. (continued)

Agent	Intravenous Dosage	Oral Dosage	Therapeutic Plasma Level	Route of Elimination	Side Effects
Class II: Action: β-blocker, slows AV conduction. *Note:* Other β-blockers may also have antiarrhythmic effects but are not yet approved for this indication in the United States.					
Indications: Supraventricular tachycardia; may prevent ventricular fibrillation.					
Esmolol	500 mcg/kg over 1–2 min; maintain at 25–200 mcg/kg/min	Other β-blockers may be used concomitantly	Not established	Hepatic	↓LVF, bronchospasm
Propranolol	1–5 mg at 1 mg/min	40–320 mg in 1–4 doses daily (depending on preparation)	Not established	Hepatic	↓LVF, bradycardia, AV block, bronchospasm
Metoprolol	2.5–5 mg	50–200 mg daily	Not established	Hepatic	↓LVF, bradycardia, AV block
Class III: Action: Prolong action potential.					
Indications: *Amiodarone:* refractory ventricular tachycardia, supraventricular tachycardia, prevention of ventricular tachycardia, atrial fibrillation, ventricular fibrillation; *dofetilide:* atrial fibrillation and flutter; *sotalol:* ventricular tachycardia, atrial fibrillation; *ibutilide:* conversion of atrial fibrillation and flutter.					
Amiodarone	150–300 mg infused rapidly, followed by 1-mg/min infusion for 6 h (360 mg) and then 0.5 mg/min	800–1600 mg/d for 7–21 days; maintain at 100–400 mg/d (higher doses may be needed)	1–5 mg/mL	Hepatic	Pulmonary fibrosis, hypothyroidism, hyperthyroidism, photosensitivity, corneal and skin deposits, hepatitis, ↑Dig, neurotoxicity, GI
Sotalol		80–160 mg every 12 h (higher doses may be used for life-threatening arrhythmias)		Renal (dosing interval should be extended if creatinine clearance is < 60 mL/min)	Early incidence of torsades de pointes, ↓LVF, bradycardia, fatigue (and other side effects associated with β-blockers)
Dofetilide		500 mcg every 12 h		Renal (dose must be reduced with renal dysfunction)	Torsades de pointes in 3%; interaction with cytochrome P-450 inhibitors
Ibutilide	1 mg over 10 min, followed by a second infusion of 0.5–1 mg over 10 min			Hepatic and renal	Torsades de pointes in up to 5% of patients within 3 h after administration; patients must be monitored with defibrillator nearby
Class IV: Action: Slow calcium channel blockers.					
Indications: Supraventricular tachycardia.					
Verapamil	10–20 mg over 2–20 min; maintain at 5 mg/kg/min	80–120 mg every 6–8 h; 240–360 mg once daily with sustained-release preparation	0.1–0.15 mg/mL	Hepatic	↓LVF, constipation, ↑Dig, hypotension
Diltiazem	0.25 mg/kg over 2 min; second 0.35-mg/kg bolus after 15 min if response is inadequate; infusion rate, 5–15 mg/h	180–360 mg daily in 1–3 doses depending on preparation (oral forms not approved for arrhythmias)		Hepatic metabolism, renal excretion	Hypotension, ↓LVF
Miscellaneous: Indications: Supraventricular tachycardia.					
Adenosine	6 mg rapidly followed by 12 mg after 1–2 min if needed; use half these doses if administered via central line			Adenosine receptor stimulation, metabolized in blood	Transient flushing, dyspnea, chest pain, AV block, sinus bradycardia; effect ↓ by theophylline, ↑ by dipyridamole
Digoxin	0.5 mg over 20 min followed by increment of 0.25 or 0.125 mg to 1–1.5 mg over 24 h	1–1.5 mg over 24–36 h in 3 or 4 doses; maintenance, 0.125–0.5 mg/d	0.7–2 mg/mL	Renal	AV block, arrhythmias, GI, visual changes

AV, atrioventricular; CNS, central nervous system; ↑Dig, elevation of serum digoxin level; GI, gastrointestinal (nausea, vomiting, diarrhea); ↓LVF, reduced left ventricular function; NAPA, *N*-acetylprocainamide; SLE, systemic lupus erythematosus; VT, ventricular tachycardia.

Table 13. Classification and management of blood pressure for adults aged 18 years or older.

BP Classification	Systolic BP, mm Hg[1]		Diastolic BP, mm Hg[1]	Lifestyle Modification	Management — Initial Drug Therapy: Without Compelling Indication	Management — Initial Drug Therapy: With Compelling Indications
Normal	< 120	and	< 80	Encourage		
Prehypertension	120–139	or	80–89	Yes	No antihypertensive drug indicated	Drug(s) for the compelling indications[2]
Stage 1 hypertension	140–159	or	90–99	Yes	Thiazide-type diuretics for most; may consider ACE inhibitor, ARB, β-blocker, CCB, or combination	Drug(s) for the compelling indications; Other antihypertensive drugs (diuretics, ACE inhibitor, ARB, β-blocker, CCB) as needed
Stage 2 hypertension	≥ 160	or	≥ 100	Yes	Two-drug combination for most (usually thiazide-type diuretic and ACE inhibitor or ARB or β-blocker or CCB)[3]	Drug(s) for the compelling indications; Other antihypertensive drugs (diuretics, ACE inhibitor, ARB, β-blocker, CCB) as needed

[1]Treatment determined by highest BP category.
[2]Treat patients with chronic kidney disease or diabetes to BP goal of < 130/80 mm Hg.
[3]Initial combined therapy should be used cautiously in those at risk for orthostatic hypotension.
ACE, angiotensin-converting enzyme; ARB, angiotensin receptor blocker; BP, blood pressure; CCB, calcium channel blocker.
Source: Chobanian AV et al. The Seventh Report of the Joint National Committee on Prevention, Detection, Evaluation, and Treatment of High Blood Pressure: the JNC 7 report. JAMA. 2003 May 21;289(19):2560–72.

Table 14. Causes of resistant hypertension.

Improper blood pressure measurement
Volume overload and pseudotolerance
   Excess sodium intake
   Volume retention from kidney disease
   Inadequate diuretic therapy
Drug-induced or other causes
   Nonadherence
   Inadequate doses
   Inappropriate combinations
   Nonsteroidal anti-inflammatory drugs; cyclooxygenase-2 inhibitors
   Cocaine, amphetamines, other illicit drugs
   Sympathomimetics (decongestants, anorectics)
   Oral contraceptives
   Adrenal steroids
   Cyclosporine and tacrolimus
   Erythropoietin
   Licorice (including some chewing tobacco)
   Selected over-the-counter dietary supplements and medicines (eg, ephedra, ma huang, bitter orange)
Associated conditions
   Obesity
   Excess alcohol intake
Identifiable causes of hypertension

Source: Chobanian AV et al. The Seventh Report of the Joint National Committee on Prevention, Detection, Evaluation, and Treatment of High Blood Pressure: the JNC 7 report. JAMA. 2003 May 21;289(19):2560–72.

Table 15. Summary of the current ACC/AHA guideline recommendations for medical management of acute coronary syndromes (ACS) and acute myocardial infarction (AMI).[1]

Medication	Acute Therapies ACS	Acute Therapies AMI	Discharge Therapies
Aspirin (ASA)	IA	IA	IA
Clopidogrel in ASA-allergic patients	IA	IC	IA
Clopidogrel, intended medical management	IA	—	IA
Clopidogrel or IIb/IIIa inhibitor, up front (prior to catheterization)	IA		
Clopidogrel, early catheterization/percutaneous coronary intervention (catheterization/percutaneous coronary intervention [cath/PCI])	IA (prior to or at time of PCI)	IB	IA
Heparin (unfractionated or low-molecular-weight)	IA	IA[2]	—
β-Blockers	IB	IA	IB
Angiotensin-converting enzyme (ACE) inhibitors	IB[3]	IA/IIaB[4]	IA
GP IIb/IIIa inhibitors for intended early cath/PCI			
Eptifibatide/tirofiban	IA	—	—
Abciximab	IA	IIaB[5]	—
GP IIb/IIIa inhibitors for high-risk patients without intended early cath/PCI			
Eptifibatide/tirofiban	IIaA	—	—
Abciximab	IIIA	—	—
Lipid-lowering agent[6]	—	—	IA
Smoking cessation counseling	—	—	IB

[1]Class I indicates treatment is useful and effective, IIa indicates weight of evidence is in favor of usefulness/efficacy, class IIb indicates weight of evidence is less well established, and class III indicates intervention is not useful/effective and may be harmful. Type A recommendations are derived from large-scale randomized trials, and B recommendations are derived from smaller randomized trials or carefully conducted observational analyses. ACC/AHA = American College of Cardiology/American Heart Association.

[2]As a class IIb, low-molecular-weight heparin (best studied is enoxaparin with tenecteplase) can be considered an acceptable alternative to unfractionated heparin for patients less than 75 years old who are receiving fibrinolytic therapy provided significant renal dysfunction is not present.

[3]For patients with persistent hypertension despite treatment, diabetes mellitus, congestive heart failure, or any left ventricular dysfunction.

[4]IA for patients with congestive heart failure or ejection fraction < 0.40, IIa for others, in absence of hypotension (systolic blood pressure < 100 mm Hg); angiotensin receptor blocker (valsartan or candesartan) for patients with ACE inhibitor intolerance.

[5]As early as possible before primary PCI.

[6]For patients with a low-density lipoprotein cholesterol level > 100 mg/dL.

Table 16. Antihypertensive drugs: diuretics.

Drugs	Proprietary Names	Initial Oral Doses	Dosage Range	Cost per Unit	Cost of 30 Days Treatment[1] (Average Dosage)	Adverse Effects	Comments
Thiazides and related diuretics							
Hydrochloro-thiazide	Esidrix, Hydro-Diuril	12.5 or 25 mg once daily	12.5–50 mg once daily	$0.08/25 mg	$2.40	$\downarrow$ K$^+$, $\downarrow$ Mg^{2+}, $\uparrow$ Ca^{2+}, $\downarrow$ Na$^+$, $\uparrow$ uric acid, $\uparrow$ glucose, $\uparrow$ LDL cholesterol, $\uparrow$ triglycerides; rash, erectile dysfunction.	Low dosages effective in many patients without associated metabolic abnormalities; metolazone more effective with concurrent renal insufficiency; indapamide does not alter serum lipid levels.
Chlorthalidone	Hygroton, Thaliton	12.5 or 25 mg once daily	12.5–50 mg once daily	$0.23/25 mg	$6.90		
Metolazone	Zaroxolyn	1.25 or 2.5 mg once daily	1.25–5 mg once daily	$1.48/5 mg	$44.40		
Indapamide	Lozol	2.5 mg once daily	2.5–5 mg once daily	$0.83/2.5 mg	$24.90		
Loop diuretics							
Furosemide	Lasix	20 mg twice daily	40–320 mg in 2 or 3 doses	$0.16/40 mg	$9.60	Same as thiazides, but higher risk of excessive diuresis and electrolyte imbalance. Increases calcium excretion.	Furosemide: Short duration of action a disadvantage; should be reserved for patients with renal insufficiency or fluid retention. Poor anti-hypertensive. Torsemide: Effective blood pressure medication at low dosage.
Ethacrynic acid	Edecrin	50 mg once daily	50–100 mg once or twice daily	$0.90/25 mg	$108.00		
Bumetanide	Bumex	0.25 mg twice daily	0.5–10 mg in 2 or 3 doses	$0.45/1 mg	$27.00		
Torsemide	Demadex	2.5 mg once daily	5–10 mg once daily	$0.70/10 mg	$21.00		
Aldosterone receptor blockers							
Spironolactone	Aldactone	12.5 or 25 mg once daily	12.5–100 mg once daily	$0.46/25 mg	$13.80	Hyperkalemia, metabolic acidosis, gynecomastia.	Can be useful add-on therapy in patients with refractory hypertension.
Amiloride	Midamor	5 mg once daily	5–10 mg once daily	$0.69/5 mg	$20.70		
Eplerenone	Inspra	25 mg once daily	25–100 mg once daily	$4.17/25 mg	$125.03		
Combination products							
Hydrochloro-thiazide and tri-amterene	Dyazide (25/50 mg); Maxzide (25/37.5 mg)	1 tab once daily	1 or 2 tabs once daily	$0.36	$10.80	Same as thiazides plus GI disturbances, hyperkalemia rather than hypokalemia, headache; triamterene can cause kidney stones and renal dysfunction; spironolactone causes gynecomastia. Hyperkalemia can occur if this combination is used in patients with renal failure or those taking ACE inhibitors.	Use should be limited to patients with demonstrable need for a potassium-sparing agent.
Hydrochloro-thiazide and amiloride	Moduretic (50/5 mg)	$^1/_2$ tab once daily	1 or 2 tabs once daily	$0.42	$12.60		
Hydrochloro-thiazide and spironolactone	Aldactazide (25/25 mg)	1 tab once daily	1 or 2 tabs once daily	$0.50	$15.00		

[1]Average wholesale price (AWP, for AB-rated generic when available) for quantity listed. Source: *Red Book Update,* Vol. 27, No. 2, February 2008. AWP may not accurately represent the actual pharmacy cost because wide contractual variations exist among institutions.
LDL, low-density lipoprotein; GI, gastrointestinal; ACE, angiotensin-converting enzyme.

Table 17. Antihypertensive drugs: β-adrenergic blocking agents.

Drug	Proprietary Name	Initial Oral Dosage	Dosage Range	Cost per Unit	Cost of 30 Days Treatment (Based on Average Dosage)[1]	Special Properties					Comments[5]
						β1 Selectivity[2]	ISA[3]	MSA[4]	Lipid Solubility	Renal vs Hepatic Elimination	
Acebutolol	Sectral	200 mg once daily	200–1200 mg in 1 or 2 doses	$1.34/400 mg	$40.20	+	+	+	+	H > R	Positive ANA; rare LE syndrome; also indicated for arrhythmias. Doses > 800 mg have β1 and β2 effects.
Atenolol	Tenormin	25 mg once daily	25–200 mg once daily	$0.83/50 mg	$24.90	+	0	0	0	R	Also indicated for angina pectoris and post-MI. Doses > 100 mg have β1 and β2 effects.
Betaxolol	Kerlone	10 mg once daily	10–40 mg once daily	$1.32/10 mg	$39.60	+	0	0	+	H > R	
Bisoprolol and hydrochlorothiazide	Ziac	5 mg/6.25 mg once daily	2.5–10 mg plus 6.25 mg	$1.14/2.5/6.25 mg	$34.20	+	0	0	0	R = H	Low-dose combination approved for initial therapy. Bisoprolol also effective for heart failure.
Carvedilol	Coreg	6.25 mg twice daily	12.5–100 mg in 2 doses	$2.13/25 mg	$127.80 (25 mg twice a day)	0	0	0	+++	H > R	α:β-Blocking activity 1:9; may cause orthostatic symptoms; effective for congestive heart failure.
Labetalol	Normodyne, Trandate	100 mg twice daily	200–1200 mg in 2 doses	$0.71/200 mg	$42.60	0	0/+	0	++	H	α:β-Blocking activity 1:3; more orthostatic hypotension, fever, hepatotoxicity.
Metoprolol	Lopressor	50 mg in 1 or 2 doses	50–200 mg in 1 or 2 doses	$0.55/50 mg	$33.00	+	0	+	+++	H	Also indicated for angina pectoris and post-MI. Approved for heart failure. Doses > 100 mg have β1 and β2 effects.
	Toprol XL (SR preparation)	50 mg once daily	50–200 mg once daily	$0.90/100 mg	$27.00						
Nadolol	Corgard	20 mg once daily	20–160 mg once daily	$1.05/40 mg	$31.50	0	0	0	0	R	
Penbutolol	Levatol	20 mg once daily	20–80 mg once daily	$2.11/20 mg	$63.30	0	+	0	++	R > H	
Pindolol	Visken	5 mg twice daily	10–60 mg in 2 doses	$0.73/5 mg	$43.80	0	++	+	+	H > R	In adults, 35% renal clearance.
Propranolol	Inderal	20 mg twice daily	40–320 mg in 2 doses	$0.51/40 mg	$30.60	0	0	++	+++	H	Once-daily SR preparation also available. Also indicated for angina pectoris and post-MI.
Timolol	Blocadren	5 mg twice daily	10–40 mg in 2 doses	$0.50/10 mg	$30.00	0	0	0	++	H > R	Also indicated for post-MI. 80% hepatic clearance.

[1]Average wholesale price (AWP, for AB-rated generic when available) for quantity listed. Source: *Red Book Update*, Vol. 27, No. 2, February 2008. AWP may not accurately represent the actual pharmacy cost because wide contractual variations exist among institutions.
[2]Agents with β1 selectivity are less likely to precipitate bronchospasm and decreased peripheral blood flow *in low doses*, but selectivity is only relative.
[3]Agents with ISA cause less resting bradycardia and lipid changes.
[4]MSA generally occurs at concentrations greater than those necessary for β-adrenergic blockade. The clinical importance of MSA by β-blockers has not been defined.
[5]Adverse effects of all β-blockers: bronchospasm, fatigue, sleep disturbance and nightmares, bradycardia and atrioventricular block, worsening of congestive heart failure, cold extremities, gastrointestinal disturbances, impotence, ↑triglycerides, ↓HDL cholesterol, rare blood dyscrasias.
ISA, intrinsic sympathomimetic activity; MSA, membrane-stabilizing activity; ANA, antinuclear antibody; LE, lupus erythematosus; MI, myocardial infarction; SR, sustained release; 0, no effect; +, some effect; ++, moderate effect; +++, most effect.

Table 18. Antihypertensive drugs: renin and ACE inhibitors and angiotensin II receptor blockers.

Drug	Proprietary Name	Initial Oral Dosage	Dosage Range	Cost per Unit	Cost of 30 Days Treatment (Average Dosage)[1]	Adverse Effects	Comments
Renin inhibitors							
Aliskiren	Tekturna	150 mg once daily	150–300 mg/d	$2.34/150 mg	$70.20	Angioedema, hypotension, hyperkalemia Contraindicated in pregnancy.	Probably metabolized by CYP3A4. Absorption is inhibited by high fat meal.
ACE inhibitors							
Benazepril	Lotensin	10 mg once daily	5–40 mg in 1 or 2 doses	$1.05/20 mg	$31.50	Cough, hypotension, dizziness, renal dysfunction, hyperkalemia, angioedema; taste alteration and rash (may be more frequent with captopril); rarely, proteinuria, blood dyscrasia. Contraindicated in pregnancy.	More fosinopril is excreted by the liver in patients with renal dysfunction (dose reduction may or may not be necessary). Captopril and lisinopril are active without metabolism. Captopril, enalapril, lisinopril, and quinapril are approved for congestive heart failure.
Captopril	Capoten	25 mg twice daily	50–300 mg in 2 or 3 doses	$0.76/25 mg	$45.60		
Enalapril	Vasotec	5 mg once daily	5–40 mg in 1 or 2 doses	$1.52/20 mg	$45.60		
Fosinopril	Monopril	10 mg once daily	10–80 mg in 1 or 2 doses	$1.19/20 mg	$35.70		
Lisinopril	Prinivil, Zestril	5–10 mg once daily	5–40 mg once daily	$1.06/20 mg	$31.80		
Moexipril	Univasc	7.5 mg once daily	7.5–30 mg in 1 or 2 doses	$1.39/7.5 mg	$41.70		
Perindopril	Aceon	4 mg once daily	4–16 mg in 1 or 2 doses	$2.48/8 mg	$74.40		
Quinapril	Accupril	10 mg once daily	10–80 mg in 1 or 2 doses	$1.68/20 mg	$50.40		
Ramipril	Altace	2.5 mg once daily	2.5–20 mg in 1 or 2 doses	$2.02/5 mg	$60.60		
Trandolapril	Mavik	1 mg once daily	1–8 mg once daily	$1.32/4 mg	$39.60		
Angiotensin II receptor blockers							
Candesartan cilexitil	Atacand	16 mg once daily	8–32 mg once daily	$1.83/16 mg	$54.90	Hyperkalemia, renal dysfunction, rare angioedema. Combinations have additional side effects. Contraindicated in pregnancy.	Losartan has a very flat dose-response curve. Valsartan and irbesartan have wider dose-response ranges and longer durations of action. Addition of low-dose diuretic (separately or as combination pills) increases the response.
Candesartan cilexitil/HCTZ	Atacand HCT	16 mg/12.5 mg once daily	8–32 mg of candesartan once daily	$2.48/16 mg/12.5 mg	$74.40		
Eprosartan	Teveten	600 mg once daily	400–800 mg in 1–2 doses	$2.52/600 mg	$75.60		
Eprosartan/HCTZ	Teveten HCT	600 mg/12.5 mg once daily	600 mg/12.5 mg or 600 mg/25 mg once daily	$2.87/600 mg/12.5 mg	$86.10		
Irbesartan	Avapro	150 mg once daily	150–300 mg once daily	$1.99/150 mg	$59.70		
Irbesartan and HCTZ	Avalide	150 mg/12.5 mg once daily	150–300 mg irbesartan daily	$2.41/150 mg	$72.30		
Losartan	Cozaar	50 mg once daily	25–100 mg in 1 or 2 doses	$1.98/50 mg	$59.40		
Losartan and hydrochlorothiazide	Hyzaar	50 mg/12.5 mg once daily	One or 2 tablets once daily	$2.06/50 mg/12.5 mg/tablet	$61.80		
Olmesartan	Benicar	20 mg once daily	20–40 mg daily	$1.86/20 mg	$55.80		
Olmesartan and HCTZ	Benicar HCT	20 mg/12.5 mg daily	20–40 mg olmesartan daily	$2.27/20 mg/12.5 mg	$68.10		
Telmisartan	Micardis	40 mg once daily	20–80 mg once daily	$2.11/40 mg	$63.30		
Telmisartan and HCTZ	Micardis HCT	40 mg/12.5 mg once daily	20–80 mg telmisartan daily	$2.26/40 mg/12.5 mg	$67.80		
Valsartan	Diovan	80 mg once daily	80–320 mg once daily	$2.26/160 mg	$67.80		
Valsartan and HCTZ	Diovan HCT	80 mg/12.5 mg once daily	80–320 mg valsartan daily	$2.46/160 mg/12.5 mg	$73.80		

[1]Average wholesale price (AWP, for AB-rated generic when available) for quantity listed. Source: *Red Book Update*, Vol. 27, No. 2, February 2008. AWP may not accurately represent the actual pharmacy cost because wide contractual variations exist among institutions.
ACE, angiotensin-converting enzyme; HCTZ, hydrochlorothiazide.

Table 19. Antihypertensive drugs: calcium channel blocking agents.

Drug	Proprietary Name	Initial Oral Dosage	Dosage Range	Cost of 30 Days Treatment (Average Dosage)[1]	Special Properties			Adverse Effects	Comments
					Peripheral Vasodilation	Cardiac Automaticity and Conduction	Contractility		
Nondihydropyridine agents									
Diltiazem	Cardizem SR	90 mg twice daily	180–360 mg in 2 doses	$74.25 (120 mg twice daily)	++	↓↓	↓↓	Edema, headache, bradycardia, GI disturbances, dizziness, AV block, congestive heart failure, urinary frequency.	Also approved for angina.
	Cardizem CD; Cartia XT	180 mg daily	180–360 mg daily	$61.50 (240 mg daily)					
	Dilacor XR	180 or 240 mg daily	180–480 mg daily	$34.50 (240 mg daily)					
	Tiazac SA	240 mg daily	180–540 mg daily	$73.40 (240 mg daily)					
Verapamil	Calan SR	180 mg daily	180–480 mg in 1 or 2 doses	$46.80 (240 mg daily)	++	↓↓↓	↓↓↓	Same as diltiazem but more likely to cause constipation and congestive heart failure.	Also approved for angina and arrhythmias.
	Isoptin SR								
	Verelan								
	Covera HS			$73.20 (240 mg daily)					
Dihydropyridines									
Amlodipine	Norvasc	5 mg daily	5–10 mg daily	$71.20 (10 mg daily)	+++	↓/0	↓/0	Edema, dizziness, palpitations, flushing, headache, hypotension, tachycardia, GI disturbances, urinary frequency, worsening of congestive heart failure (may be less common with felodipine, amlodipine).	Amlodipine, nicardipine, and nifedipine also approved for angina.
Felodipine	Plendil	5 mg daily	5–20 mg daily	$42.00 (10 mg daily)	+++	↓/0	↓/0		
Isradipine	DynaCirc	2.5 mg twice daily	2.5–5 mg twice daily	$120.00 (5 mg twice daily)	+++	↓/0	→		
	DynaCirc CR	5 mg daily	5–10 mg daily	$115.24 (10 mg daily)					
Nicardipine	Cardene	20 mg three times daily	20–40 mg three times daily	$41.20 (20 mg three times daily)	+++	↓/0	→		
	Cardene SR	30 mg twice daily	30–60 mg twice daily	$72.31 (30 mg twice daily)					
Nifedipine	Adalat CC	30 mg daily	30–120 mg daily	$65.10 (60 mg daily)	+++	→	↓↓		
	Procardia XL	30 mg daily	30–120 mg daily	$70.86 (60 mg daily)					
Nisoldipine	Sular	20 mg/d	20–60 mg/d	$83.10 (40 mg daily)	+++	↓/0	→		

[1]Average wholesale price (AWP, for AB-rated generic when available) for quantity listed. Source: *Red Book Update*, Vol. 27, No. 2, February 2008. AWP may not accurately represent the actual pharmacy cost because wide contractual variations exist among institutions.
GI, gastrointestinal; AV, atrioventricular.

Table 20. α-Adrenoceptor blocking agents, sympatholytics, and vasodilators.

Drug	Proprietary Names	Initial Dosage	Dosage Range	Cost per Unit	Cost of 30 Days Treatment (Average Dosage)[1]	Adverse Effects	Comments
α-Adrenoceptor blockers							
Prazosin	Minipress	1 mg hs	2–20 mg in 2 or 3 doses	$0.78/5 mg	$46.80 (5 mg twice daily)	Syncope with first dose; postural hypotension, dizziness, palpitations, headache, weakness, drowsiness, sexual dysfunction, anticholinergic effects, urinary incontinence; first-dose effects may be less with doxazosin.	May ↑ HDL and ↓ LDL cholesterol. May provide short-term relief of obstructive prostatic symptoms. Less effective in preventing cardiovascular events than diuretics.
Terazosin	Hytrin	1 mg hs	1–20 mg in 1 or 2 doses	$1.60/1, 2, 5, 10 mg	$48.00 (5 mg daily)		
Doxazosin	Cardura	1 mg hs	1–16 mg daily	$0.97/4 mg	$29.10 (4 mg daily)		
Central sympatholytics							
Clonidine	Catapres	0.1 mg twice daily	0.2–0.6 mg in 2 doses	$0.22/0.1 mg	$13.20 (0.1 mg twice daily)	Sedation, dry mouth, sexual dysfunction, headache, bradyarrhythmias; side effects may be less with guanfacine. Contact dermatitis with clonidine patch. Methyldopa also causes hepatitis, hemolytic anemia, fever.	"Rebound" hypertension may occur even after gradual withdrawal. Methyldopa should be avoided in favor of safer agents.
	Catapres TTS	0.1 mg/d patch weekly	0.1–0.3 mg/d patch weekly	$32.42/0.2 mg	$129.68 (0.2 mg weekly)		
Guanabenz	Wytensin	4 mg twice daily	8–64 mg in 2 doses	$0.98/4 mg	$58.80 (4 mg twice daily)		
Guanfacine	Tenex	1 mg once daily	1–3 mg daily	$0.87/1 mg	$26.10 (1 mg daily)		
Methyldopa	Aldomet	250 mg twice daily	500–2000 mg in 2 doses	$0.63/500 mg	$37.80 (500 mg twice daily)		
Peripheral neuronal antagonists							
Reserpine	Serpasil	0.05 mg once daily	0.05–0.25 mg daily	$0.48/0.1 mg	$14.40 (0.1 mg daily)	Depression (less likely at low dosages, ie, < 0.25 mg), night terrors, nasal stuffiness, drowsiness, peptic disease, gastrointestinal disturbances, bradycardia.	
Direct vasodilators							
Hydralazine	Apresoline	25 mg twice daily	50–300 mg in 2–4 doses	$0.51/25 mg	$30.60 (25 mg twice daily)	GI disturbances, tachycardia, headache, nasal congestion, rash, LE-like syndrome.	May worsen or precipitate angina.
Minoxidil	Loniten	5 mg once daily	5–40 mg once daily	$1.29/10 mg	$38.70 (10 mg once daily)	Tachycardia, fluid retention, headache, hirsutism, pericardial effusion, thrombocytopenia.	Should be used in combination with β-blocker and diuretic.

[1]Average wholesale price (AWP, for AB-rated generic when available) for quantity listed. Source: *Red Book Update,* Vol. 27, No. 2, February 2008. AWP may not accurately represent the actual pharmacy cost because wide contractual variations exist among institutions.
GI, gastrointestinal; LE, lupus erythematosus.

Table 21. Drugs for hypertensive emergencies and urgencies.

Agent	Action	Dosage	Onset	Duration	Adverse Effects	Comments
Parenteral agents (intravenous unless noted)						
Nitroprusside (Nipride)	Vasodilator	0.25–10 mcg/kg/min	Seconds	3–5 minutes	GI, CNS; thiocyanate and cyanide toxicity, especially with renal and hepatic insufficiency; hypotension.	Most effective and easily titratable treatment. Use with β-blocker in aortic dissection.
Nitroglycerin	Vasodilator	0.25–5 mcg/kg/min	2–5 minutes	3–5 minutes	Headache, nausea, hypotension, bradycardia.	Tolerance may develop. Useful primarily with myocardial ischemia.
Labetalol (Normodyne, Trandate)	β- and α-Blocker	20–40 mg every 10 minutes to 300 mg; 2 mg/min infusion	5–10 minutes	3–6 hours	GI, hypotension, bronchospasm, bradycardia, heart block.	Avoid in congestive heart failure, asthma. May be continued orally.
Esmolol (Brevibloc)	β-Blocker	Loading dose 500 mcg/kg over 1 minute; maintenance, 25–200 mcg/kg/min	1–2 minutes	10–30 minutes	Bradycardia, nausea.	Avoid in congestive heart failure, asthma. Weak antihypertensive.
Fenoldopam (Corlopam)	Dopamine receptor agonist	0.1–1.6 mcg/kg/min	4–5 minutes	< 10 minutes	Reflex tachycardia, hypotension, ↑intraocular pressure.	May protect renal function.
Nicardipine (Cardene)	Calcium channel blocker	5 mg/h; may increase by 1–2.5 mg/h every 15 minutes to 15 mg/h	1–5 minutes	3–6 hours	Hypotension, tachycardia, headache.	May precipitate myocardial ischemia.
Enalaprilat (Vasotec)	ACE inhibitor	1.25 mg every 6 hours	15 minutes	6 hours or more	Excessive hypotension.	Additive with diuretics; may be continued orally.
Furosemide (Lasix)	Diuretic	10–80 mg	15 minutes	4 hours	Hypokalemia, hypotension.	Adjunct to vasodilator.
Hydralazine (Apresoline)	Vasodilator	5–20 mg intravenously or intramuscularly (less desirable); may repeat after 20 minutes	10–30 minutes	2–6 hours	Tachycardia, headache, GI.	Avoid in coronary artery disease, dissection. Rarely used except in pregnancy.
Diazoxide (Hyperstat)	Vasodilator	50–150 mg repeated at intervals of 5–15 minutes, or 15–30 mg/min by intravenous infusion to a maximum of 600 mg	1–2 minutes	4–24 hours	Excessive hypotension, tachycardia, myocardial ischemia, headache, nausea, vomiting, hyperglycemia. Necrosis with extravasation.	Avoid in coronary artery disease and dissection. Use with β-blocker and diuretic. Mostly obsolete.
Trimethaphan (Arfonad)	Ganglionic blocker	0.5–5 mg/min	1–3 minutes	10 minutes	Hypotension, ileus, urinary retention, respiratory arrest. Liberates histamine; use caution in allergic individuals.	Useful in aortic dissection. Otherwise rarely used.
Oral agents						
Nifedipine (Adalat, Procardia)	Calcium channel blocker	10 mg initially; may be repeated after 30 minutes	15 minutes	2–6 hours	Excessive hypotension, tachycardia, headache, angina, myocardial infarction, stroke.	Response unpredictable.
Clonidine (Catapres)	Central sympatholytic	0.1–0.2 mg initially; then 0.1 mg every hour to 0.8 mg	30–60 minutes	6–8 hours	Sedation.	Rebound may occur.
Captopril (Capoten)	ACE inhibitor	12.5–25 mg	15–30 minutes	4–6 hours	Excessive hypotension.	

GI, gastrointestinal; CNS, central nervous system; ACE, angiotensin-converting enzyme.

Table 22. Common vestibular disorders: differential diagnosis based on classic presentations.

Duration of Typical Vertiginous Episodes	Auditory Symptoms Present	Auditory Symptoms Absent
Seconds	Perilymphatic fistula	Positioning vertigo (cupulolithiasis), vertebrobasilar insufficiency, cervical vertigo
Hours	Endolymphatic hydrops (Ménière syndrome, syphilis)	Recurrent vestibulopathy, vestibular migraine
Days	Labyrinthitis, labyrinthine concussion	Vestibular neuronitis
Months	Acoustic neuroma, ototoxicity	Multiple sclerosis, cerebellar degeneration

Table 23. The inflamed eye: differential diagnosis of common causes.

	Acute Conjunctivitis	Acute Anterior Uveitis	Acute Angle-Closure Glaucoma	Corneal Trauma or Infection
Incidence	Extremely common	Common	Uncommon	Common
Discharge	Moderate to copious	None	None	Watery or purulent
Vision	No effect on vision	Often blurred	Markedly blurred	Usually blurred
Pain	Mild	Moderate	Severe	Moderate to severe
Conjunctival injection	Diffuse; more toward fornices	Mainly circumcorneal	Mainly circumcorneal	Mainly circumcorneal
Cornea	Clear	Usually clear	Steamy	Clarity change related to cause
Pupil size	Normal	Small	Moderately dilated and fixed	Normal
Pupillary light response	Normal	Poor	None	Normal
Intraocular pressure	Normal	Usually normal but may be low or elevated	Markedly elevated	Normal
Smear	Causative organisms	No organisms	No organisms	Organisms found only in corneal infection

Table 24. Topical ophthalmic agents.

Agent	Cost/Size[1]	Recommended Regimen	Indications
Antibacterial Agents[2]			
Bacitracin 500 units/g ointment (various)[3]	$4.75/3.5 g	Refer to package insert (instructions vary)	Ocular surface infection involving lid, conjunctiva, or cornea.
Chloramphenicol 1% (10 mg/g) ointment (compounding pharmacy)[4]	No U.S. price		
Ciprofloxacin HCl (Ciloxan)	0.3% solution: $45.89/5 mL / 0.3% ointment: $68.64/3.5 g		
Erythromycin 0.5% ointment (various)[5]	$5.73/3.5 g		
Fusidic acid 1% in gel (Fucithalmic)	Not available in United States		
Gatifloxacin 0.3% solution (Zymar)	$62.02/5 mL		
Gentamicin sulfate 0.3% solution (various)	$9.50/5 mL		
Gentamicin sulfate 0.3% ointment (various)	$17.70/3.5 g		
Levofloxacin 0.5% solution (Iquix 1.5%)	$67.20/5 mL		
Moxifloxacin sulfate 0.5% solution (Vigamox)	$61.74/3 mL		
Norfloxacin 0.3% solution (Chibroxin)	Not available in United States		
Ofloxacin 0.3% solution (Ocuflox)	$42.17/5 mL		

(continued)

Table 24. Topical ophthalmic agents. (continued)

Agent	Cost/Size[1]	Recommended Regimen	Indications
Polymyxin B sulfate 500,000 units, powder for solution (Polymyxin B Sulfate Sterile)[6]	$15.24/500,000 units		
Tobramycin 0.3% solution (various)	$15.00/5 mL		
Tobramycin 0.3% ointment (Tobrex)	$62.64/3.5 g		
Sulfacetamide sodium 10% solution (various)	$5.08/15 mL	1 or 2 drops every 1–3 hours	
Sulfacetamide sodium 10% ointment (various)	$8.10/3.5 g	Apply small amount (0.5 inch) into lower conjunctival sac once to four times daily and at bedtime	
Antifungal Agents			
Natamycin 5% suspension (Natacyn)	$180.00/15 mL	1 drop every 1–2 hours	Fungal ocular infections.
Antiviral Agents			
Acyclovir 3% ointment (Zovirax)	Not available in United States	5 times daily	Herpes simplex virus keratitis.
Trifluridine 1% solution (Viroptic)	$121.07/7.5 mL	1 drop onto cornea every 2 hours while awake for a maximum daily dose of 9 drops until resolution occurs; then an additional 7 days of 1 drop every 4 hours while awake (minimum five times daily)	
Anti-Inflammatory Agents			
Antihistamines[7]			
Levocabastine HCl 0.05% ophthalmic solution (Livostin)	$94.59/10 mL	1 drop four times daily (up to 2 weeks)	Allergic eye disease.
Emedastine difumarate 0.05% solution (Emadine)	$67.26/5 mL	1 drop four times daily	
Mast cell stabilizers			
Cromolyn sodium 4% solution (Crolom)	$44.56/10 mL	1 drop four to six times daily	Allergic eye disease.
Ketotifen fumarate 0.025% solution (Zaditor)	$47.85/5 mL	1 drop two to four times daily	
Lodoxamide tromethamine 0.1% solution (Alomide)	$85.20/10 mL	1 or 2 drops four times daily (up to 3 months)	
Nedocromil sodium 2% solution (Alocril)	$89.40/5 mL	1 drop twice daily	
Olopatadine hydrochloride 0.1% solution (Patanol)	$87.12/5 mL	1 drop twice daily	
Nonsteroidal anti-inflammatory agents[8]			
Bromfenac 0.09% solution (Xibrom)	$99.06/2.5 mL	1 drop to operated eye twice daily beginning 24 hours after cataract surgery and continuing through first 2 postoperative weeks	Treatment of postoperative inflammation following cataract extraction.
Diclofenac sodium 0.1% solution (Voltaren)	$78.78/5 mL	1 drop to operated eye four times daily beginning 24 hours after cataract surgery and continuing through first 2 postoperative weeks	Treatment of postoperative inflammation following cataract extraction and laser corneal surgery.
Flurbiprofen sodium 0.03% solution (various)	$8.73/2.5 mL	1 drop every half hour beginning 2 hours before surgery; 1 drop to operated eye four times daily beginning 24 hours after cataract surgery	Inhibition of intraoperative miosis. Treatment of cystoid macular edema and inflammation after cataract surgery.
Ketorolac tromethamine 0.5% solution (Acular)	$81.58/5 mL	1 drop four times daily	Treatment of allergic eye disease, postoperative inflammation following cataract extraction and laser corneal surgery.
Nepafenac 0.1% suspension (Nevanac)	$81.30/3 mL	1 drop to operated eye three times daily beginning 24 hours after cataract surgery and continuing through first 2 postoperative weeks	Treatment of postoperative inflammation following cataract extraction.
Corticosteroids[9]			
Dexamethasone sodium phosphate 0.1% solution (various)	$17.31/5 mL	1 or 2 drops as often as indicated by severity; use every hour during the day and every 2 hours during the night in severe inflammation; taper off as inflammation decreases	Treatment of steroid-responsive inflammatory conditions of anterior segment.
Dexamethasone sodium phosphate 0.05% ointment (various)	$6.34/3.5 g	Apply thin coating on lower conjunctival sac three or four times daily	

(continued)

Table 24. Topical ophthalmic agents. (continued)

Agent	Cost/Size[1]	Recommended Regimen	Indications
Fluorometholone 0.1% suspension (various)[10]	$16.01/10 mL	1 or 2 drops as often as indicated by severity; use every hour during the day and every 2 hours during the night in severe inflammation; taper off as inflammation decreases	Treatment of steroid-responsive inflammatory conditions of anterior segment.
Fluorometholone 0.25% suspension (FML Forte)[10]	$38.63/10 mL		
Fluorometholone 0.1% ointment (FML S.O.P.)	$34.92/3.5 g	Apply thin coating on lower conjunctival sac three or four times daily	
Prednisolone acetate 0.12% suspension (Pred Mild)	$36.14/10 mL	1 or 2 drops as often as indicated by severity of inflammation; use every hour during the day and every 2 hours during the night in severe inflammation; taper off as inflammation decreases	
Prednisolone sodium phosphate 0.125% solution (compounding pharmacy)	No U.S. price		
Prednisolone acetate 1% suspension (various)	$23.10/10 mL		
Prednisolone sodium phosphate 1% solution (various)	$24.06/10 mL		
Rimexolone 1% suspension (Vexol)	$61.68/10 mL		

Immunomodulator

Agent	Cost/Size[1]	Recommended Regimen	Indications
Cyclosporine 0.05% emulsion (Restasis)	$3.50/unit dose	1 drop twice daily	Dry eyes and severe allergic eye disease.

Agents for Glaucoma and Ocular Hypertension

Sympathomimetics

Agent	Cost/Size[1]	Recommended Regimen	Indications
Apraclonidine HCl 0.5% solution (Iopidine)	$82.20/5 mL	1 drop three times daily	Reduction of intraocular pressure. Expensive. Reserve for treatment of resistant cases.
Apraclonidine HCl 1% solution (Iopidine)	$13.65/unit dose	1 drop 1 hour before and immediately after anterior segment laser surgery	To control or prevent elevations of intraocular pressure after laser trabeculoplasty or iridotomy.
Brimonidine tartrate 0.2% solution (Alphagan)	$32.65/5 mL	1 drop two or three times daily	Reduction of intraocular pressure.
Dipivefrin HCl 0.1% solution (Propine)[11]	$14.07/5 mL	1 drop every 12 hours	Open-angle glaucoma.

β-Adrenergic blocking agents

Agent	Cost/Size[1]	Recommended Regimen	Indications
Betaxolol HCl 0.5% solution and 0.25% suspension (Betoptic S)[12]	0.5%: $39.10/10 mL 0.25%: $97.92/10 mL	1 drop twice daily	Reduction of intraocular pressure.
Levobunolol HCl 0.25% and 0.5% solution (Betagan)[13]	0.5%: $32.25/10 mL	1 drop once or twice daily	
Metipranolol HCl 0.3% solution (OptiPranolol)[13]	$26.85/10 mL	1 drop twice daily	
Timolol 0.25% and 0.5% solution (Betimol)[13]	0.5%: $52.20/10 mL	1 drop once or twice daily	
Timolol maleate 0.25% and 0.5% solution (Timoptic) and 0.25% and 0.5% gel (Timoptic-XE)[13]	0.5% solution: $32.35/10 mL 0.5% gel: $26.40/5 mL	1 drop once or twice daily	

Miotics

Agent	Cost/Size[1]	Recommended Regimen	Indications
Pilocarpine HCl (various)[14] 1–4%, 6%, 8%, and 10%	2%: $11.80/15 mL	1 drop three or four times daily	Reduction of intraocular pressure, treatment of acute or chronic angle-closure glaucoma, and pupillary constriction.
Pilocarpine HCl 4% gel (Pilopine HS)	$51.66/4 g	Apply 0.5-inch ribbon in lower conjunctival sac at bedtime	

Carbonic anhydrase inhibitors

Agent	Cost/Size[1]	Recommended Regimen	Indications
Dorzolamide HCl 2% solution (Trusopt)	$65.96/10 mL	1 drop three times daily	Reduction of intraocular pressure.
Brinzolamide 1% suspension (Azopt)	$80.52/10 mL	1 drop three times daily	

Prostaglandin analogs

Agent	Cost/Size[1]	Recommended Regimen	Indications
Bimatoprost 0.03% solution (Lumigan)	$71.68/2.5 mL	1 drop once daily at night	Reduction of intraocular pressure.
Latanoprost 0.005% solution (Xalatan)	$68.11/2.5 mL	1 drop once or twice daily at night	
Travoprost 0.004% solution (Travatan)	$71.28/2.5 mL	1 drop once daily at night	

(continued)

Table 24. Topical ophthalmic agents. (continued)

Agent	Cost/Size[1]	Recommended Regimen	Indications
Combined preparations			
Xalacom (latanoprost 0.005% and timolol 0.5%)	Not available in United States	1 drop daily in the morning	Reduction of intraocular pressure.
Ganfort (bimatoprost 0.03% and timolol 0.5%)	Not available in United States	1 drop daily in the morning	
DuoTrav (travoprost 0.004% and timolol 0.5%)	Not available in United States	1 drop daily	
Cosopt (dorzolamide 2% and timolol 0.5%)	$123.52/10 mL	1 drop twice daily	
Combigan (brimonidine 0.2% and timolol 0.5%)	Not available in United States	1 drop twice daily	

[1]Average wholesale price (AWP, for AB-rated generic when available) for quantity listed. Source: *Red Book Update*, Vol. 27, No. 2, February 2008. AWP may not accurately represent the actual pharmacy cost because wide contractual variations exist among institutions.
[2]Many combination products containing antibacterials or antibacterials and corticosteroids are available.
[3]Little efficacy against gram-negative organisms (except *Neisseria*).
[4]Aplastic anemia has been reported with prolonged ophthalmic use.
[5]Also indicated for prophylaxis of neonatal conjunctivitis due to *Neisseria gonorrhoeae* or *Chlamydia trachomatis*.

[6]No gram-positive coverage.
[7]May produce rebound hyperemia and local reactions.
[8]Cross-sensitivity to aspirin and other nonsteroidal anti-inflammatory drugs.
[9]Long-term use increases intraocular pressure, causes cataracts and predisposes to bacterial, herpes simplex virus, and fungal keratitis.
[10]Less likely to elevate intraocular pressure.
[11]Macular edema occurs in 30% of patients.
[12]Cardioselective (β_1) β-blocker.
[13]Nonselective (β_1 and β_2) β-blocker. Monitor all patients for systemic side effects, particularly exacerbation of asthma.
[14]Decreased night vision, headaches possible.

Table 25. The Diabetes Expert Committee criteria for evaluating the standard oral glucose tolerance test.[1]

	Normal Glucose Tolerance	Impaired Glucose Tolerance	Diabetes Mellitus[2]
Fasting plasma glucose (mg/dL)	< 100	100–125	≥ 126
Two hours after glucose load (mg/dL)	< 140	≥ 140–199	≥ 200

[1]Give 75 g of glucose dissolved in 300 mL of water after an overnight fast in persons who have been receiving at least 150–200 g of carbohydrate daily for 3 days before the test.
[2]A fasting plasma glucose ≥ 126 mg/dL is diagnostic of diabetes if confirmed on a subsequent day.

Table 26. Drugs for treatment of type 2 diabetes mellitus.

Drug	Tablet Size	Daily Dose	Duration of Action
Sulfonylureas			
Tolbutamide (Orinase)	500 mg	0.5–2 g in two or three divided doses	6–12 hours
Tolazamide (Tolinase)	100, 250, and 500 mg	0.1–1 g as single dose or in two divided doses	Up to 24 hours
Acetohexamide (Dymelor)	250 and 500 mg	0.25–1.5 g as single dose or in two divided doses	8–24 hours
Chlorpropamide (Diabinese)	100 and 250 mg	0.1–0.5 g as single dose	24–72 hours
Glyburide			
(DiaβΕta, Micronase)	1.25, 2.5, and 5 mg	1.25–20 mg as single dose or in two divided doses	Up to 24 hours
(Glynase)	1.5, 3, and 6 mg	1.5–12 mg as single dose or in two divided doses	Up to 24 hours
Glipizide			
(Glucotrol)	5 and 10 mg	2.5–20 mg twice a day 30 minutes before meals	6–12 hours
(Glucotrol XL)	2.5, 5, and 10 mg	2.5 to 10 mg once a day is usual dose; 20 mg once a day is maximal dose	Up to 24 hours
Gliclazide (not available in US)	80 mg	40–80 mg as single dose; 160–320 mg as divided dose	12 hours
Glimepiride (Amaryl)	1, 2, and 4 mg	1–4 mg once a day is usual dose; 8 mg once a day is maximal dose	Up to 24 hours
Meglitinide analogs			
Repaglinide (Prandin)	0.5, 1, and 2 mg	0.5 to 4 mg three times a day before meals	3 hours
D-Phenylalanine derivative			
Nateglinide (Starlix)	60 and 120 mg	60 or 120 mg three times a day before meals	1.5 hours
Biguanides			
Metformin (Glucophage)	500, 850, and 1000 mg	1–2.5 g; 1 tablet with meals two or three times daily	7–12 hours
Extended-release metformin (Glucophage XR)	500 mg	500–2000 mg once a day	Up to 24 hours
Thiazolidinediones			
Rosiglitazone (Avandia)	2, 4, and 8 mg	4–8 mg daily (can be divided)	Up to 24 hours
Pioglitazone (Actos)	15, 30, and 45 mg	15–45 mg daily	Up to 24 hours
α-Glucosidase inhibitors			
Acarbose (Precose)	50 and 100 mg	25 to 100 mg three times a day just before meals	4 hours
Miglitol (Glyset)	25, 50, and 100 mg	25–100 mg three times a day just before meals	4 hours
Incretins			
Exenatide (Byetta)	1.2 mL and 2.4 mL cartridges containing 5 mcg and 10 mcg (subcutaneous injection)	5 mcg subcutaneously twice a day within 1 hour of breakfast and dinner. Increase to 10 mcg subcutaneously twice a day after about a month. Do not use if calculated creatinine clearance is less than 30 mL/min.	6 hours
Sitagliptin (Januvia)	25, 50, and 100 mg	100 mg once daily is usual dose; dose is 50 mg once daily if calculated creatinine clearance is 30 to 50 mL/min and 25 mg once daily if clearance is less than 30 mL/min.	24 hours
Others			
Pramlintide (Symlin)	5 mL vial containing 0.6 mg/mL (subcutaneous injection)	For insulin-treated type 2 patients, start at 60 mcg dose three times a day (10 units on U100 insulin syringe). Increase to 120 mcg three times a day (20 units on U100 insulin syringe) if no nausea for 3–7 days. Give immediately before meal.	
		For type 1 patients, start at 15 mcg three times a day (2.5 units on U100 insulin syringe) and increase by increments of 15 mcg to a maximum of 60 mcg three times a day, as tolerated.	
		To avoid hypoglycemia, lower insulin dose by 50% on initiation of therapy.	

Table 27. Insulin preparations available in the United States.[1]

Rapidly acting human insulin analogs
  Insulin lispro (Humalog, Lilly)
  Insulin aspart (Novolog, Novo Nordisk)
  Insulin glulisine (Apidra, Sanofi Aventis)
Short-acting regular insulin
  Regular insulin (Lilly, Novo Nordisk)
Intermediate-acting insulins
  NPH insulin (Lilly, Novo Nordisk)
Premixed insulins
  70% NPH/30% regular (70/30 insulin—Lilly, Novo Nordisk)
  50% NPH/50% regular (50/50 insulin—Lilly)
  70% NPL/25% insulin lispro (Humalog Mix 75/25—Lilly)
  50% NPL/50% insulin lispro (Humalog Mix 50/50—Lilly)
  70% insulin aspart protamine/30% insulin aspart (Novolog Mix 70/3—Novo Nordisk)
Long-acting human insulin analogs
  Insulin glargine (Lantus, Sanofi Aventis)
  Insulin detemir (Levemir, Novo Nordisk)

[1]All insulins available in the United States are recombinant human or human insulin analog origin. All the insulins are dispensed at U100 concentration. There is an additional U500 preparation of regular insulin.
NPH, neutral protamine Hagedorn.

Table 28. Examples of intensive insulin regimens using rapidly acting insulin analogs (insulin lispro, aspart, or glulisine) and insulin detemir, or insulin glargine in a 70-kg man with type 1 diabetes.[1–3]

	Pre-Breakfast	Pre-Lunch	Pre-Dinner	At Bedtime
Rapidly acting insulin analog	5 units	4 units	6 units	—
Insulin detemir	6-7 units			8-9 units
OR				
Rapidly acting insulin analog	5 units	4 units	6 units	—
Insulin glargine	—	—	—	15-16 units

[1]Assumes that patient is consuming approximately 75 g carbohydrate at breakfast, 60 g at lunch, and 90 g at dinner.
[2]The dose of rapidly acting insulin can be raised by 1 or 2 units if extra carbohydrate (15–30 g) is ingested or if premeal blood glucose is > 170 mg/dL.
[3]Insulin glargine or insulin detemir must be given as a separate injection.

Table 29. Total body water (as percentage of body weight) in relation to age and sex.

Age	Male	Female
18–40	60%	50%
41–60	60–50%	50–40%
Over 60	50%	40%

Table 30. Causes of hyperkalemia.

Spurious
  Leakage from erythrocytes when separation of serum from clot is delayed (plasma K^+ normal)
  Marked thrombocytosis or leukocytosis with release of intracellular K^+ (plasma K^+ normal)
  Repeated fist clenching during phlebotomy, with release of K^+ from forearm muscles
  Specimen drawn from arm with intravenous K^+ infusion
Decreased excretion
  Kidney disease, acute and chronic
  Renal secretory defects (may or may not have frank renal failure): kidney transplant, interstitial nephritis, systemic lupus erythematosus, sickle cell disease, amyloidosis, obstructive nephropathy
  Hyporeninemic hypoaldosteronism (often in diabetic patients with mild to moderate nephropathy) or selective hypoaldosteronism (some patients with AIDS)
  Drugs that inhibit potassium excretion: spironolactone, eplerenone, drospirenone, NSAIDs, ACE inhibitors, angiotensin II receptor blockers, triamterene, amiloride, trimethoprim, pentamidine, cyclosporine, tacrolimus)
Shift of K^+ from within the cell
  Massive release of intracellular K^+ in burns, rhabdomyolysis, hemolysis, severe infection, internal bleeding, vigorous exercise
  Metabolic acidosis (in the case of organic acid accumulation—eg, lactic acidosis—a shift of K^+ does not occur since organic acid can easily move across the cell membrane)
  Hypertonicity (solvent drag)
  Insulin deficiency (metabolic acidosis may not be apparent)
  Hyperkalemic periodic paralysis
  Drugs: succinylcholine, arginine, digitalis toxicity, β-adrenergic antagonists
  α-Adrenergic stimulation?
Excessive intake of K^+
  Especially in patients taking medications that decrease potassium secretion (see above)

ACE, angiotensin-converting enzyme; NSAIDs, nonsteroidal anti-inflammatory drugs.

Table 31. Primary acid-base disorders and expected compensation.

Disorder	Primary Defect	Compensatory Response	Magnitude of Compensation
Respiratory acidosis			
Acute	$\uparrow Pco_2$	$\uparrow HCO_3^-$	$\uparrow HCO_3^-$ 1 mEq/L per 10 mm Hg $\uparrow Pco_2$
Chronic	$\uparrow Pco_2$	$\uparrow HCO_3^-$	$\uparrow HCO_3^-$ 3.5 mEq/L per 10 mm Hg $\uparrow Pco_2$
Respiratory alkalosis			
Acute	$\downarrow Pco_2$	$\downarrow HCO_3^-$	$\downarrow HCO_3^-$ 2 mEq/L per 10 mm Hg $\downarrow Pco_2$
Chronic	$\downarrow Pco_2$	$\downarrow HCO_3^-$	$\downarrow HCO_3^-$ 5 mEq/L per 10 mm Hg $\downarrow Pco_2$
Metabolic acidosis	$\downarrow HCO_3^-$	$\downarrow Pco_2$	$\downarrow Pco_2$ 1.3 mm Hg per 1 mEq/L $\downarrow HCO_3^-$
Metabolic alkalosis	$\uparrow HCO_3^-$	$\uparrow Pco_2$	$\uparrow Pco_2$ 0.7 mm Hg per 1 mEq/L $\uparrow HCO_3^-$

Table 32. Hyperchloremic, normal anion gap metabolic acidoses.

	Renal Defect	Serum [K+]	Distal H+ Secretion — Urinary NH_4^+ Plus Minimal Urine pH	Distal H+ Secretion — Titratable Acid	Urinary Anion Gap	Treatment
Gastrointestinal HCO_3^- loss	None	$\downarrow$	< 5.5	$\uparrow\uparrow$	Negative	Na^+, K^+, and HCO_3^- as required
Renal tubular acidosis						
I. Classic distal	Distal H^+ secretion	$\downarrow$	> 5.5	$\downarrow$	Positive	$NaHCO_3$ (1–3 mEq/kg/d)
II. Proximal secretion	Proximal H^+	$\downarrow$	< 5.5	Normal	Positive	$NaHCO_3$ or $KHCO_3$ (10–15 mEq/kg/d), thiazide
IV. Hyporeninemic hypoaldosteronism	Distal Na^+ reabsorption, K^+ secretion, and H^+ secretion	$\uparrow$	< 5.5	$\downarrow$	Positive	Fludrocortisone (0.1–0.5 mg/d), dietary K^+ restriction, furosemide (40–160 mg/d), $NaHCO_3$ (1–3 mEq/kg/d)

Modified and reproduced, with permission, from Cogan MG. *Fluid and Electrolytes: Physiology and Pathophysiology*. McGraw-Hill, 1991.

Table 33. Metabolic alkalosis.

Saline-Responsive (U_{Cl} < 10 mEq/d)	Saline-Unresponsive (U_{Cl} > 10 mEq/d)
Excessive body bicarbonate content	**Excessive body bicarbonate content**
Renal alkalosis	Renal alkalosis
Diuretic therapy	Normotensive
Poorly reabsorbable anion therapy: carbenicillin, penicillin, sulfate, phosphate	Bartter syndrome (renal salt wasting and secondary hyperaldosteronism)
Posthypercapnia	Severe potassium depletion
Gastrointestinal alkalosis	Refeeding alkalosis
Loss of HCl from vomiting or nasogastric suction	Hypercalcemia and hypoparathyroidism
Intestinal alkalosis: chloride diarrhea	Hypertensive
Exogenous alkali	Endogenous mineralocorticoids
$NaHCO_3$ (baking soda)	Primary aldosteronism
Sodium citrate, lactate, gluconate, acetate	Hyperreninism
Transfusions	Adrenal enzyme deficiency: 11- and 17-hydroxylase
Antacids	Liddle syndrome
Normal body bicarbonate content	Exogenous mineralocorticoids
"Contraction alkalosis"	Licorice

Modified and reproduced, with permission, from Narins RG et al. Diagnostic strategies in disorders of fluid, electrolyte and acid-base homeostasis. Am J Med. 1982 Mar;72(3):496–520.

Table 34. Vitamin D preparations used in the treatment of hypoparathyroidism.

	Available Preparations	Daily Dose	Duration of Action
Ergocalciferol ergosterol, (vitamin D₂, Calciferol)	Capsules of 50,000 international units; 8000 international units/mL oral solution	2000–200,000 units	1–2 weeks
Cholecalciferol (vitamin D₃)	Capsules of 50,000 international units not available commercially in United States; may be compounded	10,000–50,000 units	4–8 weeks
Calcitriol (Rocaltrol)	Capsules of 0.25 and 0.5 mcg; 1 mcg/mL oral solution; 1 mcg/mL for injection	0.25–4 mcg	½–2 weeks

Table 35. Diagnostic criteria of different types of hypercalciuria.

	Absorptive Type I	Absorptive Type II	Absorptive Type III	Resorptive	Renal
Serum					
Calcium	N	N	N	↑	N
Phosphorus	N	N	↓	↓	N
PTH	N	N	N	↑	↑
Vitamin D	N	N	↑	↑	↑
Urinary calcium					
Fasting	N	N	↑	↑	↑
Restricted	↑	N	↑	↑	↑
After calcium load	↑	↑	↑	↑	↑

PTH, parathyroid hormone; ↑, elevated; ↓, low; N, normal.

Table 36. Causes of nausea and vomiting.

Visceral afferent stimulation	**Infections**
	Mechanical obstruction
	    Gastric outlet obstruction: peptic ulcer disease, malignancy, gastric volvulus
	    Small intestinal obstruction: adhesions, hernias, volvulus, Crohn disease, carcinomatosis
	Dysmotility
	    Gastroparesis: diabetic, medications (metformin, acarbose, pramlintide, exenatide), postviral, postvagotomy
	    Small intestine: scleroderma, amyloidosis, chronic intestinal pseudo-obstruction, familial myoneuropathies
	Peritoneal irritation
	    Peritonitis: perforated viscus, appendicitis, spontaneous bacterial peritonitis
	    Viral gastroenteritis: Norwalk agent, rotavirus
	    "Food poisoning": toxins from *Bacillus cereus*, *Staphylococcus aureus*, *Clostridium perfringens*
	    Hepatitis A or B
	    Acute systemic infections
	Hepatobiliary or pancreatic disorders
	    Acute pancreatitis
	    Cholecystitis or choledocholithiasis
	Topical gastrointestinal irritants
	    Alcohol, NSAIDs, oral antibiotics
	Postoperative
	Other
	    Cardiac disease: acute myocardial infarction, congestive heart failure
	    Urologic disease: stones, pyelonephritis

CNS disorders	**Vestibular disorders**
	    Labyrinthitis, Meniere syndrome, motion sickness, migraine
	Increased intracranial pressure
	    CNS tumors, subdural or subarachnoid hemorrhage
	Migraine
	Infections
	    Meningitis, encephalitis
	Psychogenic
	    Anticipatory vomiting, bulimia, psychiatric disorders

Irritation of chemoreceptor trigger zone	**Antitumor chemotherapy**
	Drugs and medications
	    Calcium channel blockers
	    Opioids
	    Anticonvulsants
	    Antiparkinsonism drugs
	    β-blockers, antiarrhythmics, digoxin
	    Nicotine
	    Oral contraceptives
	    Cholinesterase inhibitors
	Radiation therapy
	Systemic disorders
	    Diabetic ketoacidosis
	    Uremia
	    Adrenocortical crisis
	    Parathyroid disease
	    Hypothyroidism
	    Pregnancy
	    Paraneoplastic syndrome

NSAIDs, nonsteroidal anti-inflammatory drugs; CNS, central nervous system.

Table 37. Common antiemetic dosing regimens.

	Dosage	Route
Serotonin 5-HT₃ antagonists		
Ondansetron	Doses vary: 8 mg once or twice daily to 24–32 mg once daily	IV
	8 mg twice daily	PO
Granisetron	1 mg or 0.01 mg/kg once daily	IV
	2 mg once daily	PO
Dolasetron	100 mg or 1.8 mg/kg once daily	IV
	100 mg once daily	PO
Palonosetron	0.25 mg once as a single dose 30 min before start of chemotherapy	IV
Corticosteroids		
Dexamethasone	8–20 mg once daily	IV
	4–20 mg once or twice daily	PO
Methylprednisolone	40–100 mg once daily	IV
Dopamine receptor antagonists		
Metoclopramide	10–20 mg or 0.5 mg/kg every 6–8 hours	IV
	10–20 mg every 6–8 hours	PO
Prochlorperazine	5–10 mg every 4–6 hours	PO, IM, IV
	25 mg suppository every 6 hours	PR
Promethazine	25 mg every 4–6 hours	PO, PR, IM, IV
Trimethobenzamide	250 mg every 6–8 hours	PO
	200 mg every 6–8 hours	IM, PR
Sedatives		
Diazepam	2–5 mg every 4–6 hours	PO, IV
Lorazepam	1–2 mg every 4–6 hours	PO, IV

IV, intravenously; PO, orally; IM, intramuscularly; PR, per rectum.

Table 38. Causes of ascites.

Normal Peritoneum

Portal hypertension (SAAG ≥ 1.1 g/dL)
1. Hepatic congestion[1]
    Congestive heart failure
    Constrictive pericarditis
    Tricuspid insufficiency
    Budd-Chiari syndrome
    Veno-occlusive disease
2. Liver disease[2]
    Cirrhosis
    Alcoholic hepatitis
    Fulminant hepatic failure
    Massive hepatic metastases
    Hepatic fibrosis
    Acute fatty liver of pregnancy
3. Portal vein occlusion

Hypoalbuminemia (SAAG < 1.1 g/dL)
    Nephrotic syndrome
    Protein-losing enteropathy
    Severe malnutrition with anasarca

Miscellaneous conditions (SAAG < 1.1 g/dL)
    Chylous ascites
    Pancreatic ascites
    Bile ascites
    Nephrogenic ascites
    Urine ascites
    Myxedema (SAAG ≥ 1.1 g/dL)
    Ovarian disease

Diseased Peritoneum (SAAG < 1.1 g/dL)[2]

Infections
    Bacterial peritonitis
    Tuberculous peritonitis
    Fungal peritonitis
    HIV-associated peritonitis

Malignant conditions
    Peritoneal carcinomatosis
    Primary mesothelioma
    Pseudomyxoma peritonei
    Massive hepatic metastases
    Hepatocellular carcinoma

Other conditions
    Familial Mediterranean fever
    Vasculitis
    Granulomatous peritonitis
    Eosinophilic peritonitis

[1]Hepatic congestion usually associated with SAAG ≥ 1.1 g/dL and ascitic fluid total protein > 2.5 g/dL.
[2]There may be cases of "mixed ascites" in which portal hypertensive ascites is complicated by a secondary process such as infection. In these cases, the SAAG is ≥ 1.1 g/dL.
SAAG, serum-ascites albumin gradient.

Table 39. Treatment options for peptic ulcer disease.

Active *Helicobacter pylori*-associated ulcer

1. Treat with anti-*H pylori* regimen for 10–14 days. Treatment options:

   - Proton pump inhibitor orally twice daily[1,]
     Clarithromycin 500 mg orally twice daily[2]
     Amoxicillin 1 g orally twice daily (OR metronidazole 500 mg orally twice daily, if penicillin allergic[3])

   - Proton pump inhibitor orally twice daily[1,4]
     Bismuth subsalicylate two tablets orally four times daily
     Tetracycline 500 mg orally four times daily
     Metronidazole 250 mg orally four times daily
     (OR bismuth subcitrate potassium 140 mg/metronidazole 125 mg/tetracycline 125 mg [Pylera] three capsules orally four times daily)[5]

   - Proton pump inhibitor orally twice daily[1,6]
     Days 1–5: amoxicillin 1 g orally twice daily
     Days 6–10: clarithromycin 500 mg and metronidazole 500 mg, both orally twice daily

2. After completion of course of *H pylori* eradication therapy, continue treatment with proton pump inhibitor[1] once daily for 4–6 weeks if ulcer is large (> 1 cm) or complicated.

3. Confirm successful eradication of *H pylori* with urea breath test, fecal antigen test, or endoscopy with biopsy at least 4 weeks after completion of antibiotic treatment and 1–2 weeks after proton pump inhibitor treatment.

Active ulcer not attributable to *H pylori*

1. Consider other causes: NSAIDs, Zollinger-Ellison syndrome, gastric malignancy. Treatment options:

   - Proton pump inhibitors[1]:
     Uncomplicated duodenal ulcer: treat for 4 weeks
     Uncomplicated gastric ulcer: treat for 8 weeks

   - H_2-receptor antagonists:
     Uncomplicated duodenal ulcer: cimetidine 800 mg, ranitidine or nizatidine 300 mg, famotidine 40 mg, orally once daily at bedtime for 6 weeks
     Uncomplicated gastric ulcer: cimetidine 400 mg, ranitidine or nizatidine 150 mg, famotidine 20 mg, orally twice daily for 8 weeks
     Complicated ulcers: proton pump inhibitors are the preferred drugs

Prevention of ulcer relapse

1. NSAID-induced ulcer: prophylactic therapy for high-risk patients (prior ulcer disease or ulcer complications, use of corticosteroids or anticoagulants, age > 60 years, serious comorbid illnesses).

   Treatment options:

   Proton pump inhibitor once daily[1]
   COX-2 selective NSAID (celecoxib) (contraindicated in patients with increased risk of cardiovascular disease)
   Misoprostol 200 mcg orally 4 times daily

2. Long-term "maintenance" therapy indicated in patients with recurrent ulcers who either are *H pylori*-negative or who have failed attempts at eradication therapy: once-daily oral proton pump inhibitor[1] or oral H_2-receptor antagonist at bedtime (cimetidine 400–800 mg, nizatidine or ranitidine 150–300 mg, famotidine 20–40 mg)

[1]Oral proton pump inhibitors: omeprazole 20 mg, rabeprazole 20 mg, lansoprazole 30 mg, pantoprazole 40 mg, esomeprazole 40 mg. Proton pump inhibitors are administered before meals. Esomeprazole may be given as 40 mg orally once daily.
[2]If patient has previously been treated with macrolide antibiotic, choose another regimen.
[3]Avoid in areas of known high metronidazole resistance or in patients who have failed a course of treatment that included metronidazole.
[4]Preferred regimen in patients who have previously received a macrolide antibiotic or are penicillin allergic. Effective against metronidazole-resistant organisms.
[5]Pylera is an FDA-approved formulation containing: bismuth subcitrate 140 mg/tetracycline 125 mg/metronidazole 125 mg per capsule.
[6]Regimen requires validation in U.S. studies. Appears effective against clarithromycin-resistant organisms.
NSAIDs, nonsteroidal anti-inflammatory drugs; COX-2, cyclooxygenase-2.

Table 40. Staging of colorectal cancer.

Joint Committee Classification		TNM		Dukes Class[1]
Stage 0				
Carcinoma in situ		N0	M0	
Stage I				
Tumor invades submucosa	T1	N0	M0	Dukes A
Tumor invades muscularis propria	T2	N0	M0	Dukes B_1
Stage II				
Tumor invades into subserosa or into nonperitonealized pericolic or perirectal tissues	T3	N0	M0	Dukes B_1 or B_2
Tumor perforates the visceral peritoneum or directly invades other organs or structures	T4	N0	M0	Dukes B_2
Stage III				
Any degree of bowel wall perforation with lymph node metastasis				
One to three pericolic or perirectal lymph nodes involved	Any T	N1	M0	Dukes C_1
Four or more pericolic or perirectal lymph nodes involved	Any T	N2	M0	Dukes C_2
Metastasis to lymph nodes along a vascular trunk	Any T	N3	M0	
Stage IV				
Presence of distant metastasis	Any T	Any N	M1	Dukes D

[1]Gastrointestinal Tumor Study Group modification of Dukes classification.

Table 41. Recommendations for colorectal cancer screening.[1]

Average-risk individuals ≥ 50 years old[2]
 Annual fecal occult blood testing
 Flexible sigmoidoscopy every 5 years
 Annual fecal occult blood testing and flexible sigmoidoscopy every 5 years
 Colonoscopy every 10 years
 Double-contrast barium enema every 5 years
Individuals with a family history of a first-degree member with colorectal neoplasia[3]
Single first-degree relative with colorectal cancer diagnosed at age ≥ 60 years: Begin screening at age 40. Screening guidelines same as average-risk individual; however, preferred method is colonoscopy every 10 years.
Single first-degree relative with colorectal cancer diagnosed at age < 60 years, or multiple first-degree relatives: Begin screening at age 40 or at age 10 years younger than age at diagnosis of the youngest affected relative, whichever is first in time. Recommended screening: colonoscopy every 5 years.

[1]For recommendations for families with inherited polyposis syndromes or hereditary nonpolyposis colon cancer, see Colorectal Cancer.
[2]Colorectal cancer screening and surveillance: clinical guidelines and rationale. Gastroenterology. 2003 Feb;124(2):544–60.
[3]Screening Recommendations of American College of Gastroenterology. Am J Gastroenterol. 2000 Apr;95(4):868–77.

Table 42. Some of the "unsafe" and "probably safe" drugs used in the treatment of acute porphyrias.

Unsafe	Probably Safe
Alcohol	Acetaminophen
Alkylating agents	β-Adrenergic blockers
Barbiturates	Amitriptyline
Carbamazepine	Aspirin
Chloroquine	Atropine
Chlorpropamide	Chloral hydrate
Clonidine	Chlordiazepoxide
Dapsone	Corticosteroids
Ergots	Diazepam
Erythromycin	Digoxin
Estrogens, synthetic	Diphenhydramine
Food additives	Guanethidine
Glutethimide	Hyoscine
Griseofulvin	Ibuprofen
Hydralazine	Imipramine
Ketamine	Insulin
Meprobamate	Lithium
Methyldopa	Naproxen
Metoclopramide	Nitrofurantoin
Nortriptyline	Opioid analgesics
Pentazocine	Penicillamine
Phenytoin	Penicillin and derivatives
Progestins	Phenothiazines
Pyrazinamide	Procaine
Rifampin	Streptomycin
Spironolactone	Succinylcholine
Succinimides	Tetracycline
Sulfonamides	Thiouracil
Theophylline	
Tolazamide	
Tolbutamide	
Valproic acid	

Table 43. Yesavage Geriatric Depression Scale (short form).

1. Are you basically satisfied with your life? (no)
2. Have you dropped many of your activities and interests? (yes)
3. Do you feel that your life is empty? (yes)
4. Do you often get bored? (yes)
5. Are you in good spirits most of the time? (no)
6. Are you afraid that something bad is going to happen to you? (yes)
7. Do you feel happy most of the time? (no)
8. Do you often feel helpless? (yes)
9. Do you prefer to stay home at night, rather than go out and do new things? (yes)
10. Do you feel that you have more problems with memory than most? (yes)
11. Do you feel it is wonderful to be alive now? (no)
12. Do you feel pretty worthless the way you are now? (yes)
13. Do you feel full of energy? (no)
14. Do you feel that your situation is hopeless? (yes)
15. Do you think that most persons are better off than you are? (yes)

Score one point for each response that matches the yes or no answer after the question.
Key: Scores: 3 ± 2 = normal; 7 ± 3 = mildly depressed; 12 ± 2 = very depressed.

Table 44. Treatment of pressure ulcers.

Ulcer Type	Dressing Type and Considerations
Stage I	Polyurethane film Hydrocolloid wafer Semipermeable foam dressing
Stage II	Hydrocolloid wafers Semipermeable foam dressing Polyurethane film
Stage III/IV	For highly exudative wounds, use highly absorptive dressing or packing, such as calcium alginate Wounds with necrotic debris must be debrided Debridement can be autolytic, mechanical (wet to moist), or surgical Shallow, clean wounds can be dressed with hydrocolloid wafers, semipermeable foam, or polyurethane Deep wounds can be packed with gauze; if the wound is deep and highly exudative, an absorptive packing should be used
Heel ulcer	Do not remove eschar on heel ulcers because it can help promote healing (eschar in other locations should be debrided)

Table 45. Classification systems for Papanicolaou smears.

Numerical	Dysplasia	CIN	Bethesda System
1	Benign	Benign	Normal
2	Benign with inflammation	Benign with inflammation	Normal, ASC-US
3	Mild dysplasia	CIN I	Low-grade SIL
3	Moderate dysplasia	CIN II	High-grade SIL
3	Severe dysplasia	CIN III	
4	Carcinoma in situ		
5	Invasive cancer	Invasive cancer	Invasive cancer

CIN, cervical intraepithelial neoplasia; ASC-US, atypical squamous cells of undetermined significance; SIL, squamous intraepithelial lesion.

Table 46. FIGO[1] staging of cancer of the cervix.

Preinvasive carcinoma	
Stage 0	Carcinoma in situ.
Invasive carcinoma	
Stage I	Carcinoma strictly confined to the cervix.
IA	Invasive cancer diagnosed only by microscopy.
	IA1 Measured invasion of stroma no greater than 3 mm in depth and no wider than 7 mm.
	IA2 Measured invasion of stroma greater than 3 mm in depth and no greater than 5 mm in depth and no wider than 7 mm.
IB	Clinical lesions confined to the cervix or preclinical lesions greater than 1A. All gross lesions, even with superficial invasion, are stage IB.
	IB1 Clinical lesions no greater than 4 cm.
	IB2 Clinical lesions greater than 4 cm.
Stage II	Carcinoma extends beyond the cervix but has not extended to the pelvic wall. The carcinoma involves the vagina but not as far as the lower third.
IIA	No obvious parametrial involvement.
IIB	Obvious parametrial involvement.
Stage III	Carcinoma has extended either to the lower third of the vagina or to the pelvic sidewall. All cases of hydronephrosis.
IIIA	Involvement of lower third of vagina. No extension to pelvic sidewall.
IIIB	Extension onto the pelvic wall and/or hydronephrosis or nonfunctioning kidney.
Stage IV	Carcinoma extended beyond the true pelvis or clinically involving the mucosa of the bladder or rectum.
IVA	Spread of growth to adjacent organs.
IVB	Spread of growth to distant organs.

[1]International Federation of Gynecology and Obstetrics.

Table 47. Ovarian functional and neoplastic tumors.

Tumor	Incidence	Size	Consistency	Menstrual Irregularities	Endocrine Effects	Potential for Malignancy	Special Remarks
Follicle cysts	Rare in childhood; frequent in menstrual years; never in postmenopausal years.	< 6 cm, often bilateral.	Moderate	Occasional	Occasional anovulation with persistently proliferative endometrium	None	Usually disappear spontaneously within 2–3 months.
Corpus luteum cysts	Occasional, in menstrual years.	4–6 cm, unilateral.	Moderate	Occasional delayed period	Prolonged secretory phase	None	Functional cysts. Intraperitoneal bleeding occasionally.
Theca lutein cysts	Occurs with hydatidiform mole, choriocarcinoma; also with gonadotropin or clomiphene therapy.	To 4–5 cm, multiple, bilateral. (Ovaries may be ≥ 20 cm in diameter.)	Tense	Amenorrhea	hCG elevated as a result of trophoblastic proliferation	None	Functional cysts. Hematoperitoneum or torsion of ovary may occur. Surgery is to be avoided.
Inflammatory (tubo-ovarian abscess)	Concomitant with acute salpingitis.	To 15–20 cm, often bilateral.	Variable, painful	Menometrorrhagia	Anovulation usual	None	Unilateral removal indicated if possible.
Endometriotic cysts	Never in preadolescent or postmenopausal years. Most common in women aged 20–40 years.	To 10–12 cm, occasionally bilateral.	Moderate to softened	Rare	None	Very rare	Associated pelvic endometriosis. Medical treatment or conservative surgery recommended.
Teratoid tumors:							
Benign teratomas (dermoid cysts)	Childhood to postmenopause.	< 15 cm; 15% are bilateral.	Moderate to softened	None	None	Rare	Torsion can occur. Partial oophorectomy recommended.
Malignant teratomas	< 1% of ovarian tumors. Usually in infants and young adults.	> 20 cm, unilateral.	Irregularly firm	None	Occasionally, hCG elevated	All	Surgery alone may be curative.
Cystadenoma, cyst-adenocarcinoma	Common in reproductive years.	Serous: < 25 cm, 33% bilateral; mucinous: up to 1 cm, 10% bilateral.	Moderate to softened	None	None	> 50% for serous, about 5% for mucinous	Peritoneal implants often occur with serous, rarely with mucinous. If mucinous tumor is ruptured, pseudomyxoma peritonei may occur.
Endometrioid carcinoma	15% of ovarian carcinomas.	Moderate, 13% bilateral.	Firm	None	None	All	Adenocarcinoma of endometrium coexists in 15–30% of cases.
Fibroma	< 5% of ovarian tumors.	Usually < 15 cm.	Very firm	None	None	Rare	Ascites in 20% (rarely, pleural fluid).
Arrhenoblastoma	Rare. Average age 30 years or more.	Often small (< 10 cm), unilateral.	Firm to softened	Amenorrhea	Androgens elevated	< 20%	Recurrences are moderately sensitive to irradiation.
Theca cell tumor (thecoma)	Uncommon.	< 10 cm, unilateral.	Firm	Occasional irregularity	Estrogens or androgens elevated	< 1%	
Granulosa cell tumor	Uncommon. Usually in prepubertal girls or women older than 50 years.	May be very small.	Firm to softened	Menometrorrhagia	Estrogens elevated	15–20%	Recurrences are moderately sensitive to irradiation.
Dysgerminoma	About 1–2% of ovarian tumors.	< 30 cm, bilateral in 33%.	Moderate to softened	None	—	All	Very radiosensitive.
Brenner tumor	About 1% of ovarian tumors.	< 30 cm, unilateral.	Firm	None	—	Very rare	> 50% occur in postmenopausal years.
Secondary ovarian tumors	10% of fatal malignant disease in women.	Varies; often bilateral.	Firm to softened	Occasional	Very rare (thyroid, adrenocortical origin)	All	Bowel or breast metastases to ovary common.

Table 48. TNM staging for breast cancer.

Primary Tumor (T)	
Definitions for classifying the primary tumor (T) are the same for clinical and for pathologic classification. If the measurement is made by physical examination, the examiner will use the major headings (T1, T2, or T3). If other measurements, such as mammographic or pathologic measurements, are used, the subsets of T1 can be used. Tumors should be measured to the nearest 0.1 cm increment.	
TX	Primary tumor cannot be assessed
T0	No evidence of primary tumor
Tis	Carcinoma in situ
Tis (DCIS)	Ductal carcinoma in situ
Tis (LCIS)	Lobular carcinoma in situ
Tis (Paget)	Paget disease of the nipple with no tumor
Note: Paget disease associated with a tumor is classified according to the size of the tumor.	
T1	Tumor 2 cm or less in greatest dimension
T1mic	Microinvasion 0.1 cm or less in greatest dimension
T1a	Tumor more than 0.1 cm but not more than 0.5 cm in greatest dimension
T1b	Tumor more than 0.5 cm but not more than 1 cm in greatest dimension
T1c	Tumor more than 1 cm but not more than 2 cm in greatest dimension
T2	Tumor more than 2 cm but not more than 5 cm in greatest dimension
T3	Tumor more than 5 cm in greatest dimension
T4	Tumor of any size with direct extension to (a) chest wall or (b) skin, only as described below
T4a	Extension to chest wall, not including petoralis muscle
T4b	Edema (including peau d'orange) or ulceration of the skin of the breast, or satellite skin nodules confined to the same breast
T4c	Both T4a and T4b
T4d	Inflammatory carcinoma
Regional lymph nodes (N)	
Clinical	
NX	Regional lymph nodes cannot be assessed (eg, previously removed)
N0	No regional lymph node metastasis
N1	Metastasis to movable ipsilateral axillary lymph node(s)
N2	Metastases in ipsilateral axillary lymph nodes fixed or matted, or in clinically apparent ipsilateral internal mammary nodes in the *absence* of clinically evident axillary lymph node metastasis

N2a	Metastasis in ipsilateral axillary lymph nodes fixed to one another (matted) or to other structures
N2b	Metastasis only in clinically apparent[1] ipsilateral internal mammary nodes and in the *absence* of clinically evident axillary lymph node metastasis
N3	Metastasis in ipsilateral infraclavicular lymph node(s) with or without axillary lymph node involvement, or in clinically apparent[1] ipsilateral internal mammary lymph node(s) and in the *presence* of clinically evident axillary lymph node metastasis; or metastasis in ipsilateral supraclavicular lymph node(s) with or without axillary or internal mammary lymph node involvement
N3a	Metastasis in ipsilateral infraclavicular lymph node(s)
N3b	Metastasis in ipsilateral internal mammary lymph node(s) and axillary lymph node(s)
N3c	Metastasis in ipsilateral supraclavicular lymph node(s)
Pathologic (pN)[2]	
pNX	Regional lymph nodes cannot be assessed (eg, previously removed, or not removed for pathologic study)
pN0	No regional lymph node metastasis histologically, no additional examination for isolated tumor cells
Note: Isolated tumor cells (ITC) are defined as single tumor cells or small cell clusters not greater than 0.2 mm, usually detected only by immunohistochemical (IHC) or molecular methods but which may be verified on hematoxylin and eosin stains. ITCs do not usually show evidence of malignant activity, eg, proliferation or stromal reaction.	
pN0(i-)	No regional lymph node metastasis histologically, negative IHC
pN0(i+)	No regional lymph node metastasis histologically, positive IHC, no IHC cluster greater than 0.2 mm
pN0(mol-)	No regional lymph node metastasis histologically, negative molecular findings (RT-PCR)
pN0(mol+)	No regional lymph node metastasis histologically, positive molecular findings (RT-PCR)
pN1	Metastasis in one to three axillary lymph nodes, and/or in internal mammary nodes with microscopic disease detected by sentinel lymph node dissection but not clinically apparent[1]
pN1mi	Micrometastasis (greater than 0.2 mm, none greater than 2.0 mm)
pN1a	Metastasis in one to three axillary lymph nodes
pN1b	Metastasis in internal mammary nodes with microscopic disease detected by sentinel lymph node dissection but not clinically apparent[1]
pN1c	Metastasis in one to three axillary lymph nodes and in internal mammary lymph nodes with microscopic disease detected by sentinel lymph node dissection but not clinically apparent.[1] (If associated with greater than three positive axillary lymph nodes, the internal mammary nodes are classified as pN3b to reflect increased tumor burden)

(continued)

Table 48. TNM staging for breast cancer. (continued)

		Distant metastasis (M)		
pN2	Metastasis in four to nine axillary lymph nodes, or in clinically apparent[1] internal mammary lymph nodes in the *absence* of axillary lymph node metastasis	MX	Distant metastasis cannot be assessed	
		M0	No distant metastasis	
pN2a	Metastasis in four to nine axillary lymph nodes (at least one tumor deposit greater than 2.0 mm)	M1	Distant metastasis	
pN2b	Metastasis in clinically apparent[1] internal mammary lymph nodes in the *absence* of axillary lymph node metastasis	**Stage grouping**		
		Stage 0	Tis	N0	M0
pN3	Metastasis in 10 or more axillary lymph nodes, or in infraclavicular lymph nodes, or in clinically apparent[1] ipsilateral internal mammary lymph nodes in the *presence* of one or more positive axillary lymph nodes; or in more than three axillary lymph nodes with clinically negative microscopic metastasis in internal mammary lymph nodes; or in ipsilateral supraclavicular lymph nodes	Stage 1	T1[3]	N0	M0

Stage grouping			
Stage 0	Tis	N0	M0
Stage 1	T1[3]	N0	M0
Stage IIA	T0	N1	M0
	T1[3]	N1	M0
	T2	N0	M0
Stage IIB	T2	N1	M0
	T3	N0	M0
Stage IIIA	T0	N2	M0
	T1[3]	N2	M0
	T2	N2	M0
	T3	N1	M0
	T3	N2	M0
Stage IIIB	T4	N0	M0
	T4	N1	M0
	T4	N2	M0
Stage IIIC	Any T	N3	M0
Stage IV	Any T	Any N	M1

pN3a	Metastasis in 10 or more axillary lymph nodes (at least one tumor deposit greater than 2.0 mm), or metastasis to the infraclavicular lymph nodes
pN3b	Metastasis in clinically apparent[1] ipsilateral internal mammary lymph nodes in the *presence* of one or more positive axillary lymph nodes; or in more than three axillary lymph nodes and in internal mammary lymph nodes with microscopic disease detected by sentinel lymph node dissection but not clinically apparent[1]
pN3c	Metastasis in ipsilateral supraclavicular lymph nodes

Note: Stage designation may be changed if postsurgical imaging studies reveal the presence of distant metastases, provided that the studies are carried out within 4 months of diagnosis in the absence of disease progression and provided that the patient has not received neoadjuvant therapy.

[1]*Clinically apparent* is defined as detected by imaging studies (excluding lymphoscintigraphy) or by clinical examination or grossly visible pathologically. *Not clinically apparent* is defined as not detected by imaging studies (excluding lymphoscintigraphy) or by clinical examination.
[2]Classification is based on axillary lymph node dissection with or without sentinel lymph node dissection. Classification based solely on sentinel lymph node dissection without subsequent axillary lymph node dissection is designated (sn) for "sentinel node," eg, pN0(i+)(sn).
[3]T1 includes T1mic.
RT-PCR, reverse transcriptase/polymerase chain reaction.
Reproduced, with permission, of the American Joint Committee on Cancer (AJCC), Chicago, Illinois. *AJCC Cancer Staging Manual*, 6th edition, Springer-Verlag, 2002. www.springeronline.com.

Table 49. Prognostic factors in node-negative breast cancer.

Prognostic Factors	Increased Recurrence	Decreased Recurrence
Size	T3, T2	T1, T0
Hormone receptors	Negative	Positive
DNA flow cytometry	Aneuploid	Diploid
Histologic grade	High	Low
Tumor labeling index	< 3%	> 3%
S phase fraction	> 5%	< 5%
Lymphatic or vascular invasion	Present	Absent
Cathepsin D	High	Low
HER-2/*neu* oncogene	High	Low
Epidermal growth factor receptor	High	Low

Table 50. Agents commonly used for hormonal management of metastatic breast cancer.

Drug	Action	Dose, Route, Frequency	Major Side Effects
Tamoxifen citrate (Nolvadex)	SERM	20 mg orally daily	Hot flushes, uterine bleeding, thrombophlebitis, rash
Fulvestrant (Faslodex)	Steroidal estrogen receptor antagonist	250 mg intramuscularly monthly	Gastrointestinal upset, headache, back pain, hot flushes, pharyngitis
Toremifene citrate (Fareston)	SERM	40 mg orally daily	Hot flushes, sweating, nausea, vaginal discharge, dry eyes, dizziness
Diethylstilbestrol (DES)	Estrogen	5 mg orally three times daily	Fluid retention, uterine bleeding, thrombophlebitis, nausea
Goserelin (Zoladex)	Synthetic luteinizing hormone releasing analogue	3.6 mg subcutaneously monthly	Arthralgias, blood pressure changes, hot flushes, headaches, vaginal dryness
Megestrol acetate (Megace)	Progestin	40 mg orally four times daily	Fluid retention
Letrozole (Femara)	AI	2.5 mg orally daily	Hot flushes, arthralgia/arthritis, myalgia
Anastrozole (Arimidex)	AI	1 mg orally daily	Hot flushes, skin rashes, nausea and vomiting
Exemestane (Aromasin)	AI	25 mg orally daily	Hot flushes, increased arthralgia/arthritis, myalgia, and alopecia

SERM, selective estrogen receptor modulator; AI, aromatase inhibitor.

Table 51. Approximate survival (%) of patients with breast cancer by TNM stage.

TNM Stage	Five Years	Ten Years
0	95	90
I	85	70
IIA	70	50
IIB	60	40
IIIA	55	30
IIIB	30	20
IV	5–10	2
All	65	30

Table 52. Commonly used low-dose oral contraceptives.

Name	Progestin	Estrogen (Ethinyl Estradiol)	Cost per Month[1]
COMBINATION			
Alesse[2,3]	0.1 mg levonorgestrel	20 mcg	$34.96
Loestrin 1/20[2]	1 mg norethindrone acetate	20 mcg	$28.60
Mircette[2]	0.15 mg desogestrel	20 mcg	$54.78
Yaz	3 mg drospirenone	20 mcg	$52.06
Loestrin 1.5/30[2]	1.5 mg norethindrone acetate	30 mcg	$28.94
Lo-Ovral[2]	0.3 mg norgestrel	30 mcg	$30.52
Levlen[2]	0.15 mg levonorgestrel	30 mcg	$30.93
Ortho-Cept[2] Desogen[2]	0.15 mg desogestrel	30 mcg	$30.52 $30.52
Yasmin	3 mg drospirenone	30 mcg	$52.06
Brevicon[2] Modicon[2]	0.5 mg norethindrone	35 mcg	$32.14 $32.14
Demulen 1/35[2]	1 mg ethynodiol diacetate	35 mcg	$29.88
Ortho-Novum 1/35[2]	1 mg norethindrone	35 mcg	$29.47
Ortho-Cyclen[2]	0.25 mg norgestimate	35 mcg	$34.10
Ovcon 35[2]	0.4 mg norethindrone	35 mcg	$44.84
COMBINATION: EXTENDED-CYCLE			
Seasonale	0.15 mg levonorgestrel	30 mcg	$66.30
Seasonique	0.15 mg levonorgestrel (days 1–84)/ 0 mg levonorgestrel (days 85–91)	30 mcg (84 days)/10 mcg (7 days)	$56.54
Lybrel	90 mcg levonorgestrel	20 mcg	$52.80
TRIPHASIC			
Estrostep	1.0 mg norethindrone acetate (days 1–5) 1.0 mg norethindrone acetate (days 6–12) 1.0 mg norethindrone acetate (days 13–21)	20 mcg 30 mcg 35 mcg	$59.06
Cyclessa[2]	0.1 mg desogestrel (days 1–7) 0.125 mg desogestrel (days 8–14) 0.15 mg desogestrel (days 15–21)	25 mcg	$57.67
Ortho-Tri-Cyclen Lo	0.18 norgestimate (days 1–7) 0.21 norgestimate (days 8–14) 0.25 norgestimate (days 15–21)	25 mcg	$53.29
Triphasil[2,3]	0.05 mg levonorgestrel (days 1–6) 0.075 mg levonorgestrel (days 7–11) 0.125 mg levonorgestrel (days 12–21)	30 mcg 40 mcg 30 mcg	$27.49
Ortho-Novum 7/7/7[2,3]	0.5 mg norethindrone (days 1–7) 0.75 mg norethindrone (days 8–14) 1 mg norethindrone (days 15–21)	35 mcg	$50.70
Ortho-Tri-Cyclen[2,3]	0.18 mg norgestimate (days 1–7) 0.215 mg norgestimate (days 8–14) 0.25 mg norgestimate (days 15–21)	35 mcg	$39.32
Tri-Norinyl[2,3]	0.5 mg norethindrone (days 1–7) 1 mg norethindrone (days 8–16) 0.5 mg norethindrone (days 17–21)	35 mcg	$48.34
PROGESTIN-ONLY MINIPILL			
Ortho Micronor[2,3]	0.35 mg norethindrone to be taken continuously	None	$36.92
Ovrette	0.075 mg norgestrel to be taken continuously	None	$37.54

[1]Average wholesale price (AWP, for AB-rated generic when available) for quantity listed. Source: *Red Book Update*, Vol. 27, No. 2, February 2008. AWP may not accurately represent the actual pharmacy cost because wide contractual variations exist among institutions.
[2]Generic equivalent available.
[3]Multiple other brands available.

Table 53. Contraindications to use of oral contraceptives.

Absolute contraindications
Pregnancy
Thrombophlebitis or thromboembolic disorders (past or present)
Stroke or coronary artery disease (past or present)
Cancer of the breast (known or suspected)
Undiagnosed abnormal vaginal bleeding
Estrogen-dependent cancer (known or suspected)
Benign or malignant tumor of the liver (past or present)
Uncontrolled hypertension
Diabetes mellitus with vascular disease
Age over 35 and smoking > 15 cigarettes daily
Known thrombophilia
Migraine with aura
Active hepatitis
Surgery or orthopedic injury requiring prolonged immobilization
Relative contraindications
Migraine without aura
Hypertension
Cardiac or renal disease
Diabetes mellitus
Gallbladder disease
Cholestasis during pregnancy
Sickle cell disease (S/S or S/C type)
Lactation

Table 54. Contraindications to IUD use.

Absolute contraindications
Pregnancy
Acute or subacute pelvic inflammatory disease or purulent cervicitis
Significant anatomic abnormality of uterus
Unexplained uterine bleeding
Active liver disease (Mirena only)
Relative contraindications
History of pelvic inflammatory disease since the last pregnancy
Lack of available follow-up care
Menorrhagia or severe dysmenorrhea (copper IUD)
Cervical or uterine neoplasia

IUD, intrauterine device.

Table 58. Treatment of AIDS-related opportunistic infections and malignancies.

Infection or Malignancy	Treatment	Complications
Pneumocystis jiroveci infection[1]	Trimethoprim-sulfamethoxazole, 15 mg/kg/d (based on trimethoprim component) orally or intravenously for 14–21 days.	Nausea, neutropenia, anemia, hepatitis, drug rash, Stevens-Johnson syndrome.
	Pentamidine, 3–4 mg/kg/d intravenously for 14–21 days.	Hypotension, hypoglycemia, anemia, neutropenia, pancreatitis, hepatitis.
	Trimethoprim, 15 mg/kg/d orally, with dapsone, 100 mg/d orally, for 14–21 days.[2]	Nausea, rash, hemolytic anemia in G6PD[2]-deficient patients. Methemoglobinemia (weekly levels should be < 10% of total hemoglobin).
	Primaquine, 15–30 mg/d orally, and clindamycin, 600 mg every 8 hours orally, for 14–21 days.	Hemolytic anemia in G6PD-deficient patients. Methemoglobinemia, neutropenia, colitis.
	Atovaquone, 750 mg orally three times daily for 14–21 days.	Rash, elevated aminotransferases, anemia, neutropenia.
	Trimetrexate, 45 mg/m^2 intravenously for 21 days (given with leucovorin calcium) if intolerant of all other regimens.	Leukopenia, rash, mucositis.
Mycobacterium avium complex infection	Clarithromycin, 500 mg orally twice daily with ethambutol, 15 mg/kg/d orally (maximum, 1 g). May also add:	Clarithromycin: hepatitis, nausea, diarrhea; ethambutol: hepatitis, optic neuritis.
	Rifabutin, 300 mg orally daily.	Rash, hepatitis, uveitis.
Toxoplasmosis	Pyrimethamine, 100–200 mg orally as loading dose, followed by 50–75 mg/d, combined with sulfadiazine, 4–6 g orally daily in four divided doses, and folinic acid, 10 mg daily for 4–8 weeks; then pyrimethamine, 25–50 mg/d, with clindamycin, 2–2.7 g/d in three or four divided doses, and folinic acid, 5 mg/d, until clinical and radiographic resolution is achieved.	Leukopenia, rash.
Lymphoma	Combination chemotherapy (eg, modified CHOP, M-BACOD, with or without G-CSF or GM-CSF). Central nervous system disease: radiation treatment with dexamethasone for edema.	Nausea, vomiting, anemia, leukopenia, cardiac toxicity (with doxorubicin).
Cryptococcal meningitis	Amphotericin B, 0.6 mg/kg/d intravenously, with or without flucytosine, 100 mg/kg/d orally in four divided doses for 2 weeks, followed by:	Fever, anemia, hypokalemia, azotemia.
	Fluconazole, 400 mg orally daily for 6 weeks, then 200 mg orally daily.	Hepatitis.
Cytomegalovirus infection	Valganciclovir, 900 mg orally twice a day for 21 days with food (induction), followed by 900 mg daily with food (maintenance).	Neutropenia, anemia, thrombocytopenia.
	Ganciclovir, 10 mg/kg/d intravenously in two divided doses for 10 days, followed by 6 mg/kg 5 days a week indefinitely. (Decrease dose for renal impairment.) May use ganciclovir as maintenance therapy (1 g orally with fatty foods three times a day).	Neutropenia (especially when used concurrently with zidovudine), anemia, thrombocytopenia.
	Foscarnet, 60 mg/kg intravenously every 8 hours for 10–14 days (induction), followed by 90 mg/kg once daily. (Adjust for changes in renal function.)	Nausea, hypokalemia, hypocalcemia, hyperphosphatemia, azotemia.
Esophageal candidiasis or recurrent vaginal candidiasis	Fluconazole, 100–200 mg orally daily for 10–14 days.	Hepatitis, development of imidazole resistance.
Herpes simplex infection	Acyclovir, 400 mg orally three times daily until healed; or acyclovir, 5 mg/kg intravenously every 8 hours for severe cases.	Resistant herpes simplex with chronic therapy.
	Famciclovir, 500 mg orally twice daily until healed.	Nausea.
	Valacyclovir, 500 mg orally twice daily until healed.	Nausea.
	Foscarnet, 40 mg/kg intravenously every 8 hours, for acyclovir-resistant cases. (Adjust for changes in renal function.)	See above.
Herpes zoster	Acyclovir, 800 mg orally four or five times daily for 7 days. Intravenous therapy at 10 mg/kg every 8 hours for ocular involvement, disseminated disease.	See above.
	Famciclovir, 500 mg orally three times daily for 7 days.	Nausea.
	Valacyclovir, 500 mg orally three times daily for 7 days.	Nausea.
	Foscarnet, 40 mg/kg intravenously every 8 hours for acyclovir-resistant cases. (Adjust for changes in renal function.)	See above.

(continued)

Table 58. Treatment of AIDS-related opportunistic infections and malignancies. (continued)

Infection or Malignancy	Treatment	Complications
Kaposi sarcoma		
Limited cutaneous disease	Observation, intralesional vinblastine.	Inflammation, pain at site of injection.
Extensive or aggressive cutaneous disease	Systemic chemotherapy (eg, liposomal doxorubicin). Interferon-α (for patients with CD4 > 200 cells/mcL and no constitutional symptoms). Radiation (amelioration of edema).	Bone marrow suppression, peripheral neuritis, flu-like syndrome.
Visceral disease (eg, pulmonary)	Combination chemotherapy (eg, daunorubicin, bleomycin, vinblastine).	Bone marrow suppression, cardiac toxicity, fever.

[1]For moderate to severe *P jiroveci* infection (oxygen saturation < 90%), corticosteroids should be given with specific treatment. The dose of prednisone is 40 mg orally twice daily for 5 days, then 40 mg daily for 5 days, and then 20 mg daily until therapy is complete.
[2]When considering use of dapsone, check glucose-6-phosphate dehydrogenase (G6PD) level in black patients and those of Mediterranean origin.
CHOP, cyclophosphamide, doxorubicin (hydroxydaunomycin), vincristine (Oncovin), and prednisone; modified M-BACOD, methotrexate, bleomycin, doxorubicin (Adriamycin), cyclophosphamide, vincristine (Oncovin), and dexamethasone; G-CSF, granulocyte-colony stimulating factor (filgrastim); GM-CSF, granulocyte-macrophage colony-stimulating factor (sargramostim).

Table 59. Antiretroviral therapy.

Drug	Dose	Common Side Effects	Special Monitoring[1]	Cost[2]	Cost/Month
Nucleoside reverse transcriptase inhibitors					
Zidovudine (AZT) (Retrovir)	600 mg orally daily in two divided doses	Anemia, neutropenia, nausea, malaise, headache, insomnia, myopathy	No special monitoring	$6.08/300 mg	$365.09
Didanosine (ddI) (Videx)	400 mg orally daily (enteric-coated capsule) for persons ≥ 60 kg	Peripheral neuropathy, pancreatitis, dry mouth, hepatitis	Bimonthly neurologic questionnaire for neuropathy, K⁺, amylase, bilirubin, triglycerides	$11.50/400 mg	$344.92
Zalcitabine (ddC) (Hivid)	0.375–0.75 mg orally three times daily	Peripheral neuropathy, aphthous ulcers, hepatitis	Monthly neurologic questionnaire for neuropathy	$2.73/0.75 mg	$245.70
Stavudine (d4T) (Zerit)	40 mg orally twice daily for persons ≥ 60 kg	Peripheral neuropathy, hepatitis, pancreatitis	Monthly neurologic questionnaire for neuropathy, amylase	$7.31/40 mg	$438.61
Lamivudine (3TC) (Epivir)	150 mg orally twice daily	Rash, peripheral neuropathy	No special monitoring	$6.45/150 mg	$386.93
Emtricitabine (Emtriva)	200 mg orally once daily	Skin discoloration palms/soles (mild)	No special monitoring	$12.30/200 mg	$368.93
Abacavir (Ziagen)	300 mg orally twice daily	Rash, fever—if occur, rechallenge may be fatal	No special monitoring	$8.67/300 mg	$519.92
Nucleotide reverse transcriptase inhibitors					
Tenofovir (Viread)	300 mg orally once daily	Gastrointestinal distress	Renal function	$20.47/300 mg	$614.18
Protease inhibitors (PIs)					
Indinavir (Crixivan)	800 mg orally three times daily	Kidney stones	Cholesterol, triglycerides, bilirubin level	$3.05/400 mg	$548.12
Saquinavir hard gel (Invirase)	1000 mg orally twice daily with 100 mg ritonavir orally twice daily	Gastrointestinal distress	Cholesterol, triglycerides	$6.58/500 mg	$789.70 (plus cost of ritonavir)
Ritonavir (Norvir)	600 mg orally twice daily or in lower doses (eg, 100 mg orally once or twice daily) for boosting other PIs	Gastrointestinal distress, peripheral paresthesias	Cholesterol, triglycerides	$10.29/100 mg	$3703.20 ($617.20 in lower doses)
Nelfinavir (Viracept)	750 mg orally three times daily or 1250 mg twice daily	Diarrhea	Cholesterol, triglycerides	$2.42/250 mg $6.05/625 mg	$680.99 $726.40
Amprenavir (Agenerase)	1200 mg orally twice daily	Gastrointestinal, rash	Cholesterol, triglycerides	$0.60/50 mg	$862.20

(continued)

Table 59. Antiretroviral therapy. (continued)

Drug	Dose	Common Side Effects	Special Monitoring[1]	Cost[2]	Cost/Month
Fosamprenavir (Lexiva)	For PI-experienced patients: 700 mg orally twice daily and 100 mg of ritonavir orally twice daily. For PI-naïve patients: above or 1400 mg orally twice daily or 1400 mg orally once daily and 200 mg of ritonavir orally once daily	Same as amprenavir	Same as amprenavir	$12.24/700 mg	$734.56–$1469.12 (plus cost of ritonavir for lower dose)
Lopinavir/ ritonavir (Kaletra)	400 mg/100 mg orally twice daily	Diarrhea	Cholesterol, triglycerides	$7.02/200 mg (lopinavir)	$841.90
Atazanavir (Reyataz)	400 mg orally once daily	Hyperbilirubinemia	Bilirubin level; when used with ritonavir: cholesterol and tri-glycerides	$16.46/200 mg	$987.41
Tipranavir/ ritonavir (Aptivus/ Norvir)	500 mg of tipranavir and 200 mg of ritonavir orally twice daily	Gastrointestinal, rash	Cholesterol, triglycerides	$8.94/250 mg (tipranavir) $10.29/100 mg (ritonavir)	$2307.20 (for combination)
Darunavir/ ritonavir (Prezista/ Norvir)	600 mg of darunavir and 100 mg of ritonavir orally twice daily	Rash	Cholesterol, triglycerides	$7.50/300 mg (darunavir) $10.29/100 mg (ritonavir)	$1517.20 (for combination)
Nonnucleoside reverse transcriptase inhibitors (NNRTIs)					
Nevirapine (Viramune)	200 mg orally daily for 2 weeks, then 200 mg orally twice daily	Rash	No special monitoring	$7.73/200 mg	$463.85
Delavirdine (Rescriptor)	400 mg orally three times daily	Rash	No special monitoring	$1.69/200 mg	$303.70
Efavirenz (Sustiva)	600 mg orally daily	Neurologic disturbances	No special monitoring	$17.70/600 mg	$531.04
Entry inhibitors					
Enfuvirtide (Fuzeon)	90 mg subcutaneously twice daily	Injection site pain and allergic reaction	No special monitoring	$38.90/90 mg	$2333.93
Maraviroc (Selzentry)	150–300 mg orally daily	Cough, fever, rash	No special monitoring	$17.40/150 mg or 300 mg	$1044.00
Integrase inhibitor					
Raltegravir (Isentress)	400 mg orally twice daily	Diarrhea, nausea, headache	No special monitoring	$16.20/400 mg	$972.00

[1]Standard monitoring is complete blood count (CBC) and differential, and serum aminotransferases.
[2]Average wholesale price (AWP, for AB-rated generic when available) for quantity listed. Source: *Red Book Update, Vol. 27, No. 2,* February 2008. AWP may not accurately represent the actual pharmacy cost because wide contractual variations exist among institutions.

Table 60. *Pneumocystis jiroveci* prophylaxis.

Drug	Dose	Side Effects	Limitations
Trimethoprim-sulfamethoxazole	One double-strength tablet three times a week to one tablet daily	Rash, neutropenia, hepatitis, Stevens-Johnson syndrome	Hypersensitivity reaction is common but, if mild, it may be possible to treat through.
Dapsone	50–100 mg daily or 100 mg two or three times per week	Anemia, nausea, methemoglobinemia, hemolytic anemia	Less effective than above. Glucose-6-phosphate dehydrogenase (G6PD) level should be checked prior to therapy. Check methemoglobin level at 1 month.
Atovaquone	1500 mg daily with a meal	Rash, diarrhea, nausea	Less effective than suspension trimethoprim-sulfamethoxazole; equal efficacy to dapsone, but more expensive.
Aerosolized pentamidine	300 mg monthly	Bronchospasm (pretreat with bronchodilators); rare reports of pancreatitis	Apical *Pneumocystis jiroveci* pneumonia, extrapulmonary *P jiroveci* infections, pneumothorax.

Table 61. Diagnostic features of some acute exanthems.

Disease	Prodromal Signs and Symptoms	Nature of Eruption	Other Diagnostic Features	Laboratory Tests
Eczema herpeticum	None.	Vesiculopustular lesions in area of eczema.		Herpes simplex virus isolated in cell culture. Multinucleate giant cells in smear of lesion.
Varicella (chicken-pox)	0–1 day of fever, anorexia, head-ache.	Rapid evolution of macules to papules, vesicles, crusts; all stages simulta-neously present; lesions superficial, dis-tribution centripetal.	Lesions on scalp and mucous membranes.	Specialized complement fixation and virus neutralization in cell culture. Fluorescent antibody test of smear of lesions.
Infectious mono-nucleosis (EBV)	Fever, adenopathy, sore throat.	Maculopapular rash resembling rubella, rarely papulovesicular.	Splenomegaly, tonsillar exu-date.	Atypical lymphocytes in blood smears; het-erophil agglutination (Monospot test).
Exanthema subi-tum (HHV-6, 7; roseola)	3–4 days of high fever.	As fever falls by crisis, pink maculopap-ules appear on chest and trunk; fade in 1–3 days.		White blood count low.
Measles (rubeola)	3–4 days of fever, coryza, conjunc-tivitis, and cough.	Maculopapular, brick-red; begins on head and neck; spreads downward and out-ward, in 5–6 days rash brownish, desquamating. See atypical measles, below.	Koplik spots on buccal mucosa.	White blood count low. Virus isolation in cell culture. Antibody tests by hemagglu-tination inhibition or neutralization.
Atypical measles	Same as measles.	Maculopapular centripetal rash, becom-ing confluent.	History of measles vaccination.	Measles antibody present in past, with titer rise during illness.
Rubella	Little or no pro-drome.	Maculopapular, pink; begins on head and neck, spreads downward, fades in 3 days. No desquamation.	Lymphadenopathy, postauric-ular or occipital.	White blood count normal or low. Serologic tests for immunity and definitive diagno-sis (hemagglutination inhibition).
Erythema infectio-sum (parvovirus B19)	None. Usually in epidemics.	Red, flushed cheeks; circumoral pallor; maculopapules on extremities.	"Slapped face" appearance.	White blood count normal.
Enterovirus infections	1–2 days of fever, malaise.	Maculopapular rash resembling rubella, rarely papulovesicular or petechial.	Aseptic meningitis.	Virus isolation from stool or cerebrospinal fluid; complement fixation titer rise.
Typhus	3–4 days of fever, chills, severe headaches.	Maculopapules, petechiae, initial distri-bution centrifugal (trunk to extremi-ties).	Endemic area, lice.	Complement fixation.
Rocky Mountain spotted fever	3–4 days of fever, vomiting.	Maculopapules, petechiae, initial distri-bution centripetal (extremities to trunk, including palms).	History of tick bite.	Indirect fluorescent antibody; complement fixation.
Ehrlichiosis	Headache, malaise.	Rash in one-third, similar to Rocky Mountain spotted fever.	Pancytopenia, elevated liver function tests.	Polymerase chain reaction, immunofluores-cent antibody.
Scarlet fever	One-half to 2 days of malaise, sore throat, fever, vomiting.	Generalized, punctate, red; prominent on neck, in axillae, groin, skin folds; circu-moral pallor; fine desquamation involves hands and feet.	Strawberry tongue, exuda-tive tonsillitis.	Group A β-hemolytic streptococci in cultures from throat; antistreptolysin O titer rise.
Meningococcemia	Hours of fever, vomiting.	Maculopapules, petechiae, purpura.	Meningeal signs, toxicity, shock.	Cultures of blood, cerebrospinal fluid. High white blood count.
Kawasaki disease	Fever, adenopathy, conjunctivitis.	Cracked lips, strawberry tongue, maculo-papular polymorphous rash, peeling skin on fingers and toes.	Edema of extremities. Angii-tis of coronary arteries.	Thrombocytosis, electrocardiographic changes.
Smallpox (based on prior experience)	Fever, malaise, prostration.	Maculopapules to vesicles to pustules to scars (lesions develop at the same pace).	Centrifugal rash; fulminant sepsis in small percentage of patients, gastrointestinal and skin hemorrhages.	Contact CDC[1] for suspicious rash; EM and gel diffusion assays.

[1] http://www.bt.cdc.gov/agent/smallpox/response-plan/.
EBV, Epstein–Barr virus; HHV, human herpesvirus; EM, electron microscopy.

Table 62. Drugs of choice for suspected or proved microbial pathogens, 2008.[1]

Suspected or Proved Etiologic Agent	Drug(s) of First Choice	Alternative Drug(s)
Gram-negative cocci		
Moraxella catarrhalis	TMP-SMZ,[2] a fluoroquinolone[3]	Cefuroxime, cefotaxime, ceftriaxone, cefuroxime axetil, an erythromycin,[4] a tetracycline,[5] azithromycin, amoxicillin-clavulanic acid, clarithromycin
Neisseria gonorrhoeae (gonococcus)	Cefpodoxime proxetil, ceftriaxone	Ciprofloxacin, ofloxacin
Neisseria meningitidis (meningococcus)	Penicillin[6]	Cefotaxime, ceftriaxone, ampicillin
Gram-positive cocci		
Streptococcus pneumoniae[8] (pneumococcus)	Penicillin[6]	An erythromycin,[4] a cephalosporin,[7] vancomycin, TMP-SMZ,[2] clindamycin, azithromycin, clarithromycin, a tetracycline,[5] certain fluoroquinolones[3]
Streptococcus, hemolytic, groups A, B, C, G	Penicillin[6]	An erythromycin,[4] a cephalosporin,[7] vancomycin, clindamycin, azithromycin, clarithromycin
Viridans streptococci	Penicillin[6] ± gentamicin	Cephalosporin,[7] vancomycin
Staphylococcus, methicillin-resistant	Vancomycin ± gentamicin	TMP-SMZ,[2] doxycycline, minocycline, a fluoroquinolone,[3] linezolid, daptomycin, quinupristin-dalfopristin
Staphylococcus, non-penicillinase-producing	Penicillin[6]	A cephalosporin,[8] clindamycin
Staphylococcus, penicillinase-producing	Penicillinase-resistant penicillin[9]	Vancomycin, a cephalosporin,[7] clindamycin, amoxicillin-clavulanic acid, ticarcillin-clavulanic acid, ampicillin-sulbactam, piperacillin-tazobactam, TMP-SMZ[2]
Enterococcus faecalis	Ampicillin ± gentamicin[10]	Vancomycin ± gentamicin
Enterococcus faecium	Vancomycin ± gentamicin[10]	Linezolid, quinupristin-dalfopristin, daptomycin
Gram-negative rods		
Acinetobacter	Imipenem, meropenem	Tigecycline, minocycline, doxycycline, aminoglycosides,[11] colistin
Prevotella, oropharyngeal strains	Clindamycin	Metronidazole
Bacteroides, gastrointestinal strains	Metronidazole	Clindamycin, ticarcillin-clavulanic acid, ampicillin-sulbactam, piperacillin-tazobactam
Brucella	Tetracycline + rifampin[5]	TMP-SMZ[2] ± gentamicin; chloramphenicol ± gentamicin; doxycycline ± gentamicin
Campylobacter jejuni	Erythromycin[4] or azithromycin	Tetracycline,[5] a fluoroquinolone[3]
Enterobacter	TMP-SMZ,[2] imipenem, meropenem	Aminoglycoside, a fluoroquinolone,[3] cefepime
Escherichia coli (sepsis)	Cefotaxime, ceftriaxone	Imipenem or meropenem, aminoglycosides,[11] a fluoroquinolone[3]
Escherichia coli (uncomplicated urinary infection)	Fluoroquinolones,[3] nitrofurantoin	TMP-SMZ,[2] oral cephalosporin
Haemophilus (meningitis and other serious infections)	Cefotaxime, ceftriaxone	Aztreonam
Haemophilus (respiratory infections, otitis)	TMP-SMZ[2]	Ampicillin, amoxicillin, doxycycline, azithromycin, clarithromycin, cefotaxime, ceftriaxone, cefuroxime, cefuroxime axetil, ampicillin-clavulanate
Helicobacter pylori	Amoxicillin + clarithromycin + proton pump inhibitor (PPI)	Bismuth subsalicylate + tetracycline + metronidazole + PPI
Klebsiella	A cephalosporin	TMP-SMZ,[2] aminoglycoside,[11] imipenem or meropenem, a fluoroquinolone,[3] aztreonam
Legionella species (pneumonia)	Erythromycin[4] or clarithromycin or azithromycin, or fluoroquinolones[3] ± rifampin	Doxycycline ± rifampin
Proteus mirabilis	Ampicillin	An aminoglycoside,[11] TMP-SMZ,[2] a fluoroquinolone,[3] a cephalosporin[7]
Proteus vulgaris and other species (*Morganella, Providencia*)	Cefotaxime, ceftriaxone	Aminoglycoside,[11] imipenem, TMP-SMZ,[2] a fluoroquinolone[3]
Pseudomonas aeruginosa	Aminoglycoside[11] + antipseudomonal penicillin[12]	Ceftazidime ± aminoglycoside; imipenem or meropenem ± aminoglycoside; aztreonam ± aminoglycoside; ciprofloxacin (or levofloxacin) ± piperacillin; ciprofloxacin (or levofloxacin) ± ceftazidime; ciprofloxacin (or levofloxacin) ± cefepime
Burkholderia pseudomallei (melioidosis)	Ceftazidime	Tetracycline,[5] TMP-SMZ,[2] amoxicillin-clavulanic acid, imipenem or meropenem
Burkholderia mallei (glanders)	Streptomycin + tetracycline[5]	Chloramphenicol + streptomycin
Salmonella (bacteremia)	Ceftriaxone	A fluoroquinolone[3]
Serratia	Cefotaxime, ceftriaxone	TMP-SMZ,[2] aminoglycosides,[11] imipenem or meropenem, a fluoroquinolone[3]

(continued)

Table 62. Drugs of choice for suspected or proved microbial pathogens, 2008.[1] (continued)

Suspected or Proved Etiologic Agent	Drug(s) of First Choice	Alternative Drug(s)
Shigella	A fluoroquinolone[3]	Ampicillin, TMP-SMZ,[2] ceftriaxone
Vibrio (cholera, sepsis)	A tetracycline[5]	TMP-SMZ,[2] a fluoroquinolone[3]
Yersinia pestis (plague)	Streptomycin ± a tetracycline[5]	Chloramphenicol, TMP-SMZ[2]
Gram-positive rods		
Actinomyces	Penicillin[6]	Tetracycline,[5] clindamycin
Bacillus (including anthrax)	Penicillin[6] (ciprofloxacin or doxycycline for anthrax; see Table 71)	Erythromycin,[4] a fluoroquinolone[3]
Clostridium (eg, gas gangrene, tetanus)	Penicillin[6]	Metronidazole, clindamycin, imipenem or meropenem
Corynebacterium diphtheriae	Erythromycin[4]	Penicillin[6]
Corynebacterium jeikeium	Vancomycin	A fluoroquinolone
Listeria	Ampicillin ± aminoglycoside[11]	TMP-SMZ[2]
Acid-fast rods		
Mycobacterium tuberculosis[13]	Isoniazid (INH) + rifampin + pyrazinamide ± ethambutol (or streptomycin)	Other antituberculous drugs (see Tables 107 and 108)
Mycobacterium leprae	Dapsone + rifampin ± clofazimine	Minocycline, ofloxacin, clarithromycin
Mycobacterium kansasii	INH + rifampin ± ethambutol	Ethionamide, cycloserine
Mycobacterium avium complex	Clarithromycin or azithromycin + one or more of the following: ethambutol, rifampin or rifabutin, ciprofloxacin	Amikacin
Mycobacterium fortuitum-chelonei	Amikacin + clarithromycin	Cefoxitin, sulfonamide, doxycycline, linezolid
Nocardia	TMP-SMZ[2]	Minocycline, imipenem or meropenem, linezolid
Spirochetes		
Borrelia burgdorferi (Lyme disease)	Doxycycline, amoxicillin, cefuroxime axetil	Ceftriaxone, cefotaxime, penicillin, azithromycin, clarithromycin
Borrelia recurrentis (relapsing fever)	Doxycycline[5]	Penicillin[6]
Leptospira	Penicillin,[6] ceftriaxone	Doxycycline[5]
Treponema pallidum (syphilis)	Penicillin[6]	Doxycycline, ceftriaxone
Treponema pertenue (yaws)	Penicillin[6]	Doxycycline
Mycoplasmas	**Erythromycin[4] or doxycycline**	**Clarithromycin, azithromycin, a fluoroquinolone[3]**
Chlamydiae		
C psittaci	Doxycycline	Chloramphenicol
C trachomatis (urethritis or pelvic inflammatory disease)	Doxycycline or azithromycin	Ofloxacin
C pneumoniae	Doxycycline[5]	Erythromycin,[4] clarithromycin, azithromycin, a fluoroquinolone[3,14]
Rickettsiae	**Doxycycline[5]**	**Chloramphenicol, a fluoroquinolone[3]**

[1]Adapted, with permission, from Med Lett Drugs Ther. 2004;2:13.
[2]TMP-SMZ is a mixture of 1 part trimethoprim and 5 parts sulfamethoxazole.
[3]Fluoroquinolones include ciprofloxacin, ofloxacin, levofloxacin, moxifloxacin, and others (see text). Gemifloxacin, levofloxacin, and moxifloxacin have the best activity against gram-positive organisms, including penicillin-resistant *S pneumoniae* and methicillin-sensitive *S aureus*. Activity against enterococci and *S epidermidis* is variable.
[4]Erythromycin estolate is best absorbed orally but carries the highest risk of hepatitis; erythromycin stearate and erythromycin ethylsuccinate are also available.
[5]All tetracyclines have similar activity against most microorganisms. Minocycline and doxycycline have increased activity against *S aureus*.
[6]Penicillin G is preferred for parenteral injection; penicillin V for oral administration—to be used only in treating infections due to highly sensitive organisms.
[7]Most intravenous cephalosporins (with the exception of ceftazidime) have good activity against gram-positive cocci.
[8]Infections caused by isolates with intermediate resistance may respond to high doses of penicillin, cefotaxime, or ceftriaxone. Infections caused by highly resistant strains should be treated with vancomycin. Many strains of penicillin-resistant pneumococci are resistant to macrolides, cephalosporins, tetracyclines, and TMP-SMZ.
[9]Parenteral nafcillin or oxacillin; oral dicloxacillin, cloxacillin, or oxacillin.
[10]Addition of gentamicin indicated only for severe enterococcal infections (eg, endocarditis, meningitis).
[11]Aminoglycosides—gentamicin, tobramycin, amikacin, netilmicin—should be chosen on the basis of local patterns of susceptibility.
[12]Antipseudomonal penicillins: ticarcillin, piperacillin.
[13]Resistance is common and susceptibility testing should be done.
[14]Ciprofloxacin has inferior antichlamydial activity compared with newer fluoroquinolones.
Key: ±, alone or combined with.

Table 63. Examples of initial antimicrobial therapy for acutely ill, hospitalized adults pending identification of causative organism.

Suspected Clinical Diagnosis	Likely Etiologic Diagnosis	Drugs of Choice
(A) Meningitis, bacterial, community-acquired	Pneumococcus,[1] meningococcus	Cefotaxime,[2] 2–3 g IV every 6 hours; **or** ceftriaxone, 2 g IV every 12 hours plus vancomycin, 10 mg/kg IV every 8 hours
(B) Meningitis, bacterial, age > 50, community-acquired	Pneumococcus, meningococcus, *Listeria monocytogenes*,[3] gram-negative bacilli	Ampicillin, 2 g IV every 4 hours, plus cefotaxime **or** ceftriaxone and vancomycin as in (A)
(C) Meningitis, postoperative (or posttraumatic)	*S aureus*, gram-negative bacilli (pneumococcus, in posttraumatic)	Vancomycin, 10 mg/kg IV every 8 hours, plus ceftazidime, 3 g IV every 8 hours
(D) Brain abscess	Mixed anaerobes, pneumococci, streptococci	Penicillin G, 4 million units IV every 4 hours, plus metronidazole, 500 mg orally every 8 hours; **or** cefotaxime or ceftriaxone as in (A) plus metronidazole, 500 mg orally every 8 hours
(E) Pneumonia, acute, community-acquired, severe	Pneumococci, *M pneumoniae*, Legionella, *C pneumoniae*	Cefotaxime, 2 g IV every 8 hours (or ceftriaxone, 1 g IV every 24 hours or ampicillin 2 g IV every 6 hours) plus azithromycin 500 mg IV every 24 hours; **or** a fluoroquinolone[5] alone
(F) Pneumonia, postoperative or nosocomial	*S aureus*, mixed anaerobes, gram-negative bacilli	Cefepime, 2 g IV every 8 hours; **or** ceftazidime, 2 g IV every 8 hours; **or** piperacillin-tazobactam, 45 g IV every 6 hours; **or** imipenem, 500 mg IV every 6 hours; **or** meropenem, 1 g IV every 8 hours plus tobramycin, 5 mg/kg IV every 24 hours; **or** ciprofloxacin, 400 mg IV every 12 hours; **or** levofloxacin, 500 mg IV every 24 hours plus vancomycin, 15 mg/kg IV every 12 hours
(G) Endocarditis, acute (including injection drug user)	*S aureus*, *E faecalis*, gram-negative aerobic bacteria, viridans streptococci	Vancomycin, 15 mg/kg IV every 12 hours, plus gentamicin, 1 mg/kg every 8 hours
(H) Septic thrombophlebitis (eg, IV tubing, IV shunts)	*S aureus*, gram-negative aerobic bacteria	Vancomycin, 15 mg/kg IV every 12 hours plus ceftriaxone, 1 g IV every 24 hours
(I) Osteomyelitis	*S aureus*	Nafcillin, 2 g IV every 4 hours; **or** cefazolin, 2 g IV every 8 hours
(J) Septic arthritis	*S aureus*, *N gonorrhoeae*	Ceftriaxone, 1–2 g IV every 24 hours
(K) Pyelonephritis with flank pain and fever (recurrent urinary tract infection)	*E coli*, *Klebsiella*, *Enterobacter*, *Pseudomonas*	Ceftriaxone, 1 g IV every 24 hours; **or** ciprofloxacin, 400 mg IV every 12 hours (500 mg orally); **or** levofloxacin, 500 mg once daily (IV/PO)
(L) Fever in neutropenic patient receiving cancer chemotherapy	*S aureus*, *Pseudomonas*, *Klebsiella*, *E coli*	Ceftazidime, 2 g IV every 8 hours; **or** cefepime, 2 g IV every 8 hours
(M) Intra-abdominal sepsis (eg, postoperative, peritonitis, cholecystitis)	Gram-negative bacteria, *Bacteroides*, anaerobic bacteria, streptococci, clostridia	Piperacillin-tazobactam as in (F) or ticarcillin-clavulanate, 3.1 g IV every 6 hours; **or** ertapenem, 1 g every 24 hours

[1]Some strains may be resistant to penicillin. Vancomycin can be used with or without rifampin.
[2]Cefotaxime, ceftriaxone, ceftazidime, or ceftizoxime can be used. Most studies on meningitis have been with cefotaxime or ceftriaxone (see text).
[3]TMP-SMZ can be used to treat *Listeria monocytogenes* in patients allergic to penicillin in a dosage of 15–20 mg/kg of TMP in three or four divided doses.
[4]Depending on local drug susceptibility pattern, use tobramycin, 5 mg/kg/d, or amikacin, 15 mg/kg/d, in place of gentamicin.
[5]Levofloxacin 750 mg/d, moxifloxacin 400 mg/d.

Table 64. Initial antimicrobial therapy for purulent meningitis of unknown cause.

Population	Common Microorganisms	Standard Therapy
18–50 years	*Streptococcus pneumoniae*, *Neisseria meningitidis*	Vancomycin[1] **plus** cefotaxime or ceftriaxone[2]
Over 50 years	*S pneumoniae*, *N meningitidis*, *Listeria monocytogenes*, gram-negative bacilli	Vancomycin[1] **plus** ampicillin,[3] **plus** cefotaxime or ceftriaxone[2]
Impaired cellular immunity	*L monocytogenes*, gram-negative bacilli, *S pneumoniae*	Vancomycin[1] **plus** ampicillin[3] **plus** ceftazidime[4]
Postsurgical or posttraumatic	*Staphylococcus aureus*, *S pneumoniae*, gram-negative bacilli	Vancomycin[1] **plus** ceftazidime[4]

[1]The dose of vancomycin is 10–15 mg/kg/dose IV every 6 hours.
[2]The usual dose of cefotaxime is 2 g IV every 6 hours and that of ceftriaxone is 2 g IV every 12 hours. If the organism is sensitive to penicillin, 3–4 million units IV every 4 hours is given.
[3]The dose of ampicillin is usually 2 g IV every 4 hours.
[4]Ceftazidime is given in a dose of 50–100 mg/kg IV every 8 hours.

Table 65. Typical cerebrospinal fluid findings in various central nervous system diseases.

Diagnosis	Cells/mcL	Glucose (mg/dL)	Protein (mg/dL)	Opening Pressure
Normal	0–5 lymphocytes	45–85[1]	15–45	70–180 mm H_2O
Purulent meningitis (bacterial),[2] community-acquired	200–20,000 polymorphonuclear neutrophils	Low (< 45)	High (> 50)	Markedly elevated
Granulomatous meningitis (mycobacterial, fungal)[3]	100–1000, mostly lymphocytes[3]	Low (< 45)	High (> 50)	Moderately elevated
Spirochetal meningitis	100–1000, mostly lymphocytes[3]	Normal	Moderately high (> 50)	Normal to slightly elevated
Aseptic meningitis, viral or meningoencephalitis[4]	25–2000, mostly lymphocytes[3]	Normal or low	High (> 50)	Slightly elevated
"Neighborhood reaction"[5]	Variably increased	Normal	Normal or high	Variable

[1]Cerebrospinal fluid glucose must be considered in relation to blood glucose level. Normally, cerebrospinal fluid glucose is 20–30 mg/dL lower than blood glucose, or 50–70% of the normal value of blood glucose.
[2]Organisms in smear or culture of cerebrospinal fluid; counterimmunoelectrophoresis or latex agglutination may be diagnostic.
[3]Polymorphonuclear neutrophils may predominate early.
[4]Viral isolation from cerebrospinal fluid early; antibody titer rise in paired specimens of serum; polymerase chain reaction for herpesvirus.
[5]May occur in mastoiditis, brain abscess, epidural abscess, sinusitis, septic thrombus, brain tumor. Cerebrospinal fluid culture results usually negative.

Table 66. Acute bacterial diarrheas and "food poisoning."

Organism	Incubation Period	Vomiting	Diarrhea	Fever	Associated Foods	Diagnosis	Clinical Features and Treatment
Staphylococcus (preformed toxin)	1–8 hours	+++	±	±	Staphylococci grow in meats, dairy, and bakery products and produce enterotoxin.	Clinical. Food and stool can be tested for toxin	Abrupt onset, intense nausea and vomiting for up to 24 hours, recovery in 24–48 hours. Supportive care.
Bacillus cereus (preformed toxin)	1–8 hours	+++	±	–	Reheated fried rice causes vomiting or diarrhea.	Clinical. Food and stool can be tested for toxin	Acute onset, severe nausea and vomiting lasting 24 hours. Supportive care.
B cereus (diarrheal toxin)	10–16 hours	±	+++	–	Toxin in meats, stews, and gravy.	Clinical. Food and stool can be tested for toxin	Abdominal cramps, watery diarrhea, and nausea lasting 24–48 hours. Supportive care.
Clostridium perfringens	8–16 hours	±	+++	–	Clostridia grow in rewarmed meat and poultry dishes and produce an enterotoxin.	Stools can be tested for enterotoxin or cultured.	Abrupt onset of profuse diarrhea, abdominal cramps, nausea; vomiting occasionally. Recovery usual without treatment in 24–48 hours. Supportive care; antibiotics not needed.
Clostridium botulinum	12–72 hours	±	–	–	Clostridia grow in anaerobic acidic environment eg, canned foods, fermented fish, foods held warm for extended periods.	Stool, serum, and food can be tested for toxin. Stool and food can be cultured.	Diplopia, dysphagia, dysphonia, respiratory embarrassment. Treatment requires clear airway, ventilation, and intravenous polyvalent antitoxin (see text). Symptoms can last for days to months.
Clostridium difficile	Usually occurs after 7–10 days of antibiotics. Can occur after a single dose or several weeks after completion of antibiotics.	–	+++	++	Associated with antimicrobial drugs; clindamycin and cephalosporins most commonly implicated.	Stool tested for toxin	Abrupt onset of diarrhea that may be bloody; fever. Oral metronidazole first-line therapy. If no response, oral vancomycin can be given.
Enterohemorrhagic *Escherichia coli*, including *E coli* O157:H7 and other Shiga-toxin producing strains (STEC)	1–8 days	+	+++	–	Undercooked beef, especially hamburger; unpasteurized milk and juice; raw fruits and vegetables.	*E coli* O157:H7 can be cultured on special medium. Other toxins can be detected in stool.	Usually abrupt onset of diarrhea, often bloody; abdominal pain. In adults, it is usually self-limited to 5–10 days. In children, it is associated with hemolytic-uremic syndrome (HUS). Antibiotic therapy may increase risk of HUS.
Enterotoxigenic *E coli* (ETEC)	1–3 days	±	+++	±	Water, food contaminated with feces.	Stool culture. Special tests required to identify toxin-producing strains.	Watery diarrhea and abdominal cramps, usually lasting 3–7 days. In travelers, fluoroquinolones shorten disease.
Vibrio parahaemolyticus	2–48 hours	+	+	±	Undercooked or raw seafood.	Stool culture on special medium.	Abrupt onset of watery diarrhea, abdominal cramps, nausea and vomiting. Recovery is usually complete in 2–5 days.
Vibrio cholerae	24–72 hours	+	+++	–	Contaminated water, fish, shellfish, street vendor food.	Stool culture on special medium.	Abrupt onset of liquid diarrhea in endemic area. Needs prompt intravenous or oral replacement of fluids and electrolytes. Tetracyclines shorten excretion of vibrios.
Campylobacter jejuni	2–5 days	±	+++	+	Raw or undercooked poultry, unpasteurized milk, water.	Stool culture on special medium.	Fever, diarrhea that can be bloody, cramps. Usually self-limited in 2–10 days. Early treatment (erythromycin) shortens course. May be associated with Guillain-Barré syndrome.
Shigella species (mild cases)	24–48 hours	±	+	+	Food or water contaminated with human feces. Person to person spread.	Routine stool culture.	Abrupt onset of diarrhea, often with blood and pus in stools, cramps, tenesmus, and lethargy. Stool cultures are positive. Therapy depends on sensitivity testing, but the fluoroquinolones are most effective. Do not give opioids. Often mild and self-limited.

Organism	Incubation period				Foods	Diagnosis	Clinical features and treatment
Salmonella species	1–3 days	–	++	+	Eggs, poultry, unpasteurized milk, cheese, juices, raw fruits and vegetables.	Routine stool culture.	Gradual or abrupt onset of diarrhea and low-grade fever. No antimicrobials unless high risk (see text) or systemic dissemination is suspected, in which case give a fluoroquinolone. Prolonged carriage can occur.
Yersinia enterocolitica	24–48 hours	±	+	+	Undercooked pork, contaminated water, unpasteurized milk, tofu.	Stool culture on special medium.	Severe abdominal pain, (appendicitis-like symptoms) diarrhea, fever. Polyarthritis, erythema nodosum in children. If severe, give tetracycline or fluoroquinolone. Without treatment, self-limited in 1–3 weeks.
Rotavirus	1–3 days	++	+++	+	Fecally contaminated foods touched by infected food handlers.	Immunoassay on stool.	Acute onset, vomiting, watery diarrhea that lasts 4–8 days. Supportive care.
Noroviruses and other caliciviruses	12–48 hours	++	+++	+	Shell fish and fecally contaminated foods touched by infected food handlers.	Clinical diagnosis with negative stool cultures. PCR available on stool.	Nausea, vomiting (more common in children), diarrhea (more common in adults), fever, myalgias, abdominal cramps. Lasts 12–60 hours. Supportive care.

PCR, polymerase chain reaction.

Table 67. Recommended childhood and adolescent immunization schedule—United States, 2008.[1]

Recommended Immunization Schedule for Persons Aged 0–6 Years — UNITED STATES • 2008
For those who fall behind or start late, see the catch-up schedule

Vaccine ▸ Age	Birth	1 month	2 months	4 months	6 months	12 months	15 months	18 months	19–23 months	2–3 years	4–6 years
Hepatitis B[1]	HepB	HepB		see footnote1		HepB					
Rotavirus[2]			Rota	Rota	Rota						
Diphtheria, Tetanus, Pertussis[3]			DTaP	DTaP	DTaP	see footnote3	DTaP				DTaP
Haemophilus influenzae type b[4]			Hib	Hib	Hib[4]	Hib					
Pneumococcal[5]			PCV	PCV	PCV	PCV				PPV	
Inactivated Poliovirus			IPV	IPV		IPV					IPV
Influenza[6]						Influenza (Yearly)					
Measles, Mumps, Rubella[7]						MMR					MMR
Varicella[8]						Varicella					Varicella
Hepatitis A[9]						HepA (2 doses)				HepA Series	
Meningococcal[10]										MCV4	

■ Range of recommended ages
■ Certain high-risk groups

This schedule indicates the recommended ages for routine administration of currently licensed childhood vaccines, as of December 1, 2007, for children aged 7–18 years. Additional information is available at **www.cdc.gov/vaccines/recs/schedules.** Any dose not administered at the recommended age should be administered at any subsequent visit, when indicated and feasible. Additional vaccines may be licensed and recommended during the year. Licensed combination vaccines may be used whenever any components of the combination are indicated and other components of the vaccine are not contraindicated and if approved by the Food and Drug Administration for that dose of the series. **Providers should consult the respective Advisory Committee on Immunization Practices statement for detailed recommendations, including for high risk conditions: http://www.cdc.gov/vaccines/pubs/ACIP-list.htm.** Clinically significant adverse events that follow immunization should be reported to the Vaccine Adverse Event Reporting System (VAERS). Guidance about how to obtain and complete a VAERS form is available at **www.vaers.hhs.gov** or by telephone, **800-822-7967.**

1. Hepatitis B vaccine (HepB). *(Minimum age: birth)*
At birth:
- Administer monovalent HepB to all newborns prior to hospital discharge.
- If mother is hepatitis B surface antigen (HBsAg) positive, administer HepB and 0.5 mL of hepatitis B immune globulin (HBIG) within 12 hours of birth.
- If mother's HBsAg status is unknown, administer HepB within 12 hours of birth. Determine the HBsAg status as soon as possible and if HBsAg positive, administer HBIG (no later than age 1 week).
- If mother is HBsAg negative, the birth dose can be delayed, in rare cases, with a provider's order and a copy of the mother's negative HBsAg laboratory report in the infant's medical record.

After the birth dose:
- The HepB series should be completed with either monovalent HepB or a combination vaccine containing HepB. The second dose should be administered at age 1–2 months. The final dose should be administered no earlier than age 24 weeks. Infants born to HBsAg-positive mothers should be tested for HBsAg and antibody to HBsAg after completion of at least 3 doses of a licensed HepB series, at age 9–18 months (generally at the next well-child visit).

4-month dose:
- It is permissible to administer 4 doses of HepB when combination vaccines are administered after the birth dose. If monovalent HepB is used for doses after the birth dose, a dose at age 4 months is not needed.

2. Rotavirus vaccine (Rota). *(Minimum age: 6 weeks)*
- Administer the first dose at age 6–12 weeks.
- Do not start the series later than age 12 weeks.
- Administer the final dose in the series by age 32 weeks. Do not administer any dose later than age 32 weeks.
- Data on safety and efficacy outside of these age ranges are insufficient.

3. Diphtheria and tetanus toxoids and acellular pertussis vaccine (DTaP). *(Minimum age: 6 weeks)*
- The fourth dose of DTaP may be administered as early as age 12 months, provided 6 months have elapsed since the third dose.
- Administer the final dose in the series at age 4–6 years.

4. Haemophilus influenzae type b conjugate vaccine (Hib). *(Minimum age: 6 weeks)*
- If PRP-OMP (PedvaxHIB® or ComVax® [Merck]) is administered at ages 2 and 4 months, a dose at age 6 months is not required.
- TriHIBit® (DTaP/Hib) combination products should not be used for primary immunization but can be used as boosters following any Hib vaccine in children age 12 months or older.

5. Pneumococcal vaccine. *(Minimum age: 6 weeks for pneumococcal conjugate vaccine [PCV]; 2 years for pneumococcal polysaccharide vaccine [PPV])*
- Administer one dose of PCV to all healthy children aged 24–59 months having any incomplete schedule.
- Administer PPV to children aged 2 years and older with underlying medical conditions.

6. Influenza vaccine. *(Minimum age: 6 months for trivalent inactivated influenza vaccine [TIV]; 2 years for live, attenuated influenza vaccine [LAIV])*
- Administer annually to children aged 6–59 months and to all eligible close contacts of children aged 0–59 months.
- Administer annually to children 5 years of age and older with certain risk factors, to other persons (including household members) in close contact with persons in groups at higher risk, and to any child whose parents request vaccination.
- For healthy persons (those who do not have underlying medical conditions that predispose them to influenza complications) ages 2–49 years, either LAIV or TIV may be used.
- Children receiving TIV should receive 0.25 mL if age 6–35 months or 0.5 mL if age 3 years or older.
- Administer 2 doses (separated by 4 weeks or longer) to children younger than 9 years who are receiving influenza vaccine for the first time or who were vaccinated for the first time last season but only received one dose.

7. Measles, mumps, and rubella vaccine (MMR). *(Minimum age: 12 months)*
- Administer the second dose of MMR at age 4–6 years. MMR may be administered before age 4–6 years, provided 4 weeks or more have elapsed since the first dose.

8. Varicella vaccine. *(Minimum age: 12 months)*
- Administer second dose at age 4–6 years; may be administered 3 months or more after first dose.
- Do not repeat second dose if administered 28 days or more after first dose.

9. Hepatitis A vaccine (HepA). *(Minimum age: 12 months)*
- Administer to all children aged 1 year (i.e., aged 12–23 months). Administer the 2 doses in the series at least 6 months apart.
- Children not fully vaccinated by age 2 years can be vaccinated at subsequent visits.
- HepA is recommended for certain other groups of children, including in areas where vaccination programs target older children.

10. Meningococcal vaccine. *(Minimum age: 2 years for meningococcal conjugate vaccine [MCV4] and for meningococcal polysaccharide vaccine [MPSV4])*
- Administer MCV4 to children aged 2–10 years with terminal complement deficiencies or anatomic or functional asplenia and certain other high-risk groups. MPSV4 is also acceptable.
- Administer MCV4 to persons who received MPSV4 3 or more years previously and remain at increased risk for meningococcal disease.

The Recommended Immunizations Schedules for Persons Aged 0–18 Years are approved by the Advisory Committee on Immunization Practices (www.cdc.gov/vaccines/recs/acip), The American Academy of Pediatrics (http://www.aap.org), and the American Academy of Family Physicians (http://www.aafp.org).

(continued)

Recommended Immunization Schedule for Persons Aged 7–18 Years — UNITED STATES • 2008

For those who fall behind or start late, see the medium blue bars and the catch-up schedule

Vaccine ▸ Age	7–10 years	11–12 years	13–18 years
Diphtheria, Tetanus, Pertussis [1]	*see footnote 1*	**Tdap**	**Tdap**
Human Papillomavirus [2]	*see footnote 2*	**HPV (3 doses)**	**HPV Series**
Meningococcal [3]	**MCV4**	**MCV4**	**MCV4**
Pneumococcal [4]	**PPV**		
Influenza [5]	**Influenza (Yearly)**		
Hepatitis A [6]	**HepA Series**		
Hepatitis B [7]	**HepB Series**		
Inactivated Poliovirus [8]	**IPV Series**		
Measles, Mumps, Rubella [9]	**MMR Series**		
Varicella [10]	**Varicella Series**		

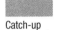 Range of recommended ages

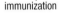 Catch-up immunization

 Certain high-risk groups

This schedule indicates the recommended ages for routine administration of currently licensed childhood vaccines, as of December 1, 2007, for children aged 7–18 years. Additional information is available at **www.cdc.gov/vaccines/recs/schedules.** Any dose not administered at the recommended age should be administered at any subsequent visit, when indicated and feasible. Additional vaccines may be licensed and recommended during the year. Licensed combination vaccines may be used whenever any components of the combination are indicated and other components of the vaccine are not contraindicated and if approved by the Food and Drug Administration for that dose of the series. **Providers should consult the respective Advisory Committee on Immunization Practices statement for detailed recommendations, including for high risk conditions: http://www.cdc.gov/vaccines/pubs/ACIP-list.htm.** Clinically significant adverse events that follow immunization should be reported to the Vaccine Adverse Event Reporting System (VAERS). Guidance about how to obtain and complete a VAERS form is available at **www.vaers.hhs.gov** or by telephone, **800-822-7967.**

1. Tetanus and diphtheria toxoids and acellular pertussis vaccine (Tdap). *(Minimum age: 10 years for BOOSTRIX® and 11 years for ADACEL™)*
- Administer at age 11–12 years for those who have completed the recommended childhood DTP/DTaP vaccination series and have not received a tetanus and diphtheria toxoids (Td) booster dose.
- 13–18-year-olds who missed the 11–12 year Tdap or received Td only are encouraged to receive one dose of Tdap 5 years after the last Td/DTaP dose.

2. Human papillomavirus vaccine (HPV). *(Minimum age: 9 years)*
- Administer the first dose of the HPV vaccine series to females at age 11–12 years.
- Administer the second dose 2 months after the first dose and the third dose 6 months after the first dose.
- Administer the HPV vaccine series to females at age 13–18 years if not previously vaccinated.

3. Meningococcal vaccine.
- Administer MCV4 at age 11–12 years and at age 13–18 years if not previously vaccinated. MPSV4 is an acceptable alternative.
- Administer MCV4 to previously unvaccinated college freshmen living in dormitories.
- MCV4 is recommended for children aged 2–10 years with terminal complement deficiencies or anatomic or functional asplenia and certain other high-risk groups.
- Persons who received MPSV4 3 or more years previously and remain at increased risk for meningococcal disease should be vaccinated with MCV4.

4. Pneumococcal polysaccharide vaccine (PPV).
- Administer PPV to certain high-risk groups.

5. Influenza vaccine.
- Administer annually to all close contacts of children aged 0–59 months.
- Administer annually to persons with certain risk factors, health-care workers, and other persons (including household members) in close contact with persons in groups at higher risk.
- Administer 2 doses (separated by 4 weeks or longer) to children younger than 9 years who are receiving influenza vaccine for the first time or who were vaccinated for the first time last season but only received one dose.
- For healthy nonpregnant persons (those who do not have underlying medical conditions that predispose them to influenza complications) ages 2–49 years, either LAIV or TIV may be used.

6. Hepatitis A vaccine (HepA).
- Administer the 2 doses in the series at least 6 months apart.
- HepA is recommended for certain other groups of children, including in areas where vaccination programs target older children.

7. Hepatitis B vaccine (HepB).
- Administer the 3-dose series to those who were not previously vaccinated.
- A 2-dose series of Recombivax HB ® is licensed for children aged 11–15 years.

8. Inactivated poliovirus vaccine (IPV).
- For children who received an all-IPV or all-oral poliovirus (OPV) series, a fourth dose is not necessary if the third dose was administered at age 4 years or older.
- If both OPV and IPV were administered as part of a series, a total of 4 doses should be administered, regardless of the child's current age.

9. Measles, mumps, and rubella vaccine (MMR).
- If not previously vaccinated, administer 2 doses of MMR during any visit, with 4 or more weeks between the doses.

10. Varicella vaccine.
- Administer 2 doses of varicella vaccine to persons younger than 13 years of age at least 3 months apart. Do not repeat the second dose if administered 28 or more days following the first dose.
- Administer 2 doses of varicella vaccine to persons aged 13 years or older at least 4 weeks apart.

The Recommended Immunizations Schedules for Persons Aged 0–18 Years are approved by the Advisory Committee on Immunization Practices (www.cdc.gov/vaccines/recs/acip). The American Academy of Pediatrics (http://www.aap.org), and the American Academy of Family Physicians (http://www.aafp.org).

(continued)

Table 67. Recommended childhood and adolescent immunization schedule—United States, 2008.[1] (continued)

Catch-up Immunization Schedule
for Persons Aged 4 Months–18 Years Who Start Late or Who Are More Than 1 Month Behind

UNITED STATES • 2008

The table below provides catch-up schedules and minimum intervals between doses for children whose vaccinations have been delayed. A vaccine series does not need to be restarted, regardless of the time that has elapsed between doses. Use the section appropriate for the child's age.

CATCH-UP SCHEDULE FOR PERSONS AGED 4 MONTHS–6 YEARS

Vaccine	Minimum Age for Dose 1	Minimum Interval Between Doses			
		Dose 1 to Dose 2	Dose 2 to Dose 3	Dose 3 to Dose 4	Dose 4 to Dose 5
Hepatitis B[1]	Birth	4 weeks	**8 weeks** (and 16 weeks after first dose)		
Rotavirus[2]	6 wks	4 weeks	4 weeks		
Diphtheria, Tetanus, Pertussis[3]	6 wks	4 weeks	4 weeks	6 months	6 months[3]
Haemophilus influenzae type b[4]	6 wks	**4 weeks** if first dose administered at younger than 12 months of age **8 weeks (as final dose)** if first dose administered at age 12-14 months **No further doses needed** if first dose administered at 15 months of age or older	**4 weeks**[4] if current age is younger than 12 months **8 weeks (as final dose)**[4] if current age is 12 months or older and second dose administered at younger than 15 months of age **No further doses needed** if previous dose administered at age 15 months or older	**8 weeks (as final dose)** This dose only necessary for children aged 12 months–5 years who received 3 doses before age 12 months	
Pneumococcal[5]	6 wks	**4 weeks** if first dose administered at younger than 12 months of age **8 weeks (as final dose)** if first dose administered at age 12 months or older or current age 24–59 months **No further doses needed** for healthy children if first dose administered at age 24 months or older	**4 weeks** if current age is younger than 12 months **8 weeks (as final dose)** if current age is 12 months or older **No further doses needed** for healthy children if previous dose administered at age 24 months or older	**8 weeks (as final dose)** This dose only necessary for children aged 12 months–5 years who received 3 doses before age 12 months	
Inactivated Poliovirus[6]	6 wks	4 weeks	4 weeks	4 weeks[6]	
Measles, Mumps, Rubella[7]	12 mos	4 weeks			
Varicella[8]	12 mos	3 months			
Hepatitis A[9]	12 mos	6 months			

CATCH-UP SCHEDULE FOR PERSONS AGED 7–18 YEARS

Vaccine	Minimum Age for Dose 1	Dose 1 to Dose 2	Dose 2 to Dose 3	Dose 3 to Dose 4	Dose 4 to Dose 5
Tetanus, Diphtheria/ Tetanus, Diphtheria, Pertussis[10]	7 yrs[10]	4 weeks	**4 weeks** if first dose administered at younger than 12 months of age **6 months** if first dose administered at age 12 months or older	**6 months** if first dose administered at younger than 12 months of age	
Human Papillomavirus[11]	9 yrs	4 weeks	**12 weeks** (and 24 weeks after the first dose)		
Hepatitis A[9]	12 mos	6 months			
Hepatitis B[1]	Birth	4 weeks	**8 weeks** (and 16 weeks after first dose)		
Inactivated Poliovirus[6]	6 wks	4 weeks	4 weeks	4 weeks[6]	
Measles, Mumps, Rubella[7]	12 mos	4 weeks			
Varicella[8]	12 mos	**4 weeks** if first dose administered at age 13 years or older **3 months** if first dose administered at younger than 13 years of age			

1. Hepatitis B vaccine (HepB).
- Administer the 3-dose series to those who were not previously vaccinated.
- A 2-dose series of Recombivax HB® is licensed for children aged 11–15 years.

2. Rotavirus vaccine (Rota).
- Do not start the series later than age 12 weeks.
- Administer the final dose in the series by age 32 weeks.
- Do not administer a dose later than age 32 weeks.
- Data on safety and efficacy outside of these age ranges are insufficient.

3. Diphtheria and tetanus toxoids and acellular pertussis vaccine (DTaP).
- The fifth dose is not necessary if the fourth dose was administered at age 4 years or older.
- DTaP is not indicated for persons aged 7 years or older.

4. *Haemophilus influenzae* type b conjugate vaccine (Hib).
- Vaccine is not generally recommended for children aged 5 years or older.
- If current age is younger than 12 months and the first 2 doses were PRP-OMP (PedvaxHIB® or ComVax® [Merck]), the third (and final) dose should be administered at age 12–15 months and at least 8 weeks after the second dose.
- If first dose was administered at age 7–11 months, administer 2 doses separated by 4 weeks plus a booster at age 12–15 months.

5. Pneumococcal conjugate vaccine (PCV).
- Administer one dose of PCV to all healthy children aged 24–59 months having any incomplete schedule.
- For children with underlying medical conditions, administer 2 doses of PCV at least 8 weeks apart if previously received less than 3 doses, or 1 dose of PCV if previously received 3 doses.

6. Inactivated poliovirus vaccine (IPV).
- For children who received an all-IPV or all-oral poliovirus (OPV) series, a fourth dose is not necessary if third dose was administered at age 4 years or older.

- If both OPV and IPV were administered as part of a series, a total of 4 doses should be administered, regardless of the child's current age.
- IPV is not routinely recommended for persons aged 18 years and older.

7. Measles, mumps, and rubella vaccine (MMR).
- The second dose of MMR is recommended routinely at age 4–6 years but may be administered earlier if desired.
- If not previously vaccinated, administer 2 doses of MMR during any visit with 4 or more weeks between the doses.

8. Varicella vaccine.
- The second dose of varicella vaccine is recommended routinely at age 4–6 years but may be administered earlier if desired.
- Do not repeat the second dose in persons younger than 13 years of age if administered 28 or more days after the first dose.

9. Hepatitis A vaccine (HepA).
- HepA is recommended for certain groups of children, including in areas where vaccination programs target older children. See *MMWR* 2006;55(No. RR-7):1–23.

10. Tetanus and diphtheria toxoids vaccine (Td) and tetanus and diphtheria toxoids and acellular pertussis vaccine (Tdap).
- Tdap should be substituted for a single dose of Td in the primary catch-up series or as a booster if age appropriate; use Td for other doses.
- A 5-year interval from the last Td dose is encouraged when Tdap is used as a booster dose. A booster (fourth) dose is needed if any of the previous doses were administered at younger than 12 months of age. Refer to ACIP recommendations for further information. See *MMWR* 2006;55(No. RR-3).

11. Human papillomavirus vaccine (HPV).
- Administer the HPV vaccine series to females at age 13–18 years if not previously vaccinated.

Information about reporting reactions after immunization is available online at **http://www.vaers.hhs.gov** or by telephone via the 24-hour national toll-free information line 800-822-7967. Suspected cases of vaccine-preventable diseases should be reported to the state or local health department. Additional information, including precautions and contraindications for immunization, is available from the National Center for Immunization and Respiratory Diseases at **http://www.cdc.gov/vaccines** or telephone, 800-CDC-INFO (800-232-4636).

Table 68. Recommended adult immunization schedule—United States, 2008.

Recommended Adult Immunization Schedule

Note: These recommendations must be read with the footnotes that follow.

Recommended adult immunization schedule, by vaccine and age group
United States, October 2007 – September 2008

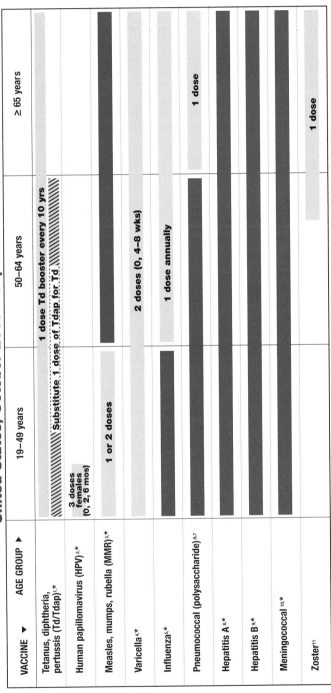

VACCINE ▼ / AGE GROUP ▶	19–49 years	50–64 years	≥ 65 years
Tetanus, diphtheria, pertussis (Td/Tdap)[1],*	Substitute 1 dose of Tdap for Td	1 dose Td booster every 10 yrs	
Human papillomavirus (HPV)[2],*	3 doses females (0, 2, 6 mos)		
Measles, mumps, rubella (MMR)[3],*	1 or 2 doses		
Varicella[4],*	2 doses (0, 4–8 wks)		
Influenza[5],*	1 dose annually	1 dose annually	
Pneumococcal (polysaccharide)[6,7]	1 dose		1 dose
Hepatitis A[8],*			
Hepatitis B[9],*			
Meningococcal[10],*			
Zoster[11]			1 dose

*Covered by the Vaccine Injury Compensation Program.

Legend:
- For all persons in this category who meet the age requirements and who lack evidence of immunity (e.g., lack documentation of vaccination or have no evidence of prior infection)
- Recommended if some other risk factor is present (e.g., on the basis of medical, occupational, lifestyle, or other indications)

Report all clinically significant postvaccination reactions to the Vaccine Adverse Event Reporting System (VAERS). Reporting forms and instructions on filing a VAERS report are available at **www.vaers.hhs.gov** or by telephone, 800-822-7967.

Information on how to file a Vaccine Injury Compensation Program claim is available at www.hrsa.gov/vaccinecompensation or by telephone, 800-338-2382. To file a claim for vaccine injury, contact the U.S. Court of Federal Claims, 717 Madison Place, N.W., Washington, D.C. 20005; telephone, 202-357-6400.

Additional information about the vaccines in this schedule, extent of available data, and contraindications for vaccination is also available at www.cdc.gov/vaccines or from the CDC-INFO Contact Center at 800-CDC-INFO (800-232-4636) in English and Spanish, 24 hours a day, 7 days a week.

Use of trade names and commercial sources is for identification only and does not imply endorsement by the U.S. Department of Health and Human Services.

(continued)

Table 68. Recommended adult immunization schedule—United States, 2008. (continued)

Vaccines that might be indicated for adults based on medical and other indications
United States, October 2007 – September 2008

VACCINE ▼ / INDICATION ▶	Pregnancy	Immuno-compromising conditions (excluding human immunodeficiency virus [HIV]), medications, radiation[13]	HIV infection[3,12,13] CD4+ T lymphocyte count <200 cells/µL	HIV infection[3,12,13] CD4+ T lymphocyte count ≥200 cells/µL	Diabetes, heart disease, chronic pulmonary disease, chronic alcoholism	Asplenia[12] (including elective splenectomy and terminal complement component deficiencies)	Chronic liver disease	Kidney failure, end-stage renal disease, receipt of hemodialysis	Health-care personnel
Tetanus, diphtheria, pertussis (Td/Tdap)[1],*	1 dose Td booster every 10 yrs — Substitute 1 dose of Tdap for Td								
Human papillomavirus (HPV)[2],*		3 doses for females through age 26 yrs (0, 2, 6 mos)							
Measles, mumps, rubella (MMR)[3],*	Contraindicated	Contraindicated			1 or 2 doses				
Varicella[4],*	Contraindicated	Contraindicated			2 doses (0, 4–3 wks)				
Influenza[5],*	1 dose TIV annually							1 dose TIV or LAIV annually
Pneumococcal (polysaccharide)[6,7]					1–2 doses				
Hepatitis A[8],*		2 doses (0, 6–12 mos, or 0, 6–18 mos)							
Hepatitis B[9],*		3 doses (0, 1–2, 4–6 mos)							
Meningococcal[10],*		1 or more doses							
Zoster[11]	Contraindicated						1 dose		

*Covered by the Vaccine Injury Compensation Program.

Legend:

□ For all persons in this category who meet the age requirements and who lack evidence of immunity (e.g., lack documentation of vaccination or have no evidence of prior infection)

■ Recommended if some other risk factor is present (e.g., on the basis of medical, occupational, lifestyle, or other indications)

These schedules indicate the recommended age groups and medical indications for which administration of currently licensed vaccines is commonly indicated for adults ages 19 years and older, as of October 1, 2007. Licensed combination vaccines may be used whenever any components of the combination are indicated and when the vaccine's other components are not contraindicated. For detailed recommendations on all vaccines, including those used primarily for travelers or that are issued during the year, consult the manufacturers' package inserts and the complete statements from the Advisory Committee on Immunization Practices (www.cdc.gov/vaccines/pubs/acip-list.htm).

The recommendations in this schedule were approved by the Centers for Disease Control and Prevention's (CDC) Advisory Committee on Immunization Practices (ACIP), the American Academy of Family Physicians (AAFP), the American College of Obstetricians and Gynecologists (ACOG), and the American College of Physicians (ACP).

Table 69. Guide to tetanus prophylaxis in wound management.

History of Absorbed Tetanus Toxoid	Clean, Minor Wounds		All Other Wounds[1]	
	Tdap or Td[2]	TIG[3]	Tdap or Td[2]	TIG[3]
Unknown or < 3 doses	Yes	No	Yes	Yes
3 or more doses	No[4]	No	No[5]	No

[1]Such as, but not limited to, wounds contaminated with dirt, feces, soil, saliva, etc; puncture wounds; avulsions; and wounds resulting from missiles, crushing, burns, and frostbite.
[2]Td indicates tetanus toxoid and diphtheria toxoid, adult form. Tdap indicates tetanous toxoid, reduced diphtheria toxoid, and acellular pertussis vaccine, which may be substituted as a single dose for Td. Unvaccinated individuals should receive a complete series of three doses, one of which is Tdap.
[3]Human tetanus immune globulin, 250 units intramuscularly.
[4]Yes if more than 10 years have elapsed since last dose.
[5]Yes if more than 5 years have elapsed since last dose. (More frequent boosters are not needed and can enhance side effects.) Tdap has been safely administered within 2 years of Td vaccination, although local reactions to the vaccine may be increased.

Table 70. Prevention regimens for infection in immunocompromised patients.

Etiology	Microorganism	Therapy	Dose/Duration
Transplant	Pneumocystis jiroveci	Trimethoprim-sulfamethoxazole (TMP-SMZ)	One double-strength tablet three times a week or one double-strength tablet twice a day on weekends or one single-strength tablet daily for 3–6 months
		In TMP-SMZ allergy:	
		Aerosolized pentamidine	300 mg once a month
		Dapsone (check glucose-6 phosphate dehydrogenase levels)	50 mg daily or 100 mg three times a week
Solid organ or bone marrow herpes simplex-seropositive patients	Herpes simplex	Acyclovir or ganciclovir	200 mg orally three times daily for 4 weeks (bone marrow transplants) or for 12 weeks (other solid organ transplants)
Cytomegalovirus (CMV)-seronegative solid organ transplant patients who receive transplants from seropositive donors	CMV	Ganciclovir	2.5–5 mg/kg intravenously twice daily during hospitalization (usually about 10 days) then oral ganciclovir, 1 g three times daily, for 3 months
CMV-seropositive solid organ transplant patients	CMV; herpesvirus	Ganciclovir	2.5–5 mg/kg intravenously twice daily during hospitalization (usually about 10 days) then oral acyclovir, 800 mg four times a day or oral ganciclovir, 1 g three times daily for 3 months
Periods of rejection	CMV	Ganciclovir	2.5–5 mg/kg intravenously twice daily during rejection therapy
Bone marrow transplant[1]			
Universal prophylaxis for all seropositive patients who receive allogeneic transplants	CMV	Ganciclovir	5 mg/kg intravenously every 12 h for a week, then oral ganciclovir, 1 g three times daily to Day 100; alternatively, patients can be followed without specific therapy and have blood sampled weekly for the presence of CMV; if CMV is detected by an antigenemia assay, preemptive therapy
Preemptive therapy; less toxic than universal prophylaxis	CMV	Ganciclovir	5 mg/kg intravenously twice daily for 7–14 days, then oral ganciclovir, 1 g three times daily to Day 100
CMV-seronegative recipients			Use of CMV-negative or leukocyte-depleted blood products
Severe hypogammaglobulinemia following bone marrow transplantation		Intravenous immunoglobulin	
Neutropenia[2–4]	Fungal	Amphotericin B	Moderate dose (0.5 mg/kg/day) and low dose (0.1–0.25 mg/kg/day)
		Liposomal preparations of amphotericin B, aerosolized amphotericin B, itraconazole (capsules and solution), voriconazole	

[1]Whether universal prophylaxis or observation with preemptive therapy is the best approach has not been determined.
[2]Routine decontamination of the gastrointestinal tract to prevent bacteremia in the neutropenic patient is not recommended.
[3]Prophylactic administration of antibiotics in the afebrile, asymptomatic neutropenic patient is controversial, though many centers have adopted this strategy.
[4]Because voriconazole appears to be more effective than amphotericin for documented aspergillus infections, one approach to prophylaxis is to use fluconazole for patients at low risk for developing fungal infections (those who receive autologous bone marrow transplants) and voriconazole for those at high risk (allogeneic transplants).

Table 71. Antimicrobial agents for treatment of anthrax or for prophylaxis against anthrax.

First-line agents and recommended doses
    Ciprofloxacin, 500 mg twice daily orally or 400 mg every 12 hours
      intravenously
    Doxycycline, 100 mg every 12 hours orally or intravenously
Second-line agents and recommended doses
    Amoxicillin, 500 mg three times daily orally
    Penicillin G, 2 mU every 4 hours intravenously
Alternative agents with in vitro activity and suggested doses
    Rifampin, 10 mg/kg/d orally or intravenously
    Clindamycin, 450–600 mg every 8 hours orally or intravenously
    Clarithromycin, 500 mg orally twice daily
    Erythromycin, 500 mg every 6 hours intravenously
    Vancomycin, 1 g every 12 hours intravenously
    Imipenem, 500 mg every 6 hours intravenously

Table 72. American Heart Association recommendations for endocarditis prophylaxis for dental procedures for patients with cardiac conditions.[1–3]

Oral	Amoxicillin	2 g 1 hour before procedure
Penicillin allergy	Clindamycin or	600 mg 1 hour before procedure
	Cephalexin or	2 g 1 hour before procedure (contraindicated if there is history of a β-lactam immediate hypersensitivity reaction)
	Azithromycin or clarithromycin	500 mg 1 hour before procedure
Parenteral	Ampicillin	2 g IM or IV 30 minutes before procedure
Penicillin allergy	Clindamycin or	600 mg IV 1 hour before procedure
	Cefazolin	1 g IM or IV 30 minutes before procedure (contraindicated if there is history of a β-lactam immediate hypersensitivity reaction)

[1]Modified and reproduced, with permission, from the American Heart Association. Circulation. 2007 Oct 9;116(15):1736–54.
[2]For patients undergoing respiratory tract procedures involving incision of respiratory tract mucosa to treat an established infection or a procedure on infected skin, skin structure, or musculoskeletal tissue known or suspected to be caused by *S aureus*, the regimen should contain an anti-staphylococcal penicillin or cephalosporin. Vancomycin can be used to treat patients unable to tolerate a β-lactam or if the infection is known or suspected to be caused by a methicillin-resistant strain of *S aureus*.
[3]See Table 73 for list of cardiac conditions.

Table 73. Cardiac conditions with high risk of adverse outcomes from endocarditis for which prophylaxis with dental procedures is recommended.[1,2]

Prosthetic cardiac valve
Previous infective endocarditis
Congenital heart disease (CHD)[3]
    Unrepaired cyanotic CHD, including palliative shunts and conduits
    Completely repaired congenital heart defect with prosthetic material or
      device, whether placed by surgery or by catheter intervention, during the
      first 6 months after the procedure[4]
    Repaired CHD with residual defects at the site or adjacent to the site of a
      prosthetic patch or prosthetic device
Cardiac transplantation recipients in whom cardiac valvulopathy develops

[1]Based on recommendations by the American Heart Association. Circulation. 2007 Oct 9;116(15):1736–54.
[2]See Table 72 for prophylactic regimens.
[3]Except for the conditions listed above, antibiotic prophylaxis is no longer recommended for other forms of CHD.
[4]Prophylaxis is recommended because endothelialization of prosthetic material occurs within 6 months after procedure.

Table 74. Recommendations for administration of bacterial endocarditis prophylaxis for patients according to type of procedure.[1]

Prophylaxis Recommended	Prophylaxis Not Recommended
Dental procedures All dental procedures that involve manipulation of gingival tissue or the periapical region of the teeth or perforation of the oral mucosa **Respiratory tract procedures** Only respiratory tract procedures that involve incision of the respiratory mucosa **Procedures on infected skin, skin structure, or musculoskeletal tissue**	**Dental procedures** Routine anesthetic injections through noninfected tissue, taking dental radiographs, placement of removable prosthodontic or orthodontic appliances, adjustment of orthodontic appliances, placement of orthodontic brackets, shedding of deciduous teeth, and bleeding from trauma to the lips or oral mucosa **Gastrointestinal tract procedures** **Genitourinary tract procedures**

[1]Based on recommendations by the American Heart Association. Circulation. 2007 Oct 9;116(15):1736–54.

Table 75. Treatment of infective endocarditis.

Condition	Standard Therapy	Remarks
Empirical regimens pending culture results	Nafcillin or oxacillin, 1.5 g intravenously every 4 h, plus penicillin, 2–3 million units every 4 h (or ampicillin, 1.5 g every 4 h), plus gentamicin, 1 mg/kg every 8 h	Should include agents active against staphylococci, streptococci, and enterococci
For penicillin allergy or if infection by methicillin-resistant staphylococci is suspected	Vancomycin, 15 mg/kg intravenously every 12 h	
Viridans streptococci		
Penicillin-susceptible viridans streptococci (ie, minimum inhibitory concentration [MIC] ≤ 0.1 μg/mL)	Penicillin G, 2–3 million units intravenously every 4 h for 4 weeks; the duration of therapy can be shortened to 2 weeks if gentamicin, 1 mg/kg every 8 h, is used with penicillin or Ceftriaxone, 2 g once daily intravenously or intramuscularly for 4 weeks	A convenient regimen for home therapy
In the penicillin-allergic patient	Vancomycin, 15 mg/kg intravenously every 12 h for 4 weeks	The 2-week regimen is not recommended for patients with symptoms of more than 3 months duration or patients with complications such as myocardial abscess or extracardiac infection; prosthetic valve endocarditis should be treated with a 6-week course of penicillin with at least 2 weeks of gentamicin
Viridans streptococci relatively resistant to penicillin (ie, MIC > 0.1 μg/mL but ≤ 0.5 μg/mL)	Penicillin G, 3 million units intravenously every 4 h for 4 weeks; combine with gentamicin, 1 mg/kg every 8 h for the first 2 weeks	
Viridans streptococci resistant to penicillin (MIC > 0.5 μg/mL)	Treat as for enterococci	
In the penicillin-allergic patient	Vancomycin, 15 mg/kg intravenously every 12 h for 4 weeks	
Enterococci	Ampicillin, 2 g intravenously every 4 h, or penicillin G, 3–4 million units every 4 h plus gentamicin, 1 mg/kg every 8 h for 4–6 weeks	The relapse rate is unacceptably high when penicillin is used alone; because aminoglycoside resistance occurs in enterococci, susceptibility should be documented; the longer duration of therapy is recommended for patients with symptoms for more than 3 months, relapse, or prosthetic valve endocarditis, though a recent retrospective study of native valve enterococcal endocarditis suggests that less than 4 weeks of an aminoglycoside may be sufficient
In the penicillin-allergic patient	Vancomycin, 15 mg/kg intravenously every 12 h, plus gentamicin, 1 mg/kg every 8 h	
Enterococci that demonstrate high-level resistance to aminoglycosides (ie, not inhibited by 500 μg/mL of gentamicin)	Ampicillin, high dose (16 g/day by continuous infusion for 8–12 weeks)	The addition of an aminoglycoside will not be beneficial. Relapse rate up to 50%. Surgery may be the only option.
Staphylococci		
For methicillin-susceptible *Staphylococcus aureus*	Nafcillin or oxacillin, 1.5 g intravenously every 4 h for 4–6 weeks	
For methicillin-resistant strain	Vancomycin, 15 mg/kg intravenously every 12 h for 4 weeks	Aminoglycoside combination regimens may be useful in shortening the duration of bacteremia; their maximum benefit is achieved at low doses (1 mg/kg every 8 h) and in the first 3–5 days of therapy, and they should not be continued beyond the early phase of therapy; for treatment of tricuspid valve endocarditis (with or without pulmonary involvement) in the injection drug user who does not have serious extrapulmonary sites of infection, the total duration of therapy can be shortened from 4 to 2 weeks if an aminoglycoside is added to an antistaphylococcal drug for the entire 2 weeks of therapy

(continued)

Table 75. Treatment of infective endocarditis. (continued)

Condition	Standard Therapy	Remarks
Staphylococci (continued)		
Coagulase-negative staphylococci	Vancomycin, 15 mg/kg intravenously for 6 weeks, plus rifampin, 300 mg orally every 8 h for 6 weeks, plus gentamicin, 1 mg/kg intravenously every 8 h for the first 2 weeks	Routinely resistant to methicillin; β-lactam antibiotics should not be used until the isolate is known to be susceptible; if the organism is sensitive to methicillin, either nafcillin or oxacillin or cefazolin can be used in combination with rifampin and gentamicin
Prosthetic valve endocarditis	Combination therapy with nafcillin or oxacillin (vancomycin for methicillin-resistant strains or patients allergic to β-lactams), rifampin, and gentamicin	
HACEK organisms (*Haemophilus aphrophilus, Haemophilus parainfluenzae, Actinobacillus actinomycetemcomitans, Cardiobacterium hominis, Eikenella corrodens,* and *Kingella kingae*)	Ceftriaxone (or some other third-generation cephalosporin), 2 g intravenously or intramuscularly once daily for 4 weeks	These organisms can produce β-lactamase; prosthetic valve endocarditis should be treated for 6 weeks
In the penicillin-allergic patient	Trimethoprim-sulfamethoxazole, quinolones, and aztreonam have in vitro activity and should be considered	

Table 76. Treatment of anaerobic intra-abdominal infections.

Oral therapy
   Moxifloxacin 400 mg every 24 hours
Intravenous therapy
   Moderate to moderately severe infections:
      Ertapenem 1 g every 24 hours
            or—
      Ceftriaxone 1 g every 24 hours (or ciprofloxacin 400 mg every 12 hours, if penicillin allergic) plus metronidazole 500 mg every 8 hours
            or—
      Tigecycline 100 mg once followed by 50 mg every 12 hours
            or—
      Moxifloxacin 400 mg every 24 hours
   Severe infections:
      Imipenem, 0.5 g every 6–8 hours; meropenem 1 g every 8 hours; doripenem 0.5 g every 8 hours; piperacillin/tazobactam 4.5 g every 8 hours

Table 77. Fecal leukocytes in intestinal disorders.

Infectious			Noninfectious
Present	**Variable**	**Absent**	**Present**
Shigella	*Salmonella*	Noroviruses	Ulcerative colitis
Campylobacter	*Yersinia*	Rotavirus	Crohn's disease
Enteroinvasive	*Vibrio para-*	*Giardia lamblia*	Radiation colitis
Escherichia	*haemolytica*	*Entamoeba histolytica*	Ischemic colitis
coli (EIEC)	*Clostridium*	*Cryptosporidium*	
	difficile	"Food poisoning"	
	Aeromonas	*Staphylococcus aureus*	
		Bacillus cereus	
		Clostridium perfringens	
		E coli	
		Enterotoxigenic (ETEC)	
		Enterohemorrhagic (EHEC)	

Table 78. Treatment of Lyme disease.

Manifestations	Drug and Dosage
Tick bite	No treatment in most circumstances (see text); observe
Erythema migrans	Doxycycline, 100 mg orally twice daily, or amoxicillin, 500 mg orally three times daily, or cefuroxime axetil, 500 mg orally twice daily—all for 2–3 weeks
Neurologic disease	
Bell palsy (without meningitis)	Doxycycline, amoxicillin, or cefuroxime axetil as above for 2–3 weeks
Other central nervous system disease	Ceftriaxone, 2 g intravenously once daily, or penicillin G, 18–24 million units daily intravenously in six divided doses, or cefotaxime, 2 g intravenously every 8 hours—all for 2–4 weeks
Cardiac disease	
Atrioventricular block and myopericarditis[1]	An oral or parenteral regimen as described above can be used
	Ceftriaxone or penicillin G as above for 30–60 days (see text)
Arthritis	
Oral dosage	Doxycycline, amoxicillin, or cefuroxime axetil as above for 28 days (see text)
Parenteral dosage	Ceftriaxone, cefotaxime, or penicillin G as above for 2–4 weeks
Acrodermatitis chronicum atrophicans	Doxycycline, amoxicillin, or cefuroxime axetil as above for 3 weeks
"Chronic Lyme disease" or "post-Lyme disease syndrome"	Symptomatic therapy

[1]Symptomatic patients, those with second- or third-degree block and those with first-degree block with a PR interval ≥ 30 milliseconds should be hospitalized for observation.

Table 79. Treatment of amebiasis.[1]

Clinical Setting	Drugs of Choice and Adult Dosage	Alternative Drugs and Adult Dosage
Asymptomatic intestinal infection	Luminal agent: Diloxanide furoate,[2] 500 mg orally three times daily for 10 days –or– Iodoquinol, 650 mg orally three times daily for 21 days –or– Paromomycin, 10 mg/kg orally three times daily for 7 days	
Mild to moderate intestinal infection	Metronidazole, 750 mg orally three times daily (or 500 mg IV every 6 hours) for 10 days –or– Tinidazole, 2 g orally daily for 3 days –plus– Luminal agent (see above)	Luminal agent (see above) plus either– Tetracycline, 250 mg orally three times daily for 10 days –or– Erythromycin, 500 mg orally four times daily for 10 days
Severe intestinal infection	Metronidazole, 750 mg orally three times daily (or 500 mg IV every 6 hours) for 10 days –or– Tinidazole, 2 g orally daily for 3 days –plus– Luminal agent (see above)	Luminal agent (see above) plus either– Tetracycline, 250 mg orally three times daily for 10 days –or– Dehydroemetine[3] or emetine,[2] 1 mg/kg SC or IM for 3–5 days
Hepatic abscess, ameboma, and other extraintestinal disease	Metronidazole, 750 mg orally three times daily (or 500 mg IV every 6 hours) for 10 days –or– Tinidazole, 2 g orally daily for 3 days –plus– Luminal agent (see above)	Dehydroemetine[3] or emetine,[2] 1 mg/kg SC or IM for 8–10 days, followed by (liver abscess only) chloroquine, 500 mg orally twice daily for 2 days, then 500 mg daily for 21 days –plus– Luminal agent (see above)

[1]See text for additional details and cautions.
[2]Not available in the United States.
[3]Available in the United States only from the CDC Drug Service, Centers for Disease Control and Prevention, Atlanta (404-639-3670).

Table 80. WHO recommendations for the treatment of malaria.

Regimen	Notes
Artemether-lumefantrine (Coartem, Riamet)[1]	Coformulated, first-line therapy in multiple African countries.
Artesunate-amodiaquine (ASAQ)[1]	Coformulated, first-line therapy in multiple African countries.
Artesunate-mefloquine	Standard therapy in parts of southeast Asia
Artesunate-sulfadoxine-pyrimethamine	Efficacy low compared with other regimens in some areas
Amodiaquine-sulfadoxine-pyrimethamine	Less expensive; efficacy varies, but remains good in some areas; recommended as an interim option when efficacy established and other regimens are not available

[1]Not available in the United States.
World Health Organization: Guidelines for the Treatment of Malaria. World Health Organization. Geneva 2006. *ISBM* 924 1546948.

Table 81. Drugs for the prevention of malaria in travelers.[1]

Drug	Use[2]	Adult Dosage (All Oral)[3]
Chloroquine	Areas without resistant *Plasmodium falciparum*	500 mg weekly
Malarone	Areas with multidrug-resistant *P falciparum*	1 tablet (250 mg atovaquone/100 mg proguanil) daily
Mefloquine	Areas with chloroquine-resistant *P falciparum*	250 mg weekly
Doxycycline	Areas with multidrug-resistant *P falciparum*	100 mg daily
Primaquine[4]	Terminal prophylaxis of *Plasmodium vivax* and *Plasmodium ovale* infections	30 mg base daily for 14 days after travel

[1]Recommendations may change, as resistance to all available drugs is increasing. See text for additional information on toxicities and cautions. For additional details and pediatric dosing, see Centers for Disease Control and Prevention's guidelines (phone: 877-FYI-TRIP; http://www.cdc.gov). Travelers to remote areas should consider carrying effective therapy (see text) for use if a febrile illness develops, and they cannot reach medical attention quickly.
[2]Areas without known chloroquine-resistant *P falciparum* are Central America west of the Panama Canal, Haiti, Dominican Republic, Egypt, and most malarious countries of the Middle East. Malarone or mefloquine is currently recommended for other malarious areas except for border areas of Thailand, where doxycycline is recommended.
[3]For drugs other than primaquine, begin 1–2 weeks before departure (except 2 days before for doxycycline and Malarone) and continue for 4 weeks after leaving the endemic area (except 1 week for Malarone). All dosages refer to salts unless otherwise indicated.
[4]Screen for glucose-6-phosphate dehydrogenase deficiency before using primaquine.
Reproduced, with permission, from Katzung BG. *Basic & Clinical Pharmacology*. 10th edition. McGraw-Hill, 2007.

Table 82. Major antimalarial drugs.

Drug	Class	Use
Chloroquine	4-Aminoquinoline	Treatment and chemoprophylaxis of infection with sensitive parasites
Amodiaquine[1]	4-Aminoquinoline	Treatment of infection with some chloroquine-resistant *Plasmodium falciparum* strains
Piperaquine[1]	4-Aminoquinoline	Treatment of *P falciparum* in fixed combination with dihydroartemisinin
Quinine	Quinoline methanol	Oral treatment of infections with chloroquine-resistant *P falciparum*
Quinidine	Quinoline methanol	Intravenous therapy of severe infections with *P falciparum*
Mefloquine	Quinoline methanol	Chemoprophylaxis and treatment of infections with *P falciparum*
Primaquine	8-Aminoquinoline	Radical cure and terminal prophylaxis of infections with *Plasmodium vivax* and *Plasmodium ovale*
Sulfadoxine-pyrimethamine (Fansidar)	Folate antagonist combination	Treatment of infections with some chloroquine-resistant *P falciparum*
Atovaquone-proguanil (Malarone)	Quinone-folate antagonist combination	Treatment and chemoprophylaxis of *P falciparum* infection
Chlorproguanil-dapsone (Lapdap)[1]	Folate antagonist combination	Treatment of multidrug-resistant *P falciparum* in Africa
Doxycycline	Tetracycline	Treatment (with quinine) of infections with *P falciparum*; chemoprophylaxis
Halofantrine[1]	Phenanthrene methanol	Treatment of infections with some chloroquine-resistant *P falciparum*
Lumefantrine[1]	Amyl alcohol	Treatment of *P falciparum* malaria in fixed combination with artemether (Coartem)
Artemisinins[1] (Artesunate, artemether, dihydroartemisinin)	Sesquiterpene lactone endoperoxides	Treatment of infection with multidrug-resistant *P falciparum*, generally in combination regimens

[1]Not available in the United States.
Modified, with permission, from Katzung BG. *Basic & Clinical Pharmacology*. 10th edition. McGraw-Hill, 2007.

Table 83. Treatment of malaria.

Clinical Setting	Drug Therapy[1]	Alternative Drugs
Chloroquine-sensitive *Plasmodium falciparum* and *Plasmodium malariae* infections	Chloroquine phosphate, 1 g, followed by 500 mg at 6, 24, and 48 hours –or– Chloroquine phosphate, 1 g at 0 and 24 hours, then 0.5 g at 48 hours	
Plasmodium vivax and *Plasmodium ovale* infections	Chloroquine (as above), then (if G6PD normal) primaquine, 30 mg base daily for 14 days	
Uncomplicated infections with chloroquine-resistant *P falciparum*	Quinine sulfate, 650 mg three times daily for 3–7 days Plus one of the following (when quinine given for < 7 days)– Doxycycline, 100 mg twice daily for 7 days –or– Clindamycin, 600 mg twice daily for 7 days	Malarone, 4 tablets (total of 1 g atovaquone, 400 mg proguanil) daily for 3 days –or– Mefloquine, 15 mg /kg once or 750 mg, then 500 mg in 6–8 hours –or– Coartem[2] (artemether 20 mg, lumefantrine 120 mg), four tablets twice daily for 3 days –or– ASAQ[2] (artesunate 100 mg, amodiaquine 270 mg), two tablets daily for 3 days
Severe or complicated infections with *P falciparum*[3]	Artesunate 2.4 mg/kg IV every 12 hours for 1 day, then daily[3,6]	Quinidine gluconate,[4-6] 10 mg/kg IV over 1–2 hours, then 0.02 mg/kg IV/min –or– Quinidine gluconate,[4-6] 15 mg/kg IV over 4 hours, then 7.5 mg/kg IV over 4 hours every 8 hours –or– Quinine dihydrochloride,[2,4-6] 20 mg/kg IV over 4 hours, then 10 mg/kg IV every 8 hours –or– Artemether,[2,6] 3.2 mg/kg IM, then 1.6 mg/kg/d IM

[1]All dosages are oral and refer to salts unless otherwise indicated. See text for additional information on all agents, including toxicities and cautions. See Centers for Disease Control and Prevention's guidelines (phone: 877-FYI-TRIP; http://www.cdc.gov) for additional information and pediatric dosing.
[2]Not available in the United States.
[3]Available in the United States only on an investigational basis through the CDC (phone: 770-488-7788).
[4]Cardiac monitoring should be in place during intravenous administration of quinidine or quinine.
[5]Avoid loading doses in persons who have received quinine, quinidine, or mefloquine in the prior 24 hours.
[6]With all parenteral regimens, change to an oral regimen (most commonly doxycycline in adults or clindamycin in children) as soon as the patient can tolerate it.
G6PD, glucose-6-phosphate dehydrogenase.
Modified, with permission, from Katzung BG. *Basic & Clinical Pharmacology*. 10th edition. McGraw-Hill, 2007.

Table 84. Guidelines for treatment of malaria in the United States.

(Based on drugs currently available for use in the United States)

CDC Malaria Hotline: (770) 488-7788 Monday-Friday 8 am to 4:30 pm EST
(770) 488-7100 after hours, weekends and holidays (ask to page the malaria person on-call)

Clinical Diagnosis/ *Plasmodium* species	Region Infection Acquired	Recommended Drug and Adult Dose[1,8]	Recommended Drug and Pediatric Dose[1,8] *Pediatric dose should NEVER exceed adult dose*
Uncomplicated malaria/ *P. falciparum* or Species not identified If "species not identified" is subsequently diagnosed as *P. vivax* or *P. ovale*: see *P. vivax* and *P. ovale* (below) regarding treatment with primaquine	**Chloroquine-sensitive** (Central America west of Panama Canal; Haiti; the Dominican Republic; and most of the Middle East)	**Chloroquine phosphate (Aralen™ and generics)** 600 mg base (=1,000 mg salt) po immediately, followed by 300 mg base (=500 mg salt) po at 6, 24, and 48 hours Total dose: 1,500 mg base (=2,500 mg salt) *2nd line alternative for treatment:* **Hydroxychloroquine (Plaquenil™ and generics)** 620 mg base (=800 mg salt) po immediately, followed by 310 mg base (=400 mg salt) po at 6, 24, and 48 hours Total dose: 1,550 mg base (=2,000 mg salt)	**Chloroquine phosphate (Aralen™ and generics)** 10 mg base/kg po immediately, followed by 5 mg base/kg po at 6, 24, and 48 hours Total dose: 25 mg base/kg *2nd line alternative for treatment:* **Hydroxychloroquine (Plaquenil™ and generics)** 10 mg base/kg po immediately, followed by 5 mg base/kg po at 6, 24, and 48 hours Total dose: 25 mg base/kg
	Chloroquine-resistant or unknown resistance[1] (All malarious regions except those specified as chloroquine-sensitive listed in the box above. Middle Eastern countries with chloroquine-resistant *P. falciparum* include Iran, Oman, Saudi Arabia, and Yemen. Of note, infections acquired in the Newly Independent States of the former Soviet Union and Korea to date have been uniformly caused by *P. vivax* and should therefore be treated as chloroquine-sensitive infections.)	**A. Quinine sulfate**[2] **plus one of the following:** **Doxycycline, Tetracycline, or Clindamycin** **Quinine sulfate:** 542 mg base (=650 mg salt)[3] po tid x 3 to 7 days **Doxycycline:** 100 mg po bid x 7 days **Tetracycline:** 250 mg po qid x 7 days **Clindamycin:** 20 mg base/kg/day po divided tid x 7 days **B. Atovaquone-proguanil (Malarone™)**[5] **Adult tab** = 250 mg atovaquone/ 100 mg proguanil 4 adult tabs po qd x 3 days	**A. Quinine sulfate**[2,3] **plus one of the following:** **Doxycycline**[4]**, Tetracycline**[4] **or Clindamycin** **Quinine sulfate:** 8.3 mg base/kg (=10 mg salt/kg)[3] po tid x 3 to 7 days **Doxycycline:** 2.2 mg/kg po every 12 hours x 7 days **Tetracycline:** 25 mg/kg/day po divided qid x 7 days **Clindamycin:** 20 mg base/kg/day po divided tid x 7 days **B. Atovaquone-proguanil (Malarone™)**[5] **Adult tab** = 250 mg atovaquone/ 100 mg proguanil **Peds tab** = 62.5 mg atovaquone/ 25 mg proguanil 5 - 8 kg: 2 peds tabs po qd x 3 d 9-10 kg: 3 peds tabs po qd x 3 d 11-20 kg: 1 adult tab po qd x 3 d 21-30 kg: 2 adult tabs po qd x 3d 31-40 kg: 3 adult tabs po qd x 3d > 40 kg: 4 adult tabs po qd x 3d
		C. Mefloquine (Lariam™ and generics)[6] 684 mg base (=750 mg salt) po as initial dose, followed by 456 mg base (=500 mg salt) po given 6-12 hours after initial dose Total dose= 1,250 mg salt *2nd line alternative for treatment:* **Chloroquine phosphate:** Treatment as above **Hydroxychloroquine:** Treatment as above	**C. Mefloquine (Lariam™ and generics)**[6] 13.7 mg base/kg (=15 mg salt/kg) po as initial dose, followed by 9.1 mg base/kg (=10 mg salt/kg) po given 6-12 hours after initial dose Total dose= 25 mg salt/kg *2nd line alternative for treatment:* **Chloroquine phosphate:** Treatment as above **Hydroxychloroquine:** Treatment as above
Uncomplicated malaria/ *P. malariae*	**All regions**	**Chloroquine phosphate:** Treatment as above *2nd line alternative for treatment:* **Hydroxychloroquine:** Treatment as above	**Chloroquine phosphate:** Treatment as above *2nd line alternative for treatment:* **Hydroxychloroquine:** Treatment as above

[1] NOTE: There are three options (A, B, or C) available for treatment of uncomplicated malaria caused by chloroquine-resistant *P. falciparum*. Options A and B are equally recommended. Because of a higher rate of severe neuropsychiatric reactions seen at treatment doses, we do not recommend option C (mefloquine) unless options A and B cannot be used. For option A, because there is more data on the efficacy of quinine in combination with doxycycline or tetracycline, these treatment combinations are generally preferred to quinine in combination with clindamycin.
[2] For infections acquired in Southeast Asia, quinine treatment should continue for 7 days. For infections acquired in Africa and South America, quinine treatment should continue for 3 days.
[3] US manufactured quinine sulfate capsule is in a 324mg dosage; therefore 2 capsules should be sufficient for adult dosing. Pediatric dosing may be difficult due to unavailability of non-capsule forms of quinine. If unable to provide pediatric doses of quinine, consider malarone (recommendation B) or mefloquine (recommendation C).
[4] Doxycycline and tetracycline are not indicated for use in children less than 8 years old. For children less than 8 years old with chloroquine-resistant *P. falciparum*, quinine (given alone for 7 days or given in combination with clindamycin) and atovaquone-proguanil are recommended treatment options; mefloquine can be considered if no other options are available. For children less than 8 years old with chloroquine-resistant *P. vivax*, quinine (given alone for 7 days) or mefloquine are recommended treatment options. If none of these treatment options are available or are not being tolerated and if the treatment benefits outweigh the risks, doxycycline or tetracycline may be given to children less than 8 years old.
[5] Give atovaquone-proguanil with food. If patient vomits within 30 minutes of taking a dose, then they should repeat the dose.
[6] Treatment with mefloquine is not recommended in persons who have acquired infections from the Southeast Asian region of Burma, Thailand, and Cambodia due to resistant strains.

Clinical Diagnosis/ Plasmodium species	Region Infection Acquired	Recommended Drug and Adult Dose[1,8]	Recommended Drug and Pediatric Dose[1,8] *Pediatric dose should NEVER exceed adult dose*
Uncomplicated malaria/ *P. vivax* or *P. ovale*	**All regions**[8] Note: for suspected chloroquine-resistant *P. vivax*, see row below	**Chloroquine phosphate plus Primaquine phosphate**[7] Chloroquine phosphate: Treatment as above Primaquine phosphate: 30 mg base po qd x 14 days *2nd line alternative for treatment:* Hydroxychloroquine plus Primaquine phosphate[7] Hydroxychloroquine: Treatment as above Primaquine phosphate: 30 mg base po qd x 14 days	**Chloroquine phosphate plus Primaquine phosphate**[7] Chloroquine phosphate: Treatment as above Primaquine phosphate: 0.5 mg base/kg po qd x 14 days *2nd line alternative for treatment:* Hydroxychloroquine plus Primaquine phosphate[7] Hydroxychloroquine: Treatment as above Primaquine phosphate: 30 mg base po qd x 14 days
Uncomplicated malaria/ *P. vivax*	**Chloroquine-resistant**[8] (Papua New Guinea and Indonesia)	**A. Quinine sulfate**[2] plus either Doxycycline or Tetracycline plus Primaquine phosphate[7] Quinine sulfate: Treatment as above Doxycycline or Tetracycline: Treatment as above Primaquine phosphate: Treatment as above **B. Mefloquine plus Primaquine phosphate**[7] Mefloquine: Treatment as above Primaquine phosphate: Treatment as above	**A. Quinine sulfate**[2,3] plus either Doxycycline[4] or Tetracycline[4] plus Primaquine phosphate[7] Quinine sulfate: Treatment as above Doxycycline or Tetracycline: Treatment as above Primaquine phosphate: Treatment as above **B. Mefloquine plus Primaquine phosphate**[7] Mefloquine: Treatment as above Primaquine phosphate: Treatment as above
Uncomplicated malaria: alternatives for pregnant women [9,10,11,12]	**Chloroquine-sensitive**[12] (see uncomplicated malaria sections above for chloroquine-sensitive *Plasmodium* species by region)	**Chloroquine phosphate**: Treatment as above *2nd line alternative for treatment:* Hydroxychloroquine: Treatment as above	Not applicable
	Chloroquine resistant *P. falciparum*[9,10,11] (see uncomplicated malaria sections above for regions with known chloroquine resistant *P. falciparum*)	**Quinine sulfate**[2] plus Clindamycin Quinine sulfate: Treatment as above Clindamycin: Treatment as above	Not applicable
	Chloroquine-resistant *P. vivax*[9,10,11,12] (see uncomplicated malaria sections above for regions with chloroquine-resistant *P. vivax*)	**Quinine sulfate** Quinine sulfate: 650 mg salt po tid x 7 days	Not applicable

[7] Primaquine is used to eradicate any hypnozoite forms that may remain dormant in the liver, and thus prevent relapses, in *P. vivax* and *P. ovale* infections. Because primaquine can cause hemolytic anemia in persons with G6PD deficiency, patients must be screened for G6PD deficiency prior to starting treatment with primaquine. For persons with borderline G6PD deficiency or as an alternate to the above regimen, primaquine may be given 45 mg orally one time per week for 8 weeks; consultation with an expert in infectious disease and/or tropical medicine is advised if this alternative regimen is considered in G6PD-deficient persons. Primaquine must not be used during pregnancy.

[8] NOTE: There are two options (A or B) available for treatment of uncomplicated malaria caused by chloroquine-resistant *P. vivax*. High treatment failure rates due to chloroquine-resistant *P. vivax* have been well documented in Papua New Guinea and Indonesia. Rare case reports of chloroquine-resistant *P. vivax* have also been documented in Burma (Myanmar), India, and Central and South America. Persons acquiring *P. vivax* infections outside of Papua New Guinea or Indonesia should be started on chloroquine. If the patient does not respond, the treatment should be changed to a chloroquine-resistant *P. vivax* regimen and CDC should be notified (Malaria Hotline number listed above). For treatment of chloroquine-resistant *P. vivax* infections, options A and B are equally recommended.

[9] For pregnant women diagnosed with uncomplicated malaria caused by chloroquine-resistant *P. falciparum* or chloroquine-resistant *P. vivax* infection, treatment with doxycycline or tetracycline is generally not indicated. However, doxycycline or tetracycline may be used in combination with quinine (as recommended for non-pregnant adults) if other treatment options are not available or are not being tolerated, and the benefit is judged to outweigh the risks.

[10] Because there are no adequate, well-controlled studies of atovaquone and/or proguanil hydrochloride in pregnant women, atovaquone-proguanil is generally not recommended for use in pregnant women. For pregnant women diagnosed with uncomplicated malaria caused by chloroquine-resistant *P. falciparum* infection, atovaquone-proguanil may be used if other treatment options are not available or are not being tolerated, and if the potential benefit is judged to outweigh the potential risks. There are no data on the efficacy of atovaquone-proguanil in the treatment of chloroquine-resistant *P. vivax* infections.

[11] Because of a possible association with mefloquine treatment during pregnancy and an increase in stillbirths, mefloquine is generally not recommended for treatment in pregnant women. However, mefloquine may be used if it is the only treatment option available and if the potential benefit is judged to outweigh the potential risks.

[12] For *P. vivax* and *P. ovale* infections, chloroquine should not be given during pregnancy. Pregnant patients with *P. vivax* and *P. ovale* infections should be maintained on chloroquine prophylaxis for the duration of their pregnancy. The chemoprophylactic dose of chloroquine phosphate is 300 mg base (=500 mg salt) orally once per week. After delivery, pregnant patients who do not have G6PD deficiency should be treated with primaquine.

(continued)

Table 84. Guidelines for treatment of malaria in the United States. (continued)

Severe malaria [13,14,15,16]	All regions
	Quinidine gluconate[14] plus one of the following: Doxycycline, Tetracycline, or Clindamycin **Quinidine gluconate:** 6.25 mg base/kg (=10 mg salt/kg) loading dose IV over 1-2 hrs, then 0.0125 mg base/kg/min (=0.02 mg salt/kg/min) continuous infusion for at least 24 hours. An alternative regimen is 15 mg base/kg (=24 mg salt/kg) loading dose IV infused over 4 hours, followed by 7.5 mg base/kg (=12 mg salt/kg) infused over 4 hours every 8 hours, starting 8 hours after the loading dose (see package insert). Once parasite density <1% and patient can take oral medication, complete treatment with oral quinine, dose as above. Quinidine/quinine course = 7 days in Southeast Asia; = 3 days in Africa or South America. **Doxycycline:** Treatment as above. If patient not able to take oral medication, give 100 mg IV every 12 hours and then switch to oral doxycycline (as above) as soon as patient can take oral medication. For IV use, avoid rapid administration. Treatment course = 7 days. **Tetracycline:** Treatment as above **Clindamycin:** Treatment as above. If patient not able to take oral medication, give 10 mg base/kg loading dose IV followed by 5 mg base/kg IV every 8 hours. Switch to oral clindamycin (oral dose as above) as soon as patient can take oral medication. For IV use, avoid rapid administration. Treatment course = 7 days. *Investigational new drug (contact CDC for information):* **Artesunate followed by one of the following:** **Atovaquone-proguanil (Malarone™),[5]** **Doxycycline (Clindamycin in pregnant women), or Mefloquine**	**Quinidine gluconate[14] plus one of the following: Doxycycline[4], Tetracycline[4], or Clindamycin** **Quinidine gluconate:** Same mg/kg dosing and recommendations as for adults. **Doxycycline:** Treatment as above. If patient not able to take oral medication, may give IV. For children <45 kg, give 2.2 mg/kg IV every 12 hours and then switch to oral doxycycline (dose as above) as soon as patient can take oral medication. For children ≥45 kg, use same dosing as for adults. For IV use, avoid rapid administration. Treatment course = 7 days. **Tetracycline:** Treatment as above **Clindamycin:** Treatment as above. If patient not able to take oral medication, give 10 mg base/kg loading dose IV followed by 5 mg base/kg IV every 8 hours. Switch to oral clindamycin (oral dose as above) as soon as patient can take oral medication. For IV use, avoid rapid administration. Treatment course = 7 days. *Investigational new drug (contact CDC for information):* **Artesunate followed by one of the following:** **Atovaquone-proguanil (Malarone™),[5]** **Clindamycin, or Mefloquine**

[13] Persons with a positive blood smear OR history of recent possible exposure and no other recognized pathology who have one or more of the following clinical criteria (impaired consciousness/coma, severe normocytic anemia, renal failure, pulmonary edema, acute respiratory distress syndrome, circulatory shock, disseminated intravascular coagulation, spontaneous bleeding, acidosis, hemoglobinuria, jaundice, repeated generalized convulsions, and/or parasitemia of > 5%) are considered to have manifestations of more severe disease. Severe malaria is practically always due to *P. falciparum*.

[14] Patients diagnosed with severe malaria should be treated aggressively with parenteral antimalarial therapy. Treatment with IV quinidine should be initiated as soon as possible after the diagnosis has been made. Patients with severe malaria should be given an intravenous loading dose of quinidine unless they have received more than 40 mg/kg of quinine in the preceding 48 hours or if they have received mefloquine within the preceding 12 hours. Consultation with a cardiologist and a physician with experience treating malaria is advised when treating malaria patients with quinidine. During administration of quinidine, blood pressure monitoring (for hypotension) and cardiac monitoring (for widening of the QRS complex and/or lengthening of the QTc interval) should be monitored continuously and blood glucose (for hypoglycemia) should be monitored periodically. Cardiac complications, if severe, may warrant temporary discontinuation of the drug or slowing of the intravenous infusion.

[15] Consider exchange transfusion if the parasite density (i.e., parasitemia) is > 10% OR if the patient has altered mental status, non-volume overload pulmonary edema, or renal complications. The parasite density can be estimated by examining a monolayer of red blood cells (RBCs) on the thin smear under oil immersion magnification. The slide should be examined where the RBCs are more or less touching (approximately 400 RBCs per field). The parasite density can then be estimated from the percentage of infected RBCs and should be monitored every 12 hours. Exchange transfusion should be continued until the parasite density is <1% (usually requires 8-10 units). IV quinidine administration should not be delayed for an exchange transfusion and can be given concurrently throughout the exchange transfusion.

[16] Pregnant women diagnosed with severe malaria should be treated aggressively with parenteral antimalarial therapy.

Courtesy of the Centers for Disease Control and Prevention.

Table 85. Stages of chronic kidney disease: a clinical action plan.[1,2]

Stage	Description	GFR (mL/min/1.73 m²)	Action[3]
1	Kidney damage with normal or ↑ GFR	≥ 90	Diagnosis and treatment. Treatment of comorbid conditions. Slowing of progression. Cardiovascular disease risk reduction.
2	Kidney damage with mildly ↓ GFR	60–89	Estimating progression.
3	Moderately ↓ GFR	30–59	Evaluating and treating complications.
4	Severely ↓ GFR	15–29	Preparation for kidney replacement therapy.
5	Kidney failure	< 15 (or dialysis)	Replacement (if uremia is present).

[1]From National Kidney Foundation, KDOQI, chronic kidney disease guidelines.
[2]Chronic kidney disease is defined as either kidney damage or GFR < 60 mL/min/1.73 m² for 3 or more months. Kidney damage is defined as pathologic abnormalities or markers of damage, including abnormalities in blood or urine tests or imaging studies.
[3]Includes actions from preceding stages.
GFR, glomerular filtration rate.

Table 86. Major causes of chronic kidney disease.

Glomerulopathies
Primary glomerular diseases
  Focal and segmental glomerulosclerosis
  Membranoproliferative glomerulonephritis
  IgA nephropathy
  Membranous nephropathy
Secondary glomerular diseases
  Diabetic nephropathy
  Amyloidosis
  Postinfectious glomerulonephritis
  HIV-associated nephropathy
  Collagen-vascular diseases
  Sickle cell nephropathy
  HIV-associated membranoproliferative glomerulonephritis
Tubulointerstitial nephritis
  Drug hypersensitivity
  Heavy metals
  Analgesic nephropathy
  Reflux/chronic pyelonephritis
  Idiopathic
Hereditary diseases
  Polycystic kidney disease
  Medullary cystic disease
  Alport syndrome
Obstructive nephropathies
  Prostatic disease
  Nephrolithiasis
  Retroperitoneal fibrosis/tumor
  Congenital
Vascular diseases
  Hypertensive nephrosclerosis
  Renal artery stenosis

Table 87. Classification and findings in glomerulonephritis: nephrotic syndromes.

	Etiology	Histopathology	Pathogenesis
Minimal change disease (nil disease; lipoid nephrosis)	Associated with allergy, Hodgkin disease, NSAIDs	**Light:** Normal (with or without mesangial proliferation) **Immunofluorescence:** No immunoglobulins **Electron microscopy:** Fusion foot processes	Unknown
Focal and segmental glomerulosclerosis	Associated with heroin abuse, HIV infection, reflux nephropathy, obesity	**Light:** Focal segmental sclerosis **Immunofluorescence:** IgM and C3 in sclerotic segments **Electron microscopy:** Fusion foot processes	Unknown
Membranous nephropathy	Associated with non-Hodgkin lymphoma, carcinoma (gastrointestinal, renal, bronchogenic, thyroid), gold therapy, penicillamine, lupus erythematosus	**Light:** Thickened GBM and spikes **Immunofluorescence:** Granular IgG and C3 along capillary loops **Electron microscopy:** Dense deposits in subepithelial area	In situ immune complex formation
Membranoproliferative glomerulonephropathy	Type I associated with upper respiratory infection	**Light:** Increased mesangial cells and matrix with splitting of GBM **Immunofluorescence:** Granular C3, C1q, C4 with IgG and IgM **Electron microscopy:** Dense deposits in subendothelium	Unknown
	Type II	**Light:** Same as type I **Immunofluorescence:** C3 only **Electron microscopy:** Dense material in GBM	Unknown

NSAIDs, nonsteroidal anti-inflammatory drugs; GBM, glomerular basement membrane.

Table 88. LDL goals and treatment cutpoints: Recommendations of the NCEP Adult Treatment Panel III.

Risk Category	LDL Goal (mg/dL)	LDL Level at Which to Initiate Lifestyle Changes (mg/dL)	LDL Level at Which to Consider Drug Therapy[1] (mg/dL)
High risk: CHD[2] or CHD risk equivalents[3] (10-year risk > 20%)	< 100 (optional goal: < 70 mg/dL)[4]	≥ 100[5]	≥ 100[6] (< 100: consider drug options)[1]
Moderately high risk: 2+ risk factors[7] (10-year risk 10% to 20%)[8]	< 130[9]	≥ 130[5]	≥ 130 (100–129; consider drug options)[10]
Moderate risk: 2+ risk factors[7] (10-year risk < 10%)[8]	< 130	≥ 130	≥ 160
Low risk: 0–1 risk factors[11]	< 160	≥ 160	≥ 190 (160–189: LDL-lowering drug optional)

[1]When LDL-lowering drug therapy is used, it is advised that intensity of therapy be sufficient to achieve at least a 30–40% reduction in LDL cholesterol levels.
[2]CHD includes history of myocardial infarction, unstable angina, coronary artery procedures (angioplasty or bypass surgery), or evidence of clinically significant myocardial ischemia.
[3]CHD risk equivalents include clinical manifestations of noncoronary forms of atherosclerotic disease (peripheral arterial disease, abdominal aortic aneurysm, and carotid artery disease [transient ischemic attacks or stroke of carotid origin with > 50% obstruction of a carotid artery]), diabetes mellitus, and ≥ 2 risk factors with 10-year risk for CHD > 20%.
[4]Very high risk favors the optional LDL cholesterol goal of < 70 mg/dL, or in patients with high triglycerides, non-high density lipoprotein (HDL) cholesterol < 100 mg/dL.
[5]Any person at high risk or moderately high risk who has lifestyle-related risk factors (eg, obesity, physical inactivity, elevated triglyceride, low HDL cholesterol, or metabolic syndrome) is a candidate for therapeutic lifestyle changes to modify these risk factors regardless of LDL cholesterol.
[6]If baseline LDL cholesterol is < 100 mg/dL, institution of an LDL-lowering drug is a therapeutic option on the basis of available clinical trial results. If a high-risk person has high triglycerides or low HDL cholesterol, combining a fibrate or nicotinic acid with an LDL-lowering drug can be considered.
[7]Risk factors include cigarette smoking, hypertension (blood pressure ≥ 140/90 mm Hg or on antihypertensive medication), low HDL cholesterol (< 40 mg/dL), family history of premature CHD (CHD in male first-degree relative < 55 years of age; CHD in female first-degree relative < 65 years of age), and age (men ≥ 45 years; women ≥ 55 years).
[8]Electronic 10-year risk calculators are available at www.nhlbi.nih.gov/guidelines/cholesterol.
[9]Optional LDL cholesterol goal < 100 mg/dL.
[10]For moderately high-risk persons, when the LDL cholesterol level is 100–129 mg/dL at baseline or on lifestyle therapy, initiation of an LDL-lowering drug to achieve an LDL cholesterol level < 100 mg/dL is a therapeutic option on the basis of available clinical trial results.
[11]Almost all people with zero or one risk factor have a 10-year CHD risk < 10%, and 10-year risk assessment in these people is thus not necessary.
LDL, low-density lipoprotein; NCEP, National Cholesterol Education Program; CHD, coronary heart disease.
Reproduced, with permission, from Grundy SM et al. Implications of recent clinical trials for the National Cholesterol Education Program Adult Treatment Panel III guidelines. Circulation. 2004 Jul 13;110(2):227–39.

Table 89. Effects of selected lipid-modifying drugs.

| Drug | Lipid-Modifying Effects | | Triglyceride | Initial Daily Dose | Maximum Daily Dose | Cost for 30 Days Treatment with Dose Listed[1] |
	LDL	HDL				
Atorvastatin (Lipitor)	–25 to –40%	+5 to 10%	↓↓	10 mg once	80 mg once	$124.64 (20 mg once)
Cholestyramine (Questran, others)	–15 to –25%	+5%	±	4 g twice a day	24 g divided	$126.65 (8 g divided)
Colesevelam (WelChol)	–10 to –20%	+10%	±	625 mg, 6–7 tablets once	625 mg, 6–7 tablets once	$205.20 (6 tablets once)
Colestipol (Colestid)	–15 to –25%	+5%	±	5 g twice a day	30 g divided	$134.44 (10 g divided)
Ezetimibe (Zetia)	–20%	+5%	±	10 mg once	10 mg once	$96.35 (10 mg once)
Fenofibrate (Tricor, others)	–10 to –15%	+15 to 25%	↓↓	48 mg once	145 mg once	$113.76 (145 mg once)
Fluvastatin (Lescol)	–20 to –30%	+5 to 10%	↓	20 mg once	40 mg once	$74.84 (20 mg once)
Gemfibrozil (Lopid)	–10 to –15%	+15 to 20%	↓↓	600 mg once	1200 mg divided	$74.80 (600 mg twice a day)
Lovastatin (Mevacor)	–25 to –40%	+5 to 10%	↓	10 mg once	80 mg divided	$71.19 (20 mg once)
Niacin (OTC, Niaspan)	–15 to –25%	+25 to 35%	↓↓	100 mg once	3–4.5 g divided	$15.28 (1.5 g twice a day, OTC) $230.83 (2 g Niaspan)
Pravastatin (Pravachol)	–25 to –40%	+5 to 10%	↓	20 mg once	40 mg once	$98.01 (20 mg once)
Rosuvastatin (Crestor)	–40 to –50%	+10 to 15%	↓↓	10 mg once	40 mg once	$103.24 (20 mg once)
Simvastatin (Zocor)	–25 to –40%	+5 to 10%	↓↓	5 mg once	80 mg once	$84.60 (10 mg once)

[1]Average wholesale price (AWP, for AB-rated generic when available) for quantity listed. Source: *Red Book Update*, Vol. 27, No. 2, February 2008. AWP may not accurately represent the actual pharmacy cost because wide contractual variations exist among institutions.
LDL, low-density lipoprotein; HDL, high-density lipoprotein; ± variable, if any; OTC, over the counter.

Table 90. Liver biochemical tests: normal values and changes in two types of jaundice.

Tests	Normal Values	Hepatocellular Jaundice	Uncomplicated Obstructive Jaundice
Bilirubin Direct Indirect	0.1–0.3 mg/dL 0.2–0.7 mg/dL	Increased Increased	Increased Increased
Urine bilirubin	None	Increased	Increased
Serum albumin/total protein	Albumin, 3.5–5.5 g/dL	Albumin decreased Total protein, 6.5–8.4 g/dL	Unchanged
Alkaline phosphatase	30–115 units/L	Increased (+)	Increased (++++)
Prothrombin time	INR of 1.0–1.4. After vitamin K, 10% increase in 24 hours	Prolonged if damage severe and does not respond to parenteral vitamin K	Prolonged if obstruction marked, but responds to parenteral vitamin K
ALT, AST	ALT, 5–35 units/L; AST, 5–40 units/L	Increased in hepatocellular damage, viral hepatitis	Minimally increased

INR, international normalized ratio; ALT, alanine aminotransferase; AST, aspartate aminotransferase.

Table 91. Common serologic patterns in hepatitis B virus infection and their interpretation.

HBsAg	Anti-HBs	Anti-HBc	HBeAg	Anti-HBe	Interpretation
+	–	IgM	+	–	Acute hepatitis B
+	–	IgG[1]	+	–	Chronic hepatitis B with active viral replication
+	–	IgG	–	+	Chronic hepatitis B with low viral replication
+	+	IgG	+ or –	+ or –	Chronic hepatitis B with heterotypic anti-HBs (about 10% of cases)
–	–	IgM	+ or –	–	Acute hepatitis B
–	+	IgG	–	+ or –	Recovery from hepatitis B (immunity)
–	+	–	–	–	Vaccination (immunity)
–	–	IgG	–	–	False-positive; less commonly, infection in remote past

[1]Low levels of IgM anti-HBc may also be detected.

Table 92. Child-Turcotte-Pugh scoring system and model for end-stage liver disease (MELD) for staging cirrhosis.

Child-Turcotte-Pugh scoring system			
	Numerical Score		
Parameter	**1**	**2**	**3**
Ascites	None	Slight	Moderate to severe
Encephalopathy	None	Slight to moderate	Moderate to severe
Bilirubin (mg/dL)	< 2.0	2–3	> 3.0
Albumin (g/dL)	> 3.5	2.8–3.5	< 2.8
Prothrombin time (seconds increased)	1–3	4–6	> 6.0

Total Numerical Score and Corresponding Child-Turcotte-Pugh Class	
Score	**Class**
5–6	A
7–9	B
10–15	C

MELD scoring system

MELD = 11.2 $\log_e$ (INR) + 3.78 $\log_e$ (bilirubin [mg/dL]) + 9.57 $\log_e$ (creatinine [mg/dL]) + 6.43. (Range 6–40).

INR, international normalized ratio.

Table 93. Diseases of the biliary tract.

	Clinical Features	Laboratory Features	Diagnosis	Treatment
Gallstones	Asymptomatic	Normal	Ultrasound	None
Gallstones	Biliary pain	Normal	Ultrasound	Laparoscopic cholecystectomy
Cholesterolosis of gallbladder	Usually asymptomatic	Normal	Oral cholecystography	None
Adenomyomatosis	May cause biliary pain	Normal	Oral cholecystography	Laparoscopic cholecystectomy if symptomatic
Porcelain gallbladder	Usually asymptomatic, high risk of gallbladder cancer	Normal	Radiograph or CT	Laparoscopic cholecystectomy
Acute cholecystitis	Epigastric or right upper quadrant pain, nausea, vomiting, fever, Murphy sign	Leukocytosis	Ultrasound, HIDA scan	Antibiotics, laparoscopic cholecystectomy
Chronic cholecystitis	Biliary pain, constant epigastric or right upper quadrant pain, nausea	Normal	Ultrasound (stones), oral cholecystography (nonfunctioning gallbladder)	Laparoscopic cholecystectomy
Choledocholithiasis	Asymptomatic or biliary pain, jaundice, fever; gallstone pancreatitis	Cholestatic liver function tests; leukocytosis and positive blood cultures in cholangitis; elevated amylase and lipase in pancreatitis	Ultrasound (dilated ducts), endoscopic ultrasound, MRCP, ERCP	Endoscopic sphincterotomy and stone extraction; antibiotics for cholangitis

HIDA, hepatic iminodiacetic acid; MRCP, magnetic resonance cholangiopancreatography; ERCP, endoscopic retrograde cholangiopancreatography.

Table 94. Ranson criteria for assessing the severity of acute pancreatitis.

Three or more of the following predicts a severe course complicated by pancreatic necrosis with a sensitivity of 60–80%

    Age over 55 years
    White blood cell count > 16,000/mcL
    Blood glucose > 200 mg/dL
    Serum lactic dehydrogenase > 350 units/L
    Aspartate aminotransferase > 250 units/L

Development of the following in the first 48 hours indicates a worsening prognosis

    Hematocrit drop of more than 10 percentage points
    Blood urea nitrogen rise > 5 mg/dL
    Arterial Po_2 of < 60 mm Hg
    Serum calcium of < 8 mg/dL
    Base deficit over 4 mEq/L
    Estimated fluid sequestration of > 6 L

Mortality rates correlate with the number of criteria present[1]

Number of Criteria	Mortality Rate
0–2	1%
3–4	16%
5–6	40%
7–8	100%

[1]An APACHE II score ≥ 8 also correlates with mortality.

Table 95. Selected pancreatic enzyme preparations.

Product	Enzyme Content per Unit Dose		
	Lipase	Amylase	Protease
Conventional preparations			
Viokase 8	8000	30,000	30,000
Pancrelipase	8000	30,000	30,000
Enteric-coated microencapsulated preparations			
Creon 10	10,000	33,200	37,500
Creon 20	20,000	66,400	75,000
Lipram CR10	10,000	33,200	37,500
Lipram UL12	12,000	39,000	39,000
Lipram PN16	16,000	48,000	48,000
Lipram UL18	18,000	58,500	58,500
Lipram CR20	20,000	66,400	75,000
Pancrease	4500	20,000	25,000
Pancrease MT 10	10,000	30,000	30,000
Pancrease MT 16	16,000	48,000	48,000
Pancrease MT 20	20,000	56,000	44,000
Ultrase MT 12	12,000	39,000	39,000
Ultrase MT 20	20,000	65,000	65,000

Source: *Martinale, The Complete Drug Reference, Pharmaceutic Press, 2006.*

Table 96. Evaluation of asthma exacerbation severity.

	Mild	Moderate	Severe	Subset: Respiratory Arrest Imminent
Symptoms				
Breathlessness	While walking	While at rest (infant—softer, shorter cry, difficulty feeding)	While at rest (infant—stops feeding)	
	Can lie down	Prefers sitting	Sits upright	
Talks in	Sentences	Phrases	Words	
Alertness	May be agitated	Usually agitated	Usually agitated	Drowsy or confused
Signs				
Respiratory rate	Increased	Increased Guide to rates of breathing in awake children: *Age* < 2 months 2–12 months 1–5 years 6–8 years	Often > 30/minute *Normal Rate* < 60/minute < 50/minute < 40/minute < 30/minute	
Use of accessory muscles; suprasternal retractions	Usually not	Commonly	Usually	Paradoxical thoracoabdominal movement
Wheeze	Moderate, often only end-expiratory	Loud; throughout exhalation	Usually loud; throughout inhalation and exhalation	Absence of wheeze
Pulse/minute	< 100	100-200 Guide to normal pulse rates in children: *Age* 2–12 months 1–2 years 2–8 years	> 120 *Normal Rate* < 160/minute < 120/minute < 110/minute	Bradycardia
Pulsus paradoxus	Absent < 10 mm Hg	May be present 10–25 mm Hg	Often present > 25 mm Hg (adult) 20–40 mm Hg (child)	Absence suggests respiratory muscle fatigue
Functional Assessment				
PEF Percent predicted or percent personal best	≥ 70%	Approx. 40–69% or response lasts < 2 hours	< 40%	< 25% Note: PEF testing may not be needed in very severe attacks
Pao_2 (on air) and/or Pco_2	Normal (test not usually necessary) < 42 mm Hg (test not usually necessary)	≥ 60 mm Hg (test not usually necessary) < 42 mm Hg (test not usually necessary)	< 60 mm Hg: possible cyanosis ≥ 42 mm Hg: possible respiratory failure	
Sao_2 percent (on air) at sea level	> 95% (test not usually necessary) Hypercapnia (hypoventilation) develops more readily in young children than in adults and adolescents.	90–95% (test not usually necessary)	< 90%	

PEF, peak expiratory low; Sao_2, oxygen saturation.
Notes:
· The presence of several parameters, but not necessarily all, indicates the general classification of the exacerbation.
· Many of these parameters have not been systematically studied, especially as they correlate with each other. Thus, they serve only as general guides.
· The emotional impact of asthma symptoms on the patient and family is variable but must be recognized and addressed and can affect approaches to treatment and follow-up.
Adapted from National Asthma Education and Prevention Program. Expert Panel Report 3: Guidelines for the Diagnosis and Management of Asthma. National Institutes of Health Pub. No. 08-4051. Bethesda, MD, 2007. www.nhlbi.nih.gov/guidelines/asthma/asthgdln.htm.

Table 97. Classifying severity of asthma exacerbations.

Note: Patients are instructed to use quick-relief medications if symptoms occur or if PEF drops below 80% predicted or personal best. If PEF is 50–79%, the patient should monitor response to quick relief medications carefully and consider contacting a clinician. If PEF is below 50%, immediate medical care is usually required. In the urgent or emergency care setting, the following parameters describe the severity and likely clinical course of an exacerbation.

	Symptoms and Signs	Initial PEF (or FEV$_1$)	Clinical Course
Mild	Dyspnea only with activity (assess tachypnea in young children)	PEV ≥ 70% predicted or personal best	• Usually cared for at home • Prompt relief with inhaled SABA • Possible short course of oral systemic corticosteroids
Moderate	Dyspnea interferes with limits of usual activity	PEF 40–69% predicted or personal best	• Usually requires office or ED visit • Relief from frequent inhaled SABA • Oral systemic corticosteroids; some symptoms last for 1-2 days after treatment is begun
Severe	Dyspnea at rest; interferes with conversation	PEF < 40% predicted or personal best	• Usually requires ED visit and likely hospitalization • Partial relief from frequent inhaled SABA • Oral systemic corticosteroids; some symptoms last for > 3 days after treatment is begun • Adjunctive therapies are helpful
Subset: Life-threatening	Too dyspneic to speak; perspiring	PEF < 25% predicted or personal best	• Requires ED/hospitalization; possible ICU • Minimal or no relief from frequent inhaled SABA • Intravenous corticosteroids • Adjunctive therapies are helpful

PEF, peak expiratory flow; FEV$_1$, forced expiratory volume in 1 second; SABA, short-acting β_2-agonist; ED, emergency department; ICU, intensive care unit. Adapted from National Asthma Education and Prevention Program. Expert Panel Report 3: Guidelines for Diagnosis and Management of Asthma. National Institutes of Health Pub. No. 08-4051. Bethesda, MD, 2007. www.nhibi.nih.gov/guidelines/asthma/asthgdln.htm.

Table 98. Assessing asthma control.

Components of control		Classification of Asthma Control (≥ 12 years of age)		
		Well Controlled	Not Well Controlled	Very Poorly Controlled
Impairment	Symptoms	≤ 2 days/week	> 2 days/week	Throughout the day
	Nighttime awakenings	≤ 2×/month	1–3×/week	≥ 4×/week
	Interference with normal activity	None	Some limitation	Extremely limited
	Short-acting β_2-agonist use for symptom control (not prevention of EIB)	≤ 2 days/week	>2 days/week	Several times/day
	FEV_1 or peak flow	> 80% predicted/personal best	60–80% predicted/personal best	< 60% predicted/personal best
	Validated questionnaires			
	ATAQ	0	1–2	3–4
	ACQ	≤ 0.75[1]	≥ 1.5	N/A
	ACT	≥ 20	16–19	≤ 15
Risk	Exacerbations requiring oral system corticosteroids	0–1/year	≥ 2/year (see note)	
		Consider severity and interval since last exacerbation		
	Progressive loss of lung function	Evaluation requires long-term follow-up care		
	Treatment-related adverse effects	Medication side effects can vary in intensity from none to very troublesome and worrisome. The level of intensity does not correlate to specific levels of control but should be considered in the overall assessment of risk.		
Recommended Action for Treatment		• Maintain current step • Regular follow-ups every 1–6 months to maintain control. • Consider step down if well controlled for at least 3 months.	• Step up 1 step and • Reevaluate in 2–6 weeks. • For side effects, consider alternative treatment options.	• Consider short course of oral systemic corticosteroids, • Step up 1–2 steps, and • Reevaluate in 2 weeks. • For side effects, consider alternative treatment options.

[1]ACQ values of 0.76–1.4 are indeterminate regarding well-controlled asthma.

EIB, exercise-induced bronchospasm; ICU, intensive care unit.

Notes:

· The stepwise approach is meant to assist, not replace, the clinical decision-making required to meet individual patient needs.

· The level of control is based on the most severe impairment or risk category. Assess impairment domain by patient's recall of previous 2–4 weeks and by spirometry or peak flow measures. Symptom assessment for longer periods should reflect a global assessment, such as inquiring whether the patient's asthma is better or worse since the last visit.

· At present, there are inadequate data to correspond frequencies of exacerbations with different levels of asthma control. In general, more frequent and intense exacerbations (eg, requiring urgent, unscheduled care, hospitalization, or ICU admission) indicate poorer disease control. For treatment purposes, patients who had ≥ 2 exacerbations requiring oral systemic corticosteroids in the past year may be considered the same as patients who have not-well-controlled asthma, even in the absence of impairment levels consistent with not-well-controlled asthma.

· Validated Questionnaires for the impairment domain (the questionnaire did not assess lung function or the risk domain).

   ATAQ = Asthma Therapy Assessment Questionnaire©

   ACQ = Asthma Control Questionnaire© (user package may be obtained at www.qoltech.co.uk or juniper@qoltech.co.uk)

   ACT = Asthma Control Test™

   Minimal Importance Difference: 1.0 for the ATAQ; 0.5 for the ACQ; not determined for the ACT.

· Before step up in therapy:

   —Review adherence to medication, inhaler.

   —If an alternative treatment option was used in a step, discontinue and use the preferred treatment for that step.

Adapted from National Asthma Education and Prevention Program. Expert Panel Report 3: Guidelines for the Diagnosis and Management of Asthma. National Institutes of Health Pub. No. 08-4051. Bethesda, MD, 2007. www.nhlbi/nih.gov/guidelines/asthma/asthgdln.htm.

Table 99. Long-term control medications for asthma.

Medication	Dosage Form	Adult Dose	Comments
Inhaled Corticosteroids (See Table 100)			
Systemic Corticosteroids			**(Applies to all three corticosteroids)**
Methylpred-nisolone	2, 4, 6, 8, 16, 32 mg tablets	7.5–60 mg daily in a single dose in AM or every other day as needed for control	• For long-term treatment of severe persistent asthma, administer single dose in AM either daily or on alternate days (alternate-day therapy may produce less adrenal suppression). Short courses or "bursts" are effective for establishing control when initiating therapy or during a period of gradual deterioration.
Prednisolone	5 mg tablets, 5 mg/5 mL, 15 mg/5 mL	Short-course "burst": to achieve control, 40–60 mg per day as single or 2 divided doses for 3–10 days	• There is no evidence that tapering the dose following improvement in symptom control and pulmonary function prevents relapse.
Prednisone	1, 2.5, 5, 10, 20, 50 mg tablets; 5 mg/mL, 5 mg/mL		
Inhaled Long-Acting β_2-Agonists			**Should not be used for symptom relief or exacerbations. Use with inhaled corticosteroids.**
Salmeterol	DPI 50 mcg/blister	1 blister every 12 hours	• Decreased duration of protection against EIB may occur with regular use.
			• Decreased duration of protection against EIB may occur with regular use.
Formoterol	DPI 12 mcg/single-use capsule	1 capsule every 12 hours	• Each capsule is for single use only; additional doses should not be administered for at least 12 hours.
			• Capsules should be used only with the Aerolizor™ inhaler and should not be taken orally.
Combined Medication			
Fluticasone/ Salmeterol	DPI 100 mcg/50 mcg, 250 mcg/50 mcg, or 500 mcg/50 mcg HFA 45 mcg/21 mcg 115 mcg/21 mcg 230 mcg/21 mcg	1 inhalation twice daily; dose depends on severity of asthma	• 100/50 DPI or 45/21 HFA for patient not controlled on low- to medium-dose inhaled corticosteroids • 250/50 DPI or 115/21 HFA for patients not controlled on medium- to high-dose inhaled corticosteroids
Budesonide/ Formoterol	HFA MDI 80 mcg/4.5 mcg 160 mcg/4.5 mcg	2 inhalations twice daily; dose depends on severity of asthma	• 80/4.5 for patients who have asthma not controlled on low- to medium-dose inhaled corticosteroids • 160/4.5 for patients who have asthma not controlled on medium- to high-dose inhaled corticosteroids
Cromolyn and Nedocromil			
Cromolyn	MDI 0.8 mg/puff	2 puffs four times daily	• 4–6 week trial may be needed to determine maximum benefit.
	Nebulizer 20 mg/ampule	1 ampule four times daily	• Dose by MDI may be inadequate to affect hyperresponsiveness.
Nedocromil	MDI 1.75 mg/puff	2 puffs four times daily	• One dose before exercise or allergen exposure provides effective prophylaxis for 1–2 hours. Not as effective for EIB as SABA. • Once control is achieved, the frequency of dosing may be reduced.
Leukotriene Modifiers			
Leukotriene Receptor Antagonists			
Montelukast	4 mg or 5 mg chewable tablet 10 mg tablet	10 mg each night at bedtime	• Montelukast exhibits a flat dose-response curve. Doses > 10 mg will not produce a greater response in adults.
Zafirlukast	10 or 20 mg tablet	40 mg daily (20 mg tablet twice daily)	• For zafirlukast, administration with meals decreases bioavailability; take at least one hour before or 2 hours after meals. • Monitor for signs and symptoms of hepatic dysfunction.
5-Lipoxygenase inhibitor			
Zileuton	600 mg tablet	2400 mg daily (600 mg four times daily)	• For zileuton, monitor hepatic enzymes (ALT).

(continued)

Table 99. Long-term control medications for asthma. (continued)

Medication	Dosage Form	Adult Dose	Comments
Methylxanthines			
Theophylline	Liquids, sustained-release tablets, and capsules	Starting dose 10 mg/kg/d up to 300 mg maximum; usual maximum 800 mg/d	• Adjust dosage to achieve serum concentration of 5–15 mcg/mL at steady-state (at least 48 hours on same dosage). • Due to wide interpatient variability in theophylline metabolic clearance, routine serum theophylline level monitoring is important. • See below for factors that can affect theophylline levels.
Immunomodulators			
Omalizumab	Subcutaneous injection, 150 mg/1.2 mL following reconstitution with 1.4 mL sterile water for injection	150–375 mg SC every 2–4 weeks, depending on body weight and pretreatment serum IgE level	• Do not administer more than 150 mg per injection site. • Monitor for anaphylaxis for 2 hours following at least the first 3 injections.

Factor[1,2]	Decreases Theophylline Concentrations	Increases Theophylline Concentrations	Recommended Action
Food	↓ or delays absorption of some sustained-release theophylline (SRT) products	↑ rate of absorption (fatty foods)	Select theophylline preparation that is not affected by food.
Diet	↑ metabolism (high protein)	↓ metabolism (high carbohydrate)	Inform patients that major changes in diet are not recommended while taking theophylline.
Systemic, febrile viral illness (eg, influenza)		↓ metabolism	Decrease theophylline dose according to serum concentration. Decrease dose by 50% if serum concentration measurement is not available.
Hypoxia, cor pulmonale, and decompensated congestive heart failure, cirrhosis		↓ metabolism	Decrease dose according to serum concentration.
Age	↑ metabolism (1–9 years)	↓ metabolism (< 6 months, elderly)	Adjust dose according to serum concentration.
Phenobarbital, phenytoin, carbamazepine	↑ metabolism		Increase dose according to serum concentration.
Cimetidine		↓ metabolism	Use alternative H_2 blocker (eg, famotidine or ranitidine).
Macrolides: erythromycin, clarithromycin, troleandomycin		↓ metabolism	Use alternative macrolide antibiotic, azithromycin, or alternative antibiotic or adjust theophylline dose.
Quinolones: ciprofloxacin, enoxacin, pefloxacin		↓ metabolism	Use alternative antibiotic or adjust theophylline dose. Circumvent with ofloxacin if quinolone therapy is required.
Rifampin	↑ metabolism		Increase dose according to serum concentration.
Ticlopidine		↓ metabolism	Decrease dose according to serum concentration.
Smoking	↑ metabolism		Advise patient to stop smoking; increase dose according to serum concentration.

[1]Factors affecting serum theophylline concentration.
[2]This list is not all inclusive; for discussion of other factors, see package inserts.
DPI, dry powder inhaler; EIB, exercise-induced bronchospasm; HFA, hydrofluoroalkane; IgE, immunoglobulin E; MDI, metered-dose inhaler; SABA, short-acting β_2-agonist.
Adapted from National Asthma Education and Prevention Program. Expert Panel Report 3: Guidelines for the Diagnosis and Management of Asthma. National Institutes of Health Pub. No. 08-4051. Bethesda, MD, 2007. www.nhlbi.nih.gov/guidelines/asthma/asthgdln.htm.

Table 100. Quick-relief medications for asthma.

Medication	Dosage Form	Adult Dose	Comments
Inhaled Short-Acting β₂-Agonists			
	MDI		
Albuterol CFC	90 mcg/puff, 200 puffs/canister	2 puffs 5 minutes before exercise	• An increasing use or lack of expected effect indicates diminished control of asthma.
Albuterol HFA	90 mcg/puff, 200 puffs/canister	2 puffs every 4–6 hours as needed	• Not recommended for long-term daily treatment. Regular use exceeding 2 days/week for symptom control (not prevention of EIB) indicates the need to step up therapy.
Pirbuterol CFC	200 mcg/puff, 400 puffs/canister		• Differences in potency exist, but all products are essentially comparable on a per puff basis.
Levalbuterol HFA	45 mcg/puff, 200 puffs/canister		• May double usual dose for mild exacerbations.
			• Should prime the inhaler by releasing four actuations prior to use.
			• Periodically clean HFA activator, as drug may block/plug orifice.
			• Nonselective agents (ie epinephrine, isoproterenol, metaproterenol) are not recommended due to their potential for excessive cardiac stimulation, especially in high doses.
	Nebulizer solution		
Albuterol	0.63 mg/3 mL 1.25 mg/3 mL 2.5 mg/3 mL 5 mg/mL (0.5%)	1.25–5 mg in 3 mL of saline every 4–8 hours as needed	• May mix with budesonide inhalant suspension, cromolyn or ipratropium nebulizer solutions. May double dose for severe exacerbations.
Levalbuterol (R-albuterol)	0.31 mg/3 mL 0.63 mg/3 mL 1.25 mg/0.5 mL 1.25 mg/3 mL	0.63 mg–1.25 mg every 8 hours as needed	• Compatible with budesonide inhalant suspension. The product is a sterile-filled, preservative-free, unit dose vial.
Anticholinergics			
	MDI		
Ipratropium HFA	17 mcg/puff, 200 puffs/canister	2–3 puffs every 6 hours	• Evidence is lacking for anticholinergics producing added benefit to β₂-agonists in long-term control asthma therapy.
	Nebulizer solution		
	0.25 mg/mL (0.025%)	0.25 mg every 6 hours	
	MDI		
Ipratropium with albuterol	18 mcg/puff of ipratropium bromide and 90 mcg/puff of albuterol 200 puffs/canister	2–3 puffs every 6 hours	
	Nebulizer solution		
	0.5 mg/3 mL ipratropium bromide and 2.5 mg/3 mL albuterol	3 mL every 4–6 hours	• Contains EDTA to prevent discolorations of the solution. This additive does not induce bronchospasm.
Systemic Corticosteroids			
Methylprednisolone	2, 4, 6, 8, 16, 32 mg tablets	Short course "burst": 40–60 mg/d as single or 2 divided doses for 3–10 days	• Short courses or "bursts" are effective for establishing control when initiating therapy or during a period of gradual deterioration.
Prednisolone	5 mg tablets, 5 mg/5 mL, 15 mg/5 mL		• The burst should be continued until symptoms resolve and the PEF is at least 80% of personal best. This usually requires 3–10 days but may require longer. There is no evidence that tapering the dose following improvements prevents relapse.
Prednisone	1, 2.5, 5, 10, 20, 50 mg tablets; 5 mg/mL, 5 mg/5mL		• May be used in place of a short burst of oral corticosteroids in patients who are vomiting or if adherence is a problem.
	Repository injection		
(Methylprednisolone acetate)	40 mg/mL 80 mg/mL	240 mg IM once	

CFC, chlorofluorocarbon; EIB, exercise-induced bronchospasm; HFA, hydrofluoroalkane; IM, intramuscular; MDI, metered-dose inhaler; PEF, peak expiratory flow.

Adapted from National Asthma Education and Prevention Program. Expert Panel Report 3: Guidelines for the Diagnosis and Management of Asthma. National Institutes of Health Pub. No. 08-4051. Bethesda, MD, 2007. www.nhlbi.gov/guidelines/asthma/asthgdln.htm.

Table 101. Patterns of disease in advanced COPD.

	Type A: Pink Puffer (Emphysema Predominant)	Type B: Blue Bloater (Bronchitis Predominant)
History and physical examination	Major complaint is dyspnea, often severe, usually presenting after age 50. Cough is rare, with scant clear, mucoid sputum. Patients are thin, with recent weight loss common. They appear uncomfortable, with evident use of accessory muscles of respiration. Chest is very quiet without adventitious sounds. No peripheral edema.	Major complaint is chronic cough, productive of mucopurulent sputum, with frequent exacerbations due to chest infections. Often presents in late 30s and 40s. Dyspnea usually mild, though patients may note limitations to exercise. Patients frequently overweight and cyanotic but seem comfortable at rest. Peripheral edema is common. Chest is noisy, with rhonchi invariably present; wheezes are common.
Laboratory studies	Hemoglobin usually normal (12–15 g/dL). Pa_{O_2} normal to slightly reduced (65–75 mm Hg) but Sa_{O_2} normal at rest. Pa_{CO_2} normal to slightly reduced (35–40 mm Hg). Chest radiograph shows hyperinflation with flattened diaphragms. Vascular markings are diminished, particularly at the apices.	Hemoglobin usually elevated (15–18 g/dL). Pa_{O_2} reduced (45–60 mm Hg) and Pa_{CO_2} slightly to markedly elevated (50–60 mm Hg). Chest radiograph shows increased interstitial markings ("dirty lungs"), especially at bases. Diaphragms are not flattened.
Pulmonary function tests	Airflow obstruction ubiquitous. Total lung capacity increased, sometimes markedly so. $D_{L_{CO}}$ reduced. Static lung compliance increased.	Airflow obstruction ubiquitous. Total lung capacity generally normal but may be slightly increased. $D_{L_{CO}}$ normal. Static lung compliance normal.
Special evaluations		
$\dot{V}/\dot{Q}$ matching	Increased ventilation to high $\dot{V}/\dot{Q}$ areas, ie, high dead space ventilation	Increased perfusion to low $\dot{V}/\dot{Q}$ areas.
Hemodynamics	Cardiac output normal to slightly low. Pulmonary artery pressures mildly elevated and increase with exercise.	Cardiac output normal. Pulmonary artery pressures elevated, sometimes markedly so, and worsen with exercise.
Nocturnal ventilation	Mild to moderate degree of oxygen desaturation not usually associated with obstructive sleep apnea.	Severe oxygen desaturation, frequently associated with obstructive sleep apnea.
Exercise ventilation	Increased minute ventilation for level of oxygen consumption. Pa_{O_2} tends to fall, Pa_{CO_2} rises slightly.	Decreased minute ventilation for level of oxygen consumption. Pa_{O_2} may rise; Pa_{CO_2} may rise significantly.

$D_{L_{CO}}$, single-breath diffusing capacity for carbon monoxide; $\dot{V}/\dot{Q}$, ventilation-perfusion.

Table 102. Home oxygen therapy: requirements for Medicare coverage.[1]

Group I (any of the following):
1. $Pa_{O_2} \leq 55$ mm Hg or $Sa_{O_2} \leq 88\%$ taken at rest breathing room air, while awake.
2. During sleep (prescription for nocturnal oxygen use only):
   a. $Pa_{O_2} \leq 55$ mm Hg or $Sa_{O_2} \leq 88\%$ for a patient whose awake, resting, room air Pa_{O_2} is ≥ 56 mm Hg or $Sa_{O_2} \geq 89\%$,
      or
   b. Decrease in $Pa_{O_2} > 10$ mm Hg or decrease in $Sa_{O_2} > 5\%$ associated with symptoms or signs reasonably attributed to hypoxemia (eg, impaired cognitive processes, nocturnal restlessness, insomnia).
3. During exercise (prescription for oxygen use only during exercise):
   a. $Pa_{O_2} \leq 55$ mg Hg or $Sa_{O_2} \leq 88\%$ taken during exercise for a patient whose awake, resting, room air Pa_{O_2} is ≥ 56 mm Hg or $Sa_{O_2} \geq 89\%$,
      and
   b. There is evidence that the use of supplemental oxygen during exercise improves the hypoxemia that was demonstrated during exercise while breathing room air.

Group II[2]:
$Pa_{O_2} = 56$–59 mm Hg or $Sa_{O_2} = 89\%$ if there is evidence of any of the following:
1. Dependent edema suggesting congestive heart failure.
2. P pulmonale on ECG (P wave > 3 mm in standard leads II, III, or aVF).
3. Hematocrit > 56%.

[1]Health Care Financing Administration, 1989.
[2]Patients in this group must have a second oxygen test 3 months after the initial oxygen set-up.

Table 103. Characteristics and treatment of selected pneumonias.

Organism; Appearance on Smear of Sputum	Clinical Setting	Complications	Laboratory Studies	Antimicrobial Therapy[1,2]
Streptococcus pneumoniae (pneumococcus). Gram-positive diplococci.	Chronic cardiopulmonary disease; follows upper respiratory tract infection	Bacteremia, meningitis, endocarditis, pericarditis, empyema	Gram stain and culture of sputum, blood, pleural fluid	Preferred[3]: Penicillin G, amoxicillin. Alternative: Macrolides, cephalosporins, doxycycline, fluoroquinolones, clindamycin, vancomycin, TMP-SMZ, linezolid.
Haemophilus influenzae. Pleomorphic gram-negative coccobacilli.	Chronic cardiopulmonary disease; follows upper respiratory tract infection	Empyema, endocarditis	Gram stain and culture of sputum, blood, pleural fluid	Preferred[3]: Cefotaxime, ceftriaxone, cefuroxime, doxycycline, azithromycin, TMP-SMZ. Alternative: Fluoroquinolones, clarithromycin.
Staphylococcus aureus. Plump gram-positive cocci in clumps.	Residence in chronic care facility, hospital-acquired, influenza epidemics; cystic fibrosis, bronchiectasis, injection drug use	Empyema, cavitation	Gram stain and culture of sputum, blood, pleural fluid	For methicillin-susceptible strains: Preferred: A penicillinase-resistant penicillin with or without rifampin, or gentamicin. Alternative: A cephalosporin; clindamycin, TMP-SMZ, vancomycin, a fluoroquinolone. For methicillin-resistant strains: Vancomycin with or without gentamicin or rifampin, linezolid.
Klebsiella pneumoniae. Plump gram-negative encapsulated rods.	Alcohol abuse, diabetes mellitus; hospital-acquired	Cavitation, empyema	Gram stain and culture of sputum, blood, pleural fluid	Preferred: Third-generation cephalosporin. For severe infections, add an aminoglycoside. Alternative: Aztreonam, imipenem, meropenem, β-lactam/β-lactamase inhibitor, an aminoglycoside, or a fluoroquinolone.
Escherichia coli. Gram-negative rods.	Hospital-acquired; rarely, community-acquired	Empyema	Gram stain and culture of sputum, blood, pleural fluid	Same as for *Klebsiella pneumoniae.*
Pseudomonas aeruginosa. Gram-negative rods.	Hospital-acquired; cystic fibrosis, bronchiectasis	Cavitation	Gram stain and culture of sputum, blood	Preferred: An antipseudomonal β-lactam plus an aminoglycoside. Alternative: Ciprofloxacin plus an aminoglycoside or an antipseudomonal β-lactam.
Anaerobes. Mixed flora.	Aspiration, poor dental hygiene	Necrotizing pneumonia, abscess, empyema	Culture of pleural fluid or of material obtained by transtracheal or transthoracic aspiration	Preferred: Clindamycin, β-lactam/β-lactamase inhibitor, imipenem.
Mycoplasma pneumoniae. PMNs and monocytes; no bacteria.	Young adults; summer and fall	Skin rashes, bullous myringitis; hemolytic anemia	PCR. Culture.[4] Complement fixation titer.[5] Cold agglutinin serum titers are not helpful as they lack sensitivity and specificity.	Preferred: Doxycycline or erythromycin. Alternative: Clarithromycin; azithromycin, or a fluoroquinolone.
Legionella species. Few PMNs; no bacteria.	Summer and fall; exposure to contaminated construction site, water source, air conditioner; community-acquired or hospital-acquired	Empyema, cavitation, endocarditis, pericarditis	Direct immunofluorescent examination or PCR of sputum or tissue; culture of sputum or tissue.[4] Urinary antigen assay for *L pneumophila* serogroup 1.	Preferred: A macrolide with or without rifampin; a fluoroquinolone. Alternative: Doxycycline with or without rifampin, TMP-SMZ.
Chlamydophila pneumoniae. Nonspecific.	Clinically similar to *M pneumoniae*, but prodromal symptoms last longer (up to 2 weeks). Sore throat with hoarseness common. Mild pneumonia in teenagers and young adults.	Reinfection in older adults with underlying COPD or heart failure may be severe or even fatal	Isolation of the organism is very difficult. Serologic studies include microimmunofluorescence with TWAR antigen. PCR at selected laboratories.	Preferred: Doxycycline. Alternative: Erythromycin, clarithromycin, azithromycin, or a fluoroquinolone.
Moraxella catarrhalis. Gram-negative diplococci.	Preexisting lung disease; elderly; corticosteroid or immunosuppressive therapy	Rarely, pleural effusions and bacteremia	Gram stain and culture of sputum, blood, pleural fluid	Preferred: A second- or third-generation cephalosporin; a fluoroquinolone. Alternative: TMP-SMZ, amoxicillin-clavulanic acid, or a macrolide.
Pneumocystis jiroveci. Nonspecific.	AIDS, immunosuppressive or cytotoxic drug therapy, cancer	Pneumothorax, respiratory failure, ARDS, death	Methenamine silver, Giemsa, or DFA stains of sputum or bronchoalveolar lavage fluid	Preferred: TMP-SMZ or pentamidine isethionate plus prednisone. Alternative: Dapsone plus trimethoprim; clindamycin plus primaquine; trimetrexate plus folinic acid.

[1]Antimicrobial sensitivities should guide therapy when available. (Modified from: The choice of antibacterial drugs. Med Lett Drugs Ther 2004;43:69, and from Bartlett JG et al: Practice guidelines for the management of community-acquired pneumonia in adults. Clin Infect Dis 2000;31:347.)

[2]For additional antimicrobial therapy information, see Infectious Disease: Antimicrobial Therapy: Table 62 (drugs of choice).

[3]Consider penicillin resistance when choosing therapy. See text.

[4]Selective media are required.

[5]Fourfold rise in titer is diagnostic.

TMP-SMZ, trimethoprim-sulfamethoxazole; PCR, polymerase chain reaction; COPD, chronic obstructive pulmonary disease; ARDS, acute respiratory distress syndrome.

Table 104. Scoring system for risk class assignment for PORT prediction rule.

Patient Characteristic	Points Assigned[1]
Demographic factor	
Age: men	Number of years
Age: women	Number of years minus 10
Nursing home resident	10
Comorbid illnesses	
Neoplastic disease[2]	30
Liver disease[3]	20
Congestive heart failure[4]	10
Cerebrovascular disease[5]	10
Renal disease[6]	10
Physical examination finding	
Altered mental status[7]	20
Respiratory rate $\geq$ 30 breaths/min	20
Systolic blood pressure < 90 mm Hg	20
Temperature $\leq$ 35 °C or $\geq$ 40 °C	15
Pulse $\geq$ 125 beats/min	10
Laboratory or radiographic finding	
Arterial pH < 7.35	30
Blood urea nitrogen $\geq$ 30 mg/dL	20
Sodium < 130 mEq/L	20
Glucose > 250 mg/dL	10
Hematocrit < 30%	10
Arterial Po_2 < 60 mm Hg	10
Pleural effusion	10

[1]A total point score for a given patient is obtained by summing the patient's age in years (age minus 10 for women) and the points for each applicable characteristic.

[2]Any cancer except basal or squamous cell of the skin that was active at the time of presentation or diagnosed within 1 year before presentation.

[3]Clinical or histologic diagnosis of cirrhosis or another form of chronic liver disease.

[4]Systolic or diastolic dysfunction documented by history, physical examination and chest radiograph, echocardiogram, MUGA scan, or left ventriculogram.

[5]Clinical diagnosis of stroke or transient ischemic attack or stroke documented by MRI or CT scan.

[6]History of chronic renal disease or abnormal blood urea nitrogen and creatinine concentration documented in the medical record.

[7]Disorientation (to person, place, or time, not known to be chronic), stupor, or coma.

Modified and reproduced, with permission, from Fine MJ et al. A prediction rule to identify low-risk patients with community-acquired pneumonia. N Engl J Med. 1997;336:243. Copyright © 1997 Massachusetts Medical Society. All rights reserved.

Table 105. PORT risk class 30-day mortality rates and recommendations for site of care.

Number of Points	Risk Class	Mortality at 30 days (%)	Recommended Site of Care
Absence of predictors	I	0.1–0.4	Outpatient
≤ 70	II	0.6–0.7	Outpatient
71–90	III	0.9–2.8	Outpatient or brief inpatient
91–130	IV	8.2–9.3	Inpatient
≥ 130	V	27.0–31.1	Inpatient

Data from Fine MJ et al. A prediction rule to identify low-risk patients with community-acquired pneumonia. N Engl J Med. 1997;336:243. Copyright © 1997 Massachusetts Medical Society. All rights reserved.

Table 106. Classification of positive tuberculin skin test reactions.[1]

Reaction Size	Group
≥ 5 mm	1. HIV-positive persons. 2. Recent contacts of individuals with active tuberculosis. 3. Persons with fibrotic changes on chest x-rays suggestive of prior tuberculosis. 4. Patients with organ transplants and other immunosuppressed patients (receiving the equivalent of > 15 mg/d of prednisone for 1 month or more).
≥ 10 mm	1. Recent immigrants (< 5 years) from countries with a high prevalence of tuberculosis (eg, Asia, Africa, Latin America). 2. HIV-negative injection drug users. 3. Mycobacteriology laboratory personnel. 4. Residents of and employees[2] in the following high-risk congregate settings: correctional institutions; nursing homes and other long-term facilities for the elderly; hospitals and other health care facilities; residential facilities for AIDS patients; and homeless shelters. 5. Persons with the following medical conditions that increase the risk of tuberculosis: gastrectomy, ≥ 10% below ideal body weight, jejunoileal bypass, diabetes mellitus, silicosis, chronic renal failure, some hematologic disorders, (eg, leukemias, lymphomas), and other specific malignancies (eg, carcinoma of the head or neck and lung). 6. Children < 4 years of age or infants, children, and adolescents exposed to adults at high risk.
≥ 15 mm	1. Persons with no risk factors for tuberculosis.

[1]A tuberculin skin test reaction is considered positive if the transverse diameter of the *indurated* area reaches the size required for the specific group. All other reactions are considered negative.
[2]For persons who are otherwise at low risk and are tested at entry into employment, a reaction of > 15 mm induration is considered positive.
Source: Screening for tuberculosis and tuberculosis infection in high-risk populations: recommendations of the Advisory Council for the Elimination of Tuberculosis. MMWR Morb Mortal Wkly Rep 1995;44(RR-11):19.

Table 107. Characteristics of antituberculous drugs.

Drug	Most Common Side Effects	Tests for Side Effects	Drug Interactions	Remarks
Isoniazid	Peripheral neuropathy, hepatitis, rash, mild CNS effects.	AST and ALT; neurologic examination.	Phenytoin (synergistic); disulfiram.	Bactericidal to both extracellular and intracellular organisms. Pyridoxine, 10 mg orally daily as prophylaxis for neuritis; 50–100 mg orally daily as treatment.
Rifampin	Hepatitis, fever, rash, flu-like illness, gastrointestinal upset, bleeding problems, renal failure.	CBC, platelets, AST and ALT.	Rifampin inhibits the effect of oral contraceptives, quinidine, corticosteroids, warfarin, methadone, digoxin, oral hypoglycemics; aminosalicylic acid may interfere with absorption of rifampin. Significant interactions with protease inhibitors and nonnucleoside reverse transcriptase inhibitors.	Bactericidal to all populations of organisms. Colors urine and other body secretions orange. Discoloring of contact lenses.
Pyrazinamide	Hyperuricemia, hepatotoxicity, rash, gastrointestinal upset, joint aches.	Uric acid, AST, ALT.	Rare.	Bactericidal to intracellular organisms.
Ethambutol	Optic neuritis (reversible with discontinuance of drug; rare at 15 mg/kg); rash.	Red-green color discrimination and visual acuity (difficult to test in children under 3 years of age).	Rare.	Bacteriostatic to both intracellular and extracellular organisms. Mainly used to inhibit development of resistant mutants. Use with caution in renal disease or when ophthalmologic testing is not feasible.
Streptomycin	Eighth nerve damage, nephrotoxicity.	Vestibular function (audiograms); BUN and creatinine.	Neuromuscular blocking agents may be potentiated and cause prolonged paralysis.	Bactericidal to extracellular organisms. Use with caution in older patients or those with renal disease.

AST, aspartate aminotransferase; ALT, alanine aminotransferase; CBC, complete blood count; BUN, blood urea nitrogen.

Table 108. Recommended dosages for the initial treatment of tuberculosis.

Drugs	Daily	Cost[1]	Twice a Week[2]	Cost[1]/wk	Three Times a Week[2]	Cost[1]/wk
Isoniazid	5 mg/kg Max: 300 mg/dose	$0.13/300 mg	15 mg/kg Max: 900 mg/dose	$0.78	15 mg/kg Max: 900 mg/dose	$1.17
Rifampin	10 mg/kg Max: 600 mg/dose	$3.80/600 mg	10 mg/kg Max: 600 mg/dose	$7.60	10 mg/kg Max: 600 mg/dose	$11.40
Pyrazinamide	15–30 mg/kg Max: 2 g/dose	$4.64/2 g	50–70 mg/kg Max: 4 g/dose	$18.56	50–70 mg/kg Max: 3 g/dose	$20.88
Ethambutol	5–25 mg/kg Max: 2.5 g/dose	$11.27/2.5 g	50 mg/kg Max: 2.5 g/dose	$22.54	25–30 mg/kg Max: 2.5 g/dose	$33.81
Streptomycin	15 mg/kg Max: 1 g/dose	$9.10/1 g	25–30 mg/kg Max: 1.5 g/dose	$36.40	25–30 mg/kg Max: 1.5 g/dose	$54.60

[1]Average wholesale price (AWP, for AB-rated generic when available) for quantity listed. Source: *Red Book Update,* Vol. 27, No. 2, February 2008. AWP may not accurately represent the actual pharmacy cost because wide contractual variations exist among institutions.
[2]All intermittent dosing regimens should be used with directly observed therapy.

Table 109. TNM staging for lung cancer.

Stage	T	N	M	Description
0	Tis			Carcinoma in situ
IA	T1	N0	M0	Limited local disease without nodal or distant metastases
IB	T2	N0	M0	
IIA	T1	N1	M0	Limited local disease with ipsilateral hilar or peribronchial nodal involvement but not distant metastases
IIB	T2	N1	M0	or
	T3	N0	M0	Locally invasive disease without nodal or distant metastases
IIIA	T3	N1	M0	Locally invasive disease with ipsilateral or peribronchial nodal involvement but not distant metastases or
	T1–3	N2	M0	Limited or locally invasive disease with ipsilateral mediastinal or subcarinal nodal involvement but not distant metastases
IIIB	Any T	N3	M0	Any primary with contralateral mediastinal or hilar nodes, or ipsilateral scalene or supraclavicular nodes or
	T4	Any N	M0	Unresectable local invasion with any degree of adenopathy but no distant metastases; malignant pleural effusion
IV	Any T	Any N	M1	Distant metastases

Primary Tumor (T)

TX	Primary tumor cannot be assessed; or tumor proved by the presence of malignant cells in sputum or bronchial washings but not visualized by imaging or bronchoscopy.
T0	No evidence of primary tumor.
Tis	Carcinoma in situ.
T1	A tumor ≤ 3 cm in greatest dimension, surrounded by lung or visceral pleura, and without evidence of invasion proximal to a lobar bronchus at bronchoscopy.
T2	A tumor > 3.0 cm in greatest dimension, or a tumor of any size that either involves a main bronchus (but is ≥ 2 cm distal to the carina), invades the visceral pleura, or has associated atelectasis or obstructive pneumonitis extending to the hilar region. Any associated atelectasis or obstructive pneumonitis must involve less than an entire lung.
T3	A tumor of any size with direct extension into the chest wall (including superior sulcus tumors), the diaphragm, the mediastinal pleura, or the parietal pericardium; or a tumor in the main bronchus < 2 cm distal to the carina without involving the carina; or associated atelectasis or obstructive pneumonitis of the entire lung.
T4	A tumor of any size with invasion of the mediastinum, heart, great vessels, trachea, esophagus, vertebral body, or carina; or with a malignant pleural or pericardial effusion; or with satellite tumor nodules within the ipsilateral lobe of the lung containing the primary tumor.

Regional Lymph Nodes (N)

NX	Regional lymph nodes cannot be assessed.
N0	No demonstrable metastasis to regional lymph nodes.
N1	Metastasis to lymph nodes in the peribronchial or the ipsilateral hilar region, or both, including direct extension.
N2	Metastasis to ipsilateral mediastinal lymph nodes and/or subcarinal lymph nodes.
N3	Metastasis to contralateral mediastinal lymph nodes, contralateral hilar lymph nodes, ipsilateral or contralateral scalene or supraclavicular lymph nodes.

Distant Metastases (M)

MX	Presence of distant metastasis cannot be assessed.
M0	No (known) distant metastasis.
M1	Distant metastasis present.

Adapted, with permission, from Mountain CF. Revisions in the international system for staging lung cancer. Chest. 1997;111:1710.

Table 110. Approach to staging of patients with lung cancer.

Part A: Recommended tests for all patients
Complete blood count
Electrolytes, calcium, alkaline phosphatase, albumin, AST, ALT, total bilirubin, creatinine
Chest radiograph
CT of chest through the adrenal glands[1,2]
Pathologic confirmation of malignancy[3]

Part B: Recommended tests for selected but not all patients	
Test	**Indication**
CT with contrast of liver or liver ultrasound	Elevated liver function tests; abnormal non-contrast-enhanced CT of liver or abnormal clinical evaluation
CT with contrast of brain or MRI of brain	CNS symptoms or abnormal clinical evaluation
Whole body ^{18}F-fluoro-deoyx-D-glucose positron emission tomography scan (FDG-PET)	To evaluate the mediastinum in patients who are candidates for surgery
Radionuclide bone scan	Elevated alkaline phosphatase (bony fraction), elevated calcium, bone pain, or abnormal clinical evaluation
Pulmonary function tests	If lung resection or thoracic radiotherapy planned
Quantitative radionuclide perfusion lung scan or exercise testing to evaluate maximum oxygen consumption	Patients with borderline resectability due to limited cardiovascular status

[1]May not be necessary if patient has obvious M1 disease on chest x-ray or physical examination.
[2]Intravenous iodine contrast enhancement is not essential but is recommended in probable mediastinal invasion.
[3]While optimal in most cases, tissue diagnosis may not be necessary prior to surgery in some cases where the lesion is enlarging or the patient will undergo surgical resection regardless of the outcome of a biopsy.
Modified and reproduced, with permission, from Pretreatment evaluation of non-small cell lung cancer. Consensus Statement of the American Thoracic Society and the European Respiratory Society. Am J Respir Crit Care Med. 1997;156:320.

Table 111. Approximate survival rates following treatment for lung cancer.

Non–Small Cell Lung Cancer: Mean 5-Year Survival Following Resection		
Stage	**Clinical Staging**	**Surgical Staging**
IA (T1N0M0)	60%	74%
IB (T2N0M0)	38%	61%
IIA (T1N1M0)	34%	55%
IIB (T2N1M0, T3N0M0)	23%	39%
IIIA	9–13%	22%
IIIB[1]	3–12%	
IV[1]	4%	

Small Cell Lung Cancer: Survival Following Chemotherapy		
Stage	**Mean 2-Year Survival**	**Median Survival**
Limited	15–20%	14–20 months
Extensive	< 3%	8–13 months

[1]Independent of therapy, generally not surgical patients.
Data from multiple sources. Modified and reproduced, with permission, from Reif MS et al. Evidence-based medicine in the treatment of non-small cell cancer. Clin Chest Med. 2000;21:107.

Table 112. Differential diagnosis of interstitial lung disease.

Drug-related
    Antiarrhythmic agents (amiodarone)
    Antibacterial agents (nitrofurantoin, sulfonamides)
    Antineoplastic agents (bleomycin, cyclophosphamide, methotrexate, nitrosoureas)
    Antirheumatic agents (gold salts, penicillamine)
    Phenytoin
Environmental and occupational (inhalation exposures)
    Dust, inorganic (asbestos, silica, hard metals, beryllium)
    Dust, organic (thermophilic actinomycetes, avian antigens, *Aspergillus* species)
    Gases, fumes, and vapors (chlorine, isocyanates, paraquat, sulfur dioxide)
    Ionizing radiation
    Talc (injection drug users)
Infections
    Fungus, disseminated (*Coccidioides immitis, Blastomyces dermatitidis, Histoplasma capsulatum*)
    Mycobacteria, disseminated
        Pneumocystis jiroveci
    Viruses
Primary pulmonary disorders
    Cryptogenic organizing pneumonitis (COP)
    Idiopathic fibrosing interstitial pneumonia: Acute interstitial pneumonitis, desquamative interstitial pneumonitis, nonspecific interstitial pneumonitis, usual interstitial pneumonitis, respiratory bronchiolitis-associated interstitial lung disease
    Pulmonary alveolar proteinosis
Systemic disorders
    Acute respiratory distress syndrome
    Amyloidosis
    Ankylosing spondylitis
    Autoimmune disease: Dermatomyositis, polymyositis, rheumatoid arthritis, systemic sclerosis (scleroderma), systemic lupus erythematosus
    Chronic eosinophilic pneumonia
    Goodpasture syndrome
    Idiopathic pulmonary hemosiderosis
    Inflammatory bowel disease
    Langerhans cell histiocytosis (eosinophilic granuloma)
    Lymphangitic spread of cancer (lymphangitic carcinomatosis)
    Lymphangioleiomyomatosis
    Pulmonary edema
    Pulmonary venous hypertension, chronic
    Sarcoidosis
    Wegener granulomatosis

Table 113. Idiopathic fibrosing interstitial pneumonias.

Name and Clinical Presentation	Histopathology	Radiographic Pattern	Response to Therapy and Prognosis
Usual interstitial pneumonia (UIP) Age 55-60, slight male predominance. Insidious dry cough and dyspnea lasting months to years. Clubbing present at diagnosis in 25-50%. Diffuse fine late inspiratory crackles on lung auscultation. Restrictive ventilatory defect and reduced diffusing capacity on pulmonary function tests. ANA and RF positive in ~25% in the absence of documented collagen-vascular disease.	Patchy, temporally and geographically nonuniform distribution of fibrosis, honeycomb change, and normal lung. Type I pneumocytes are lost, and there is proliferation of alveolar type II cells. "Fibroblast foci" of actively proliferating fibroblasts and myofibroblasts. Inflammation is generally mild and consists of small lymphocytes. Intra-alveolar macrophage accumulation is present but is not a prominent feature.	Diminished lung volume. Increased linear or reticular bibasilar and subpleural opacities. Unilateral disease is rare. High-resolution CT scanning shows minimal ground-glass and variable honeycomb change. Areas of normal lung may be adjacent to areas of advanced fibrosis. Between 2% and 10% have normal chest radiographs and high-resolution CT scans on diagnosis.	No randomized study has demonstrated improved survival compared with untreated patients. Inexorably progressive. Response to corticosteroids and cytotoxic agents at best 15%, and these probably represent misclassification of histopathology. Median survival approximately 3 years, depending on stage at presentation. Current interest in antifibrotic agents.
Respiratory bronchiolitis-associated interstitial lung disease (RB-ILD)[1] Age 40-45. Presentation similar to that of UIP though in younger patients. Similar results on pulmonary function tests, but less severe abnormalities. Patients with respiratory bronchiolitis are invariably heavy smokers.	Increased numbers of macrophages evenly dispersed within the alveolar spaces. Rare fibroblast foci, little fibrosis, minimal honeycomb change. In RB-ILD the accumulation of macrophages is localized within the peribronchiolar air spaces; in DIP,[1] it is diffuse. Alveolar architecture is preserved.	May be indistinguishable from UIP. More often presents with a nodular or reticulonodular pattern. Honeycombing rare. High-resolution CT more likely to reveal diffuse ground-glass opacities and upper lobe emphysema.	Spontaneous remission occurs in up to 20% of patients, so natural history unclear. Smoking cessation is essential. Prognosis clearly better than that of UIP: median survival greater than 10 years. Corticosteroids thought to be effective, but there are no randomized clinical trials to support this view.
Acute interstitial pneumonitis (AIP) Clinically known as Hamman-Rich syndrome. Wide age range, many young patients. Acute onset of dyspnea followed by rapid development of respiratory failure. Half of patients report a viral syndrome preceding lung disease. Clinical course indistinguishable from that of idiopathic ARDS.	Pathologic changes reflect acute response to injury within days to weeks. Resembles organizing phase of diffuse alveolar damage. Fibrosis and minimal collagen deposition. May appear similar to UIP but more homogeneous and there is no honeycomb change—though this may appear if the process persists for more than a month in a patient on mechanical ventilation.	Diffuse bilateral airspace consolidation with areas of ground-glass attenuation on high-resolution CT scan.	Supportive care (mechanical ventilation) critical but effect of specific therapies unclear. High initial mortality: fifty to 90 percent die within 2 months after diagnosis. Not progressive if patient survives. Lung function may return to normal or may be permanently impaired.
Nonspecific interstitial pneumonitis (NSIP) Age 45-55. Slight female predominance. Similar to UIP but onset of cough and dyspnea over months, not years.	Nonspecific in that histopathology does not fit into better-established categories. Varying degrees of inflammation and fibrosis, patchy in distribution but uniform in time, suggesting response to single injury. Most have lymphocytic and plasma cell inflammation without fibrosis. Honeycombing present but scant. Some have advocated division into cellular and fibrotic subtypes.	May be indistinguishable from UIP. Most typical picture is bilateral areas of ground-glass attenuation and fibrosis on high-resolution CT. Honeycombing is rare.	Treatment thought to be effective, but no prospective clinical studies have been published. Prognosis overall good but depends on the extent of fibrosis at diagnosis. Median survival greater than 10 years.
Cryptogenic organizing pneumonitis (COP, formerly bronchiolitis obliterans organizing pneumonia [BOOP]) Typically age 50-60 but wide variation. Abrupt onset, frequently weeks to a few months following a flu-like illness. Dyspnea and dry cough prominent, but constitutional symptoms are common: fatigue, fever, and weight loss. Pulmonary function tests usually show restriction, but up to 25% show concomitant obstruction.	Included in the idiopathic interstitial pneumonias on clinical grounds. Buds of loose connective tissue (Masson bodies) and inflammatory cells fill alveoli and distal bronchioles.	Lung volumes normal. Chest radiograph typically shows interstitial and parenchymal disease with discrete, peripheral alveolar and ground-glass infiltrates. Nodular opacities common. High-resolution CT shows subpleural consolidation and bronchial wall thickening and cilation.	Rapid response to corticosteroids in two-thirds of patients. Long-term prognosis generally good for those who respond. Relapses are common.

[1]Includes desquamative interstitial pneumonia (DIP).
ANA, antinuclear antibody; RF, rheumatoid factor; UIP, usual interstitial pneumonia; ARDS, acute respiratory distress syndrome.

Table 114. Frequency of specific symptoms and signs in patients at risk for pulmonary thromboembolism.

	UPET[1] PE+ (n = 327)	PIOPED[2] PE+ (n = 117)	PIOPED[2] PE− (n = 248)
Symptoms			
Dyspnea	84%	73%	72%
Respirophasic chest pain	74%	66%	59%
Cough	53%	37%	36%
Leg pain	nr	26%	24%
Hemoptysis	30%	13%	8%
Palpitations	nr	10%	18%
Wheezing	nr	9%	11%
Anginal pain	14%	4%	6%
Signs			
Respiratory rate ≥ 16 UPET, ≥ 20 PIOPED I	92%	70%	68%
Crackles (rales)	58%	51%	40%[3]
Heart rate ≥ 100/min	44%	30%	24%
Fourth heart sound (S_4)	nr	24%	13%[3]
Accentuated pulmonary component of second heart sound (S_2P)	53%	23%	13%[3]
T ≥ 37.5 °C UPET, ≥ 38.5 °C PIOPED	43%	7%	12%
Homans sign	nr	4%	2%
Pleural friction rub	nr	3%	2%
Third heart sound (S_3)	nr	3%	4%
Cyanosis	19%	1%	2%

[1]Data from the Urokinase-Streptokinase Pulmonary Embolism Trial, as reported in Bell WR, Simon TL, DeMets DL. The clinical features of submassive and massive pulmonary emboli. Am J Med. 1977;62:355.
[2]Data from patients enrolled in the PIOPED I study, as reported in Stein PD et al. Clinical, laboratory, roentgenographic, and electrocardiographic findings in patients with acute pulmonary embolism and no preexisting cardiac or pulmonary disease. Chest. 1991;100:598.
[3]$P < .05$ comparing patients in the PIOPED I study.
PE+, confirmed diagnosis of pulmonary embolism; PE−, diagnosis of pulmonary embolism ruled out; nr, not reported.

Table 115. Selected methods for the prevention of venous thromboembolism.

Risk Group	Recommendations for Prophylaxis
Surgical patients	
General surgery	
Low-risk: Minor procedures, age under 40, and no clinical risk factors	Early ambulation
Moderate risk: Minor procedures with additional thrombosis risk factors; age 40–60, and no other clinical risk factors; or major operations with age under 40 without additional clinical risk factors	ES, or LDUH, or LMWH, or IPC; plus early ambulation if possible
Higher risk: Major operation, over age 40 or with additional risk factors	LDUH, or LMWH, or IPC
Higher risk plus increased risk of bleeding	ES or IPC
Very high risk: Multiple risk factors	LDUH, or higher-dose LMWH, plus ES or IPC
Selected very high risk	Consider ADPW, INR 2.0–3.0, or postdischarge LMWH
Orthopedic surgery	
Elective total hip replacement surgery	Subcutaneous LMWH, or ADPW, or adjusted-dose heparin started preoperatively; plus IPC or ES
Elective total knee replacement surgery	LMWH, or ADPW, or IPC
Hip fracture surgery	LMWH or ADPW
Neurosurgery	
Intracranial neurosurgery	IPC with or without ES; LDUH and postoperative LMWH are acceptable alternatives; IPC or ES plus LDUH or LMWH may be more effective than either modality alone in high-risk patients.
Acute spinal cord injury	LMWH; IPC and ES may have additional benefit when used with LMWH. In the rehabilitation phase, conversion to full-dose warfarin may provide ongoing protection.
Trauma	
With an identifiable risk factor for thromboembolism	LMWH; IPC or ES if there is a contraindication to LMWH; consider duplex ultrasound screening in very high risk patients; IVC filter insertion if proximal DVT is identified and anticoagulation is contraindicated.
Medical patients	
Acute myocardial infarction	Subcutaneous LDUH, or full-dose heparin; if heparin is contraindicated, IPC and ES may provide some protection.
Ischemic stroke with impaired mobility	LMWH or LDUH or danaparoid; IPC or ES if anticoagulants are contraindicated
General medical patients with clinical risk factors; especially patients with cancer, congestive heart failure, or severe pulmonary disease	Low-dose LMWH, or LDUH
Cancer patients with indwelling central venous catheters	Warfarin, 1 mg/d, or LMWH

Recommendations assembled from Geerts WH et al. Prevention of venous thromboembolism. Chest. 2001 Jan;119(1 Suppl):132S–175S.
ADPW, adjusted-dose perioperative warfarin: begin 5–10 mg the day of or the day following surgery; adjust dose to INR 2.0–3.0; DVT, deep venous thrombosis; ES, elastic stockings; IPC, intermittent pneumatic compression; IVC, inferior vena cava; LDUH, low-dose unfractionated heparin: 5000 units subcutaneously every 8–12 hours starting 1–2 hours before surgery; LMWH, low-molecular-weight heparin. See Table 116 for dosing regimens.

Table 116. Selected low-molecular-weight heparin and heparinoid regimens to prevent venous thromboembolism.

Risk Group	Drug	Subcutaneous Dose[1]	Administration Regimen	Cost[2]
General surgery, moderate risk	Dalteparin (Fragmin)	2500 units	1–2 h preop and qd postop	$18.08/dose
	Enoxaparin (Lovenox)	20 mg	1–2 h preop and qd postop	$23.38/dose
	Nadroparin (Fraxiparin)	2850 units	2–4 h preop and qd postop	No price available: Not available in U.S.
	Tinzaparin (Innohep)	3500 units	2 h preop and qd postop	$14.11/dose
General surgery, high risk	Dalteparin (Fragmin)	5000 units	8–12 preop and qd postop	$29.34/dose
	Danaparoid (Organ)	750 units	1–4 h preop and q12 h postop	No price available: Not available in U.S.
	Enoxaparin (Lovenox)	40 mg	1–2 h preop and qd postop	$31.17/dose
	Enoxaparin (Lovenox)	30 mg	q12 h starting 8–12 h postop	$23.38/dose
Orthopedic surgery	Dalteparin (Fragmin)	5000 units	8–12 h preop and qd starting 12–24 h postop	$29.34/dose
	Dalteparin (Fragmin)	2500 units	6–8 h postop then 5000 units qd	$18.08/dose
	Danaparoid (Organ)	750 units	1–4 preop and q12 h postop	No price available: Not available in U.S.
	Enoxaparin (Lovenox)	30 mg	q12 h starting 12–24 h postop	$23.38/dose
	Enoxaparin (Lovenox)	40 mg	qd starting 10–12 h preop	$31.17/dose
	Nadroparin (Fraxiparin)	38 units/kg	12 h preop, 12 h postop, and qd on postop days 1, 2, 3; then increase to 57 units/kg qd	No price available: Not available in U.S.
	Tinzaparin (Innohep)	75 units/kg	qd starting 12–24 h postop	$18.14/dose (60 kg pt)
	Tinzaparin (Innohep)	4500 units	12 h preop and qd postop	$18.14/dose
Major trauma	Enoxaparin (Lovenox)	30 mg	q12h starting 12–36 h postinjury if hemostatically stable	$23.38/dose
Acute spinal cord injury	Enoxaparin (Lovenox)	30 mg	q12h	$23.38/dose
Medical conditions	Dalteparin (Fragmin)	2500 units	qd	$18.08/dose
	Danaparoid (Organ)	750 units	q12h	No price available: Not available in U.S.
	Enoxaparin (Lovenox)	40 mg	qd	$31.17/dose
	Nadroparin (Fraxiparin)	2850 units	qd	No price available: Not available in U.S.

[1]Dose expressed in anti-Xa units; for enoxaparin, 1 mg = 100 anti-Xa units.
[2]Average wholesale price (AWP, for AB-rated generic when available) for quantity listed. Source: *Red Book Update*, Vol. 26, No. 3, March 2007. AWP may not accurately represent the actual pharmacy cost because wide contractual variations exist among institutions.
preop, preoperatively; postop, postoperatively; qd, once daily.
Modified and reproduced with permission, from Geerts WH et al. Prevention of venous thromboembolism. Chest. 2001 Jan;119(1 Suppl):132S–175S.

Table 117. Intravenous heparin dosing based on body weight.

Initial dosing	
1. Load with 80 units/kg IV, then	
2. Initiate a maintenance infusion at 18 units/kg/h	
3. Check activated partial thromboplastin time (aPTT) in 6 hours	

Dose adjustment schedule based on aPTT results	
< 35 s (< 1.2 × control)	Rebolus with 80 units/kg; increase infusion by 4 units/kg/h
35–45 s (1.2–1.5 × control)	Rebolus with 40 units/kg; increase infusion by 2 units/kg/h
46–70 s (1.5–2.3 × control)	No change
71–90 s (2.3–3 × control)	Decrease infusion rate by 2 units/kg/h
> 90 s (> 3 × control)	Stop infusion for 1 hour, then decrease infusion by 3 units/kg/h

Repeat aPTT every 6 hours for the first 24 hours. If the aPTT is 46–70 s after 24 hours, then recheck once daily every morning. If the aPTT is outside this therapeutic range at 24 hours, continue checking every 6 hours until it is 46–70 s. Once it has been in the therapeutic range on two consecutive measurements after 24 hours, check once daily every morning.

Adapted, with permission, from Raschke RA et al. The weight-based heparin dosing nomogram compared with a "standard care" nomogram. Ann Intern Med. 1993 Nov 1;119(9):874–81.

Table 118. Selected low-molecular-weight heparin anticoagulation regimens.

Drug	Suggested Treatment Dose[1] (Subcutaneous)
Dalteparin	200 units/kg once daily (not to exceed 18,000 units/dose)
Enoxaparin	1.5 mg/kg once daily (single dose not to exceed 180 mg)
Nadroparin	86 units/kg twice daily for 10 days, or 171 units/kg once daily (single dose not to exceed 17,000 units)
Tinzaparin	175 units/kg once daily

[1]Dose expressed in anti-Xa units; for enoxaparin, 1 mg = 100 anti-Xa units. Modified and reproduced with permission, from Hyers TM et al. Antithrombotic therapy for venous thromboembolic disease. Chest. 2001 Jan;119 (1 Suppl):176S–193S.

Table 119. Selected causes of hypersensitivity pneumonitis.

Disease	Antigen	Source
Farmer's lung	*Micropolyspora faeni, Thermoactinomyces vulgaris*	Moldy hay
"Humidifier" lung	Thermophilic actino-mycetes	Contaminated humidifi-ers, heating systems, or air conditioners
Bird fancier's lung ("pigeon-breeder's disease")	Avian proteins	Bird serum and excreta
Bagassosis	*Thermoactinomyces sac-chari* and *T vulgaris*	Moldy sugar cane fiber (bagasse)
Sequoiosis	Graphium, Aureobasid-ium, and other fungi	Moldy redwood sawdust
Maple bark stripper's disease	*Cryptostroma (Coniospo-rium) corticale*	Rotting maple tree logs or bark
Mushroom picker's disease	Same as farmer's lung	Moldy compost
Suberosis	*Penicillium frequentans*	Moldy cork dust
Detergent worker's lung	*Bacillus subtilis* enzyme	Enzyme additives

Table 120. Causes of pleural fluid transudates and exudates.

Transudates	Exudates
Congestive heart failure (> 90% of cases)	Pneumonia (parapneumonic effusion)
Cirrhosis with ascites	Cancer
Nephrotic syndrome	Pulmonary embolism
Peritoneal dialysis	Bacterial infection
Myxedema	Tuberculosis
Acute atelectasis	Connective tissue disease
Constrictive pericarditis	Viral infection
Superior vena cava obstruction	Fungal infection
Pulmonary embolism	Rickettsial infection
	Parasitic infection
	Asbestos
	Meigs syndrome
	Pancreatic disease
	Uremia
	Chronic atelectasis
	Trapped lung
	Chylothorax
	Sarcoidosis
	Drug reaction
	Post-myocardial infarction syndrome

Table 121. Characteristics of important exudative pleural effusions.

Etiology or Type of Effusion	Gross Appearance	White Blood Cell Count (cells/mcL)	Red Blood Cell Count (cells/mcL)	Glucose	Comments
Malignant effusion	Turbid to bloody; occasionally serous	1000 to < 100,000 M	100 to several hundred thousand	Equal to serum levels; < 60 mg/dL in 15% of cases	Eosinophilia uncommon; positive results on cytologic examination
Uncomplicated parapneumonic effusion	Clear to turbid	5000–25,000 P	< 5000	Equal to serum levels	Tube thoracostomy unnecessary
Empyema	Turbid to purulent	25,000–100,000 P	< 5000	Less than serum levels; often very low	Drainage necessary; putrid odor suggests anaerobic infection
Tuberculosis	Serous to serosanguineous	5000–10,000 M	< 10,000	Equal to serum levels; occasionally < 60 mg/dL	Protein > 4.0 g/dL and may exceed 5 g/dL; eosinophils (> 10%) or mesothelial cells (> 5%) make diagnosis unlikely
Rheumatoid effusion	Turbid; greenish yellow	1000–20,000 M or P	< 1000	< 40 mg/dL	Secondary empyema common; high LD, low complement, high rheumatoid factor, cholesterol crystals are characteristic
Pulmonary infarction	Serous to grossly bloody	1000–50,000 M or P	100 to > 100,000	Equal to serum levels	Variable findings; no pathognomonic features
Esophageal rupture	Turbid to purulent; red-brown	< 5000 to > 50,000 P	1000–10,000	Usually low	High amylase level (salivary origin); pneumothorax in 25% of cases; effusion usually on left side; pH < 6.0 strongly suggests diagnosis
Pancreatitis	Turbid to serosanguineous	1000–50,000 P	1000–10,000	Equal to serum levels	Usually left-sided; high amylase level

M, mononuclear cell predominance; P, polymorphonuclear leukocyte predominance; LD, lactate dehydrogenase.

Table 122. Selected disorders associated with ARDS.

Systemic Insults	Pulmonary Insults
Trauma	Aspiration of gastric contents
Sepsis	Embolism of thrombus, fat, air, or amniotic fluid
Pancreatitis	Miliary tuberculosis
Shock	Diffuse pneumonia (eg, SARS)
Multiple transfusions	Acute eosinophilic pneumonia
Disseminated intravascular coagulation	Cryptogenic organizing pneumonitis
Burns	Upper airway obstruction
Drugs and drug overdose	Free-base cocaine smoking
Opioids	Near-drowning
Aspirin	Toxic gas inhalation
Phenothiazines	Nitrogen dioxide
Tricyclic antidepressants	Chlorine
Amiodarone	Sulfur dioxide
Chemotherapeutic agents	Ammonia
Nitrofurantoin	Smoke
Protamine	Oxygen toxicity
Thrombotic thrombocytopenic purpura	Lung contusion
Cardiopulmonary bypass	Radiation exposure
Head injury	High-altitude exposure
Paraquat	Lung reexpansion or reperfusion

ARDS, acute respiratory distress syndrome; SARS, severe acute respiratory syndrome.

Table 123. Frequency (%) of autoantibodies in rheumatic diseases.[1]

	ANA	Anti-Native DNA	Rheumatoid Factor	Anti-Sm	Anti-SS-A	Anti-SS-B	Anti-SCL-70	Anti-Centromere	Anti-Jo-1	ANCA
Rheumatoid arthritis	30–60	0–5	80	0	0–5	0–2	0	0	0	0
Systemic lupus erythematosus	95–100	60	20	10–25	15–20	5–20	0	0	0	0–1
Sjögren syndrome	95	0	75	0	65	65	0	0	0	0
Diffuse scleroderma	80–95	0	30	0	0	0	33	1	0	0
Limited scleroderma (CREST syndrome)	80–95	0	30	0	0	0	20	50	0	0
Polymyositis/dermatomyositis	80–95	0	33	0	0	0	0	0	20–30	0
Wegener granulomatosis	0–15	0	50	0	0	0	0	0	0	93–96[1]

[1]Frequency for generalized, active disease.
ANA, antinuclear antibodies; Anti-Sm, anti-Smith antibody; anti-SCL-70, anti-scleroderma antibody; ANCA, antineutrophil cytoplasmic antibody; CREST, calcinosis cutis, Raynaud phenomenon, esophageal motility disorder, sclerodactyly, and telangiectasia.

Table 124. Examination of joint fluid.

Measure	(Normal)	Group I (Noninflammatory)	Group II (Inflammatory)	Group III (Purulent)
Volume (mL) (knee)	< 3.5	Often > 3.5	Often > 3.5	Often > 3.5
Clarity	Transparent	Transparent	Translucent to opaque	Opaque
Color	Clear	Yellow	Yellow to opalescent	Yellow to green
WBC (per mcL)	< 200	200–300	2000–75,000[1]	> 100,000[2]
Polymorphonuclear leukocytes	< 25%	< 25%	50% or more	75% or more
Culture	Negative	Negative	Negative	Usually positive[2]

[1]Gout, rheumatoid arthritis, and other inflammatory conditions occasionally have synovial fluid WBC counts > 75,000/mcL and < 100,000/mcL.
[2]Most purulent effusions are due to septic arthritis. Septic arthritis, however, can present with group II synovial fluid, particularly if infection is caused by organisms of low virulence (eg, *Neisseria gonorrhoeae*) or if antibiotic therapy has been started.
WBC, white blood cell count.

Table 125. Neurologic testing of lumbosacral nerve disorders.

Nerve Root	Motor	Reflex	Sensory Area
L4	Dorsiflexion of foot	Knee jerk	Medial calf
L5	Dorsiflexion of great toe	None	Medial forefoot
S1	Eversion of foot	Ankle jerk	Lateral foot

Table 126. AHRQ criteria for lumbar radiographs in patients with acute low back pain.

Possible fracture
Major trauma
Minor trauma in patients > 50 years
Long-term corticosteroid use
Osteoporosis
> 70 years
Possible tumor or infection
> 50 years
< 20 years
History of cancer
Constitutional symptoms
Recent bacterial infection
Injection drug use
Immunosuppression
Supine pain
Nocturnal pain

AHRQ, Agency for Healthcare Research and Quality.
Modified and reproduced, with permission, from Suarez-Almazov ME et al. Use of lumbar radiographs for the early diagnosis of low back pain. JAMA. 1997 227(22):1782–88. © 1997 American Medical Association. All rights reserved.

Table 127. Drugs associated with lupus erythematosus.

Definite association	
Chlorpromazine	Methyldopa
Hydralazine	Procainamide
Isoniazid	Quinidine
Possible association	
β-Blockers	Nitrofurantoin
Captopril	Penicillamine
Carbamazepine	Phenytoin
Cimetidine	Propylthiouracil
Ethosuximide	Sulfasalazine
Levodopa	Sulfonamides
Lithium	Trimethadione
Methimazole	
Unlikely association	
Allopurinol	Penicillin
Chlorthalidone	Phenylbutazone
Gold salts	Reserpine
Griseofulvin	Streptomycin
Methysergide	Tetracyclines
Oral contraceptives	

Modified and reproduced, with permission, from Hess EV et al. Drug-related lupus. Bull Rheum Dis. 1991;40(4):1–8.

Table 128. Criteria for the classification of SLE. (A patient is classified as having SLE if any 4 or more of 11 criteria are met.)

1. Malar rash
2. Discoid rash
3. Photosensitivity
4. Oral ulcers
5. Arthritis
6. Serositis
7. Renal disease
   a. > 0.5 g/d proteinuria, or—
   b. ≥ 3+ dipstick proteinuria, or—
   c. Cellular casts
8. Neurologic disease
   a. Seizures, or—
   b. Psychosis (without other cause)
9. Hematologic disorders
   a. Hemolytic anemia, or—
   b. Leukopenia (< 4000/mcL), or—
   c. Lymphopenia (< 1500/mcL), or—
   d. Thrombocytopenia (< 100,000/mcL)
10. Immunologic abnormalities
    a. Positive LE cell preparation, or—
    b. Antibody to native DNA, or—
    c. Antibody to Sm, or—
    d. False-positive serologic test for syphilis
11. Positive ANA

SLE, systemic lupus erythematosus; ANA, antinuclear antibody.
Modified and reproduced, with permission, from Tan EM et al. The 1982 revised criteria for the classification of systemic lupus erythematosus. Arthritis Rheum. 1982 Nov;25(11):1271–7. Reprinted with permission of Wiley-Liss, Inc., a subsidiary of John Wiley & Sons, Inc.

Table 129. Clinical features associated with acute headache that warrant urgent or emergent neuroimaging.

Prior to lumbar puncture
Abnormal neurologic examination
Abnormal mental status
Abnormal funduscopic examination (papilledema; loss of venous pulsations)
Meningeal signs
Emergent (conduct prior to leaving office or emergency department)
Abnormal neurologic examination
Abnormal mental status
Thunderclap headache
Urgent (scheduled prior to leaving office or emergency department)
HIV-positive patient[1]
Age > 50 years (normal neurologic examination)

[1]Use CT with or without contrast or MRI if HIV positive.
Source: American College of Emergency Physicians. Clinical Policy: critical issues in the evaluation and management of patients presenting to the emergency department with acute headache. Ann Emerg Med. 2002 Jan;39(1):108–22.

Table 130. Prophylactic treatment of migraine.

Drug	Usual Adult Daily Dose	Common Side Effects
Propranolol[1]	80–240 mg	Fatigue, lassitude, depression, insomnia, nausea, vomiting, constipation.
Amitriptyline	10–150 mg	Sedation, dry mouth, constipation, weight gain, blurred vision, edema, hypotension, urinary retention.
Imipramine	10–150 mg	Similar to those of amitriptyline (above).
Sertraline	50–200 mg	Anxiety, insomnia, sweating, tremor, gastrointestinal disturbances.
Fluoxetine	20–60 mg	Similar to those of sertraline (above).
Cyproheptadine	12–20 mg	Sedation, dry mouth, epigastric discomfort, gastrointestinal disturbances.
Clonidine	0.2–0.6 mg	Dry mouth, drowsiness, sedation, headache, constipation.
Verapamil[2]	80–160 mg	Headache, hypotension, flushing, edema, constipation. May aggravate atrioventricular nodal heart block and congestive heart failure.

[1]Other β-blockers (eg, timolol and metoprolol) have also been used.
[2]Other calcium channel antagonists (eg, nimodipine, nicardipine, and diltiazem) have also been used.
Botulinum toxin type A injected locally into the scalp is effective for prophylaxis in some patients. The antiseizure agents valproic acid (500–1500 mg), gabapentin (900–2400 mg), and topiramate (50–200 mg) are also effective and are detailed in Table 133. Valproic acid should be avoided during pregnancy.

Table 131. Features of the major stroke subtypes.

Stroke Type and Subtype	Clinical Features	Diagnosis	Treatment
Ischemic stroke			
Lacunar infarct	Small (< 5 mm) lesions in the basal ganglia, pons, cerebellum, or internal capsule; less often in deep cerebral white matter; prognosis generally good; clinical features depend on location, but may worsen over first 24–36 hours.	CT may reveal small hypodensity but is often normal.	Aspirin; long-term management is to control risk factors (hypertension and diabetes mellitus).
Carotid circulation obstruction	See text—signs vary depending on occluded vessel.	Noncontrast CT to exclude hemorrhage but findings may be normal during first 6–24 hours of an ischemic stroke; when available, diffusion-weighted MRI plus gradient-echo sequences and FLAIR may also be used; electrocardiography, blood glucose, complete blood count, and tests for hypercoagulable states, hyperlipidemia are indicated; echocardiography or Holter monitoring in selected instances; carotid duplex studies, MR angiography and conventional angiography in selected cases.	Select patients for intravenous thrombolytics or intra-arterial mechanical thrombolysis; aspirin (325 mg/d orally) combined with sustained-release dipyridamole (200 mg twice daily) is first-line therapy; anticoagulation with heparin for cardioembolic strokes when no contraindications exist.
Vertebrobasilar occlusion	See text—signs vary based on location of occluded vessel.	As for carotid circulation obstruction.	As for carotid circulation obstruction.
Hemorrhagic stroke			
Spontaneous intracerebral hemorrhage	Commonly associated with hypertension; also with bleeding disorders, amyloid angiopathy. Hypertensive hemorrhage is located commonly in the basal ganglia and less commonly in the pons, thalamus, cerebellum, or cerebral white matter.	Noncontrast CT is superior to MRI for detecting bleeds of < 48 hours duration; laboratory tests to identify bleeding disorder; angiography may be indicated to exclude aneurysm or AVM. Do not perform lumbar puncture.	Most managed supportively, but cerebellar bleeds or hematomas with gross mass effect may require urgent surgical evacuation.
Subarachnoid hemorrhage	Present with sudden onset of worst headache of life, may lead rapidly to loss of consciousness; signs of meningeal irritation often present; etiology usually aneurysm or AVM, but 20% have no source identified.	CT to confirm diagnosis, but may be normal in rare instances; if CT negative and suspicion high, perform lumbar puncture to look for red blood cells or xanthochromia; angiography to determine source of bleed in candidates for treatment.	See sections on AVM and aneurysm.
Intracranial aneurysm	Most located in the anterior circle of Willis and are typically asymptomatic until subarachnoid bleed occurs; 20% rebleed in first 2 weeks.	CT indicates subarachnoid hemorrhage, and angiography then demonstrates aneurysms; angiography may not reveal aneurysm if vasospasm present.	Prevent further bleeding by clipping aneurysm or coil embolization; nimodipine helps prevent vasospasm; reverse vasospasm by intravenous fluids and induced hypertension after aneurysm has been obliterated, if no other aneurysms are present; angioplasty may also reverse symptomatic vasospasm.
AVMs	Focal deficit from hematoma or AVM itself.	CT reveals bleed, and may reveal the AVM; may be seen by MRI. Angiography demonstrates feeding vessels and vascular anatomy.	Surgery indicated if AVM has bled or to prevent further progression of neurologic deficit; other modalities to treat nonoperable AVMs are available at specialized centers.

AVMs, arteriovenous malformations.

Table 132. Seizure classification.

Seizure Type	Key Features	Other Associated Features
Partial seizures	Involvement of only restricted part of brain; may become secondarily generalized	
Simple partial	Consciousness preserved	May be manifested by focal motor, sensory, or autonomic symptoms
Complex partial	Consciousness impaired	Above symptoms may precede, accompany, or follow
Generalized seizures	Diffuse involvement of brain at onset	
Absence (petit mal)	Consciousness impaired briefly; patient often unaware of attacks	May be clonic, tonic, or atonic components (ie, loss of postural tone); autonomic components (eg, enuresis); or accompanying automatisms. Almost always begin in childhood and frequently cease by age 20
Atypical absences	May be more gradual onset and termination than typical absence	More marked changes in tone may occur
Myoclonic	Single or multiple myoclonic jerks	
Tonic-clonic (grand mal)	Tonic phase: Sudden loss of consciousness, with rigidity and arrest of respiration, lasting < 1 minute. Clonic phase: Jerking occurs, usually for < 2–3 minutes. Flaccid coma: Variable duration	May be accompanied by tongue biting, incontinence, or aspiration; commonly followed by postictal confusion variable in duration
Status epilepticus	Repeated seizures without recovery between them, a fixed and enduring epileptic condition lasting 30 minutes	

Table 133. Drug treatment for seizures in adults.

Drug	Usual Adult Daily Dose	Minimum No. of Daily Doses	Time to Steady State Drug Levels	Optimal Drug Level	Selected Side Effects and Idiosyncratic Reactions
Generalized tonic-clonic (grand mal) or partial (focal) seizures					
Phenytoin	200–400 mg	1	5–10 days	10–20 mcg/mL	Nystagmus, ataxia, dysarthria, sedation, confusion, gingival hyperplasia, hirsutism, megaloblastic anemia, blood dyscrasias, skin rashes, fever, systemic lupus erythematosus, lymphadenopathy, peripheral neuropathy, dyskinesias.
Carbamazepine (extended-release formulation)	600–1200 mg	2–3 (2)	3–4 days	4–8 mcg/mL	Nystagmus, dysarthria, diplopia, ataxia, drowsiness, nausea, blood dyscrasias, hepatotoxicity, hyponatremia. May exacerbate myoclonic seizures.
Valproic acid	1500–2000 mg	2–3	2–4 days	50–100 mcg/mL	Nausea, vomiting, diarrhea, drowsiness, alopecia, weight gain, hepatotoxicity, thrombocytopenia, tremor, pancreatitis.
Phenobarbital	100–200 mg	1	14–21 days	10–40 mcg/mL	Drowsiness, nystagmus, ataxia, skin rashes, learning difficulties, hyperactivity.
Primidone	750–1500 mg	3	4–7 days	5–15 mcg/mL	Sedation, nystagmus, ataxia, vertigo, nausea, skin rashes, megaloblastic anemia, irritability.
Lamotrigine[1,2,5]	100–500 mg	2	4–5 days	?	Sedation, skin rash, visual disturbances, dyspepsia, ataxia.
Topiramate[1-4]	200–400 mg	2	4 days	?	Somnolence, nausea, dyspepsia, irritability, dizziness, ataxia, nystagmus, diplopia, glaucoma, renal calculi, weight loss, hypohidrosis, hyperthermia.
Oxcarbazepine[1,3]	900–1800 mg	2	2–3 days	?	As for carbamazepine.
Levetiracetam[1,2]	1000–3000 mg	2	2 days	?	Somnolence, ataxia, headache, behavioral changes.
Zonisamide[1]	200–600 mg	1	10 days	?	Somnolence, ataxia, anorexia, nausea, vomiting, rash, confusion, renal calculi. Do not use in patients with sulfonamide allergy.
Tiagabine[1]	32–56 mg	2	2 days	?	Somnolence, anxiety, dizziness, poor concentration, tremor, diarrhea.
Pregabalin[1]	150–300 mg	2	2–4 days	?	Somnolence, dizziness, poor concentration, weight gain, thrombocytopenia, skin rashes, anaphylactoid reactions.
Gabapentin[1]	900–3600 mg	3	1 day	?	Sedation, fatigue, ataxia, nystagmus, weight loss.
Felbamate[1,3,6]	1200–3600 mg	3	4–5 days	?	Anorexia, nausea, vomiting, headache, insomnia, weight loss, dizziness, hepatotoxicity, aplastic anemia.
Absence (petit mal) seizures					
Ethosuximide	100–1500 mg	2	5–10 days	40–100 mcg/mL	Nausea, vomiting, anorexia, headache, lethargy, unsteadiness, blood dyscrasias, systemic lupus erythematosus, urticaria, pruritus.
Valproic acid	1500–2000 mg	3	2–4 days	50–100 mcg/mL	See above.
Clonazepam	0.04–0.2 mg/kg	2	?	20–80 ng/mL	Drowsiness, ataxia, irritability, behavioral changes, exacerbation of tonic-clonic seizures.
Myoclonic seizures					
Valproic acid	1500–2000 mg	3	2–4 days	50–100 mcg/mL	See above.
Clonazepam	0.04–0.2 mg/kg	2	?	20–80 ng/mL	See above.

[1]Approved as adjunctive therapy for partial-onset seizures.
[2]Approved as adjunctive therapy for primary generalized tonic-clonic seizures.
[3]Approved as initial monotherapy for partial-onset seizures.
[4]Approved as initial monotherapy for primary generalized tonic-clonic seizures.
[5]Approved as monotherapy (after conversion from another drug) in partial-onset seizures.
[6]Not to be used as a first-line drug; when used, blood counts should be performed regularly (every 2–4 weeks). Should be used only in selected patients because of risk of aplastic anemia and hepatic failure. It is advisable to obtain written informed consent before use.

Table 134. Primary intracranial tumors.

Tumor	Clinical Features	Treatment and Prognosis
Glioblastoma multiforme	Presents commonly with nonspecific complaints and increased intracranial pressure. As it grows, focal deficits develop.	Course is rapidly progressive, with poor prognosis. Total surgical removal is usually not possible. Radiation therapy and chemotherapy may prolong survival.
Astrocytoma	Presentation similar to glioblastoma multiforme but course more protracted, often over several years. Cerebellar astrocytoma may have a more benign course.	Prognosis is variable. By the time of diagnosis, total excision is usually impossible; tumor may be radiosensitive and chemotherapy may also be helpful. In cerebellar astrocytoma, total surgical removal is often possible.
Medulloblastoma	Seen most frequently in children. Generally arises from roof of fourth ventricle and leads to increased intracranial pressure accompanied by brainstem and cerebellar signs. May seed subarachnoid space.	Treatment consists of surgery combined with radiation therapy and chemotherapy.
Ependymoma	Glioma arising from the ependyma of a ventricle, especially the fourth ventricle; leads to early signs of increased intracranial pressure. Arises also from central canal of cord.	Tumor is best treated surgically if possible. Radiation therapy may be used for residual tumor.
Oligodendroglioma	Slow-growing. Usually arises in cerebral hemisphere in adults. Calcification may be visible on skull x-ray.	Treatment is surgical and usually successful. Radiation and chemotherapy may be used if tumor has malignant features.
Brainstem glioma	Presents during childhood with cranial nerve palsies and then with long tract signs in the limbs. Signs of increased intracranial pressure occur late.	Tumor is inoperable; treatment is by irradiation and shunt for increased intracranial pressure.
Cerebellar hemangioblastoma	Presents with disequilibrium, ataxia of trunk or limbs, and signs of increased intracranial pressure. Sometimes familial. May be associated with retinal and spinal vascular lesions, polycythemia, and renal cell carcinoma.	Treatment is surgical. Radiation is used for residual tumor.
Pineal tumor	Presents with increased intracranial pressure, sometimes associated with impaired upward gaze (Parinaud syndrome) and other deficits indicative of midbrain lesion.	Ventricular decompression by shunting is followed by surgical approach to tumor; irradiation is indicated if tumor is malignant. Prognosis depends on histopathologic findings and extent of tumor.
Craniopharyngioma	Originates from remnants of Rathke pouch above the sella, depressing the optic chiasm. May present at any age but usually in childhood, with endocrine dysfunction and bitemporal field defects.	Treatment is surgical, but total removal may not be possible. Radiation may be used for residual tumor.
Acoustic neurinoma	Ipsilateral hearing loss is most common initial symptom. Subsequent symptoms may include tinnitus, headache, vertigo, facial weakness or numbness, and long tract signs. (May be familial and bilateral when related to neurofibromatosis.) Most sensitive screening tests are MRI and brainstem auditory evoked potential.	Treatment is excision by translabyrinthine surgery, craniectomy, or a combined approach. Outcome is usually good.
Meningioma	Originates from the dura mater or arachnoid; compresses rather than invades adjacent neural structures. Increasingly common with advancing age. Tumor size varies greatly. Symptoms vary with tumor site—eg, unilateral proptosis (sphenoidal ridge); anosmia and optic nerve compression (olfactory groove). Tumor is usually benign and readily detected by CT scanning; may lead to calcification and bone erosion visible on plain x-rays of skull.	Treatment is surgical. Tumor may recur if removal is incomplete.
Primary cerebral lymphoma	Associated with AIDS and other immunodeficient states. Presentation may be with focal deficits or with disturbances of cognition and consciousness. May be indistinguishable from cerebral toxoplasmosis.	Treatment is high-dose methotrexate followed by radiation therapy. Prognosis depends on CD4 count at diagnosis.

Table 135. Some anticholinergic antiparkinsonian drugs.

Drug	Usual Daily Dose
Benztropine mesylate (Cogentin)	1–6 mg
Biperiden (Akineton)	2–12 mg
Orphenadrine (Disipal, Norflex)	150–400 mg
Procyclidine (Kemadrin)	7.5–30 mg
Trihexyphenidyl (Artane)	6–20 mg

Modified, with permission, from Aminoff MJ: Pharmacologic management of parkinsonism and other movement disorders. In: *Basic & Clinical Pharmacology*, 10th ed. Katzung BG (editor). McGraw-Hill, 2007.

Table 136. Acute cerebral sequelae of head injury.

Sequelae	Clinical Features	Pathology
Concussion	Transient loss of consciousness with bradycardia, hypotension, and respiratory arrest for a few seconds followed by retrograde and posttraumatic amnesia. Occasionally followed by transient neurologic deficit.	Bruising on side of impact (coup injury) or contralaterally (contrecoup injury).
Cerebral contusion or laceration	Loss of consciousness longer than with concussion. May lead to death or severe residual neurologic deficit.	Cerebral contusion, edema, hemorrhage, and necrosis. May have subarachnoid bleeding.
Acute epidural hemorrhage	Headache, confusion, somnolence, seizures, and focal deficits occur several hours after injury and lead to coma, respiratory depression, and death unless treated by surgical evacuation.	Tear in meningeal artery, vein, or dural sinus, leading to hematoma visible on CT scan.
Acute subdural hemorrhage	Similar to epidural hemorrhage, but interval before onset of symptoms is longer. Treatment is by surgical evacuation.	Hematoma from tear in veins from cortex to superior sagittal sinus or from cerebral laceration, visible on CT scan.
Cerebral hemorrhage	Generally develops immediately after injury. Clinically resembles hypertensive hemorrhage. Surgical evacuation is sometimes helpful.	Hematoma, visible on CT scan.

Table 137. The muscular dystrophies.[1]

Disorder	Inheritance	Age at Onset (years)	Distribution	Prognosis	Genetic Locus
Duchenne type	X-linked recessive	1–5	Pelvic, then shoulder girdle; later, limb and respiratory muscles.	Rapid progression. Death within about 15 years after onset.	Xp21
Becker	X-linked recessive	5–25	Pelvic, then shoulder girdle.	Slow progression. May have normal life span.	Xp21
Limb-girdle (Erb)	Autosomal recessive, dominant or sporadic	10–30	Pelvic or shoulder girdle initially, with later spread to the other.	Variable severity and rate of progression. Possible severe disability in middle life.	Multiple
Facioscapulo-humeral	Autosomal dominant	Any age	Face and shoulder girdle initially; later, pelvic girdle and legs.	Slow progression. Minor disability. Usually normal life span.	4q35
Emery-Dreifuss	X-linked recessive or autosomal dominant	5–10	Humeroperoneal or scapuloperoneal.	Variable.	Xq28, 1q21.2
Distal	Autosomal dominant or recessive	40–60	Onset distally in extremities; proximal involvement later.	Slow progression.	2p13, 14q12
Ocular	Autosomal dominant (may be recessive)	Any age (usually 5–30)	External ocular muscles; may also be mild weakness of face, neck, and arms.		
Oculopharyngeal	Autosomal dominant	Any age	As in the ocular form but with dysphagia.		14q11.2-q13
Myotonic dystrophy	Autosomal dominant	Any age (usually 20–40)	Face, neck, distal limbs.	Slow progression.	19q13.2-q13.3; 3q13.3-q24

[1]Not all possible genetic loci are shown.

Table 138. Common drugs that are teratogenic or fetotoxic.[1]

ACE inhibitors	Hypoglycemics, oral (older drugs)
Alcohol	Isotretinoin
Amantadine	Lithium
Androgens	Methotrexate
Anticonvulsants	Misoprostol
Aminoglutethimide	NSAIDs (third trimester)
Carbamazepine	Opioids (prolonged use)
Phenytoin	Progestins
Valproic acid	Radioiodine (antithyroid)
Aspirin and other salicylates (third trimester)	Reserpine
	Ribavirin
Benzodiazepines	SSRIs
Carbarsone (amebicide)	Sulfonamides (third trimester)
Chloramphenicol (third trimester)	Tetracycline (third trimester)
Cyclophosphamide	Thalidomide
Diazoxide	Tobacco smoking
Diethylstilbestrol	Trimethoprim (third trimester)
Disulfiram	Warfarin and other coumarin anti-
Ergotamine	coagulants
Estrogens	
Griseofulvin	

[1]Many other drugs are also contraindicated during pregnancy. Evaluate any drug for its need versus its potential adverse effects. Further information can be obtained from the manufacturer or from any of several teratogenic registries around the country.
ACE, angiotensin-converting enzyme; NSAIDs, nonsteroidal anti-inflammatory drugs; SSRIs, selective serotonin reuptake inhibitors.

Table 139. Indicators of mild to moderate versus severe preeclampsia-eclampsia.

Site	Indicator	Mild to Moderate	Severe
Central nervous system	Symptoms and signs	Hyperreflexia Headache	Seizures Blurred vision Scotomas Headache Clonus Irritability
Kidney	Proteinuria Uric acid Urinary output	0.3–5 g/24 h ↑ > 4.5 mg/dL > 20–30 mL/h	> 5 g/24 h or catheterized urine with 4+ protein ↑↑ > 4.5 mg/dL < 20–30 mL/h
Liver	AST, ALT, LDH	Normal	Elevated LFTs Epigastric pain Ruptured liver
Hematologic	Platelets Hemoglobin	> 100,000/mcL Normal range	< 100,000/mcL Elevated
Vascular	Blood pressure Retina	< 160/110 mm Hg Arteriolar spasm	> 160/110 mm Hg Retinal hemorrhages
Fetal-placental unit	Growth restriction Oligohydramnios Fetal distress	Absent May be present Absent	Present Present Present

AST, aspartate aminotransferase; ALT, alanine aminotransferase; LDH, lactate dehydrogenase; LFTs, liver function tests.

Table 140. Screening and diagnostic criteria for gestational diabetes mellitus.

Screening for gestational diabetes mellitus
1. 50-g oral glucose load, administered between the 24th and 28th weeks, without regard to time of day or time of last meal. Universal blood glucose screening is indicated for patients who are of Hispanic, African, Native American, South or East Asian, Pacific Island, or Indigenous Australian ancestry. Other patients who have no known diabetes in first-degree relatives, are under 25 years of age, have normal weight before pregnancy, and have no history of abnormal glucose metabolism or poor obstetric outcome do not require routine screening.
2. Venous plasma glucose measure 1 hour later.
3. Value of 130 mg/dL (7.2 mmol/L) or above in venous plasma indicates the need for a full diagnostic glucose tolerance test.
Diagnosis of gestational diabetes mellitus
1. 100-g oral glucose load, administered in the morning after overnight fast lasting at least 8 hours but not more than 14 hours, and following at least 3 days of unrestricted diet (> 150 g carbohydrate) and physical activity.
2. Venous plasma glucose is measured fasting and at 1, 2, and 3 hours. Subject should remain seated and should not smoke throughout the test.
3. Two or more of the following venous plasma concentrations must be equaled or exceeded for a diagnosis of gestational diabetes: fasting, 95 mg/dL (5.3 mmol/L); 1 hour, 180 mg/dL (10 mmol/L); 2 hours, 155 mg/dL (8.6 mmol/L); 3 hours, 140 mg/dL (7.8 mmol/L).

Table 141. Drugs and substances that require a careful assessment of risk before they are prescribed for breast-feeding women.[1]

Category	Specific Drugs or Compounds
Analgesic drugs	Meperidine, oxycodone
Antiarthritis drugs	Gold salts, methotrexate, high-dose aspirin
Anticoagulant drugs	Phenindione[2]
Antidepressant drugs and lithium	Fluoxetine, doxepin, lithium[2]
Antiepileptic drugs	Phenobarbital, ethosuximide, primidone
Antimicrobial drugs	Chloramphenicol, tetracycline
Anticancer drugs	All (eg, cyclophosphamide,[2] methotrexate,[2] doxorubicin[2])
Anxiolytic drugs	Diazepam, alprazolam
Cardiovascular and antihypertensive drugs	Acebutolol, amiodarone, atenolol, nadolol, sotalol
Endocrine drugs and hormones	Estrogens, bromocriptine[2]
Immunosuppressive drugs	Cyclosporine,[2] azathioprine
Respiratory drugs	Theophylline
Radioactive compounds	All
Drugs of abuse	All
Nonmedicinal substances	Ethanol, caffeine, nicotine
Miscellaneous compounds	Iodides and iodine, ergotamine,[2] ergonovine

[1]Reproduced with permission from Dershewitz RA, ed. *Ambulatory Pediatric Care*, LWW, 1999. Drugs for which there is no information are not included, although a careful risk assessment is necessary before such drugs are prescribed.
[2]The use of this drug or these drugs by breast-feeding women is contraindicated according to the American Academy of Pediatrics

Table 142. Currently available cyanide (CN) antidote kits.

Antidote	Contents	Action
Conventional cyanide antidote kit[1]	Amyl nitrite, 0.3 mL aspirol for inhalation; sodium nitrite 300 mg in a 10-mL vial; sodium thiosulfate 12.5 g in a 50-mL vial	Nitrites induce methemoglobinemia, which binds CN; thiosulfate hastens CN conversion to less toxic thiocyanate
Cyanokit[2]	Hydroxocobalamin 5 g in two 2.5-g vials	Converts CN to cyanocobalamin (vitamin B_{12})

[1]In the United States, manufactured by Taylor Pharmaceuticals.
[2]Manufactured by EMD Pharmaceuticals.

Table 143. Common seafood poisonings.

Type of Poisoning	Mechanism	Clinical Presentation
Ciguatera	Reef fish ingest toxic dinoflagellates, whose toxins accumulate in fish meat. Commonly implicated fish in the United States are barracuda, jack, snapper, and grouper.	1–6 hours after ingestion, victims develop abdominal pain, vomiting, and diarrhea accompanied by a variety of neurologic symptoms, including paresthesias, reversal of hot and cold sensation, vertigo, headache, and intense itching. Autonomic disturbances, including hypotension and bradycardia, may occur.
Scombroid	Improper preservation of large fish results in bacterial degradation of histidine to histamine. Commonly implicated fish include tuna, mahimahi, bonita, mackerel, and kingfish.	Allergic-like (anaphylactoid) symptoms are due to histamine, usually begin within 15–90 minutes, and include skin flushing, itching, urticaria, angioedema, bronchospasm, and hypotension as well as abdominal pain, vomiting, and diarrhea.
Paralytic shellfish poisoning	Dinoflagellates produce saxitoxin, which is concentrated by filter-feeding mussels and clams. Saxitoxin blocks sodium conductance and neuronal transmission in skeletal muscles.	Onset is usually within 30–60 minutes. Initial symptoms include perioral and intraoral paresthesias. Other symptoms include nausea and vomiting, headache, dizziness, dysphagia, dysarthria, ataxia, and rapidly progressive muscle weakness that may result in respiratory arrest.
Puffer fish poisoning	Tetrodotoxin is concentrated in liver, gonads, intestine, and skin. Toxic effects are similar to those of saxitoxin. Tetrodotoxin is also found in some North American newts and Central American frogs.	Onset is usually within 30–40 minutes but may be as short as 10 minutes. Initial perioral paresthesias are followed by headache, diaphoresis, nausea, vomiting, ataxia, and rapidly progressive muscle weakness that may result in respiratory arrest.

Table 144. Screening for alcohol abuse.

A. CAGE screening test[1]	
Have you ever felt the need to	Cut down on drinking?
Have you ever felt	Annoyed by criticism of your drinking?
Have you ever felt	Guilty about your drinking?
Have you ever taken a morning	Eye opener?

INTERPRETATION: Two "yes" answers are considered a positive screen. One "yes" answer should arouse a suspicion of alcohol abuse.

B. The Alcohol Use Disorder Identification Test (AUDIT).[2] (Scores for response categories are given in parentheses. Scores range from 0 to 40, with a cutoff score of ≥ 5 indicating hazardous drinking, harmful drinking, or alcohol dependence.)

1. How often do you have a drink containing alcohol?

(0) Never	(1) Monthly or less	(2) Two to four times a month	(3) Two or three times a week	(4) Four or more times a week

2. How many drinks containing alcohol do you have on a typical day when you are drinking?

(0) 1 or 2	(1) 3 or 4	(2) 5 or 6	(3) 7 to 9	(4) 10 or more

3. How often do you have six or more drinks on one occasion?

(0) Never	(1) Less than monthly	(2) Monthly	(3) Weekly	(4) Daily or almost daily

4. How often during the past year have you found that you were not able to stop drinking once you had started?

(0) Never	(1) Less than monthly	(2) Monthly	(3) Weekly	(4) Daily or almost daily

5. How often during the past year have you failed to do what was normally expected of you because of drinking?

(0) Never	(1) Less than monthly	(2) Monthly	(3) Weekly	(4) Daily or almost daily

6. How often during the past year have you needed a first drink in the morning to get yourself going after a heavy drinking session?

(0) Never	(1) Less than monthly	(2) Monthly	(3) Weekly	(4) Daily or almost daily

7. How often during the past year have you had a feeling of guilt or remorse after drinking?

(0) Never	(1) Less than monthly	(2) Monthly	(3) Weekly	(4) Daily or almost daily

8. How often during the past year have you been unable to remember what happened the night before because you had been drinking?

(0) Never	(1) Less than monthly	(2) Monthly	(3) Weekly	(4) Daily or almost daily

9. Have you or has someone else been injured as a result of your drinking?

(0) No	(2) Yes, but not in the past year	(4) Yes, during the past year

10. Has a relative or friend or a doctor or other health worker been concerned about your drinking or suggested you cut down?

(0) No	(2) Yes, but not in the past year	(4) Yes, during the past year

[1]Source: Mayfield D et al. The CAGE questionnaire: validation of a new alcoholism screening instrument. Am J Psychiatry. 1974;131:1121. With permission from BMJ Publishing Group, Ltd.
[2]Adapted, with permission, from Piccinelli M et al. Efficacy of the alcohol use disorders identification test as a screening tool for hazardous alcohol intake and related disorders in primary care: a validity study. BMJ. 1997 Feb 8;314(7078):420–4.

Table 145. Commonly used antianxiety and hypnotic agents.

Drug	Usual Daily Oral Doses	Usual Daily Maximum Doses	Cost for 30 Days Treatment Based on Maximum Dosage[1]
Benzodiazepines (used for anxiety)			
Alprazolam (Xanax)[2]	0.5 mg	4 mg	$117.87
Chlordiazepoxide (Librium)[3]	10–20 mg	100 mg	$40.82
Clonazepam (Klonopin)[3]	1–2 mg	10 mg	$177.68
Clorazepate (Tranxene)[3]	15–30 mg	60 mg	$260.94
Diazepam (Valium)[3]	5–15 mg	30 mg	$28.13
Lorazepam (Ativan)[2]	2–4 mg	4 mg	$73.27
Oxazepam (Serax)[2]	10–30 mg	60 mg	$95.41
Benzodiazepines (used for sleep)			
Estazolam (Prosom)[2]	1 mg	2 mg	$29.70
Flurazepam (Dalmane)[3]	15 mg	30 mg	$10.40
Midazolam (Versed IV)[4]	5 mg IV		$1.66/dose
Quazepam (Doral)[3]	7.5 mg	15 mg	$138.11
Temazepam (Restoril)[2]	15 mg	30 mg	$26.54
Triazolam (Halcion)[5]	0.125 mg	0.25 mg	$20.25
Miscellaneous (used for anxiety)			
Buspirone (Buspar)[2]	10–30 mg	60 mg	$218.10
Phenobarbital[3]	15–30 mg	90 mg	$3.15
Miscellaneous (used for sleep)			
Chloral hydrate (Noctec)[2]	500 mg	1000 mg	$9.41
Eszopiclone (Lunesta)[5]	2–3 mg	3 mg	$138.24
Hydroxyzine (Vistaril)[2]	50 mg	100 mg	$18.81
Zolpidem (Ambien)[5]	5–10 mg	10 mg	$138.59
Zaleplon (Sonata)[6]	5–10 mg	10 mg	$111.20
Ramelteon (Rozerem)	8 mg	8 mg	$106.25

[1]Average wholesale price (AWP, for AB-rated generic when available) for quantity listed. Source: *Red Book Update*, Vol. 27, No. 2, February 2008. AWP may not accurately represent the actual pharmacy cost because wide contractual variations exist among institutions.
[2]Intermediate physical half-life (10–20 hours).
[3]Long physical half-life (> 20 hours).
[4]Intravenously for procedures.
[5]Short physical half-life (1–6 hours).
[6]Short physical half-life (about 1 hour).

Table 146. Commonly used antipsychotics.

Drug	Usual Daily Oral Dose	Usual Daily Maximum Dose[1]	Cost per Unit	Cost for 30 Days Treatment Based on Maximum Dosage[2]
Phenothiazines				
Chlorpromazine (Thorazine; others)	100–400 mg	1 g	$1.05/200 mg	$157.50
Thioridazine (Mellaril)	100–400 mg	600 mg	$.67/100 mg	$120.60
Mesoridazine (Serentil)	50–200 mg	400 mg		Not available in United States
Perphenazine (Trilafon)[3]	16–32 mg	64 mg	$1.54/16 mg	$184.80
Trifluoperazine (Stelazine)	5–15 mg	60 mg	$1.63/10 mg	$293.60
Fluphenazine (Permitil, Prolixin)[3]	2–10 mg	60 mg	$1.25/10 mg	$225.00
Thioxanthenes				
Thiothixene (Navane)[3]	5–10 mg	80 mg	$0.65/10 mg	$156.00
Dihydroindolone				
Molindone (Moban)	30–100 mg	225 mg	$4.03/50 mg	$544.05
Dibenzoxazepine				
Loxapine (Loxitane)	20–60 mg	200 mg	$2.57/50 mg	$308.40
Dibenzodiazepine				
Clozapine (Clozaril)	300–450 mg	900 mg	$3.42/100 mg	$923.40
Butyrophenone				
Haloperidol (Haldol)	2–5 mg	60 mg	$2.76/20 mg	$248.40
Benzisoxazole				
Risperidone[4] (Risperdal)	2–6 mg	10 mg	$7.59/2 mg	$946.16
Thienobenzodiazepine				
Olanzapine (Zyprexa)	5–10 mg	10 mg	$13.09/10 mg	$392.69
Dibenzothiazepine				
Quetiapine (Seroquel)	200–400 mg	800 mg	$7.37/200 mg	$681.16
Benzisothiazolyl piperazine				
Ziprasidone (Geodon)	40–160 mg	160 mg	$7.02/80 mg	$421.44
Dipiperazine				
Aripiprazole (Abilify)	10–15 mg	30 mg	$19.80/30 mg	$594.10

[1]Can be higher in some cases.
[2]Average wholesale price (AWP, for AB-rated generic when available) for quantity listed. Source: *Red Book Update*, Vol. 27, No. 2, February 2008. AWP may not accurately represent the actual pharmacy cost because wide contractual variations exist among institutions.
[3]Indicates piperazine structure.
[4]For risperidone, daily doses above 6 mg increase the risk of extrapyramidal syndrome. Risperidone 6 mg is approximately equivalent to haloperidol 20 mg.

Table 147. Relative potency and side effects of antipsychotics.

Drug	Chlorpromazine: Drug Potency Ratio	Anticholinergic Effects[1]	Extrapyramidal Effect[1]
Phenothiazines			
Chlorpromazine	1:1	4	1
Thioridazine	1:1	4	1
Mesoridazine	1:2	3	2
Perphenazine	1:10	2	3
Trifluoperazine	1:20	1	4
Fluphenazine	1:50	1	4
Thioxanthene			
Thiothixene	1:20	1	4
Dihydroindolone			
Molindone	1:10	2	3
Dibenzoxazepine			
Loxapine	1:10	2	3
Butyrophenone			
Haloperidol	1:50	1	4
Dibenzodiazepine			
Clozapine	1:1	4	—
Benzisoxazole			
Risperidone	1:50	1	1
Thienobenzodiazepine			
Olanzapine	1:20	1	1
Dibenzothiazepine			
Quetiapine	1:1	1	—
Benzisothiazolyl piperazine			
Ziprasidone	1:1	1	1
Dipiperazine			
Aripiprazole	1:20	1	0

[1]4, strong effect; 1, weak effect.

Table 148. Commonly used antidepressants.

Drug	Usual Daily Oral Dose (mg)	Usual Daily Maximum Dose (mg)	Sedative Effects[1]	Anticholinergic Effects[1]	Cost per Unit	Cost for 30 Days Treatment Based on Maximum Dosage[2]
SSRIs						
Fluoxetine (Prozac, Sarafem)	5–40	80	< 1	< 1	$2.67/20 mg	$320.40
Fluvoxamine (Luvox)	100–300	300	1	< 1	$2.64/100 mg	$237.60
Nefazodone (Serzone)	300–600	600	2	< 1	$1.60/200 mg	$144.00
Paroxetine (Paxil)	20–30	50	1	1	$2.73/20 mg	$163.80
Sertraline (Zoloft)	50–150	200	< 1	< 1	$2.72/100 mg	$163.20
Citalopram (Celexa)	20	40	< 1	1	$2.53/40 mg	$75.78
Escitalopram (Lexapro)	10	20	< 1	1	$2.98/20 mg	$89.39
Tricyclic and clinically similar compounds						
Amitriptyline (Elavil)	150–250	300	4	4	$1.16/150 mg	$69.60
Amoxapine (Asendin)	150–200	400	2	2	$1.67/100 mg	$200.40
Clomipramine (Anafranil)	100	250	3	3	$1.48/75 mg	$158.92
Desipramine (Norpramin)	100–250	300	1	1	$1.50/100 mg	$135.00
Doxepin (Sinequan)	150–200	300	4	3	$1.00/100 mg	$90.00
Imipramine (Tofranil)	150–200	300	3	3	$1.22/50 mg	$219.60
Maprotiline (Ludiomil)	100–200	300	4	2	$1.14/75 mg	$136.50
Nortriptyline (Aventyl, Pamelor)	100–150	150	2	2	$1.52/50 mg	$136.62
Protriptyline (Vivactil)	15–40	60	1	3	$2.95/10 mg	$531.00
Monoamine oxidase inhibitors						
Phenelzine (Nardil)	45–60	90	. . .	. . .	$0.66/15 mg	$119.55
Tranylcypromine (Parnate)	20–30	50	. . .	. . .	$0.97/10 mg	$145.53
Selegiline transdermal (Emsam)	6 (skin patch)	12			$16.42/6 mg patch	$985.34
Other compounds						
Venlafaxine XR (Effexor)	150–225	225	1	< 1	$4.09/75 mg	$367.73
Duloxetine (Cymbalta)	40	60	2	3	$4.24/60 mg	$127.20
Mirtazapine (Remeron)	15–45	45	4	2	$2.80/30 mg	$85.50
Bupropion XL (Wellbutrin XL)	300[3]	450[3]		< 1	$5.87/300 mg	$309.75
Bupropion SR (Wellbutrin SR)	300	400[4]		< 1	$3.83/200 mg	$229.98
Trazodone (Desyrel)	100–300	400	4	< 1	$0.73/100 mg	$87.60
Trimipramine (Surmontil)	75–200	200	4	4	$4.40/100 mg	$264.00

[1]4, strong effect; 1, weak effect.

[2]Average wholesale price (AWP, for AB-rated generic when available) for quantity listed. Source: *Red Book Update*, Vol. 27, No. 2, February 2008. AWP may not accurately represent the actual pharmacy cost because wide contractual variations exist among institutions.

[3]Wellbutrin XL is a once-daily form of bupropion. Bupropion is still available as immediate release, and, if used, no single dose should exceed 150 mg.

[4]200 mg twice daily.

SSRIs, serotonin selective reuptake inhibitors.

Table 149. Etiology of delirium and other cognitive disorders.

Disorder	Possible Causes
Intoxication	Alcohol, sedatives, bromides, analgesics (eg, pentazocine), psychedelic drugs, stimulants, and household solvents.
Drug withdrawal	Withdrawal from alcohol, sedative-hypnotics, corticosteroids.
Long-term effects of alcohol	Wernicke-Korsakoff syndrome.
Infections	Septicemia; meningitis and encephalitis due to bacterial, viral, fungal, parasitic, or tuberculous organisms or to central nervous system syphilis; acute and chronic infections due to the entire range of microbiologic pathogens.
Endocrine disorders	Thyrotoxicosis, hypothyroidism, adrenocortical dysfunction (including Addison disease and Cushing syndrome), pheochromocytoma, insulinoma, hypoglycemia, hyperparathyroidism, hypoparathyroidism, panhypopituitarism, diabetic ketoacidosis.
Respiratory disorders	Hypoxia, hypercapnia.
Metabolic disturbances	Fluid and electrolyte disturbances (especially hyponatremia, hypomagnesemia, and hypercalcemia), acid-base disorders, hepatic disease (hepatic encephalopathy), renal failure, porphyria.
Nutritional deficiencies	Deficiency of vitamin B_1 (beriberi), vitamin B_{12} (pernicious anemia), folic acid, nicotinic acid (pellagra); protein-calorie malnutrition.
Trauma	Subdural hematoma, subarachnoid hemorrhage, intracerebral bleeding, concussion syndrome.
Cardiovascular disorders	Myocardial infarctions, cardiac arrhythmias, cerebrovascular spasms, hypertensive encephalopathy, hemorrhages, embolisms, and occlusions indirectly cause decreased cognitive function.
Neoplasms	Primary or metastatic lesions of the central nervous system, cancer-induced hypercalcemia.
Seizure disorders	Ictal, interictal, and postictal dysfunction.
Collagen-vascular and immunologic disorders	Autoimmune disorders, including systemic lupus erythematosus, Sjögren syndrome, and AIDS.
Degenerative diseases	Alzheimer disease, Pick disease, multiple sclerosis, parkinsonism, Huntington chorea, normal pressure hydrocephalus.
Medications	Anticholinergic drugs, antidepressants, H_2-blocking agents, digoxin, salicylates (long-term use), and a wide variety of other over-the-counter and prescribed drugs.

Table 150. Useful topical dermatologic therapeutic agents.

Agent	Formulations, Strengths, and Prices[1]	Apply	Potency Class	Common Indications	Comments
Corticosteroids					
Hydrocortisone acetate	Cream 1%: $3.00/30 g Ointment 1%: $3.00/30 g Lotion 1%: $6.29/120 mL	Twice daily	Low	Seborrheic dermatitis Pruritus ani Intertrigo	Not the same as hydrocortisone butyrate or valerate! Not for poison oak! OTC lotion (Aquinil HC) OTC solution (Scalpicin, T Scalp)
	Cream 2.5%: $8.95/30 g	Twice daily	Low	As for 1% hydrocortisone	Perhaps better for pruritus ani Not clearly better than 1% More expensive Not OTC
Alclometasone dipropionate (Aclovate)	Cream 0.05%: $28.31/15 g Ointment 0.05%: $59.06/45 g	Twice daily	Low	As for hydrocortisone	More efficacious than hydrocortisone Perhaps causes less atrophy
Clocortolone (Cloderm)	Cream 0.1%: $75.00/30 g	Three times daily	Medium	Contact dermatitis Atopic dermatitis	Does not cross react with other corticosteroids chemically and can be used in patients allergic to other corticosteroids
Desonide	Cream 0.05%: $15.47/15 g Ointment 0.05%: $39.88/60 g Lotion 0.05%: $32.83/60 mL	Twice daily	Low	As for hydrocortisone For lesions on face or body folds resistant to hydrocortisone	More efficacious than hydrocortisone Can cause rosacea or atrophy Not fluorinated
Prednicarbate (Dermatop)	Emollient cream 0.1%: $26.38/15 g Ointment 0.1%: $25.13/15 g	Twice daily	Medium	As for triamcinolone	May cause less atrophy No generic formulations Preservative-free
Triamcinolone acetonide	Cream 0.1%: $3.60/15 g Ointment 0.1%: $3.60/15 g Lotion 0.1%: $42.44/60 mL	Twice daily	Medium	Eczema on extensor areas Used for psoriasis with tar Seborrheic dermatitis and psoriasis on scalp	Caution in body folds, face Economical in 0.5-lb and 1-lb sizes for treatment of large body surfaces Economical as solution for scalp
	Cream 0.025%: $3.00/15 g Ointment 0.025%: $5.25/80 g	Twice daily	Medium	As for 0.1% strength	Possibly less efficacy and few advantages over 0.1% formulation
Fluocinolone acetonide	Cream 0.025%: $3.05/15 g Ointment 0.025%: $4.20/15 g	Twice daily	Medium	As for triamcinolone	
	Solution 0.01%: $11.00/60 mL	Twice daily	Medium	As for triamcinolone solution	
Mometasone furoate (Elocon)	Cream 0.1%: $27.00/15 g Ointment 0.1%: $24.00/15 g Lotion 0.1%: $55.71/60 mL	Once daily	Medium	As for triamcinolone	Often used inappropriately on the face or in children Not fluorinated
Diflorasone diacetate	Cream 0.05%: $36.78/15 g Ointment 0.05%: $51.86/30 g	Twice daily	High	Nummular dermatitis Allergic contact dermatitis Lichen simplex chronicus	
Amcinonide (Cyclocort)	Cream 0.1%: $18.42/15 g Ointment 0.1%: $27.46/30 g	Twice daily	High	As for betamethasone	
Fluocinonide (Lidex)	Cream 0.05%: $9.00/15 g Gel 0.05%: $21.01/15 g Ointment 0.05%: $21.25/15 g Solution 0.05%: $27.27/60 mL	Twice daily	High	As for betamethasone Gel useful for poison oak	Economical generics Lidex cream can cause stinging on eczema Lidex emollient cream preferred
Betamethasone dipropionate (Diprolene)	Cream 0.05%: $7.80/15 g Ointment 0.05%: $9.40/15 g Lotion 0.05%: $30.49/60 mL	Twice daily	Ultra-high	For lesions resistant to high-potency corticosteroids Lichen planus Insect bites	Economical generics available
Clobetasol propionate (Temovate)	Cream 0.05%: $24.71/15 g Ointment 0.05%: $24.71/15 g Lotion 0.05%: $51.26/50 mL	Twice daily	Ultra-high	As for betamethasone dipropionate	Somewhat more potent than diflorasone Limited to 2 continuous weeks of use Limited to 50 g or less per week Cream may cause stinging; use "emollient cream" formulation Generic available

(continued)

Table 150. Useful topical dermatologic therapeutic agents. (continued)

Agent	Formulations, Strengths, and Prices[1]	Apply	Potency Class	Common Indications	Comments
Halobetasol propionate (Ultravate)	Cream 0.05%: $31.49/15 g Ointment 0.05%: $31.49/15 g	Twice daily	Ultra-high	As for clobetasol	Same restrictions as clobetasol Cream does not cause stinging Compatible with calcipotriene (Dovonex)
Flurandrenolide (Cordran)	Tape: $68.17/80" × 3" roll Lotion 0.05%: $117.60/60 mL	q12h	Ultra-high	Lichen simplex chronicus	Protects the skin and prevents scratching
Nonsteroidal anti-inflammatory agents					
Tacrolimus[2] (Protopic)	Ointment 0.1%: $94.68/30 g Ointment 0.03%: $94.68/30 g	Twice daily	N/A	Atopic dermatitis	Steroid substitute not causing atrophy or striae Burns in ≥ 40% of patients with eczema
Pimecrolimus[2] (Elidel)	Cream 1%: $74.08/30 g	Twice daily	N/A	Atopic dermatitis	Steroid substitute not causing atrophy or striae
Antibiotics (for acne)					
Clindamycin phosphate	Solution 1%: $12.09/30 mL Gel 1%: $38.13/30 mL Lotion 1%: $53.06/60 mL Pledget 1%: $46.40/60	Twice daily	N/A	Mild papular acne	Lotion is less drying for patients with sensitive skin
Erythromycin	Solution 2%: $7.53/60 mL Gel 2%: $25.19/30 g Pledget 2%: $44.34/60	Twice daily	N/A	As for clindamycin	Many different manufacturers Economical
Erythromycin/ Benzoyl peroxide (Benzamycin)	Gel: $30.57/23.3 g Gel: $161.18/46.6 g	Twice daily	N/A	As for clindamycin Can help treat comedonal acne	No generics More expensive More effective than other topical antibiotic Main jar requires refrigeration
Clindamycin/ Benzoyl peroxide (BenzaClin)	Gel: $86.60/25 g Gel: $147.84/50 g	Twice daily	N/A	As for benzamycin	No generic More effective than either agent alone
Antibiotics (for impetigo)					
Mupirocin (Bactroban)	Ointment 2%: $44.65/22 g Cream 2%: $44.84/15 g	Three times daily	N/A	Impetigo, folliculitis	Because of cost, use limited to tiny areas of impetigo Used in the nose twice daily for 5 days to reduce staphylococcal carriage
Antifungals: *Imidazoles*					
Clotrimazole	Cream 1%: $4.25/15 g OTC Solution 1%: $7.40/10 mL	Twice daily	N/A	Dermatophyte and *Candida* infections	Available OTC Inexpensive generic cream available
Econazole (Spectazole)	Cream 1%: $17.60/15 g	Once daily	N/A	As for clotrimazole	No generic Somewhat more effective than clotrimazole and miconazole
Ketoconazole	Cream 2%: $16.46/15 g	Once daily	N/A	As for clotrimazole	No generic Somewhat more effective than clotrimazole and miconazole
Miconazole	Cream 2%: $3.20/30 g OTC	Twice daily	N/A	As for clotrimazole	As for clotrimazole
Oxiconazole (Oxistat)	Cream 1%: $34.77/15 g Lotion 1%: $64.25/30 mL	Twice daily	N/A		
Sertaconazole (Ertaczo)	Cream 2%: $61.68/30 g	Twice daily	N/A	Refractory tinea pedis	By prescription More expensive
Sulconazole (Exelderm)	Cream 1%: $13.92/15 g Solution 1%: $29.95/30 mL	Twice daily	N/A	As for clotrimazole	No generic Somewhat more effective than clotrimazole and miconazole
Other antifungals					
Butenafine (Mentax)	Cream 1%: $45.03/15 g	Once daily	N/A	Dermatophytes	Fast response; high cure rate; expensive Available OTC
Ciclopirox (Loprox) (Penlac)	Cream 0.77%: $51.10/30 g Lotion 0.77%: $96.15/60 mL Solution 8%: $181.81/6.6 mL	Twice daily	N/A	As for clotrimazole	No generic Somewhat more effective than clotrimazole and miconazole

(continued)

Table 150. Useful topical dermatologic therapeutic agents. (continued)

Agent	Formulations, Strengths, and Prices[1]	Apply	Potency Class	Common Indications	Comments
Naftifine (Naftin)	Cream 1%: $52.07/30 g Gel 1%: $91.68/60 mL	Once daily	N/A	Dermatophytes	No generic Somewhat more effective than clotrimazole and miconazole
Terbinafine (Lamisil)	Cream 1%: $8.15/12 g OTC	Once daily	N/A	Dermatophytes	Fast clinical response OTC
Antipruritics					
Camphor/ menthol	Compounded lotion (0.5% of each)	Two to three times daily	N/A	Mild eczema, xerosis, mild contact dermatitis	
Pramoxine hydrochloride (Prax)	Lotion 1%: $14.78/120 mL OTC	Four times daily	N/A	Dry skin, varicella, mild eczema, pruritus ani	OTC formulations (Prax, Aveeno Anti-Itch Cream or Lotion; Itch-X Gel) By prescription mixed with 1% or 2% hydrocortisone
Doxepin (Zonalon)	Cream 5%: $91.70/30 g	Four times daily	N/A	Topical antipruritic, best used in combination with appropriate topical corticosteroid to enhance efficacy	Can cause sedation
Emollients					
Aveeno	Cream, lotion, others	Once to three times daily	N/A	Xerosis, eczema	Choice is most often based on personal preference by patient
Aqua glycolic	Cream, lotion, shampoo, others	Once to three times daily	N/A	Xerosis, ichthyosis, keratosis pilaris Mild facial wrinkles Mild acne or seborrheic dermatitis	Contains 8% glycolic acid Available from other makers, eg, Alpha Hydrox, or generic 8% glycolic acid lotion May cause stinging on eczematous skin
Aquaphor	Ointment: $7.50/50 g	Once to three times daily	N/A	Xerosis, eczema For protection of area in pruritus ani	Not as greasy as petrolatum
Carmol	Lotion 10%: $11.03/180 mL Cream 20%: $11.08/90 g	Twice daily	N/A	Xerosis	Contains urea as humectant Nongreasy hydrating agent (10%); debrides keratin (20%)
Complex 15	Lotion: $6.48/240 mL Cream: $4.82/75 g	Once to three times daily	N/A	Xerosis Lotion or cream recommended for split or dry nails	Active ingredient is a phospholipid
DML	Cream, lotion, facial moisturizer: $5.32/240 mL	Once to three times daily	N/A	As for Complex 15	Face cream has sunscreen
Eucerin	Cream: $5.10/120 g Lotion: $5.10/240 mL	Once to three times daily	N/A	Xerosis, eczema	Many formulations made Eucerin Plus contains alphahydroxy acid and may cause stinging on eczematous skin Facial moisturizer has SPF 25 sunscreen
Lac-Hydrin-Five	Lotion: $10.12/240 mL OTC	Twice daily	N/A	Xerosis, ichthyosis, keratosis pilaris	Rx product is 12%
Lubriderm	Lotion: $5.03/300 mL	Once to three times daily	N/A	Xerosis, eczema	Unscented usually preferred
Neutrogena	Cream, lotion, facial moisturizer: $7.39/240 mL	Once to three times daily	N/A	Xerosis, eczema	Face cream has titanium-based sunscreen
Ceratopic Cream	Cream: $39.50/4 oz	Twice daily	N/A	Xerosis, eczema	Contains ceramide; anti-inflammatory and non-greasy moisturizer
U-Lactin	Lotion: $7.13/240 mL OTC	Once daily	N/A	Hyperkeratotic heels	Moisturizes and removes keratin

[1]Average wholesale price (AWP, for AB-rated generic when available) for quantity listed. AWP may not accurately represent the actual pharmacy cost because wide contractual variations exist among institutions. Source: *Red Book Update*, Vol. 27, No. 2, February 2008.
[2]Topical tacrolimus and pimecrolimus should only be used when other topical treatments are ineffective. Treatment should be limited to an area and duration to be as brief as possible. Treatment with these agents should be avoided in persons with known immunosuppression, HIV infection, bone marrow and organ transplantation, lymphoma, at high risk for lymphoma, and those with a prior history of lymphoma.
OTC, over-the-counter; N/A, not applicable.

Table 151. Staging system for classifying pressure ulcers.

Grade	Description
1	Intact skin. Fixed erythema (pink, red, or mottled) after pressure is relieved.
2	Loss of epidermis or dermis. Resembles blister, abrasion, or shallow crater. Necrotic tissue may overlie ulcer.
3	Ulceration through the epidermis and dermis with damage to the underlying subcutaneous fat. Ulcer may extend to the fascia.
4	Full thickness skin loss with extension of the ulcer to bone, muscle, tendon, or joint.
5	Closed cavity communicating through a small sinus.

Table 152. Skin reactions due to systemic drugs.

Reaction	Appearance	Distribution and Comments	Common Offenders
Toxic erythema	Morbilliform, maculopapular, exanthematous reactions.	The most common skin reaction to drugs. Often more pronounced on the trunk than on the extremities. In previously exposed patients, the rash may start in 2–3 days. In the first course of treatment, the eruption often appears about the seventh to ninth days. Fever may be present.	Antibiotics (especially ampicillin and trimethoprim-sulfamethoxazole), sulfonamides and related compounds (including thiazide diuretics, furosemide, and sulfonylurea hypoglycemic agents), and barbiturates.
Erythema multiforme major	Target-like lesions. Bullae may occur. Mucosal involvement.	Usually trunk and proximal extremities.	Sulfonamides, anticonvulsants, and NSAIDs.
Erythema nodosum	Inflammatory cutaneous nodules.	Usually limited to the extensor aspects of the legs. May be accompanied by fever, arthralgias, and pain.	Oral contraceptives.
Allergic vasculitis	Inflammatory changes may present as urticaria that lasts over 24 hours, hemorrhagic papules ("palpable purpura"), vesicles, bullae, or necrotic ulcers.	Most severe on the legs.	Sulfonamides, phenytoin, propylthiouracil.
Exfoliative dermatitis and erythroderma	Red and scaly.	Entire skin surface.	Allopurinol, sulfonamides, isoniazid, anticonvulsants, gold, or carbamazepine.
Photosensitivity: increased sensitivity to light, often of ultraviolet A wavelengths, but may be due to UVB or visible light as well	Sunburn, vesicles, papules in photodistributed pattern.	Exposed skin of the face, the neck, and the backs of the hands and, in women, the lower legs. Exaggerated response to ultraviolet light.	Sulfonamides and sulfonamide-related compounds (thiazide diuretics, furosemide, sulfonylureas), tetracyclines, phenothiazines, sulindac, amiodarone, voriconazole, and NSAIDs.
Drug-related lupus erythematosus	May present with a photosensitive rash, annular lesions or psoriasis on upper trunk.	Less severe than systemic lupus erythematosus, sparing the kidneys and central nervous system. Recovery often follows drug withdrawal.	Diltiazem, etanercept, hydrochlorothiazide, infliximab, lisinopril.
Lichenoid and lichen planus-like eruptions	Pruritic, erythematous to violaceous polygonal papules that coalesce or expand to form plaques.	May be in photo- or nonphotodistributed pattern.	Carbamazepine, furosemide, gold salts, hydroxychloroquine, methyldopa, phenothiazines, propranolol, quinidine, quinine, sulfonylureas, tetracyclines, thiazides, and triprolidine.
Fixed drug eruptions	Single or multiple demarcated, round, erythematous plaques that often become hyperpigmented.	Recur at the same site when the drug is repeated. Hyperpigmentation, if present, remains after healing.	Numerous drugs, including antimicrobials, analgesics, barbiturates, cardiovascular drugs, heavy metals, antiparasitic agents, antihistamines, phenolphthalein, ibuprofen, and naproxen.
Toxic epidermal necrolysis	Large sheets of erythema, followed by separation, which looks like scalded skin.	Rare.	In adults, the eruption has occurred after administration of many classes of drugs, particularly anticonvulsants (lamotrigine and others), antibiotics, sulfonamides, and NSAIDs.

(continued)

701

Table 152. Skin reactions due to systemic drugs. (continued)

Reaction	Appearance	Distribution and Comments	Common Offenders
Urticaria	Red, itchy wheals that vary in size from < 1 cm to many centimeters. May be accompanied by angioedema.	Chronic urticaria is rarely caused by drugs.	Acute urticaria: penicillins, NSAIDs, sulfonamides, opiates, and salicylates. Angioedema is common in patients receiving ACE inhibitors.
Pigmentary changes	Flat hyperpigmented areas.	Forehead and cheeks (chloasma, melasma). The most common pigmentary disorder associated with drug ingestion. Improvement is slow despite stopping the drug.	Oral contraceptives are the usual cause.
	Blue-gray discoloration.	Light-exposed areas.	Chlorpromazine and related phenothiazines.
	Brown or blue-gray pigmentation.	Generalized.	Heavy metals (silver, gold, bismuth, and arsenic). Arsenic, silver, and bismuth are not used therapeutically, but patients who receive gold for rheumatoid arthritis may show this reaction.
	Yellow color.	Generalized.	Usually quinacrine.
	Blue-black patches on the shins.		Minocycline, chloroquine.
	Blue-black pigmentation of the nails and palate and depigmentation of the hair.		Chloroquine.
	Slate-gray color.	Primarily in photoexposed areas.	Amiodarone.
	Brown discoloration of the nails.	Especially in more darkly pigmented patients.	Zidovudine (azidothymidine; AZT), hydroxyurea.
Psoriasiform eruptions	Scaly red plaques.	May be located on trunk and extremities. Palms and soles may be hyperkeratotic. May cause psoriasiform eruption or worsen psoriasis.	Chloroquine, lithium, β-blockers, tumor necrosis factor (TNF)-inhibitors, and quinacrine.
Pityriasis rosea–like eruptions	Oval, red, slightly raised patches with central scale.	Mainly on the trunk.	Barbiturates, bismuth, captopril, clonidine, gold salts, methopromazine, metoprolol, metronidazole, and tripelennamine.

NSAIDs, nonsteroidal anti-inflammatory drugs; ACE, angiotensin-converting enzyme.

Table 153. American Urological Association symptom index for benign prostatic hyperplasia.[1]

Questions to Be Answered	Not at All	Less Than One Time in Five	Less Than Half the Time	About Half the Time	More Than Half the Time	Almost Always
1. Over the past month, how often have you had a sensation of not emptying your bladder completely after you finish urinating?	0	1	2	3	4	5
2. Over the past month, how often have you had to urinate again less than 2 hours after you finished urinating?	0	1	2	3	4	5
3. Over the past month, how often have you found you stopped and started again several times when you urinated?	0	1	2	3	4	5
4. Over the past month, how often have you found it difficult to postpone urination?	0	1	2	3	4	5
5. Over the past month, how often have you had a weak urinary stream?	0	1	2	3	4	5
6. Over the past month, how often have you had to push or strain to begin urination?	0	1	2	3	4	5
7. Over the past month, how many times did you most typically get up to urinate from the time you went to bed at night until the time you got up in the morning?	0	1	2	3	4	5

[1]Sum of seven circled numbers equals the symptom score. See text for explanation.
Reproduced, with permission, from Barry MJ et al. The American Urological Association symptom index for benign prostatic hyperplasia. J Urol. 1992 Nov;148(5):1549–57.

Orientation *(Score 1 for each correct; max = 10)*

Where are you? Name this place (building or hospital)
What floor are you on now?
What state are you in?
What country are you in?
(If not in a country, score correct if city is correct.)
What city are you in (or near) now?

What is the date today? What year is it?
What season is it?
What month is it?
What is the day of the week?
What is the date today?

Registration *(Score 1 for each object correctly repeated; max = 3)*

Name three objects (ball, flag, and tree) and have the patient repeat them.
(Say objects at about 1 word per second. If patient misses object, ask patient to repeat them after you until he/she learns them. Stop at 6 repeats.)

Attention and calculation *(Score 1 for each correct to 65; max = 5)*

Subtract 7s from 100 in a serial fashion to 65
(Alternatively, subtract serial 3s from 20 or spell WORLD backwards.)

Recall *(Score 1 for each object recalled; max = 3)*

Do you recall the names of the three objects?

Language *(max = 8)*

Ask the patient to provide names of a watch and pen as you show them to him/her
(Score 1 for each object correct; max = 2)
Repeat "No ifs, ands, or buts."
(Only one trial. Score 1 if correct; max = 1)
Give the patient a piece of plain blank paper and say, "Take the paper in your right hand (1), fold it in half (2), and put it on the floor (3)."
(Score 1 for each part done correctly; max = 3)
Ask the patient to read and perform the following task written on paper: Close your eyes.
(Score 1 if patient closes eyes; max = 1)
Ask the patient to write a sentence on a piece of paper.
(Score total of 1 if sentence has a subject, object and verb; max = 1)

Construction

Ask patient to copy the two interlocking pentagons.
(Score total of 1, if all 10 angles are present and the two angles intersect. Ignore tremor and rotation; max = 1)

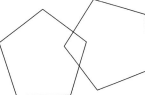

Total Score *(Maximum = 30, likely organic < 27)*

▲ **Figure 1.** Mini-mental State Exam. (Adapted from Folstein MF et al: Mini-mental state: a practical method for grading the cognitive state of patients for the clinician. J Psychiatr Res 1975;12:189.)

Standard algorithm

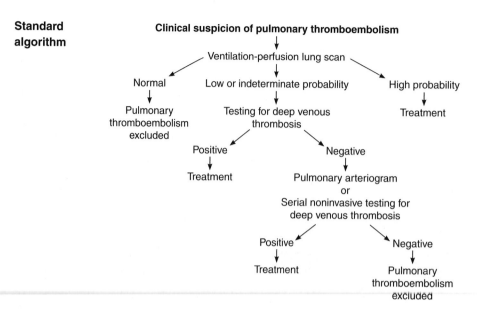

Clinical suspicion of pulmonary thromboembolism

↓

Ventilation-perfusion lung scan

- Normal → Pulmonary thromboembolism excluded
- Low or indeterminate probability → Testing for deep venous thrombosis
  - Positive → Treatment
  - Negative → Pulmonary arteriogram or Serial noninvasive testing for deep venous thrombosis
    - Positive → Treatment
    - Negative → Pulmonary thromboembolism excluded
- High probability → Treatment

Emerging practice algorithm

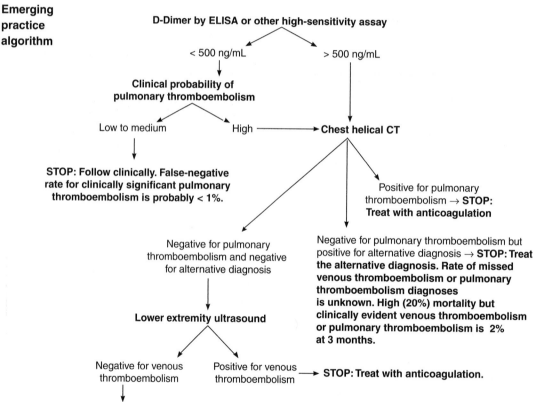

D-Dimer by ELISA or other high-sensitivity assay

- < 500 ng/mL → Clinical probability of pulmonary thromboembolism
  - Low to medium → STOP: Follow clinically. False-negative rate for clinically significant pulmonary thromboembolism is probably < 1%.
  - High → Chest helical CT
- > 500 ng/mL → Chest helical CT

Chest helical CT:
- Positive for pulmonary thromboembolism → STOP: Treat with anticoagulation
- Negative for pulmonary thromboembolism but positive for alternative diagnosis → STOP: Treat the alternative diagnosis. Rate of missed venous thromboembolism or pulmonary thromboembolism diagnoses is unknown. High (20%) mortality but clinically evident venous thromboembolism or pulmonary thromboembolism is 2% at 3 months.
- Negative for pulmonary thromboembolism and negative for alternative diagnosis → Lower extremity ultrasound
  - Negative for venous thromboembolism
  - Positive for venous thromboembolism → STOP: Treat with anticoagulation.

STOP: Follow clinically. Overall mortality rate is approximately 4% at 12 weeks, but risk of death for undiagnosed pulmonary thromboembolism appears to be very low. If the prior probability of pulmonary thromboembolism is high, if there is no alternative diagnosis, or if there is a high risk of morbid event from undiagnosed pulmonary thromboembolism, then repeat lower extremity ultrasound on day 4. In rare circumstances, with high-risk patients, consider pulmonary arteriogram.

▲ **Figure 2.** Two simple algorithms to guide evaluation of suspected venous thromboembolism. The standard algorithm is based on the results of ventilation-perfusion lung scanning using PIOPED data. Management of patients with ventilation-perfusion lung scans of low and indeterminate probability must always be guided by clinical judgment based upon cumulative clinical information and the degree of suspicion of pulmonary thromboembolism. The second algorithm uses D-dimer, helical CT, and venous ultrasonography to describe an evidence-based, efficient evaluation that reflects emerging practice. This second algorithm is not based on the experience of the standard ventilation-perfusion approach but anticipates a shift toward use of helical CT as the primary diagnostic test in pulmonary thromboembolism.

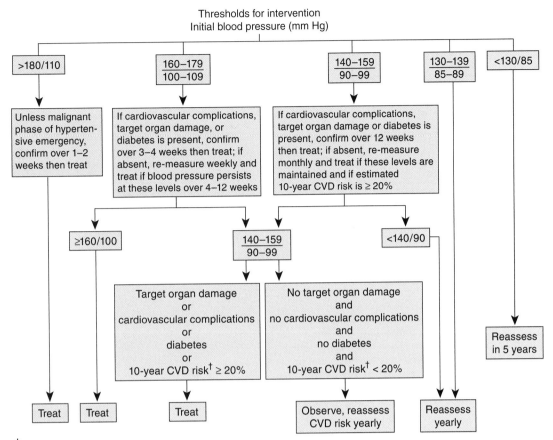

Thresholds for intervention
Initial blood pressure (mm Hg)

> 180/110

160–179
100–109

140–159
90–99

130–139
85–89

< 130/85

Unless malignant phase of hypertensive emergency, confirm over 1–2 weeks then treat

If cardiovascular complications, target organ damage, or diabetes is present, confirm over 3–4 weeks then treat; if absent, re-measure weekly and treat if blood pressure persists at these levels over 4–12 weeks

If cardiovascular complications, target organ damage or diabetes is present, confirm over 12 weeks then treat; if absent, re-measure monthly and treat if these levels are maintained and if estimated 10-year CVD risk is ≥ 20%

≥ 160/100

140–159
90–99

< 140/90

Target organ damage
or
cardiovascular complications
or
diabetes
or
10-year CVD risk[†] ≥ 20%

No target organ damage
and
no cardiovascular complications
and
no diabetes
and
10-year CVD risk[†] < 20%

Reassess in 5 years

Treat   Treat   Treat

Observe, reassess CVD risk yearly

Reassess yearly

[†]Assessed with CVD risk chart

▲ **Figure 3.** British Hypertension Society algorithm for diagnosis and treatment of hypertension, incorporating total cardiovascular risk in deciding which "pre-hypertensive" patients to treat. CVD = cardiovascular disease. (Reproduced with permission from: Guidelines for management of hypertension: report of the fourth working party of the the British Hypertension Society, 2004-BHS IV. J Hum Hypertens 2004 Mar;18(3):139–85. [PMID: 14973512]. Reprinted by permission from Macmillan Publishers, Ltd.)

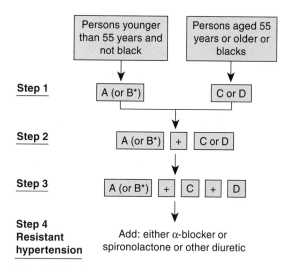

Step 1

Step 2

Step 3

Step 4
Resistant
hypertension

Persons younger than 55 years and not black

Persons aged 55 years or older or blacks

A (or B*)

C or D

A (or B*) + C or D

A (or B*) + C + D

Add: either α-blocker or spironolactone or other diuretic

*Combination therapy involving B and D may induce more new-onset diabetes compared with other combination therapies.

▲ **Figure 4.** The British Hypertension Society's recommendations for combining blood pressure lowering drugs. The "ABCD" rule. A = Angiotensin-converting enzyme inhibitor or angiotensin receptor blocker; B = β-blocker (the parentheses indicate that β-blockers should no longer be considered ideal first-line agents); C = calcium channel blockers; D = diuretic (thiazide). (J Human Hypertens 2004;18:139–185. Reprinted by permission from Macmillan Publishers, Ltd.)

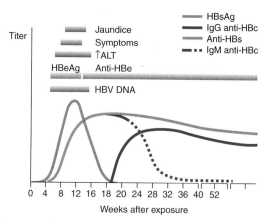

▲ **Figure 6.** The typical course of acute type B hepatitis. HBsAg = hepatitis B surface antigen; anti-HBs = antibody to HBsAg; HBeAg = hepatitis Be antigen; anti-HBe = antibody to HBeAg; anti-HBc = antibody to hepatitis B core antigen; ALT = alanine aminotransferase. (Reprinted from Koff RS: Acute viral hepatitis. In: *Handbook of Liver Disease.* Friedman LS, Keeffe EB [editors], 2nd ed. © 2004, with permission from Elsevier.)

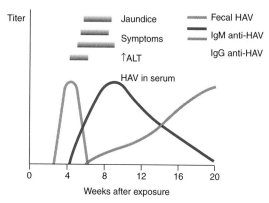

▲ **Figure 5.** The typical course of acute type A hepatitis. HAV = hepatitis A virus; anti-HAV = antibody to hepatitis A virus; ALT = alanine aminotransferase. (Reprinted from Koff RS: Acute viral hepatitis. In: *Handbook of Liver Disease.* Friedman LS, Keeffe EB [editors], 2nd ed. © 2004, with permission from Elsevier.)

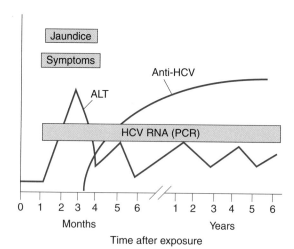

▲ **Figure 7.** The typical course of acute and chronic hepatitis C. ALT = alanine aminotransferase; Anti-HCV = antibody to hepatitis C virus by enzyme immunoassay; HCV RNA [PCR] = hepatitis C viral RNA by polymerase chain reaction.

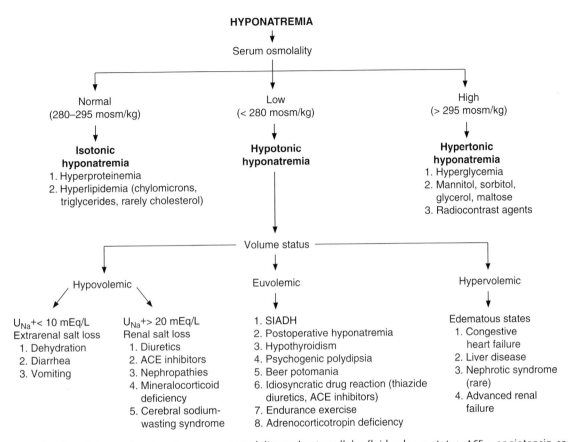

HYPONATREMIA

Serum osmolality

| Normal
(280–295 mosm/kg) | Low
(< 280 mosm/kg) | High
(> 295 mosm/kg) |

Isotonic hyponatremia
1. Hyperproteinemia
2. Hyperlipidemia (chylomicrons, triglycerides, rarely cholesterol)

Hypotonic hyponatremia

Hypertonic hyponatremia
1. Hyperglycemia
2. Mannitol, sorbitol, glycerol, maltose
3. Radiocontrast agents

Volume status

Hypovolemic

$U_{Na}+< 10$ mEq/L
Extrarenal salt loss
1. Dehydration
2. Diarrhea
3. Vomiting

$U_{Na}+> 20$ mEq/L
Renal salt loss
1. Diuretics
2. ACE inhibitors
3. Nephropathies
4. Mineralocorticoid deficiency
5. Cerebral sodium-wasting syndrome

Euvolemic
1. SIADH
2. Postoperative hyponatremia
3. Hypothyroidism
4. Psychogenic polydipsia
5. Beer potomania
6. Idiosyncratic drug reaction (thiazide diuretics, ACE inhibitors)
7. Endurance exercise
8. Adrenocorticotropin deficiency

Hypervolemic
Edematous states
1. Congestive heart failure
2. Liver disease
3. Nephrotic syndrome (rare)
4. Advanced renal failure

▲ **Figure 8.** Evaluation of hyponatremia using serum osmolality and extracellular fluid volume status. ACE = angiotensin-converting enzyme; SIADH = syndrome of inappropriate antidiuretic hormone. (Adapted, with permission, from Narins RG et al: Diagnostic strategies in disorders of fluid, electrolyte and acid-base homeostasis. Am J Med 1982;72:496.)

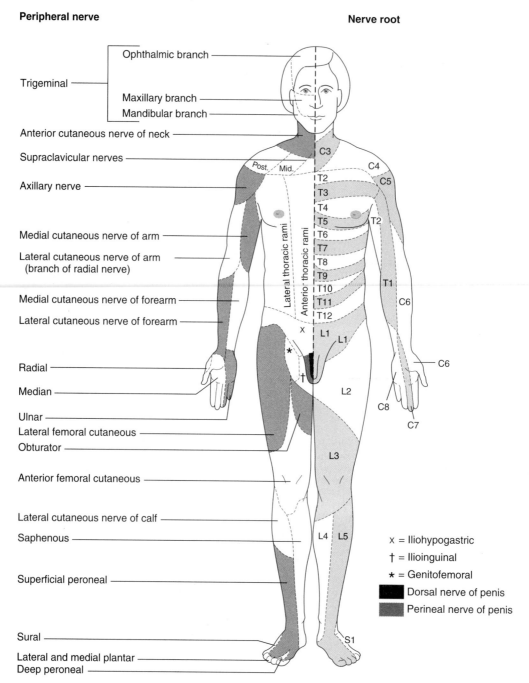

Peripheral nerve

- Trigeminal
  - Ophthalmic branch
  - Maxillary branch
  - Mandibular branch
- Anterior cutaneous nerve of neck
- Supraclavicular nerves
- Axillary nerve
- Medial cutaneous nerve of arm
- Lateral cutaneous nerve of arm (branch of radial nerve)
- Medial cutaneous nerve of forearm
- Lateral cutaneous nerve of forearm
- Radial
- Median
- Ulnar
- Lateral femoral cutaneous
- Obturator
- Anterior femoral cutaneous
- Lateral cutaneous nerve of calf
- Saphenous
- Superficial peroneal
- Sural
- Lateral and medial plantar
- Deep peroneal

Nerve root

C3 C4 C5 T2 T3 T4 T5 T6 T7 T8 T9 T10 T11 T12 L1 L2 L3 L4 L5 S1
T1 T2 C6 C7 C8

Post. Mid.
Lateral thoracic rami
Anterior thoracic rami

x = Iliohypogastric
† = Ilioinguinal
★ = Genitofemoral
Dorsal nerve of penis
Perineal nerve of penis

▲ **Figure 9.** Cutaneous innervation. The segmental or radicular (root) distribution is shown on the left side of the body and the peripheral nerve distribution on the right side. **Above:** anterior view; **facing page:** posterior view. (Reproduced, with permission, from Simon RP, Aminoff MJ, Greenberg DA: Clinical Neurology, 4th ed. McGraw-Hill, 1999.)

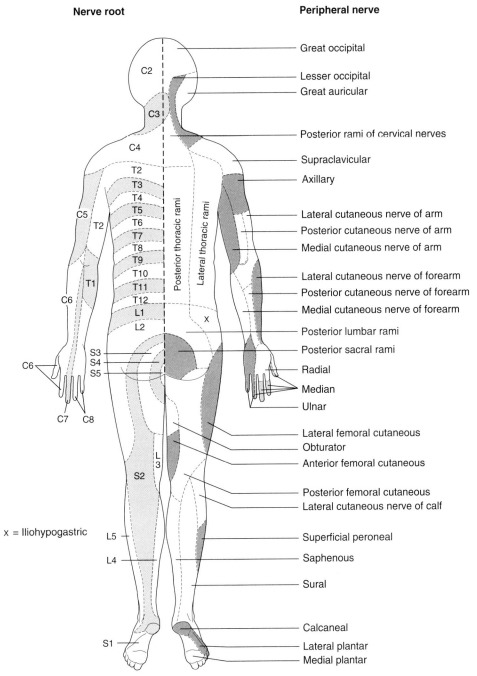

Nerve root

Peripheral nerve

- Great occipital
- Lesser occipital
- Great auricular
- Posterior rami of cervical nerves
- Supraclavicular
- Axillary
- Lateral cutaneous nerve of arm
- Posterior cutaneous nerve of arm
- Medial cutaneous nerve of arm
- Lateral cutaneous nerve of forearm
- Posterior cutaneous nerve of forearm
- Medial cutaneous nerve of forearm
- Posterior lumbar rami
- Posterior sacral rami
- Radial
- Median
- Ulnar
- Lateral femoral cutaneous
- Obturator
- Anterior femoral cutaneous
- Posterior femoral cutaneous
- Lateral cutaneous nerve of calf
- Superficial peroneal
- Saphenous
- Sural
- Calcaneal
- Lateral plantar
- Medial plantar

C2, C3, C4, T2, T3, T4, T5, T6, T7, T8, T9, T10, T11, T12, L1, L2, C5, T2, C6, T1, S3, S4, S5, C6, C7, C8, S2, L3, L5, L4, S1

Posterior thoracic rami

Lateral thoracic rami

x = Iliohypogastric

▲ **Figure 9.** Continued.

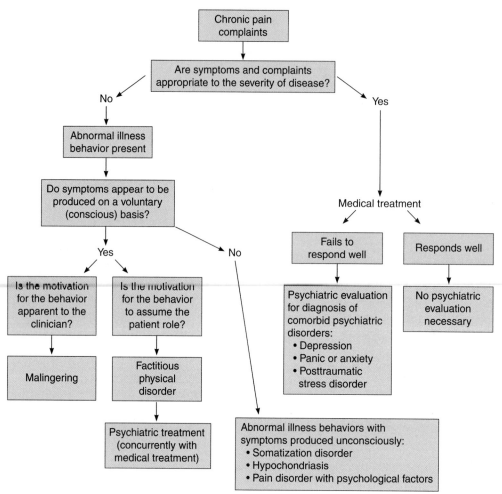

▲ **Figure 10.** Algorithm for assessing psychiatric component of chronic pain. (Modified and reproduced, with permission, from Eisendrath SJ: Psychiatric aspects of chronic pain. Neurology 1995;45[Suppl 9]:S26.)

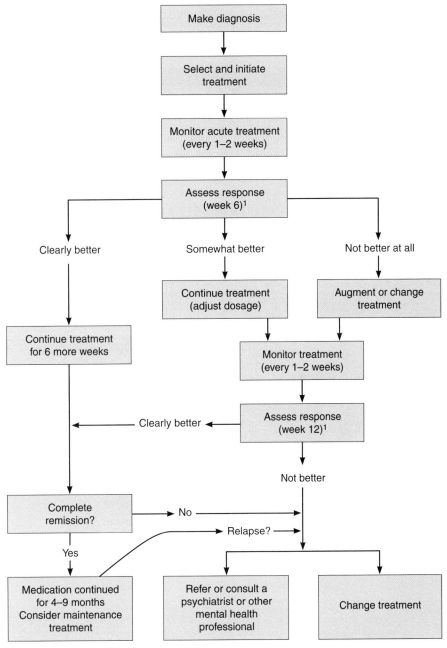

¹Times of assessment (weeks 6 and 12) rest on very modest data. It may be necessary to revise the treatment plan earlier for patients not responding at all.

▲ **Figure 11.** Overview of treatment for depression. (Reproduced, with permission, from Agency for Health Care Policy and Research: *Depression in Primary Care. Vol. 2: Treatment of Major Depression.* United States Department of Health and Human Services, 1993.)

APPENDIX OF ON-LINE RESOURCES

Government Centers

Agency for Healthcare Research and
Quality
http://www.ahrq.gov/

California Poison Control System
http://www.calpoison.org/

Centers for Disease Control and Prevention
http://www.cdc.gov/

MedlinePlus
http://medlineplus.gov/

National Cancer Institute
http://www.cancer.gov/

National Center for Biotechnology
Information
http://www.ncbi.nlm.nih.gov/

National Center for Infectious Diseases
http://www.cdc.gov/ncidod/

National Cholesterol Education Program
http://www.nhlbi.nih.gov/about/ncep/
index.htm

National Diabetes Information
Clearinghouse
http://diabetes.niddk.nih.gov/

National Digestive Diseases Clearinghouse
http://digestive.niddk.nih.gov/

National Heart Lung and Blood Institute
http://www.nhlbi.nih.gov/

National Institute for Occupational
Safety and Health
http://www.cdc.gov/NIOSH/

National Institute of Allergy and Infectious
Diseases
http://www3.niaid.nih.gov/

National Institute of Arthritis and
Musculoskeletal and Skin Diseases
http://www.niams.nih.gov/

National Institute of Child Health &
Human Development
http://www.nichd.nih.gov/

National Institute of Diabetes and
Digestive & Kidney Disease
http://www2.niddk.nih.gov/

National Institute of Environmental
Health Sciences
http://www.niehs.nih.gov/

National Institute of Mental Health
http://www.nimh.nih.gov/

National Institute of Neurological
Disorders and Stroke
http://www.ninds.nih.gov/

National Institute on Aging
http://www.nia.nih.gov/

National Institute on Alcohol Abuse and
Alcoholism
http://www.niaaa.nih.gov/

National Institute on Deafness and Other
Communication Disorders
http://www.nidcd.nih.gov/

National Kidney and Urologic Diseases
http://kidney.niddk.nih.gov/

National Library of Medicine
http://www.nlm.nih.gov/

National Women's Health Information
Center
http://www.4woman.gov/

NIH
http://www.nih.gov/

NIH AIDS Information
http://www.aidsinfo.nih.gov/

OSHA
http://www.osha.gov/

US Department of Health and Human
Services
http://www.hhs.gov/

US Food and Drug Administration
http://www.fda.gov/

World Federation of Hemophilia
http://www.wfh.org/index.asp?lang=EN

Worldwide Education and Awareness for
Movement Disorders
http://www.wemove.org/

Associations

AARP Guide to Internet Resources on
Aging
http://www.aarp.org/internetresources/

Acromegaly.org
http://www.acromegaly.org/

Alcoholics Anonymous
http://www.aa.org/?Media=PlayFlash

Alzheimer's Association
http://www.alz.org/index.asp

Alzheimer's Disease Education and
Referral Center
http://www.nia.nih.gov/Alzheimers/

Alzheimer's Family Relief Program
http://www.ahaf.org/AFRP_March31_
2007.html

American Association for Study of Liver
Diseases
http://www.aasld.org/Pages/Default.aspx

American Association of Clinical
Chemistry Lab Tests On Line
http://www.labtestsonline.org/

American Cancer Society
http://www.cancer.org/docroot/home/
index.asp

American Diabetes Association
http://www.diabetes.org/home.jsp

American Geriatrics Association
http://www.americangeriatrics.org/

American Liver Foundation
http://www.liverfoundation.org/

American Lung Association
http://www.lungusa.org/

American Lyme Disease Foundation
http://www.aldf.com/

American Obesity Association
http://www.obesity.org/

American Pancreatic Association
http://www.american-pancreatic-
association.org/

American Red Cross
http://www.redcross.org/

American Social Health Association
http://www.ashastd.org/

American Speech-Language-Hearing
Association
http://www.asha.org/default.htm

Amyloidosis Support Network
http://www.amyloidosis.org/

Ankylosing Spondylitis International
Federation
http://www.asif.rheumanet.org/

Aplastic Anemia & MDS International
Foundation
http://www.aamds.org/aplastic/

Arthritis Foundation
http://www.arthritis.org/

Cystic Fibrosis Foundation
http://www.cff.org/

Depression and Bipolar Support Alliance
http://www.dbsalliance.org/site/
PageServer?pagename=home

Diabetes Insipidus Foundation
http://www.diabetesinsipidus.org/

Divers Alert Network
http://www.diversalertnetwork.org/

Epilepsy Foundation
http://www.epilepsyfoundation.org/

Huntington's Disease Society of America
http://www.hdsa.org/

International Foundation for Functional
Gastrointestinal Disorders
http://www.iffgd.org/

International Myeloma Foundation
http://myeloma.org/

International Pemphigus Foundation
http://www.pemphigus.org/

Leukemia & Lymphoma Society
http://www.leukemia-lymphoma.org/
hm_lls

Lupus Foundation of America
http://www.lupus.org/newsite/index.html

March of Dimes
http://www.marchofdimes.com/

Myositis Association
http://www.myositis.org/template/index.
cfm

National Abortion Federation
http://www.prochoice.org/

National Adrenal Disease Foundation
http://www.nadf.us/

National Association of Anorexia Nervosa
& Associated Disorders
http://www.anad.org/

National Eating Disorders Association
http://www.nationaleatingdisorders.org/

National Eczema Association for Science
& Education
http://www.nationaleczema.org/home.
html

National Hemophilia Foundation
http://www.hemophilia.org/

National Infertility Association
http://www.resolve.org/site/PageServer

National Kidney Foundation
http://www.kidney.org/

National Lymphedema Network
http://www.lymphnet.org/

National Multiple Sclerosis Society
http://www.nationalmssociety.org/index.
aspx

National Organization of Rare Disorders
http://www.rarediseases.org/

National Osteoporosis Foundation
http://www.nof.org/

National Primary Immunodeficiency
Resource Center
http://www.jmfworld.com/

National Uterine Fibroids Foundation
http://www.nuff.org/

Nemours Foundation
http://www.nemours.org/index.html

North American Menopause Society
http://www.menopause.org/

Pituitary Foundation
http://www.pituitary.org.uk/

Pituitary Network Association
http://www.pituitary.org/

Platelet Disorder Support Association
http://www.pdsa.org/

Regional Cancer Center
http://www.trcc.org/

Skin Cancer Foundation
http://www.skincancer.org/

Vestibular Disorders Association
http://www.vestibular.org/

Medical Associations

American Academy of Allergy Asthma
and Immunology
http://www.aaaai.org/

American Academy of Dermatology
http://www.aad.org/

American Academy of Family Physicians
http://www.aafp.org/online/en/home.
html

American Academy of Neurology
http://www.aan.com/

American Academy of Ophthalmology
http://www.aao.org/

American Academy of Orthopaedic
Surgeons
http://www.aaos.org/

American Academy of Otolaryngology
http://www.entnet.org/

American Association of Clinical
Endocrinologists
http://www.aace.com/

American Association of Diabetes
Educators
http://www.diabeteseducator.org/

American College of Allergy, Asthma and
Immunology
http://www.acaai.org/

American College of Cardiology
http://www.acc.org/

American College of Chest Physicians
http://www.chestnet.org/

American College of Emergency
Physicians
http://www.acep.org/

American College of Gastroenterology
http://www.acg.gi.org/

American College of Obstetricians &
Gynecologists (ACOG)
http://www.acog.org/

American College of Physicians
http://www.acponline.org/

American College of Rheumatology
http://www.rheumatology.org/

American Heart Association
http://www.americanheart.org

American Medical Association
http://www.ama-assn.org/

American Osteopathic College of
Dermatology
http://www.aocd.org/

American Physical Therapy Association
http://www.apta.org//AM/Template.
cfm?Section=Home

American Psychiatric Association
http://www.psych.org/

American Society for Reproductive
Medicine
http://www.asrm.org/

American Thyroid Association
http://www.thyroid.org/

American Urological Association
http://www.auanet.org/

Society of Thoracic Surgeons
http://www.sts.org/